Nursing Assistant
A Nursing Process Approach

TENTH EDITION

Barbara R. Hegner, MSN, RN
(deceased)

Barbara Acello, MS, RN
Independent nurse consultant
and educator

Esther Caldwell, MA, PhD
Consultant in Vocational
Education

THOMSON

DELMAR LEARNING

Australia Canada Mexico Singapore Spain United Kingdom United Sta

p. 581

THOMSON

DELMAR LEARNING

Nursing Assistant: A Nursing Process Approach
Tenth Edition
by Barbara R. Hegner, Barbara Acello, and Esther Caldwell

Vice President, Health Care Business Unit:
William Brottmiller

Director of Learning Solutions:
Matthew Kane

Managing Editor:
Marah Bellegarde

Acquisitions Editor:
Matthew Seeley

Product Manager:
Jadin Babin-Kavanaugh

Editorial Assistant:
Megan Tarquinio

Marketing Director:
Jennifer McAvey

Senior Marketing Manager:
Lynn Henn

Marketing Manager:
Michele McTighe

Marketing Coordinator:
Chelsey Iaquinta

Technology Director:
Laurie Davis

Technology Product Manager:
Mary Colleen Liburdi

Technology Project Manager:
Carolyn Fox

Production Director:
Carolyn Miller

Content Project Manager:
Kenneth McGrath

Senior Art Director:
Jack Pendleton

Library of Congress Cataloging-in-Publication Data
Hegner, Barbara R.
  Nursing assistant : a nursing process approach / Barbara R. Hegner, Barbara Acello, Esther Caldwell.—10th ed.
    p. ; cm.
  Includes bibliographical references and index.
  ISBN-10: 1-4180-6606-0 (softcover)
  ISBN-13: 978-1-4180-6606-2
  ISBN-10: 1-4180-6607-9 (hardcover)
  ISBN-13: 978-1-4180-6607-9

  1. Nurses' aides. 2. Care of the sick.
I. Acello, Barbara. II. Caldwell, Esther. III. Title.
  [DNLM: 1. Nurses' Aides. 2. Nursing Care. WY 193 H4644n 2008]
  RT84.H45 2008
  610.7306'98--dc22

                                    2007022078

NOTICE TO THE READER

brief TABLE OF CONTENTS

LIST *of* PROCEDURES

Icon Key: **OBRA** = OBRA   🖐 = PPE   💿 = DVD icon   💻 = online

WWW.

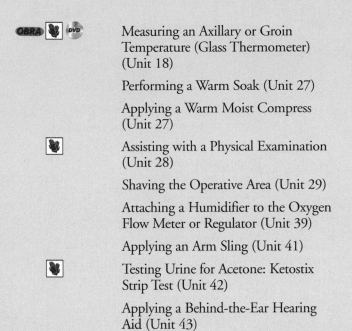

LIST *of* TABLES

CONTENTS

SECTION 6

MEASURING AND RECORDING VITAL SIGNS, HEIGHT, AND WEIGHT 305

SECTION 10

OTHER HEALTH CARE SETTINGS 555

SECTION 11

BODY SYSTEMS, COMMON DISORDERS, AND RELATED CARE PROCEDURES 645

SECTION 12

EXPANDED ROLE OF THE NURSING ASSISTANT 837

SECTION 13

SECTION 14

BARBARA R. HEGNER

Barbara Robinson Hegner, RN, MSN, was a graduate of a three-year diploma nursing program where direct and total care was the focus. She earned a BSN at Boston College and an MS in nursing from Boston University, with a minor in biologic sciences. She was Professor Emerita of Nursing and Life Sciences at Long Beach City College, Long Beach (CA).

Throughout her professional career, she had a deep interest in both hospital-based and long-term care nursing.

It was Ms. Hegner's belief that to ensure the rights and well-being of all patients and residents requires the care of competent, caring nursing assistants under the supervision of professional nurses. The nursing assistants who provide this care should be thoroughly trained and consistently encouraged, evaluated, and given the opportunity for continued learning. Providing the tools to prepare these health care providers in the most effective and efficient way is the goal of *Nursing Assistant, A Nursing Process Approach*, 10th edition.

BARBARA ACELLO

Barbara Acello, MS, RN, is an independent nurse consultant and educator in Denton, Texas. She is a member of the Texas Nurses' Association, Association of Nurses in AIDS Care, National Association of Directors of Nursing in Long Term Care, and American College of Healthcare Administrators. Mrs. Acello is a proponent and supporter of CNAs. She has written many textbooks, journal articles, and other materials related to nursing assistant education. She believes the nursing assistant is the most important caregiver in the health care facility.

INTRODUCTION

The passage of the Omnibus Budget Reconciliation Act (OBRA) of 1987, which included the Nursing Home Reform Act, was the first federal legislation to address standards for certification of nursing assistants as health care providers in long-term care. This legislation has influenced both the education and practice of all nursing assistants.

Following the enactment of OBRA, the National Council of State Boards of Nursing Inc. developed the Nurse Aide Competency Evaluation Program as the guideline for evaluating nursing assistant education to meet the specific needs of health care consumers. Individual states have developed training programs that meet and, in many cases, exceed the minimum requirements of the federal government.

Nursing assistants are important members of the nursing team (one part of the interdisciplinary health care team that plans and provides care to patients). Nursing assistants make valuable contributions to the nursing process that the professional nurse follows in assessing the patient's needs, planning interventions, implementing care, and evaluating outcomes. Nursing assistants must be helped to see the vital role their accurate observations, reporting skills, and careful attention to instructions plays in the overall success of the nursing care plan. Only then can they recognize their full value as part of the nursing team.

Previous editions of this best-selling text emphasized the importance of treating those entrusted to care as total individuals who possess dignity, have value, and deserve respect. The continuing goal of this text and supplement package is to provide the tools that instructors can use to teach nursing assistants to meet high standards of care. This will enable them to help patients achieve a desirable level of comfort, restoration, and wellness while protecting and respecting patients' rights as health care consumers.

THE FUTURE

The ways in which health care is provided in the United States continue to change. Emphasis continues to be placed on maintaining wellness, limiting length of stay in acute care facilities, controlling costs through managed care, providing short- and long-term rehabilitation and restorative care in more cost-effective settings, and increasing home care services. In addition, the population of the United States is aging, with the greatest increase in the number of people over 65. As a result, restorative care and home care services will be major components in health care. Nursing assistants will provide much of this service. It is essential that nursing assistants be prepared to assume these vital responsibilities.

TENTH EDITION

Numerous revisions were made in the 10th edition to keep pace with the evolution of health care. New health care settings, new and improved technology, shorter acute care stays, an aging population, and drug-resistant microorganisms are some of the factors that are changing the ways in which care is provided. These factors also affect the way in which nursing assistants provide care.

The following updated and enhanced content addresses the changing character of nursing assistant responsibilities:

- Introduction to the HIPAA laws
- Expanded information about computerized documentation
- The effects of noise and how loud noise affects patients and hospital staff
- An introduction to pathogens that are problematic in the United States, including *Klebsiella, Listeria, Acinetobacter baumannii, Aspergillis,* Streptococcus A and necrotizing fasciitis, *Rotavirus* and *Norovirus,* and Severe acute respiratory syndrome (SARS), and parasites
- CDC guidelines for personal protective equipment
- Ultraviolet Germicidal Irradiation (UVGI)
- Expanded focus on ergonomics and manual patient handling
- Procedure for sliding board transfers
- Family dynamics on hospital admission
- Updated nutrition information including revised food pyramid
- Preventing foodborne illness
- Care of patients who have had spinal surgery
- Working with doulas
- The mental health chapter was rewritten and updated to include common anxiety disorders, affective disorders, eating disorders, substance abuse, defense mechanisms, and maladaptive behaviors.
- Bariatrics has become an area of concern related to employee injury. A chapter has been added on care of the bariatric patient.
- Care of patients who are mechanically ventilated, or who have oral or nasal airways
- Standardized designations for code emergencies
- CPR and obstructed airway procedures have been updated to 2005 changes

- Text box alerts were updated with pertinent information on infection control, OSHA, communication, age-appropriate care, legal implications, safety, culture, difficult situations and patient care, and patient care tips. Clinical Information alerts were added.
- URLS were updated for further information and research.

EXTENSIVE TEACHING AND LEARNING PACKAGE

Thomson Delmar Learning has provided a complete learning package to accompany the tenth edition of *Nursing Assistant: A Nursing Process Approach.*
Each supplement has been extensively revised to reflect the changes in the tenth edition textbook.

Student Resources

The following resources were developed to help students learn and practice the information essential to becoming certified as a skilled nursing assistant:

StudyWare CD-ROM is included in the back of this text and features quizzes, games, and case studies for each unit. Students can take the quizzes in Practice Mode to improve mastery of the material; instant feedback tells whether an answer is right or wrong, and explains why. Quiz Mode allows students to test themselves and keep a record of their scores. StudyWare games, flashcards, and image labeling exercises reinforce unit content, and the unique critical thinking case studies help synthesize and apply unit topics to real-world scenarios.

Student Workbook
ISBN 1418066095
The student workbook has been updated with new content and directly correlates to the textbook. This competency-based supplement includes challenging items such as word games, puzzles, and exercises to help students understand essential content and master defining and spelling key terms. A new section on studying for the state written and competency examination has been added to the workbook, designed to help students who will be taking a state certification exam.

Online Companion
ISBN 1418066109
The Online Companion is new to this edition and features additional resources to supplement book content, plus up-to-date information on ever-changing practices and standards in nursing assisting, as well as additional unit content.

On the Job: the Essentials of Nursing Assisting
ISBN 1418066125
This on-the-job companion is a handy pocket-reference designed to keep critical nursing care information at the fingertips of practicing nursing assistants. Many safety and infection control alerts, as well as suggested responses to common situations are easily referenced using this book.

Instructor Resources
The following comprehensive tools are available to instructors to enhance the planning and implementation of their instructional program.

Instructor's Manual
ISBN 1418066087
Contains answer keys to all text and student workbook exercises, in addition to lesson plans, student and instructor resources, quizzes and testing material, performance competency checklists for procedures, and numerous images to use as transparency masters and student handouts. The Instructor's Manual is available in print, and is also available electronically both on the Electronic Classroom Manager CD-ROM as well as the instructor's side of the Online Companion.

Electronic Classroom Manager CD-ROM
ISBN 1418066117
This supplement is new to the tenth edition and features a **Computerized Test Bank** with over 1,700 questions in *ExamView ® Pro* test generator software, and 700 **PowerPoint**™ slides with illustrations from the text. It also includes electronic versions of both the Instructor's Manual and Instructor's Resource Kit.

Instructor's Resource Kit
The Instructor's Resource Kit is available electronically on both the Electronic Classroom Manager and the Online Companion. This kit provides you with in-depth resources to help simplify the planning and implementation of a nursing assisting instructional program. It integrates the use of the text, Student Workbook, Electronic Classroom Manager, Instructor's Manual, and skills videos to help you develop an efficient instructional plan. The Instructor's Resource Kit includes comprehensive teaching resources, course syllabi, unit outlines, and lesson plans with supplemental materials.

Online Companion
ISBN 1418066109
This key resource is available for the first time with the tenth edition, and includes additional procedures and skills checklists, as well as additional unit content. For your convenience, the Online Companion will also include electronic versions of both the Instructors' Manual and the Instructor's Resource Kit.

WebTutor™
WebCT ISBN 1418066133, BlackBoard ISBN 1418066141
This course cartridge for Blackboard and WebCT can be used to supplement on-campus course delivery or as the course management platform for an online course. WebTutor™ provides communication tools to instructors and students, including a course calendar, chat, e-mail, and threaded discussions. Each unit contains the following items:

- Advance Preparation—details what a student should do before starting each online unit

- Unit Objectives—alert the student to what is expected as outcomes for each unit
- Class Notes—are helpful tips that provide further clarification and expansion of text content
- Frequently Asked Questions (FAQs)—provide answers to questions that students commonly ask
- Glossary of terms—is specific to the unit and is also rolled into a comprehensive glossary for the course
- Discussion Topics—provide interactive classroom discussion by means of a threaded bulletin board
- Learning Links—require students to search the Web for information to reinforce and expand learning; students report back findings to instructors through e-mail
- Online Exercises—provide further reinforcement of learning with immediate feedback

WebTutor™ also includes a midterm test and a final test.

Nursing Assisting: Basic Skills DVD-ROM
ISBN 141806615X

Finally, skills-based videos to accompany many of the procedures in the text! Each of the 76 core procedures is presented step-by-step for maximum effectiveness. In addition to the procedures, general guidelines are included for lifting and moving, ambulation, handling clean or soiled linen, and observation and reporting. These videos are great for in-class demonstration to help prepare students for exams or for clinical rotations. This series includes the following modules:

Module 1	Obstructed Airway, Handwashing, Beginning and Completion Procedure Actions, Communication Skills
Module 2	Personal Protective Equipment, Standard Precautions, and Transmission Based Precautions
Module 3	Positioning, Transfers, and Ambulation
Module 4	Bedmaking and Bathing
Module 5	Bladder, Bowel, and Perineal Care
Module 6	Personal Care
Module 7	Dressing, Meal Care, and Restraints
Module 8	Vital Signs, Height, and Weight
Module 9	Observation/Reporting Guidelines and Postmortem Care
Module 10	Range of Motion and Mechanical Lift

For your convenience, a DVD icon appears in the text on every procedure that has a corresponding video clip.

ACKNOWLEDGMENTS

Each new edition brings with it the pleasant task of acknowledging the contributions of a number of individuals.

First, my husband Francis and son Jon have given greatly of themselves while I worked on this manuscript. I appreciate their love and support.

The following individuals provided valuable information and resources for new content:
- Leah Schoettmer, Hill-Rom, Inc.
- Stacey Grandinetti, HoverTech International
- Dan Plyman, Medline Industries, Inc.
- Arnie Silverman, Skil-Care, Inc.
- Paula Schneider, MS, RN
- Lois Stotter, MS, RNC
- Donna Wong, PhD, RN, PNP, FAAN

A book of this size represents an enormous investment of time and talent by many dedicated individuals. I sincerely appreciate the support and assistance of the following individuals at Delmar Learning: Jadin Babin-Kavanaugh, product manager, whose support was invaluable in manuscript construction and development; Matthew Seeley, acquisitions editor, whose vision and tolerance of my idiosyncrasies is sincerely appreciated; Nicole Bruno, editorial assistant, who coordinated the many facets of manuscript review. I am always delighted when Brooke Graves lends her many copyediting talents to my projects.

REVIEWERS

The revision was aided by a dedicated group of instructors who reviewed content at different stages of the revision process. For their valuable suggestions and insights, the publisher and author would like to thank the following:

Marty Bachman, PhD, RN
Program Chair
Front Range Community College
Fort Collins, Colorado

Suzanne Barnes, RN
Allied Health Technology Instructor
Bridgman High School
Bridgman, Michigan

Lee W. Bell, RN, BSN
Instructor
Clayton State University Continuing Education
Morrow, Georgia

Carol Brueggeman, RN, BSN
Nursing Assisting Instructor
Blackhawk Technical College
Janesville, Wisconsin

Helen Bruner, RN
Entry-level Health Care Programs Manager
Century College
White Bear Lake, Minnesota

Patricia Burkett, RN, BSN, MEd
Allied Health Educator
Wallingford Public Schools
Wallingford, Connecticut

Theresa Ann Cairns, RN, BSN, MEd
Health Occupations and Nurse Aide Programs
Coordinator
Beaver County AVTS
Monaca, Pennsylvania

Betty Earp, RN, BSN
Program Coordinator
Mesa Community College
Mesa, Arizona

Michele Emond, RN, MSN
Department Head, Allied Health
Worcester Technical High School
Worcester, Massachusetts

Catherine V. English, RN
Adult Education Instructor
Polaris Career Center
Middleburg Heights, Ohio

Ellen Gerrity, RN, MA
Program Manager
Palm Beach Community College
Lake Worth, Florida

Yolanda Hampel, PhD, RN, BC
Professor
Tidewater Community College
Virginia Beach, Virginia

Coleen Linn, RN
Health Care Science Technology Instructor
Gordon Central High School
Calhoun, Georgia

JoAnne McCarthy, RN
Instructor/Coordinator
Luzerne County Community College

Robin Nabity, RN
Program Coordinator
Southwest Skill Center at Estrella Mountain Community
College
Avondale, Arizona

Janice M. Roberts, RN
Instructor
Caddo Career & Technology Center
Shreveport, Louisiana

Linda A. Robertshaw, RN, MSN
Instructor
Community College of Southern Nevada
Boulder City, Nevada

Mary Kate Shore, RN, MS
CNA Program Coordinator
Highland Community College
Freeport, Illinois

Ann Sims, RN, BSN
Program Director
Albuquerque TVI Community College
Albuquerque, New Mexico

Pamela Smith, RN, MSN
Program Director
Front Range Community College
Fort Collins, Colorado

Lois R. Stotter, MS, RNC
Medical Programs Coordinator
Dorsey Schools–The Career Connection
Madison Heights, MI

Valerie Taylor, RN, C., BSN, MEd.
Nurse Aide Program Director
Lorain County Community College
Elyria, Ohio

HOW TO *use this* TEXTBOOK

TABLE OF CONTENTS

The tenth edition of *Nursing Assistant: A Nursing Process Approach* has been carefully designed and updated to make the study of nursing assistant tasks and responsibilities easier and more productive. For best results, you may want to become familiar with the features incorporated into this text and accompanying learning tools.

TABLE OF CONTENTS

For each unit, the table of contents lists the unit title, major topic headings, general guidelines for specific areas of care and topics of importance to the nursing assistant, and patient care procedures.

UNIT OPENING PAGE

Each unit opening page contains objectives and vocabulary terms.

The **objectives** help you know what is expected of you as you read the text. Your success in mastering each objective is measured by the review questions at the end of each unit.

The **vocabulary** list alerts you to new terms presented in the unit. When each term is first used in the unit, it is highlighted in boldface and color. Each term is defined at this point in the unit. Read the definition of the term and note the context in which it is used so that you will feel comfortable in using the term. Note that the glossary at the back of the book also defines these highlighted terms.

TEXT ALERTS

The alerts provide important content on infection control, OSHA, communication, age-appropriate care, legal implications, safety, difficult situations, and clinical information related to patient care. These alerts make the learner aware of best practices in patient care, include practical tips based on experience, and highlight critical infection control, safety, and other OSHA workplace guidelines.

PHOTOGRAPHS AND ILLUSTRATIONS

Numerous color illustrations and photos help to clarify and reinforce the unit content. Many figures are used in the procedures to help you visualize critical step-by-step information. Full-color anatomy drawings help you to locate body components and understand body organization.

GUIDELINES

These guidelines highlight important points that you need to remember for specific situations or types of care. They are presented in an easy-to-use format that you can refer to repeatedly until you know the actions you must take when confronted with the situation.

PROCEDURES

The textbook contains 140 clinical procedures in a step-by-step format. Each procedure reminds you to perform both beginning and completion actions. Any notes or cautions about performing the procedure are given. The steps take you carefully through the procedure, emphasizing at all times the need to work safely and to protect the patient's privacy. Each procedure contains icons which help you to easily identify those procedures that contain key OBRA and PPE standards, as well as those procedures for which there is a corresponding video available on *Delmar's Basic Core Skills for Nursing Assistants* video series.

UNIT REVIEWS AND TESTING MATERIAL

A variety of review questions at the end of each unit test your understanding of the unit content. Each review contains a Nursing Assistant Challenge that presents a typical clinical situation and asks questions about your response to the situation. These questions help you master critical thinking skills and require you to integrate what you have learned to arrive at an appropriate solution or set of actions.

FIGURE 8-1 Medicine and nursing each have a separate focus, but both are essential for patients' well-being if positive outcomes are to be achieved.

* Implementation
* Evaluation

Assessment involves the collection of data (information) about the patient. The nurse coordinates assessment with other members of the interdisciplinary team. The data are entered on a special form contained in the patient's medical record. Information is obtained from:

* Interviewing the patient
* The medical record
* The patient's family if the patient is unable to communicate
* Physical examination (Figure 8-2)
* collection of measurable data and information such as weight and vital signs
* observations made by members of the nursing team

Proper use of the nursing process is a key element in the delivery of effective health care. Nursing...

The nursing assistant is responsible for collection of data by making and reporting observations. This is explained later in the unit. After the assessment is finished, the nurse analyzes the data, identifies the patient's problems, and formulates nursing diagnoses. A nursing diagnosis is the statement of a patient problem and the cause of the problem. For example, the nursing diagnosis may be impaired physical mobility (the problem) related to hemiplegia due to stroke (the cause of the problem). Nursing diagnoses may reflect actual clinical problems, the risk that certain problems will develop, or wellness objectives. The nursing diagnoses provide the foundation for nursing care to achieve outcomes for which nurses are accountable. Table 8-1 gives a few examples of nursing diagnoses and what they mean.

Planning the care of the patient (developing a care plan) is done after the nursing diagnoses are made. The purpose of planning is to:

* Identify possible solutions to the problems (nursing diagnoses).
* Develop approaches (what team members are going to do) that will help the patient solve the problems. Approaches may also be called interventions.
* Establish measurable goals for the patient (a goal is an outcome) so that caregivers will know whether the approaches are successful and whether the problems are being resolved.

Planning may be done at a care plan conference (Figure 8-3). This is a meeting of the members of the interdisciplinary team who are directly involved in the care of the patient. The patient and/or the family (if the patient consents) should be invited to attend the conference. The care plan developed at the conference contains a list of the nursing diagnoses, the approaches, and the patient's goals (Figures 8-4A and 8-4B). The care plan may be kept in the patient's medical record or in a file called a Kardex

8-3 The care plan is developed during a care [conferen]ce involving the patient and family member (if [present]) and members of the interdisciplinary team.

GUIDELINES for Preventing Infection

* Assist patients to maintain adequate fluid intake. This helps prevent urinary tract and respiratory tract infections and keeps the skin healthier.
* Assist patients to maintain adequate nutritional intake. Report to the nurse when patients eat less or refuse food.
* Assist patients to carry out exercise programs established by the nurse or physical therapist. Follow positioning schedules and orders for range-of-motion exercises and ambulation. Exercise improves breathing and circulation.
* Toilet patients who need assistance. This keeps the bladder empty and also assures patients that they will receive help when they need to urinate.
* When cleaning the perineal area of patients, be sure to wipe women from front to back. This avoids contaminating the urethra (bladder opening) with stool or vaginal excretions.
* Perform catheter care as directed. Avoid opening the drainage system.
* Observe patients carefully and report any unusual signs or changes, such as:
  – Changes in frequency of urination or amount of urine voided
  – Complaints of pain or burning on urination
  – Changes in character of urine
  – Coughing or respiratory problems

* Confusion or disorientation that was not present before or that has increased
* Drainage or discharge from any body opening or skin wound
* Changes in skin color
* Complaints of pain, discomfort, or nausea
* Elevated temperature
* Red, swollen areas on body
* Keep patients clean.
* Staff members who have an infectious disease should not be on duty. Caring for your own health is vital in preventing illness in patients. Friends and [relatives] should be advised not to visit [patients if you notice a visitor]

diarrhea, especially in immunosuppressed people... is no specific treatment.

BIOTERRORISM

Bioterrorism is the use of biological agents, ... ogenic organisms or agricultural pests, for ... poses. Since October 2001, state, local, and ... health authorities have been investigating ... rorism-related illness. Specifically, some in... from inhalation ... powdery substa... sent through the... developed the... Cutaneous and... from one pe... through cont...

PROCEDURE

① HANDWASHING

1. Check that there is an adequate supply of soap and paper towels. A waste container lined with a plastic bag should be in the area near you.
2. Remove rings, if possible, or be sure to lather soap underneath.
3. Remove watch, or push up over wrist.
4. Turn on the faucet.
5. Adjust water to a warm temperature. Once used, drop the paper towel in the waste container.

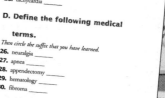

Stand back from the sink so you do not contaminate your uniform. Wet your hands, keeping your fingertips pointed downward (Figure 13-1).

6. Apply soap and lather over your hands and wrists, between fingers, and under rings. Use friction and interlace your fingers (Figure 13-2). Work lather over every part of your hands and wrists. Clean your fingernails by rubbing them against the palm of the other hand to force soap under the nails for 15 to 20 seconds (Figure 13-3).
7. Rinse hands with your fingertips pointed down. Do not shake water from hands.
8. Dry hands thoroughly with a clean paper towel.
9. Turn off the faucet with a paper towel (Figure 13-4); drop the towel in the waste container.

...an, dry ...cets off.

REVIEW

A. Matching.

Match the abbreviations in Column I with their meanings in Column II.

Column I	Column II
1. _____ a.c.	a. three times a day
2. _____ b.i.d.	b. whenever necessary
3. _____ OR	c. head of bed
4. _____ PRN	d. before meals
5. _____ NPO	e. operating room
6. _____ stat	f. nothing by mouth
7. _____ HOB	g. after meals
8. _____ c̄	h. without
9. _____ ung.	i. twice a day
10. _____ s̄	j. at once
	k. ointment
	l. with

B. Matching.

Match the prefixes in Column I with their meanings in Column II.

Column I	Column II
11. _____ ur (o)	a. bile
12. _____ cardi (o)	b. ear
13. _____ chol (e)	c. lung
14. _____ dermat (o)	d. child
15. _____ gastr (o)	e. muscle
16. _____ ot (o)	f. pharynx
17. _____ ped (o)	g. stomach
18. _____ pneum (o)	h. larynx
19. _____ my (o)	i. heart
20. _____ pharyng (o)	j. urine
	k. chest
	l. skin

C. Define the following med... ...

24. hypertension _____
25. tachycardia _____

D. Define the following medical terms.

Then circle the suffix that you have learned.

26. neuralgia _____
27. apnea _____
28. appendectomy _____
29. hematology _____
30. fibroma _____

E. Write the medical term that means the following.

31. kidney stones _____
32. examination of the rectum using an instrument _____
33. incision into thorax _____
34. inflammation of the stomach _____
35. white blood cell _____

F. In each of the following, circle the prefix and underline the suffix.

36. anemia
37. neuritis
38. pharyngitis
39. pandemic
40. tracheotomy

Dedication

This text is dedicated to the memory of Barbara R. Hegner. Barbara was a visionary who saw the need for formalized instructional materials to help educate and develop skilled nursing assistants. She was committed to this unique and important group of health care professionals.

Introduction to Nursing Assisting

UNIT 1

Community Health Care

OBJECTIVES

After completing this unit, you will be able to:

- Spell and define terms.
- List the five basic functions of health care facilities.
- Describe four changes that have taken place in health care in the past few years.
- Describe the differences between acute care and long-term care.

- Name the departments within a hospital.
- Describe the functions of the departments within a hospital.
- Explain three ways by which health care costs are paid.
- State the purpose of health care facility surveys.

VOCABULARY

Learn the meaning and the correct spelling of the following words and phrases:

acute illness
certification
chronic illness
citation
client
community
diagnosis related groups (DRG)
facility
health care consumer
health maintenance organization (HMO)
hospice

hospital
Joint Commission (JayCo)
license
long-term acute care hospital (LTACH)
Magnet Program for Excellence in Nursing Services
managed care
Medicaid
Medicare
obstetric

Occupational Safety and Health Administration (OSHA)
occupational therapy
orthopedic
pathology
patient
patient-focused care
pediatric
physical therapy
post-anesthesia recovery (PAR)
postpartum

prenatal
psychiatric
quality assurance (QA)
rehabilitation
resident
respiratory therapy
skilled care facility
speech therapy
survey
surveyor

INTRODUCTION

Nursing assistants play an important role in the care of people who are ill or injured. You will give care to these persons under the direction and supervision of licensed, professional health care workers, such as doctors and nurses. Care is provided in various types of health care facilities. The term **facility** refers to the place in which care is given. A **hospital** is a complex organization that provides a full range of health care services. Highly sophisticated equipment and treatments are available there. Some hospitals provide general care for patients with many conditions. Others provide only specialized services, such as treatment for cancer or rehabilitation care. A **skilled care facility** provides care to persons whose conditions are stable but who need monitoring, nursing care, and treatments. All health care facilities have five basic functions:

1. Providing services for the ill and injured (Figure 1-1).
2. Preventing disease.
3. Promoting individual and community health.
4. Educating health care workers (Figure 1-2).
5. Promoting research in medicine and nursing.

OVERVIEW OF HEALTH CARE

Health care today emphasizes **patient-focused care**. This care focus is based on the fact that each patient is a unique individual and has different needs. Attention must be given to the physical, mental, and emotional aspects of

FIGURE 1-2 Health care changes frequently, and education is an important objective for personnel.

the person's being if that person is to lead a fulfilling and satisfying life.

Because people are living longer, quality of life has become an important consideration in health care delivery. Some health care decisions are made with the patient's future quality of life in mind. Quality-of-life policies and requirements focus on creating and maintaining an environment that humanizes and individualizes each patient. In some situations, preserving the quality of the patient's life is viewed as more important than increasing the length or duration of life.

Many changes have occurred in health care within the past few years. There are several reasons for these changes:

- People are living longer. As people age, their need for health care increases, so more services are needed (Figure 1-3).

FIGURE 1-1 Health care facilities provide routine, emergency, and surgical services to many different types of patients. ("Be All You Can Be," Courtesy United States Government, as represented by the Secretary of the Army)

FIGURE 1-3 An aging population needs more health care services to manage illness and disability.

Infection Control ALERT

The development of infection is dangerous for the patient and is very costly to insurance companies and the hospital. Prevention of infection is a major nursing assistant function. ▪

- Advanced technology means that more lives are saved. Although life is maintained, some of these individuals need continuing health care.
- The cost of health care has increased tremendously because of the demand for services and because of advances in technology.
- Science has created many ethical (moral) questions that must be answered by health care providers and consumers.

To reduce the cost of health care, patients are discharged earlier from hospitals. These patients may still require health care. This care can be given more economically in skilled care facilities and in the patient's home. More diagnostic tests and procedures are provided in outpatient facilities to further decrease costs. Surgicenters, urgent care centers, and clinics are examples of such facilities. It is less expensive, for example, to receive treatment for a throat infection in an urgent care center than in a hospital emergency room.

Most health care is paid for with insurance. Insurance companies use **managed care** to provide the services in the most efficient manner at the lowest cost. Briefly, this means that the insurance company will:

- Not permit certain procedures or diagnostic tests until they have been approved by the insurer.
- Negotiate with specific physicians, hospitals, pharmacies, and other care providers to render services at a lower cost to the company's members.
- Approve only a certain number of days of hospitalization for specific diagnoses. A woman giving birth, for example, may be allowed up to 48 hours of hospitalization.
- Require that specific procedures be done on an outpatient basis rather than having the patient admitted to the hospital.

NEEDS OF THE COMMUNITY

People who live in a common area and share common health needs form a **community**. Provisions for disposal of wastes, assurance of safe drinking water, availability of healthful foods, protection from disease, and health care are important to every person within a community. Public health laws regulate these services and are enforced by government agencies.

Health care is needed throughout life. The care may be short-term or long-term and includes:

- Preventive care
  - **Prenatal** care (care of the mother during pregnancy).
  - Well-baby checkups and immunizations.
  - Health education to teach individuals how to avoid disease and injury.
  - Physical examinations throughout life.
- Emergency care
  - Short-term care for sudden illness or injury.
- Surgery
  - To repair an injured body part or remove a diseased organ.
- Rehabilitation
  - To help a patient to regain abilities after illness or injury.
- Long-term care
  - For patients who have chronic or incurable conditions.
- **Hospice** care
  - For patients who are dying and their families.

Persons receiving health care are called **health care consumers**. They are also identified by the type of care they need:

- **Patient** is a term used for persons in acute care facilities such as hospitals.
- **Client** is a term used for persons receiving care in their own homes.
- **Resident** is a term for people in long-term care facilities.

COMMUNITY HEALTH CARE SERVICES

There are two main types of health care facilities: those that provide short-term care and those that provide long-term care (Table 1-1). Short-term care is given to patients who have a routine or minor problem, such as a urinary tract infection. The care may be given in the physician's office, an outpatient clinic, or an urgent care center. Uncomplicated surgeries, such as hernia repair, require only short-term care and may be done in a surgicenter. General hospitals provide short-term care for acute illnesses. An **acute illness** or injury comes on suddenly and requires intense, immediate treatment. Heart attacks, severe burns, strokes, and uncontrolled diabetes are examples of acute conditions.

Long-term care is necessary for persons who have chronic conditions. A **chronic illness** is one that is treatable but not curable and is expected to require lifelong care. This care may be given in a skilled care facility, adult day-care setting, respite care facility, assisted living facility, or the patient's home (Figure 1-4). Cardiovascular disease (heart

TABLE 1-1 TYPES OF HEALTH CARE FACILITIES

Short-Term Care	Long-Term Care
Hospitals	Long-term acute care hospitals
	Subacute and transitional care facilities
	Skilled care facilities
Urgent care facilities	Adult day care
Surgicenters	Assisted living facilities
	Rehabilitation centers
	Psychiatric hospitals
Outpatient clinics	Respite care
Psychiatric hospitals	
Physician's offices	Home care

and blood vessels), Alzheimer's disease, multiple sclerosis, Parkinson's disease, and diabetes are examples of chronic illnesses. Additional information about long-term care is given in Section 10.

FIGURE 1-4 Home health care services are given in the client's home, eliminating the need for facility admission and reducing the cost of care.

Hospitals

Most hospitals are licensed to care for patients of all ages and for patients with a variety of problems. Some hospitals take care of patients with special conditions or care for specific age groups:

- **Pediatric** hospitals care only for children from birth to 18 years of age.
- **Psychiatric** hospitals provide care for persons with mental illness.
- **Rehabilitation** hospitals provide restorative services to patients following disease, illness, or injury. These services are designed to help the patient regain the ability to function at the highest level possible, considering the patient's illness or injury.
- **Long-term acute care hospitals (LTACH)** are a rapidly growing segment of the health care market in the United States. The facility is licensed as a hospital but is designed for patients who are expected to have a lengthy stay. To be accepted in an LTACH, the patient must have a medically complex condition, need acute care services, and have a good chance of improvement. The level of care is higher than provided in long-term care facilities (nursing homes) or subacute care facilities.

Hospital Organization

Hospitals are organized in ways that provide the most efficient delivery of service. Major departments are established within each facility to meet the needs of patients with specific conditions (Figure 1-5). These units provide nursing care 24 hours a day, 7 days a week.

- Medical department: cares for patients with medical conditions such as pneumonia or heart disease.

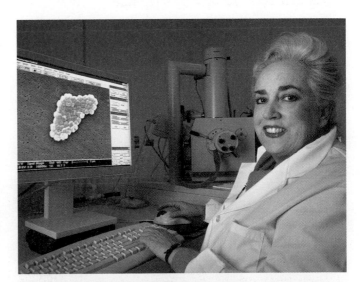

FIGURE 1-5 Many departments meet the needs of patients. Some require special equipment and are highly technical. This microbiologist is studying an electronic image of bacteria that can not be seen with the eye. (Courtesy of Centers for Disease Control and Prevention.)

- Surgical department: cares for patients before, during, and after surgery. There may be many operating rooms where surgical procedures are performed, and a **post-anesthesia recovery (PAR)** area where patients are closely monitored after surgery. Patients remain in this area until they are stable enough to leave the surgical department.
- Pediatric department: cares for sick or injured children.
- **Obstetric** department: cares for newborns and their mothers. This department includes the labor and delivery unit, the **postpartum** unit (for mothers who have given birth), and the nursery for the newborns (Figure 1-6).
- Emergency department: cares for victims of trauma, natural disasters (tornadoes, for example), or medical emergencies.
- Critical care department: cares for seriously ill patients who require constant monitoring and care.

Larger hospitals have many specialized units staffed by nurses and therapists who provide care for persons with problems such as cancer, cardiovascular disease, or kidney disease, or for those requiring **orthopedic** (bones and muscles) surgery. Specialized health care workers provide direct or indirect services to the patients in these units. Specialized services include:

- Dietary services. A registered dietitian plans the meals for all patients and provides educational services to patients on special diets. The hospital's food service department prepares meals and delivers them to patients.
- Pharmacy services. Registered pharmacists prepare and provide all medications and intravenous therapy solutions.

- Diagnostic services.
  - **Pathology** (study of disease). Diagnostic tests are done on specimens taken from body tissue to help the doctor make a diagnosis.
  - Diagnostic imaging and radiology. X-rays and other specialized procedures are done to help make a diagnosis.
  - Laboratory. A department that is equipped to perform diagnostic tests and investigative procedures. Various specimens are sent to the laboratory for analysis. The results of the tests are used by physicians and others in the care of patients.
- Rehabilitation services.
  - **Physical therapy** assists patients to regain mobility skills.
  - **Occupational therapy** helps patients to regain self-care skills.
  - **Speech therapy** helps patients to regain the ability to communicate and works with patients who have swallowing disorders.
  - **Respiratory therapy** provides care for patients who have disorders of the cardiopulmonary system, respirations, and sleep disorders that affect the patient's breathing.
- Social services. Staff members provide counseling for patients and their families, help needy families get financial assistance, plan for patient discharge, and arrange for patient transfers from one facility to another (Figure 1-7).
- Environmental services.
  - Housekeeping is responsible for the overall cleaning of the hospital (Figure 1-8).

FIGURE 1-6 The obstetric department cares for mothers and newborn infants.

FIGURE 1-7 The social worker is responsible for ensuring that patients' discharge plans are complete and the necessary resources are available in the community.

FIGURE 1-8 The housekeeping department keeps the facility clean and sanitary.

- Maintenance cares for and repairs equipment.
- Laundry services provide and clean all hospital linens.
● Business services are responsible for patient billing, employee payroll, and other financial matters.
● Medical records department transcribes and catalogs all patient records.
● Volunteers provide services free of charge and perform tasks such as delivering mail and flowers, running the gift shop, directing visitors, and raising funds for the facility (Figure 1-9).
● Pastoral care helps meet patients' religious and spiritual needs and provides counseling.

Patients may be transferred from one unit to another within a hospital. For example, a patient having surgery

FIGURE 1-9 Volunteers give of their time and provide many valuable services to the facility and its patients.

will go from the operating room to the PAR room and then to the surgical nursing unit.

FINANCING HEALTH CARE

Health care is paid for by:
● Insurance. Employers may offer a group insurance plan, or persons may buy individual insurance. Premiums are expensive—employers may pay all or a portion of the cost of a group insurance plan. **Health maintenance organizations (HMO)** are one type of prepaid insurance. The HMO is a group of health care providers and hospitals. HMO members must see only certain doctors and go only to designated hospitals, except in emergencies.
● Out-of-pocket payments by the health care consumer who has no insurance or for expenses not covered by insurance.
● **Medicare** is a federal government program that pays a portion of health care costs for persons 65 years and over and for younger persons who are permanently disabled and who qualify for the benefit.
● Medicare payment is made based on **diagnosis related groups (DRGs)**. The actual cost of care is not considered. Rather, studies were done to determine the average length of stay required for various medical diagnoses, procedures, and treatments. Medicare set the payment rates based on these data. Although a hospital may charge variable rates for patient care, Medicare pays only the fixed amount that it has determined is fair for care based on the DRG.
● **Medicaid** is a state and federal government program that pays health care costs for persons of any age who do not have financial resources for health care.

Cost containment is a priority, which means that the maximum benefit of health care must be achieved for every dollar spent. Each care provider must do everything possible to avoid waste and to keep expenditures down.

REGULATORY AGENCIES

Many external agencies regulate health care facilities. Some regulatory agencies are branches of the state and federal government, but several are voluntary, private organizations.

Health care facilities must meet certain quality standards to operate. The various agencies inspect the facility periodically to ensure that it meets health and safety regulations and complies with accepted standards. A **survey** is a review and evaluation to ensure that facilities are maintaining acceptable standards of practice. Many different agencies establish quality standards for health care facilities. Different types of facilities must meet different quality standards.

Each facility holds a state **license**, which permits it to conduct business. Most facilities also possess a **certification**. Certification is necessary to collect Medicare and Medicaid payments. Licensure and certification surveys are done by the state health department or human services agency. During a survey, a number of **surveyors** inspect conditions in the facility. Surveyors are representatives of the agency that reviews the facility.

The Joint Commission

The **Joint Commission (JayCo)**, formerly known as the Joint Commission on Accreditation of Healthcare Organizations (JCAHO), is an agency that inspects and accredits health care providers. Participation in the accreditation process is voluntary. However, hospitals are not eligible to receive Medicare payment unless they are JayCo accredited. Medicare is an important source of revenue, and most hospitals could not survive financially without it. JayCo sets very high standards that the facility must meet to become accredited and to keep that accreditation. To ensure quality care, JayCo surveyors visit periodically to ensure that the facility meets these standards.

JayCo standards state that employees must be competent to carry out their responsibilities. The facility is required to periodically evaluate staff competence, and maintain a record of these checks. Surveyors also review age-related care appropriate for the patients on each unit. Staff must participate in ongoing educational programs. Surveyors may ask staff how their competency was evaluated. They may also ask how you would operate a piece of equipment or perform a specific procedure.

Surveyors review facility policies and procedures and determine whether staff is following them. Emphasis is placed on making sure that employees know and follow facility policies and procedures when caring for patients.

During a JayCo survey, the survey team evaluates the health care organization's level of compliance with the JayCo standards. After the survey is completed, a report is issued to the facility detailing areas in which the agency's performance must improve. Accreditation is granted if the survey is acceptable. If significant problems are identified, accreditation will be awarded if the facility's administration agrees to correct the problems promptly. If severe deficiencies are identified, JayCo will follow up with the facility to check its progress in making corrections.

OSHA Surveys

The **Occupational Safety and Health Administration (OSHA)** also surveys health care facilities. OSHA is a government agency that protects the health and safety of employees. OSHA inspectors review infection control, isolation practices, employee tuberculin testing, material safety data sheets, and other policies and facility practices. An OSHA survey involves interviews with employees and a tour of all areas of the facility. The inspector will ask questions about health and safety practices. OSHA inspectors will make recommendations for correcting unsafe conditions. If the inspector notes dangerous or unsafe conditions during the survey, the agency may receive a **citation** or fine. A *citation* is a written notice that informs the facility of the violation of OSHA rules. The employer must post the written report of each citation, at or near the place where the violation occurred, for three days, or until the unsafe condition is corrected.

Magnet Hospitals

According to the American Hospital Association (AHA), 95% of all hospital care is given by nursing personnel. In recent years, the quality of nursing services has been closely studied and recognized for its effect on patient care. Negative outcomes are reduced in facilities that promote and adhere to the American Nurses' Association (ANA) standards of practice. The **Magnet Program for Excellence in Nursing Services** is based on quality indicators and standards of nursing practice. This voluntary program recognizes hospitals for nursing excellence. Its three main purposes are to:

- Elevate the status of the nursing profession.
- Recognize excellence in nursing practice on many levels, from staff nurse to management.
- Validate excellence in patient care given by the facility.

Attaining magnet designation is not easy. Out of more than 6,000 hospitals in the United States, approximately 3% had achieved magnet status by 2006. Magnet status is reviewed every four years.

Because the magnet program recognizes quality patient care and nursing excellence, it is a coveted award in the nursing community and among acute care hospitals. Hospitals that have been awarded magnet status are usually very progressive, desirable places to work. Nurses and others like to work in an environment that recognizes their professional status and contributions.

QUALITY ASSURANCE

All health care facilities have a program called **quality assurance (QA)**. Some facilities call this program Continuous Quality Improvement (CQI). You may be asked to participate on the quality assurance committee. The purpose of quality assurance is to conduct internal reviews to identify problems and find ways to improve. The quality assurance committee meets periodically to evaluate care provided and practices in the facility. Restraint use, infections, pressure ulcers, and infection control are some of the areas commonly reviewed. Committee members audit practices on each unit and make recommendations to administration to improve care. Patient care should be continuously reevaluated by the facility and adjusted to meet patient needs. The quality assurance program performs this important function.

The quality assurance committee is very important to the operation of the facility and to the facility's success in surveys. The committee identifies problems and corrects them. This self-improvement process prevents problems with regulatory agencies and improves the quality of care delivered.

REVIEW

A. True/False.

Mark the following true or false by circling T or F.

1. T F Nursing assistants work under the supervision of licensed professional health care workers.

2. T F Hospitals provide a full range of health care services.

3. T F Skilled care facilities provide care to persons who require monitoring, nursing care, and treatments.

4. T F The only function of a health care facility is to provide services for the ill and injured.

5. T F Patient-focused care means treating all patients as unique individuals.

6. T F Patients can remain in the hospital until they feel well enough to go home.

7. T F Persons receiving care in the hospital are called residents.

8. T F People who live in a common area and share common health needs form a community.

9. T F Many procedures and treatments are done on an outpatient basis to reduce costs.

10. T F A chronic illness comes on suddenly and is usually curable.

B. Multiple Choice.

Select the one best answer for each of the following.

11. The general term for a person needing health care is
    a. patient.
    b. resident.
    c. health care consumer.
    d. health care provider.

12. Psychiatric hospitals provide care only to
    a. children.
    b. persons with mental illness.
    c. persons with contagious diseases.
    d. dying persons.

13. Health care facilities
    a. treat most patients on an outpatient basis rather than admitting them.
    b. must always obtain approval from the insurer before rendering emergency care.
    c. provide a variety of health care services to ill and injured persons.
    d. allow patients to stay as long as they want if they cannot care for themselves.

14. Health care has changed because
    a. there is less demand for services.
    b. people are living longer.
    c. the death rate is increasing.
    d. it is too expensive for most people.

15. Hospice care is provided to people who
    a. are dying.
    b. need rehabilitation.
    c. need surgery.
    d. are pregnant.

16. Managed care means that insurance companies
    a. are more generous than private insurers in approving length of the patient's stay.
    b. negotiate with health care providers to render service at a lower cost.
    c. require all surgery to be done on an outpatient basis.
    d. approve only patients with certain medical conditions.

17. The obstetrics department of the hospital cares for patients
    a. with heart disease.
    b. before, during, and after childbirth.
    c. with conditions of the bones and muscles.
    d. who are mentally ill.

18. Social services staff provides
    a. nursing care 24 hours a day.
    b. diagnostic testing.
    c. counseling for patients.
    d. activities to relieve boredom.

19. Environmental services include
    a. nursing.
    b. housekeeping.
    c. therapy.
    d. surgery.

20. One type of prepaid health care insurance is
    a. Medicare.
    b. Medicaid.
    c. health maintenance organization.
    d. out-of-pocket payment.

21. The organization that accredits most health care facilities is the
    a. OSHA.
    b. Medicare.
    c. JayCo.
    d. quality assurance committee.

22. Medicare payment is made based on
    a. diagnosis related groups.
    b. services needed by the patient.
    c. actual charges billed to the government.
    d. medical supplies used.

23. The purpose of quality assurance is to
    a. guarantee quality to the government.
    b. identify and correct problems, thereby improving care.
    c. ensure that the facility receives payment for services.
    d. pass the accreditation inspection.

C. Word Choice.

Choose the correct word or phrase from the following list to complete each statement in questions 24–33.

hospitals	physical therapy
Medicare	prenatal
occupational therapy	residents
pathology	skilled care facility
patient-focused care	surgicenter

24. A _____ provides care to persons whose conditions are stable but require monitoring, nursing care, and treatments.

25. _____ are complex organizations that provide a full range of health care services.

26. _____ is given when the patient is considered a unique individual with specific needs.

27. _____ care is given to a mother during her pregnancy.

28. Persons living in a skilled care facility are usually called _____.

29. Uncomplicated surgeries may be performed in a _____.

30. _____ means the study of disease.

31. _____ helps patients regain self-care skills.

32. _____ helps patients regain mobility skills.

33. A federal program that pays health care costs for persons 65 years of age and older is called _____.

D. Nursing Assistant Challenge.

Mrs. Hernandez is pregnant with her first child. She wants to do everything she can to make sure that she has a safe and uncomplicated pregnancy, labor, and delivery, and that her baby is healthy. Consider how Mrs. Hernandez will move through the health care system to achieve this goal.

34. What is the first type of care that Mrs. Hernandez needs to help her meet the goal of an uncomplicated pregnancy?

35. In your community, where is this type of care provided?

36. What programs are offered to pregnant women in your community?

37. From which hospital departments do you think Mrs. Hernandez will receive services when she delivers her baby?

38. After the baby is born, what health care will the baby need?

UNIT 2

Role of the Nu
Assis

OBJECTIVES

After completing this unit, you will be able to:
- Spell and define terms.
- Identify the members of the interdisciplinary health care team.
- Identify the members of the nursing team.
- List the job responsibilities of the nursing assistant.
- Make a chart showing your facility's lines of authority.
- Describe the legal importance of working within the established scope of nursing assistant practice.
- Discuss the potential for career growth and advancement, and identify opportunities for expanding the scope of nursing assistant practice.
- Describe the importance of good human relationships and list ways of building productive relationships with patients, families, and staff.
- List the rules of personal hygiene and explain the importance of a healthy mental attitude.
- Describe the appropriate dress for the job.

VOCABULARY

Learn the meaning and the correct spelling of the following words and phrases:

attitude	interpersonal	Nurse Aide Competency	Omnibus Budget
burnout	relationships	Evaluation Program	Reconciliation Act
cross-trained	licensed practical nurse	(NACEP)	(OBRA)
empathy	(LPN)	nursing assistant	partners in practice
interdisciplinary health	licensed vocational nurse	nursing team	registered nurse (RN)
care team	(LVN)		scope of practice

THE INTERDISCIPLINARY HEALTH CARE TEAM

The nursing assistant is an important member of the **interdisciplinary health care team** (Figure 2-1). This team includes the patient, members of the patient's family, the physician, the nursing team, and other specialists trained to meet both general and specific patient needs (Figure 2-2). The physician names the condition or illness (makes a diagnosis) and prescribes treatment. Physicians frequently specialize in one area of medical practice. Table 2-1 lists common medical specialties, the name for the physician who practices each specialty, and a description of the care provided by each specialist.

The **nursing team** provides skilled nursing care. The team consists of registered nurses, licensed practical (or

FIGURE 2-1 The interdisciplinary team members are like the links in a chain; they work together in providing services to patients.

FIGURE 2-2 Each member of the health care team makes important contributions to the overall operation of the facility and well-being of patients.

TABLE 2–1 MEDICAL SPECIALTIES

Specialty	Physician	Type of Care
Allergy	Allergist	Diagnoses and treats patients with hypersensitivities.
Cardiovascular diseases	Cardiologist	Diagnoses and treats patients with disorders of the heart and blood vessels.
Critical care	Intensivist	Specializes in intensive care and treats critically ill and injured patients.
Dermatology	Dermatologist	Diagnoses and treats patients with disorders of the skin.
Endocrinology	Endocrinologist	Specializes in diabetes; diagnoses and treats other disorders of the endocrine system and glands that make hormones.
Gastroenterology	Gastroenterologist	Diagnoses and treats patients with disorders of the digestive system.
Gerontology	Gerontologist	Diagnoses and treats disorders of the aging person.
Gynecology	Gynecologist	Diagnoses and treats disorders related to the female reproductive tract.
Hematology	Hematologist	Diagnoses and treats patients with disorders of the blood and blood-forming organs.
Hospital care	Hospitalist	Specializes in hospital care. The primary practice of these doctors is in the hospital rather than an office. The doctor admits patients through the emergency department and directs, manages, and reports on the hospital course of treatment to the patient's primary physician.
Internal medicine	Internist	Diagnoses and treats patients with disorders of the internal organs.

continues

TABLE 2-1 *CONTINUED*

Specialty	Physician	Type of Care
Neurology	Neurologist	Diagnoses and treats patients with disorders of the nervous system.
Obstetrics	Obstetrician	Provides care to women during pregnancy, childbirth, and immediately thereafter.
Oncology	Oncologist	Diagnoses and treats patients with cancerous tumors.
Ophthalmology	Ophthalmologist	Diagnoses and treats patients with disorders of the eyes.
Pediatrics	Pediatrician	Diagnoses, treats, and prevents disorders in children.
Psychiatry	Psychiatrist	Diagnoses and treats disorders of the mind.
Radiology	Radiologist	Diagnoses and treats disorders with X-rays and other forms of imaging technology.
Urology	Urologist	Diagnoses and treats disorders of the urinary tract and male reproductive tract.

vocational) nurses, and nursing assistants. Registered nurses plan and direct the nursing care of patients according to the physician's orders. All members of the team provide direct patient care.

Care provider specialists who may also be part of the team include the dietitian, physical therapist, occupational therapist, speech therapist, respiratory therapist, and pharmacist. Table 2-2 provides details of the basic education and certification or licensure requirements for the members of the health care team mentioned here, as well as others.

TABLE 2-2 INTERDISCIPLINARY HEALTH CARE TEAM MEMBERS

Each of these disciplines requires a specified course of study (many require a minimum of a college degree and clinical experience). Most require either licensing by a state agency or certification from a professional association. Requirements may vary from state to state for some disciplines.

Patient	The most important member of the interdisciplinary team. The patient has input into the planning and implementation of care. The family may participate with the patient or in place of the patient if the patient is unable to do so.
Physician	Licensed by the state to diagnose and treat disease and to prescribe medications. Many specialty areas within medicine require additional education.
Clinical Nurse Specialist (CNS)	An advanced-practice registered nurse with a master's degree whose care focuses on a very specific patient population (e.g., medical, surgical, diabetic, cardiovascular, operating room, emergency room, critical care, geriatric, neonatal, etc.).
Nurse Practitioner (NP)	A registered nurse with advanced academic and clinical experience, which enables the NP to diagnose and manage common acute and chronic illnesses, either independently or as part of a health care team. A nurse practitioner provides some care previously offered only by physicians, and in most states has the ability to prescribe medications.
Physician Assistant (PA)	A health care professional licensed to practice medicine with physician supervision. PAs conduct physical exams, diagnose and treat illnesses, order and interpret tests, counsel on preventive health care, assist in surgery, and in most states can write prescriptions. Because of the close working relationship the PAs have with physicians, PAs are educated in the medical model designed to complement physician practice.

continues

TABLE 2-2 *CONTINUED*

Registered Nurse (RN)	Licensed by the state to make assessments and plan, implement, and evaluate nursing care. Supervises other nursing staff and may coordinate the interdisciplinary health care team. Many specialty areas within nursing require additional education.
Licensed Practical Nurse (LPN or LVN)	Licensed by the state to provide direct patient care under the supervision of a registered nurse. Called *licensed vocational nurse* in Texas and California.
Nursing Assistant	Has completed at least 75 hours of a state-approved course, passed a competency examination, and is certified to provide direct patient care under the supervision of a licensed nurse.
Nutrition Assistant (Feeding Assistant)	This position was created by the federal government in 2003. After completing a state-approved class, this worker may assist stable, long-term care facility residents with food and fluids, under the direction of a licensed nurse.
Medication Aide (MA)	A certified nursing assistant who has taken additional classes in medication administration methods and completed a state certification examination. Allowed to pass medications in nursing facilities and home health care in some states under the supervision of a licensed nurse.
Restorative Assistant (RNA)	A certified nursing assistant who has additional education in restorative nursing care. Delivers care designed to assist the patient to attain and maintain his or her highest level of function, and prevent physical deformities.
Specialty Services	
Chaplain	Provides services to meet the religious and spiritual needs of patients. Provides emotional support.
Dietitian	Licensed by the state to assess nutritional needs; plans menus and therapeutic diets and provides food services for patients.
Occupational Therapist (OT)	Licensed to provide rehabilitative services to evaluate and treat persons with physical injury or illness, psychosocial problems, or developmental disabilities. Occupational therapy assistants and aides have completed specified courses of study and work under the supervision of a physical occupational therapist. Most care is directed toward improving fine motor skills and activities of daily living.
Orthotist	Licensed by the state to design and fit braces and splints for the extremities.
Physical Therapist (PT)	Licensed by the state to provide rehabilitative services to evaluate and treat persons with physical injury or illness, psychosocial problems, or developmental disabilities. Physical therapy assistants and aides have completed specified courses of study and work under the supervision of a physical therapist. Most care is directed toward restoring gross motor skills, mobility, and ambulation.
Respiratory Therapist (also called respiratory care practitioner or RCP)	Licensed to evaluate and treat diseases and problems associated with breathing and the respiratory tract.
Social Worker	Licensed by the state to assess and provide services to meet the nonmedical, psychosocial needs of patients.
Speech Therapist (also called speech-language pathologist or SLP)	Licensed by the state to provide services to individuals with speech and swallowing disorders caused by acute and chronic illness and trauma.

continues

TABLE 2-2 *CONTINUED*

Ancillary Clinical	
Pharmacist	Licensed by the state to fill prescriptions for medications as ordered by the physician. Acts as information resource to nurses and physicians for updates on new medications and for maintaining safe drug therapy for patients.
Phlebotomist	Individuals who are trained to use needles to puncture a vein for the purpose of drawing blood.
Laboratory Technician	Laboratory worker who prepares specimens, operates automated analyzers, and performs manual tests.
Laboratory Technologist	Individual who has a bachelor's degree; performs complex laboratory tests and microscopically examines blood, tissue, and other body substances.

In addition to these members of the interdisciplinary health care team, other employees in the health care facility provide services that benefit patients.

Administrator—Provides general administration and supervision.

Environmental Services—Maintain a clean and comfortable environment.

Volunteers—Provide personal services such as delivering mail, doing errands, and providing reading materials.

THE NURSING TEAM

The Registered Nurse

The **registered nurse (RN)** becomes registered by passing a national licensure examination given by the state. The nurse has a four-year college education with a baccalaureate degree, or an associate in applied science degree from a two-year community college or technical school program, or a diploma from a hospital school of nursing. Because they have taken and successfully passed a licensing examination and are registered, all these nurses use the initials RN after their names.

Registered nurses have been educated to assess, plan for, evaluate, and coordinate the many aspects of patient care. Registered nurses teach patients and their families about good health practices. They also provide nursing care and supervise any duties they delegate to others.

Nurses may specialize in a specific area of nursing practice. Some of the common nursing specialties are:

- Maternal and child health
- Anesthesiology
- Gerontology
- Oncology
- Administration
- Public health
- Teaching
- Telemetry
- Surgery
- Home care
- Cardiac care
- Independent practice (nurse practitioner)
- Research
- Infection control

The Licensed Practical/ Vocational Nurse

The **licensed practical** or **licensed vocational nurse** has generally completed a 1-year to 18-month training program and has passed a national licensure examination administered by the state. She or he is identified by the initials LPN or LVN. This nurse works under the supervision of the registered nurse, a physician, or a dentist. The LPN is able to provide most of the care when the patient's nursing needs are not complex, and also assists the RN in more complicated situations.

The Nursing Assistant

The **nursing assistant** assists with the care of patients under the supervision of either an RN or an LPN (Figure 2-3). Because the assistant's responsibilities and skills are not as great as those of the RN or LPN/LVN, the basic preparation is shorter. However, growth and learning will continue throughout your career. In the health care facility, the assistant is called by one of the following names:

- Patient care attendant
- Nurse's aide, nurse assistant, or nursing assistant

FIGURE 2-3 A professional nurse heads the nursing team and supervises nursing assistants and other team members.

- Clinical support associate
- Nurse extender
- Health care assistant
- Personal care assistant
- Patient care technician
- Unlicensed assistive personnel (UAP)
- _____ care technician; the first word of the title designates the unit on which the assistant works, such as critical care technician, surgical care technician, and so forth.

ORGANIZATION OF NURSING CARE

Each facility selects a method of providing nursing care to meet its patients' needs. No single delivery system is ideal. Each facility determines job duties and the model of care based on cost-effectiveness and maximum patient benefit. The education, competency, and teamwork of nursing assistant staff are key to the success of these systems.

Nursing care is commonly organized in one of several ways:

- Primary nursing
- Functional nursing
- Team nursing
- Partners in practice

The nursing assistant has a functional role in each.

Primary Nursing

In primary nursing, care is given by a registered nurse. This nurse is responsible for an assigned patient's care for that patient's entire hospitalization. Licensed staff and assistants help with the care when the RN is not on duty. The nurse plans and coordinates the nursing care, teaches, carries out treatments, gives direct nursing care, and plans for the patient's discharge. Patients appreciate primary nursing because it enables them to relate directly to one specific nurse. Each RN is assigned to and responsible for six to eight patients in the primary nursing situation.

Functional Nursing

Functional nursing is a task-oriented way to organize care. It is an older method that is once again being used more frequently. In this method of practice, the charge nurse is the one person responsible for all patients. All other staff members are assigned specific tasks, such as giving medications, administering treatments, or providing hygienic care. Patients may find this type of nursing confusing because many people are involved in their care. However, some facilities feel that this method uses available, qualified personnel to best advantage.

Team Nursing

Team nursing is one of the most common methods of delivering nursing care. In this system, a registered nurse team leader determines the nursing needs of all the patients assigned to the team for care. In some work settings, the LPN or LVN is a team leader. He or she is supervised by a registered nurse. Team members receive instructions and assignments from, and report back to, the team leader.

The team approach is successful when:

- Team members understand the philosophy, goals, and purposes of restorative care. Restorative care helps patients reach their highest possible level of functioning.
- Team members understand their responsibilities.
- All team members, including the patient, and family members if the patient desires, attend the care plan conference.

Partners in Practice

In the **partners in practice** method of providing care, a registered nurse or primary nurse is paired with a nursing assistant or other team member. The team members work together to meet the needs of their assigned patients. In many facilities, they work on the same schedule.

There are many variations in this type of care. All involve partnering a registered nurse with a nursing assistant. In some hospitals, the assistants are taught to perform advanced clinical skills, such as drawing blood. In others, they provide only assistance with activities of daily living. The partners in practice and other similar methods of care combine positive aspects of team nursing and primary nursing into the partnership model. This method of care delivery is effective for providing patient care, communicating with physicians and staff from other departments, and coordinating care among staff members.

Teamwork

The various alternative models of patient care are successful because they emphasize and promote cooperation and teamwork, and provide many opportunities for personal growth. Learning to work with others as a member of a team is one of the most important skills to master during your nursing assistant education.

PATIENT-FOCUSED CARE

In addition to the models of care described here, the trend in health care has moved toward the patient-focused method of care delivery. This method of care emphasizes the needs of the patient rather than the convenience of the various departments involved with patient care. Team members on the unit make decisions jointly, and plan and deliver care promptly to meet patient needs. This is faster and involves fewer individuals than other methods of care that require coordination of service among different departments. Thus, the patient is the focus of the service.

The patient is a fully functional member of the team. Nursing staff build caring relationships with each patient. Nurses work with patients to teach them to be fully in control of and responsible for their own health and health care. Even the medical records are patient-focused instead of occupationally oriented. When care is patient-centered, nursing personnel focus on the caring aspects of their jobs. The goals of patient-focused care are to:

- Limit the number of people involved in patient care.
- Contain costs.
- Meet patients' needs efficiently.

Staff members are prepared as multiskilled workers by cross-training them to perform special skills. This enables staff to carry out selected duties that are usually performed by other workers, such as drawing blood, giving special treatments, working in specialty departments, and using more sophisticated instruments to perform tests. For example, a multiskilled nursing assistant may be **cross-trained** to draw blood, give respiratory treatments, or perform an electrocardiogram. These tasks can be done without calling a technician from another department or moving the patient out of the unit.

You can be an effective member of the interdisciplinary team by:

- Recognizing the importance of all team members.
- Appreciating each member's contribution to the team.
- Learning as much as possible about patients and their families, to help you understand their feelings and concerns.

- Attending care plan conferences and giving the team your observations and ideas.
- Attending in-service sessions to increase your knowledge.
- Becoming cross-trained, if possible, to increase your skills.
- Cooperating with other team members to provide patient-focused care.

Scope of nursing assiant

REGULATION OF NURSING ASSISTANT PRACTICE

Nursing assistants must understand the scope of the specific tasks they will be expected to carry out. They should also know the state regulations that govern their clinical practice. Federal regulations require that all states spell out the duties and responsibilities of the assistant, as well as the basic education and level of competency required for practice.

In 1987, a federal law was passed that regulates the education and certification of nurse aides. The law is called the **Omnibus Budget Reconciliation Act (OBRA)**. OBRA established the minimum requirements for nurse aide competency evaluation programs.

Effective October 1, 1990, all persons working as nurse aides had to complete a competency evaluation program or approved course. The education of nursing assistants is under individual state jurisdiction, guided by federal regulations.

The National Council of State Boards of Nursing, Inc., then developed the **Nurse Aide Competency Evaluation Program (NACEP)**. NACEP meets the requirements of OBRA. NACEP is a guide for individual programs that register and award credentials to nursing assistants. NACEP specifies the minimum skills to be achieved. Programs may exceed these minimums.

Nursing assistants who wish to be certified must complete a minimum of 75 hours of theory and practice. Some states require a minimum of 80 to 150 program hours in written or oral and clinical skills in several areas. These areas include:

- Basic nursing skills, including infection control
- Basic restorative services
- Mental health and social service needs
- Personal care skills
- Resident rights and good communication
- Safety and emergency care

Other rules that guide nursing assistant practice require:

- Completion of a competency evaluation program by October 1, 1990, of all persons who were working as nurse aides prior to July 1989.
- At least three opportunities for noncertified nursing assistants to meet requirements.
- Completion of a new training and competency program or retesting by persons who wish to work as nursing

Scope of Practice

assistants but who have not given nursing care for pay for a continuous 24-month period after completing a basic nursing assistant program.

- Continuing education (12 to 48 hours per year, in some states).

The OBRA regulations are important because they:

- Give nursing assistants recognition through registration.
- Help define the scope of nursing assistant practice.
- Provide better uniformity in the care provided by nursing assistants.
- Promote educational standards for nursing assistants.

Be sure you are familiar with any specific state laws that relate to your role as an assistant.

LINES OF AUTHORITY

Nursing assistants receive their assignments from the team leader or charge nurse, nurse manager, or unit manager. When they finish their assignments, they report to this same person. This represents the assistant's immediate line of authority and communication.

The assistant will work with a team whose leader is a licensed practical nurse or a registered nurse. In this case, the assistant's immediate superior is the team leader. The team leaders receive their instructions from the charge nurse. The charge nurse is responsible for the total care of a certain number of patients. Sometimes this includes all the patients on a wing, a unit, or a floor of the facility. Supervisors are responsible for several charge nurse units. They receive their authority and direction from the director of nursing. Health care facilities vary in the complexity of their staffing.

Assistants should learn the lines of authority in their health care facility, as shown in Figure 2-4. As a student, your immediate authority is your teacher or the person designated as your supervisor.

The physician directs the patient's medical care. The registered nurse carries out the physician's orders and plans the patient's nursing care. The authority for nursing care passes from the registered nurse supervisor to the charge nurse, to the team leader, and then to the nursing assistant. When you accept the responsibility for an assignment, you must fully understand the assignment and be capable of handling it. *If there is any doubt, you should discuss it with the team leader or charge nurse* (Figure 2-5).

GUIDELINES FOR THE NURSING ASSISTANT

Only perform tasks that you have been taught to do. If you are unsure how to carry out a procedure, inform the nurse. Do not feel embarrassed. It is better to ask for help than to make an error and injure a patient.

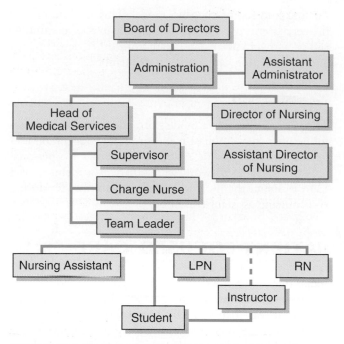

FIGURE 2-4 Typical model of the nursing department lines of authority. The diagram may vary slightly from one facility to the next.

FIGURE 2-5 If you have a question, consult your supervisor.

Seeking Higher Authority

Sometimes a report you make to your immediate supervisor is not taken seriously. Make very sure of your facts and try again to make your supervisor understand. If you fail and your information is very important, you can move up the chain of command.

For example, if you report that a person is being harmed by a coworker's inattention, but your supervisor does not listen to your report of the situation, for your patient's safety you must try again. If the second attempt also fails, the next step is to bring the problem to the attention of the next level of authority. This situation should not occur often if there are good staff relations, but it can happen.

Scope of Practice

Scope of practice means the skills the nursing assistant is legally permitted to perform by state regulations and facility policies. If another worker asks you to perform a task that is clearly out of your scope of practice, such as giving medications, be prepared to refuse. Explain in a courteous manner that this is a task for which you have not been technically or legally prepared. Report the incident to your charge nurse so that your scope of duties can be clearly understood by all staff members.

For the same reason, nursing assistants do not take orders from doctors or tell families about the contents of patient care plans or records. These actions are not within the scope of nursing assistant practice.

Nevertheless, be willing to learn new skills under the close supervision of your nurse. If the new skill is within the scope of nursing assistant practice, this will increase your ability to provide good, safe nursing care. If, for example, your nurse suggests a new way to lift a patient that is different from the way you learned in your program, listen and watch carefully as the instruction is given. Seek supervision as you practice the new technique until both you and your supervisor feel you can do it safely on your own.

Safety ALERT

Doing only tasks that you have been instructed to do, and doing things in the way that you were taught, protects patients from injury. It also protects you from injury, legal exposure, and liability. ■

Legal ALERT

Scope of practice is a very important legal concept. Your scope of practice is described in the job description given to you by your employer. The policy and procedure manuals are an additional resource. Functioning within this scope of practice protects the nursing assistant and the facility. ■

THE ROLE AND RESPONSIBILITIES OF THE NURSING ASSISTANT

The nursing assistant works directly with the patient, giving physical care and emotional support. This care is always given under the direction of the licensed nurse. The nursing assistant has an important role and can con-

tribute much to the patient's comfort and safety. Observations made during the delivery of care are reported to the nurse and are recorded on the patient's chart.

Tasks commonly assigned to nursing assistants are listed in Table 2-3. Remember that not all health care facilities assign the same tasks to nursing assistants.

Not everyone can be a nursing assistant. Nursing assistants are special people: they are interested in others, they take pride in themselves, and they are willing to learn the skills necessary to care for those who are ill.

This interest in and caring for people can be a valuable asset to the entire nursing team. You are the person the patient sees most often. This means that you have the chance to observe and hear many things that the other team members will not. By transmitting these observations to your charge nurse, you are likely to give the other team members valuable insight into the patient's illness and attitude toward that illness. For example, you may see that the patient's attitude toward the attending doctor or nurse is much less relaxed than it is with you, the nursing assistant. For that same reason, the patient is far more likely to tell you of "minor complaints" that may not be minor at all. Competent, caring nursing assistants make a valuable contribution to the comfort and safety of the patients.

EXPANDED SCOPE OF PRACTICE

In many states and facilities, persons who have completed the nursing assistant program and have experience in clinical practice can expand their scope of practice by taking additional classes to learn new skills and gain job responsibilities. These programs provide the opportunity for career advancement. Some of these programs are given by the employer, and enable the assistant to perform additional skills while at work in the facility. Other classes are held by private companies that sponsor seminars for nursing assistants. Other programs are recognized by the state. These are normally given by community colleges. Successfully completing the program enables the assistant to practice the advanced skills anywhere in the state.

Types of classes vary widely. Common types of classes include those that:

- Prepare students to provide advanced nursing skills, such as drawing blood, inserting a urinary catheter, or performing an electrocardiogram.
- Teach the nursing assistant how to give medications in the long-term care facility.
- Expand clinical responsibilities by learning clerical skills, unit management, supply and inventory management, or mentoring new workers.
- Provide specialized information and additional certification in specialized subjects, such as geriatric care, therapy or restorative nursing care, or end-of-life care.

TABLE 2-3 TYPICAL JOB DESCRIPTION FOR A NURSING ASSISTANT

Nursing assistants commonly participate in the nursing process by carrying out the activities listed. **Note:** Use standard precautions while providing care.

1. Assist with patient assessment and care planning.
   a. Check and record vital signs
   b. Measure height and weight
   c. Measure intake and output
   d. Collect specimens
   e. Test urine and feces
   f. Observe patient response to care given
   g. Report and record observations of patients' conditions
2. Assist patients in meeting nutritional and elimination needs.
   a. Check food trays
   b. Pass food trays
   c. Feed patients
   d. Provide fresh drinking water and nourishments
   e. Assist with bedpans, urinals, and commodes
   f. Empty urine collection bags
   g. Assist with colostomy care
   h. Give enemas
   i. Observe feces and urine
3. Assist patients with mobility.
   a. Turn and position
   b. Provide range-of-motion exercises
   c. Transfer to wheelchair or stretcher
   d. Assist with ambulation
4. Assist patients with personal hygiene and grooming.
   a. Bathe patients
   b. Provide nail and hair care
   c. Give oral hygiene
   d. Provide denture care
   e. Shave patients
   f. Assist with dressing and undressing

5. Assist with patient comfort and anxiety relief.
   a. Protect patient privacy and maintain confidentiality
   b. Keep call signal within patient's reach
   c. Answer call signal promptly
   d. Provide orientation to the room or unit and to other patients and visitors
   e. Assist patients with communications
   f. Protect personal possessions
   g. Provide diversional activities
   h. Give backrubs
   i. Prepare hot and cold applications
6. Assist in promoting patient safety and environmental cleanliness.
   a. Use side rails and restraints appropriately
   b. Keep patient unit clean and clutter-free
   c. Make beds
   d. Clean and care for equipment
   e. Carry out isolation precautions
   f. Observe oxygen precautions
   g. Assist in keeping recreational and nonpatient areas clean and free of hazards
   h. Participate in fire drills and patient evacuation procedures
7. Assist with unit management and efficiency.
   a. Transport patients
   b. Take specimens to lab
   c. Assist with special procedures
   d. Do errands as required
   e. Assist with cost-containment measures
   f. Answer the telephone
   g. Document care provided and assist with unit recordkeeping

As you can see, there are many opportunities for qualified health care workers. Take advantage of classes in which you will learn new information and skills. Many facilities have special programs, such as career ladders for career growth and enhancement. You will find that you have chosen a career with unlimited opportunities for personal growth and satisfaction.

PERSONAL VOCATIONAL ADJUSTMENTS

You will have to make some personal adjustments to your new work situation. Health care facility rules and orders

from supervisors must be obeyed promptly, even if you do not agree with them. Rules are written for the protection and welfare of both the patient and the health care provider. You must also learn to accept constructive criticism and profit by it. It means you are willing to learn and grow.

You show your maturity in many ways. You demonstrate:

- Dependability and accuracy by reporting for duty on time (Figure 2-6) and completing your assignments carefully.
- Respect for your coworkers and the place you share together on the nursing team when you are ready to help.
- Understanding of human relationships by being empathetic, patient, and tactful with others.

FIGURE 2-6 Reporting for work on time is a sign of responsibility and demonstrates dependability.

FIGURE 2-7 A positive attitude and spirit of cooperation are employee attributes that make the workplace pleasant.

Interpersonal Relationships

Interpersonal relationships are simply interactions between people. You develop interpersonal relationships with everyone you know. Some relationships are deep and lasting, and some are only casual. But to some degree, you react to others and they react to you. Friendship is a good example of an interpersonal relationship that is satisfactory to two people.

Much of the satisfaction that a nursing assistant gets from work comes from the quality of the relationships that are developed with other staff members and patients. Some people call this the ability to get along with others.

Similarly, good relationships with others begin with your own personality and attitudes. If you are a warm and accepting person with positive attitudes, others will respond in the same way. If you walk down the street and someone smiles at you, without thinking, your reaction is to smile back. Most human relationships are like this.

It is not necessary for you personally to like someone else to be pleasant and cooperative with him or her as you carry out your duties (Figure 2-7).

Attitude

Perhaps the most important single characteristic that you bring to your job is your **attitude**. Your attitude is developed throughout your lifetime, and it is shaped by the experiences you have had. Some people think having an "attitude" means being negative or opinionated, but all people show attitude through their behavior. Sometimes the attitude demonstrated is good and sometimes it is poor.

All the other characteristics described are an outer reflection of your inner feelings—of your attitude toward yourself and others. Your attitude should reflect:

- Caring
- Courtesy
- Cooperation
- Emotional control
- **Empathy** (understanding)
- Tact
- Patience

Patients have the right and need to be cared for in a calm, unhurried atmosphere by people with a caring attitude.

Patient Relationships

Patients come in all sizes and shapes and ages: young, old, and in between. Some have major, complicated illnesses. Others have physical problems that can be helped with rest and medication. Some patients are in the health facility to begin their lives. Others will end their lives there. A good nursing assistant shows empathy for the patient by being eager to serve and by using a gentle touch.

Every patient entering a health care facility presents a unique set of problems and concerns to the staff. These problems and concerns are important. As you compare the conditions of many patients in your own mind, however, it might seem that one has more serious problems than another. Because patients do not share your knowledge, they will not know this. Never forget that, to the patient, her or his own problems are the most important.

Meeting the Patient's Needs

Patients' personalities are shaped by their life experiences, which are now complicated by illness. Their social, spiritual, and physical needs must continue to be met even though they are in a different, more confined setting. The restrictions imposed by illness limit, to some degree, their ability to satisfy these needs through the normal channels. This is naturally frustrating and puts great strain on the patient's ability to establish and maintain good interpersonal relationships.

Some patients become irritable, complaining, and uncooperative because of:

- Fears about their diagnosis, disfigurement, disability, and death
- Pain
- Unrealistic perceptions of activities around them
- Uncertainties about the future
- Worries about family
- The loss or lack of social support systems
- Dependence on others
- Financial concerns

Offer emotional support (Figure 2-8), listen carefully, and report these concerns to the nurse.

Meeting the Family's Needs

Families and friends are very concerned when one of their loved ones is in a health care facility, especially when that person may have a life-threatening illness. This puts stress in their lives too. They need to be reassured. Their anxiety sometimes makes them demanding and uncooperative.

The nursing assistant who understands human behavior makes allowances for these stresses and realizes that ill people, coworkers, and families under stress may be touchy and not always on their best behavior. This is why

FIGURE 2-9 Concerned family members also need support from staff.

sensitivity and awareness of the needs of others are most important at this time (Figure 2-9). It is in these situations that patience and tact are most needed. Sometimes just quietly listening to another or rephrasing your sentences can change an entire interaction. Try to be aware not only of the words used but also of the body language. As with words, clues such as the tone of a voice or a hand movement reveal much about the inner feelings of other people. Always keep in mind that people are three-dimensional. They are physical beings, emotional beings, and social beings.

Staff Relationships

You are part of the staff of a health care facility. All workers share a single goal: to help the patient. This single purpose welds you together into a unit that must work smoothly if your goal is to be accomplished. Good interpersonal relationships will make your working hours satisfying and productive. Good relationships can be formed if you:

- Remember that each of you has a specific role to fulfill and jobs to carry out.
- Do not overstep your authority or criticize others.
- Listen to instructions from your supervisor carefully. Phrase questions about your assignment in such a way that your supervisor knows you are looking for clarification—not challenging authority.
- Remember that your tone of voice and body language can change the message you are trying to convey.
- Promptly carry out orders and report any work that you are unable to finish.
- Offer help to others and accept help when you need it. Coworkers can often help one another when a task is particularly difficult or physically taxing (for example, lifting a heavy patient or moving equipment). Simply being available when another member of the team gets behind in his or her work is a great help.

FIGURE 2-8 A worried patient is reassured by gentle touch.

- Have a cheerful, positive attitude. This is as important for staff members' relationships as it is in establishing rapport (sympathetic understanding) with patients.
- Extend the same dignity and courtesy to every staff member that you would to patients.
- Always keep your common goal in mind. Recognize coworkers as important members of the total team.

Professional and personal adjustments are made easier if the nursing assistant:

- Understands and follows facility policies and procedures.
- Treats patients, coworkers, and visitors with respect.
- Practices proper hygiene and grooming, good nutrition, and stress reduction.

PERSONAL HEALTH AND HYGIENE

Good personal grooming is essential, because the assistant is in close contact with patients (Figure 2-10). Because the work of the assistant, although rewarding, can be physically challenging, it is important that all body odors be controlled. The nursing assistant is often the last to know that he or she has bad breath or body odor. A daily shower or bath and the use of an antiperspirant/deodorant are essential. The mouth and teeth must be kept clean. The nursing assistant should also recognize that strong perfumes, aftershave lotions, and cigarette odors are often offensive to patients.

Hair should be clean and either short or tied back in a controlled style. Fingernails should be kept short and clean. If nail polish is used, it should be clear, not colored. Stockings and socks should be freshly laundered. Shoes and shoelaces should be cleaned daily. Fatigue will be lessened if shoes give proper support to the feet and are well-fitted.

Jewelry is not part of the nursing assistant's uniform, as it is a ready medium for bacterial growth. Jewelry may also injure the patient or the assistant, especially if the patient is confused or is a young child. Long, dangling earrings can be especially dangerous to the assistant, because they are easily caught in linen or pulled out by a combative patient. Most health care agencies permit members of the nursing staff to wear wedding rings and small earrings. Watches with second hands are used to monitor the condition of patients and to measure vital signs.

Infection Control ALERT

Your hair is like a magnet for germs. Keeping it short makes it easier to care for. Washing your hair regularly is best. Long fingernails, artificial nails, and chipped nail polish are also good hiding places for germs. Avoid acrylic and artificial nails. Keep your natural nails short and clean. Jewelry also harbors germs. Sharp stones and settings can injure patients and tear gloves. Only simple jewelry, such as a plain wedding band, should be worn when on duty. ■

Safety ALERT

Keeping long hair pulled back reduces the risk of injury from hair becoming entangled in equipment or being inadvertently pulled by a patient. Small stud-type pierced earrings also reduce your risk of injury from an earring being pulled or caught. ■

Uniforms

Many health care facilities allow health care workers great leeway in selecting the type and style of their uniforms. Traditionally, patients were able to identify the various types of health care workers by their uniforms, including caps. Today, it can be very difficult to distinguish between a physical therapist, registered nurse, physician, or social worker. It is no wonder that newly admitted patients are

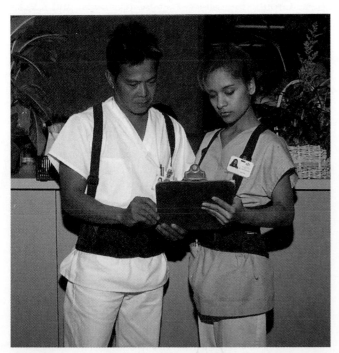

FIGURE 2-10 Well-groomed caregivers instill confidence in patients.

often confused as to whom they should approach for information or help. To help avoid this confusion, some states and many health care facilities require personnel to wear a name badge or photo identification tag at all times while on the job. The name badge may state only your first name and title. Some facilities do not list the last name of a worker on the name badge, as a protective security measure.

If your health care facility requires that you wear a uniform, you should wear it only while you are on duty. If your health care agency does not provide facilities for changing your uniform before and after going on duty, be sure to wear a cover-up as you travel to and from work so you will not spread germs. When you get home, remove your uniform, fold it inside out, and put it into the laundry. This helps keep the dirtiest part of your uniform away from the other clothes in the laundry. Wearing a fresh uniform every day should become a habit. It should be clean and in good condition. Torn hems and missing buttons should be repaired and replaced.

Above all, remember that your patients' safety and comfort are your main concerns. Try to keep in mind their needs and feelings. After all, would you feel confident if you were ill and the assistant caring for you had long fingernails that could scratch you, or that could collect dirt and possibly infect your surgical incision? How would you feel if the assistant who was preparing you for surgery kept having to push the hair out of his eyes? Or if the assistant assigned to give you a backrub wore clanking bracelets on her wrists?

Remember, too, that how you look reflects the pride you have in yourself and in your work. Well-groomed nursing assistants who pay attention to the details of their person and appearance show others, especially their patients and coworkers, that they are likely to have the same pride and caring attitude in their work. If you are well groomed and have good personal habits, patients will feel more secure and confident, and other staff members will regard you as mature and reliable. As you develop good health habits, you become a role model for your family, friends, and coworkers.

Reducing Stress

Your work as a nursing assistant is physically and emotionally demanding because you must give so much of yourself to those in your care. To stay healthy and do your best, you will need:

- Sufficient rest
- Good nutrition
- Satisfying leisure activities (Figure 2-11)
- Ways to reduce stress

Burnout is total mental, emotional, and sometimes physical exhaustion. Burnout is common among those working in health care facilities. You can reduce the stress that leads to burnout by balancing your work with rest and recreation.

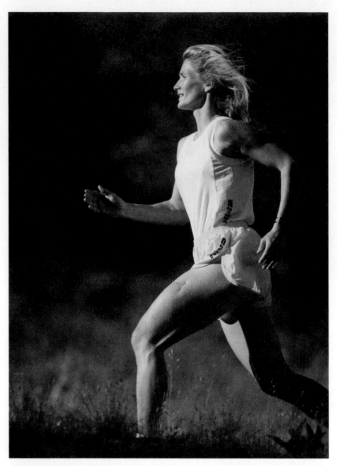

FIGURE 2-11 Strive to balance your life between work, recreational activities, and family responsibilities.

Some facilities offer programs to help employees reduce stress. Group discussions, exercise programs, and special counseling are available for general stress management and to meet special circumstances, such as when a patient dies or when individual interstaff conflicts arise. Death is always a possibility, but the staff usually focus on improvement and recovery. The loss of a patient, especially a child, can be very stressful. Caring for an abused child can take a great toll on the staff as they try to work with the child and family.

Occasionally personality conflicts are aggravated by the daily close contact. Stress caused by these situations can often be handled through a stress management group discussion.

Change

Experienced health care workers will tell you that change is ongoing in the health care industry. New competitors build facilities and take away established customers (patients); technology changes constantly; legislation changes the way services must be delivered; patients have increasing expectations as they learn, grow, and become more knowledgeable. Change is never really finished. In one way or other, it is ongoing. Change can be very disruptive and unpredictable, and uncertainty about change can be difficult for everyone. Venturing into unknown territory can be threatening. Workers faced with change may feel insecure, believing that change will expose their shortcomings and deficits. Because of this, many people resist change. When workers are resistant to change, negative attitudes cause additional turmoil for others.

The ability to adapt to change is an asset that all workers must master. Try these strategies to cope with change successfully:

- Learn all you can about the change and your responsibilities.
- Try to understand the need for and value of the change.
- Find ways to adapt and accommodate to the change.
- Try to be open-minded and flexible.
- Cooperate with others and be a team player.
- Adjust your attitude. Look forward to the change as an opportunity for new challenges, growth, and accomplishment.
- Try to keep your sense of humor. Make change fun. Although you may take change seriously, try to have a good time in spite of any discomfort you feel.
- Compensate for the stress and pressure you feel by making time for activities you enjoy when you are off duty.

Remember the old adage, "Change is inevitable, but growth is optional." View each workplace change as an opportunity for growth. Doing so will do more than help you survive. Having a positive attitude and using change as an opportunity for growth will help you thrive in the ever-changing health care workplace.

Personal Stress Reduction

You can learn personal stress-reducing techniques. Food, alcohol, or other drugs are used by some people to reduce stress, but these substances can cause serious health problems. For example, some people use chemicals or drugs to reduce stress. This is dangerous because chemicals and drugs alter the body's chemistry, causing serious changes to thought and behavior. In some cases, drug use becomes addictive and can cause death.

There are better and safer ways to prevent burnout and relieve stress. To reduce stress:

- Talk to your supervisor; a team conference may help.
- Try sitting for a few moments with your feet up.
- Shut your eyes and take some deep breaths.
- With your eyes shut, picture a special place you like and, in your mind, take yourself there.
- Take a warm, relaxing bath.
- Listen to some quiet music.
- Carry out a specific relaxation exercise.
- Make yourself a cup of herbal tea and drink it slowly.
- Exercise.
- Devote time to hobbies such as sewing, painting, woodworking, or playing a musical instrument.
- Go for a walk.
- Take advantage of available stress reduction programs.

REVIEW

A. True/False.

Mark the following true or false by circling T or F.

1. T F The registered nurse plans and directs the nursing care of patients.

2. T F Interdisciplinary health care providers work as a team.

3. T F The LVN has completed a four-year college-based program.

4. T F The nursing assistant gives physical care and emotional support to patients under the direction of the licensed nurse.

5. T F The nursing assistant is an important member of the nursing team.

6. T F Patients enjoy primary nursing because it allows them to relate directly to one specific registered nurse.

7. T F Team nursing is a common way of providing patient care.

8. T F It is all right to perform a task even if you are unsure how to do it.

9. T F Nursing assistants are special people.

10. T F Nursing assistants should be willing to learn and practice new skills under the supervision of the nurse.

11. T F Caring about people is a valuable asset for a nursing assistant.

12. T F It is not important for the nursing assistant to be well groomed.

13. T F Patients may find strong perfumes or after-shave lotions offensive.

14. T F Hair and fingernails should be kept short and clean.

15. T F It is all right to wear your uniform when you go grocery shopping.

16. T F How you look reflects the pride you feel in yourself.

17. T F Patient safety and comfort are main concerns for all caregivers.

18. T F Being a nursing assistant can be very stressful.

19. T F Smoking and eating are the best ways to reduce stress.

20. T F One of the most important characteristics you bring to your job is a positive attitude.

B. Multiple Choice.

Select the one best answer for each of the following.

21. The interdisciplinary team member who writes the medical orders for patient care is the
  a. registered nurse.
  b. social worker.
  c. physician.
  d. dietitian.

22. The nursing care approach that is task-oriented is
  a. primary nursing.
  b. functional nursing.
  c. team nursing.
  d. patient-focused care.

23. A nursing assistant who has a question regarding an assignment should properly ask the
  a. physician.
  b. charge nurse.
  c. physiotherapist.
  d. administrator.

24. A patient tells you that he has difficulty making a fist because his hand feels weak. He did not mention this fact to the nurse. You must
  a. ignore it. The patient should have told the nurse.
  b. tell another assistant.
  c. tell the nurse.
  d. tell the physician.

25. You demonstrate maturity by
  a. rushing assignments.
  b. being disrespectful to coworkers.
  c. "bending" the rules.
  d. reporting for duty on time.

C. Matching.

Match the interdisciplinary team member and his or her function.

26. _____ Licensed to fill prescriptions for medications.

27. _____ Qualified to test hearing.

28. _____ Provides services to meet spiritual needs.

29. _____ Licensed to fit and design braces and splints for extremities.

30. _____ Licensed to provide rehabilitative services and to evaluate and treat persons with physical injury or illness, psychosocial problems, or developmental disabilities.

  a. orthotist
  b. pharmacist
  c. chaplain
  d. occupational therapist
  e. audiologist

D. Completion.

Complete the following.

31. Why is it improper for nursing assistants to take orders directly from the physician? _____

32. The benefits of a nursing assistant certification are:
  a. _____
  b. _____
  c. _____
  d. _____ **E. Nursing Assistant Challenge.**

Read each clinical situation and answer the questions.

33. Enrique is given his assignment and has questions.
  a. He must check his assignment with _____.
  b. One of his assignments is to bathe patients. Is this appropriate? _____
  c. One of his assignments is to give medications. Is this appropriate? _____

34. Felicia once worked as a part-time assistant to an elderly woman but was never certified as a nursing assistant. What can you tell her about the requirements?
  a. Is a competency evaluation program required? _____
  b. How many opportunities are there to meet requirements? _____
  c. How much continuing education is required once certification is granted? _____

35. Peggy reported for duty wearing bracelets, long earrings, and pale pink nail polish. Her uniform was clean and crisp but the hem was hanging down on one side. Her shoes were dirty. State ways in which her appearance can be improved.

UNIT 3

Consumer Rights and Responsibilities in Health Care

OBJECTIVES

After completing this unit, you will be able to:

- Spell and define terms.
- Explain the purpose of health care consumer rights.
- Describe six items that are common to Residents' Rights, the Patients' Bill of Rights, and the Clients' Rights in Home Care.

- List three specific rights from each of the three documents.
- Describe eight responsibilities of health care consumers.

VOCABULARY

Learn the meaning and the correct spelling of the following words and phrases:

advance directives
Clients' Rights
corporal punishment

grievance
informed consent
involuntary seclusion

Patients' Bill of Rights
Residents' Rights

CONSUMER RIGHTS

All citizens in the United States have certain rights (for example, the right to vote) that are guaranteed by law. Health care consumers have rights to ensure that they will receive quality patient care. There are different documents for patient rights, depending on where care is given. In each setting, if the health care consumer is unable to read or understand the document, the law makes provisions to ensure that he or she is informed of these rights. For example, facilities are required to have the bill of rights translated into languages that are common in the community. If the patient cannot understand the information because of a mental condition, the bill of rights is given to

his or her family. Staff are expected to be familiar with and protect each patient's rights. A copy of the **Residents' Rights** is given to each person before he or she is admitted to a skilled care facility (Figure 3-1). The rights of residents in skilled care facilities were legislated by the federal government in the Omnibus Budget Reconciliation Act (OBRA) of 1987. The resident must sign a form indicating that the resident and/or the resident's family have received the document. The **Patients' Bill of Rights** is given to patients upon admission to a hospital. Persons receiving care in their homes are given a copy of the **Clients' Rights** by the nurse on the first visit to the home. The client is asked to sign a form indicating that he or she received the document.

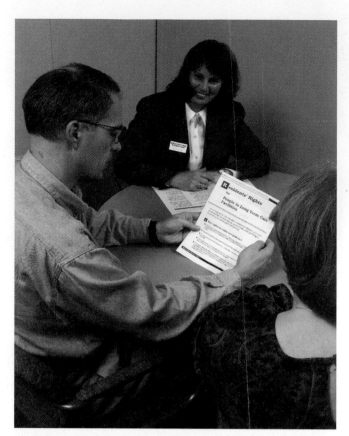

FIGURE 3-1 The Residents' Bill of Rights is presented to each resident (or the resident's legally responsible party) upon long-term care facility admission.

FIGURE 3-2 Informed consent is necessary for some procedures.

All persons working in health care should be familiar with the document that pertains to the facility they work in. Supporting the rights of the health care consumer contributes to more effective care. Each of these documents is similar and emphasizes the right of the patient, resident, or client to:

- Be treated in a respectful, dignified manner—this includes the right to privacy and to confidentiality.
- Have the benefit of open and honest communication with caregivers.
- Have a role in decision making for treatment choices and planning of care. **Informed consent** means that the consumer gives permission for care or procedures after full disclosure of the purpose of the care or procedure, the benefits, and risks involved (Figure 3-2).
- Be advised of their rights about **advance directives** (documents that give instructions about the consumer's wishes for treatment if the consumer is terminally ill or unable to communicate).
- Receive continuity of care.
- Be informed of resources for resolving conflicts or grievances. A **grievance** is a situation in which the consumer feels there are grounds for complaint.

Each rights document is reproduced in this unit (Figures 3-3, 3-4, and 3-5).

RESPONSIBILITIES OF HEALTH CARE CONSUMERS

Providing for the rights of the consumer will not ensure quality care unless consumers are willing to fulfill certain responsibilities. These responsibilities include:

- Maintaining personal health care records so information is readily available when needed.
- Communicating openly and honestly with the physician and other caregivers and being willing to give a complete health and family history.
- Providing information regarding past hospitalizations and medications.
- Informing the physician and other caregivers if they anticipate problems with following prescribed treatment.
- Learning how to manage their own health (Figure 3-6).
- Asking for clarification if they do not fully understand instructions or explanations.
- Living a healthy lifestyle and avoiding unnecessary risks of illness or injury.
- Accepting financial responsibility for payment of health care and providing information for insurance claims.

The rights of health care consumers have both a legal and an ethical basis. Legal and ethical aspects are discussed in Unit 4.

Residents' Rights

OBRA (handwritten)

This is an abbreviated version of the Residents' Rights as set forth in the Omnibus Budget Reconciliation Act. This document must be given to all residents and/or their families prior to admission to a long-term care facility.

1. The resident has the right to free choice, including the right to:
   - choose an attending physician
   - full advance information about changes in care or treatment
   - participate in the assessment and care planning process
   - self-administer medications if the resident is able to safely do so
   - consent to participate in experimental research
2. The resident has the right to freedom from abuse and restraints, including freedom from:
   - physical, sexual, mental abuse
   - **corporal punishment** (the use of physical force) and **involuntary seclusion** (isolating a resident without a medical reason)
   - physical and chemical restraints
3. The resident has the right to privacy, including privacy for:
   - treatment and nursing care
   - receiving/sending mail
   - telephone calls
   - visitors
4. The resident has the right to confidentiality of personal and clinical records.
5. The resident has the right to accommodation of needs, including:
   - choices about life
   - receiving assistance in maintaining independence

6. The resident has the right to voice grievances.
7. The resident has the right to organize and participate in family and resident groups.
8. The resident has the right to participate in social, religious, and community activities, including the right to:
   - vote
   - keep religious items in the room
   - attend religious services
9. The resident has the right to examine survey results and correction plans.
10. The resident has the right to manage personal funds.
11. The resident has the right to information about eligibility for Medicare/Medicaid funds.
12. The resident has the right to file complaints about abuse, neglect, or misappropriation of property.
13. The resident has the right to information about advocacy groups.
14. The resident has the right to immediate and unlimited access to family or relatives.
15. The resident has the right to share a room with the spouse if they are both residents in the same facility.
16. The resident has the right to perform or not perform work for the facility if it is medically appropriate for the resident to work.
17. The resident has the right to remain in the facility except in certain circumstances.
18. The resident has the right to use personal possessions.
19. The resident has the right to notification of change in condition.

FIGURE 3-3 Residents' Bill of Rights

Ombudsman – paid position to advocate for the resident (handwritten)

The Patients' Bill of Rights

Introduction

Effective health care requires collaboration between patients and physicians and other health care professionals. Open and honest communication, respect for personal and professional values, and sensitivity to differences are integral to optimal patient care. As the setting for the provision of health services, hospitals must provide a foundation for understanding and respecting the rights and responsibilities of patients, their families, physicians, and other caregivers. Hospitals must ensure a health care ethic that respects the role of patients in decision making about treatment choices and other aspects of their care. Hospitals must be sensitive to cultural, racial, linguistic, religious, age, gender, and other differences as well as the needs of persons with disabilities.

The American Hospital Association presents *The Patients' Bill of Rights* with the expectation that it will contribute to more effective patient care and be supported by the hospital on behalf of the institution, its medical staff, employees, and patients. The American Hospital Association encourages health care institutions to tailor this bill of rights to their patient community by translating and/or simplifying the language of this bill of rights as may be necessary to ensure that the patients and their families understand their rights and responsibilities.

Bill of Rights*

1. The patient has the right to considerate and respectful care.

2. The patient has the right to and is encouraged to obtain from physicians and other direct caregivers relevant, current, and understandable information concerning diagnosis, treatment, and prognosis.

   Except in emergencies when the patient lacks decision-making capacity and the need for treatment is urgent, the patient is entitled to the opportunity to discuss and request information related to the specific procedures and/or treatments, the risks involved, the possible length of recuperation, and the medically reasonable alternatives and their accompanying risks and benefits.

   Patients have the right to know the identity of physicians, nurses, and others involved in their care, as well as when those involved are students, residents, or other trainees. The patient also has the right to know the immediate and long-term financial implications of treatment choices, insofar as they are known.

3. The patient has the right to make decisions about the plan of care prior to and during the course of treatment and to refuse a recommended treatment or plan of care to the extent permitted by law and hospital policy and to be informed of the medical consequences of this action. In case of such refusal, the patient is entitled to other appropriate care and services that the hospital provides or transfer to another hospital. The hospital should notify patients of any policy that might affect patient choice within the institution.

4. The patient has the right to have an advance directive (such as a living will, health care proxy, or durable power of attorney for health care) concerning treatment or designating a surrogate decision maker with the expectation that the hospital will honor the intent of that directive to the extent permitted by law and hospital policy.

   Health care institutions must advise patients of their rights under state law and hospital policy to make informed medical choices, ask if the patient has an advance directive, and include that information in patient records. The patient has the right to timely information about hospital policy that may limit its ability to implement fully a legally valid advance directive.

5. The patient has the right to every consideration of privacy. Case discussion, consultation, examination, and treatment should be conducted so as to protect each patient's privacy.

These rights can be exercised on the patient's behalf by a designated surrogate or proxy decision maker if the patient lacks decision-making capacity, is legally incompetent, or is a minor.

The Patients' Bill of Rights was first adopted by the American Hospital Association in 1973. This revision was approved by the AHA Board of Trustees on October 21, 1992.

© 1992 by the American Hospital Association, 840 North Lake Shore Drive, Chicago, Illinois 60611. Printed in the U.S.A. All rights reserved. Catalog no. 157759.

FIGURE 3-4 Patients' Bill of Rights

6. The patient has the right to expect that all communications and records pertaining to his/her care will be treated as confidential by the hospital, except in cases such as suspected abuse and public health hazards when reporting is permitted or required by law. The patient has the right to expect that the hospital will emphasize the confidentiality of this information when it releases it to any other parties entitled to review information in these records.

7. The patient has the right to review the records pertaining to his/her medical care and to have the information explained or interpreted as necessary, except when restricted by law.

8. The patient has the right to expect that, within its capacity and policies, a hospital will make reasonable response to the request of a patient for appropriate and medically indicated care and services. The hospital must provide evaluation, service, and/or referral as indicated by the urgency of the case. When medically appropriate and legally permissible, or when a patient has so requested, a patient may be transferred to another facility. The institution to which the patient is to be transferred must first have accepted the patient for transfer. The patient must also have the benefit of complete information and explanation concerning the need for, risks, benefits, and alternatives to such a transfer.

9. The patient has the right to ask and be informed of the existence of business relationships among the hospital, educational institutions, other health care providers, or payers that may influence the patient's treatment and care.

10. The patient has the right to consent to or decline to participate in proposed research studies or human experimentation affecting care and treatment or requiring direct patient involvement, and to have those studies fully explained prior to consent. A patient who declines to participate in research or experimentation is entitled to the most effective care that the hospital can otherwise provide.

11. The patient has the right to expect reasonable continuity of care when appropriate and to be informed by physicians and other caregivers of available and realistic patient care options when hospital care is no longer appropriate.

12. The patient has the right to be informed of hospital policies and practices that relate to patient care, treatment, and responsibilities. The patient has the right to be informed of available resources for resolving disputes, grievances, and conflicts, such as ethics committees, patient representatives, or other mechanisms available in the institution. The patient has the right to be informed of the hospital's charges for services and available payment methods.

The collaborative nature of health care requires that the patients, or their families/surrogates, participate in their care. The effectiveness of care and patient satisfaction with the course of treatment depend, in part, on the patient fulfilling certain responsibilities. Patients are responsible for providing information about past illnesses, hospitalizations, medications, and other matters related to health status. To participate effectively in decision making, patients must be encouraged to take responsibility for requesting additional information or clarification about their health status or treatment when they do not fully understand information and instructions. Patients are also responsible for ensuring that the health care institution has a copy of their written advance directive if they have one. Patients are responsible for informing their physicians and other caregivers if they anticipate problems in following prescribed treatment.

Patients should also be aware of the hospital's obligation to be reasonably efficient and equitable in providing care to other patients and the community. The hospital's rules and regulations are designed to help the hospital meet this obligation. Patients and their families are responsible for making reasonable accommodations to the needs of the hospital, other patients, medical staff, and hospital employees. Patients are responsible for providing necessary information for insurance claims and for working with the hospital to make payment arrangements, when necessary.

A person's health depends on much more than health care services. Patients are responsible for recognizing the impact of their life-style on their personal health.

Conclusion

Hospitals have many functions to perform, including the enhancement of health status, health promotion, and the prevention and treatment of injury and disease; the immediate and ongoing care and rehabilitation of patients; the education of health professionals, patients, and the community; and research. All these activities must be conducted with an overriding concern for the values and dignity of patients.

Clients' Rights in Home Care

The persons receiving home health care services or their families possess basic rights and responsibilities. As the client, you have:

The right to:
1. be treated with dignity, consideration, and respect
2. have your property treated with respect
3. receive a timely response from the agency to requests for service
4. be fully informed on admission of the care and treatment that will be provided, how much it will cost, and how payment will be handled
5. know in advance if you will be responsible for any payment
6. be informed in advance of any changes in your care
7. receive care from professionally trained personnel, and to know their names and responsibilities
8. participate in planning care
9. refuse treatment and be told the consequences of your action
10. expect confidentiality of all information
11. be informed of anticipated termination of service
12. be referred elsewhere if you are denied services solely based on your inability to pay
13. know how to make a complaint or recommend a change in agency policies and services

The responsibility to:
1. remain under a doctor's care while receiving services
2. provide the agency with a complete health history
3. provide the agency all requested insurance and financial information
4. sign the required consents and releases for insurance billing
5. participate in your care by asking questions, expressing concerns, and stating if you do not understand
6. provide a safe home environment in which care can be given
7. cooperate with your doctor, the staff, and other caregivers
8. accept responsibility for any refusal of treatment
9. abide by agency policies that restrict the duties our staff may perform
10. advise agency administration of any dissatisfaction or problems with your care

FIGURE 3-5 Clients' Rights in Home Care

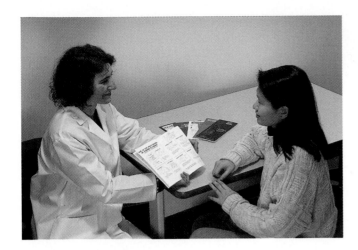

FIGURE 3-6 The RN develops a plan to teach the patient how to manage her own health.

REVIEW

A. True/False.

Mark the following true or false by circling T or F.

1. T F The rights of health care consumers are important only to patients in hospitals.

2. T F All United States citizens have certain rights that are guaranteed by law.

3. T F The Clients' Bill of Rights is given to persons receiving home care.

4. T F The Patients' Bill of Rights was legislated by OBRA of 1987.

5. T F Health care consumers in any setting have the right to prepare advance directives.

B. Multiple Choice.

Select the one best answer for each of the following.

6. Resident's Rights are given to persons before they are admitted to
  a. home care.
  b. a skilled care facility.
  c. the hospital.
  d. hospice services.

7. All types of consumer rights state that the consumer has the right to
  a. be treated in a respectful, dignified manner.
  b. select the individuals assigned to provide health care to them.
  c. private-duty nursing care, if desired by the patient or family.
  d. withhold personal information describing his or her medical condition.

8. The purpose of advance directives is to
  a. allow individuals to give instructions about their care should they become unable to do so.
  b. give individuals the right to choose their caregivers.
  c. provide a resource for resolving conflicts.
  d. permit the physician to prescribe treatment without conferring with the individual.

9. Health care consumers are responsible for
  a. leaving their bad habits at home when they are admitted to a health care facility.
  b. reading and studying medical books to learn all there is to know about their conditions.
  c. making treatment decisions in keeping with their physician's wishes.
  d. communicating openly and honestly with their physician and caregivers.

C. Completion.

Choose the correct word from the following list to complete each statement in questions 10–15.

advance directive	involuntary seclusion
grievance	privacy
informed consent	respect

10. _____ means that the consumer gives permission for care or procedures after full disclosure.

11. A _____ exists when the consumer feels there are grounds for complaint.

12. A document that gives instructions about the consumer's wishes for treatment if the consumer is unable to communicate is called a[an]_____.

13. Isolating a resident without a medical reason is called _____ .

14. By not opening and reading the consumer's mail, you are respecting the consumer's right to _____.

15. All health care consumers have the right to be treated with _____.

D. Nursing Assistant Challenge.

Mr. Delmonico was admitted to General Hospital for surgery to repair a fractured hip. After a few days in the hospital, he will be transferred to Memorial Nursing Center, a skilled care facility, for additional rehabilitation. After discharge from Memorial, it is expected that he will need home care for four to six weeks. Briefly explain how the different rights of each document will affect Mr. Delmonico's care.

16. Consider Mr. Delmonico's diagnosis and the services he will need for recovery. Which aspects of the Patients' Bill of Rights are especially important to his hospital care?

17. Discuss the statements in the Residents' Rights document that pertain specifically to rehabilitation and independence.

18. For which items in the Clients' Rights document would the nursing assistant be responsible?

UNIT 4

Ethical Issues t...

SECTION 1

36

The ethical stan...
to ensure that o...
these standards...
rules that g...
legal actio...

ET

OBJECTIVES

After completing this unit, you will be able to:

- Spell and define terms.
- Discuss ethical and legal situations in health care.
- Describe the legal and ethical responsibilities of the nursing assistant concerning patient information.
- Describe tactful ways to refuse a tip offered by a patient.

- Describe the legal responsibilities of a nursing assistant.
- Describe how to protect patients' right to privacy.
- Define sexual harassment and give examples of activities that may be perceived as being sexually harassing.

VOCABULARY

Learn the meaning and the correct spelling of the following words and phrases:

abuse
aiding and abetting
assault
battery
coercion
confidential
defamation

ethical standards
false imprisonment
informed consent
invasion of privacy
involuntary seclusion
legal standards
liable

libel
malpractice
neglect
negligence
physical abuse
Platinum Rule
psychological abuse

sexual abuse
sexual harassment
slander
theft
verbal abuse

ETHICAL STANDARDS AND LEGAL STANDARDS

Each day, as you carry out your work and relate to patients, coworkers, families, and others from the community, you will be faced with decisions to make about your actions. Some of these decisions involve the moral right or wrong of an action. Other decisions involve the legality of your behavior.

Two sets of rules help govern the moral and legal actions you will take.

1. **Ethical standards**. These are guides to moral behavior. People who give health care voluntarily agree to live up to these standards. When these rules are not followed, the nursing assistant fails to live up to the promise to give safe, correct care and to do no harm.

2. **Legal standards**. These are guides to lawful behavior. When laws are not obeyed, the nursing assistant may be prosecuted and found **liable** (held responsible) for injury or damage. Legal guilt can result in the payment of fines or imprisonment.

...ds and legal standards are established ...ly safe, quality care is given. Following ... also protects the caregiver. Sometimes the ...vern moral actions and the laws that govern ...ns cover the same area.

...HICS QUESTIONS

Probably at no other time in history have the questions of medical ethics been under such scrutiny. Questions health care providers ask include:

- When is life gone from a person on a life support system?
- How much lifesaving or resuscitation effort should be given in situations of terminal illness?
- When does human life actually begin?
- How much assistance should be given to the conception process?
- Should the body organs of a brain-dead person be harvested for transplants for the living?
- Does an unborn baby have rights?
- Is assisting a patient during or after an abortion right or wrong?
- Is euthanasia (assisted death) ever justified?
- Should animals be used in research of potential value to human life?
- Should food and water be withheld to speed death when the patient has expressed the desire to die?
- Who makes decisions about removing life support systems when there is no direct expression of the patient's wishes or there is conflict within the family?
- How will a choice be made when two or more people could benefit from an organ transplant but only one organ is available?
- How should the limited money available be spent when many serious disease conditions ought to be researched?
- Who has the final authority over whether a woman will carry a pregnancy to term?
- Should marijuana be used for medicinal purposes?

Many facilities have ethics committees (Figure 4-1) that advise the staff on ethical matters. The members of ethics committees often include staff, clergy, interested community members, and advocates for the sick and elderly. The committee reviews the ethical problems and principles involved to help guide the staff and family. The committee may be asked to make difficult decisions, such as when doctors recommend removing life support and the patient's family members disagree with the decision.

The law permits physicians and hospitals to refuse to comply with advance directives and treatment decisions in some circumstances. An example is when the physician believes that care that prolongs the patient's life is inappropriate or futile. In situations like this, the family always has the option of moving the patient to another

FIGURE 4-1 The ethics committee often discusses complex patient situations and sometimes must make difficult decisions. (Courtesy of Photodisc)

facility within a given time frame, such as 10 days. In some states, facilities may not be required to provide a grace period in which to make arrangements. The burden is placed on family members to petition the court to obtain an extension. Finding placement is often very difficult and time-consuming. The required care is usually highly technical and very expensive. Resources are almost always limited, and most communities do not have a variety of facilities that are qualified or able to provide the necessary care. A facility that is qualified and willing to accept the patient may be hundreds of miles away or in another state, placing further strain on the family.

The ethics committee is responsible for resolving disputes such as this, in which one or both opposing parties may be unhappy with the decision. As you can see, these committees carry great responsibility, making their members' jobs difficult, sensitive, and very important to the operation of the facility. Respect for patients and their wishes is the primary concern. Part of this respect for life is shown by having patients actively involved in decisions about their care and future.

As a nursing assistant, you will take directions from the legal and ethical guidelines established by your facility.

RESPECT FOR LIFE

One of the most basic rules of ethics is that life is precious.

Everyone involved in the care of patients has the promotion of health and the quality of life as primary goals (Figure 4-2). Death, however, is a natural progression of life. When death is certain, the objective is to keep the dying person comfortable. Today, there is a greater appreciation of individual wishes and the quality of life expected. One fact remains clear: the major responsibility of medicine and all members of the health care team is to maintain quality of life and make comfortable those whose lives are limited.

FIGURE 4-2 Promoting good health and the highest possible quality of life are primary goals.

RESPECT FOR THE INDIVIDUAL

Respect for each patient as a unique individual is another ethical principle.

This uniqueness is demonstrated by differences in:

- Age
- Race
- Religion
- Gender
- Sexual preference
- Culture
- Attitudes
- Background
- Response to illness

You may find the differences that make the patient so special also make dealing with the patient challenging or difficult. If you respect each patient as a valuable person, you can learn to accept and work with each one in the best possible way.

You probably learned the Golden Rule, "Do unto others as you would have them do unto you," when you were young. The Golden Rule reflects your intent to provide proper care. However, your good intentions are effective only when you act on them. To provide proper care, you also have the ethical responsibility to maintain competence in your practice. An alternative to the Golden Rule is the **Platinum Rule**: "Treat others the way they want to be treated." The Platinum Rule shifts the focus from treating everyone alike to providing highly individualized care. Find out what patients want and give it to them, as much as possible, in keeping with their plans of care.

Use both principles to guide your practice. There will be times when personal comfort and convenience could interfere with the care you give. By placing patients' interests ahead of your own, you are fulfilling the ethical and legal obligations of your practice, protecting patient safety, enhancing patient comfort and satisfaction with care, and reducing your personal risk of legal exposure.

PATIENT INFORMATION

The ethical code asserts that information about patients is privileged and must not be shared with others (Figure 4-3).

1. Discuss patient information only in appropriate places.
   a. It is unwise to discuss a patient's condition while in the patient's room, even if the patient is unresponsive. The patient may be able to hear everything that is said. This could cause unnecessary worry.
   b. Never discuss the patients in your care with your family or others in the community.

FIGURE 4-3 Patient information is always confidential and must never be discussed casually.

c. Never discuss patients during lunch or coffee breaks, even with your coworkers.

2. Discuss information only with the proper people.

   a. At times you will be approached by others requesting information about a patient. For example, you might be asked for such information by other patients, family members, or members of the public, such as news reporters.

   b. Discuss patients and their personal concerns only with your supervisor during conference or report. Make sure you will not be overheard by visitors or other patients.

   c. Learn to evade inquiries tactfully by:
      – Stating that you do not know all the details of the treatment or the patient's condition.
      – Redirecting inquirers to the proper authority.
      – Firmly, but politely, indicating that you do not have the authority to provide the answers.

3. Refer patient requests for information about laboratory results, the patient's condition, or course of the illness to the nurse or doctor.

4. Let the nurse or doctor relay information about a patient's death. Never give information concerning the death of a patient to the patient's family. When done tactfully, a refusal of this kind is rarely resented by the family.

5. Follow the ethical code to ensure respect of patients' personal religious beliefs. People of all faiths or beliefs and those with no proclaimed faith are admitted for care. These differences must be respected. You show your respect when you:

   a. Inform the nurse of requests for clergy visits.

   b. Know correct information about the type of chaplain services available in your facility.

   c. Know if a chapel is open for use by patients and families.

   d. Respectfully treat patients' religious articles, such as a Bible, crucifix, Koran, or holy pictures.

   e. Avoid imposing your own religious beliefs on patients.

   f. Assist patients to practice their religious beliefs and rituals, if requested.

   When the clergy visits (Figure 4-4), you should:

   a. Be helpful and courteous.

   b. Escort the clergyperson to the patient's bedside.

   c. Draw the curtains or close the door for privacy.

   d. Leave the room.

TIPPING

If you follow the ethical code, the service you give will depend on need. It will *not* depend on the patient's race,

FIGURE 4-4 People who are sick typically have many spiritual needs. A private visit from a clergyperson can be very comforting.

creed, color, or ability to pay. There is no place for tipping within the health care system (Figure 4-5).

Patients are charged for the services they receive while in the hospital. The salary you are paid is included in that charge.

Sometimes patients will offer a "little something" to you. A firm but courteous refusal of the money is usually all that is necessary to assure the patient of your meaning.

As you can see, the ethical code ensures that each patient is treated with dignity and respect in ways that always promote safe care.

LEGAL ISSUES

Laws are passed by governments (local, state, and federal) and are to be obeyed by citizens. Anyone who fails to obey a law may be liable (responsible) for fines or imprisonment.

You need not fear breaking these laws if you are careful to:

- Stay within your scope of practice and do not overstep your authority.
- Do only those things that you have been taught and that are within the scope of nursing assistant practice.
- Carry out procedures carefully and as you were taught.
- Keep your skills and knowledge up to date.
- Request guidance from the proper person before you take action in a questionable situation.
- Always keep the safety and well-being of the patient foremost in your mind, and act accordingly.
- Make sure you thoroughly understand directions for the care you are to give.

FIGURE 4-5 Tips must be courteously refused.

- Perform your job according to facility policy.
- Stay within OBRA guidelines.
- Maintain in-service requirements of OBRA.
- Do no harm to the patient.
- Respect the patient's belongings (property).

Situations you must avoid are negligence, theft, defamation, false imprisonment, assault and battery, abuse, neglect, and invasion of privacy.

Negligence

Negligence is failure to exercise the degree of care considered reasonable under the circumstances, when that failure results in an unintended injury to a patient. Simply put, negligence is carelessness, which is often caused by hurrying or not focusing on the task at hand. Negligence may be accidental or deliberate. It may be the result of an action or an omission (failure to act). For example, not feeding a confused patient lunch because she is a slow eater and you are short on time is considered negligence. However, forgetting to give a lunch tray to a confused patient who feeds himself is also a negligent act. Either way, the patient is not given the expected level of care.

Nursing assistants are qualified care providers and are expected to perform in certain ways. You would be guilty of negligence if you injured a patient by:

- Not performing your work as taught. For example, a patient is burned by an enema solution that you prepared and was too hot.
- Not carrying out your job in a conscientious manner. For example, your facility has a policy that two workers are necessary to transfer a patient with the mechanical lift, but you fail to ask another worker to assist you in moving a patient. The lift tips and the patient is injured.

Malpractice is improper, negligent, or unethical conduct that results in harm, injury, or loss to a patient. Practicing within your scope of practice, following facility policies

and procedures, and doing things in the way you were taught will help protect your patients from injury. Being discreet, respecting confidentiality, and avoiding gossip will help protect you from inadvertently harming a patient emotionally. Be kind and polite to patients. If a patient complains about something you have done, apologize and promptly correct the problem without becoming defensive.

Theft

Taking anything that does not belong to you makes you guilty of **theft**. The patients' and residents' rights documents refer to this action as the "misappropriation of property."

If you see someone stealing something and do not report it, you are guilty of **aiding and abetting** the crime.

Because of the nature of their work, people working in facilities must be honest and dependable. Despite careful screening, dishonest people are sometimes hired and things do disappear. These things range from washcloths, money, and patients' personal belongings to drugs.

Sometimes workers are reluctant to report things that they see other people doing. Remember, however, that you are responsible for your own actions and must do the right thing. For a nursing assistant, opportunities for poor practice, illegal activities, and neglect are always present. Resist the temptation to lower your standards. Honesty and integrity are the hallmarks of the sincere and conscientious nursing assistant.

Defamation

If you make false statements about someone to a third person and the character of the first person is injured, you are guilty of **defamation**. This is true if you make the statement verbally (**slander**) or in writing (**libel**). For example, if you inaccurately tell a coworker that a patient has AIDS, you have slandered that patient. If you write the same untrue information in a note, you are guilty of libel.

False Imprisonment

Restraining a person's movements or actions without proper authorization constitutes unlawful or **false imprisonment**. For example, patients have the right to leave the hospital *with or without* the physician's permission. You may not interfere with this right. If you do interfere, you will be guilty of false imprisonment.

If you learn of a patient's intention to leave the hospital without permission, inform your supervisor. The supervisor will handle the situation.

Using physical restraints, or even threatening to do so, in order to make a patient cooperate can also constitute false imprisonment. Restraints may be in the form of physical devices or chemical agents. A physical restraint is any manual method or physical or mechanical device, material, or equipment attached or adjacent to the patient's body that:

- A patient cannot easily remove.
- Restricts a patient's movement.
- Does not allow the patient normal access to his or her own body.

Examples of physical restraints include:

- Wrist/arm and ankle/leg restraints
- Vests
- Jackets
- Hand mitts
- Geriatric and cardiac chairs
- Wheelchair safety belts and bars
- Bed rails, which are considered physical restraints if they meet the definition listed

In general, many devices and practices meet the definition of physical restraints if the patient does not have the physical or mental ability to remove the device. Examples of other practices that constitute restraint are:

- Tucking in, tying, or using Velcro to hold a sheet, fabric, or clothing tightly so that a patient's movement is restricted.
- Using devices in conjunction with a chair (such as trays, tables, bars, or belts) that the patient cannot remove easily and that keep the patient from rising.
- Placing a patient in a chair that prevents the patient from rising.
- Placing a chair or bed so close to a wall that the wall prevents the patient from rising out of the chair or voluntarily getting out of bed.

Psychoactive medications are considered chemical restraints because they affect the patient's mobility. The use of restraints is discussed further in Unit 14.

Sometimes it is necessary to support and restrain the movement of patients. Supports and restraints cannot be used without a physician's order. This order indicates the type of restraint or support to be used, when it is to be used, and the reason for it.

Assault and Battery

Assault and battery are serious legal matters. **Assault** means intentionally attempting to touch the body of a person or even threatening to do so. **Battery** means actually touching a person without that person's permission.

The care we provide is given with the patient's permission or **informed consent**. This means the patient must know and agree to what we plan to do before we start. Consent may be withdrawn at any time. For example, you are assigned to give a patient a warm foot soak. Despite your explanation of the reasons for the order, the patient refuses. You may not force the patient to submit. Doing so would make you guilty of battery. You commit assault

if you threaten the patient by telling her that you will get others to assist you if she refuses.

Either situation could make you liable for legal charges. You can avoid this legal pitfall by:

- Informing the patient of what you plan to do.
- Making sure the patient understands.
- Pausing before starting, to give the patient an opportunity to ask questions or refuse.
- Reporting refusal of care to your supervisor and documenting the facts.
- Never carrying out a treatment on your own against the patient's wishes.

Coercion means forcing the patient to do something against his wishes. Refusal of treatment creates a dilemma for the nursing assistant when the patient is mentally confused. In general, a family member or other responsible person consents to treatment and hospital care for patients who are confused. In this situation, we presume that the patient would agree to the care if he were mentally able to do so. The patient may refuse a procedure, such as a bath, but the legally responsible person has already consented to the procedure, so you may perform it. Gaining the patient's cooperation and trust is always best. You may be able to perform the procedure if you wait a while, then return. Avoid forcing the patient. If in doubt about how to handle refusals of care, consult your supervisor.

Abuse

Abuse of a patient (doing harm to a patient) violates ethical principles and makes you liable for legal prosecution. Ethical standards require that you do no harm to patients. Legal standards enforce this through laws, with penalties if you are found guilty.

Abuse is defined as any act or failure to act that is nonaccidental and causes or could cause harm or death to a patient. Some forms of abuse are subtle but nevertheless cause the patient physical harm or mental anguish. Abuse can occur in several forms, including verbal, sexual, physical, and mental abuse and involuntary seclusion.

Verbal abuse may be directed toward the patient or expressed about the patient. You are guilty of verbally abusing a patient if you:

- Use profanity (swearing) in dealing with the patient.
- Raise your voice in anger at the patient.
- Call the patient unpleasant names.
- Tease or embarrass the patient.
- Use threatening or obscene gestures.
- Make written threats or abusive statements.
- Use inappropriate words to describe a person's race or nationality.

Sexual abuse is the use of physical means or verbal threats to force a patient to perform sexual acts. In many states, sexual abuse is any behavior that is seductive, sexu-

Legal ALERT

Most states have laws prohibiting abuse of children and elderly adults. These laws often require mandatory reporting of suspected patient abuse to police and state agencies. You are not responsible for determining whether abuse has occurred. If you suspect that a patient has been abused, inform your supervisor, who will assess the situation and take the proper action. The penalties for abusing a patient can be severe, and may include imprisonment.

Caregiver stress is frequently the cause of patient abuse. Learning and practicing methods of reducing stress is best for your mental, emotional, and physical health. Recognize signs of stress, including difficulty sleeping, irritability, feelings of sadness, anxiety, guilt, indecisiveness, loss of appetite, loss of interest in sexual activity, isolation, loss of interest in work, hopelessness, drug or alcohol misuse, and inability to concentrate. If a combination of these symptoms is present, seek help in managing your stress. ■

FIGURE 4-6 Handling a patient roughly is physical abuse.

FIGURE 4-7 Making fun of a patient is psychological abuse.

ally demeaning, harassing, or reasonably interpreted as sexual by the patient. Examples of sexual abuse include:

- Tormenting or teasing a patient with sexual gestures or words.
- Touching a patient in a sexual way.
- Suggesting that the patient engage in sexual acts with you.

Physical abuse does actual physical harm to the patient. Examples of physical abuse include:

- Handling a patient roughly (Figure 4-6).
- Hitting, slapping, pushing, kicking, or pinching the patient.
- Performing the wrong treatment on the patient, such as ambulating a patient who should remain in bed.

Psychological abuse includes:

- Making the patient fearful of you, such as threatening not to respond when the patient calls.
- Threatening the patient with harm.
- Threatening to tell something to others that the patient does not want known.
- Threatening to withhold care.
- Making fun of or belittling the patient in any way (Figure 4-7). Calling the patient by names such as "honey" and "grandma" is another way of belittling the patient.
- Calling the attention of others to a patient's behavior.

Involuntary seclusion is the separation of a patient from others against the patient's will. Examples of involuntary seclusion are:

- Shutting the door to the patient's room when the patient is confined to bed and wants the door open.
- Continually placing a patient's gerichair far from others.
- Leaving a patient without a form of communication, such as a signal cord or call bell.

Separation may be permitted if it is part of a therapeutic plan to reduce agitation. The decision to use seclusion must be made by the nurse. This form of seclusion requires accurate documentation and a plan of care. The seclusion must be effective. Note: When describing a patient's behavior, avoid the use of words such as *uncooperative, belligerent,* or *hostile.* Instead, describe the exact actions that you observed. Often, so-called uncooperative behavior is a problem caused by faulty communication on the part of the health care provider. People should not be unfairly labeled.

Abuse by Others

If you suspect that a person in your care is being abused by others, discuss this matter with your supervisor. Laws require a health care provider who suspects abuse to report the situation so the patient can be protected. In some states, a person who does not report the abuse is held as guilty as the abusing person.

It may be difficult to understand why anyone would abuse a person who is weak or infirm, but it happens. A few people may take satisfaction out of feeling that they have control of others. Most abuse, however, probably originates in feelings of frustration or fatigue.

Anyone can be abused, but the old and the young are the most vulnerable. Usually, the caregiver or a family member is the abuser.

- Some families provide loving, capable care for older, dependent relatives for many years without assistance. After providing care for a long period, they may be physically and emotionally exhausted and may also have depleted their financial resources.
- In some cases, one spouse has abused the other for a long time.
- Self-abuse may occur when a disabled person is unable to adequately carry out activities of daily living and is unwilling to accept help.

It is not the responsibility of the nursing assistant to determine if an individual has been abused or what type of abuse has been inflicted. It *is* the nursing assistant's responsibility to report to the supervisor any signs or symptoms that might be the result of abuse. This includes:

- Statements by the patient that reflect neglect or abuse.
- Unexplained bruises or wounds.
- Signs of neglect such as poor personal hygiene.
- A change in personality.

Remember, these do not necessarily indicate that the person is being abused. However, they may indicate a need for further investigation by your supervisor. Any observed abusive behavior toward patients, whether inside or outside a facility, must be reported to the appropriate authority.

When Your Patience Is Stressed

If you feel that your own tolerance level is being tested, you need to find ways to safeguard the patient and release your own stress. You might:

- Try to identify the exact cause of your irritation.
- Talk with your supervisor about your feelings.
- Consider asking to be assigned to another patient.
- Try to reduce your overall stress and fatigue so that you are more positive and patient on the your job.
- Request counseling through an employee assistance program.

Neglect

Neglect is the failure to provide the services or care necessary to avoid physical harm, mental anguish, or mental illness. Neglect can be deliberate or accidental, such as forgetting an assignment and not providing care. Neglect is also a violation of the law. The nursing assistant is not expected to determine if neglect has occurred. You *are* responsible for reporting signs of neglect to your supervisor, who will investigate the situation. Examples of neglect include:

- Failing to turn the patient as often as needed, causing impaired circulation and pressure ulcers.
- Failing to perform regular exercises so that the patient experiences pain when unused joints are finally moved.
- Failing to carry out proper hygiene, such as not shaving the patient regularly.
- Failing to provide mealtime assistance to a patient who cannot eat independently.
- Failing to provide water to a patient who is on bedrest and has an order to encourage fluids.

Invasion of Privacy

Patients have a right to have their person and personal affairs kept **confidential**. To do otherwise is an **invasion of privacy**. Invading the privacy of another is against the law.

You can protect the patient's privacy by:

- Protecting the patient from exposure of the body.
- Knocking and pausing before entering a room.
- Drawing curtains when providing care.
- Leaving while visitors are with the patient.
- Not listening as patients make telephone calls.
- Abiding by the rules of confidentiality.
- Not trying to force a patient to accept your personal beliefs or views.
- Not discussing the patient's condition with anyone outside of work.

SEXUAL HARASSMENT

Some people are unaware of or are insensitive to the fact that their words or behavior constitute **sexual harassment**. A simple definition of *sexual harassment* is unwelcome sexual advances, requests for sexual favors, and other verbal or physical conduct of a sexual nature. The action may be physical, verbal, or nonverbal. The other party may be a patient or coworker, of the same gender or the opposite gender as the harasser.

Sexual harassment is illegal. Most facilities have orientation and in-service programs to reduce the risk of sexual harassment in the workplace. However, it sometimes occurs despite the employer's best efforts. The facility has a duty to protect both patients and staff from sexual harassment. Facilities must respond promptly and appropriately when patients or employees make a claim of sexual harassment, whether the source of the harassment is another employee, an independent contractor, a patient, visitor, guest, or other person who was invited to the facility by the employer. If the conduct of another person unreasonably interferes with the employee's work performance or subjects the employee to an intimidating, hostile, or offensive work environment, and the facility has reason to know about it, the facility must take some immediate corrective action. Your facility will have policies and procedures regarding actions to take and penalties if harassment occurs.

Upon being informed that an incident of sexual harassment has occurred, the facility is responsible for investigating the situation. During the investigation, the facility must protect the victim from further harassment. Exam-

ples of actions that may be considered sexual harassment include:

- Making comments about anatomy, such as the size or shape of the breasts, genitals, or areas of the body considered sexual
- Making suggestions of a sexual nature
- Staring at a person's body
- Unwanted touching, holding, grabbing, hugging, fondling, kissing, or pinching
- "Accidental" collisions or brushing up against another person
- Making lewd or sexually suggestive comments
- Using offensive gestures or motions
- Telling offensive graphic jokes or using offensive language
- Making threats or comments, or asking questions about a person's sexual orientation or personal sexual practices or behavior
- Displaying or circulating sexually suggestive material (written or pictorial, including cartoons)

If you believe you are being sexually harassed, or suspect that a patient is being sexually harassed, notify your supervisor promptly. Avoid conversations, gestures, and other behavior that may be offensive and perceived to be sexually harassing by patients and coworkers.

REVIEW

A. Multiple Choice.

Select the one best answer for each of the following.

1. You overhear another assistant raise his voice when speaking to Mrs. Ryan. The assistant is guilty of
   a. negligence.
   b. theft.
   c. abuse.
   d. invasion of privacy.

2. Mr. Deonne offers you two dollars for picking up a newspaper for him. Your response should be to
   a. ignore the money and pretend not to see it.
   b. take the money—you earned it.
   c. report the matter to the supervisor.
   d. politely refuse because tipping is not allowed.

3. Mr. Chan's daughter is visiting and wants to know what her father's blood pressure reading is. Your best response is to
   a. tell her.
   b. say you don't know.
   c. refer her to the nurse.
   d. refer her to another assistant who measured blood pressure this morning.

4. You observe another assistant slipping a patient's rosary into her pocket. Your response is to
   a. know you are not required to do anything.
   b. report the matter to your supervisor.
   c. tell the patient.
   d. tell the patient's family.

5. You notice that every time a patient makes a telephone call, one nursing assistant stands so that she can hear the conversation. That assistant is guilty of
   a. invasion of privacy.
   b. defamation.
   c. negligence.
   d. libel.

6. An assistant forgets that she is assigned to care for Mr. Huynh, a mentally confused patient. The nurse discovers that Mr. Huynh has developed a pressure ulcer. This is an example of
   a. abuse.
   b. libel.
   c. involuntary seclusion.
   d. neglect.

7. Mrs. Rosario has very fragile skin that tears and bruises easily. The nurse instructed Tony, a nursing assistant, to handle the patient gently to prevent injury. Tony is in a hurry and bumps Mrs. Rosario's leg against the side rail, causing a large skin tear. This is an example of

   a. slander.

   b. invasion of privacy.

   c. libel.

   d. negligence.

8. Mr. McNally tells you he is tired and does not want his bath right now. You should

   a. tell him you will not have time to bathe him later.

   b. ask him when he would like you to return to assist him.

   c. advise him that the doctor insists that he bathe.

   d. forget the bath for today.

9. Mr. Strong, a mentally confused patient, has a visitor. After he leaves, you discover a large bruise on the patient's arm that was not there previously. You should

   a. notify the charge nurse of your observations.

   b. call the police.

   c. do nothing, as this is not your responsibility.

   d. inform the nurse that the visitor abused Mr. Strong.

10. A patient with cancer tells you that she no longer wants to live. She confides that she is collecting her medicine so she can take an overdose and die. You should

    a. respect the patient's right to confidentiality and tell no one.

    b. notify the patient's husband when he visits.

    c. inform your supervisor immediately.

    d. ask a more experienced assistant to reason with the patient.

B. True/False.

Mark the following true or false by circling T or F.

11. T F A patient may not refuse any treatment prescribed by the physician.

12. T F You may learn much about a patient's personal life as you provide care.

13. T F Lunchtime is the best time to discuss your patients with others.

14. T F If you accept a tip, you are guilty of abuse.

15. T F Your patient has an order to encourage fluid intake, and you fail to do this. You are guilty of neglect.

16. T F You forget to put side rails up when ordered, and a patient falls. You are guilty of negligence.

17. T F Failure to report your observation of an illegal act makes you guilty of aiding and abetting the action.

18. T F Leaving a patient unnecessarily exposed is an invasion of the patient's privacy.

19. T F Jackets, belts, vests, straps, and side rails can be considered unlawful restraints.

20. T F Ethics relates to moral rights and wrongs of behavior.

21. T F Anxiety can sometimes make a person very demanding.

22. T F People give up their right to privacy when they are admitted to health care facilities.

23. T F If an error occurs as you give care, it is important to report it immediately.

24. T F Patients should not question the cost of care.

25. T F Every patient has the right to considerate, respectful care.

26. T F Honesty and integrity are the hallmarks of a conscientious nursing assistant.

27. T F Telling an off-color joke to a patient of the opposite gender may be considered malpractice.

28. T F If a patient resists you, you may apply restraints to make sure the treatment is given.

29. T F Patients may not be subjected to either verbal or physical abuse.

C. Nursing Assistant Challenge.

In each of the following situations, describe the correct nursing assistant action.

30. Ms. Harvey is dying. Her doctors believe that she will live only a few days. What is your responsibility to this patient? _____

31. Mrs. Wybok insists on saying her prayers every morning just as breakfast is ready. _____

32. Mr. Bishop's daughter asks you what medicine the doctor ordered for her father's heart condition.

    _____

SECTION 2

Scientific Principles

UNIT 5

Medical Terminology and Body Organization

OBJECTIVES

After completing this unit, you will be able to:

- Spell and define terms.
- Recognize the meanings of common prefixes, suffixes, and root words.
- Build medical terms from word parts.
- Write the abbreviations commonly used in health care facilities.

- Describe the organization of the body, from simple to complex.
- Name four types of tissues and their characteristics.
- Name and locate major organs as parts of body systems, using proper anatomic terms.

VOCABULARY

Learn the meaning and the correct spelling of the following words and phrases:

abbreviation	dorsal	nerve cell	skeletal (voluntary) muscle
anatomic position	epithelial cell	nervous tissue	smooth (involuntary) muscle
anatomy	epithelial tissue	organ	suffix
anterior	health	pericardium	superior
cardiac muscle	inferior	peritoneum	synovial membranes
cavity	lateral	physiology	system
cell	medial	pleura	tissue
combining form	membranes	posterior	umbilicus
connective tissue	meninges	prefix	ventral
connective tissue cell	mucous membrane	proximal	word root
cutaneous membrane	mucus	quadrant	
disease	muscle cell	serous membrane	
distal	muscle tissue		

MEDICAL TERMINOLOGY

Medical science and health care have a special language called *medical terminology*. In this language, the terms are formed by building on common word parts (Figure 5-1). Terms are developed by combining:

- **Word root**—the foundation of a medical term. A word root usually, but not always, refers to the part of the body or condition that is being treated, studied, or named by the term.
- **Combining form**—a vowel may be added to the end of the word root to make it easier to form medical

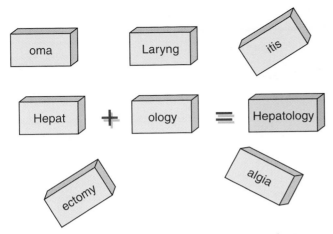

FIGURE 5-1 New words can be formed by combining different prefixes and suffixes.

words. This combination of the word root and vowel is called a combining form.

- **Prefix**—word part added to the beginning of a word to change or add to its meaning.
- **Suffix**—word part added to the end of a word to change or add to its meaning.
- **Abbreviation**—shortened form of a word (often letters). You already know the abbreviation RN (registered nurse). You will soon become familiar with additional abbreviations that are common to the world of medicine and health care.

Each health care facility also has special abbreviations that it uses (Figure 5-2). Check the procedure or policy manual of your facility to determine which abbreviations have been approved for use. A good medical dictionary is also a helpful tool.

FIGURE 5-2 Documentation is a very important responsibility.

Each facility will also have a list of abbreviations that should *not* be used. The facility adds abbreviations to the list every three months, so you must check it regularly. Abbreviations on the "do not use" list are usually those that were formerly common and accepted. However, they did not withstand the test of time. Over the years, the abbreviations on this list have been found to cause confusion and errors. Because this list affects patient safety, it is very important.

Legal ALERT

Documentation is a means of communication. Abbrevations must be clear, and others must know their meanings, if the communication is to be effective and meaningful. ■

MEDICAL WORD PARTS

Word Roots

Familiarity with the important word parts comes from study and repeated usage. You will gain experience with the word parts as you practice reporting and charting, and by communicating with your coworkers.

A single medical word root can sometimes be placed in different parts of a word and still have a specific meaning. For example, the root *cyte* means cell:

- *cyt*ology—the study of cells
- a leuko*cyte*—a white blood cell
- poly*cyt*osis—an illness in which there are too many red and white blood cells

No matter where the form *cyte* occurs in a medical word, it refers to cells. It may be a prefix, a suffix, or a word root. Word roots are often derived from Greek or Latin. For example, the word root *nephro* is derived from the word for kidney. This root may be used to form a variety of medical terms. For example:

- Nephroma—a tumor of the kidney
- Nephrectomy—surgical excision of the kidney
- Nephrolithiasis—presence of kidney stones

Give special attention to the exercises and activities in this unit. Learning the new words and parts of words in this unit will make it easier for you to recognize meanings of medical terms.

Table 5-1 lists combining forms (word roots plus vowel).

Prefixes and Suffixes

Many medical words have common beginnings (prefixes) or common endings (suffixes). By learning some of the more common prefixes (Table 5-2) and suffixes (Table 5-3), you can put together many new words.

TABLE 5-1 COMBINING FORMS

Combining Form	Meaning	Example	Meaning
abdomin (o)	abdomen	abdominal	portion of body between the thorax and pelvis
aden (o)	gland	adenoma	a glandular tumor
angi (o)	vessel	angioedema	recurrent large areas of subcutaneous edema of sudden onset, commonly an allergic reaction to foods or drugs
arteri (o)	artery	arteriogram	X-ray of an artery after injection of contrast medium (dye)
arthr (o)	joint	arthritis	inflammation of a joint
bronch (i) (o)	bronchus bronchi	bronchiectasis	one of the larger passages conveying air to and within the lungs becomes abnormally enlarged
cardi (o)	heart	cardialgia	pain in the region of the heart
cephal (o)	head	cephaloma	soft or encephaloid tumor
cerebr (o)	brain	cerebrovascular accident	another name for a stroke
chol (e)	bile	cholecystitis	inflammation of the gallbladder
col (o)	colon, large intestine	colectomy	excision of the colon
crani (o)	skull	craniotomy	opening of the skull
cyst (o)	bladder, cyst	cystitis	inflammation of the bladder
cyt (o)	cell	cytology	study of cells
dent (i) (o)	tooth	dentist	person licensed to practice dentistry
dermat (o)	skin	dermatitis	inflammation of the skin
encephal (o)	brain	encephaloma	herniation of brain substance
enter (o)	small intestine	enteritis	inflammation of the intestines
erythr (o)	red	erythroblastosis	presence of many red blood cells
fibr (o)	fiber	fibroadenoma	benign growth commonly occurring in breast tissue
gastr (o)	stomach	gastritis	inflammation of the lining of the stomach
geront (o)	elderly	gerontology	scientific study of process and problems related to aging
gloss (o)	tongue	glossodynia	burning or painful tongue
glyc (o)	sugar	glycosuria	urinary excretion of sugar

continues

Patricia Coulka

TABLE 5-1 *CONTINUED*

Combining Form	Meaning	Example	Meaning
gynec (o)	female	gynecomastia	excessive development of male mammary glands
hem (o)	blood	hematuria	discharge of blood in urine
hepat (o)	liver	hepatitis	inflammation of the liver
hydr (o)	water	hydrocephalus	enlargement of the cranium caused by abnormal accumulation of fluid
hyster (o)	uterus	hysterectomy	surgical removal of the uterus
lapar (o)	abdomen, flank, loin	laparoscopy	examination of the contents of the abdomen through a scope passed through the abdominal wall
laryng (o)	larynx	laryngectomy	partial or total removal of the larynx by surgery
lith (o)	stone	lithiasis	formation of stones in any hollow structure of the body
mamm (o)	breast	mammography	imaging examination of the breasts
mast (o)	breast	mastitis	inflammation of the breast
men (o)	menstruation	menorrhagia	excessive menstrual flow
my (o)	muscle	myalgia	muscular pain
myel (o)	bone marrow, spinal cord	myelocele	protrusion of the spinal cord
nephr (o)	kidney	nephrolithiasis	presence of renal calculi (kidney stones)
neur (o)	nerve	neuropathy	any disease of the nervous system
ocul (o)	eye	oculodynia	pain in the eyeball
ophthalm (o)	eye	ophthalmoscope	instrument used to view the inside of the eye
oste (o)	bone	osteitis	inflammation of the bone
ot (o)	ear	otitis media	inflammation of the middle ear
ped (i) (o)	child	pedodontics	dental care of children
pharyng (o)	throat, pharynx	pharyngitis	inflammation of the pharynx
phleb (o)	vein	phlebitis	inflammation of a vein
pneum (o)	lung, air, gas	pneumonectomy	resection of lung tissue
proct (o)	rectum	proctoscopy	rectal exam with a proctoscope
psych (o)	mind	psychology	study of human behavior
pulm (o)	lung	pulmonary	pertaining to the lungs
py (o)	pus	pyogenic	producing pus

continues

TABLE 5-1 *CONTINUED*

Combining Form	Meaning	Example	Meaning
rect (o)	rectum	rectocele	hernial protrusion of part of the rectum into the vagina
rhin (o)	nose	rhinorrhea	discharge from nasal mucous membrane
splen (o)	spleen	splenoma	enlarged spleen
stern (o)	sternum	sternotomy	incision into or through the sternum
thorac (o)	chest	thoracotomy	opening of the chest
thromb (o)	clot	thrombocytopenia	abnormally small number of platelets in the circulating blood
tox (o)	poison	toxoplasmosis	disease produced by a parasite; can cause birth defects if acquired during pregnancy
trache (i) (o)	trachea	tracheotomy	incision of the trachea for exploration
ur (o)	urine, urinary tract, urination	urinalysis	analysis of the urine
urethr (o)	urethra	urethralgia	pain in the urethra
urin (o)	urine	urinometer	an instrument for determining the specific gravity of urine
uter (i) (o)	uterus	uterotonic	drugs that give tone to uterine muscle
ven (o)	vein	venostat	any instrument used to suppress venous bleeding

TABLE 5-2 COMMON PREFIXES

Prefix	Meaning	Example	Meaning
a-	without	asepsis	without infection
brady-	slow	bradycardia	slow heart rate
dys-	pain or difficulty	dysuria	painful urination
hyper-	above, excessive	hypertension	high blood pressure
hypo-	low, deficient	hypotension	low blood pressure
pan-	all	pandemic	widespread epidemic
poly-	many	polyuria	excessive urine
post-	after	postoperative	after surgery
pre-	before	premenstrual	before the menses
retro-	behind, backward	retrograde	moving backward, degenerating
tachy-	fast	tachycardia	pulse rate above normal

TABLE 5-3 COMMON SUFFIXES

Suffix	Meaning	Example	Meaning	Suffix	Meaning	Example	Meaning
-algia	pain	arthralgia	pain in the joints	-oma	tumor	fibroma	a tumor containing fibrous tissue
-ectomy	removal of	appendectomy	removal of the appendix	-otomy	incision	tracheotomy	incision of trachea
-emia	blood	anemia	lacking sufficient quality or quantity of blood	-plegia	paralysis	hemiplegia	paralysis of one side of the body
				-pnea	breathing, respiration	apnea	temporary absence of respirations
-gram	record	electro-cardiogram	record produced by electro-cardiography	-scope	examination instrument	otoscope	instrument for inspecting
-itis	inflammation	appendicitis	inflammation of the appendix	-scopy	examination using a scope	proctoscopy	rectal exam with a proctoscope
-logy	study of	hematology	study of blood				

Common Abbreviations

Table 5-4 lists abbreviations and their meanings. They have been grouped according to most common usage for easier learning. Other abbreviations are presented in following units, within the context in which they are most often used.

TABLE 5-4 COMMON ABBREVIATIONS

Body Parts					
ABCs	airways, breathing, circulation	sh	shoulder	CA	cancer
abd	abdomen	vag	vagina, vaginal	CAD	coronary artery disease
ant	anterior	**Diagnosis**		CBC	complete blood count
ax	axillary	AFB	acid-fast bacillus	CHD	coronary heart disease
bld	blood	AIDS	acquired immune deficiency syndrome	CHF	congestive heart failure
BLE	both lower extremities	AKA	above knee amputation	COPD	chronic obstructive pulmonary disease
GI	gastrointestinal	AMI	acute myocardial infarction	CVA	cerebrovascular accident; stroke
GU	genitourinary	ASCVD	arteriosclerotic cardiovascular disease	DJD	degenerative joint disease
int	internal	ASHD	arteriosclerotic heart disease	DVT	deep vein thrombosis
lt	left	BKA	below knee amputation	ESRD	end-stage renal disease
rt	right	BPH	benign prostatic hypertrophy (hyperplasia)	FUO	fever of unknown origin
quad	quadrant			Fx	fracture

continues

TABLE 5-4 *CONTINUED*

Diagnosis *continued*

GERD	gastroesophageal reflux disease
HBV	hepatitis B virus (infection)
HCV	hepatitis C virus (infection)
HIV	human immunodeficiency virus (infection)
HTN	hypertension
IDDM	insulin-dependent diabetes mellitus
IH	infectious hepatitis
KS	Kaposi's sarcoma
LBP	low back pain
MD	muscular dystrophy
MI	myocardial infarction (refers to the death of tissues due to loss of blood supply)
MRSA	methicillin-resistant *Staphylococcus aureus*
MS	multiple sclerosis
NB	newborn
NIDDM	non–insulin-dependent diabetes mellitus
NSU	nonspecific urethritis
OA	osteoarthritis
OBS	organic brain syndrome
PID	pelvic inflammatory disease
PUD	peptic ulcer disease
PVD	peripheral vascular disease
RF	renal failure
RO, R/O	rule out
SDAT	senile dementia of Alzheimer's type

STD	sexually transmitted disease
TIA	transient ischemic attack
URI	upper respiratory infection
UTI	urinary tract infection
VRE	vancomycin-resistant *Enterococcus*

Patient Orders and Charting

$\bar{a}$	before
AAROM	active assistive (assisted) range of motion
abd.	abduction; abdomen
ACT	active, actively, activities
add.	adduction
ADL	activities of daily living
ad lib.	as desired
adm	admission; administer; administrator
ADT	admission, discharge, transfer
AEB	as evidenced by
AFO	ankle foot orthosis
aka	also known as
AMA	against medical advice
amb	ambulate, ambulatory
AROM	active range of motion
ASAP	as soon as possible
assist	assistance
as tol	as tolerated
B, (B), Ⓑ	bilateral, both
BB	bed bath
bilat	bilateral
BLE	both lower extremities

B.M., bm	bowel movement
BP, B/P	blood pressure
BPM	beats per minute
B.R.	bedrest; bathroom
BRP	bathroom privileges
BS	blood sugar
BSC	bedside commode
BSE	breast self-examination
BUE	both upper extremities
$\bar{c}$	with
cal	calorie
cath	catheterize, catheter
CBB	complete bed bath
CBR	complete bed rest
ck or √	check
ck freq or √ freq	check frequently
cl liq	clear liquid
c/o	complains of
CP	care plan; chest pain
CPG	clinical practice guidelines
CPM	continuous passive motion
CPR	cardiopulmonary resuscitation
DAT	diet as tolerated
dehyd	dehydration
dep	dependent
disch	discharge
DNR	do not resuscitate
DOA	dead on arrival

continues

TABLE 5-4 *CONTINUED*

Patient Orders and Charting *continued*					
doc	document, documentation	H	hydrogen	N/C, no c/o	no complaints
Dr	doctor	H₂O	water	neg, ⊖	negative
drsg	dressing	H₂O₂	hydrogen peroxide	NG	nasogastric
DSD	dry sterile dressing	HOB	head of bed	NKA	no known allergies
Dx	diagnosis	HOH	hard of hearing	NN	nurses' notes
E, en	enema	ht	height	NPO	nothing by mouth
EHR	electronic health record	Hx	history	N/S, NSS	normal saline solution
EMR	electronic medical record	①, ind.	independent	N & V	nausea and vomiting
EOL	end of life	I&O	intake and output	NVD	nausea, vomiting, diarrhea
EOLC	end-of-life care	IM	intramuscular	NWB	no weight bearing
et	and	irrig	irrigation	O₂	oxygen
ETOH	ethanol (used to refer to alcoholic beverages)	isol	isolation	occ	occasional
Eval	evaluation	IV	intravenous	OOB	out of bed
ex	exercise, example	JT	jejunostomy tube	O, OS	oral; mouth
exam	examination	K⁺	potassium	P	poor, pulse
ext.	extension; extremity; external	Kcal	kilocalorie, calorie	PB, PBB	partial bath, partial bed bath
F	fair	L	left, liter	per	by
FB	foreign body	lat	lateral	p.o.	by mouth
FE	Fleet's enema	LBP	low back pain	postop	postoperative
flex	flexion	lg, lge, L	large	preop	preoperative
FM	flow meter	liq	liquid	prep	prepare
FU, f/u	follow-up	L/min, LPM	liters per minute	PRN	whenever necessary
FUO	fever of unknown origin	LOC	loss of consciousness	prog	progress; prognosis
FWB	full weight bearing	max	maximum	PROM	passive range of motion
G	good	min	minimum	PWB	partial weight bearing
g/c, GC	geriatric chair	meds	medications	Px	prognosis (prog)
GT, g/t	gastrostomy tube	mmHg	millimeters of mercury	q̄	each, every
		mod	moderate	q.s.	sufficient quantity
		NA, N/A	nursing assistant also means "not applicable"	qt	quiet

continues

TABLE 5-4 *CONTINUED*

Patient Orders and Charting
continued

R	rectal; respiration; right
re:	regarding
rehab	rehabilitation
resp	respiration
rot	rotated, rotation
rt (R)	right; routine
r/t	related to
RT	respiratory therapy
Rx	treatment; prescription
s̄	without
s/s, S & S	signs and symptoms
sm	small
SOB	short(ness) of breath
SBA	standby assistance
SSE	soapsuds enema
stat	at once; immediately
std prec	standard precautions
Sx	symptoms
T, temp	temperature
TIAN	toilet in advance of need
TKO	to keep open
TLC	tender loving care
TPN	total parenteral nutrition
TPR	temperature, pulse, respirations
trach	tracheostomy
TSE	testicular self-examination

TWE	tap water enema
Tx	treatment
ung oint	ointment
vc	verbal cues
VS	vital signs
w/c	wheelchair
WB	weight bearing
WBAT	weight bearing as tolerated
wt	weight

Physical and History

CC	chief complaint
DOB	date of birth
EENT	eye, ear, nose, throat
ENT	ear, nose, throat
FH	family history
H & P	history and physical
LMP	last menstrual period
L & W	living and well
M & F	mother and father
MH	marital history
NB	newborn
PE	physical examination
PI	present illness
PMH	past medical history
R/O	rule out
SOB	short(ness) of breath
UCD	usual childhood diseases
UK	unknown
WDWN	well-developed,

	well-nourished
WFL	within functional limits
WNL	within normal limits
Y/O	years old
YOB	year of birth

Tests

ABG	arterial blood gas study
BS	blood sugar
C & S	culture and sensitivity
CBC	complete blood count
CXR	chest X-ray
FBS	fasting blood sugar
FSBS	fingerstick blood sugar
H & H	hemoglobin and hematocrit
spec	specimen
UA, U/A	urinalysis

Places or Departments

CS	central supply
DR, D/R	delivery room; dining room
ED/ER	emergency department/ emergency room
ECG, EKG	electrocardiogram
EEG	electroencephalogram
EENT	eye, ear, nose, throat
GYN	gynecology
ICCU	intensive coronary care unit
IDT	interdisciplinary team
Lab	laboratory

continues

TABLE 5-4 *CONTINUED*

Places or Departments
continued

LTC	long-term care
MRD	medical record department
OPD	outpatient department
OR	operating room
OT	occupational therapy
PAR	post-anesthesia recovery
Peds, pedi	pediatrics
PT	physical therapy
RR	recovery room
RT	respiratory therapy
SNU, SNF	skilled nursing unit, skilled nursing facility
ST	speech therapy
XR, X/R	X-ray

Process Improvement

assess	assess, assessment
BNE	board of nurse examiners
BON	board of nursing
CE	continuing education
CEU	continuing education unit
CQI	continuous quality improvement
EBDM	evidence-based decision making
EBR	evidence-based recommendations
eval	evaluate, evaluation
HC	health care
HCI	health care improvement

HCQ	health care quality
ID	identify, identification
IDT	interdisciplinary team
info	information
IT	information technology
NAR	nurse aide registry, nursing assistant registry
NP	nursing practice, nurse practitioner
NPA	nurse practice act
PI	performance improvement, process improvement
PRO	professional improvement organization, process improvement organization
QA	quality assessment, quality assurance
QHC	quality health care
QI	quality improvement, quality initiative
QIO	quality improvement organization
QM	quality management
QR	quality review
RCA	root cause analysis
SIQ	sharing innovations in quality
SOC	standard(s) of care
SOP	standard(s) of practice
std, stds	standard, standards
TQM	total quality management

Time Abbreviations

a.c.	before meals
AM	morning
b.i.d.	twice a day
d	day
h	hour
noc, noct	night
OC, oc	on call
$\bar{p}$	after
$\bar{p.c.}$	after meals
PM	evening or afternoon
$\bar{q}$h	every hour
$\bar{q}$4h	every four hours
q.i.d.	four times a day
t.i.d.	three times a day
WA, W/A	while awake
x, X	times
x2, x3	two times, three times, . . .

Roman Numerals

I	1
II	2
III	3
IV	4
V	5
VI	6
VII	7
VIII	8
IX	9
X	10

continues

TABLE 5-4 *CONTINUED*

Other Common Numbers					
1°	first; primary; first degree	VS, vitals	vital signs	O	oral
				R	rectal
2°	second; secondary to; second degree	**Weight/Height**		**Symbols**	
		cm	centimeter	♂	male
3°	third; tertiary; third degree	ft	feet	♀	female
		ht	height	↑	up, increase
1x, 2x,	one time, one person; two times, two people, . . .	kg	kilogram	↓	down, decrease
		lb	pounds	//	parallel
Measurements and Volume		in	inches	Δ	change to, change in
		oz	ounce	Ø	zero, none, nothing
amt.	amount	wt	weight	＊	important
gtt	drop	**Temperature**			
mL	milliliter	°	degree		
L	liter	Ax	axillary		
oz	ounce	F	Fahrenheit		
Vital Signs		C	Celsius		
TPR	temperature, pulse, respirations				

BODY ORGANIZATION

All nursing care is directed toward helping patients reach optimum health and independence. **Health** is a state of well-being in which all parts of the body and mind are functioning properly. **Disease** is any change from the healthy state. Disease takes many forms. Medical science is the study of disease and its effects on the human body. These effects are easier to understand when you have a clear picture in your mind of a normal and properly functioning body. The first step is to understand the organization of the body.

ANATOMIC TERMS

The **anatomy** (structure) and **physiology** (function) of the body are most easily understood and learned if they are studied in an orderly manner. Special terms are used to describe the relationship of one body part to another. Whenever we describe the relationship of the body parts, we refer to the **anatomic position** (Figure 5-3), which is:

- Standing erect with feet together or slightly separated
- Facing the observer
- Arms at the sides with the palms forward

In our own minds, we should always position the body in this way before describing any body part or area. This gives everyone the same frame of reference.

Notice as you look at a patient's body or the pictures in the book that you are seeing a mirror image of yourself. The patient's right side is opposite to your left and your left is opposite to the right of the patient or the picture.

Descriptive Terms

Imaginary lines drawn through the body (Figure 5-4) provide us with other reference terms.

- A line drawn down the center of the body from head to foot (the *midline*) divides the body into equal right and left sides. Note that the body has the same parts on either side. For example, there is an arm, a leg, an eye, and half of a nose on each side of the line.
- Parts close to this line are **medial** to the line.
- Parts farther away from the line are **lateral** to the line.

For example, in the anatomic position, the thumbs are more lateral to the line and the little fingers are more medial to the line.

FIGURE 5-3 All references to body parts are made in relationship to the anatomic position.

Another line drawn parallel to the floor divides the body into upper and lower parts. This line can be drawn at any level on the body as long as it is parallel to the floor.

- Parts located above this line are **superior** to the line.
- Parts located below this line are **inferior** to the line.

For example, if the line is drawn between the knees and ankles, the knees are superior to the ankles and the ankles are inferior to the knees.

A third line can be drawn to divide the body into front and back.

- Parts in front of this line are **anterior** or **ventral** to the line.
- Parts in back of this line are **posterior** or **dorsal** to the line.

Points of Attachment

The arms and legs are called the *extremities* of the body. The arms are attached to the body at the shoulders. The

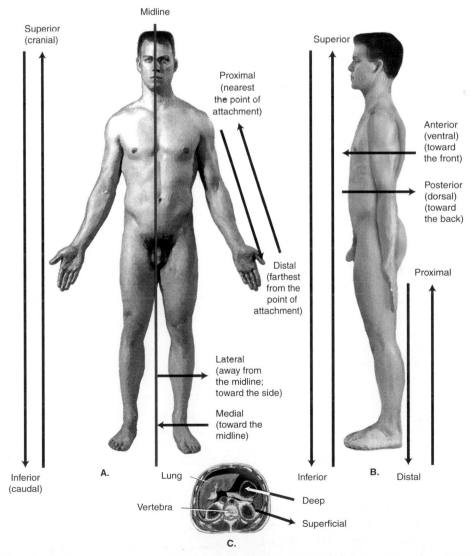

FIGURE 5-4 Imaginary lines are used to section the body to make it easier to locate parts. Directional terms relating to the anatomic position. (A) anatomic position; (B) lateral views of the body; (C) directional terms *deep* and *superficial*.

legs are attached to the body at the hips. Two terms are used to describe the relationship between the parts of the extremities and their points of attachment to the body.

- **Proximal**—means closest to the point of attachment
- **Distal**—means farthest away from the point of attachment

Because the upper arm is closest to the shoulder, where it is attached, this part is described as *proximal* when compared to the fingers, which are farthest away. The fingers are *distal* or farthest away from the point of attachment of the upper extremity.

Abdominal Regions

The abdomen is divided into four **quadrants**, with the **umbilicus** (navel) at the central point (Figure 5-5A). The abdomen can also be divided into nine regions (Figure 5-5B). Knowing these regions will be important as you report and document your observations.

ORGANIZATION OF THE BODY

All parts of the body are interdependent. The basic unit of the body is the **cell**. Groups of similar cells are organized into **tissues**. Different tissues form **organs**. The organs are organized into **systems** that perform the body functions.

Cells

Each cell performs the same basic functions that the total body performs, but on a smaller scale. These functions are breathing (respiration), reproduction, nutrition, and excretion (eliminating wastes). Some cells perform different kinds of work necessary for the body as a whole to function. Some of the various specialized types of cells are:

- Epithelial cells
- Nerve cells
- Muscle cells
- Connective tissue cells

Epithelial cells, which are very close together, form protective coverings and sometimes produce body fluids.

Nerve cells carry electrical messages to and from the different parts of the body, coordinating activities and making us aware of changes in the environment.

Muscle cells are special in their ability to shorten or lengthen, changing their shape and the position of parts to which they are attached. They also surround body openings, such as the mouth, to control the size of these openings.

Connective tissue cells are present throughout the body in many different types. They support and connect body parts.

Tissues

Groups of similar cells are organized into tissues. The basic tissue types are:

- Epithelial tissue
- Connective tissue
- Nervous tissue
- Muscle tissue

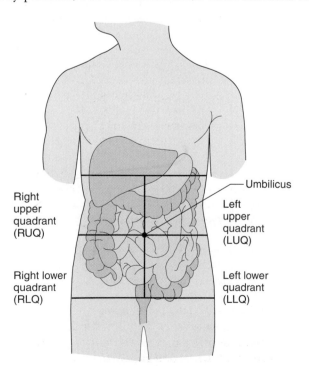

FIGURE 5-5A Division of the abdomen into four quadrants

FIGURE 5-5B Nine regions of the thorax and abdomen

Epithelial tissue is specialized in its ability to absorb, secrete (produce) fluids, excrete (eliminate) waste products, and protect.

Nervous tissue forms the brain and spinal cord and the nerves throughout the body. This tissue is also found in the special sense organs such as the eyes, ears, and taste-buds. The activities of the rest of the body are directed and coordinated through the nervous tissues.

Three kinds of **muscle tissue** are found in the body:

- **Skeletal (voluntary) muscle** is attached to bones for movement.
- **Cardiac muscle** forms the heart wall.
- **Smooth (involuntary) muscle** (visceral) forms the walls of body organs such as the stomach and intestines.

Connective tissue forms blood, bone, and fibrous and elastic tissues to hold the skin on the body, attach muscles to bones, and support delicate cells throughout the body. Generally, connective tissues support and form connections for other tissue types.

Organs

Each organ is made up of more than one kind of tissue and performs special functions that contribute to the function of the body systems. Some organs, like the kidneys, are found in pairs. Some single organs contribute to more than one system. For example, the pancreas contributes secretions to both the endocrine and digestive systems.

Systems

The body has 10 major body systems. Table 5-5 lists the organs that contribute to the function of each system. Notice that some organs are included with more than one

TABLE 5-5 SYSTEMS OF THE BODY

System	Function	Structures
Cardiovascular (Circulatory)	Transports materials around the body; carries oxygen and nutrients to the cells and carries waste products away; part of the immune system that provides protective cells and chemicals to fight current infections and protect against future infections	Heart, arteries, capillaries, veins, spleen, lymph nodes, lymphatic vessels, blood, lymph
Endocrine	Produces hormones that regulate body processes	Pituitary gland, thyroid gland, parathyroid glands, thymus gland, adrenal glands, testes, ovaries, pineal body, islets of Langerhans in pancreas
Gastrointestinal (Digestive)	Digests, transports food, absorbs nutrients, and eliminates wastes	Mouth, esophagus, pharynx, stomach, small intestine, large intestine, salivary glands, teeth, tongue, liver, gallbladder, pancreas
Integumentary	Protects the body from injury and against infection, regulates body temperature, eliminates some wastes	Skin, hair, nails, sweat and oil glands
Muscular	Protects organs by forming body walls, forms walls of some organs, assists in movement by changing position of bones at joints	*Smooth* muscles—form walls of organs *Skeletal* muscles—attached to bones *Cardiac* muscles—form wall of heart
Nervous	Coordinates body functions	Brain, spinal cord, spinal nerves, cranial nerves, special sense organs such as eyes and ears
Reproductive	Reproduces the species, fulfills sexual needs, develops sexual identity	*Male:* Testes, epididymis, urethra, seminal vesicles, ejaculatory duct, prostate gland, bulbourethral glands, penis, spermatic cord *Female:* Breasts, ovaries, oviducts, uterus, vagina, Bartholin glands, vulva

continues

TABLE 5-5 *CONTINUED*

System	Function	Structures
Respiratory	Brings in oxygen and eliminates carbon dioxide	Sinuses, nose, pharynx, larynx, trachea, bronchi, lungs
Skeletal	Supports and protects body parts, produces blood cells, acts as lever in movement	Bones, joints
Urinary	Manages fluids and electrolytes of body, eliminates liquid wastes	Kidneys, ureters, urinary bladder, urethra

system. For example, the ovaries contribute to the endocrine system by producing female hormones and to the reproductive system by producing the egg.

Membranes

Membranes are sheets of epithelial tissues supported by connective tissues. Membranes:

- Cover the body
- Line body cavities
- Produce some body fluids

Important membranes include:

- **Mucous membranes**
  - Produce a fluid called **mucus**
  - Line body cavities that open to the outside

Because the respiratory, digestive, and genitourinary systems all open to the outside, they are lined with mucous membranes. The eyelids are also lined with a mucous membrane; a mucous membrane covers the eyeballs.

- **Synovial membranes**
  - Produce synovial fluid
  - Line joint cavities

The synovial fluid is a clear fluid resembling the white of an egg. It reduces the friction between the bones of active joints and the tendons.

- **Serous membranes**
  - Produce serous fluid
  - Cover the organs and line the closed cavities of the body

Serous fluid reduces friction as the organs work and move. Important serous membranes are the:

- **Pericardium**—surrounds the heart
- **Pleura**—surround the lungs and line the thoracic cavity
- **Meninges**—cover the brain and spinal cord and line the dorsal cavity
- **Peritoneum**—covers the digestive organs and lines the abdominal cavity
- **Cutaneous membrane** (skin)
  - Protects the body
  - Covers the entire body
  - Helps to control body temperature
  - Eliminates wastes through sweat glands
  - Produces vitamin D when exposed to sunlight

Special epithelial cells in this membrane, called *glands*, secrete perspiration and oils.

Cavities

The body seems like a solid structure, but **cavities** (spaces) within it contain the organs. Table 5-6 lists the two main cavities, the dorsal cavity and the ventral cavity. Each of these cavities is lined by and divided into other cavities by serous membranes. These other cavities are also listed in the table, as are the organs contained in each.

Figure 5-6 is a simple drawing of the location of these cavities.

TABLE 5-6 BODY CAVITIES AND THE ORGANS CONTAINED WITHIN EACH CAVITY

Cavity	Organs	
Dorsal Cavity		
Cranial	Brain, pineal body, pituitary gland	
Spinal	Nerves, spinal cord	
Ventral Cavity		
Thoracic	Lungs, heart, great blood vessels, thymus gland	
Abdominal Peritoneal	Stomach, small intestine, most of large intestine, liver, gallbladder, pancreas, spleen	
Pelvic	*Male*	*Female*
	Seminal vesicles, prostate gland, ejaculatory ducts, urinary bladder, urethra, rectum	Uterus, oviducts, ovaries, urinary bladder, urethra, rectum
Retroperitoneal space	Kidneys, adrenal glands, ureters	

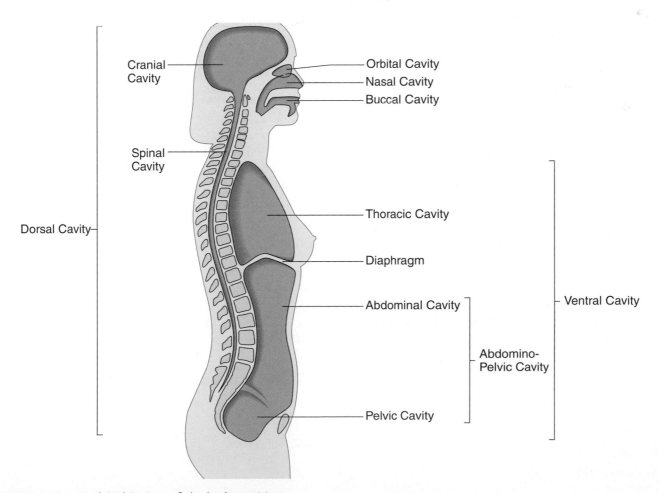

FIGURE 5-6 Lateral (side) view of the body cavities

REVIEW

A. Matching.

Match the abbreviations in Column I with their meanings in Column II.

Column I

1. _____ a̅.c̅.
2. _____ b.i.d.
3. _____ OR
4. _____ PRN
5. _____ NPO
6. _____ stat
7. _____ HOB
8. _____ c̅
9. _____ ung.
10. _____ s̅

Column II

a. three times a day
b. whenever necessary
c. head of bed
d. before meals
e. operating room
f. nothing by mouth
g. after meals
h. without
i. twice a day
j. at once
k. ointment
l. with

B. Matching.

Match the prefixes in Column I with their meanings in Column II.

Column I

11. _____ ur (o)
12. _____ cardi (o)
13. _____ chol (e)
14. _____ dermat (o)
15. _____ gastr (o)
16. _____ ot (o)
17. _____ ped (o)
18. _____ pneum (o)
19. _____ my (o)
20. _____ pharyng (o)

Column II

a. bile
b. ear
c. lung
d. child
e. muscle
f. pharynx
g. stomach
h. larynx
i. heart
j. urine
k. chest
l. skin

C. Define the following medical terms.

Then circle the prefix that you have learned.

21. dysuria _____
22. apnea _____
23. craniotomy _____
24. hypertension _____
25. tachycardia _____

D. Define the following medical terms.

Then circle the suffix that you have learned.

26. neuralgia _____
27. apnea _____
28. appendectomy _____
29. hematology _____
30. fibroma _____

E. Write the medical term that means the following.

31. kidney stones _____
32. examination of the rectum using an instrument _____
33. incision into thorax _____
34. inflammation of the stomach _____
35. white blood cell _____

F. In each of the following, circle the prefix and underline the suffix.

36. anemia

37. neuritis

38. pharyngitis

39. pandemic

40. tracheotomy

G. Measurements.

Print the abbreviations for the following.

41. milliliter _____
42. kilogram _____

43. pound _____

44. Fahrenheit _____

45. inches _____

H. Print the Roman numerals for each of the following.

46. 2 _____

47. 5 _____

48. 6 _____

49. 9 _____

50. 10 _____

I. Multiple Choice.

Select the one best answer for each of the following.

51. When describing the relationship of the hand to the elbow, you should refer to the hand as being
  a. proximal.
  b. posterior.
  c. distal.
  d. anterior.

52. The appendix is located in which quadrant of the abdomen?
  a. URQ
  b. RLQ
  c. ULQ
  d. LLQ

53. Which membrane covers the lungs?
  a. pleura
  b. pericardium
  c. peritoneum
  d. meninges

54. Which organs are located in the dorsal cavity?
  a. heart and liver
  b. kidney and spleen
  c. brain and spinal cord
  d. uterus and testes

55. Which organ pumps blood throughout the body?
  a. lungs
  b. heart
  c. liver
  d. adrenal glands

56. Which of the following is part of the skeletal system?
  a. ureters
  b. sternum
  c. gallbladder
  d. testes

57. The breasts are part of which system?
  a. muscular
  b. urinary
  c. cardiovascular
  d. reproductive

58. Membranes that line body cavities that open to the outside are called
  a. mucous membranes.
  b. basilar membranes.
  c. serous membranes.
  d. fibrous membranes.

59. The eye and ear are part of which system?
  a. endocrine
  b. nervous
  c. cardiovascular
  d. digestive

60. The endocrine system
  a. reproduces the species.
  b. brings in oxygen.
  c. transports blood.
  d. produces hormones.

J. True/False.

Mark the following true or false by circling T or F.

61. T F The urinary bladder and gallbladder are the same structure.

62. T F The pancreas functions in both the digestive and endocrine systems.

63. T F Muscular tissue enables the body to move.

64. T F Structures of different tissues acting together to carry out a specific function are called organs.

K. Nursing Assistant Challenge.

Examine the sample care plan and use your understanding of medical science and terminology to define each medical term and abbreviation used on the plan.

1.	**Patient Name**	Bruce Tratt	**Age** 47	**Rel** Prot		#876-3291-7	
2.	**Physician**	R. Morgan M.D.	**Dx** Splenomegaly—Diabetes Mellitus				
3.			**Orders**				
4.	**Preop orders**	3/18	on call for OR at 8 am 3/19				
5.	Stat CBC, ABG, FBS						
6.	UA						
7.	NG Tube at 6 am 3/19						
8.	Foley cath this pm.						
9.	Surg Prep.						
10.	NPO p̄ midnight						
11.	SSE at 9 pm.						
12.	Amb ad lib. this pm.						
13.							
14.	Anesthesiologist will call preop meds.						
15.							

UNIT 6

Classification of Disease

OBJECTIVES

After completing this unit, you will be able to:
- Spell and define terms.
- Define disease and list some possible causes.
- Distinguish between signs and symptoms.
- List six major health problems.
- Identify disease-related terms.
- List ways in which a diagnosis is made.
- Describe malignant and benign tumors.

VOCABULARY

Learn the meaning and the correct spelling of the following words and phrases:

acute disease	congenital	malignant	risk factor
acute exacerbation	etiology	medical diagnosis	sarcoma
antibodies	genetic	metastasize	signs
autoimmune	hypersensitivity	neoplasm	symptoms
benign	immune response	noninvasive	therapy
cachexia	infection	obstruction	trauma
carcinoma	inflammation	predisposing factor	tumor
chronic disease	invasive	prognosis	vaccine
complication	ischemia	protocol	

INTRODUCTION

The nurse values your observations and uses them when making evaluations and planning nursing care for patients, as part of the nursing process. The better you understand the basic principles of disease, the more accurate information you can provide.

DISEASE

The body is a complex chemical factory that depends upon all of its parts to perform efficiently. It is subject to external and internal forces and stress that can threaten its ability to function properly (Figure 6-1).

Disease is any change from a healthy state. The disease (illness) may be a change in structure or function, or it may be failure of a part of the body to develop properly. Each illness has

- An **etiology**—cause of the illness or abnormality.
- A usual set of indications that the illness is in progress. These are called signs and symptoms.
- A usual course or disease progression.
- A **prognosis** or probable outcome of the process.

Predisposing factors to disease are general conditions, such as malnutrition, that may contribute to the development of illness. Some diseases have related risk factors. **Risk factors** are specific behaviors or conditions that tend to promote certain diseases (Figure 6-2). For example,

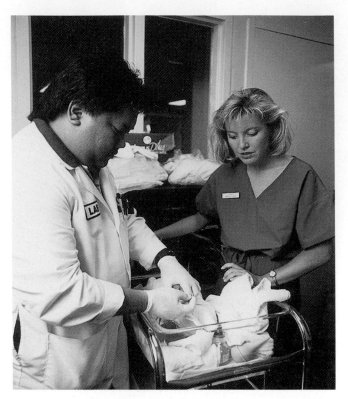

FIGURE 6-1 The laboratory technician draws blood from the heel of this newborn.

FIGURE 6-2 Advanced age is a risk factor that predisposes people to some diseases.

smoking is a risk factor that increases the likelihood that the person will develop lung disease. Other risk factors and associated diseases include:

- Excess weight—high blood pressure, strokes, heart attack, diabetes
- Poor nutrition—infections, skin breakdown
- Lack of exercise—osteoporosis
- High-fat, low-fiber diet—cancer of the colon
- Unprotected sex—hepatitis, AIDS, gonorrhea
- Family history—breast cancer, heart disease, diabetes mellitus

Age-Appropriate Care ALERT

As a nursing assistant, you will be caring for patients of all ages. You must learn how to provide age-appropriate care to each age group. This means that you will meet the patient's age-related needs for communication, safety and security, and personal care and comfort. You will find that these measures vary slightly for each age group. Avoid treating adults as children, or children as adults. Meet each patient on his or her own level. ■

A young child who is malnourished and underweight is much more likely to develop an infection than one who is well nourished. The germs causing the infection are the actual cause of the illness, but the age and nutritional state of the child contribute to the development of the infectious process. Table 6-1 lists common causes of disease (both external and internal) and a number of risk factors for disease.

Signs and Symptoms

Signs of a disease can be seen by others. The color or condition of the skin is an example of a sign of disease (Figure 6-3). **Symptoms** are felt by the patient, who tells us about them. Pain is a symptom common to many illnesses (Figure 6-4).

The Course (Pattern) of Disease

The development and course of different illnesses vary greatly. **Acute disease** develops suddenly, progresses rapidly, and lasts for a predictable period, and then the person recovers (or dies). For example, the signs and symptoms of an infected finger may develop rapidly and last a relatively short period. Then, as the body controls the process, recovery is seen.

TABLE 6–1 COMMON CAUSES OF DISEASE AND PREDISPOSING FACTORS

External Etiology	Internal Etiology	Predisposing Factors
traumas	metabolic disorders	age
radiation	congenital abnormalities	malnutrition
microorganisms	tumors	heredity
chemical agents		previous illness

FIGURE 6-3 A maculopapular rash is characteristic of skin changes is measles (rubeola). (Courtesy of Centers of Disease Control and Prevention)

FIGURE 6-4 Sometimes patients communicate pain through their body language.

Long term

With a **chronic disease**, there are often periods when the patient experiences the signs and symptoms and periods when evidence of the disease is less pronounced or disappears altogether. Rheumatoid arthritis is such a disease. At times the affected joints are red, hot to the touch, swollen, and painful. At other times, the signs and symptoms seem to go away. An **acute exacerbation** of a chronic disease is when the severity of signs and symptoms increases.

Sudden

Complications

A **complication** makes the original condition more serious. For example, if a child has measles and develops pneumonia (a serious lung condition), the pneumonia is a complication that makes it more difficult for the child to recover.

MAJOR CONDITIONS

Some of the major conditions or illnesses that can affect the body's ability to function are:

- **Ischemia**—the lack of adequate blood supply to a body tissue, which prevents delivery of essential oxygen and nutrients. For example, a blood clot (thrombus) that

has formed within a blood vessel wall can block the blood vessel.

- **Congenital** abnormalities—abnormalities that are present at birth (Figure 6-5). Some abnormalities occur while the baby is growing in the mother's uterus. Examples include:
  - Spina bifida—a defect in the formation of the vertebral column
  - Cleft lip—an imperfection in the formation of the upper lip
  - Agenesis of a kidney—one kidney fails to develop, so the baby is born with only one functioning kidney
  - Talipes (club foot)—the child's foot is turned or twisted out of its normal position

Some abnormalities are due to defects in the **genetic** information passed from the parents to the child. Examples include:

- Sickle cell anemia—the red blood cells are improperly formed so they do not maintain their normal disc shape
- Color blindness—the person is unable to distinguish between certain colors
- Hemophilia—there is a lack of an important blood component needed for proper blood clotting.

- **Infection**—Infectious organisms or their products cause infection, including pneumonias, scarlet fever, and abscesses. Inflammation is usually part of the infectious process.

- **Inflammation** is a localized protective reaction of tissue to irritation, injury, or infection. It is characterized by pain, redness, swelling, a feeling of heat on the skin, and loss of function. Inflammations that develop for reasons other than infection include:
  - **Autoimmune** reactions—Mechanisms that are designed to protect the body turn against the body and cause damage, resulting in conditions such as rheumatoid arthritis, systemic lupus erythematosus, and multiple sclerosis.

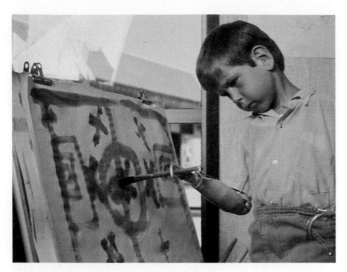

FIGURE 6-5 This child has phocomelia. His hands did not develop before birth because a drug his mother took during early pregnancy interfered with limb development. (Photo courtesy of the March of Dimes—Birth Defects Foundation)

- **Hypersensitivity** reactions—Allergic types of reactions such as hay fever, skin rashes, and asthma.
- Irritations—May be caused by seeds in the intestinal tract, stones in the gallbladder or kidney, or redness of the skin due to chemical exposure.
- Metabolic imbalances—Conditions of fluid and electrolyte imbalance include malnutrition, edema, scurvy, alcoholism, and diabetes mellitus.
- **Obstruction**—Tubes throughout the body carry a variety of materials that must continue to flow. Obstructions impede the flow. Examples of obstructions include blood clots in blood vessels, stones in the bile ducts or the kidneys, and blockages that occur when the tube structures become twisted, as in an intestinal obstruction.
- **Trauma**—Injuries that cause tissue damage resulting from a blow to the body, such as an auto accident. Exposure to unusual pressure or extremes of temperature also causes trauma.
- Neoplasm—The word **neoplasm** means new growth. It is another term for **tumor**. Neoplasms are an important kind of disease. There are two types of neoplasms: benign or nonmalignant tumors and malignant tumors. Sometimes benign tumors can change and become malignant. People with a malignant tumor or a malignancy are said to have cancer. Neoplasms are discussed later in this unit.

DIAGNOSIS

The **medical diagnosis** (the process of identifying and naming the disease) is made by the physician. To do this, the patient is examined, a history of previous illness is taken and reviewed, and various laboratory and diagnostic tests are performed. The physician compiles the information, matches it to possible diseases, and then names the process to establish the medical diagnosis.

Diagnostic Studies

Laboratory tests (Figure 6-6) and diagnostic studies give the physician valuable information for naming the disease process and for planning proper treatment for the patient. The nursing staff prepares the patient for the ordered tests and cares for the patient after the tests are completed. The nursing assistant helps give this care and may be assigned to collect certain specimens.

Protocols are procedural standards and standards of care developed for the preparation and care of the patient for each test or study. Protocols must be followed carefully to achieve satisfactory results. Improper patient preparation can result in:

- Inability to perform the test
- Inaccurate test results
- Delayed diagnosis
- Increased costs
- Increased patient anxiety, pain, or discomfort
- Slower recovery

Noninvasive Tests

Some tests and studies are **noninvasive**. This means that the techniques used do not break the skin or damage body tissues. For example, X-rays do not break the skin, but do give information about internal body structures. Commonly ordered noninvasive tests include:

- Ultrasound—sound waves are bounced against the body to measure variations in tissue density (Figure 6-7). For example, the Doppler ultrasound probe measures the blood flow in blood vessels. Sonograms of a pregnant woman's uterus give information about the growing fetus.

FIGURE 6-6 Blood tests provide information about body chemistry and contribute to a correct medical diagnosis.

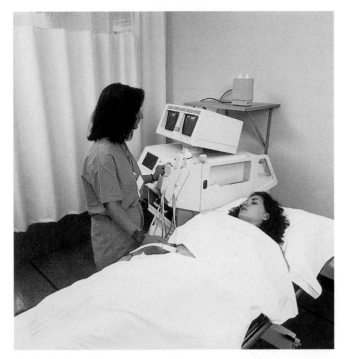

FIGURE 6-7 A sonogram of the uterus provides useful information about the developing fetus.

- Thermography—measures the temperature in different body tissues. Thermograms of the breast indicate increased temperature in tumorous tissue.
- X-ray and fluoroscopy—use short-wavelength electromagnetic radiation to examine internal tissues. X-ray techniques are sophisticated. One of the newest techniques is computerized axial tomography (CT scan or CAT scan). This procedure gives a three-dimensional view of the internal structures of the body. A computer records and prints out information.
- Magnetic resonance imaging (MRI)—an imaging technique that provides excellent pictures (images) with minimal risk to the patient (Figure 6-8). The body is placed in a strong magnetic field. Radio frequency pulses cause certain chemicals (ions) in body tissues to change position. When the radio waves are discontinued, the ions return to their original positions. As they go back to normal, the energy given off is recorded. All of this occurs without the patient feeling any of it.
- Recording of the electrical activity occurring in different body organs. A recording of this activity is made on paper or on a screen for viewing. Such examinations include:
  - Electrocardiogram (EKG or ECG) to record electrical activity of the cardiac cycle
  - Electroencephalogram (EEG) to record electrical activity of the brain
  - Electromyogram (EMG) to record electrical activity of muscles

Invasive Tests

Some tests and studies actually penetrate body surfaces and thus are known as **invasive** tests. Examples of invasive tests include taking tissue samples, introducing contrast media, and probing deeply into body cavities.

A sternal puncture is a procedure in which a needle pierces the sternum to draw a sample of blood-producing cells. For some invasive examinations, iodine dyes, barium compounds, or air may be introduced into a body cavity to produce contrast when making recordings and pictures.

Most of these invasive techniques are carried out in special areas, such as laboratories, that are designed for this purpose. Also, patient specimens usually are examined in laboratories.

Some special invasive procedures include:

- Direct visualization procedures—to examine body parts with instruments (scopes) introduced into the body. For example, the proctoscope, inserted in the anus, allows direct observation of the interior rectum. Other direct visualization procedures are:
  - Cystoscopy to observe the bladder
  - Laryngoscopy to observe the larynx
  - Sigmoidoscopy to observe the colon
- Dye studies—dyes are introduced into the body to outline body parts so that they will show up on X-rays. Some examples are:
  - Upper GI series (barium swallow)—the patient swallows a barium solution and then X-rays or fluoroscopy show the structures highlighted.
  - Lower GI series (barium enema)—the patient is given the barium rectally. The patient holds the solution while X-rays are taken.
  - Myelogram—dye is introduced into the spinal canal and then X-rays are taken.

FIGURE 6-8 An MRI shows the body in great detail. (Courtesy of GE Medical Systems)

- Cardiac catheterization—a catheter (small sterile tube) is introduced into the vascular system and delivers a dye. A monitor shows the dye flowing through the cardiovascular system.

Other Techniques

Chemical and microscopic studies examine samples of various body tissues and secretions. Getting some samples requires invasive procedures. Other sampling requires noninvasive procedures. The most common samples are:

- Blood
- Urine
- Sputum from the lungs
- Cultures from infected tissues
- Gastric secretions
- Feces (Figure 6-9)

THERAPY

Once the medical diagnosis is confirmed, it is possible to predict the course of the disease and a probable prognosis (likely outcome or course of the disease process). Then the most appropriate **therapy** (treatment) is determined.

There are four basic approaches to therapy. They may be used alone or in different combinations.

1. Surgery: This form of therapy may remove unhealthy tissue (Figure 6-10), replace unhealthy parts, or repair injured, malformed, or congenitally defective areas. Prostatectomies remove unhealthy prostate glands. Coronary bypasses replace blocked arteries with other arteries. Herniorrhaphies repair weakened muscle walls.

2. Chemotherapy: This form of therapy uses drugs and chemicals to promote and improve body functions and to control pain (Figure 6-11). For example, the patient with a fever is given an antipyretic, such as acetaminophen (Tylenol), to reduce the temperature.

3. Radiation: This form of therapy uses controlled radioactivity or X-rays to destroy tumor cells.

4. Supportive (palliative) care: This form of therapy is designed to support the patient's body in its attempt to stay healthy or return to health. For example, positioning a person upright makes it easier for him to breathe when he is having an asthmatic attack. Pain control, rest, proper nutrition, fluid intake, and good hygiene all aid the body's own attempt to control the effects of illness.

FIGURE 6-10 This patient's leg was amputated because of peripheral vascular disease.

FIGURE 6-11 The nursing assistant reports the patient's complaint to the nurse, who will further assess the patient and provide pain medication.

FIGURE 6-9 Stool specimens may be examined for occult blood.

NEOPLASMS

Tumors can affect almost any organ of the body. Tumor cells do not follow the normal laws of growth and reproduction and may not stay within the normal boundaries. Excess numbers of cells and abnormal cells crowd out the normal cells and compete with them for nutrients.

Types of Tumors

Different types of tumors are more common among certain groups of people. Children have more tumors of the nervous system, urinary system, and blood vessels. Adults have more tumors of the reproductive organs, lungs, and colon.

The two major types of tumors are classified as benign or malignant. Each type has its own characteristics.

Benign or nonmalignant tumors:

- Usually grow slowly
- Do not spread
- Are usually encapsulated (surrounded by a capsule)
- Do not cause death unless located in a vital area such as the brain
- Are usually named by stating the part of the body involved and adding the suffix -oma. For example, *osteoma* names a benign bone tumor.

Malignant tumors or cancerous growths:

- Grow relatively rapidly
- Spread to other body parts (**metastasize**)
- If untreated, cause death
- May be named sarcoma or carcinoma or have special names like leukemia.
  - **Carcinomas** are spread primarily by way of the lymph system to the lymph nodes. They occur more commonly in people over 40 years of age.
  - **Sarcomas** are spread primarily by way of the bloodstream. They occur more commonly in people under 40 years of age.

Early Detection

Early detection of cancer can often result in a cure. The sooner the cancer is found, the higher the rate of cure. Pain is usually a late symptom.

Early Signs and Symptoms. Early signs and symptoms of malignancies include:

Change in bowel or bladder habits

A sore that does not heal

Unusual bleeding or discharge

Thickening or lump in breast or elsewhere

Indigestion or difficulty in swallowing

Obvious change in wart or mole

Nagging cough or hoarseness

> **Note:** The first letters of these early signs and symptoms spell **CAUTION**.

Late Signs and Symptoms. Late signs and symptoms of malignancies include:

- Fever of unknown origin
- **Cachexia** or general wasting of the body tissues with loss of weight
- Anemia
- Pain due to pressure, obstruction, and ischemia
- Hormonal irregularities
- Inflammations of the skin

BODY DEFENSES

The body has a natural line of defense against disease. These defenses include:

- Unbroken skin and mucous membranes, which act as mechanical barriers
- Mucus, which traps foreign particles, and cilia (small hairlike structures), which propel them out of the body
- The acidity of certain body secretions such as perspiration, saliva, and stomach juices, which slows the growth of microorganisms
- White blood cells, which surround and destroy anything foreign that enters the body
- Inflammation
- The immune response

Inflammation

The process of inflammation, which we often associate with infections such as boils and abscesses, is really an important part of the body's natural defenses. When anything foreign enters the body, small blood vessels (capillaries) in the area get bigger (dilate), bringing more blood to the infected part. In the blood are white blood cells and other protective substances. Fluid (serum) and white blood cells pass through the capillary walls into the area and a wall is gradually built up around the foreign object. As the white blood cells try to destroy the invader, pressure builds up to force the material to the surface of the body. The inflammatory process takes place to some extent in the body whenever injury occurs. The signs and symptoms of acute inflammation are:

- Redness
- Swelling
- Heat
- Loss of function
- Pain

Immune Response

Immune response (immunity) protects the body against specific infections by producing special chemicals called **antibodies**. For example, a person exposed to the measles virus may become ill with the disease. After recovery, the antibodies formed by the person against the measles virus will protect him from becoming sick again with the same disease.

Vaccines (altered germs or their products) may be given before exposure to a disease. The body can then produce antibodies before actual exposure occurs.

REVIEW

A. Matching.

Match the statements in questions 1–10 with the correct terms in the list a–j.

1. _____ Probable outcome
2. _____ Color of the skin
3. _____ Cause of disease
4. _____ Noncancerous tumor
5. _____ Pain as reported by the patient
6. _____ Illness with sudden onset and short course
7. _____ Injury
8. _____ Inflammation
9. _____ Condition transmitted from one generation to another
10. _____ Cancer

  a. acute   **f.** malignancy
  b. benign   **g.** prognosis
  c. a natural body **h.** sign
     defense   **i.** symptom
  d. etiology   **j.** trauma
  e. genetic

B. Fill-In.

For each of the items in questions 11–15, mark which is a sign and which is a symptom.

11. _____ dry, flushed skin
12. _____ nausea
13. _____ dizziness
14. _____ rapid pulse
15. _____ elevated temperature

C. Matching.

Match the abnormality with its classification by matching Column I with Column II.

Column I   **Column II**

16. _____ abscessed tooth   **a.** ischemia
17. _____ adenosarcoma   **b.** congenital
18. _____ renal stones   **c.** infectious

19. _____ thrombosis   **d.** inflammation
20. _____ strep throat   **e.** metabolic imbalance
21. _____ frostbite   **f.** trauma
22. _____ osteoma   **g.** neoplasm
23. _____ rheumatoid arthritis **h.** obstruction
24. _____ spina bifida
25. _____ sickle cell anemia

D. True/False.

Mark the following true or false by circling T or F.

26. T F The medical diagnosis is made by the supervising nurse.
27. T F Nursing assistants may be assigned to collect certain specimens.
28. T F Protocols are drugs given in diagnostic testing.
29. T F Proper patient preparation contributes to the success of diagnostic testing.
30. T F Improper patient preparation may cause faulty results.
31. T F Ultrasound is used to give information about a growing fetus.
32. T F Thermography uses radio waves to test the electrical current of tissues.
33. T F An upper GI series is an X-ray of the gallbladder.
34. T F Nursing assistants may be asked to deliver specimens.
35. T F Nursing assistants may contribute to the diagnostic testing process by offering emotional support to the patient.

E. Completion.

Write out the early signs of possible malignancies.

36. C _____
37. A _____
38. U _____
39. T _____
40. I _____
41. O _____
42. N _____

F. Nursing Assistant Challenge.

Read each clinical situation and answer the questions.

43. Your patient is 82 years old, poorly nourished, and has a diagnosis of pneumonia.

   a. Name two factors that might predispose your patient to pneumonia. _____

   b. Will these factors make recovery more or less difficult? _____

   c. How would you classify the illness pneumonia? _____

44. Your patient is six years old and has a broken leg. He also has a condition that he inherited from his parents. This condition makes his bones brittle so they break more easily.

   a. What word would you use to describe his inherited condition? _____

   b. What term would you use to classify his inability to make strong bones? _____

   c. Do you think this kind of injury might occur often? _____

45. Your patient is 45 years old, 40 pounds overweight, and gets little exercise. Her diagnosis is high blood pressure. She is scheduled for an ECG.

   a. What factors might contribute to her diagnosis? _____

   b. For what conditions is she at risk? _____

   c. What information will the ECG provide? _____

Basic Human Needs and Communication

Communication Skills

OBJECTIVES

After completing this unit, you will be able to:

- Spell and define terms.
- Explain the types of verbal and nonverbal communication.
- Describe and demonstrate how to answer the telephone while on duty.

- Describe four tools of communication for staff members.
- Describe the guidelines for communicating with patients with impaired hearing, impaired vision, aphasia, and disorientation.
- State the guidelines for working with interpreters.

VOCABULARY

Learn the meaning and the correct spelling of the following words and phrases:

aphasia	disorientation	memo	sender
assignment	ethnic	message	shift report
body language	feedback	nonverbal communication	sign language
braille	hand-off communication	organizational chart	staff development
care plan	interpreter	paraphrasing	symbols
communication	medical chart	receiver	verbal communication

INTRODUCTION

Communication is a two-way process. It is the way in which information—whether facts or feelings—is shared. Information can be sent orally, in writing, and through body language. Nursing assistants communicate with their patients, with visitors, with their coworkers, and with their supervisors when they are working. As a nursing assistant, you will need to receive and send information about your:

- Observations and care of patients
- Interactions with patients and visitors
- Patients' feelings

This information is received and sent through the process of communication.

Elements of Communication

Understanding the elements of communication will help you communicate effectively. Each message has four parts (Figure 7-1):

- **sender**—the person who originates the communication
- **message**—the information the sender wants to communicate
- **receiver**—the person for whom the communication is intended

FIGURE 7-1 Nursing assistants communicate with patients in many different ways. However, all messages have a sender, message, and receiver. Feedback is a method of ensuring that the message was received as intended.

• **feedback**—confirmation that the message was received as intended

The *channel* is the medium through which the message is sent. Feedback may be verbal or nonverbal. An example of verbal feedback is saying something in response. An example of nonverbal feedback is a nod of the head indicating understanding.

COMMUNICATION IN HEALTH CARE

Communication between staff members must be effective if patients are to receive the safest and best care. Communication with patients and their visitors is also important. You and your patients must understand each other.

Verbal Communication

Verbal communication uses words. They may be spoken or written. Written communication also depends on the use of **symbols**. Traffic signs are an example of symbols. You will use words to explain to patients what you plan to do in carrying out a procedure and how they can help. Your nurse or team leader will use words to explain your assignment. You will use words to report your observations (Figure 7-2), as well as written communication in your charting. You will use words to answer visitors' questions. Choose words carefully so that your message is clear. Avoid using slang or words with more than one meaning. Avoid sound-alike words such as *haul* and *hall*. Use words that the receiver is likely to be familiar with. Speak slowly and clearly. Look at the receiver when speaking.

Paraphrasing. Paraphrasing is an effective method of showing that you understand what has been said. When using paraphrasing, restate your understanding of what was said. Listening to the message and paraphrasing provides feedback and shows that you are sincerely interested in the conversation. Tone of voice, choice of words, and hand movements give clues to the real meaning of the

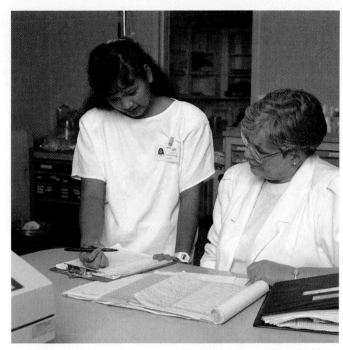

FIGURE 7–2 Verbal communication is the most common way of reporting observations to the nurse. In some cases, you may also provide written information, such as a piece of paper listing a patient's vital signs.

message. Listen carefully to the message and watch the sender's facial expressions and body language.

Nonverbal Communication

Nonverbal communication is a message that is sent through the use of one's body, rather than through speech or writing. This kind of communication, called **body language**, can tell you a great deal. Often nonverbal messages send even stronger signals than verbal messages.

When speaking with others, always remember the impact of nonverbal communication (Figure 7-3). Your words represent only 7% of your message. The remainder of the message is conveyed and interpreted through facial expressions, gestures, and overall body language. Your tone of voice represents 38% of the meaning. If the tone and pitch of your voice contradict the spoken words, the tone and pitch will overshadow the message. Be aware of the effect that the tone, pitch, and quality of your voice have on the way your message is interpreted. Gestures, facial expressions, and other body language represent 55% of your total communication.

Eye contact makes the biggest impression and will be remembered best (Figure 7-4). You create a positive atmosphere by looking at the other person. In North America, eye contact is very important to communication. This is not true in all cultures. Be sensitive to cultural differences of patients and coworkers. In North America, people who do not make eye contact may be considered dishonest or fearful. Making eye contact can

> Your message is:
>
> 7% words + 38% tone of voice
> + 55% body language
> _____
> = Total Communication

FIGURE 7-3 Make sure your body language and the tone, pitch, and quality of voice match the message you intend to send.

open communication channels and create a bond between two people. During conversation, eye contact communicates interest, concern, warmth, trust, feelings, and credibility. Eye contact can send many different messages.

A patient who is in pain may protect the affected area. Tears or an unwillingness to make eye contact with you may be a sign of depression. Some of the other ways your patients may "talk" to you through their body language include:

- Posture
- Hand and body movements
- Activity level
- Facial expressions
- Overall appearance
- Body position

COMMUNICATING WITH STAFF MEMBERS

In Unit 2 you learned that each health care facility has a line of authority and communication. The **organizational chart** is a guide for communication and spells out the line of authority. Each facility has an organizational chart that illustrates how a department relates to other departments. Some of the larger departments, such as nursing, have their own charts that indicate the line of authority within the department (Figure 7-5). As a nursing assistant, you will need to communicate with other staff members in nursing and other departments.

Oral Communications

Oral reports are used frequently to communicate information about patients. When you first come on duty, you will listen to the **shift report**. The nurse who worked the previous shift will report to oncoming staff. In some facilities, the shift report is tape-recorded. This report will include:

- Changes in patients' conditions
- Information about new patients
- Names of patients who were discharged or died
- Any incidents that occurred to patients
- New physicians' orders
- Special events for patients that will occur during your shift

Listen carefully to the report because it will help you plan your **assignment** (Figure 7-6). Your assignment tells you:

- Which patients you will care for during your shift
- The procedures you will need to do for these patients

Your supervising nurse will give you additional information about your assignment based on the shift report.

Messengers

They express anger; That is easily detected. They express hopelessness; When we feel dejected.

They express delight; When we achieve. They express sorrow; When we grieve.

They express victory; When we win. They express forgiveness; For an imagined sin.

They express confusion; When we don't perceive. They express appreciation; For what we receive.

They express happiness; For all we hold dear. They express fright; When we encounter a fear.

They express disappointment; When we lose. They express indecision; When we must choose.

They express patience; For a child. They express excitement; When our imagination runs wild.

They express love; It's perfectly clear. They speak a language; For all to hear.

In one fluid motion; As they part. The hands become Messengers of the heart.

To really know a person; If this is your goal. Look deep into their eyes; The Messengers of the soul.

An original poem by Marilyn Sossaman, LPN. Used with permission.

FIGURE 7-4 An original poem by Marilyn Sossaman, LPN. Used with permission.

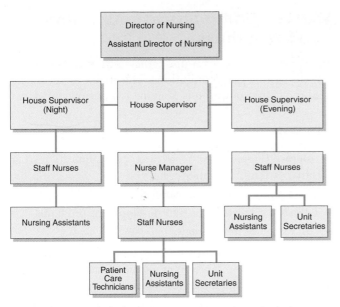

FIGURE 7-5 Nursing department organizational chart

This information may include orders to complete procedures for specific patients:

- Take temperature, pulse, respirations, and blood pressures on designated patients
- Obtain weights on designated patients
- Allow a patient to remain in bed because of a change in condition

- Make observations of a patient who has had a recent change in condition

During your shift, you will give oral reports to the nurse about procedures you have completed and observations you have made. At the end of the shift, you will summarize your assignment to the nurse so that the information can be included in the shift report to the employees coming on duty after you. When you leave the nursing unit for any reason during your shift, always report to the nurse before you go. Unit 8 gives additional information about oral reports.

Hand-Off Communication

Hand-off communication is essential communication that must occur when patient care is transferred from one worker or department to another worker or department. This is a very vulnerable time for the patient and is one of the most likely places for errors to occur. Information in the hand-off communication includes:

- The patient's situation and background
- Relevant observations and findings
- Recommendations for continuity of ongoing care

Hand-off communication must be accurate, clear, and complete. It should also include an opportunity to ask questions. As a nursing assistant, you will be on the giving and receiving end of hand-off information. Write down information about patients, if necessary, and refer to your

								ADL		
Rm.	Resident	Bath	Pos. Sched.	ROM	V.S.	WT.	B+B	Prog.	Transfer	Safety
101ᴬ	J. Damski	X	X	X			X	X	2+TB	X
101ᴮ	G. Jones		X	X	X	X			Mech Lift	
102ᴬ	C. Hernandez	X				X			Indep.	
102ᴮ	R. Lattini	X	X	X			X		2+TB	X
103	N. Goldberg	X			X	X	X		SBA	
104ᴬ	M. Welch		X	X					Mech Lift	
104ᴮ	L. Ordoni		X	X			X	X	1+TB	X
105	B. Brinzoski	X			X		X		Indep.	
106ᴬ	A. Feinstein	X				X		X	1+TB	
106ᴮ	D. Farmell		X	X	X		X	X	2+TB	
107	T. Green	X	X	X		X	X		2+TB	
108ᴬ	H. Johnson	X	X	X	X			X	2+TB	
108ᴮ	B. Miller		X	X		X			1+TB	X

CNA ASSIGNMENT SHEET **DATE** 4-18-XX

FIGURE 7-6 The assignment sheet provides an overview of patient needs and activities.

notes to make sure you all pass on the necessary information when providing hand-off communication.

Answering the Telephone

Many telephone calls come into a health care facility. Families call to inquire about the condition of a loved one. Physicians call to leave new medical orders. The laboratory may call to give test results. Remember that nursing assistants are not allowed to take physicians' orders, to take results of diagnostic tests, or to give information to families. You must call the nurse to do this. If you answer the telephone:

- Identify the nursing unit: "third floor, north," for example.
- Identify yourself and your position: "Mary Smith, nursing assistant."
- Ask the caller's name and ask the caller to wait while you locate the person called.
- If the person is unavailable, take a message (Figure 7-7) and write down the following information:
  - date and time of call
  - caller's name and telephone number
  - message left by caller
  - whether the person is to return the call or whether the caller will telephone again later
  - your signature

Some facilities have more complex telephone systems. You will be taught how to transfer calls or to voice-page. Most facilities do not allow employees to make or receive personal telephone calls while they are on duty, except in an emergency.

Written Communications Among Staff Members

In many situations, you and other staff members must rely on written communications. The ability to accurately read the communication is essential to your patient care.

Memos

A **memo** (Figure 7-8) is a brief communication that informs or reminds employees of:

- Changes in policies or procedures
- Upcoming meetings or staff development programs
- Admission of new patients
- Promotions of staff members

Be sure you know where memos are posted so that you will be aware of the facility activities.

Manuals

All facilities have several manuals that provide information about policies and procedures (Figure 7-9). These may include:

- Employee Personnel Handbook—Describes all personnel policies and benefits.
- Safety and Disaster Manual—Gives directions for actions to take in case of fire or other disasters.
- Procedure Manual—Gives directions on how all procedures should be performed for patients.
- Nursing Policy Manual—Describes rules and regulations pertaining to the care of patients.
- Material Safety Data Sheet (MSDS) Manual— Contains information on safe use and handling of substances used in the facility.

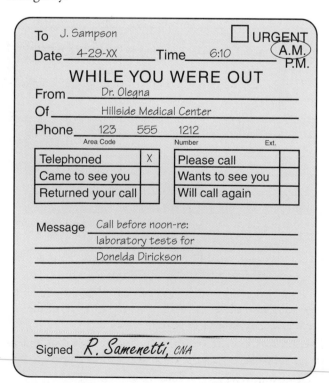

FIGURE 7-7 Telephone message

MEMO

Date: April 21, XXXX
From: Jane Sowalski, RN Director of Nursing
To: All nursing staff

Please note that the Nursing Procedure Manual has been updated and revised. The list of changes is attached. Please read the indicated procedures and sign the attached page.

Thank you.

FIGURE 7-8 Memos provide important information.

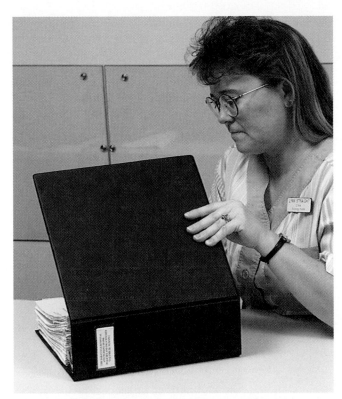

FIGURE 7-9 Manuals are an excellent source of information.

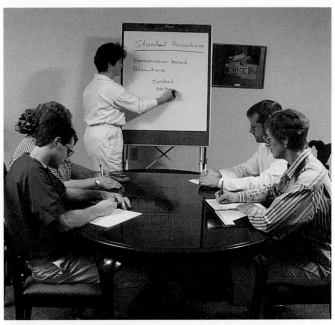

FIGURE 7-10 Attending regular staff development classes helps nursing assistants learn the most current information.

- Recent health findings from research
- How to use new equipment

The Patient Care Plan

The interdisciplinary health care team develops an individualized **care plan** for each patient. Unit 8 presents more information on the patient care plan.

The Patient's Medical Chart

Each patient has a **medical chart** or record. The medical chart contains:

- The physician's medical orders for that patient: medications, treatments, diagnostic tests
- The medical history of the patient: summary of all past illnesses and surgeries
- Results of physical examinations
- Results of all diagnostic tests: blood tests and X-rays
- Progress notes from the physician and from all disciplines involved in the patient's care: brief, periodic descriptions of the patient's condition and response to treatment
- Assessments from all disciplines: the assessment identifies the patient's problems
- Nursing notes: information that describes the patient's condition, nursing care that has been given, and the patient's response to the care

The information entered into the chart is called *documentation*. The chart is a legal document. It may be used to:

- Determine payments by insurance companies
- Determine settlement of lawsuits

Legal ALERT

Becoming familiar with the location and contents of facility policy and procedure manuals will help you do your job and practice within your scope of responsibility, in keeping with state and federal laws. You must perform procedures according to the guidelines in these manuals. They may be slightly different from those of other facilities. Following your facility policies and procedures will ensure that you give good patient care, and will reduce your risk of legal exposure. ■

There may be other manuals for infection control and quality assurance. You are not expected to memorize all the information in these manuals, but you should know where they are kept on the nursing unit and be able to look up information when you need to.

Staff Development

Staff development is a process used to educate staff from all departments in the facility (Figure 7-10). Classes may be given to inform staff of:

- New rules and regulations
- New procedures

Unit 8 gives instructions for documenting (making notations) on the patient's chart.

Other Methods of Communication

Modern technology has increased opportunities for communication. You will see computers at the nurses' station and throughout the building.

Most facilities will have at least one desktop computer in each department. In the nursing department, computers are used to document patient care, to maintain databases, to communicate with physicians' offices, and to maintain records of supplies and equipment. Some facilities have computers in every patient room. Nursing staff can then document appropriate information before they leave the bedside.

If you will be expected to use a computer and have had very little experience doing so, remember:

- Do not be intimidated by the computer. You have the ability to learn how to use one. You do not have to be a computer expert to use a computer.
- Learn from classes, from manuals, and from other users. Be creative and try to figure out some things on your own.
- Be patient, be determined, and do not panic. Do not be afraid to ask questions. You will not learn everything right away, but your confidence will grow quickly as you master new tasks.

You will be given special training if you will be expected to use a computer (Figure 7-11).

Fax machines are common in health care facilities (Figure 7-12). They are used to send and receive information from physicians and laboratories.

COMMUNICATING WITH PATIENTS

Your skill in communicating with patients will develop with experience. It is not always the words we choose that are important, but the way in which we say them. Tone of voice, facial expression, and even the way you touch a patient all communicate a sense of honest caring to the patient. Looking directly at patients as you speak and addressing them respectfully by name are also indications of caring.

Culture ALERT

Some cultures value periods of silence during talks. Allow adequate time. Learn to overcome your personal discomfort with periods of silence. ■

Listening actively is a special skill requiring more than just being physically present. When you listen actively, all your attention is focused on the speaker. You maintain eye contact and do not interrupt while the other person is speaking. You ask questions that encourage the speaker to

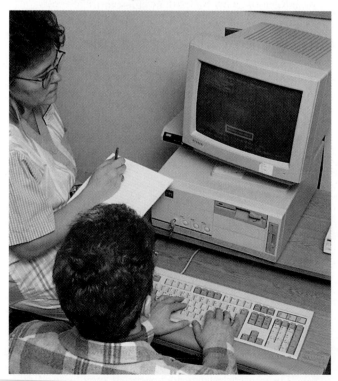

FIGURE 7-11 Most health care facilities depend on computers for data management, patient documentation, and communication.

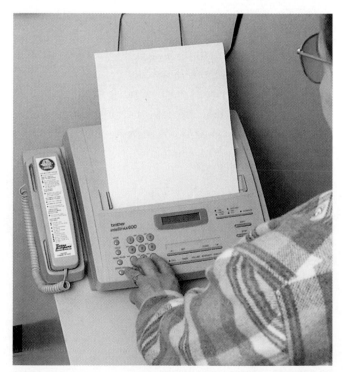

FIGURE 7-12 Fax machines are a convenient means of communication. Remember to protect patient privacy with fax transmissions.

continue and respond to specific questions that he or she asks. Follow these guidelines to communicate effectively with patients.

Communicating with Patients Who Have Special Needs

There are many reasons why communication with patients may be impaired. The patient may:

- Be hearing impaired
- Be vision impaired
- Have aphasia
- Be disoriented
- Be from a culture different from the nursing assistant's

These patients have special communication needs that should be addressed on the care plan. Always check the care plan before attempting to communicate with a patient who has special communication needs. Specific approaches may be established for all staff members to use with the patient. Lack of consistency in use of these approaches is confusing and frustrating to the patient.

Communication HIGHLIGHT

Remember that one of the most important and powerful messages you send to patients is that you care about them. You do this in many ways, including your demeanor when you enter the room, your body language, your tone of voice, and your touch. Verbal communication with some patients will be very limited. Use nonverbal communication to send the message that you care to all patients. ▪

Communicating with Patients Who Have Hearing Impairments

1. Get the patient's attention first.
   – Make sure the patient sees you.

GUIDELINES *for*
Communicating with Patients

- Be sure you have the patient's attention.
- Avoid chewing gum, eating, or covering your mouth with your hand when you speak.
- Use nonthreatening words and gestures.
- Speak clearly and courteously.
- Use a pleasant tone of voice.
- Use appropriate body language.
- Be alert to the patient's needs to communicate with you—allow time for the patient to talk and respond. Show interest and concern (Figure 7-13).
- Do not speak about the patient in front of the patient or other patients.
- Do not interrupt the patient.
- Reflect the patient's feelings and thoughts by rewording his or her statements into questions.
- Ask for clarification if you are unsure of what the patient is saying.
- Give the patient only factual information—not your personal feelings, opinions, or beliefs.
- Information concerning the patient's condition, medications, and treatments should be given by the physician or nurse.
- Do not argue with patients.

- Avoid using slang or cultural terms that are not familiar to the patient, and may be misinterpreted.
- Do not try to provide false reassurance, such as, "Everything will be all right." The patient will not trust you when she learns you were not sincere.
- Wait long enough for a reply. Patients who are elderly, hard of hearing, or under the effects of certain medications may take longer to process a message and respond.

FIGURE 7-13 Recognize the patient's need to communicate with you.

    – Touch the patient lightly to indicate that you wish to speak.

    – Recognize that individuals who are hard of hearing hear less well when they are tired or ill.

2. If the patient uses a hearing aid, be sure that the patient is wearing it and that the hearing aid is on.

3. If the patient has a "good" ear, stand or sit on that side.

4. Do not chew gum, eat, or cover your mouth while talking.

5. Keep the light behind the patient, so your face can be clearly seen (Figure 7-14).

6. Face the patient; many people with hearing impairments can read lips or interpret your facial expressions.

7. Reduce outside distractions. Speak in a quiet, calm manner.

8. Start conversations with a key word or phrase so the patient has some clues as to what you are saying (context).

9. Avoid abrupt changes of subject, because your hard-of-hearing listener depends heavily on context to understand what you are saying. Also, do not interrupt your conversation with "small talk."

10. Keep your voice pitch low.

11. Speak slowly, distinctly, and naturally.

12. Form words carefully, use familiar words, and keep sentences short.

13. Pronounce words clearly. If the patient who has a hearing impairment has difficulty with letters and numbers, say: "M as in Mary," "2 as in twins," "B as in boy." Say each number separately: "five six" instead of fifty-six. Remember that *m, n,* and *2, 3, 56, 66,* and *b, c, d, e, t,* and *v* are groups that sound alike.

14. Rephrase words as needed.

15. Avoid shouting, mouthing, or exaggerating words, or speaking very slowly. This only makes it harder for the patient to understand you.

16. Keep a notepad handy and write your words if the patient does not understand.

17. Use facial expressions, gestures, and body language to help express your meanings.

18. Some patients with hearing impairment use **sign language**.

    – Signing depends upon hand and finger movements and facial expressions.

    – This skill requires learning and practice (Figure 7-15).

    – There are different forms of sign language, just as there are different spoken languages.

    – There are some basic signs that may be helpful (Figure 7-16).

19. Patients who have been hearing impaired for several years may have speech that is difficult to understand.

20. Some hearing-impaired people are embarrassed to tell you when they do not understand you.

21. People who cannot hear may appear confused when they are not.

22. Never walk away leaving a patient who has a hearing impairment puzzling over what you said and thinking that you do not care. Avoid speaking from another room, when walking away, or with your back turned to the patient.

Information and guidelines on caring for patients who use hearing aids are found in Unit 43.

FIGURE 7-14 The light source should be behind the patient so that it lights your face. Make sure the light does not shine directly in the patient's face.

FIGURE 7-15 Learning sign language takes special education and practice with the signs.

| HURT, PAIN, ACHE, SORE | NO | HELLO, HI! | GOOD MORNING |

FIGURE 7-16 Basic signs

Communicating with Patients Who Have Visual Impairments

Patients who have visual impairments may have problems communicating because they are unable to see the sender or the sender's facial expressions and body language.

1. When approaching a person who is visually impaired, address the person by name and then touch lightly on the hand or arm to avoid startling.
2. After you speak to the patient, identify yourself and explain why you are there. "Hello, Mr. Smith. My name is Mary Jones and I would like to take your blood pressure."
3. Be specific when giving directions. "I am putting your call light on the right side of your bed."
4. When giving directions on how to find an area in the building, tell the patient how many doors he or she will pass and when to turn right or left.
5. When you leave the patient, make sure you announce your departure. "I am leaving your room now. Can I get you anything else?"
6. Offer to read mail to visually impaired patients.
7. If the patient has a telephone, make sure he or she can use it. The patient can count the numbers or buttons on the dial or number pad to make calls.
8. Tactfully inform a person who has visual impairment if clothing is soiled, mismatched, or in need of repair.
9. Encourage the patient to listen to the radio or television to keep up with news and current events.
10. Make sure the patient is aware of talking-book machines. Inform Social Services if the patient wishes to use one.
11. Describe the environment and objects around the patient so a frame of reference is established. This helps avoid disorientation related to vision impairment. Never change the location of items or furniture without discussing it with the patient.
12. Some patients may read **braille**, a system that uses a series of raised dots to represent letters and words (Figure 7-17). The patient reads the letters and words by moving his or her fingertips over them.

Communicating with Patients Who Have Aphasia

Patients who have had a stroke or brain damage due to an injury may have aphasia. **Aphasia** means that the patient cannot understand spoken or written language, or cannot express spoken or written language, or both. Trying to communicate with patients who have aphasia can be frustrating for both the patient and the caregiver.

1. Face the patient and make eye contact before speaking.
2. Say the patient's name and give a social greeting before asking questions or giving instructions.
3. Speak slowly and clearly. Use short, complete sentences.
4. Pause between sentences to allow the patient time to comprehend and interpret what you said.
5. Check the patient's comprehension before you proceed. Ask a question based on information you just gave the patient.

a 1	b 2	c 3	d 4	e 5	f 6	g 7
h 8	i 9	j 0	k	l	m	n
o	p	q	r	s	t	u
v	w	x	y	z	Capital sign	Numeral sign

FIGURE 7-17 Many persons with visual impairment use braille.

6. Use nonverbal cues to augment spoken communication. Use gestures, facial expressions, or pictures.

7. Ask questions that require only short responses or that can be answered nonverbally.

8. Repeat what the patient just said to help him keep focused on the conversation.

9. Find out if the speech therapist has devised methods of nonverbal communication, such as communication boards or picture books (Figure 7-18).

10. Do not avoid talking to a person with aphasia. Speak in a normal tone of voice. Do not shout to try to make her understand.

11. If you sense frustration, let the patient know that you are aware of the frustration. Suggest that you talk about something else for a while and then try again.

12. Accept responsibility for being unable to understand. The patient is doing his best. He is probably more frustrated than you are. Do not discourage or blame him for the breakdown in communication.

Communicating with Disoriented Patients

Some patients you care for may be disoriented. **Disorientation** means that the patient is confused about time, place (his physical location), or person (who he is). Dis-

orientation can be caused by Alzheimer's disease, stroke, or other disorders or injuries of the brain.

1. Begin conversation by identifying yourself and calling the patient by name. Do not ask the patient if she remembers you or if she knows who you are.

2. Talk to the patient at eye level and maintain eye contact.

3. Maintain a pleasant facial expression while you are talking and listening.

4. Place a hand on the patient's arm or hand, unless this causes agitation (Figure 7-19).

5. Make sure the patient can hear you. Avoid distractions of noise and activity.

6. Use a lower tone of voice.

7. Use short, common words and short, simple sentences.

8. Give the patient time to respond.

9. Ask only one simple question at a time. If you must repeat it, say it exactly the same.

10. Ask the patient to do only one task at a time.

11. Patients with dementia will eventually be unable to comprehend verbal communication.
    - Use pictures, and point, touch, or hand her things.
    - Demonstrate an action when you want her to complete a task.

12. The patient may use word substitutes. If these are consistent, find out what they mean. Use them yourself to see if the patient understands you better.

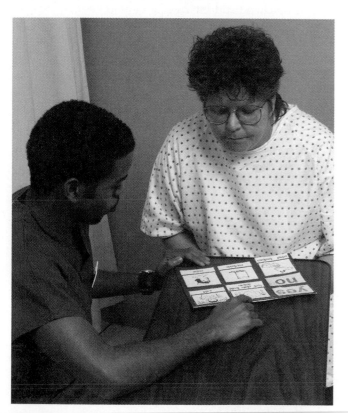

FIGURE 7-18 Patients with aphasia often use special communication boards and cards to make their needs known.

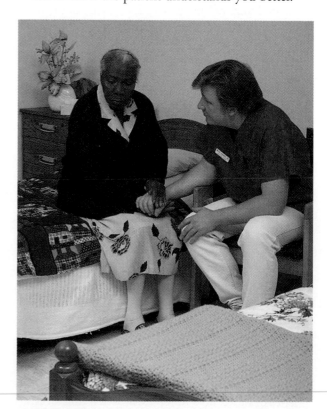

FIGURE 7-19 Gently touching a patient's hand or arm may be comforting.

13. Avoid abstract, common expressions. For example, "You can hop into bed now" means just that to the patient.

14. Repeat the patient's last words to help him stay on track during conversation.

15. Do not try to "make" the patient understand. Avoid lengthy explanations and excessive verbal communication. This tends to agitate most people with dementia.

16. Use nonverbal praise freely and always respect the patient's feelings.

Communicating with Patients from a Different Culture

The persons you care for may come from many different cultures or have different **ethnic** backgrounds. This means people who come from other countries and who have different customs, languages, and traditions. For example, in some countries it is considered a sign of disrespect to maintain eye contact when speaking with another person. If you are assigned to someone from a different ethnic background, you should be given specific communication guidelines.

Additional information about culturally competent care can be found in Unit 11.

Culture ALERT

Patients who are able to speak and read about their care in their native language usually feel more at ease and understand their care better. ■

WORKING WITH INTERPRETERS

Occasionally, you will care for a patient who does not speak your language, and communication may be limited. Gestures and body language can be helpful, but they are not universal. For example, in the United States, we shake the head up and down to mean yes. We move the head from side to side to signify no. In India, gestures are just the opposite. Moving the head from side to side means yes, and shaking it up and down means no. Because of differences in culture and language, there may be times when you need the assistance of a communication professional.

Suggestions for Working with Interpreters

An **interpreter** is a communication professional who mediates between speakers of different languages. Interpretation is an activity that consists of establishing, either simultaneously or consecutively, oral or gestural communications between two or more persons who do not speak the same language. Some interpreters speak. Others use sign language to establish communication between a hearing person and a nonhearing person.

Facilities will use medical interpreters when they are available in the community. Try to avoid using patients' minor children or grandchildren as interpreters. This may upset the child or family social order. The child's language skills and social experience may not be well developed in either language, causing inaccurate translation. Some medical subject matter may frighten children. Using a layperson as an interpreter may also cause problems. Persons who are unfamiliar with medical terms and procedures may not be able to interpret them correctly. A qualified interpreter is very familiar with the language, cultural values, beliefs, gestures, body language, and verbal and nonverbal expressions that are used in the languages he or she is interpreting. As you can see, this is a great responsibility. In health care, the terminology and technical information are complex. Health care interpreters receive special education to ensure that communication is accurate.

The facility is required to furnish interpreters in certain situations, according to federal law. Some facilities use a telephone service for interpreting, so communication is not face-to-face. This service fills an important need, because interpreters are "on call" personnel. The local interpreter may not be quickly available when services are needed.

REVIEW

A. Multiple Choice.

Select the one best answer for each of the following.

1. Successful communication is essential for
   a. body language to be meaningful.
   b. patients only.
   c. staff only.
   d. safe care.

2. Verbal communication includes
   a. talking and listening.
   b. facial expressions.
   c. reading reports.
   d. using a fax machine.

3. For successful communication to occur, all of the following elements must be present except
   a. receiver.
   b. hearing.
   c. feedback.
   d. sender.

4. Examples of nonverbal communication include
   a. reading and using the patient's care plan.
   b. answering the telephone.
   c. listening to the shift report.
   d. conversing with patients.

5. A nursing assistant may give or take which information over the telephone?
   a. report of a patient's condition
   b. physician's orders
   c. results of laboratory tests
   d. name of person leaving the message

6. The shift report is given by the
   a. administrator.
   b. physician.
   c. nurse who worked the previous shift.
   d. director of nursing.

7. The purpose of the shift report is to
   a. give information about all the patients on the nursing unit.
   b. discuss the social activities of the staff.
   c. tell the nursing assistants when they are scheduled for days off.
   d. rest before starting work.

8. You must report to the nurse when you
   a. prepare to take vital signs.
   b. complete each patient's care.
   c. begin your documentation.
   d. leave the unit for any reason.

9. One purpose of a memo is to inform staff of
   a. meetings or educational programs.
   b. patients' conditions.
   c. new physician's orders for specific patients.
   d. weather warnings.

10. Examples of manuals that are found on nursing units include
   a. computer manual, administrative policy manual, quality assurance manual.
   b. procedure manual, infection control manual, disaster manual.
   c. employee assistance program manual, personnel manual, benefits manual.
   d. isolation manual, X-ray manual, nuclear medicine manual.

11. The patient's care plan provides information for
   a. the nursing assistant assignments.
   b. employee benefits.
   c. the procedure for fire drills.
   d. licensed personnel only.

12. The patient's medical record or chart is
   a. used only by the physician.
   b. used by all members of the interdisciplinary health care team.
   c. a temporary record.
   d. a report of the nursing assistant's competencies.

13. The patient grimaces and holds his right arm close to his body when he moves. You suspect he may
   a. be right-handed.
   b. not want to get out of bed.
   c. be tired.
   d. be having pain.

14. If a patient is disoriented, it means that the patient is
   a. mentally ill.
   b. unaware of the environment and the time.
   c. unable to communicate with you.
   d. unable to hear.

15. Aphasia means that the patient
   a. has an infection of the respiratory tract.
   b. is hearing impaired.
   c. is disoriented.
   d. is unable to speak or to understand the spoken language of others.

16. When working with patients who have hearing impairments, you should
   a. get the patient's attention before speaking.
   b. talk louder.
   c. avoid speaking if possible.
   d. speak very slowly.

17. When working with patients who have aphasia, it is best to
   a. use only hand gestures to communicate.
   b. speak louder.
   c. avoid communication if at all possible.
   d. face the patient and make eye contact.

18. Persons with visual impairment should
   a. stay in their rooms to avoid getting lost in the facility.
   b. have identification on their clothing so everyone knows who they are.
   c. learn to use sign language.
   d. be given directions for locating various areas in the building.

19. When working with disoriented patients, you should
  a. ask the patient if she remembers you or knows who you are.
  b. try to make the patient understand you.
  c. avoid distractions of noise and activity when communicating with them.
  d. get as close as possible to the patient when talking or giving care.

20. Touching the patient can be a successful method of communication if you
  a. ask the family's permission.
  b. are not offended by touch.
  c. are gentle and caring.
  d. always grasp the patient firmly.

B. Completion.

Choose the correct word from the following list to complete each statement in questions 21–31.

aphasia	medical chart
body language	memo
braille	nonverbal communication
care plan	shift report
disorientation	verbal communication
interpreter	

21. Persons who cannot express themselves verbally or understand verbal communication have _____.

22. Loss of recognition of time, place, location, or person is called _____.

23. The exchange of information given by the nurse going off duty to those coming on duty is called the _____.

24. The _____ is a legal document.

25. A brief, written message that provides information is a _____.

26. _____ is an example of nonverbal communication.

27. The record that contains a description of the patient's problems, the goals for resolving the problems, and the approaches used is the _____.

28. Sign language is an example of _____.

29. Talking orally is _____.

30. _____ is used by persons with visual impairment.

31. An _____ is a professional who mediates between people who speak different languages.

C. Nursing Assistant Challenge.

Miss Johnson is one of your patients. She is visually impaired and in the hospital because she has a heart problem. Miss Johnson can feed herself and can give herself a bath, brush her teeth, and comb her own hair if she has adequate assistance. Think about suggestions presented in this unit for communicating with persons with visual impairment.

32. What can you do to set up meal trays so that Miss Johnson can feed herself?

33. How can you prepare bath items so that she can give herself her bath?

34. What can you do to enable her to comb her own hair and brush her teeth?

35. What other actions can you take to help this patient maintain as much independence as possible?

Observation, Reporting, and Documentation

OBJECTIVES

After completing this unit, you will be able to:
- Spell and define terms.
- List the components of the nursing process.
- Explain the responsibilities of the nursing assistant for each component of the nursing process.
- Describe two observations to make for each body system.
- Describe the purpose of the care plan.

- List three times when oral reports are given.
- Describe the information given when reporting.
- Describe the purpose of the patient's medical record.
- Explain the rules for documentation.
- State the purpose of the HIPAA laws.
- List at least 10 guidelines for computerized documentation.

VOCABULARY

Learn the meaning and the correct spelling of the following words and phrases:

approaches	evaluation	intervention	oral report
assessment	flow sheet	Kardex	personal digital assistant
care plan conference	goal	nurse's notes	(PDA)
charting	Health Insurance Porta-	nursing diagnosis	planning
critical (clinical) path-	bility and Account-	nursing process	subjective observation
ways	ability Act (HIPAA)	objective observation	tablet PC (TPC)
document	implementation	observation	

INTRODUCTION

One of the responsibilities of the nursing assistant is to collect and communicate information about patients. Information is collected by making observations of the patient. Information is communicated to other team members by reporting and documenting. The mechanism used to carry out these actions is called the **nursing process**.

NURSING PROCESS

An understanding of the basic difference between nursing care and medical care is necessary to understand the focus of this chapter. Both medicine and nursing are necessary for positive patient outcomes (Figure 8-1). The physician collects information to diagnose and treat human illnesses. Nurses collect information, then use it to diagnose and treat the *human response to illness*.

The registered nurse is responsible for achieving patient-focused care by using the nursing process. The nurse coordinates care and delegates responsibilities to other caregivers in an effort to achieve this goal. The nursing process consists of five steps:

- Assessment
- Problem identification
- Planning

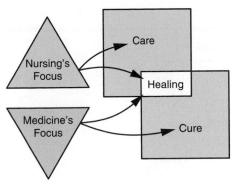

FIGURE 8-1 Medicine and nursing each have a separate focus, but both are essential for patients' well-being if positive outcomes are to be achieved.

- Implementation
- Evaluation

Assessment involves the collection of data (information) about the patient. The nurse coordinates assessment with other members of the interdisciplinary team. The data are entered on a special form contained in the patient's medical record. Information is obtained from:

- Interviewing the patient
- The medical record
- The patient's family if the patient is unable to communicate
- Physical examination (Figure 8-2)
- collection of measurable data and information such as weight and vital signs
- observations made by members of the nursing team

Proper use of the nursing process is a key element in the delivery of effective health care. Nursing units run more efficiently and effectively if all staff understand and adhere to this model of care. If there is a breakdown of the nursing process, patients are at high risk of negative outcomes and the facility and its personnel are at high risk of legal exposure. Understanding and fulfilling your role in the nursing process is an important responsibility.

The nursing assistant is responsible for collection of data by making and reporting observations. This is explained later in the unit. After the assessment is finished, the nurse analyzes the data, identifies the patient's problems, and formulates nursing diagnoses. A **nursing diagnosis** is the statement of a patient problem and the cause of the problem. For example, the nursing diagnosis may be impaired physical mobility (the problem) related to hemiplegia due to stroke (the cause of the problem). Nursing diagnoses may reflect actual clinical problems, the risk that certain problems will develop, or wellness objectives. The nursing diagnoses provide the foundation for nursing care to achieve outcomes for which nurses are accountable. Table 8-1 gives a few examples of nursing diagnoses and what they mean.

Planning the care of the patient (developing a care plan) is done after the nursing diagnoses are made. The purpose of planning is to:

- Identify possible solutions to the problems (nursing diagnoses).
- Develop **approaches** (what team members are going to do) that will help the patient solve the problems. Approaches may also be called **interventions**.
- Establish measurable **goals** for the patient (a goal is an outcome) so that caregivers will know whether the approaches are successful and whether the problems are being resolved.

Planning may be done at a **care plan conference** (Figure 8-3). This is a meeting of the members of the interdisciplinary team who are directly involved in the care of the patient. The patient and/or the family (if the patient consents) should be invited to attend the conference. The care plan developed at the conference contains a list of the nursing diagnoses, the approaches, and the patient's goals (Figures 8-4A and 8-4B). The care plan may be kept in the patient's medical record or in a file called a **Kardex**

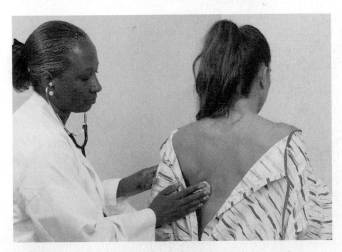

FIGURE 8-2 Part of the nursing assessment involves physical examination. The nurse is auscultating (listening to) the patient's lungs. The admission data are used as a basis for comparison of different assessments.

FIGURE 8-3 The care plan is developed during a care conference involving the patient and family member (if desired), and members of the interdisciplinary team.

TABLE 8-1 EXAMPLES OF NURSING DIAGNOSES AND OBSERVATIONS TO MAKE

Nursing Diagnosis	Observations to Make
Altered nutrition; less than body requirements	• Food/fluid intake • Weight loss • Inability to eat, dislike or refusal of food or fluids • Pain in abdomen or mouth • Sores in mouth
Constipation	• Lack of bowel movement or hard, dry stools • Complaints of feeling full • Abdomen distended and firm • Passing flatus (gas)
Impaired Urinary Elimination	• Involuntary loss of urine associated with a strong sense of urinary urgency • Abrupt and strong desire to void • When the urge to void occurs, patient must go immediately and cannot suppress the urine • Once the bladder begins to empty, patient is unable to stop or control the urine flow • Signs or symptoms of urinary infection, including incontinence, frequency, foul odor, pain, burning • Mucus, sediment, or blood in the urine • Voiding frequently in small amounts • Urine leakage after patient drinks small amounts of liquid or hears water running • Patient uses the bathroom many times each day; may get up at night to urinate
Decreased cardiac output	• Changes in B/P, irregular pulse, fatigue, difficulty breathing
Risk for aspiration	• Difficulty in swallowing, depressed cough and gag reflex, reduced level of consciousness
Impaired skin integrity	• Redness or destruction of skin
Impaired verbal communication	• Inability or difficulty with speaking, difficulty breathing, disorientation
Ineffective coping	• Change in usual communication patterns • Inability to cope or meet basic needs • Change in behavior
Impaired adjustment	• Disbelief, anger, inability to solve problems
Impaired physical mobility	• Ability to move in bed, range of motion, balance, coordination, endurance
Activity intolerance	• Fatigue, weakness, shortness of breath • Irregular pulse
Disturbed sleep pattern	• Inability to sleep at night, or wakes frequently • Abnormal daytime sleepiness as a result of not sleeping at night • Changes in behavior or speech
Anxiety	• Shakiness, quivering voice, increased movements • Poor eye contact, helplessness

NURSING DIAGNOSIS	NURSING INTERVENTIONS	EVALUATION
Ineffective breathing pattern R/T operative site/incisional pain.	1. Auscultate breath sounds q̄ 4h. & PRN. 2. Assist pt. to turn, cough, and deep breathe q̄ 2h while awake.	1. Lungs clear on auscultation. 2. "It doesn't hurt as much to cough today."
Risk for infection R/T surgical incision & indwelling catheter.	Assess for s/s of infection q̄ 4h	T 100.2°, incision site warm & pink, non-edematous. "It really hurts under the bandage."
Risk for constipation R/T abdominal surgery.	1. Restart oral fluids gradually. Offer clear liquids frequently. 2. Observe for abd. distension & evaluate tolerance when pt. begins taking fluid/foods.	Unable to tolerate oral fluids — vomited p̄ taking ice chips.

FIGURE 8-4A A handwritten care plan, such as the kind used on the Kardex

PLAN OF CARE

PC: ABDOMINAL SURGERY

PB: TD:____/____Ineffective breathing pattern r/t: op site/incision pain.

EO: Respiratory rate & effort WNL with good chest expansion.

  1: Auscultate breath sounds Q4H & PRN. Note diminished/absent sounds, rales, wheezing, crackles, rhonchi. DOCUMENT IN NURSE'S NOTES.

  2: Assist pt to turn, cough, and deep breathe Q2H while awake. Support incision. DOCUMENT RESPONSE & EFFORT.

PB: TD:____/____Risk for infection r/t surgical incision/indwelling cath.

EO: Surgical incision healing w/out s/s of infection.

  1: Assess for s/s of infection Q4H: (fever, chills, swelling, redness, pain, drainage, increased WBC, etc) DOCUMENT IN NURSE'S NOTES.

PB: TD:____/____Acute pain r/t_____ surgical incision/operative site.

EO: Pt reports pain relieved/ controlled.

  1: Implement Patient Controlled Analgesia (PCA) Protocol and PCA Teaching Protocol.

PB: TD:____/____Risk for constipation r/t_____surgery.

EO: Pt's bowel elimination is normal within limits of surgical procedure.

  1: Restart oral fluids gradually. Offer clear liquids frequently.

  2: Observe for abdominal distention & evaluate tolerance when pt begins taking fluid/foods post-op. DOCUMENT IN NURSE'S NOTES.

INT   SIGNATURE

FIGURE 8-4B A computer-generated care plan. Some programs list approaches based on the nursing diagnoses, but the nurse entering the data can reject them or modify them if they are not appropriate. The nurse can also add any relevant personal data to the plan. (Courtesy of St. Tammany Parish Hospital, Covington, LA)

(Figures 8-5A and 8-5B) at the nurses' station. The nursing assistant is responsible for contributing information (observations) that will help the team develop a workable care plan. Some facilities invite nursing assistants to attend the care plan conference.

Implementation is the activation of the care plan. It means carrying out the approaches listed on the care plan in an effort to resolve the problems (nursing diagnoses) and to help the patient reach the goals (Figure 8-6). The approach states:

- Who is to carry out the approach
- When the approach is carried out
- How the approach is carried out

See Figure 8-4 for examples of approaches. The nursing assistant is responsible for knowing when and how the approach is to be carried out and for implementing the approach correctly.

Evaluation is the final step of the nursing process, but it is an ongoing procedure. The evaluation determines:

- Whether the patient is reaching the goals on the care plan
- Why the goals are not being reached, if the patient is not successful in meeting the goals
- What should be done to assist the patient to reach the goals
- When goals are reached, whether they should be extended; for example if the patient reaches the goal of walking 200 feet, it may be increased to 250 feet

The nursing assistant is responsible for reporting to the nurse when the:

- Approach cannot be carried out for any reason
- Patient is having problems with the approach
- Patient has met a goal

Critical (Clinical) Pathways

The DRG method of payment has affected many health care practices and shortened hospital stays. Many hospitals

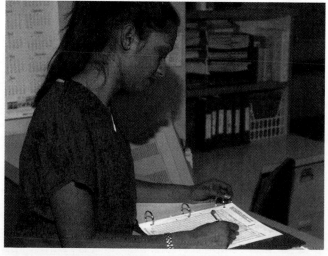

FIGURE 8-5A Care plans are often kept in the Kardex at the nurses' station.

Case Presentation

Mrs. White is admitted with medical diagnoses of hyperglycemia, ketoacidosis, and a history of diabetes mellitus (DM), all diagnostic indicators of diabetic ketoacidosis (DKA). Mrs. White is having labored breathing, vomiting, and weakness. Mr. White states that his wife takes insulin for her diabetes, she doesn't follow her diet, and she has been complaining of thirst and frequent urination. On examination, the patient complains of weakness and abdominal pain, and she has an acetone breath.

White, Mary   F 56
MR#: 000135039   ACCT#: 9710144268
Dr: J. Smith   2/W 402–XX
DX: Diabetic Ketoacidosis (DKA)   DATE: 12/14/XX

SUMMARY: 12/14   0701 to 1501

CILIENT INFORMATION

10/14	ADVANCE DIRECTIVES: No. Advance directive does not exist
10/14	ORGAN DONOR: Unknown
10/14	ADMIT DX: Diabetic Ketoacidosis (DKA)
10/14	ALLERGIES: None Known
10/14	ISOLATION: Not at this time

MISC. CLIENT DATA

10/14   History of Diabetes Mellitus (DM): Insulin-Dependent Diabetic

MEDICAL DIAGNOSES

10/14   PROBLEM # 1: Hyperglyccmia
10/14   PROBLEM # 2: Ketoacidosis
10/14   PROBLEM # 3: Hyperventilation
10/14   PROBLEM # 4: Hypovolemia, Hypernatremia
10/14   PROBLEM # 5: Hypotension
10/14   PROBLEM # 6: Hypokalemia

NURSING DIAGNOSES

10/14   PROBLEM 1: Deficient fluid volume r/t osmotic diuresis associated
          with hyperglycemia
10/14   PROBLEM 2: Ineffective breathing pattern: Kussmaul respirations/air
          hunger r/t metabolic acidosis associated with DKA
10/14   PROBLEM 3: Decreased cardiac output r/t hypokalemia associated
          with metabolic acidosis
10/14   PROBLEM 4: Risk for injury: circulatory collapse, renal shutdown,
          and coma r/t persistent, untreated hyperglycemia
10/14   PROBLEM 5: Risk for injury: seizure susceptibility if hyperglycemia
          is corrected too abruptly
10/14   PROBLEM 6: Ineffective airway clearance: aspiration r/t presence of
          vomiting and altered level of conciousness
10/14   PROBLEM 7: Risk for infection r/t invasive procedures
10/14   PROBLEM 8: Altered nutrition: less than body requirements r/t anorexia,
          nausea, or vomiting associated with ketoacidosis and hypokalemia
10/14   PROBLEM 9: Deficient knowledge: prevention of DKA r/t proper
          management of DM
10/14   PROBLEM 10: Ineffective therapeutic regimen management r/t
          inadequate motivation for incorporating strategies for prevention of
          DKA into daily living

FIGURE 8-5B Sample computerized care plan, based in part on information from the case presentation. (From Springhouse. (2001). *Mastering documentation*. Springhouse, PA: Springhouse; Reiner, A. (Ed.). (2001). *Manual of patient care standards*. Gaithersburg, MD: Aspen; Williams, S. M. (2001). *Decision making in critical care nursing*. Philadelphia, PA: Decker).

ALL CURRENT MEDICAL ORDERS

NURSING ORDERS:

10/14   Activity: Bedrest
         VS: Q15" first 2 Hours, then Q30" until within normal limits, then Q1H
10/14   Telemetry
10/14   Daily Weight: 0600
10/14   Intake & Output: Q 15 min. first 2 hours, then Q 30 min. until output stable at
         30 mL/H, then Q1H
10/14   Urine: Specific Gravity Q1H
10/14   Measure blood glucose levels: Q1H, notify physician when serum
         glucose is less than 300 mg percent
10/14   Oral Hygiene: Q1H
10/14   Monitor for s/s of infection: IV site, triple-lumen, central
         line, right subclavian and indwelling Foley catheter
10/14   Institute fall precautions

SUMMARY: 10/14   0701 to 1501

DIET:

10/14   NPO; Diabetic: 1600 cal., start with breakfast tomorrow

IVS:

10/14   Central line #1...0.9 percent normal saline, 1000 mL @ rate of 1 L/H
         for first 2 H, infusion pump; then decrease infusion of 0.9 percent
         normal saline, 500 mL @ rate of 500 mL/H for the next 2 H; then
         decrease infusion of 0.9 percent normal saline, 250 mL @ rate of 250 mL/H
10/14   Central line #2...50 U of regular insulin to 500 mL normal saline to produce
         a concentration of 0.1 U/mL, infuse @ 7 U/kg per hour, infusion pump
10/14   Administer KCL IV: If serum K^+ is <3.5 give 40 mEq/H; 3.5–5.5 give
         20 mEq/H; >5.5 give no K^+

SCHEDULED MEDICATIONS:

10/14   None

STAT/NOW MEDICATIONS:

10/14   IV bolus of regular insulin of 0.2 U/kg

PRN MEDICATIONS:

10/14   None

LABORATORY:

10/14   Stat Chem Profile 23
         Blood Glucose Q1H
         Stat Arterial Blood Gases
         Urinalysis Now

ANCILLARY:

10/14   Stat EKG
10/14   FSBS PRN s/s hypo/hyperglycemia

Last Page

FIGURE 8-6 Nursing assistants are responsible for implementing many of the care plan approaches.

are using **critical (clinical) pathways** to direct care. The pathways are written documents that detail the expected course of treatment and expected outcomes for a DRG. New goals are set each day during the patient's stay. The pathway lists nursing actions to help the patient achieve the goal. The nursing assistant is responsible for many of these interventions. Review the Kardex containing the patient's care plan or critical pathway at the beginning of each shift to help plan your day.

MAKING OBSERVATIONS

An **observation** is information that is obtained by using one's senses: seeing, hearing, smelling, or feeling. This information can help the care team determine:

- A change in the patient's physical condition. *Example:* a patient with diabetes may be having an insulin reaction.
- A new condition that is developing. *Example:* a pressure ulcer may be noted.
- A change in the patient's mental condition. *Example:* a patient who has shown no signs of disorientation is now wandering about, saying he does not know where he is.
- A change in the patient's emotional condition. *Example:* a patient is crying and says she "does not want to continue living."

- The effectiveness of a medication or treatment. *Example:* a patient may be taking an antibiotic for a urinary tract infection. If the signs and symptoms of the infection are not going away, then the medication may not be effective and the physician will need to change the order.

There are two types of observations: subjective and objective. An **objective observation** is one that is factual or measurable in some way. For example, blood in the urine is factual. Blood pressure, temperature, pulse, and respirations are measurable. A **subjective observation** is a statement or complaint made by the patient. For example, "I have a headache," or "I feel sick to my stomach" are subjective observations.

You make observations by using your senses.

- Your *eyes* to *see* observations:
  - blood in the urine
  - bruises or breaks in the skin (Figure 8-7)
  - the patient crying
  - a change in the way the patient walks
- Your *ears* to *hear* observations:
  - wheezing when the patient breathes
  - pulse or blood pressure with a stethoscope
  - comments from the patient, such as "I am very tired today"
- Your *nose* to *smell* observations:
  - body odor
  - discharge from a wound or body cavity
  - stool or urine when the patient is incontinent
- Your *hands and fingers* to *feel* observations:
  - a lump under the patient's skin (Figure 8-8)
  - radial pulse
  - warmth or coolness of the patient's skin

FIGURE 8-7 The nursing assistant observes the skin for bruised, red, or open areas while giving a backrub.

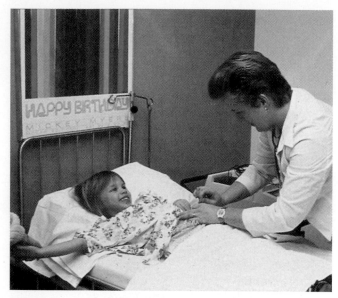

FIGURE 8-8 Lumps under the skin may be felt using the sense of touch. Abnormalities are often identified during routine care. (Photo courtesy of Henrietta Egleston Hospital for Children, Atlanta, GA. Photograph by Ginger Lovering)

Remember that observations must be:
- Accurate and timely
- Reported to the nurse in a timely manner
- Documented in the patient's record, either by you or the nurse

Making Initial Observations

To make accurate observations, you must first know what is expected or normal for an individual. For this reason, baseline information is collected when the patient is admitted to the facility. If you help admit a patient, make observations while you are completing your assignment. It is especially important to note any possible signs of injury or skin breakdown. Think of the body systems as described in the following list. This information will give you a basis for making future comparisons. For example, one patient may have a blood pressure of 110/68 on admission. If you take the patient's blood pressure later and it is 140/88, you should report this to the nurse, because this is not the usual blood pressure for this person. Try to establish a routine way of making observations. Keep in mind the age and known illnesses of the patients. It may be helpful to think of each body system and note the following:
- Integumentary system (skin, nails)
  - Color: flushed, pale, jaundiced (yellow color), or cyanotic (bluish, ashen, gray color); nails pale, pink, or cyanotic
  - Temperature: warm, hot, cool
  - Moisture: dry, moist, perspiring
  - Abnormalities: rashes, bruises, scars, pressure ulcers, areas of redness

- Musculoskeletal system (muscles, bones, joints)
  - Posture: stooped, curled up in bed, straight
  - Mobility: ability to move in bed, to get out of bed, to stand, to walk, and to maintain balance
  - Range of motion: ability to move all joints (Figure 8-9)
- Circulatory system (heart, blood vessels, blood)
  - Pulse: strength, regularity, rate
  - Skin: (see integumentary system)
  - Nails: (see integumentary system)
  - Blood pressure
- Respiratory system (nose, throat, trachea, bronchi, lungs)
  - Respirations (breathing): rate, regularity, depth, difficulty in breathing, shortness of breath upon exertion or while still, wheezing or crackling heard
  - Cough: frequency; dry, loose, productive. Color and consistency of sputum (if any)
- Nervous system (brain, spinal cord, nerves)
  - Mental status: orientation to time, place, person. Ability to make verbal or nonverbal responses
  - Coordination: tremors, reaction time
- Senses (eyes, ears, nose, sense of touch)
  - Eyes: reddened, drainage, pupils equal in size
  - Ears: drainage
  - Nose: drainage, bleeding
  - Sense of touch: ability to feel pressure and pain

FIGURE 8-9 Report to the nurse if there is a change in the patient's ability to move the joints.

- Urinary system (kidneys, ureters, bladder, urethra)
  - Urination: frequency, amount, color, clarity, odor, presence of blood or sediment (Figure 8-10); ability to hold urine, incontinence
  - Pain on urination (dysuria)
- Digestive system (mouth, teeth, throat, esophagus, stomach, large and small intestines, gallbladder, liver, pancreas)
  - Full or partial dentures
  - Dental caries (cavities)
  - Appetite: amount of fluids and food consumed (Figure 8-11), tolerance to foods, belching or burping
  - Eating: difficulty chewing or swallowing
  - Nausea and/or vomiting
  - Bowel elimination: frequency, amount, consistency, color of stools; diarrhea, constipation, incontinence, flatus; difficulty in passing stool
- Endocrine system (glands)
  - Signs and symptoms of diabetes (hypoglycemia, hyperglycemia)
- Reproductive system (male and female internal and external sex organs)

  Female

  Breasts: condition of nipples, presence of lumps, discolorations
  - Menstrual periods: frequency, amount, and character of bleeding; cramping
  - Vaginal drainage: amount, odor, and character

  Male
  - Testes: lumps
  - Penis: amount and character of drainage

In addition to the body systems observations, you also need to note facts related to pain, behavior, and function.

- Pain: location, type of pain (sharp, dull, aching), constant or intermittent or related to specific activities, time pain started
- Behavior: actions, conduct
- Function: ability to move about and complete tasks such as bathing

When reporting behavior, avoid using "labels" based on your judgment of the patient. Report only what you see and hear.

FIGURE 8-11 Monitor and record the amount of food and fluid consumed.

You may make additional observations related to the patient's medical diagnoses. For example, if a patient has a kidney condition, you would look for edema (swelling) of the face, hands, and ankles (Figure 8-12). You would also

FIGURE 8-12 Patients with heart, circulatory, or kidney problems may develop edema of the lower extremities. (The patient's shoes have been removed so the edema could be pictured. Never get a patient up in a chair without proper foot covering.)

FIGURE 8-10 Check the urine before discarding it. If you observe abnormalities, save it for the nurse to view.

monitor the person's fluid intake and output. You will learn more about observations related to medical diagnoses as you study these conditions.

In some situations, you may be expected to report "normal" observations. This information tells the nurse and physician whether the patient's condition is improving.

For example, if a patient has had a respiratory tract infection and the signs and symptoms have diminished, it is important to report "no coughing or respiratory distress is noted." Abnormal observations that should be reported to the nurse are listed in Table 8-2.

TABLE 8-2 OBSERVATION AND REPORTING GUIDELINES

General signs and symptoms of illness that should be reported to the nurse

Chest pain	Nausea or vomiting	Lethargy
Shortness of breath	Diarrhea	Unusual drainage from a wound or body cavity
Difficulty breathing	Cough	Changes in vital signs
Weakness or dizziness	Cyanosis or change in color	Profuse sweating
Headache	Change in mental status	
Pain	Excessive thirst	

System or Problem	Observation to Report	System or Problem	Observation to Report
Signs/symptoms of infection	Elevated temperature Sweating Chills Skin hot or cold to touch Skin flushed, red, gray, or blue Inflammation of skin as evidenced by redness, edema, heat, or pain Drainage from wounds or body cavities Any unusual body discharge, such as mucus or pus	Cardiovascular system, *continued*	Chest pain that radiates to neck, jaw, or arm Shortness of breath Headache, dizziness, weakness, vomiting Cold, blue, or gray appearance Cold, blue, painful feet or hands Shortness of breath, dyspnea, or abnormal respirations Feeling faint or lightheaded
Evidence of pain	Chest pain Pain that radiates Pain upon movement Pain during urination Pain when having a bowel movement (Pain is not normal; all complaints of pain should be reported to the nurse)	Respiratory system	Respiratory rate below 12 or above 20 Irregular respirations Noisy, labored respirations Dyspnea Shortness of breath Gasping for breath Wheezing Coughing Retractions Blue color of lips, nail beds, or mucous membranes
Cardiovascular system	Abnormal pulse below 60 or above 100 Blood pressure below 100/60 or above 140/90 Unable to palpate pulse or hear blood pressure Chest pain	Integumentary system	Rash Redness in the skin that does not go away within 30 minutes after pressure is relieved New, abnormally dark areas in patients with dark skin

continues

TABLE 8-2 *CONTINUED*

System or Problem	Observation to Report	System or Problem	Observation to Report
Integumentary system, *continued*	Pressure ulcers, blisters Irritation Bruises Skin discoloration Swelling Lumps Abnormal sweating Excessive heat or coolness to touch Open areas/skin breakdown Drainage Foul odor Complaints such as numbness, burning, tingling, only itching Signs of infection Unusual skin color, such as blue or gray color of the skin, lips, nail beds, roof of mouth, or mucous membranes Abrasions, skin tears, lacerations Skin growths Poor skin turgor/tenting of skin Sunken, dark appearance around eyes	Genitourinary system	Urinary output too low Oral intake too low Fluid intake and output not reasonably balanced Abnormal appearance of urine: dark, concentrated, red, cloudy Unusual material in urine: blood, pus, particles, mucus Complaints of difficulty urinating Complaints of pain, burning, urgency, frequency, pain in lower back Urinating frequently in small amounts Sudden-onset incontinence Edema, signs of fluid retention Sudden weight loss or gain Respiratory distress Change in mental status
Gastrointestinal system	Sores or ulcers inside the mouth Difficulty chewing or swallowing food Unusual or abnormal appearance of bowel movement Blood, mucus, or other unusual substances in stool Unusual color of bowel movement Hard stool, difficulty passing stool Complaints of pain, constipation, diarrhea, bleeding Frequent belching Changes in appetite Excessive thirst Fruity smell to breath Complaints of indigestion or excessive gas Nausea, vomiting Choking Abdominal pain Abdominal distention Coffee-ground appearance of emesis or stool	Nervous system	Change in level of consciousness, orientation, awareness, or alertness Feeling faint or light-headed Increasing mental confusion Progressive lethargy Loss of sensation Numbness, tingling Change in pupil size; unequal pupils Abnormal or involuntary motor function Loss of ability to move a body part Loss or lack of coordination
		Musculoskeletal system	Pain Obvious deformity Edema Immobility Inability to move arms and legs Inability to move one or more joints Limited/abnormal range of motion Jerking or shaky movements Weakness Sensory changes Changes in ability to sit, stand, move, or walk Pain upon movement

continues

TABLE 8-2 *CONTINUED*

System or Problem	Observation to Report	System or Problem	Observation to Report
Mental status	Change in level of consciousness, awareness, or alertness Changes in mood or behavior Change in ability to express self or communicate Mental confusion Excessive drowsiness	Mental status, *continued*	Sleepiness for no apparent reason Sudden onset of mental confusion Threats of harm to self or others

PAIN

It is important that you be very factual in reporting observations of pain and behavior. Never try to judge whether a patient really has pain or how severe the pain is. Some individuals are very expressive about pain and others are very stoical (they try not to show their discomfort). A person's culture may also affect his or her response to pain. Never compare patients. One person may seem to have more pain than another person with the same diagnosis. It is not appropriate to think that they should both respond in the same way.

Pain is never normal. Always report patient complaints of pain to the nurse. Determining whether pediatric or cognitively impaired patients are in pain may be difficult because they may be unable to describe the nature of the problem. Pain is discussed in greater detail in Unit 10.

REPORTING

Giving an **oral report** is one method used to relay information from one person to another. The nursing assistant may participate in oral reports several times on a shift. Oral reports are given by the:

- Nurse going off duty to the staff coming on duty (Figure 8-13) (in some facilities the nurse may give a report only to the charge nurse of the oncoming shift)—this is called a shift report. Some facilities leave a taped report for the next shift.
- Nursing assistant to the nurse when leaving the nursing unit for any reason (such as lunch break).
- Nursing assistant to the nurse at the end of the shift.
- Nursing assistant to the nurse if any unusual or new observations are made.

Be specific when you report your observations. If you are relaying a subjective observation (something the patient has told you), repeat it exactly the way the patient told it to you. Here are some examples:

- Mr. Jones in 249 says it hurts every time he urinates.
- Mrs. Goldberg was wandering around in the hall and said she did not know where she was.

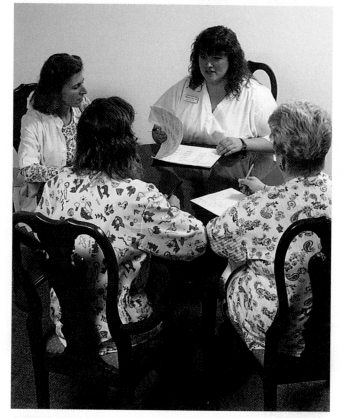

FIGURE 8-13 Report is given to the oncoming shift by the nurse who worked the previous shift.

To report objective observations, state your measurement or fact:

- Mrs. Dominick's blood pressure is 142/86.
- Mr. Hernandez ate 50% of his meal at lunch time.

When you report off duty at the end of your shift, report to the nurse:

- The condition of each of the patients you were assigned to
- The care you gave each patient
- Observations you made while giving care

Communication HIGHLIGHT

You will learn when to report your observations about patients as you gain experience. In general, high-priority items for reporting include abnormal vital signs, chest pain, difficulty breathing, change in color, change in mental status, bleeding, and pain. If you are in doubt about the urgency of reporting to the nurse, report your observation immediately. If the patient's condition changes after you have reported your observations, inform the nurse again. ■

DOCUMENTATION

In some facilities you may be expected to record your observations on the patient's medical record (chart) (Figure 8-14). The medical record is a **document**. A document is a legal record. The process of recording the patient's care, response to treatment, and progress in the patient's chart is called **charting** or *documentation*. Nursing assistants may document on **flow sheets** (Figure 8-15) in the chart or on the **nurse's notes** (Figure 8-16) (sometimes called nurse's progress notes). The charting must:

- Address the problems listed in the patient's care plan or critical pathway.
- Describe the approaches (interventions) listed in the care plan or critical pathway and note whether the interventions are effective.
- Indicate the progress the patient is making toward meeting the goals on the care plan or critical pathway.

Charting Guidelines

A patient's medical record (chart) is a legal document and may be used in court as evidence. It is important that everything be correct and legible. All charting and records must be in clear, simple, and accurate language. Entries must be printed or written carefully so that there can be no misunderstanding of the meaning. If you follow the established rules of charting, there will be no problem.

Each chart relates only to one patient, so it is unnecessary to use the term *patient* or to use the patient's name. Use phrases rather than full sentences, and do not make erasures or leave empty spaces on the record. All entries are made in black ink because the chart is a permanent record; no erasable ink or correction fluid is allowed.

If you use medical terms in your charting, make sure you are using the correct words and that spelling is correct. Use a medical dictionary if you are not sure. Abbreviations are allowed, but they must be approved for use by your facility. Do not make up your own abbreviations. You must chart only for yourself and only when the procedure or assignment has been completed.

The time of entry must be noted when the entry is made. Most health care facilities use international time (Table 8-3) to avoid confusion between AM and PM. With international time, the 24 hours of each day are identified by the numbers 0100 (1:00 AM) through 2400 (12:00 AM, midnight). The last two digits indicate the minutes of each hour (from 01 to 59). Thus, 0101 would be one minute after 1:00 AM; 1210 would be ten minutes after 12 PM (noon); 1658 would be 4:58 PM, and so on.

Many health care facilities are using flow sheets for documenting patient care. Flow sheets save nursing time and simplify the documentation process. However, there are some things you should be aware of to avoid problems:

- Understand what you are supposed to be documenting. Read the flow sheet carefully.
- Never initial any procedure or observation that you did not do.
- Initial for the right procedure, on the right day, on the right shift.
- Put your complete signature on each flow sheet (usually at the bottom of the page).
- Remember that flow sheets are legal records just like the other forms in the medical record.
- Chart after an event occurs or care is given. Never chart in advance.
- Notify the RN if something is missing from a computerized flow sheet. The RN will add missing information that is listed on the patient's care plan or critical pathway. For example, your facility routinely charts that patients are turned and repositioned every two hours. You routinely turn and reposition Ms. Avilla, according to her critical pathway. However, there is no place to document this important care on the flow sheet.
- If you forget to chart something or make an error, follow your facility policy for making a late entry note or correcting the error.

FIGURE 8-14 Observations are recorded in the patient's medical record.

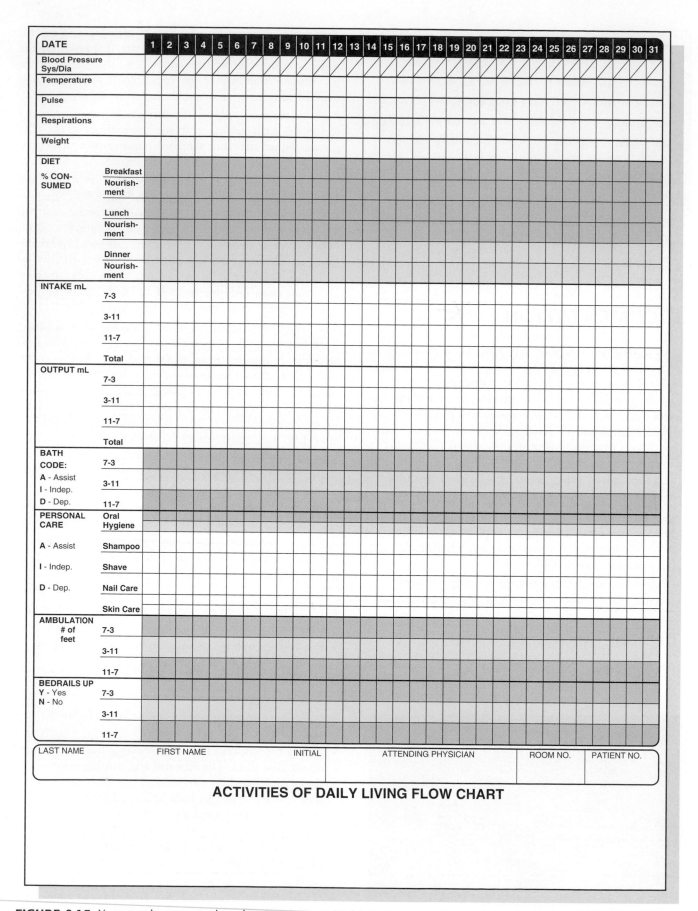

FIGURE 8-15 You may be expected to document your care and observations on a flow sheet. (Courtesy of Briggs Corporation)

DATE		1	2	3	4	5	6	7	8	9	10	11	12	13	14	15	16	17	18	19	20	21	22	23	24	25	26	27	28	29	30	31
UP IN CHAIR	7-3																															
A - Assist I - Indep. D - Dep.	3-11																															
	11-7																															
ROM Exercises A - Active	7-3																															
P - Passive	3-11																															
POSITION changed	7-3																															
A - Assist I - Indep. D - Dep.	3-11																															
	11-7																															
BLADDER **ACTION**	7-3																															
C - Continent I - Incontinent F - Foley # x's	3-11																															
	11-7																															
BOWEL **ACTION**	7-3																															
C - Continent I - Incontinent # x's	3-11																															
	11-7																															
CONSISTENCY	7-3																															
L - Liquid S - Soft formed	3-11																															
H - Hard formed	11-7																															
PERI CARE	7-3																															
A - Assist I - Indep. D - Dep.	3-11																															
	11-7																															
RESTRAINT P - Pelvic W - Waist	7-3																															
B - Belt G - Geri Chair	3-11																															
Check q 1/2 Hr. Release q 2 hrs.	11-7																															
Nursing Assistant's Initials	A.M.																															
	P.M.																															
	NOC.																															
Licensed Nurse Initials	A.M.																															
	P.M.																															
	NOC.																															

Nursing Assistant's Initials and Signature

_____ _____   _____ _____   _____ _____

_____ _____   _____ _____   _____ _____

_____ _____   _____ _____   _____ _____

Licensed Nurse Initials and Signature

_____ _____   _____ _____   _____ _____

_____ _____   _____ _____   _____ _____

_____ _____   _____ _____   _____ _____

LAST NAME	FIRST NAME	INITIAL	ATTENDING PHYSICIAN	ROOM NO.	PATIENT NO.

FIGURE 8-15 *CONTINUED*

NURSE'S PROGRESS NOTES

DATE AND TIME	NURSING CARE NOTES	SIGNATURE
3-16-XX	2200 Found lying on floor beside bed. Responds verbally. States was "trying to get to the bathroom." Nurse notified immediately	C. Simmons CNA
	2205 ROM satisfactory. Denies having pain. No injuries noted. ROM wnl. No obvious deformities. Assisted back to bed. Call light within reach. Instructed to use call light when having to go to B.R. Pulse 86, strong and regular. B/P 136/84. Oriented to time, place, person. Incontinent after fall. Pajamas chgd. Dr. Stone & responsible party notified.	
	2300 Sleeping s̄ distress	B. Selici RN
3-17-XX	2400-0200 Sleeping soundly. Respirations regular. Pulse 78 strong and regular.	
	0230 Awake. c/o "arthritis pain" in both hips. Acetaminophen 500 mg tabs ī̄ given with water. Assisted to bathroom. Voided large amt. clear urine.	
	0230-0630 Slept soundly. Pulse 72 strong and regular. B/P 128/80. T 98⁶(0). Denies pain anywhere. No other c/o distress.	P. Hernandez RN
3-17-XX	0710 Up to B.R. c̄ assistance ——Error ES	E. Seldes LPN

FIGURE 8-16 The nurse's notes are a narrative record of patient care and observations.

TABLE 8-3 INTERNATIONAL TIME

Standard Clock	Int'l. Time	Standard Clock	Int'l. Time
AM 12 midnight	2400	PM 12 noon	1200
1	0100	1	1300
2	0200	2	1400
3	0300	3	1500
4	0400	4	1600
5	0500	5	1700
6	0600	6	1800
7	0700	7	1900
8	0800	8	2000
9	0900	9	2100
10	1000	10	2200
11	1100	11	2300

Confidentiality and Privacy

As you know, each patient has a right keep his or her medical information private. The medical record is a private and confidential document. All staff are responsible for protecting patient information and data from access by unauthorized persons. Likewise, you should not be reading patient charts out of curiosity. Medical records and other patient data should be accessed only by those with a need to know the information.

In 1996, Congress passed the **Health Insurance Portability and Accountability Act (HIPAA)**. This law has many provisions. One portion applies to privacy, confidentiality, and medical records. The HIPAA rules:

- Increase patient control over personal medical records
- Restrict the use and disclosure of patient information
- Make facilities accountable for protecting patient data
- Require the facility to implement and monitor their information release policies and procedures

The HIPAA regulations protect all individually identifiable health information in any form. The rules apply to paper, verbal, and electronic documentation, billing records, and clinical records. Because of this, patient information is provided to staff on a "need to know" basis. Information is disclosed only if staff needs it to carry out their duties. For example, the dietary department would need to know if a patient was on a diabetic diet. They would not need to know that the patient has an infectious disease. The nursing assistant would need to know about both the diabetes and the infection. Facilities must monitor how and where they use patient information. Policies must protect patient charts, conversations and reports about patient information, transmission of patient documents, and disclosure of other personal information.

The HIPAA rules ask providers to analyze how and where patient information is used and develop procedures for protecting confidential data. This includes the areas where patient charts are stored, the places where patient information is discussed, and how patients' personal health information is distributed. The HIPAA policies and procedures for each facility are individualized to the facility.

Legal ALERT

Reporting and recording your observations of patients are key nursing assistant responsibilities. Pay attention to details. Practice good communication skills. You will learn which observations must be reported immediately and which can wait until the end of the shift. An alert, observant CNA is invaluable in protecting patients' safety and well-being. ■

Handheld Computers

Handheld computers were first introduced in 1995. Since then, they have become essential tools to many health care workers, because they greatly enhance the ability to communicate.

Two major classes of portable computing devices are being used with increasing frequency by health care workers: **personal digital assistants (PDAs)** and **tablet PCs (TPCs).** Many hospitals are using these small, handheld computers as an integral part of their services, and professional and paraprofessional staff members have purchased them for individual use. In addition to using the computer as an information resource at work, most individuals use them to hold personal information, such as their appointments and list of phone numbers. Most PDAs also have a calculator function. Using a computer has many benefits, and the portability of handheld models has made them a popular alternative.

Handheld computers use wireless Internet technology to transmit data. In many hospitals, handheld computers are used to transmit nursing notes and vital signs to the hospital's mainframe computer. Before handheld computer technology was available, nursing personnel often scribbled notes on the backs of their hands, on paper towels, and scraps of paper. If the data were not subsequently lost, they were transferred to patient charts later in the shift. By using the handheld computer, personnel can record important data, then transmit it to the main computer immediately.

The keypad on the handheld computer is tiny and is operated with a stylus. Light pens and touch-screen data entry are also useful tools with some models. Data such as vital signs, intake and output values, and pain scale ratings can be readily entered by using the keypad. However, for longer narrative notes, the keypad may not be practical. The handheld computer may be plugged into a larger keyboard, which is easier and faster to use.

Handheld computers are battery operated. If not regularly charged and maintained, they will lose data. *Hot-syncing* is a term that refers to linking the handheld computer to a full-size computer to update the information on both. Data are commonly transferred by placing the PDA into a cradle, which will upload data to the mainframe. This is essential for data preservation, especially if the handheld computer battery runs low. Many PDAs use rechargeable batteries, and placing the unit into the cradle also charges the battery.

Radio Frequency Emitting Devices. Radio frequency emitting devices have the potential to interfere with patient care and diagnostic, life support, and laboratory equipment. Your facility will have strict policies and procedures regarding the types of devices that may be used, and when and where they may be used. Become familiar with these policies and follow them. Most hospitals have banned cell phones or restricted their use to certain areas (Figure 8-17). The same is true of handheld computing devices. Some hospitals prohibit their use in highly instrumented clinical areas, such as the intensive care unit. Others prohibit their use within five feet of patient care and diagnostic equipment.

FIGURE 8-17 Cell phones and other electronic devices may interfere with medical equipment.

Computers and HIPAA Compliance.

HIPAA affects all health care communication, especially information technology (IT). Because of this, hospital systems have layers of access to patient medical records. For example, you will be able to access the records for only those patients listed in your assignment. Information will be limited to that which is essential to patient care. The IT department can track who is accessing any patient's record and can readily identify misuse of the system. Most PDAs have the ability to access the Internet, so the hospital will construct a firewall to ensure that sensitive patient data are not being broadcast into cyberspace.

Advantages of Using Computers

There are many advantages to using computers in health care. These include:

- Rapid information access
- Ready source of decision trees, reference material, other and information
- Provides warning messages, such as drug, allergy, and food interactions, alerting staff to potential negative side effects
- Faster, less time-consuming documentation
- Ability to manage patient and procedure information
- Bedside data entry, before information is forgotten
- Data available for research and teaching
- Improved team communication
- Ability to charge for supplies and services; charges are not lost
- Ability to create bar codes and other patient identification labels (Figure 8-18) to track laboratory specimens, medications, and other items; using bar codes and scanners reduces the risk of errors and patient injuries
- Convenience of finding information without reading many handwritten pages
- No need to hunt for a patient's chart
- No need to wait for others to finish using the chart you need

FIGURE 8-18 Many hospitals use bar codes to charge supplies, track laboratory specimens, and reduce the risk of errors.

- Ability to check personal work schedule and assignment
- Consistency in terminology and abbreviations
- Information transferred easily from one department to another
- Available as worksheets or Kardex
- Ability to check critical pathway and care plan information
- Ability to create checklists and worksheets, such as a list of patient schedules for the day
- Individual field data can be generated and database searches done (such as a list of baths, labs, surgery, and therapy)
- Not as easily lost as written patient records
- Legible and easy to read
- Portable and easy to use
- Helpful to check information at the bedside without going to the desk
- Reduce errors and improve patient safety

Having ready access to key nursing information is critical. Because of this, nursing diagnoses and classifications such as the Nursing Interventions Classification (NIC) and Nursing Outcomes Classification (NOC) are fully computerized, and data are readily available to nursing staff.

Legal ALERT

In health care, there is a saying, "If it's not charted, it wasn't done." Although some facilities use a system called "charting by exception," most adhere to the time-tested maxim and chart all care given. The purpose of documentation is to communicate care given and the patient's response. Documentation is a true record of patient care, and is the first line of defense in proving accountability for excellent care. Never chart care that you did not provide. For example, some assistants will chart that a patient was "turned every two hours" because they know that this is the care that is supposed to be given. Document only the facts. If you are unable to turn the patient every two hours, inform the nurse early in the shift. Always chart after giving care. Never document on the medical record in advance. If you forget to document, follow your facility policy for making a late entry. Specify the exact date and time the entry was recorded, as well as the exact date and time the event occurred. Clearly mark your documentation as a late entry. ■

GUIDELINES *for*

Documentation on the Computerized Medical Record

- Do not be afraid of computerized charting. When documenting on a specific patient, double-check to make sure you have entered the correct identification code.

- Do not give your identification code or password to others.

- Select a password that is not easily deciphered, such as a combination of numbers and letters. Your employer may ask that you write down your name and password, seal it in an envelope, and give the envelope to your supervisor.

  - Do not inform others of your password. Do not write it down or leave it where it is easily found, such as under the mouse pad, keyboard, or in an electronic file. Regularly change your password. Change it immediately if you suspect it has been compromised.

  - Never let someone look over your shoulder when you are signing in or accessing patient data.

  - Turn or position the monitor so it is not visible to others.

- Access only information you are authorized to obtain.

- Document only in areas you are authorized to use.

- Remember that audit trails track the computer, user, date, time, and exactly which medical records are accessed, based on your user identification data.

- The electronic record must note whether manual records are also being used. If this is the case (such as during a storm or electronic system failure), the records must cross-reference each other. Most hospitals have policies about using paper documentation if the computer is down for a period of time.

- Many computer programs place expert reminders or error codes on the screen. Read and follow the directions.

- Do not print information unnecessarily. If your facility policy requires you to retain hard copies of your documentation, print it at the end of your

shift, or according to facility policy (Figure 8-19). Printing after each entry may result in an excess of partial, unusable documents that must subsequently be destroyed. You must destroy printed copies that are not part of the permanent record. Placing them in the wastebasket is prohibited in many facilities because of privacy laws. Records are commonly destroyed by shredding them in a paper shredder.

- Never delete information from the electronic medical record.

- The procedure for late entry and addendum documentation will be different than it is in a narrative system. Know and follow your facility policies for this type of charting.

- Electronic documentation must be signed by the person giving care. Your facility will have a procedure for providing electronic signatures. These are valid as long as they are accessible only to the person identified by that signature.

- Protect patient data transmitted electronically, such as by using an e-mail encryption service. Never transmit insecure, identifiable patient information.

- Always log off when you have finished using the computer.

- Wash your hands after using the computer. Many people use it, so the keyboard is a huge potential source of cross-contamination.

  - Some facilities cover the keyboard with a plastic cover. Users type through the plastic. If this is done in your workplace, routinely disinfect the cover with the recommended product.

  - Avoid products containing alcohol when cleaning the computer and accessories. Use only products that are recommended for the surface being cleaned.

- Stay current. Attend continuing education programs to learn how to maximize the use of computerized charting and information systems.

GUIDELINES *continued*

```
                                    Longmeadow Subacute Care
Age/Sex: 70 F        Attending:                                                    Page 2
 Unit #: H000133357  Account #: M00850678608
Location: M.C4S      Admitted: 08/01/XX at 2005        **LIVE**          Printed 08/07/XX at 0152
Room/Bed: M. 486-B     Status: ADM IN            NURSING DAILY SUMMARY   24 hours ending 08/06/XX at 2359
```

	08/06 0332 KSB	08/06 0800 CIB	08/06 1200 CIB	08/06 2231 JRS
PATIENT CARE				
DIET				
Meal	Snack	Breakfast	Lunch	Supper
Diet	Soft	Soft	Soft	Soft
% Eaten	100	90	75	65
How Taken	Assisted by Famil	Assisted by Famil	Assisted by Famil	Total Feed by Sta
Diet Intake <50 % x	Y	Y	Y	
HYGIENE				
Bath		Sponge	Sponge	
Assistance		x1 Staff	x1 Staff	
Oral Care	Staff	Staff	Staff	Staff
Skin Care	Staff	Staff	Staff	Staff
Peri Care	Staff	Staff	Staff	Staff
Catheter Care	Not Applicable	Not Applicable	Not Applicable	Not Applicable
ACTIVITY				
Activity	Bedrest	Bedrest	Bedrest	Bedside Commode
Assistance		x1 Staff	x1 Staff	x1 Staff
Time: Hours		5	5	
Minutes				
Distance (ft)				
Tolerated		Good	Good	Fair
Repositioned	Staff	Staff	Staff	Staff
TCDB	Y	Y	Y	
SAFETY				
Siderails	Up X 4	Up X 4	Up X 4	Up X 4
Bed Low Position	Y	Y	Y	Y
Protective/Supporta	N	N	N	N
Call Light in Reach	Y	Y	Y	Y

```
  Recorded       Occurred                                    Notes: All Categories
Date    Time    Date   Time  By                                           Category

08/06/XX 0440 08/06/XX 0436 LRR                                      Nursing Notes
   INCONTINENT OF SOFT STOOL. HAD PRUNE JUICE AT HS. COOPERATIVE WITH CARE.
08/06/XX 1524 08/06/XX 0800 MW                                      Nursing Notes
   DISORIENTED X3. RESPONDS TO VEBRA STIMULI BUT SPEECH SOFT AND UNCLEAR AT TIMES.
08/06/XX 1526 08/06/XX 0800 MW                                      Nursing Notes
   GENERALIZED WEAKNESS AND REQUIRES ASSIST WITH ALL TRANSFERS.
08/06/XX 1529 08/06/XX 0800 MW                                      Nursing Notes
   UP IN CHAIR AT BEDSIDE TOL. FAIR.
08/06/XX 1529 08/06/XX 1030 MW                                      Nursing Notes
   BACK TO BED POSITIONED FOR COMFORT.
08/06/XX 1554 08/06/XX 1552 KM                                  Social Service Notes
   ORDERS REC FOR HH TO FOLLOW PT AFTER DISMISSAL. SPOKE W/PT AND REVIEWED CHART. SHE WOULD LIKE SERVICES
   ARRANGED W/HOME CARE. ORDERS AND INFO WILL BE GIVEN TO AGENCY OF PT PREFERENCE CLOSER TO TIME OF DC.
08/06/XX 1732 08/06/XX 1729 BGB                                 Social Service Notes
   TEAM CONFERENCE HELD ON 8-5-XX TO DISCUSS PATIENT'S CARE PLAN AND DISCHARGE NEEDS. PATIENT IS HERE FOR THERAPY
   SERVICES FOR HER ACUTE EPISODE OF WEAKNESS RELATED TO PARKINSON'S DISEASE. SHE IS CURRENTLY IN A PROGRESSIVE
   DISEASE PROCESS.. AND IS AT TIMES NOT ORIENTED TO TIME AND PLACE. ORDERS WERE WRITTEN TODAY FOR PATIENT TO
   RETURN HOME WITH HER HUSBAND, SON, AND OTHER FAMILY AND CHURCH MEMBERS TO ASSIST WITH HER CARE. THE FAMILY HAD
   CONSIDERED ASSISTED LIVING PLACEMENT. BUT DECIDED AGAINST THIS. PATIENT WILL BE TRANSPORTED HOME ON FRIDAY BY
   AMBULANCE.
```

FIGURE 8-19 Print a hard copy of your documentation at the end of the shift, or according to facility policy. Avoid making extra or incomplete copies that subsequently must be destroyed.

GUIDELINES *for*

Charting

- Check for: right patient, right chart, right form, right room.

- Fill out new headings completely.

- Use correct color of ink.

- Date and time each entry.

- Chart entries in correct sequence.

- Make entries brief, objective, and accurate.

- Print or write clearly.

- Spell each word correctly.

- Leave no blank spaces or lines between entries.

- Do not use the term *patient*.

- Do not use ditto marks.

- Sign each entry with your first initial, last name, and job title.

- Make corrections by drawing one line through the entry; then print the word "error" on the line and your initials above.

REVIEW

A. True/False.

Mark the following true or false by circling T or F.

1. T F The nursing process is a method used by the nurse to supervise the work of others.

2. T F The nursing assistant is responsible for completing an assessment on all patients assigned to him or her.

3. T F Assessment involves the collection of data.

4. T F A statement of a patient's medical condition is called a nursing diagnosis.

5. T F An approach is sometimes called an intervention.

6. T F The patient's goal is called an outcome.

7. T F The care plan is developed at the care plan conference.

8. T F Nursing assistants are not responsible for the development or implementation of the care plan.

9. T F Taking a patient's weight is an example of an objective observation.

10. T F The patient's chart is a legal document.

B. Multiple Choice.

Select the one best answer for each of the following.

11. The purpose of the nursing process is to
   a. make a medical diagnosis.
   b. achieve patient-focused care.
   c. make assignments.
   d. cure illness.

12. The nursing assistant contributes to the nurse's assessment of the patient by
   a. listening to the heart and lungs.
   b. keeping the environment neat and tidy.
   c. establishing goals for the patient.
   d. reporting observations and vital signs.

13. The statement of a patient's problem and its cause is called
   a. a medical diagnosis.
   b. an approach.
   c. an assessment.
   d. a nursing diagnosis.

14. The purpose of evaluation is to determine whether the
   a. patient is reaching the goals on the care plan.
   b. laboratory tests are accurate.

c. patient agrees with the critical pathway.
   d. family understands the patient's condition.

15. The purpose of making observations is to
   a. make sure the nurse gets along with the patient.
   b. inform the doctor of how the patient's family is doing.
   c. note changes in condition or new problems developing.
   d. see if the medical diagnosis is accurate.

16. An example of an objective observation is that the patient
   a. complains of abdominal pain.
   b. says she is feeling sad.
   c. has a pulse of 72.
   d. says she is not hungry.

17. When you offer to give Mrs. Jones a bath, she says, "Get out of here and don't come back." You report this to the nurse and say
   a. "Mrs. Jones told me to leave her room and not come back."
   b. "Mrs. Jones is angry today."
   c. "Mrs. Jones is not cooperating with me."
   d. "Mrs. Jones does not want a bath today."

18. The form on which nurses enter daily information about the patient is called the
   a. progress notes.
   b. nurse's notes.
   c. nurse's daily flow log.
   d. document.

19. Charting should always be
   a. done in pencil.
   b. done after the procedure is completed.
   c. signed at least once each day.
   d. done before care is given.

20. In international time, midnight would be called
   a. 12:00 AM
   b. 2400
   c. 1200
   d. 12:00 PM

21. The HIPAA rules
   a. make it easier to share patient information with other health care workers.
   b. prohibit the sharing of patient information with unlicensed workers.
   c. empower the physician to specify information to disclose.
   d. restrict the use and disclosure of patient information.

22. The device that prevents patient information from being inadvertently transmitted over the Internet is the
  a. firewall.
  b. PDA.
  c. hot-sync.
  d. radio frequency emitting device.

23. Audit trails
  a. are used only if the computer is down.
  b. are done each day to identify and correct missing documentation.
  c. track the computer, user, date, time, and which records are accessed.
  d. are very difficult to establish and are seldom necessary.

24. Medical records and other patient data
  a. may be accessed by nursing employees who are curious about the patient.
  b. should be accessed only by those with a need to know the information.
  c. should be accessed only by the physician and the RN.
  d. may be accessed by the patient's family members, if desired.

C. Nursing Assistant Challenge.

Mr. Fensten is a 47-year-old patient on the medical floor. He has had a stroke. These events occur while you are taking care of him:

- He has trouble walking because of hemiplegia (paralysis) on the right side of his body and almost falls while you are walking him to the bathroom.
- He refuses to eat his breakfast.
- He throws the washcloth across the room when you help him with his bath.
- His B/P is 146/88.
- He smiles and hugs his wife when she comes to visit.
- You do range-of-motion exercises on all joints without any problem.
- You notice a persistent reddened area on his coccyx (tailbone).

For each of these observations, write out the documentation exactly as you would on the patient's medical record.

Think about these observations and consider how many examples of verbal and nonverbal communication are given.

Do any of these situations involve Mr. Fensten's rights as a patient? If so, describe them.

UNIT 9

Meeting Basic Human Needs

OBJECTIVES

After completing this unit, you will be able to:
- Spell and define terms.
- Describe the stages of human growth and development.
- List five physical needs of patients.
- Define self-esteem.
- Describe how the nursing assistant can meet the patient's emotional needs.
- List nursing assistant actions to ensure that patients have the opportunity for intimacy.
- Discuss methods of dealing with the fearful patient.
- List the guidelines to assist patients in meeting their spiritual needs.

VOCABULARY

Learn the meaning and the correct spelling of the following words and phrases:

adolescence	growth	personality	tasks
bisexuality	heterosexuality	preadolescence	tasks of personality
celibate	homosexuality	reflex	development
coitus	intimacy	self-esteem	toddler
continuum	masturbation	self-identity	
development	neonate	sexuality	

INTRODUCTION

Each of us has things that we need to live successfully. These are called *needs* simply because we cannot get along without them. When a patient is admitted to the hospital, his or her needs come too. The difference now is in the way those needs are expressed and fulfilled. Expression and fulfillment have to be different because of the hospital environment and the illness. Remember that the basic needs remain the same, regardless of how they are expressed or how they have to be met because of an individual's level of development or state of health.

Age-Appropriate Care ALERT

Each patient is an individual with his or her own:
- Likes and dislikes
- Feelings, thoughts, and beliefs
- Limitations and abilities
- Life experiences

Avoid stereotyping patients based on their age. Treat each patient as an individual. A key part of your job is learning to recognize each patient's unique needs and abilities. ■

HUMAN GROWTH AND DEVELOPMENT

Human beings change as they age, through the processes of growth and development. **Growth** involves the changes that take place in the body. It is usually measured by height and weight and degree of system maturation. **Development** involves the changes that take place on a social, emotional, and psychological level. Developmental levels are shown in behavior and interpersonal skills.

People move from one level of development to the next (Table 9-1). At each level, they change in both the way they look and the way they think and act (Figure 9-1). Each level presents tasks that must be mastered before the person can move on to the next level.

The **tasks** to be mastered are those things that lead to healthy and satisfactory participation in society. The tasks are defined by the needs of the individual and the pressures of society.

Sometimes growth spurts occur and developmental skills must catch up. Both growth and development progress from simple to complex. Each depends on the other to achieve the orderly progression. For example, a child cannot be toilet trained until the nerve pathways have matured.

Age-Appropriate Care ALERT

Your communication must be appropriate for the patient's age. ■

TABLE 9-1 STAGES OF GROWTH AND DEVELOPMENT

Neonate	Birth to 1 month
Infancy	1 month to 2 years
Toddler	2 years to 3 years
Preschool	3 years to 5 years
School Age	5 years to 12 years
Preadolescence	12 years to 14 years
Adolescence	14 years to 20 years
Adulthood	20 years to 49 years
Middle Age	50 years to 64 years
Later Maturity	65 years to 75 years
Old Age	75 years and beyond

FIGURE 9-1 The characteristics of different age groups are reflected in this family picture.

Growth and development follow a set of basic principles of progression:

- There is a continuous movement from simple to more complex. For example, baby sounds progress to speech patterns.
- Development and growth move from head to feet and from torso to limbs. The infant first raises the head, then sits, stands, and finally walks.
- Each stage of development has a specific set of tasks that the person must master before he or she can successfully move on to the next level. For example, the child learns to catch big balls before she can catch a baseball.
- Progression moves forward in an orderly manner, but the rate varies for each person. There are growth spurts in the preschool and teen years, but not all children grow to the same extent or at the same rate.
- Growth patterns progress at their own individual rate.

Neonatal and Infant Period (Birth to Two Years)

The neonatal and infant period extends through the first two years of life. It is a time of rapid physical growth and development (Table 9-2). The infant gradually learns to:

- Sit
- Crawl
- Stand
- Take first steps

Other changes also occur during this period:

- Emotional attachments move from self-awareness and parental or caregiver attachment toward ties with other family members.
- Systems that are relatively immature at birth become more stabilized.
- Alertness and activity increase.
- Teeth appear (erupt).

TABLE 9-2 HEIGHT/WEIGHT FOR THE FIRST YEAR OF LIFE (BOYS)

Age (Months)	Height (Inches)	Weight (Pounds)
Birth	20	7–8
1 month	21 1/4	7 1/2
2 months	22 1/2	10
3 months	23 3/4	11 1/2
4 months	24 3/4	12 1/2
5 months	25 1/2	14
6 months	26	15
7 months	26 3/4	16 3/4
8 months	27 1/2	18
9 months	28	19
10 months	28 1/2	20
11 months	29	20 3/4
12 months	29 1/2	21 1/2

Remember that the figures are averages only.

- Food intake progresses from milk to solid food.
- Verbal skills begin to develop.

Age-Appropriate Care ALERT

Communicate with an infant (newborn to 12 months) by smiling, being gentle, hugging, rocking, and touching. Speak softly and slowly or sing quietly during care. Introduce yourself to the parents and explain procedures to them. Allow parents to remain nearby when you are providing care. ■

The mother or primary caregiver of the infant is the central figure of emotional attachment. Growth and development progress so rapidly that changes can be seen each month.

The **neonate** (newborn) (Figure 9-2):
- Weighs 7–8 pounds.
- Is approximately 20–21 inches long.

FIGURE 9-2 Newborn infant (neonate)

- Has a head that seems disproportionately large compared to the body.
- Has skin that is wrinkled, thin, and red.
- Has an abdomen that seems to stick out (protrude).
- Has dark blue eyes.

In the newborn, the:
- Conversion of cartilage to bone (ossification) is not complete. This can be seen in the soft spots (fontanels) and suture lines (joints) of the skull.
- The nervous system is not fully developed, so muscular activities are uncoordinated.
- Vision is not clear, but hearing and taste are developed. Certain **reflexes** (automatic responses) are also developed. They are the:
  - Moro reflex—when a loud noise startles the infant, the arms are spread across the chest, the legs are extended, and the head is thrust back. This response is also called the *startle reflex*.
  - Grasp reflex—touching the infant's palm causes the fingers to flex in a grasping motion.
  - Rooting (sucking) reflex—stroking the cheek or side of the lips stimulates the infant to turn its head in the direction of the stroking. This is important in finding the nipple to suck the milk.
- Diet is milk or milk substitute.
- Routine is largely sleeping, eating, and eliminating.

The neonate is completely dependent on the caregiver for all needs. The infant is unable to support her head, so the newborn must be handled carefully and be well supported when held.

The three-month-old infant:
- Has gained enough muscular coordination to hold her head up and raise her shoulders.
- Has lost the Moro, rooting, and grasp reflexes.

- Produces real tears.
- Can follow objects with his eyes.
- Can smile and coo at the caregiver.

The six-month-old infant:

- Has learned to roll over.
- Can sit for short periods of time.
- Holds things with both hands and directs them toward his mouth.
- Responds with verbal sounds when a caregiver speaks.
- Is beginning to cut front teeth.
- Eats finger foods and strained fruits and vegetables.
- Recognizes family members.
- Develops fear of strangers.

The nine-month-old infant:

- Crawls and may begin to stand when supported.
- Has more teeth erupt.
- Can respond to her name.
- Says one- and two-syllable words such as "mama."
- Shows a preference for right- or left-hand control.
- Eats junior baby foods.

The one-year-old infant:

- Understands simple commands such as "No."
- Begins to take steps—supported at first, then independently.
- Eats table foods and can hold her own cup.
- Weighs three times what he weighed at birth (refer to Table 9-2).

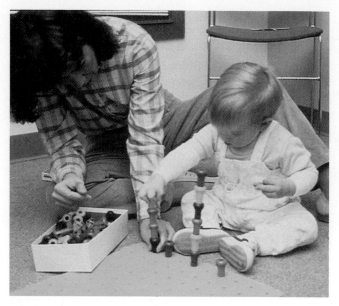

FIGURE 9-3 The toddler begins to develop gross motor skills. (Photo courtesy of Henrietta Egleston Hospital for Children, Atlanta, GA. Photograph by Ginger Lovering)

Age-Appropriate Care ALERT

When caring for the one- to three-year-old, tell the child who you are. Call him or her by name. Introduce yourself to the parents and explain procedures to them. Have them explain the procedure to the child, or do so yourself using simple terms. Allow the child to handle equipment with supervision. Communicate by using simple words and commands. Smile, be gentle, and speak to the child during care. Avoid prolonged separation from the parents, if possible. Allow the child to be as independent as possible. ■

Toddler Period (Two to Three Years)

The **toddler** period is a busy, active phase. It is a time when exploration and investigation are the main activities. It is also a period in which motor abilities develop (Figure 9-3) and vocabulary and comprehension increase.

During this period, the toddler:

- Learns to control elimination.
- Begins to become aware of right and wrong.
- Often reacts with frustration and negative responses to attempts at socialization and discipline as she becomes more aware of herself as a separate person.
- Tolerates brief periods of separation from the mother, but the mother still remains the source of security and comfort.
- May play in the company of other children but with no interaction. This age group is very possessive. "No" and "mine" are a major part of their vocabularies.

Reaching the end of this period, the toddler is able to:

- Walk and run.
- Display motor (manual) skills that include feeding himself and riding toys.
- Put words together and speak more clearly. The average vocabulary of a two-year-old is about 300 words.

Preschool Years (Three to Five Years)

The three- to five-year-old (Figure 9-4) builds on the motor and verbal skills developed as a toddler. During this period, the preschooler:

- Grows less reliant on the mother. Children in this age group begin to recognize their position as members of the family unit and their uniqueness from other members.
- Develops rivalries with siblings and develops greater attachments to the father or alternate caregiver.

FIGURE 9-4 This child is expanding her awareness of the world.

FIGURE 9-5 School-age children like to play in peer groups.

- Gradually increases cooperative play.
- Improves language skills and asks many questions.
- Develops a more active imagination.
- Becomes more sexually curious.

By the end of this period, children have become far more socialized than they were as toddlers. They are more cooperative. They seem almost eager to follow established rules within limits. They enjoy interacting with family members and peers.

Age-Appropriate Care ALERT

Communicate with the three- to five-year-old child by calling her by name. Tell the child who you are. Explain procedures to the child in simple language. Tell her what you will do each time. Do not expect her to remember. Demonstrate procedures on a doll or stuffed animal, whenever possible. Use simple words and short sentences. Smile often. Use familiar times, such as "before lunch" or "after dinner," rather than stating the time. Reward the child for positive behavior with attention and special treats, as allowed. Allow her to be as independent as possible. ∎

School-Age Children (5 to 12 Years)

The school-age child (Figure 9-5):
- Is able to communicate.
- Has developed small (fine) motor skills. With these skills, the child is able to master tasks such as writing.

- Develops an increased sense of self.
- Establishes peer relationships.
- Reinforces proper social behavior through games, simple tasks, and play.
- Chooses sex-differentiated friends.
- Joins groups like Scouts. This serves to further identify the individual as a person of a particular gender.
- Begins to show concern for other living things (Figure 9-6).

Preadolescence (12 to 14 Years)

Preadolescence is a transitional stage. It is a period of great uncertainty. During this period:
- Hormonal changes stimulate the secondary sex characteristics.
- The individual feels on the threshold of tremendous change, though not yet in a period of sexual functioning.

FIGURE 9-6 Young children learn to reach out and have concern for others.

Age-Appropriate Care ALERT

Introduce yourself to the school-age child and call her by name. Explain procedures in simple terms, but use proper names for body parts. Encourage the child to ask questions. Allow the child to make decisions, as appropriate. Set limits on behavior, if necessary. Reason with the child, if necessary. Always speak during care. Allow the child to call friends on the phone, if desired. Be aware that the child may try to delay procedures. Stay with the child during painful procedures and provide comfort and reassurance. Distraction may be effective during procedures. Give the child as much control as possible. ■

- Mood swings and feelings of insecurity are common.
- There is a growing awareness of and interest in the opposite sex.
- Arms and legs seem out of proportion to the rest of the body.

Age-Appropriate Care ALERT

When caring for the 12- to 18-year-old, introduce yourself. Children of this age are sensitive to the caregiver's body language; make sure it is appropriate. Explain procedures in adult terms. Avoid talking down to the child, but simplify and clarify information if necessary. Spend time talking with the child. Maintain a nonthreatening demeanor. Avoid power struggles. Ensure that the child informs you of his whereabouts, if he leaves the unit. Be as flexible as possible. ■

Adolescence (14 to 20 Years)

Adolescence is marked by:
- The gradual development of sexual maturity.
- A greater appreciation of the individual's own identity as a male or a female person.
- Conflicting desires for the freedom of independence and the security of dependence. Because of these conflicting desires, this is often a troublesome period.
- The establishment of personal coping systems and the ability to make independent judgments and decisions.

- Gradual success in mastering the developmental tasks of the age. The adolescent is able to make comparisons between the values she has been taught and reality.

Age-Appropriate Care ALERT

When caring for adults (ages 20 through 64), introduce yourself. Address the patient by title and last name unless she instructs you otherwise. Avoid demeaning names, such as "honey" and "dear." Be sensitive to the patient's need to communicate and allow time to talk. Be a good listener. Explain procedures honestly. Treat the patient with respect. Allow the patient to set her own routine, as much as possible. Adjust room temperature to the patient's preference. Control environmental noise. Inform the patient about policies, services, and routines, as appropriate. ■

Adulthood (20 to 49 Years)

Early adulthood is marked by:
- Independence and personal decision making.
- The choice of a mate.
- Establishment of a career and family life.
- Optimal health.
- The choice of friends to form a support group.

Middle Age (50 to 64 Years)

Middle age is associated with:
- Final career advancement, ending in retirement.
- Children who were reared during the period of adulthood leaving home to enter their own adult period.
- Health that is usually still at good levels, though some slowing may be seen.
- More time that can be spent on leisure activities.
- More time and money to pursue personal interests.
- Revitalizing one's relationship with a mate.
- Enjoying grandchildren.
- For some middle-aged persons, being a member of the "sandwich" generation—caring for both their own parents and their children or grandchildren.

Later Maturity (65 to 75 Years)

Later maturity is marked by:
- A gradual loss of vitality and stamina.
- Physical changes that signal the aging process. For example, sight and hearing diminish.

- Chronic conditions that develop and persist.
- A period of gradual losses: loss of mate, friends, self-esteem, some independence.
- Examination of a lifetime.
- More time to pursue personal interests.
- Fewer responsibilities related to raising a family and holding a job.
- Increased wisdom.

Old Age (75 Years and Beyond)

Old age is frequently characterized by:

- Failing physical health and growing dependency (Figure 9-7).
- The need to deal with illness, loneliness, loss of friends and loved ones, and the realization of mortality.

Success in this final period depends on the mechanisms of coping that the older adult has developed over the years. The extent of available emotional and physical support is also important.

Aging is a gradual process that begins at birth. Old age can be a period of development and enjoyment.

BASIC HUMAN NEEDS

Developmental skills and physical growth may vary during the life span. The basic human needs, however, are much the same for every individual.

Basic human needs are the things and activities required by all persons to successfully and satisfactorily live their lives. The needs are the same for all people at all ages. Cultural backgrounds influence the way in which individ-

FIGURE 9-7 Physical status often declines in old age.

Age-Appropriate Care ALERT

When caring for elderly adults (age 65 and older), introduce yourself. Address the patient by title and last name unless he instructs you otherwise. Avoid demeaning names, such as "honey" and "dear." Speak slowly and clearly, making good eye contact. Be alert to vision and hearing problems. Do not assume that the patient is mentally impaired. Make adaptations for impaired vision and hearing as necessary, such as cleaning glasses and providing a pad and pen for written communication. Allow adequate time for the patient to respond to you. Be sensitive to the patient's need to communicate and allow time to talk. Be a good listener. Explain procedures honestly. Treat the patient with respect. Allow the patient to set his own routine, as much as possible. Adjust room temperature to the patient's preference. Control environmental noise. Inform the patient about policies, services, and routines, as appropriate. Avoid rapid changes in position. Allow the patient to dangle at the bedside prior to transfer and ambulation. Maintain a well-lighted, safe environment. ∎

uals express these basic needs. *Culture* refers to those customs and practices that are common to groups of people that become ingrained beliefs, habits, and responses. Culture embraces language, dietary habits, health practices, expressions of spirituality, and ways of celebrating. These cultural patterns are part of the uniqueness of each individual and must be considered when providing the person's care.

Abraham Maslow and Erik Erikson are two leaders in the field of human behavior. They have helped us understand basic needs and how people go about satisfying them.

Personality

Exactly how each person goes about satisfying personal psychological needs reflects his personality. **Personality** is the sum of ways we react to the events in our lives. It is gradually formed through experience and molded by cultural heritage.

Erikson suggested that our personalities are formed as we mature from infancy to old age. He believed that we pass through eight growing stages in search of who we really are (**self-identity**). During each stage, there are choices to be made before moving on to the next task. He called these the **tasks of personality development** (Table 9-3).

TABLE 9-3 TASKS OF PERSONALITY DEVELOPMENT ACCORDING TO THE STAGES DEFINED BY ERIKSON

Physical Stage	Year of Occurrence	Tasks to Be Mastered
Oral-sensory	Birth–1 year (infant)	To learn to trust (Trust)
Muscular-anal	1–3 years (toddler)	To recognize self as being independent from mother (Autonomy)
Locomotor	3–5 years (preschool years)	To recognize self as a family member (Initiative)
Latency	6–11 years (school-age years)	To demonstrate physical and mental skills/abilities (Industry)
Adolescence	12–18 years	To develop a sense of individuality as a sexual human being (Identity)
Young Adulthood	19-35 years	To establish intimate personal relationships with a mate (Intimacy)
Adulthood	35–50 years	To live a satisfying and productive life
Maturity	50+ years	To review life's events and examine how they have influenced the development of a unique individual (Ego integrity)

Maslow described human needs as physical, psychological, and sociological. He placed the needs on a **continuum** in which physical needs had to be satisfied first. The psychological or sociological needs can be met only after the physical needs have been satisfied (Figure 9-8). The progression of needs is called a *hierarchy of needs*.

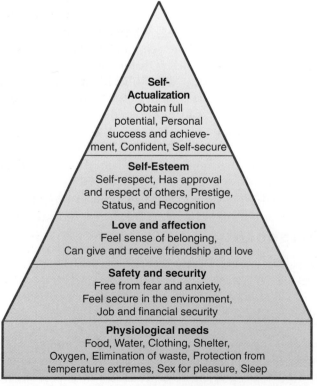

FIGURE 9-8 Maslow's hierarchy of needs. Lower-level needs must be satisfied before higher-level needs become important.

Physical Needs

The most basic human needs are physical needs. They include:

- Nutrition
- Rest
- Oxygen
- Shelter
- Elimination
- Activity
- Sexuality

Illness at any age creates stresses that make meeting the needs a challenge for both patient and caregivers.

Meeting the Patient's Physical Needs

You will need to provide for the physical needs of your patients. These are the need to be sheltered, to breathe, to eat, to sleep, and to eliminate waste products.

Shelter. In the health care facility, the need to be sheltered is met when the proper environment is maintained. Some examples include making sure that:

- A comfortable room temperature is maintained.
- Needed repairs are reported, such as a leaking faucet.

Oxygen. Most of us take breathing for granted. We hardly give it more than a passing thought until it becomes difficult. There are many reasons why people have trouble breathing. When they do have difficulty, though, the need is always the same. The body cannot live without oxygen, which is found in the air. It may be necessary, therefore, to give the patient extra oxygen to ensure that body tissues receive enough oxygen. Oxygen delivered by cannula, mask, or another device may be used for this purpose (Figure 9-9). Sometimes this need can be met by adjusting the overbed table in such a way that the patient, supported by pillows, is able to lean on it, making breathing easier.

Food. Patients may lose their appetites when they are in the hospital. Decreased appetite and intake of fluids may be due to:

- Inactivity
- Hospital odors
- Effects of some medications
- Pain
- Fear and anxiety
- Types of food served
- Illness itself
- Age of the patient

Some patients have to be fed because of their conditions. Some may be given only special foods. Some are unable to take food in the usual way. Some patients are given liquid nourishment through a feeding tube. Fluid replacement may also be given through a sterile tube into the veins.

Because patients receive nourishment in such a variety of ways, you must meet the special needs of each individual. There are, however, some general points to keep in mind:

- Patients will eat better and will be more comfortable if allowed or assisted to use the bathroom before meals.
- Appetites improve when food is served at the proper temperature in pleasant surroundings.
- Bathroom doors should be closed and unpleasant odors eliminated.
- Cultural preferences should be considered.
- Patients should be prepared by allowing them to wash hands and face. Help them sit up in bed or get out of bed, if permitted.

FIGURE 9-9 Allowing a child to play with the equipment before she has to use it is a good approach to take to decrease fear.

- The tray should be offered in a calm, pleasant manner, even if the food is not what you like. Even a bland diet offered in this way is more acceptable.
- Patients should be allowed to do as much as they are able for themselves. Be available, however, to assist if needed.

Sleep. See Unit 10 for a discussion of the patient's sleep and rest needs.

Elimination. To stay healthy, the body must be able to rid itself of perspiration, urine, and feces. Elimination is promoted by:

- Bathing, which helps get rid of perspiration and keeps the skin healthy.
- Encouraging the patient to drink six to eight glasses of fluids and, if possible, to eat foods high in fiber.
- Providing additional help, if needed, to relieve the patient's body of waste. A sterile tube (catheter) can be inserted into the urinary bladder to drain the urine out. The sterile catheter may be left in the bladder to provide constant drainage. The tube is then attached to a bag that collects the urine. Enemas, laxatives, and suppositories help the bowels get rid of solid wastes in the form of feces.
- Helping patients who are unable to use the usual toilet facilities, by providing them with bedpans, urinals, and bedside commodes.

Physical Activity. People, by nature, are active beings. When illness occurs, it often limits activity. Sometimes the patient must stay in bed for a long time. The staff must find ways to promote appropriate activity for these individuals. The capability of the patient and the goals of treatment must be kept in mind when the activity level of any patient is established.

The complications resulting from inactivity and actions to take to avoid these complications are presented in Units 41 and 48.

Activity promotes improved functioning of all systems. Circulation and respiration are increased. Muscles, bones, and joints function more efficiently. The body as a whole responds in a positive way to activity.

When patients are unable to carry out activity, such as walking, getting into and out of bed, and using the bedpan or commode independently, you may have to help them (Figure 9-10). Be sure you are aware of the patient's limitations, as well as the degree and type of activity allowed. Encourage patients to do as much as possible, but do not allow them to become either overstressed or tired.

Security and Safety Needs

If physical needs are not being met, the individual has no energy to be concerned about safety. For example, a mother whose children are starving may risk her life to provide food. Once physical needs are provided for, safety

FIGURE 9-10 This patient needs minimal assistance with ambulation.

and security become priorities. Security and safety for patients are provided by:

- Maintaining a safe environment (see Units 14 and 15).
- Knowing how to respond to medical emergencies, such as patient falls.
- Knowing how to respond to facility emergencies, such as fire.
- Implementing the patient's care plan as indicated.

Emotional Needs

The third and fourth levels of Maslow's hierarchy are related to emotional needs, including the need for love and belonging and the need for esteem. There is a need:

- To give love
- To feel love
- To be loved
- To be treated with respect and dignity
- To feel that self-esteem (our opinion of ourselves) is protected

All individuals—you, your coworkers, and your patients —have in their own minds an idea of how they appear and wish to appear to others. This idea is referred to as

self-esteem. A person's self-esteem must be protected at all costs.

For example, a person might visualize and project to others the image of a very self-reliant person, capable of making important decisions and able to care for self and family. Suddenly that same person is scantily dressed in a hospital bed. A stranger is taking care of her most intimate physical functions. Even the times to eat and bathe are decided for her. This set of circumstances threatens even the most secure person's self-esteem.

A patient's response to this threat to self-esteem depends on two things. First, it depends on how often the patient has had these feelings of helplessness before, and how well he has dealt with them. Second, it depends on you and your ability to appreciate those feelings.

One patient may feel frustrated and angry. He may not even know that these feelings are based on fear. The patient may act out these feelings by complaining about the hospital, the staff, roommates, you, or the food. In fact, every aspect of the care may be cause for complaint. Be open and receptive to these actions, recognizing the underlying feelings.

Still another patient may react quite differently to the same emotional stress. That person may be quiet and withdrawn. She may be completely cooperative and noncomplaining (Figure 9-11). The behavior shown is a false front. It hides the patient's feelings of not being able to cope with the situation. The nursing assistant must be aware of these feelings and the need for caring support.

Intimacy and Sexuality

Intimacy is a feeling of closeness with another human (Figure 9-12). It is a relationship marked by feelings of love and affection. It is an integral part of human response.

Sexuality is a lifelong characteristic that defines the maleness or femaleness of each person. This definition may be different for each person. All individuals are sexual, whether or not they have physical sexual relations. Sexuality has to do with the ability to develop relationships, to

FIGURE 9-11 Patience may be necessary to break through a wall of fear and frustration.

FIGURE 9-12 Everyone needs intimacy and human touch. This is important regardless of the patient's age or appearance. If in doubt about the patient's response, ask her permission to touch or hug her.

give of oneself to others, and to appreciate the giving by others. Intimacy is one aspect of sexuality.

Intimacy may be shared between friends or lovers. Also, a degree of intimacy is established when patient and caregiver learn to trust and have confidence in each other.

Intimate relationships may be sexual and expressed in different ways. Humans express sexual intimacy depending on orientation, preference, opportunity, and moral standards. Sexual behavior is a personal choice, but intimacy is an important aspect of the human sexual experience.

Each intimate relationship has an element of commitment. Sometimes this commitment includes a sexual aspect and sometimes it does not. For example, a loving couple may choose not to have sexual intercourse. Despite remaining **celibate** (no sexual intercourse), they still share an intimacy and commitment that is natural and fulfilling.

Being old, ill, or disabled does not diminish human sexuality. However, our society tends to associate youth, beauty, and physical agility with sexuality. By these standards, persons who are old or disabled are not considered to be sexual beings. It is important to remember that the person within a human being does not change. Although the hair is gray, or the body is not so agile, the person inside still has feelings and longing for love, affection, and intimacy. As a nursing assistant, there are several actions you can take to help patients maintain their sexuality:

- Give attention to the patient's grooming and appearance.
- Give sincere compliments on their appearance.
- Converse with patients on an adult level.

It is important to recognize that not everyone has the same orientation, preference, opportunities, or moral standards. This does not mean that differences make one

person wrong and another right. As a caregiver, you must be understanding of others who do not share your personal views.

Some terms related to human sexual expression are:

- **Heterosexuality**—sexual attraction between opposite sexes.
- **Homosexuality**—sexual attraction between persons of the same sex. Female partners are called lesbians. Male partners are often referred to as being gay.
- **Bisexuality**—sexual attraction to members of both sexes.
- **Masturbation**—self-stimulation for sexual pleasure.

The range of ways to express love is enormous. Genital and nongenital caressing, exchange of loving gestures, talking, hugging, and touching are all ways love is expressed between people. **Coitus** (intercourse), although an enjoyable part of many relationships, is not always necessary for satisfaction.

Providing opportunities for patients to meet sexual and intimate needs in a health care setting is not always easy. However, there are some actions that nursing assistants can do to help patients meet these needs:

- Respect patients' privacy. Always knock and wait before opening a closed door.
- Speak before opening curtains drawn around the bed.
- Do not judge behaviors and preferences that are different from yours as wrong.
- Do not discuss personal sexual information about a patient with others.
- Provide privacy if a patient is masturbating, and avoid passing judgment on this activity.
- Discourage patients who make sexual advances to you. State in a calm, matter-of-fact way that you are not interested and move on to other work. If a patient persists, report the matter to the nurse.
- Recognize that the need for intimacy is a basic human need that is expressed in many ways.

Human Touch

The need for human touch should not be overlooked. Pleasure and satisfaction are felt by a parent and child as they touch one another. The same human feelings are also experienced by adults.

As people grow older, they tend to reserve touching for intimate friends and family members. When circumstances change and opportunities for touching become fewer, people often feel deprived and lonely. This is especially true when one lives alone or is a resident in long-term care.

A friendly hug and smile, a pat on the shoulder, a clasp of a hand, and a backrub are ways that nursing assistants can satisfy the patient's need for human contact. Never force your attentions on a patient, but be open to nonsexual touching. It can mean much to the lives of those in your care.

You will learn that wearing gloves is sometimes necessary for the procedures you must do. Sometimes caregivers apply gloves as soon as they enter the room and wear gloves for all care. There are times when this is necessary, but wearing gloves is not necessary or desirable for most patient care situations. Wearing gloves may send a message that the patient is undesirable, untouchable, or highly infectious. Avoid offending patients with unnecessary use of gloves. Always remember the powerful need for human contact. Balance your infection control precautions with patients' emotional needs for love, belonging, and acceptance.

Dealing with the Fearful Patient

The experienced nursing assistant does not take remarks personally. The assistant realizes that the patient's complaints and refusal to cooperate may be a way of saying, "I need to be reassured and protected." Give the patient an opportunity to talk. Listen carefully to everything that is said (Figure 9-13). You may be able to convince the fearful patient to assume some personal care whenever possible. If help in feeding, shaving, elimination, or other such personal matters is needed, act in a very gentle, efficient manner and assure the patient's privacy at all times.

To handle these situations successfully, the nursing assistant must:

- Recognize that this patient is a person with individual likes and dislikes.
- Give the quality of care that considers these likes and dislikes. Honoring the patient's preference will cause her to be more satisfied with the care. Meeting the patient's needs at this level is an excellent way of giving person-centered, individualized care.
- Help the patient find ways to fill the time while in the hospital (Figure 9-14). Boredom alone can lead to irritability. Some hospitals have volunteers who bring books and other activities directly to the bedside.

Patient Privacy

Patients in the hospital give up a good bit of control over their lives. They put their lives and well-being into the

FIGURE 9-14 Activities help pass the time during convalescence.

hands of caregivers. In exchange, patients assume that certain of their rights will be assured. These rights include the right to privacy.

Patients must feel certain that their privacy will be protected. Even though you perform the most intimate procedures for them, you must do so in a way that neither exposes them unnecessarily nor embarrasses them. Privacy may be provided by means of:

- Curtains or screens placed around the bed.
- Knocking and saying the patient's name before entering a room.
- Speaking to the patient before entering a screened area. Privacy must be provided for the patient who is:
  - bathing
  - using the bedpan
  - receiving treatments
  - being visited by clergy

Be prompt at other times to recognize a patient's need for privacy and to provide it.

Patients must also be certain that personal information they share with you will not be told to others. You add to patients' sense of security if you always treat them with the courtesy you would extend to a guest in your home.

Understanding what patients are really trying to tell us is one of the most difficult parts of giving care. When we are successful, it is probably the most rewarding. With this in mind, always remember to treat each patient as a unique individual.

Spiritual Needs

Spiritual beliefs are deeply held by some patients and disregarded by others. When beliefs are strongly held, they are apt to guide a patient's actions and responses in direct ways, such as praying, reading religious writings, and participating in ceremonies and celebrations. Some personal items may have special religious significance and must be treated with respect.

Patients' spiritual needs are often greater when they are fearful and ill (Figure 9-15). Be prepared to act on

FIGURE 9-13 Successful communication is a two-way exchange.

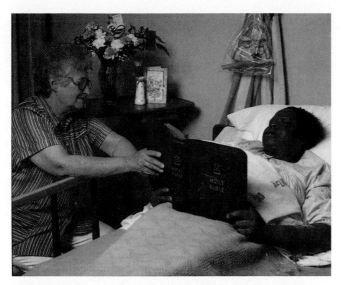

FIGURE 9-15 Spiritual needs may be greater during illness.

requests for clergy visits and spiritual support. Do not impose your beliefs on the patient.

There is always the temptation to share your personal religious faith with others. This is especially true when the patient directly asks your opinion. To handle such a situation appropriately is a challenge. Here are some guidelines to assist you.

- Remember that each person has a right to believe in any faith system or to deny the existence of any beliefs.
- Listen to the patient's thoughts and keep them confidential.
- Your role is to reflect the patient's ideas. Do not try to convince the patient of your ideas. For example, if the patient asks you if you believe in God, reflect the patient's thinking with a statement such as "You have been thinking about God," or "Would you like to talk?"

The patient may want to visit with a familiar clergy member, or may ask about the chaplain or clergy service available at the health care facility.

Some health care facilities ask clergy from the community to make visits to patients who want such a visit but who do not know a particular minister, priest, or rabbi. Larger facilities have chaplain educational residencies for people preparing for careers in the clergy. The residencies serve patients' spiritual needs while offering training for the chaplains.

Chapels are open in some facilities. Both visitors and ambulatory patients often find comfort in visiting them. Religious services are sometimes broadcast to patients' rooms from these chapels.

Know what services are available to your patients. When asked, share this information, but do not recommend any particular service. Patients should be free to make their own choices. You should always be ready and willing to support the choice.

Social Needs

When primary physical, psychological, and spiritual needs have been met, the person is free to pursue the third level of social needs and activities that are unique to the individual. These activities make one feel good as a person and increase self-esteem. They give a sense of accomplishment. Sociological needs are met by interactions with others and opportunities for free personal expression.

One of the most basic needs of all people is the need to understand others and to be understood. We achieve this sense of understanding when we communicate successfully with others. We usually try to communicate verbally. Sometimes we do this also by the:

- Words we choose
- Way we say the words
- Tone of voice
- Facial expression
- Form of touch

Even the way we stand or reach out says a lot. We know it is not always easy to find the right words to express our thoughts and feelings. Thus, caregivers must be constantly aware of the patient's need to communicate effectively, too.

Volunteers and visitors, as well as television and reading, can provide entertainment and diversion for the patient who is confined. Try to find out about patients' special interests. Look for ways to support them in these interests.

If all care providers are interested and unhurried in talking with patients, they make it easier for patients to say what they need. This approach also makes it easier for the staff to find proper ways to fulfill these needs.

REVIEW

A. True/False.

Mark the following true or false by circling T or F.

1. T F Growth and development go from the simple to the complex.

2. T F Body development proceeds from the head toward the feet.

3. T F All individuals move through the stages of growth.

4. T F Growth and development progression are interdependent.

5. T F Ossification of bones is not complete at birth.

6. T F The Moro reflex occurs when the infant's palm is touched.

7. T F The sucking reflex occurs when the infant is startled.

8. T F The three-month-old infant cries real tears.

9. T F The six-month-old infant can walk if well supported.

10. T F First teeth begin to erupt about the sixth month of life.

11. T F The one-year-old infant has progressed to eating table foods.

12. T F During the toddler period, children interact freely and play well with one another.

13. T F Between the ages of three and five years, the child seems to have an endless list of questions.

14. T F The school-age child is interested in and chooses members of the same sex as close friends.

15. T F One of the developmental tasks of old age is to learn to deal successfully with loss.

16. T F Basic human needs are the same at all ages, but different ways must be found to satisfy them.

17. T F Erikson believed that one of the developmental tasks of infancy is learning to trust.

18. T F Erikson states that the developmental task of the middle years is to integrate life's experiences.

19. T F Patients who are fearful often show anger or frustration.

20. T F Spiritual needs are part of basic human needs.

21. T F Culture has no influence over how basic human needs are met.

B. Matching.

Match the appropriate chronologic age to the life time period by matching Column I and Column II.

Column I		Column II
22. _____ old age		**a.** 65 years old
23. _____ adolescence		**b.** 16 years old
24. _____ later maturity		**c.** 7 years old
25. _____ school age		**d.** 35 years old
26. _____ adulthood		**e.** 80 years old

C. Multiple Choice.

Select the one best answer for each of the following.

27. Growth and development
  a. move from limbs to torso and feet to head.
  b. involve more complex tasks during growth spurts.
  c. can proceed normally even if tasks are not mastered.
  d. have specific tasks that must be mastered at each stage.

28. The main activity (activities) of the toddler period is (are)
  a. exploration and investigation.
  b. cooperative play.
  c. establishing peer relationships.
  d. showing concern for others.

29. Preschoolers are
  a. less reliant on their mothers.
  b. able to join groups like Scouts.
  c. able to choose sex-differentiated friends.
  d. unable to tolerate brief separation from the mother.

30. The ways in which we react to the events in our lives are called
  a. personality.
  b. self-identity.
  c. tasks of personality development.
  d. hierarchy of needs.

D. Nursing Assistant Challenge.

Mrs. McClendon is a 35-year-old patient with a diagnosis of breast cancer. She recently had a radical mastectomy. She has lost most of her hair and has no appetite as a result of chemotherapy. Mrs. McClendon has lost weight and has occasional severe pain. She has a husband and three young children. Consider the needs that all people have and think about Mrs. McClendon.

31. Which physical needs may be difficult to meet? What can the nursing staff do to help Mrs. McClendon meet these needs?

32. Do you think her need for safety and security will be met? What information do you have indicating that she has reason to feel fear and anxiety?

33. How might Mrs. McClendon's condition affect her relationship with her husband and children?

34. How do you think her sexuality may be affected?

35. Maslow states that human needs are on a hierarchy. Describe how this hierarchy may change throughout the day for Mrs. McClendon.

UNIT 10

Comfort, Pain, Rest, and Sleep

OBJECTIVES

After completing this unit, you will be able to:

- Spell and define terms.
- Explain how loud noise affects patients and hospital staff.
- Explain why nursing comfort measures are important to patients' well-being.
- List six observations to make and report for patients having pain.

- State the purpose of the pain rating scale and briefly describe how a pain scale is used.
- Describe nursing assistant measures to increase comfort and relieve pain.
- List nursing comfort measures that promote rest.
- Describe the phases of the sleep cycle and the importance of each.
- List nursing measures to promote sleep.

VOCABULARY

Learn the meaning and the correct spelling of the following words and phrases:

analgesic	insomnia	rapid eye movement	sleep deprivation
bruxism	narcolepsy	(REM) sleep	somnambulism
comfort	nonrapid eye movement	rest	
enuresis	(NREM) sleep	sleep	
hypersomnia	pain	sleep apnea	

PATIENT COMFORT

All humans need comfort, rest, and sleep for physical and emotional well-being, health, and wellness. **Comfort** is a state of physical and emotional well-being. The patient is calm and relaxed, and is not in pain or upset. Assisting patients with their comfort needs is a major nursing assistant responsibility. In fact, assisting patients with physical or emotional comfort needs is at the heart of nursing care. Many factors affect patients' comfort. Environmental factors that interfere with comfort are unfamiliar environment, lack of privacy, noise, odor, temperature, lighting, and ventilation. Personal and uncontrollable factors that may increase or contribute to discomfort include age, activity, injury, illness, surgery, stress, and pain.

As a rule, patients are uncomfortable when their physical and emotional needs are not met. Unmet needs cause tension and anxiety, and interfere with comfort and rest (Figure 10-1). Using basic nursing measures to meet patients' needs promotes comfort, aids in relaxation, and provides a sense of well-being.

NOISE CONTROL

Florence Nightingale is considered the founder of modern nursing. In *Notes on Nursing*, she wrote, "Unnecessary noise is the most cruel abuse of care which can be inflicted on either the sick or the well. For, in all these remarks, the sick are only mentioned as suffering in a

FIGURE 10-1 This patient's body language betrays the anxiety she is feeling.

greater proportion than the well from precisely the same causes. Such unnecessary noise has undoubtedly induced or aggravated delirium in many cases. Again, one nurse cannot open the door without making everything rattle. Or she opens the door unnecessarily often, for want of remembering all the articles that might be brought in at once. A good nurse will always make sure that no door or window in her patient's room shall rattle or creak; that no blind or curtain shall, by any change of wind through the open window, be made to flap—especially will she be careful of all this before she leaves her patients for the night. If you wait till your patients tell you, or remind you of these things, where is the use of their having a nurse? There are more shy than exacting patients, in all classes; and many a patient passes a bad night, time after time, rather than remind his nurse every night of all the things she has forgotten. If there are blinds to your windows, always take care to have them well up, when they are not being used. A little piece slipping down, and flapping with every draught, will distract a patient. The fidget of silk and of crinoline, the rattling of keys, the creaking of stays and of shoes, will do a patient more harm than all the medicines in the world will do him good. A nurse who rustles (I am speaking of nurses professional and unprofessional) is the horror of a patient, though perhaps he does not know why" (1859, pp. 25–30).[1] Miss Nightingale would be aghast at the high-tech world of the 21st century. Although the pants worn with uniforms and scrubs are quiet when we move, we have alarms on most medical equipment and electronic technology that did not exist in the 19th century.

Comfort, rest, and sleep are important for patient well-being. Excessive noise has been shown to delay healing, impair immune function, and increase heart rate and blood pressure. Patients may feel very stressed or anxious, and may not realize that noise is the cause of their distress. Patients who do not sleep well at night may be unhappy with care, and be unable to stay awake during the day for meals and therapy. Some patients become

OSHA ALERT

OSHA is a government agency that protects the health and safety of employees and surveys health care facilities. The inspectors review infection control, isolation practices, tuberculin testing, material safety data sheets, and other policies and facility practices. The OSHA surveyor interviews employees, tours the facility, and asks questions about health and safety practices. If unsafe conditions are found, the inspector will make recommendations for correction. ■

confused and agitated when deprived of sleep. Confused patients may begin wandering to escape the noise.

The Occupational Safety and Health Administration (OSHA) has established noise standards for employee safety. These standards state that workers should not be exposed to 90 decibels of sound for more than eight hours. Average noise levels are listed in Table 10-1. The Environmental Protection Agency (EPA) recommends that hospital noise levels not exceed 45 decibels during the day. Examples of various types of noise are pictured in Figure 10-2.

A study done by the staff of one hospital unit has direct implications for nursing assistant practice.[2] In this study, nurse researchers were admitted to the hospital as patients. Noise levels were measured with special instruments during the night. The workers who were on duty did not know of the study or that noise was being measured. During the study, decibel levels as high as 113 were recorded at night. The noisiest time was at shift change, when more visitors, physicians, and nursing staff were entering or leaving the unit. Two nurses who acted as patients noted that this noise prevented them from falling asleep. They also found that noise from equipment alarms, phones, carts, X-ray machines, opening and closing doors, the paging and intercom systems, roommates, and nursing personnel interrupted their sleep. Noises that were tolerable during the day were more disruptive at night.

[1]Nightingale, F. (1859). *Notes on nursing*. London: Harrison and Sons.

[2]Cmiel, C. A. et al. (2004). Noise control: A nursing team's approach to sleep promotion. *American Journal of Nursing, 104*(2), 40–48.

TABLE 10-1 AVERAGE NOISE LEVELS

Noise in Decibels (dB)	Source (range in dB)
194	loudest tone possible
180	rocket launch
165	12-gauge shotgun
140	jet engine at takeoff
120	ambulance siren
119	pneumatic percussion drill
110	chainsaw
108	continuous miner
105	bulldozer, spray painter
98	hand drill
96	tractor
93	belt sander
90	hair dryer, power lawn mower
80	ringing telephone
60	normal conversation
30	whisper
0	weakest sound heard by the average human ear

Modified from National Institute for Occupational Safety and Health (NIOSH). (2001). General estimates of work-related noises. Retrieved November 15, 2004, from http://www.cdc.gov/niosh/01-104.html

An uncomfortable noise level has been called an invasion of privacy by some patients. This is a concern because the patient is powerless to control the disturbing noise. Noise inside the facility has been called an "invisible pollutant." Noise should never interfere with patients' ability to hear, cause distress or anxiety, or make patients feel as if the noise is an invasion of their privacy.

A 1960 study at Johns Hopkins Hospital revealed that the average noise level was 57 decibels. A repeat study in 2005 found that the noise had increased to 72 decibels.[3] In 1995, the World Health Organization (WHO) recommended keeping noise levels below 35 decibels in hospi-

[3]Britt, R. R. (2005). Hospitals getting noisier, threatening patient safety. *Live Science*. Retrieved November 22, 2005, from http://www.livescience.com/othernews/051121_noisy_hospitals.html

FIGURE 10-2 Sound intensity generated by various activities. One study showed that hospital noises during the night were as loud as jackhammers and chainsaws, making it difficult for patients to sleep. Simple steps, such as closing doors to patients' rooms and muffling the clatter of clipboards and metal charts, help reduce noise.

tals. However, a Houston area long-term care facility study in 2005 revealed noise levels from 70 to 101 decibels.

Staff must speak louder to be heard over background noise. Some people call this the "cocktail party effect," because everyone speaks more loudly to be heard as the noise level around them increases. Most of the staff complained of feeling agitated and irritable, and were prone to making errors when the environment was noisy.[4] Surprisingly, noise is listed as a contributing factor to stress and exhaustion. Active listening requires focusing on the conversation. Hospital workers must be active listeners, whether they are listening to patients or coworkers. Active listening is work. Having to talk louder and having to be more attentive when listening to others is considered one of the leading causes of fatigue in hospital staff.

Reducing noise improves working conditions for staff and quality of care for patients. The effects of noise and sleep deprivation are areas in which additional study is needed, but it is safe to say that research proves that nighttime

[4]McClaugherty, L., Valibhai, F., & Womack, S. (2005). Physiological and psychological effects of noise on healthcare professionals and residents in long-term care facilities and enhancing quality of life. *The Director, 13*(2). Retrieved August 30, 2005, from http://www.nadona.org/noise.htm

noise is disruptive. In keeping with your facility policies, do all you can to reduce and manage noise.

PAIN

Pain (Figure 10-3) is a state of discomfort that is unpleasant for the patient. Pain is always a warning that something is wrong. It interferes with the patient's optimal level of function and self-care. Patients may limit movement when they are having pain. Unrelieved pain contributes to complications of immobility, increasing the risk of pneumonia, skin breakdown, and other problems. Pain decreases quality of life, and may cause hopelessness, anxiety, depression, and a feeling of helplessness. Pain may cause acting out, crying, and other strange, belligerent, or combative behavior in both children and adults. Pain is a major preventable public health problem that slows recovery in individuals with acute illness and increases health care costs.

Relieving pain has always been an important nursing responsibility. Nursing staff must identify patients who are having pain, and those who are at risk for pain, then take the appropriate action to ensure that all patients are made as comfortable as possible.

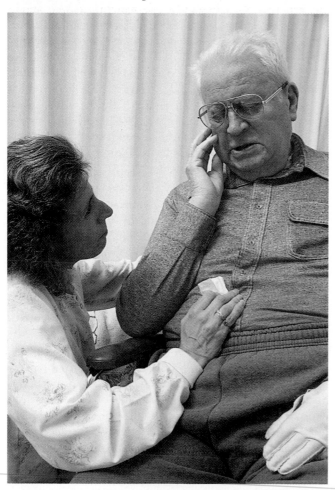

FIGURE 10-3 This patient's body language suggests that he is having severe pain.

Age-Appropriate Care ALERT

The golden rule for pain relief is that whatever is painful to adults is painful to children unless proven otherwise. Pain control should be based on scientific facts, not personal beliefs or opinions. Never lie to a child when asked if a procedure will hurt. Admit that it will, but assure the child that you will be there and that the child will be made as comfortable as possible. ■

Patients' Responses to Pain

Patients' responses to pain vary widely. Some individuals do not feel pain as acutely as others. Some try to ignore pain. Other patients may try to deny pain because they are afraid of what it means. Ignoring or denying pain increases the risk of injury because the normal warning that pain provides goes unrecognized or unheeded.

Never ignore body language or other signs of pain in patients. Use nursing measures to make the patient comfortable. Always report pain to the nurse. Your observations are a valuable contribution to the nursing assessment and patients' comfort.

Patients' responses to pain may be related to culture. People from some cultures are very emotional when they are in pain. Others are very stoic. Some think that showing pain is a sign of weakness. Some believe that pain is a punishment from a deity or higher power.

Pain causes stress and anxiety, interfering with comfort, rest, and sleep (Figure 10-4). Rest and sleep are necessary for the body to repair itself and to restore strength and energy. Insomnia (inability to sleep), restlessness, and disturbed sleep may be caused by pain.

FIGURE 10-4 Although her expression is stoic, the patient cannot sleep because of pain and anxiety.

Identifying Patients in Pain and at Risk for Pain

Pain is a serious condition that affects well-being and quality of life. Patients have the right to timely pain assessment and management. Many factors affect patients' reactions to pain. The reactions may be different from one moment to the next and from one patient to another. Four types of pain are listed in Table 10-2. Monitor patients' body language for signs of pain.

Body language is often the first clue that a patient is having pain. This may be the only clue in some pediatric and cognitively impaired patients, those from other cultures, and patients who are comatose. Look for pain upon movement, facial expressions, crying, moaning, rigid posture, and guarded positioning. The patient may withdraw when he or she is touched or repositioned. Watch for restlessness, irregular or erratic respirations, intermittent breath holding, dilated pupils, and sweating. The patient may favor one extremity. He or she may become irritable, fatigued, or withdrawn. The patient may refuse to eat for no apparent reason. Often, the patient acts opposite of normal. For example:

- A cognitively impaired geriatric patient who is normally very quiet may become noisy.
- A pediatric patient may cry for no apparent reason.
- A patient with garbled speech may accurately describe his or her pain.

TABLE 10-2 TYPES OF PAIN

Type of Pain	Description
Acute pain	Occurs suddenly and without warning. Acute pain is usually the result of tissue damage, caused by conditions such as injury or surgery. Typically, acute pain decreases over time, as healing takes place.
Persistent pain (Chronic pain)	Persistent pain lasts longer than six months. It may be intermittent or constant. Persistent pain may be caused by multiple medical conditions.
Phantom pain	Phantom pain occurs as a result of an amputation. For example, the patient has had a leg removed, but complains of pain in the toes. The pain is real, not imaginary.
Radiating pain	Radiating pain moves from the site of origin to other areas. For example, when a patient is having a heart attack, the pain may radiate from the chest to the jaw or arm.

- The agitated and combative patient may become quiet and nonverbal.
- A friendly and outgoing patient may begin to cry easily and withdraw.
- The patient who is normally active may become still and quiet.

Always suspect pain if the patient's behavior changes. Report your observations to the nurse compared with the normal behavior for the patient. If the behavior changes back to normal after the nurse administers an **analgesic** (pain) medication, this confirms that the change in body language or behavior was caused by pain.

Although many patients with pain display outward signs through their body language and behavior, avoid making assumptions about the presence or absence of pain if the patient is laughing, talking, or sleeping. For example, some health care workers assume that patients who are smiling or laughing cannot be in pain. These workers believe that patients who are having pain should be grimacing, frowning, or crying. This is untrue. Some patients may appear comfortable even while they are having severe pain. Vital signs may be normal.

Avoid judging the patient or making assumptions about the patient's pain. Regularly ask patients if they are in pain. Some will not volunteer this information if not asked directly. A patient may not display an outward appearance of pain, so asking if he is having pain is the best way to find out. *The patient's self-report is the most accurate and reliable indicator of the existence and intensity of pain, and should be respected and believed.* Never question the validity of a patient's complaints. Simply notify the nurse of the patient's complaint of pain.

Pain management is an important part of patient care. Take complaints of pain very seriously. Respect and support the patients' right to pain assessment and management without judgment or disbelief. You are responsible for reporting the information to the nurse, who will assess the patient and take the appropriate action. Avoid passing judgment on patients who take narcotic medications to control their pain. Many health care workers try to discourage patients from taking these drugs because of the potential for addiction. Studies have shown that very few patients with severe pain become addicted to the drugs.

When asking patients about pain, make sure the patient can see and hear you. Allow enough time for the patient to process your questions and respond. Be patient. Use language that is appropriate for the patient's age and mental status. Remember that patients may use different words for pain, such as "hurt," "sore," or "tender." Children and patients who are mentally confused may surprise you. Some can describe their pain accurately. Always ask patients who are crying, who display body language suggesting pain, or whose behavior suggests pain.

Observing and Reporting Signs and Symptoms of Pain

Pain always requires further intervention. It should never be ignored. Always report verbal complaints of pain, describing the pain in the patient's exact words. Be aware of signs and symptoms of pain in patients who have difficulty communicating, such as infants, children, patients who cannot speak, and patients with cognitive impairments. Clues that the patient is having pain include:

- Facial expressions
- Grimacing
- Refusing to move
- Stiff, rigid, or limited movements
- Moaning, crying, yelling, or screaming

Report your observations to the nurse.

A nursing assessment of pain involves many different factors. Your observations contribute to this assessment and the patient's well-being. Other important information you may see, hear, and observe that should be reported to the nurse includes:

- Vital signs
- Skin color
- Location of pain (specific site of pain on the body)
- Radiation (movement of pain to other areas)
- Time of onset (when the pain began)
- Duration (how long the pain lasts)
- Frequency (how often it occurs)
- Pain quality (nature and type of pain)
- Pain intensity (strength and description of pain, in the patient's own words)
- Aggravating and alleviating factors (things that improve or worsen the pain)
- Character (properties, features, characteristics)
- Variation or patterns of pain (changes in pain or cycles of pain)
- Pain management history, if any (things the patient tells you about past history of pain and things that make it better or worse)

- Present pain management regimen, if any, and its effectiveness (things the patient does to relieve pain, including response to comfort measures and medications)
- Effect of pain on activities of daily living, sleep, appetite, relationships, emotions, concentration, and the like
- Direct observation of abnormalities at the site of the pain
- Other observations, such as facial expressions, body language, movements, nausea or vomiting
- Side effects of analgesic (pain-relieving) medications, if applicable
- Response to pain medications and other forms of treatment, if applicable.

Pain Assessment Scales

The nurse may use a pain scale to help assess and manage the patient's pain. The scale is a tool for communication. The patient selects the scale that best helps her describe the pain. Most facilities have several different pain scales available. Different scales may be used for children and adults. Using a pain scale prevents subjective opinions, and keeps everyone informed as to the level and intensity of the patient's pain. The patient and nurse may have established a pain management goal using the scale. The patient may refer to the goal in conversation with you, so you should become familiar with the scales used at your facility.

Many different pain scales are used in health care. The scales shown in Figures 10-5A and 10-5B are for example only. Your facility may use similar or different tools for evaluating pain. Pain scales use pictures, words, or numbers to help the patient describe pain intensity. Most scales range from no pain to very severe pain. Picture scales use a range from smiling faces and neutral faces to frowns and tears.

Although you will not directly assess patients' pain, you must understand the purpose of the scales used in your facility and how they are interpreted. Many facilities use a 0 to 10 scale, with 0 meaning no pain and 10 meaning intolerable pain. If the patient tells you that she is having

	0	1	2	3	4	5
	NO HURT	HURTS LITTLE BIT	HURTS LITTLE MORE	HURTS EVEN MORE	HURTS WHOLE LOT	HURTS WORST
Alternate Coding	0	2	4	6	8	10

FIGURE 10-5A Each patient will select the pain rating scale that best helps describe the level and intensity of pain. The FACES scale is excellent for children needs adults, as well as patients who do not speak English. (FACES Pain Rating Scale from Hockenberry, M. J., Wilson, D., & Winkelstein, M. L. (2005). *Wong's essentials of pediatric nursing,* ed. 7. St. Louis: Mosby, p. 1259. Used with permission. Copyright © Mosby)

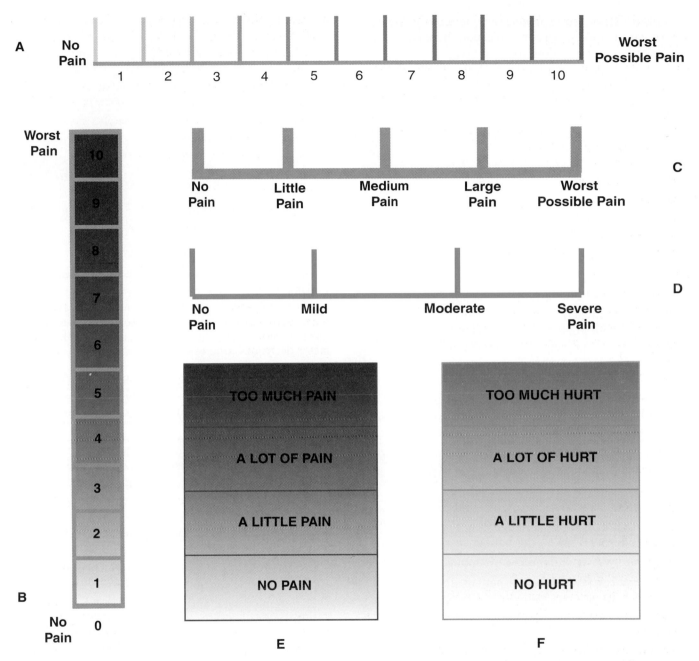

FIGURE 10-5B (A) Horizontal numeric pain scale (B) Vertical numeric pain scale (C) Verbal descriptor pain scale (D) Verbal pain scale (E) Verbal pain scale (F) Verbal pain scale

pain at "level 5," for example, you must know what this means and report the problem to the nurse. Likewise, if the patient complains of pain at "level 9" an hour after receiving pain medication, this suggests a potentially serious problem and must be reported immediately.

Some patients may not complain of pain and may appear to be comfortable. Asking them if they are having pain is not offensive. Always ask instead of assuming. Likewise, if a patient has been medicated for pain, but continues to complain, inform the nurse. Do not assume that the pain has been relieved after a medication has been given, even if the patient is laughing or talking. Ask the patient. If he or she admits to continued pain, the nurse must assess the patient further.

Managing Pain

Many facilities have a strong commitment to relieving patients' pain and suffering. They consider pain assessment and management a legal right of each person. This is because unrelieved pain has the potential to affect all areas of a patient's life. Pain is promptly assessed on admission. Pain assessment and management continue aggressively throughout the patient's stay. It is also a focus of patient teaching for discharge. Because of the importance of this care, many consider pain assessment the "fifth vital sign."

Unrelieved pain has a negative effect on the patient's health and functional status. Notify the nurse as soon as the patient complains, before pain becomes severe or out of control. Report your observations objectively. Observe the patient carefully after pain medications have been given, and report your observations to the nurse.

Sometimes the physician orders several different medications for a patient's pain. The nurse will select which drug to use based on an assessment of the patient (Figure 10-6). Your observations, the patient's self-report of pain intensity, and physical assessment findings are all considered when the nurse determines which medication to administer, when more than one is ordered. If the first drug does not relieve the pain, the nurse may have the option of administering another, so always report unrelieved pain. The quality of pain control is influenced by the education, experience, and attitude of the health care providers who are caring for the patient.

Although you as a nursing assistant are not directly responsible for pain management, your observations and nursing care are very important, because you work so closely and intimately with the patients. Understanding the responsibilities that health care providers have regarding pain relief will help you provide nursing comfort measures, monitor for signs and symptoms of pain, and report your observations to the nurse.

Nursing Assistant Comfort Measures. Relieving discomfort helps reduce pain and anxiety. Nursing

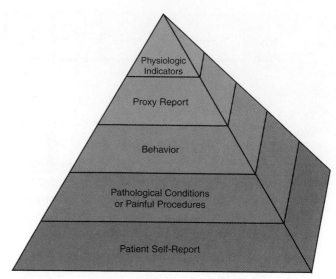

FIGURE 10-6 The hierarchy of pain assessment lists factors the health professional considers when evaluating pain. Factors at the bottom of the scale are given the most consideration. The importance and weight of each factor decreases progressively to the top.

assistants can use many basic nursing measures to make a patient more comfortable. These include:

- Telling patients what you plan to do and how you will do it
- Providing privacy
- Assisting the patient to assume a comfortable position (Figure 10-7)
- Repositioning the patient to relieve pain and muscle spasms
- Changing the angle of the bed to relieve tension on surgical sites or injured areas
- Avoiding sudden, jerking movements when moving or positioning the patient
- Performing passive range-of-motion exercises to reduce stiffness and maintain mobility
- Using pillows to support the affected body part(s) (Figure 10-8)
- Providing extra pillows and blankets for comfort and support
- Straightening the bed and linen
- Giving a backrub
- Washing the patient's face and hands
- Placing a cool, damp washcloth on the patient's forehead
- Providing oral hygiene
- Providing fresh water, food, or beverages as permitted
- Playing soft music to distract the patient
- Listening to patients' concerns
- Providing emotional support
- Maintaining a comfortable environmental temperature
- Providing a quiet, dark environment
- Eliminating unpleasant sights, sounds, and odors from the environment

Difficult SITUATIONS

Pain is very personal and subjective. One doctor tells a story of asking a patient to rate his pain using a 1 to 10 scale. The patient responded that the pain was a little more than level 2. When probed for information, the patient discussed his experiences in military service. He explained that his pain was a 2 when his finger was cut off with a dull knife. He described level 3 pain as the pain he felt when his leg was accidentally shot and the bones shattered in a friendly-fire incident. He said level 8 was like having dengue fever, an unusual disease that causes severe muscle and joint pain, feeling similar to bones breaking. He could not describe a level 10 pain. The point here is that everyone is different, and sometimes nurses must ask probing questions and consider many factors to rate the patient's pain intensity correctly. Even though a pain scale is used, avoid making judgments about the patient's pain. What is important is the patient's interpretation of the pain scale, which may differ from your own. ■

Difficult SITUATIONS

For many years, backrubs were almost a sacred part of routine nursing care. Over time, we have become much more dependent on technology. When we are busy or staffing is short, it seems as if there is no time for backrubs. Yet, calming the agitated patient who cannot sleep is time-consuming. The pregnant mother with a backache may use the call signal frequently. The patient with spasticity cannot get into a comfortable position. You may find that taking a few minutes to give a backrub will save you a great deal of time in caring for your patient. A good backrub is comforting and relaxing. Agitated patients often calm down. Uncomfortable patients become more comfortable and demand less attention. Do not omit this important part of nursing care—it pays dividends in patient comfort and satisfaction. Over time, it may even make your job easier. ■

FIGURE 10-7 Assisting the patient into a comfortable position will enable him to relax and rest.

FIGURE 10-8 Support the arm and leg with pillows to relieve discomfort.

- Waiting at least 30 minutes after the nurse administers pain medication before moving the patient, performing procedures, or undertaking activities
- Timing patient care to coincide with pain medication

Regularly incorporate these steps into your patient care. Follow the directions on the individual patient's care plan. The nurse may also direct you to apply warm or cold applications (see Unit 27) to make the patient more comfortable.

REST

Rest is a state of mental and physical comfort, calmness, and relaxation. The patient's basic needs of hunger, thirst, elimination, and pain must be met before effective rest is possible. He or she should be dressed comfortably, and feel fresh and clean. The patient may sit or lie down, or may do things that are pleasant and relaxing (Figure 10-9). Some patients have rituals, such as reciting the rosary.

The environment should be calm and quiet to promote rest. If basic care is tiring for the patient, allow him or her to rest before continuing. Some patients feel refreshed

Age-Appropriate Care ALERT

Children will often rest better if they have a personal comfort or security item with them, such as a special blanket, stuffed animal, doll, or toy. Treat this item with respect. Avoid making fun of the item, and do not make fun of the child for using it. ■

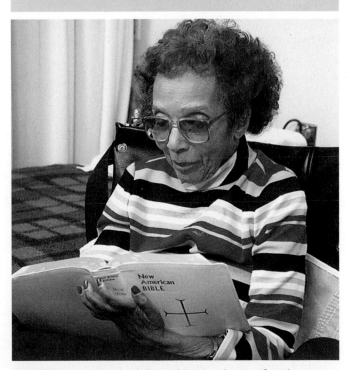

FIGURE 10-9 Reading the Bible is relaxing for this patient.

after 15 minutes of rest. Others need more time. Some patients must rest frequently throughout the day. Plan your schedule and activities to allow for rest periods. Providing a backrub, nursing comfort measures, or other relaxation activities may assist the patient to rest. Follow the care plan and the nurse's instructions.

SLEEP

Sleep is a period of continuous or intermittent unconsciousness in which physical movements are decreased. Sleep is a basic need of all humans, as it allows the mind and body to rest. Adequate sleep is necessary for the body and mind to function properly.

Sleep occurs in a cycle that lasts for several hours at a time. The body repairs itself during sleep. Because movement and activity are limited, the body's metabolic needs are reduced. The patient may become cold and need a blanket because he or she is not moving. It is common for vital signs to decrease during sleep.

The need for sleep decreases as a person ages. Elderly patients require less sleep than younger adults or middle-aged patients. Infants and children require more sleep than adults. In fact, newborns may sleep as much as 20 hours a day. Sleep needs by age group are listed in Table 10-3. Weight loss may decrease the need for sleep, whereas weight gain often increases the need for sleep.

Many factors affect sleep. Sleep problems often result from a combination of several factors. Obvious problems that may interfere with the quality and quantity of sleep are:

- Pain
- Hunger
- Thirst
- Need to eliminate
- Illness
- Exercise
- Noise
- Temperature
- Ventilation
- Light intensity
- Physical discomfort
- Some medications
- Caffeine intake
- Alcohol and/or drug use
- Some foods and beverages
- Lifestyle changes
- Anxiety, stress, fear, emotional problems
- Changes in the environment, unfamiliar environment
- Treatments and therapies
- Staff providing routine care

Worry is another factor that interferes with comfort, rest, and sleep. Patients worry about many things, such as:

TABLE 10-3 SLEEP NEEDS THROUGHOUT THE LIFE CYCLE

- Newborn infants sleep in 3- to 4-hour intervals for a total of 16–20 hours of sleep a day
- Infants require 12 to 16 hours of sleep a day
- Toddlers require 12 to 14 hours of sleep a day, usually broken into 10 to 12 hours of sleep at night, with one or more daytime naps
- Preschool children require 10 to 12 hours a day
- Elementary-school children require 10 to 12 hours a day
- Adolescents require 8 to 10 hours a day
- Young adults aged 18 to 40 require about 7 to 8 hours a day
- Middle-aged adults aged 40 to 65 require about 7 hours a day
- Elderly adults over the age of 65 require about 5 to 7 hours a day

- What the future will bring
- How much the hospitalization will cost
- Who is taking care of their home and work responsibilities

You will not have the answers to all these pressing concerns. You can listen, however. Share these concerns with the nurse. This is not gossiping. The nurse and the other members of the staff may be able to help the patient solve the problems. With worries reduced, the patient will rest better.

The Sleep Cycle

Each person has a sleep–wake cycle. An internal biological clock tells the person when it is time to sleep and wake up. The sleep cycle (Figure 10-10) includes two types of sleep:

- **Nonrapid eye movement (NREM) sleep** has four phases, progressing from light to very deep. This part of the sleep cycle begins when the patient first falls asleep. In the first two phases, the patient is easily aroused. As he or she progresses through the cycle, arousal becomes more difficult and sleep becomes deeper.
- **Rapid eye movement (REM) sleep** restores mental function. If you look closely, you will see the patient's eyes moving behind closed lids during this phase. Avoid awakening a patient who is in REM sleep, whenever possible. This is the part of the cycle in which dreams occur. The patient passes into REM

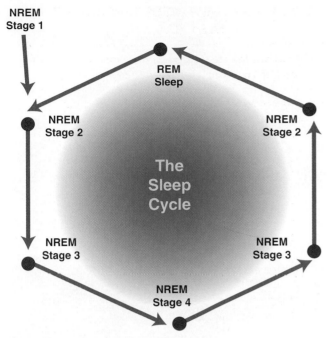

NREM
Stage 1

REM
Sleep

NREM
Stage 2

NREM
Stage 2

The
Sleep
Cycle

NREM
Stage 3

NREM
Stage 3

NREM
Stage 4

FIGURE 10-10 The sleep cycle

Clinical Information ALERT

You may be surprised to find that patients who are ill have a higher fever in the evening and at night than they do during the day. Asthma, ulcers, and certain forms of arthritis worsen at night. Heart attacks and strokes may begin at night and become fully symptomatic in the morning. The study of how the time of day affects body functions is called *chronobiology*. This is still a very new field. Science has much to learn about these body changes. If you notice a change in a patient's condition when he or she is resting or asleep, inform the nurse. ∎

sleep within approximately 60 to 90 minutes after falling asleep. Hospitalized patients may not experience prolonged periods of sleep time, so total REM time is less than normal. They awaken feeling less rested and may be more tired during the day.

The stages of the sleep cycle are further described in Table 10-4. This cycle usually repeats itself four or five times each night. Stages 1 and 2 are light sleep, whereas 3 and 4 are heavier. The four stages are followed by REM sleep. When the patient first goes to bed, each sleep cycle (four stages) takes about an hour. By the end of the night, the cycle lasts about 2 hours.

TABLE 10-4 THE SLEEP CYCLE

Stage 1: NREM Sleep

- Lasts a brief time; a few minutes
- Lightest sleep; patient is easily awakened
- Vital signs decrease progressively
- Body metabolism gradually slows
- Patient feels relaxed and drowsy
- If aroused during this phase, patient may feel as if he or she had been daydreaming

Stage 2: NREM Sleep

- Relaxation progresses, but patient remains easy to arouse
- Progresses into sound sleep
- Body functions and vital signs continue to decrease
- Lasts 10 to 20 minutes

Stage 3: NREM Sleep

- First stage of deep sleep
- Patient is difficult to arouse
- Little to no body movement
- Muscles are completely relaxed
- Vital signs continue to decrease
- Lasts 15 to 30 minutes

Stage 4: NREM Sleep

- Patient is very difficult to arouse
- Deepest stage of sleep cycle
- Body rest and restoration occur
- Vital signs significantly reduced compared with waking values
- Sleepwalking and enuresis (bedwetting)/incontinence may occur during this stage
- Lasts about 15 to 30 minutes

REM Sleep

- Rapid eye movements may be seen through closed eyelids
- Begins about 50 to 90 minutes after first falling asleep
- Full-color dreaming
- Blood pressure, pulse, respirations vary
- Limited or no voluntary movement
- Patient is very difficult to arouse
- Mental restoration occurs
- Lasts about 20 minutes

Sleep and the Older Adult

The need for sleep decreases with age. In older adults, the NREM stage takes longer to complete, and they do not get as much REM sleep as younger adults. When the older adult first falls asleep, the REM cycle lasts as long as it does in younger adults. However, by the end of the sleep cycle, younger adults may increase the length of their REM sleep by as much as 300%, but older adults experience much less. A 50% increase is more common. Also, older adults experience much more light stage 1 and 2 sleep, and deep sleep decreases. This helps explain why older patients awaken much more easily to even the slightest noise, whereas younger adults sleep through it. Older patients often have trouble falling asleep, awaken several times during the night, then wake up earlier in the morning than their younger counterparts.

Sleep is important to prevent feelings of fatigue, and for healing of medical and surgical problems. Getting enough sleep and rest allows patients to function at their highest level. Moving through the stages of the sleep cycle uninterrupted is important. Some patients become irritable if they do not have enough sleep. Elderly patients who do not sleep well may become disoriented (Figure 10-11). This correctable problem may be mistaken for confusion! It is easily corrected by allowing uninterrupted sleep. Other signs and symptoms of inadequate sleep are:

- Slow mental and physical responses
- Decreased attention span
- Forgetfulness or difficulty remembering things
- Reduced reasoning and judgment
- Puffy, red, swollen eyes
- Dark circles under eyes
- Disorientation
- Mood swings, moodiness
- Lethargy, sleepiness, fatigue
- Agitation, restlessness
- Clumsiness or lack of coordination
- Difficulty finding the right word
- Slurred speech
- Hallucinations in severe sleep deprivation

Sleep Disorders

Sleep has been studied extensively. Some facilities have units and clinics specializing in the diagnosis and treatment of sleep disorders. The most common sleep disorders are:

- **Insomnia**, a chronic deprivation of quality or quantity of sleep because sleep is ended or interrupted prematurely.
- **Hypersomnia**, a disorder characterized by sleeping very late in the morning and napping during the day. Causes can be physical or psychological.
- **Narcolepsy**, a condition in which patients have sudden, uncontrollable, unpredictable urges to fall asleep during the daytime hours. These individuals also get adequate sleep at night.

FIGURE 10-11 Lack of sleep can increase confusion and disorientation in elderly adults.

- **Sleep apnea**, a potentially serious condition in which air flow stops for 10 seconds or more. Untreated, this condition leads to severe medical problems.
- **Sleep deprivation**, which is prolonged sleep loss (inadequate quality or quantity of REM or NREM sleep).

High-Risk Conditions. Abnormal physiological problems cause several complications of the sleep cycle in some patients. These are:

- **Bruxism** (grinding of the teeth)
- **Enuresis** (bedwetting)
- **Somnambulism** (sleepwalking)

Patients with these problems are at high risk of injury when they are asleep. Special monitoring and safety measures will be listed on care plans of patients with these conditions, to reduce the risk of incidents and injuries.

Clinical Information ALERT

The gastrointestinal tract secretes more acid when the patient first goes to sleep. As a result, ulcer pain may worsen during this time, waking the patient up. ■

Difficult SITUATIONS

Patients always rest better if they are comfortable. Many elderly patients are uncomfortable in a cool environment. Other problems, such as the hospital gown, lack of a blanket, incontinence, and some treatments, increase the feeling of coldness. The discomfort increases restlessness and muscle tension, aggravates pain, and decreases patient satisfaction with care. Most hospitals have commercial warmers that are used to warm IV solutions and bath blankets. Although these are usually in the perioperative department, they may be in other areas as well. (Avoid warming blankets in a microwave, which may cause hot spots and increase the risk of burns.) Warmth appears to promote comfort, rest, and sleep, and reduces pain in elderly persons. Because of this, nurse researchers studied the effects of applying warmed blankets to patients (ages 65 to 98) who were cold, anxious, or uncomfortable. They measured the level of comfort before and one hour after applying a warm blanket. They found that the patients were more comfortable after receiving the warm blanket.[5] Patients who could describe how they felt said they were more comfortable. Nonverbal patients had fewer behavior problems and less body language suggesting discomfort.

Offering patients a warmed blanket is a simple nursing measure that the nursing assistant can implement at any time. Helping to relieve pain and suffering is an important part of nursing assistant care. By using simple measures such as a warmed blanket to increase patient comfort, you will be rewarded with improved patient satisfaction, quality of care, and quality of life. ∎

[5]Robinson, S., & Benton, G. (2002). Warmed blankets: An intervention to promote comfort for elderly hospitalized patients. *Geriatric Nursing, 23,* 320–323.

Nursing Assistant Measures to Promote Comfort, Rest, and Sleep

Basic nursing comfort measures, such as those used to relieve pain, are also effective in helping patients to rest

and sleep. Specific measures for each patient will be listed in the care plan. Measures that promote comfort, rest, and sleep are the following:

- Help the patient into loose-fitting, comfortable clothing or nightwear.
- Assist with toileting, cleanliness, oral care, and personal hygiene needs.
- Provide a warm bath or shower, if permitted.
- Avoid serving beverages containing caffeine after the evening meal.
- Provide a snack, if desired.
- Straighten the bed.
- Assist the patient into a comfortable position and provide pillows and props as needed for comfort.
- Provide a comfortable environmental temperature and ventilation.
- Provide an extra blanket, if desired.
- Eliminate unpleasant odors.
- Eliminate noise.
- Adjust the lighting to a comfortable level, darkening the room as much as possible for sleep, and provide a nightlight if desired (Figure 10-12).
- Provide nursing comfort measures, such as a backrub or repositioning the patient into a more comfortable position.
- Report pain to the nurse.
- If the patient is having pain, wait at least 30 minutes after pain medication is administered before performing procedures.
- If the patient is anxious, listen to what he or she says. Eliminate the cause of the anxiety, if possible (Figure 10-13).
- Avoid startling the patient.

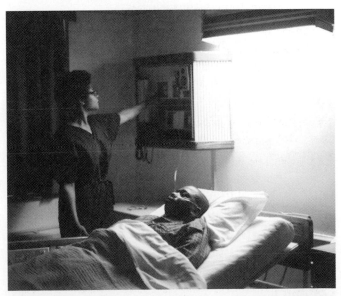

FIGURE 10-12 After the patient is comfortable and settled, turn the light off.

FIGURE 10-13 Listening to the patient's concerns provides emotional support and relieves anxiety.

- Handle the patient gently during care.
- Organize routine care to allow the patient uninterrupted sleep or rest.
- Avoid physical activity or activities that may upset the patient before bedtime.
- Assist with personal bedtime rituals, if any.
- Allow the patient to select his or her own bedtime.
- Allow the patient to read, watch television, or listen to the radio, if desired.
- Read to the patient from a favorite book.
- Assist with relaxation exercises and activities, as directed.
- If the patient receives a sleeping medication, make sure the patient is ready for sleep before the nurse administers the medication.
- Close the door to the patient's room.

REVIEW

A. True/False.

Mark the following true or false by circling T or F.

1. T F Comfort is a state of self-actualization.
2. T F Lack of privacy can affect a patient' comfort.
3. T F Unrelieved pain can lead to complications of immobility.
4. T F Chronic pain never lasts longer than one month.
5. T F Acute pain results from tissue damage.
6. T F Phantom pain is imaginary pain.
7. T F Radiating pain always encircles the area in which the pain originates.
8. T F You can assume that the patient is not in pain if he does not complain.
9. T F Rest and sleep are necessary for the body to repair itself and restore strength and energy.
10. T F Pain always indicates that something is wrong.
11. T F Culture has no effect on patients' responses to pain.
12. T F The patient's self-report of pain is the most accurate indicator of the existence and intensity of pain.

B. Matching.

Choose the correct word from Column II to match the phrases in Column I.

Column I

13. _____ sleeping all morning
14. _____ air flow stops for 10 seconds or more
15. _____ teeth grinding
16. _____ restores mental function
17. _____ bedwetting
18. _____ uncontrolled daytime sleeping
19. _____ chronic sleep deprivation
20. _____ state of discomfort

Column II

a. insomnia   **e.** hypersomnia
b. narcolepsy   **f.** bruxism
c. REM sleep   **g.** pain
d. sleep apnea   **h.** enuresis

C. Completion.

Complete the statements in questions 21 to 26 by writing in the correct word from the following list.

comfort	REM
hypersomnia	sleep apnea
narcolepsy	somnambulism

21. Full-color dreaming occurs during _____ the phase of the sleep cycle.
22. _____ is a state of well-being.
23. A patient with _____ sleeps very late in the morning.
24. A patient with _____ may suddenly fall asleep at work during the day.
25. A patient with _____ stops breathing for 10 seconds or more.
26. The medical term for sleepwalking is _____.

D. Multiple Choice.

Select the one best answer for each of the following.

27. The WHO recommends a noise level of _____ decibels in hospitals.
    a. 21
    b. 35
    c. 79
    d. 122

28. The "cocktail party effect"
    a. occurs when patients play loud, popular music.
    b. occurs when someone has the TV turned up too loud.
    c. is a form of active listening used to improve communication.
    d. occurs when workers speak louder to be heard.

29. Loud noise
    a. causes worker stress and fatigue.
    b. is to be expected in large facilities.
    c. can never be controlled.
    d. is therapeutic for most patients.

30. Pain is
    a. not the nursing assistant's responsibility.
    b. a sign of something wrong.
    c. an objective sign.
    d. a normal part of illness.

31. Pain
    a. does not normally interfere with rest and sleep.
    b. is not stressful or worrisome.
    c. negatively affects well-being.
    d. can usually be ignored.

32. If a patient expresses her problems and worries, the nursing assistant should
    a. stay out of the patient's business.
    b. not tell the nurse about the patient's concerns.
    c. allow her to talk about it and be a good listener.
    d. provide answers to the problems.

33. Aggravating and alleviating factors are
    a. things that worsen or improve pain.
    b. the strength and intensity of pain.
    c. the areas to which pain radiates.
    d. properties and characteristics of all pain.

34. Pain assessment is considered to be the
    a. first vital sign.
    b. frequency at which pain is evaluated.
    c. measurement of the "fifth vital sign."
    d. effectiveness of pain medication.

35. A state of mental calmness, comfort, and relaxation is
    a. comfort.
    b. sleep.
    c. leisure.
    d. rest.

36. A period of continuous or intermittent unconsciousness in which physical movements are decreased is
    a. relaxation.
    b. comfort.
    c. sleep.
    d. diversion.

37. When a patient is sleeping,
    a. vital signs may be lower than usual.
    b. temperature increases.
    c. movement increases.
    d. the pulse decreases and respirations increase.

38. During the REM sleep cycle, the patient
    a. dreams.
    b. awakens readily.
    c. progresses through four sleep phases.
    d. may feel hot to the touch.

E. Nursing Assistant Challenge.

Mr. Huynh is grimacing and supporting his right side with his hands when you enter the room. He smiles and nods at you. Complete the following statements regarding this patient.

39. Can Mr. Huynh smile if he is having pain?

40. If Mr. Huynh's right side hurts, you may be able to position him for comfort and support by using

    _____.

41. Should Mr. Huynh's body language be reported to the nurse?

42. Should you ask Mr. Huynh if he is having pain?

43. List six nursing assistant measures you can take to make Mr. Huynh more comfortable.

UNIT 11

Developing Cultural Sensitivity

OBJECTIVES

After completing this unit, you will be able to:

- Spell and define terms.
- Name six major cultural groups in the United States.
- Describe ways the major cultures differ in their family organization, communication, need for personal space, health practices, religion, and traditions.
- List ways nursing assistants can develop sensitivity about cultures other than their own.
- List ways the nursing assistant can help patients in practicing rituals appropriate to their cultures.
- State ways the nursing assistant can demonstrate appreciation of and sensitivity to other cultures.

VOCABULARY

Learn the meaning and the correct spelling of the following words and phrases:

ablutions	dialect	ritual	stereotype
acupuncture	ethnicity	sensitivity	talisman
amulet	mores	shaman	tradition
belief	personal space	spirituality	
culture	race	standard	

INTRODUCTION

America is a nation of people whose ancestors came primarily from other countries. Each group brought its own cultural heritage with its language, beliefs, and customs. These people are your patients. Each one is a unique individual whose development is the result of his or her own culture, current lifestyle and community participation, and personal experiences. As a health care provider, you are expected to show sensitivity to the individuality and cultural heritage of each patient. **Sensitivity** is the ability to be aware of and to appreciate the personal characteristics of others.

When members of different groups must live and work together in a community, it is easy for members of each group to form specific beliefs about the other groups. When these beliefs are rigid and are based on generalizations, they are called **stereotypes**. For example, others may view people of Asian heritage as present-focused (thinking about immediate rather than long-term goals), not self-expressive, and reluctant to make eye contact. These traits are stereotypes when applied to an entire group without consideration of the traditions of the group and individual characteristics. In contrast to these stereotypes, Van (whose heritage is Vietnamese) (Figure 11-1) is outgoing, looks directly at a person speaking to her, has a quick smile, and is future-oriented as she studies to become a health care provider.

Health care providers must be careful not to make assumptions about their patients based on stereotypes of

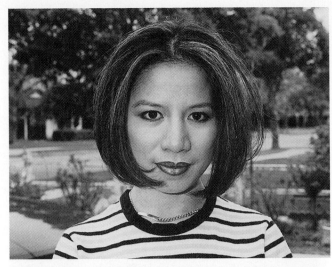

FIGURE 11-1 This young woman, whose parents were Vietnamese immigrants, has absorbed aspects of her parents' culture and the American culture in which she lives.

Culture ALERT

Treat each patient as an individual. Always consider culture. However, you must also:

- Avoid stereotyping.
- Consider other factors that may also affect care, such as age.
- Learn about the patient's unique views on health care.

Always consider the patients' cultural views on health. This is the patients' right, and considering culture shows your respect for the patient. Patients respond better to care when their culture is considered. ■

the group of which the patient is a part. The longer a group is associated with the American culture, the less its members rely on the cultural values and traditions of the country of origin. Young immigrants and second- or third-generation residents of the United States are much closer to American culture than to their original culture. Older people and new immigrants tend to cling more closely to the customs of their homeland.

RACE, ETHNICITY, AND CULTURE

The terms *race, ethnicity,* and *culture* are used to describe groups of people. **Race** is the classification of people according to shared physical characteristics such as skin color, bone structure, facial features, hair texture, and blood type.

Ethnicity

Ethnicity refers to special groups within a race as defined by national origin and/or culture. Members of an ethnic group share common:

- Heritage
- National origin
- Social customs
- Language

Six ethnic groups predominate in the United States (see Table 11-1):

- Caucasians—those of European and Scandinavian descent
- African Americans—those of African, Haitian, or Dominican Republic descent
- Hispanics—those whose ancestors came from Spanish-speaking countries
- Asians/Pacific—those whose ancestors came from the islands and countries of the Pacific Rim
- Native Americans—those who descended from one of the more than 600 tribes of North America
- Middle Easterners/Arabs—those whose ancestors came from Middle Eastern countries

TABLE 11-1 MAJOR ETHNIC GROUPS IN AMERICA

Group	Some Countries and Areas of Origin
Caucasian	England, Scotland, Ireland, Poland, Scandinavia, Italy, Russia
African American	Africa, Haiti, Jamaica, Dominican Republic
Hispanic	Cuba, Puerto Rico, Mexico, Latin and South America
Asian/Pacific	China, Japan, Philippines, Vietnam, Cambodia, Korea, Hawaii, Samoa
Native American	Hundreds of tribes, such as Cherokee, Apache, Navajo, Blackfoot, Inuit (Alaskan)
Middle Eastern	Egypt, Iran, Yemen, Pakistan, India, Jordan, Saudi Arabia, Kuwait

Culture

Culture refers to the way a particular group views the world and the set of traditions that are passed on from generation to generation. Culture enforces the **standards** (rules) established by the group based on the values and beliefs of the group. Cultural differences among ethnic groups may exist regarding:

- Family organization
- Personal space needs
- Communication
- Beliefs about health/illness and health care practices
- Religions
- Traditions

Cultural **mores** (customs) influence the way people will interact. Ethnicity and culture contribute to an individual's sense of self-identity as he or she relates to the group and to other cultures. Cross-cultural nursing recognizes the individual within an ethnic and cultural group and provides nursing care that assures cultural as well as individual acceptance and comfort.

Culture ALERT

Classes sometimes exist within a cultural group, based on income and other factors. The patient's practices and beliefs may be related to class. Financial hardship and social status may prevent a patient from seeking or following treatment. ■

FIGURE 11-2 An extended family

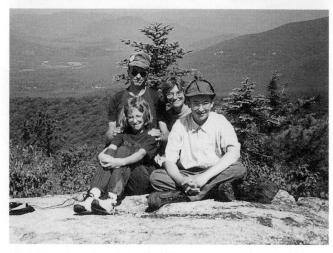

FIGURE 11-3 A nuclear family

Family Organization. Families form the basic cultural social groups, but their structure varies from culture to culture. The family organization determines who will be the decision makers and who is responsible for providing health care. In some families, the father or oldest male is the authority figure. In others, both the mother and father make decisions. In Hispanic and Middle Eastern families, the father is the dominant person, whereas in many African American households the mother has the strongest influence. In Caucasian families, the highest wage earner is often given the greatest respect and authority.

Health care may be a family responsibility. Figure 11-2 shows an extended family and Figure 11-3 a nuclear family. For example, in Asian families the elderly are given great respect, and caring for them is considered a duty and privilege by all family members. In Asian, Hispanic, and Native American cultures, extended families are common, and may include grandparents, aunts, and uncles. In these cases, caregiving is personal and shared by family members. Caucasian families tend to be structured as more independent units consisting of mother, father, and children. In this case, care of the elderly is more likely to be given over to others.

Personal Space Needs. **Personal space** refers to the actual physical closeness that one person is comfortable with during social interaction with others. Personal space can be invaded by standing too close to another person, patterns of eye contact, and touching.

Caucasians prefer to stand and speak at a distance of about 18 to 36 inches from one another. African Americans are comfortable standing closer to another person (5 to 10 inches). Space is important to Native Americans but has no specific boundaries. Asians tend to be uncomfortable if standing too close to another person.

Eye contact travels through the visual personal space and is interpreted differently by different cultures (Table 11-2). Asians consider eye contact inappropriate. The averted eyes and shifting gaze perceived as respectful in Asian cultures may be interpreted by Americans as inattention or insincerity. The direct eye contact of Caucasians and African Americans may be considered an invasion of visual space by an Asian patient. Members of Hispanic cultures make direct eye contact when speaking but consider prolonged contact disrespectful.

TABLE 11-2 CULTURAL INTERPRETATION OF NONVERBAL COMMUNICATION AND PERSONAL SPACE

Culture	Nonverbal Communication
American (U.S.)	Personal space 18 to 36 inches. Eye contact is acceptable. Lack of eye contact may be interpreted as lack of self-esteem or not telling the truth.
African American	Eye contact is acceptable; close personal space.
American Indian	*See* Native American.
Arab American	Women usually avoid eye contact with males and others whom they do not know well. Close personal space.
Asian	Varies. Eye contact is acceptable in some cultures; close personal space, but avoid touching.
Brazilian	Lack of eye contact is viewed by some as a sign of respect. Close personal space.
Cambodian	Eye contact is acceptable; women may lower eyes slightly; close personal space.
Chinese American	Avoid eye contact with authority figures as a sign of respect; will make eye contact with family and friends. Distant personal space.
Columbian	May avoid eye contact in presence of an authority figure. Close personal space.
Cuban	Eye contact expected during conversation. Close personal space with friends and family.
Ethiopian	Avoid eye contact with those perceived to be in authority. Close personal space with family and friends.
European	Eye contact acceptable; distant personal space.
Filipino	May avoid eye contact with authority figures. Close personal space.
Gypsy (Romany)	Facial expressions reflect mood. Close personal space with family members. Generally avoid contact with non-Gypsies. Also avoid surfaces considered unclean (areas that lower body has touched).
Haitian	Avoid eye contact with those perceived to be in authority.
Hmong	Avoid prolonged eye contact, which is considered rude.
Iranian	Make eye contact only with equals and close family and friends. Close personal space.
Japanese American	Little eye contact. Touching may be considered offensive.
Korean	Little direct eye contact. Touching is considered offensive. Although Koreans maintain close personal space with family, invading their personal space is a sign of disrespect.
Mexican American	Avoid eye contact with those perceived to be in authority. Some may consider touch by strangers to be disrespectful or offensive. Very close personal space.
Native American	Eye contact avoided as a sign of respect. Distant personal space is considered respectful.
Puerto Rican	Personal space varies with age group; generally closer with younger women, more distant with older women.
Russian	Close personal space with family and friends. Direct eye contact acceptable during conversation.
South Asian	May consider direct eye contact with elderly individuals offensive or rude. Close personal space with family members.
Vietnamese	Avoid eye contact with those perceived to be in authority. Distant personal space.
West Indian	Eye contact is avoided. Distant personal space.

Culture ALERT

Culture affects the type of care the patient expects to receive in the hospital. In some cultures, patients are comfortable doing self-care, if able. However, patients from other cultures may expect you to provide total care, even if they are physically able to do some things. Their feeling is that if they are sick, they should not expend energy in caring for themselves. In some cultures, family members are expected to care for the patient. In other cultures, only caregivers of the same gender may care for the patient. The care plan should guide you in culturally sensitive care. Consult the nurse if necessary. ■

Personal Care. Touching a person is considered an invasion of personal space in some cultures. A handshake is traditional in the United States for both men and women. In Middle Eastern countries, however, only men may greet other men in this manner. Greeting with handshakes and hugs is common in Hispanic cultures. Persons from Asian cultures are less likely to shake hands, especially with women.

Touching the body of another person may be even more restricted than the touching of hands in greeting. In Middle Eastern countries, men may not touch females who are not members of their immediate family. Uncovering the body is considered disrespectful in some cultures and is forbidden for women in others. For example, Muslim women may be completely veiled (Figure 11-4). Uncovering the shoulders of a person from India may be considered disrespectful. The mode of dress and body covering

FIGURE 11-4 Traditional Muslim culture requires women to be completely veiled from head to toe.

is very important to an individual's modesty. In some cultures, caregivers cannot care for members of the opposite sex.

Nursing assistants care for patients during very personal and private moments. Workers may not think about or be troubled by patients' bodies being exposed. However, many patients are very modest, and having the body exposed is very traumatic. Cultural beliefs about keeping the body covered will affect the care you give. In some cultures, female patients must be fully covered, even when in bed. Hospital gowns are not adequate. Some hospitals have long-sleeved gowns available that cover the patient from the neck to the ankles. However, these are not available in all facilities. Do whatever you can to keep patients covered and respect their modesty. The beliefs of patients from these religions and cultures require various garments:

- Amish—women must be covered from neck to ankles; a head covering is also worn.
- Gypsies—Most avoid hospitals, if at all possible. However, if they are hospitalized they may wear a special amulet around the neck. It should not be removed, if possible.
- Mormons—Adults of both genders who have attained religious status wear a short-legged, long-underwear-type garment at all times. Although the garment may be removed for hygiene, some patients believe it must be in contact with the body at all times because it is associated with God's protection.
- Muslims—Males are always covered from waist to knee. Women must be covered from neck to ankles; a head covering may also be worn; some patients cover all but the eyes, while others show the full face.
- Native Americans—Members of various Native American tribes in the United States wear medicine bags around their necks. Avoid removing the bag, if possible.
- Sikhs—Adults of both genders wear short pants called *Kachhn(a)* to symbolize modesty and morality. They may also wear bracelets called *Kara* on the right wrist, symbolizing restraint from evil actions and unity with God and other Sikhs. Men wear turbans. Males and females do not cut their hair or remove body hair.

Patients who are members of Islamic, Hindu, or Sikh religions have beliefs about ritualistic washing, water, and personal hygiene. Spiritual **ablutions** and washing are required at certain times of the day. Ablution is the practice of removing sins and diseases and cleansing negative energy from the body, mind, and spirit through the use of ritual washing. Physical cleanliness is associated with spiritual purity. Showering is preferable to a bath. The patient may refuse to eat until he or she has washed. Water for washing should be available to the patient whenever possible. Members of some cultures use the right hand for eating. The left hand is always used for personal hygiene after toileting.

As you care for patients from cultures other than your own, remember that the customs of the individual's culture greatly influence the acceptance of the person giving care and how the care is given, the amount of disrobing that is permitted, and the degree of touch that is comfortable for and accepted by the patient. Ask the nurse for guidance. You can also learn much about the patient's desires by watching the interactions of the patient with family and with other staff members.

Communication. Touching and eye contact are nonverbal forms of communication. A common verbal language is one characteristic of an ethnic group. Silence may be an important part of the language. For example, some Native American groups consider silence to be essential to understanding. Silence does not always mean that the listener has not heard or is inattentive to the speaker.

Communication HIGHLIGHT

Sickness, medication, anesthesia, pain, aging, culture, and disease can affect the patient's ability to communicate. Some patients may have trouble seeing, hearing, or speaking. Some do not speak English. Practice empathy with patients who have difficulty communicating by putting yourself in the patient's shoes and understanding how it feels. Imagine how frustrating it would be if you were unable to make your needs known and communicate with others! Be patient when communicating with patients who do not speak English. Do not assume that patients who are unable to speak are mentally confused. Patients who cannot speak often understand what is said to them. Some have limited writing skills or dictionaries to assist them in making their needs known. Communicate caring through your body language and demeanor. Treat all patients with dignity and respect. ■

An ethnic group may share a common language, but local terminology and usage may vary (a **dialect**). For example, Hispanic Americans may have originated in Puerto Rico, Mexico, Cuba, or Central or South America. The basic language of all of these people is Spanish, but there are many dialects depending on the country of origin or even a portion of a country. The Spanish you speak may differ in certain ways from the Spanish your patients speak.

Patients may be bilingual and speak both their native language and English. Some of your patients, however, may have only a minimal understanding of English. Older people and the newest immigrants will be most comfortable communicating in their own language. The desire to return to that which is familiar and most comfortable is especially strong when people are ill or frightened. Com-

municating in a patient's own language adds greatly to her sense of security. It is helpful to have an interpreter present, but if this is not possible, some form of communication is required if good nursing care is to be given.

Patients are pleased when a caregiver can speak even a few words in the patient's own language. If many of your patients share a common language, it would be helpful for you to learn some common words and phrases. Remember, too, that body language, gestures, and facial expression can be used to express thoughts and words when verbal language is inadequate.

When communicating:

- Use a normal tone.
- Speak slowly.
- Use simple words.
- Look directly at the listener even if someone is interpreting (be sensitive to any discomfort this may cause the patient because of cultural variations).
- Try to obtain feedback from the patient to determine the level of understanding.

You may wish to go back to Unit 7 to review other ways to communicate.

Culture ALERT

Ask questions to avoid stereotyping related to culture. You probably already have a general knowledge about common cultures in your community. However, you must also consider each person within that culture as an individual. Remember that differences exist among members of the same cultural group. Also, cultures change over time. War, climate, lack of available health care, natural disasters, and other factors affect culture and also the health of individuals within the culture. ■

Beliefs About Health, Illness, and Health Care Practices. **Beliefs** are based on commonly held opinions, knowledge, and attitudes about the world and life. These beliefs will influence the person's feelings about illness and the kind of health care he will choose. Members of a culture share beliefs about:

- The nature and cause of illness
- Types of health care practices
- Their relationship to a higher power

People tend to view the causes of health and illness in one of three ways, or in a combination of these ways. Some people hold magical beliefs, in which the causes of illness are supernatural forces. Others hold scientific beliefs, relating health and illness to causes such as infectious agents, the wear and tear on the body caused by daily living and stress, environmental agents, or injury. Still others have holistic beliefs that view the person and the environment as continuously exchanging energy and matter with one another. In this belief system, the mind and body must be in harmony to ensure health.

Those who believe that illness and pain are a penance from a higher power, as punishment for wrongdoing, will be less willing to complain of suffering and to seek relief through medication and scientific medicine. They rely more on the use of charms, chants or holy words, and rituals. Some cultures turn to folk healers or shamans to help bring their bodies back into balance with nature. (A **shaman** is a traditional spiritual leader, healer, or medicine man. In some societies, the shaman is expected to heal the sick, escort the souls of the dead into heaven, and meet with gods by taking on the shape or language of an animal or bird.) They believe that the imbalance is the cause of their discomfort. The balance is achieved by eating certain foods, taking natural medicines, or through the power of healing ceremonies.

Those who see illness as the result of environmental factors, infectious agents, or injury are more likely to seek scientifically based medical help. Asian cultures, which have traditional health and illness beliefs, use traditional medications such as herbs, **acupuncture** (placement of metal needles in the body), and mind-body practices such as tai chi and meditation to achieve balance and wellness.

Arabs who believe that some illnesses are the "Will of Allah" use **amulets** (charms against evil) and verses from the Koran (a holy book) written on turquoise stones to help them. Native Americans believe illness develops when the harmony between body, mind, and spirit is disrupted. Sand paintings are used in healing rituals to diagnose conditions and prescribe treatment. Hispanics believe that illness is caused when an imbalance exists in the four body fluids. They may use native healers, candles, prayers, and the wearing of medals as methods of treatment and to restore balance. Hot and cold conditions (illnesses) are identified and "hot" and "cold" foods and medicines, similar to those recognized in Asian cultures, are used in treatment. Cold remedies are given to balance a hot condition and vice versa. See Table 11-3 for hot and cold conditions and remedies.

Religious Practices. **Spirituality** is the part of a person that gives a sense of wholeness by fulfilling the human need to feel connected with the world and to a power greater than oneself. For many, spirituality is expressed in religious practice. *Religion* is an organized system of belief in a deity (higher power). Spirituality and religion are products of an individual's cultural background and experience. Spiritual values and religious beliefs form the rules of what a person considers to be right or wrong.

Religious beliefs provide a person with guidelines for moral behavior. Religious preferences are highly personal and can vary within a given culture. For example, Hispan-

TABLE 11-3 HOT AND COLD CONDITIONS AND REMEDIES

Hot Conditions	Cold Conditions
Constipation	Cancer
Fever	Colds
Infections	Headache
Sore throat	Pneumonia
Ulcers	Tuberculosis

Cold Food Remedies	Hot Food Remedies
Dairy products	Cereals
Milk	Eggs
Lima beans	Beef
Vegetables	Oils
Honey	Spicy foods
Chicken	Wine
Raisins	

Cold Medical Remedies	Hot Medical Remedies
Bicarbonate of soda	Aspirin
Milk of magnesia	Cinnamon
Orange flower water	Cod liver oil
Sage	Garlic
	Penicillin

ics are traditionally Roman Catholic. However, it is not unusual to find a Protestant church of Hispanics in the same community.

The major religions of the United States include:

- Protestantism (various denominations)
- Roman Catholicism
- Judaism
- Islam
- Hinduism

Religious items and **rituals** (solemn and ceremonial acts that reinforce faith) are especially meaningful to practitioners. They must be treated with respect. For example, the crucifix, Bible, and religious medals are important to Roman Catholics. The prayer rug is significant to the

Islamic, who pray five times each day in the direction of their holy city, Mecca. Amulets and special charms are important to the religious beliefs of Native Americans and to some peoples in the Middle East. **Talismans** are engraved stones, rings, or other objects that are used to ward off evil. Copper or silver bracelets and religious medals are important and sacred to some cultures.

If a patient requests a visit from clergy, be sure the request is promptly relayed to the nurse. When the clergy visits, be sure to provide privacy. It is also important to provide privacy when the patient is engaged in a religious act such as praying. Table 11-4 lists five religious faiths common in the United States and some of their beliefs and religious items. Special religious rituals and practices related to dying, death, and care of the body after death are discussed in Unit 32.

Foods are important in some religions. For example, those of the Orthodox Jewish faith may not be served milk and meat products at the same time. Roman Catholics restrict food intake on specific dates and some Baptists, Muslims, and others are not permitted to drink alcohol. Other food restrictions are discussed in Unit 26.

An understanding of some of the major belief systems will help you be more sensitive to your patient's needs. You can support your patient's spirituality and religious practices by:

- Being a willing listener
- Respecting the patient's belief system
- Never trying to convert the patient to your belief system
- Respecting religious symbols
- Not interrupting during religious rituals
- Reading aloud the patient's favorite passages from religious books

- Providing privacy during prayers and meditation or when clergy visits

TRADITIONS

Traditions are customs and practices followed by members of a culture and passed from generation to generation. Often traditions are related to religious rituals and holiday celebrations. Foods are particularly traditional at holidays. Think about ham at Easter, corned beef and

Culture ALERT

Learn about your own cultural beliefs and practices. Consider how your culture, the way you were raised, and family traditions affect you. For example, you may have opinions and beliefs about:

- How to be polite, how to greet someone in a polite manner, and use good manners in conversation with others.
- Where and how often to seek medical care.
- Punctuality (being on time).
- Preferred gender of caregiver.
- Methods of expressing pain.
- How children and elderly persons should be treated. ◼

TABLE 11-4 SOME COMMON BELIEF SYSTEMS (RELIGIOUS)

Religion	Belief in a Deity	Value of Prayer	Belief in Hereafter	Special Practices or Symbols
Protestant	Yes	Important	Yes	Baptism, Holy Communion, cross, Bible
Roman Catholic	Yes	Important	Yes	Baptism, Holy Communion, Anointing of the Sick, Reconciliation, Bible, medals, pictures and statues of saints, rosaries, crucifix
Orthodox Judaism	Yes	Important	Yes	Torah, yarmulke (cap), tallith, menorah
Hinduism	Yes (many forms)	Important	Yes	No sacraments
Buddhism	Yes	Important	Yes	No sacraments
Islam (Muslim)	Yes	Important	Yes	Koran, prayer rug

Within the framework of each belief system, there are individual differences in the depth of belief and extent of practice.

cabbage on St. Patrick's Day, and traditional tacos, tamales, and enchiladas on Cinco de Mayo.

Families carry out traditions from generation to generation. For example, it is a Chinese tradition to have a celebration accompanied by a colorful procession with a dragon to welcome in the Chinese New Year. People all over America watch fireworks to celebrate the Fourth of July. Holidays specific to cultures are celebrated each year.

Many traditions involve the coming to maturity of young people and are related to religious practice. For example, young Jewish boys have a bar mitzvah as they reach puberty. Many Protestant churches present Bibles to chil-dren when they are in the third grade of school and are able to read on their own.

Honoring and practicing traditions gives people a sense of stability and continuity. Traditions help to bind the people of a culture closer together.

Nursing assistants have a unique opportunity to learn about other cultures directly from their patients. There are ways to make this process easier for yourself and your patient (see the following guidelines). Always remember that even though a person is part of an identifiable culture, he or she must always be recognized as an individual within the culture.

GUIDELINES *for*
Developing Cultural Sensitivity

- Review your own belief systems.
- Consider how your own culture influences your behavior.
- Always view patients as individuals within a culture.
- Recognize that patients are a combination of heritage, culture, and community.
- Understand that culture influences how people behave and interact with others.
- Remember that personal space needs, eye contact, and ways of communicating are often culturally related.
- Recognize that some cultures have beliefs about health, wellness, and illness that are different from your own.
- Be willing to modify care according to the patient's cultural background and practices.
- Do not expect all members of a cultural group to behave in exactly the same manner.

- Remember that patients' health practices related to culture, values, and belief system are deeply ingrained and not easily changed.
- Avoid stereotyping people within a culture.
- Check with the nurse to learn special ways to deal with patients of different cultural backgrounds.
- Treat religious articles with respect.
- Provide privacy when a spiritual advisor is visiting the patient or the patient is practicing a devotional act.
- Try to learn about the practices, beliefs, and cultural heritage of the people who are most likely to be your patients. A library and the Internet are good sources.
- Ask patients politely about practices that are unfamiliar.
- Attend staff development classes designed to promote cultural sensitivity.

REVIEW

A. Matching.

Match each word with its definition.

1. _____ amulet
2. _____ mores
3. _____ sensitivity
4. _____ standard
5. _____ tradition

a. rules of conduct
b. charms against evil
c. passed from generation to generation
d. awareness and appreciation of
e. customs

B. Completion.

Complete the following sentences by choosing the correct word.

6. Rigid, biased ideas about people are called _____. (stereotypes) (characteristics)

7. Classification by shared physical characteristics is based on _____. (ethnicity) (race)

8. The way a group views the world, and the group's traditions, are the foundation of a _____.
(race) (culture)

9. Commonly held opinions, knowledge, and attitudes about life are called _____.
(standards) (beliefs)

10. Solemn and ceremonial acts that reinforce faith are called _____.
(rituals) (traditions)

C. Multiple Choice.

Select the one best answer for each of the following.

11. The cultural language common to most Hispanics is
   a. English.
   b. French.
   c. Spanish.
   d. German.

12. You may expect that a new black immigrant was born in
   a. Egypt.
   b. Russia.
   c. China.
   d. Poland.

13. The nuclear family is most commonly seen in
   a. African American culture.
   b. Asian culture.
   c. Hispanic culture.
   d. Caucasian culture.

14. Caucasians prefer to stand and speak about
   a. 6 inches apart.
   b. 18 inches apart.
   c. 4 feet apart.
   d. 5 feet apart.

15. A Middle Eastern man may greet another man by
   a. nodding.
   b. shaking hands.
   c. kissing on either cheek.
   d. hugging.

16. Your patient has a prayer rug and prays five times a day. You believe he is from which culture?
   a. Middle Eastern
   b. Mexican
   c. Asian
   d. Native American

17. Your Asian patient looks down and says little when you speak. This is
   a. rude in his culture.
   b. respectful in his culture.

   c. his way of showing anger.
   d. his way of showing fear.

18. Your patient makes direct and prolonged eye contact as you speak. He probably is of what culture?
   a. Asian
   b. Native American
   c. Hispanic
   d. Caucasian

19. Your patient speaks only a few words of English. When you speak to him, you should
   a. raise your voice.
   b. speak slowly.
   c. use slang.
   d. look away.

20. People from this culture believe that illness develops when harmony between the mind, body, and spirit is disrupted.
   a. Asian
   b. Hispanic
   c. Native American
   d. African American

D. Short Answer.

21. You have a Catholic patient. Briefly explain how you can show sensitivity to her religious beliefs.

22. Name your own culture. List two traditions that are common to your culture.

23. List two ways you can improve your cultural sensitivity to a new patient who has a culture different from your own.

E. Nursing Assistant Challenge.

You have a patient who is a new immigrant from Iran. He is Islamic and 60 years old. Mark the following true or false.

24. T F The Torah is his holy book.

25. T F He will wish to pray once daily.

26. T F He will be the person most likely to make his own medical decisions.

27. T F He probably feels his condition is due to the "Will of Allah."

28. T F He would celebrate Easter and Christmas if he were at home.

Infection and Infection Control

UNIT 12

Infection

OBJECTIVES

After completing this unit, you will be able to:

- Spell and define terms.
- Identify the most common microbes and describe some of their characteristics.
- List the links in the chain of infection.
- List the ways that infectious diseases are spread.
- Name and briefly describe five serious infectious diseases.

- Identify the causes of several important infectious diseases.
- Define spores and explain how spores differ from other pathogens.
- Describe common treatments for infectious disease.
- List natural body defenses against infections.
- Explain why patients are at risk for infections.

VOCABULARY

Learn the meaning and the correct spelling of the following words and phrases:

abscess
acquired immune deficiency syndrome (AIDS)
airborne transmission
allergy
antibiotic
antibody
antigen
bacillus, bacilli
bacteremia
bacteria, bacterium
bedbugs
bioterrorism
carrier
causative agent
chain of infection
coccus, cocci
colony
contact transmission
contagious
contaminated
culture and sensitivity
diplo-

distended
droplet transmission
dysentery
Escherichia coli (E. coli) O157:H7
flora
fomites
fungi, fungus
hantavirus
head lice
hemoptysis
hepatitis
host
human immunodeficiency virus (HIV)
immune response
immunity
immunization
immunosuppression
incubation
infection
infectious
inflammation
jaundice

listeriosis
methicillin-resistant *Staphylococcus aureus* (MRSA)
microbe
microorganism
mite
mold
necrotizing fasciitis
nits
nonpathogen
organism
parasite
pathogen
petechiae
phagocyte
portal of entry
portal of exit
protozoa, protozoan
pseudomembranous colitis
reservoir
risk factor
scabies

seizure
seropositive
severe acute respiratory syndrome (SARS)
source
spirillum, spirilla
spores
staphylo-
strepto-
Streptococcus A
toxin
transmission
tubercle
tuberculosis disease
tuberculosis infection
vaccine
vancomycin-resistant enterococci (VRE)
vector
virus
yeast

INTRODUCTION

Humans are surrounded by a world of tiny **organisms** (living beings). These beings cannot be seen with the naked eye. They make their presence known only by their effect, in much the same way we become aware of the wind. We cannot see the wind, but we do see its effect on the trees, which bend and sway.

These organisms can be seen only with a microscope. They are everywhere—in us, on us, and around us. They are:

- On our skin
- In our mouths
- Within our bodies
- In and on the food we eat
- On what we touch or handle

Micro means small. Because these organisms (agents) are so tiny, they are called **microorganisms** or **microbes**. The organisms live in relationship to us and to each other.

Many of these microbes are useful to us. They are called **nonpathogens** because they do not produce disease. They help in the

- Processing of cheese, beer, and yogurt
- Curing of leather
- Baking of bread

Other microbes are not useful. Microbes that cause disease in humans are called **pathogens** or pathogenic organisms. Pathogens grow best:

- At body temperature
- Where light is limited

Clinical Information ALERT

Human skin has about 100,000 bacteria per square centimeter. Ten percent of human dry weight is attributed to bacteria. The normal flora that live on the skin help to protect the person from harmful bacteria. The eyelashes and eyebrows shield the eyes from sun, dust, and perspiration. Nasal hairs protect the person from inhaling dust, pathogens, and other foreign bodies. ■

- Where there is moisture
- Where there is a food supply
- Where oxygen needs can be met

Infections occur when the pathogens invade the body and cause disease.

MICROBES

There are many different types of microbes (Figure 12-1), many of which are pathogenic to human beings. Microbes are classified as:

- Bacteria
- Viruses
- Fungi
- Protozoa

Bacteria

Bacteria (singular: **bacterium**) are simple one-celled microbes. They are named according to their shapes and arrangement. They cause infections in the skin, respiratory tract, urinary tract, and bloodstream.

Shapes. In the following list, the first term is the singular form of the word. The word in parentheses is the plural form.

- **Coccus** (**cocci**)—round or spherical
- **Bacillus** (**bacilli**)—straight rod
- **Spirillum** (**spirilla**)—spiral, corkscrew, or slightly curved

Arrangements. Bacteria grow in groups called **colonies**. If we look at a small part of a colony under a microscope, we see that the bacteria typically are arranged in pairs, clusters, or chains.

- Single
- Pairs (**diplo-**)
- Chains (**strepto-**)
- Clusters (**staphylo-**)

The shape and group arrangement of bacteria are important factors in identification. For example, round microorganisms grouped in chains are called streptococci. A very important member of this family is the *Streptococcus hemolyticus*. It causes septic sore throat and rheumatic fever.

FIGURE 12-1 Various types of microbes

Round organisms grouped in a cluster are called staphylo-cocci. An example of this family is *Staphylococcus aureus*. Staphylococci cause many infections, such as:

- Surgical wound infections
- Abscesses
- Boils
- Toxic shock syndrome

Round organisms in pairs are called diplococci. A diplo-coccus, the *Neisseria gonorrhoeae*, causes gonorrhea.

Fungi

Two groups of **fungi** (singular: **fungus**) are most com-monly associated with infection in humans:

- **Yeasts**—single-celled budding forms of a fungus. Yeast can infect areas of the body such as:
  - Mouth/vagina: *Candida albicans*
  - Skin: *Tinea capitis* (ringworm)
  - Feet: *Tinea pedis* (athlete's foot)
- **Molds**—A common mold that can cause infection in the lungs of humans is *Aspergillus*.

Yeasts and molds are known as opportunistic parasites. (A **parasite** (Figure 12-2) is an organism that lives in or on another organism without benefiting the host organism.) Under normal conditions, the organisms are harmless. However, when the human immune system is impaired and unable to protect the body, these organisms can invade the body and cause severe infections. For example, a patient with AIDS is very susceptible to fungal infec-tions because the immune system is not working properly.

Viruses

A **virus** is the smallest microbe. Viruses come in a variety of shapes. Ways viruses are classified include:

- Type of nucleic acid core (DNA or RNA)

FIGURE 12-2 This female mosquito is a parasite. Females bite as part of the reproduction process. The mosquito is taking a blood meal by pumping the ingested blood through her *labrum*, which is visible here as a thin, red, needle-like structure between the mos-quito's head and the skin. The mosquito is so full that clear fluid is spilling from the other end, enabling her to make room for more ingested blood. (Courtesy of Cen-ters for Disease Control and Prevention)

- Clinical properties

Common viral infections include:

- Hepatitis
- Herpes
- Human immune deficiency syndrome (HIV)
- Acquired immune deficiency syndrome (AIDS)
- Chickenpox
- Influenza
- Common cold
- Measles
- Mumps

Protozoa

Protozoa (singular: **protozoan**) are simple one-celled organisms that live on living matter. These organisms have a true nucleus. They are classified by the way in which they move. For example, some move by whiplike tails, oth-ers by hairlike projections. They cause diseases such as:

- Malaria
- Toxoplasmosis
- African sleeping sickness
- Amebiasis

Some signs and symptoms of diseases caused by protozoa include:

- Diarrhea
- **Dysentery** (infection in the lower bowel)
- Inflammation of the brain (encephalitis)

THE CHAIN OF INFECTION

Infections occur when certain conditions exist. These con-ditions are called the **chain of infection** (Figure 12-3A) and include:

- Causative agent (pathogen) that causes the disease
- Reservoir or source (where the pathogen can live and reproduce)

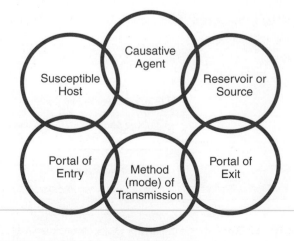

FIGURE 12-3A The chain of infection

- Portal of exit (manner in which the pathogen leaves the body)
- Method or mode of transmission (manner in which the pathogen is carried to another person)
- Portal of entry (manner in which the pathogen enters another person)
- Susceptible host (a person who will become ill from the entry of pathogens into the body)

Pathogens cause disease by entering the body through a portal of entry. They spread disease to others by leaving the body through a portal of exit and being transmitted to another person. They enter the other person's body and can again cause disease. The object of infection control is to disrupt the chain of infection. Breaking one link in the chain of infection (Figure 12-3B) is all that is needed to prevent the spread of disease.

Pathogens enter and leave the body through body openings such as:

- Eyes, ears, nose, or mouth
- Breaks in the skin, hand contact with mouth and other mucous membranes (Figure 12-4)
- Penis, vagina, urinary meatus (bladder opening), or rectum

Infection Control ALERT

Breaking one link in the chain of infection will stop the infection from spreading. ■

Causative Agent

The **causative agent** is the microorganism that can produce the disease in humans. The most common biological agents of infectious disease are:

- Bacteria
- Viruses
- Fungi
- Protozoa

Reservoir

The **reservoir** or **source** is where pathogens can survive. They may or may not multiply in the reservoir. The four most common reservoirs are:

1. Humans—active cases and carriers

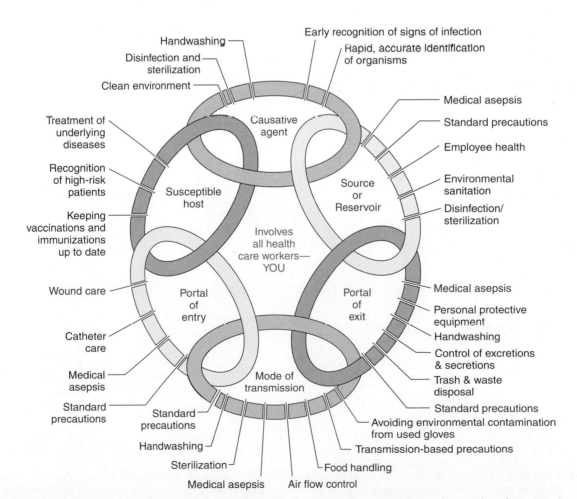

FIGURE 12-3B If one link in the chain is broken, infection cannot be transmitted to others. This diagram shows the chain of infection, with examples of various ways health care workers break each link.

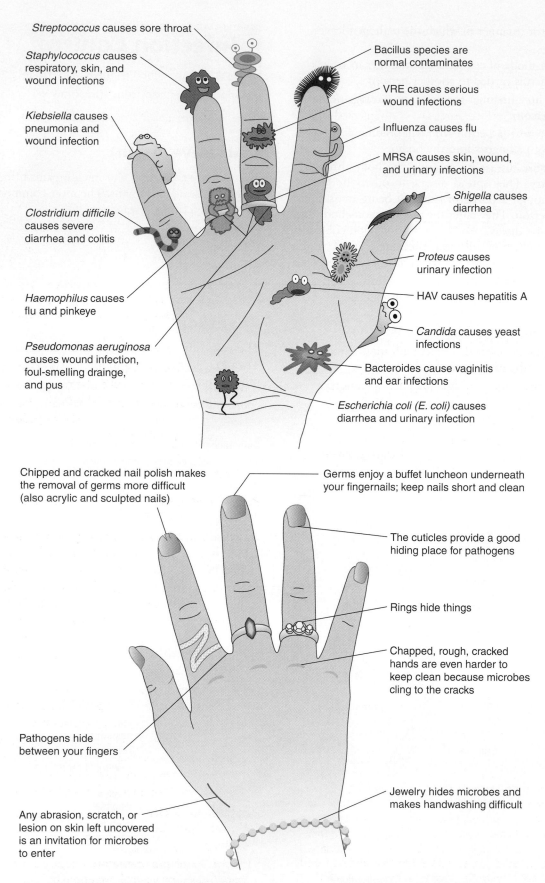

Streptococcus causes sore throat

Staphylococcus causes respiratory, skin, and wound infections

Klebsiella causes pneumonia and wound infection

Clostridium difficile causes severe diarrhea and colitis

Haemophilus causes flu and pinkeye

Pseudomonas aeruginosa causes wound infection, foul-smelling drainge, and pus

Bacillus species are normal contaminates

VRE causes serious wound infections

Influenza causes flu

MRSA causes skin, wound, and urinary infections

Shigella causes diarrhea

Proteus causes urinary infection

HAV causes hepatitis A

Candida causes yeast infections

Bacteroides cause vaginitis and ear infections

Escherichia coli (E. coli) causes diarrhea and urinary infection

Chipped and cracked nail polish makes the removal of germs more difficult (also acrylic and sculpted nails)

Pathogens hide between your fingers

Any abrasion, scratch, or lesion on skin left uncovered is an invitation for microbes to enter

Germs enjoy a buffet luncheon underneath your fingernails; keep nails short and clean

The cuticles provide a good hiding place for pathogens

Rings hide things

Chapped, rough, cracked hands are even harder to keep clean because microbes cling to the cracks

Jewelry hides microbes and makes handwashing difficult

FIGURE 12-4 (A) Many pathogens find their way to workers' hands. These are transferred to patients and environmental surfaces through touch. The worker can introduce them to his own body by touching his eyes, nose, mouth, or other mucous membranes. (B) Jewelry worn on hands provides an additional hiding place for pathogens. Practicing good handwashing and not wearing jewelry are the best methods of protecting both workers and patients.

2. Insects and animals (Figure 12-5)

3. Environment

4. Fomites—objects that become **contaminated** with infectious material that contains the microbe. Fomites are anything that comes in direct contact with the excretions or secretions of an infected person. This includes:

  – Bedpans and urinals

  – Doorknobs, faucet handles

  – Linens

  – Instruments

  – Containers with specimens for laboratory analysis

In the health care setting, the reservoirs include the:

- Patient
- Health care workers
- Environment
- Equipment

Human Reservoirs. The two major human reservoirs are cases and carriers.

- Cases—people with acute illness including obvious signs and symptoms. An example is a person with chickenpox (Figure 12-6).

- **Carriers**—persons who are infectious and can give a disease to others. The person may not know of the infection. He or she may not have symptoms or show evidence of disease. The condition is not harmful to the carrier, but may be harmful to others. Another type

FIGURE 12-6 This child has an active case of chickenpox (varicella). It is highly contagious, and spreads via coughing or sneezing. (Courtesy of Centers for Disease Control and Prevention)

of carrier is one in whom the organisms are multiplying (**incubating**) before signs and symptoms develop.

Specific diseases can persist in humans for an indefinite period of time, such as salmonella, hepatitis B, hepatitis C, HIV disease, and typhoid.

Portals of Entry or Exit

Portals of Entry. Organisms enter the body through the following **portals of entry:**

- Breaks in the skin or mucous membranes—Many organisms that are part of the normal flora, such as staphylococci, enter through breaks in the skin.

- Respiratory tract—Organisms that cause the common cold and many childhood communicable diseases (such as mumps and measles) may enter this way.

- Genitourinary tract—Organisms that cause syphilis, AIDS, gonorrhea, and other sexually transmitted diseases enter this way.

- Gastrointestinal tract—Salmonellosis, typhoid fever, and hepatitis A are examples of diseases caused by organisms that enter the digestive tract.

- Circulatory system—Malaria, yellow fever, and meningitis are diseases that can enter the body directly into the blood through the bite of insects.

- Transplacental (mother to fetus) (AIDS and hepatitis B).

Portals of Exit. Infectious organisms leave the reservoir of the host through body secretions (**portals of exit**), including:

- Excretions of the respiratory tract (sputum) or genital tract (semen or vaginal excretions)

- Draining wounds

- Urine

- Feces

Supella supellectilium
(Brown-banded cockroach)

Male   Female

FIGURE 12-5 Insects and animals can transmit pathogens from place to place. Many different types of cockroaches have adapted to U.S. environments, and are now commonly found living inside human habitations. They live in sewers and bathrooms as well as kitchens, dining areas, or other areas where food is prepared and stored. They are known for contaminating food, and have been implicated in the spread of salmonellosis (food poisoning), gastroenteritis, staphylococcus infections, generalized diarrhea, and typhoid fever. (Courtesy of Centers for Disease Control and Prevention)

- Blood and other body fluids
- Saliva
- Tears

In infected persons, these products must be considered **infectious** or capable of transmitting the disease agent.

Transmission of Disease

Transmission (spread) of infectious organisms may happen in one of three ways (Table 12-1):

- **Airborne transmission.** Small particles remain suspended in the air and move with air currents, or become trapped in dust, which is also carried in air currents. The patient breathes in pathogens carried in this manner.
- **Droplet transmission.** Droplets are moist particles produced by people coughing, sneezing, talking, laughing, or singing. Pathogens are transmitted into the air with the droplets. Droplets usually stay within three feet of the source.
- **Contact transmission.** Direct contact occurs with a person who is the reservoir of the pathogens. Indirect contact occurs when a person touches an item contaminated with pathogens, such as soiled linen.

Not all organisms are transmitted in the same way, and some organisms may be transmitted in more than one way.

Host

The person who harbors infectious organisms is called a **host**. This person does not have enough resistance to the infectious agent. An infection develops in the host when infectious organisms:

- Penetrate the body
- Begin to multiply
- Cause damage to the host

Risk Factors. Risk factors are conditions that indicate a problem may develop, causing the patient's health to worsen. Some risk factors increase the likelihood that the patient will develop an infection. Factors that increase the risk of infection are:

- Number and strength of the infectious organisms
- General health of the individual
- Age, sex, and heredity of the individual
- Condition of the person's immune system

Emotional stress and fatigue also play a role in the progress of an infectious disease.

TYPES OF INFECTIONS

Infections can be:

- Local (confined to one area)—such as a boil or skin abscess

TABLE 12-1 WAYS IN WHICH MICROBES ARE SPREAD FROM ONE PERSON TO OTHERS

Airborne Transmission

- Pathogens carried by moisture or dust particles in air; can be carried long distances

Droplet Transmission

- Droplet spread within approximately 3 feet (no personal contact) of infected person by:
  - Coughing–Whistling
  - Sneezing–Spitting
  - Talking
  - Laughing
  - Singing

Contact Transmission

- Direct contact with infected person:
  - Touching
  - Sexual contact
  - Blood
  - Body fluids (drainage, urine, feces, sputum, saliva, vomitus)

- Indirect contact with infected person:
  - Clothing
  - Dressings
  - Equipment used in care and treatment
  - Bed linens
  - Personal belongings
  - Specimen containers
  - Instruments used in treatment
  - Food
  - Water

Note that pathogens can also be carried by insects and animals (**vectors**) and passed to humans.

- Generalized—such as pneumonia (in the lungs)
- Systemic—widespread through the bloodstream (**bacteremia**)

BODY FLORA

Different microbes live in and on our body surfaces. These microbes are called the normal body **flora**. The flora are not the same in all body areas. For example, the organisms making up the flora of the intestinal tract are different from those of the respiratory tract. Healthy individuals live in harmony with the normal body flora. However, the balance may be disturbed by:

- Pathogenic organisms
- Normal flora organisms that become pathogenic
- Flora from one area being transferred into a different body area where they do not usually reside
- Drugs such as antibiotics that upset the normal balance of organisms within the body flora, allowing one group to flourish

When the organisms of one normal flora, such as those in the intestinal tract, remain within their normal environment, the body functions properly. However, when microbes from the intestines are transferred into the urinary tract, a serious urinary tract infection can result. Organisms that are non-pathogenic in their own environment may become pathogenic when they enter a different environment.

HOW PATHOGENS AFFECT THE BODY

The potential for infection depends on the risk factors listed previously. Two major factors are the susceptibility of the host and the amount of infectious agent that finds a portal of entry into the host. Even then, an infection may not occur unless all elements of the chain of infection are present.

Microbes act in different ways to produce disease in the human body. Some pathogens:

- Attack and destroy the cells they invade. For example, the microscopic protozoan that causes malaria invades the red blood cells and eventually causes them to split. The person experiences chills and fever.
- Produce poisons called **toxins** that harm the body. For example, the rabies and botulism organisms produce toxins that travel to and damage the nervous system.
- Cause sensitivity responses called **allergies**. For example, the person may have a runny nose and watery eyes but no rise in temperature. This same response occurs when pollens or dust irritate the respiratory membranes.

BODY DEFENSES

The body has some natural defenses to protect it from infections. There are several natural external defenses. The most important of these is the skin. Intact skin acts as a mechanical barrier against the entry of pathogens. Other defenses include:

- Mucous membranes lining the respiratory, reproductive, gastrointestinal, and urinary tracts. The mucus is sticky and traps foreign materials before they can cause damage.
- Cilia (fine microscopic hairs) lining the respiratory tract propel the mucus and trapped microbes out of the body.
- Coughing and sneezing remove foreign materials from the respiratory tract.

- Hydrochloric acid, a strong chemical that is produced in the stomach, destroys many microbes.
- Eyes are protected by tears that provide a flushing action to remove most microbes that enter the eyes.

The body also has a number of internal defenses against infectious agents, including:

- Fever.
- Special cells in the blood called **phagocytes** that destroy microbes,
- **Inflammation**—a process that brings blood and phagocytes to the area of infection (Figure 12-7). A skin infection, for example, causes the skin area to become swollen, hot, and painful, signs that inflammation is occurring.
- Temperature—an elevated temperature is believed to increase the body's ability to fight infection.
- **Immune response**—the body develops protective proteins after having an infectious disease.

IMMUNITY

Immunity is the ability to fight off disease caused by microbes. A pathogenic microbe that enters the body is an **antigen**. In response to this, the blood develops substances called **antibodies**. These antibodies provide immunity (resistance) to the disease caused by that particular antigen. For example, if an individual has had antigens in the bloodstream from measles, he or she will form antibodies in the blood that prevent the occurrence of measles a second time.

IMMUNIZATIONS

Artificial defenses called **immunizations** protect against specific pathogens. Immunization is provided by **vaccines**.

FIGURE 12-7 Redness, swelling, heat, pain, and loss of function are signs of the inflammatory process. A sore throat is an excellent example of painful inflammation. (Courtesy of Centers for Disease Control and Prevention)

These are artificial or weakened antigens that help the body develop protective antibodies before the need arises. Vaccines are available to prevent most childhood diseases, such as measles, rubella (German measles), meningitis, mumps, polio, diphtheria, chickenpox, whooping cough, and tetanus. Pneumonia vaccine and influenza vaccine are frequently given to elderly people. Health workers who have direct contact with patients are advised to take hepatitis B vaccine. Federal legislation requires that employers provide this vaccine without charge to employees who are considered at risk.

IMMUNOSUPPRESSION

Immunosuppression occurs when the body's immune system is inadequate and fails to respond to the challenge of infectious disease organisms that it normally would fight successfully. The individual becomes more likely to develop a variety of infections. A number of factors can lead to this condition, including:

- Advanced age
- Frailty
- Chemotherapy
- Infection with human immunodeficiency virus (HIV)
- Injury or removal of the spleen
- Radiation therapy

SERIOUS INFECTIONS IN HEALTH CARE FACILITIES

Serious bacterial and viral infections are increasing in health care facilities as well as in the general public. Ill patients, especially those who are elderly or frail, are particularly susceptible to infectious diseases, as are the very young and those with compromised (poorly functioning) immune systems.

BACTERIAL INFECTIONS

Bacteria are often the cause of serious skin, respiratory, urinary, and gastrointestinal infections in patients. If the physician suspects that a patient has a bacterial infection, a **culture and sensitivity** test may be ordered. This test can be done on urine, drainage from a wound, blood, or other body fluid. The culture tells the physician what type of microbe is causing the infection. The sensitivity tells the physician which **antibiotic** (antibacterial drug) should be used to treat the infection.

When an antibiotic is prescribed, it is important for the patient to take all the medication prescribed for the stated length of time. If the patient stops taking the antibiotic too soon, some of the microbes may remain and develop a resistance to the antibiotic.

Certain infectious microbes have become resistant to the antibiotics most commonly used against them. This is a serious problem for infection control in health care facilities. The antibiotics that are still effective often are more expensive and may have serious side effects compared with the previously preferred antibiotics. It is possible that, in time, these infectious microbes may become resistant to these newer antibiotics as well.

MRSA and VRE

Two groups of organisms have become resistant to two powerful antibiotics, methicillin and vancomycin. These organisms are:

- **Methicillin-resistant *Staphylococcus aureus* (MRSA)**. Staphylococci are normally found on skin and mucous membranes. (See the online Appendix at the Online Companion for this textbook.)
- **Vancomycin-resistant enterococci (VRE)**. Enterococci are found in the gastrointestinal tract. They are a major cause of infections acquired in health care facilities. Most strains are highly resistant to many antibiotics. Newer strains are resistant to vancomycin.

Other Bacterial Pathogens

Serious infections are also caused by the following types of bacteria:

- *Pseudomonas aeruginosa*—this organism is found in water and on other environmental surfaces. It causes urinary tract infections. This bacterium also causes respiratory system infections, dermatitis, soft tissue infections, bacteremia, bone and joint infections, gastrointestinal infections, and a variety of systemic infections, especially in patients with cystic fibrosis, burns, cancer, and AIDS. The pathogen can infect any body tissue. It usually exploits a break in the host defenses to start an infection. It is rapidly becoming drug-resistant.
- *Escherichia coli*—bacterium commonly found in the intestinal tract, where it is normally nonpathogenic. Outside the intestinal tract, however, it can cause urinary tract infections or infections in pressure ulcers.
- *Klebsiella*—a bacterium that is a major cause of pneumonia, urinary tract, and wound infections. The most common infection caused by *Klebsiella* bacteria outside the hospital is pneumonia. The bacteria are quickly becoming drug-resistant. *Klebsiella* normally resides in the colon, where it is used for normal bowel function. If it escapes from the colon and enters an area where it does not belong, serious infection occurs. *Klebsiella* usually infects patients with weakened immune systems. The infection typically occurs when the patient is hospitalized for another reason.
- Salmonella—a group of bacteria that cause mild to life-threatening intestinal infections, including "food poisoning."

- *Listeria monocytogenes*—**listeriosis** is caused by ingesting these bacteria in contaminated food. The bacterium is found in some raw foods, such as uncooked meats and vegetables, hot dogs, cold cuts, and soft cheeses. Unpasteurized (raw) milk may contain the bacteria. *Listeria* is killed by pasteurization and cooking, but in some foods, such as hot dogs, contamination may occur after cooking but before packaging.

- *Acinetobacter baumannii*—a bacterium that was contracted by many soldiers in Iraq. It is a common cause of pneumonia, including nosocomial pneumonia in 7% of hospital-acquired cases. The mortality rates for this pneumonia can be 20% or more. This pathogen also causes infections of the bone, bloodstream, and internal organs, which require complicated patient care. There are few drugs to treat it, and no new medicines are in development. Carriers have been returning from Iraq with this pathogen on their skin, although they show no signs of infection. Because of the prevalence of the pathogen, all soldiers entering military hospitals upon return from Iraq have been cultured for the bacteria. This was the second most prevalent infection for soldiers in Vietnam, but the military was surprised to see it in Iraq. Some of the most fragile patients in U.S. military hospitals have contracted the bacteria and died. Containing the spread of this infection has been very difficult.

Tuberculosis

Mycobacterium tuberculosis is the bacterium that causes tuberculosis. Before the development of antibiotics, tuberculosis was a widespread disease with a high fatality rate. In the 1950s, the use of antibiotics effective against tuberculosis caused the numbers of cases and deaths to drop sharply. Since 1985, the number of people infected with tuberculosis has increased, in part because new strains of *Mycobacterium tuberculosis* are resistant to several antibiotics used to treat tuberculosis. There has also been an increase in the number of people who are at risk for infection, including those who:

- Are HIV positive
- Are infected but fail to take their medication for the full treatment period
- Live in poverty and are malnourished
- Have immigrated to the United States from countries where tuberculosis is still common
- Have had inactive tuberculosis but have grown older and experience increased disability

Tuberculosis Infection. **Tuberculosis infection** occurs when the bacterium that causes the disease enters the body. The lungs are the most common site of infection. The body usually responds to the infection by creating a barrier that prevents the spread of pathogens to other parts of the body. This barrier is called a **tubercle**. As long as the tubercle remains intact and no other tuberculosis

bacteria enter the body, the infection is called inactive or controlled. In this state the person is not **contagious** (capable of passing the infection to others). If the person is immunocompromised, the tubercle may not form and the person develops active tuberculosis disease.

Tuberculosis Disease. **Tuberculosis disease** develops if the tubercle breaks down or more tuberculosis bacteria enter the body. The bacteria multiply, tissue damage increases, and the bacteria may spread to other parts of the body. As the disease progresses, the person will show one or more of the following signs and symptoms:

- Fatigue
- Loss of appetite and weight
- Weakness
- Elevated temperature in the afternoon and evening
- Night sweats
- Spitting up blood (**hemoptysis**)
- Coughing

The person with tuberculosis in the lungs can spread it to others through droplets in respiratory secretions.

Diagnosis. The presence of tuberculosis bacterium in the body can be shown by:

- A sputum culture—grows the organisms from a specimen of secretions from the person's lungs
- Chest X-rays—show the extent of the disease process in the lungs
- A positive skin test (Mantoux test)—shows the presence of antibodies to the tuberculosis organisms in the body (Figure 12-8)

Most health care workers must undergo a skin test for tuberculosis before employment.

Treatment. A person with tuberculosis is treated with a selected antibiotic or combination of antibiotics. Because many disease organisms have become resistant to specific drugs, a combination of drugs must be used to control them. Once antitubercular drug therapy starts, the patient usually becomes noncontagious (cannot spread the disease organism) within two to three weeks. The therapy, however, continues for six months to two years.

Streptococcus A

Streptococcus A is a bacterium that produces very powerful enzymes that destroy tissue and blood cells. Incidences of this pathogen have increased. At least 15% of people carry group A strep in their respiratory secretions. Most have no symptoms. They pass the infection to others by coughing or sneezing, or by touching a susceptible person or environmental surface without washing their hands. *Strep A* causes a serious skin infection called **necrotizing fasciitis** (Figure 12-9A). This condition is often called "flesh-eating" or "man-eating" strep. It occurs when bacteria enter the body through minor trauma or a break in the skin. The pathogen can enter a break as tiny as a

FIGURE 12-8 A positive Mantoux test shows redness and induration (swelling) 48 to 72 hours after the test.

paper cut. Occasionally, the patient has no known break in the skin. Once inside the body, the patient develops flu-like illness. The toxin destroys muscle tissue. Pain in the area of the broken skin is often severe, out of proportion to the injury. The injury worsens rapidly over several days. Pain increases, and severe swelling and redness develop on the skin. At this point, it can spread as much as an inch an hour, causing tissue death. Blood cannot reach or nourish the dead tissue. The wound turns black and gangrenous (Figure 12-9B), requiring amputation. *Strep A* can be so serious that although the patient survives, he or she is scarred and has as many as all four extremities amputated.

Every system of the body can fail as a result of the severe infection and toxicity of the pathogen. In addition to the tissue decay, the bacteria spread throughout the body, causing massive shock, heart and respiratory failure, low blood pressure, and renal failure. *Strep A* has also been showing up in increasing numbers of head and neck abscesses in pediatric patients. An **abscess** (Figure 12-9C)

FIGURE 12-9B Gangrene occurs due to loss of blood supply to a body part. Amputation is the usual treatment. (Courtesy of Centers for Disease Control and Prevention)

FIGURE 12-9A *Strep A* is also called flesh-eating strep. This serious condition spreads rapidly, and often results in the need for amputation. (Courtesy of Centers for Disease Control and Prevention)

FIGURE 12-9C An abscess is a collection of pus in tissues, organs, or confined spaces in the body. It is usually swollen and inflamed and indicates that an infection is present. This abscess has erupted and is draining. It was caused by MRSA. (Courtesy of Centers for Disease Control and Prevention)

is a collection of pus in the tissue, usually in a confined space. Abscesses can occur anywhere in the body. They are an uncommon complication of upper respiratory infections. Once developed, they can progress rapidly to airway obstruction, vision loss, brain infections, and death.

Good handwashing helps reduce the risk of infection. Although *Strep A* is treated with antibiotics and surgery, the results are not always good. Prompt diagnosis and treatment of this condition are essential because of the speed with which the infection spreads. Unfortunately, symptoms are often mistaken for the flu, so most people delay treatment. About 25% of cases result in death.

Escherichia coli O157:H7

You have learned that *Escherichia coli (E. coli)* can cause serious problems outside the intestinal tract. Another strain, *E. coli O157:H7*, has caused outbreaks resulting in serious illness and death. This form of the bacterium is found in the intestines of some cattle. A small amount of these bacteria can contaminate a large amount of meat, particularly ground beef. It is transmitted in contaminated and undercooked meat, produce that has been exposed to water or fertilizer contaminated with feces, or by a person who has been handling contaminated food. It has been found on cutting boards and utensils. The bacteria have been found in unpasteurized milk and apple juice, as well as pools and lakes contaminated with fecal matter. The best way to prevent its spread is to use good handwashing and food preparation practices. Ground beef (hamburger) should be cooked until it is well done in the center. The high temperature required to cook meat to well done will kill the pathogen.

Signs and Symptoms. When *E. coli O157:H7* enters the human intestinal tract (for example, when a person eats contaminated food), the bacterium multiplies rapidly, producing large amounts of toxins. One to two days later, the person develops watery diarrhea, nausea, vomiting, and cramping. In another day or two, the diarrhea becomes bloody. The abdomen becomes **distended** (enlarged) and very tender. The patient may show signs of dehydration, swelling, and **petechiae**, small purplish spots on the body surface, caused by minute hemorrhages. The diarrhea may subside in five to seven days, but the condition injures the mucous membranes, allowing the pathogen to escape into the bloodstream. This creates a situation in which blood flow to the brain, kidneys, and other organs is endangered. The patient develops signs and symptoms of serious illness, such as:

- Decreased urine output that may progress to complete renal failure
- Mental confusion
- **Seizures** (convulsions)
- Muscle weakness
- Pain and numbness of the feet and legs

Treatment. In some conditions, the risk of transmitting infection is highest before the diagnosis is made. Because of this, many facilities place patients in contact precautions (Unit 13) until the condition is diagnosed. Diapered and incontinent patients remain in contact precautions for the duration of illness. Standard precautions (Unit 13) may safely be used for other patients.

E. coli O157:H7 can be deadly, particularly to infants, children, and others with weakened immune systems. Care for this condition is supportive, and the patient requires careful monitoring. Unfortunately, many drugs increase the risk of kidney damage. Water intake is very important, but liquid intake will require very close observation because of the potential for kidney damage. Careful monitoring of the patient's vital signs is required.

Pseudomembranous Colitis

Many bacteria live in the bowel of a healthy person. Most of them are harmless, and some friendly bacteria help with digestion. A few of these have the potential to be troublemakers if they get out of control. Most of the time, the bad bacteria are outnumbered by the good bacteria, and no harm comes to the person. Taking antibiotics can upset the balance in the colon. Many people develop a brief bout of diarrhea because the balance is upset, but the condition resolves quickly on its own.

Pseudomembranous colitis is a very serious condition in which diarrhea is caused by a bacterium called *Clostridium difficile (C. difficile)*. It is often called by its nickname, "C. Diff." This condition develops in patients who have been on antibiotic therapy. The friendly (good) bacteria die as a result of the antibiotic, and the harmful (bad) bacteria grow out of control. Pseudomembranous colitis occurs because the antibiotics destroy the normal bowel flora except for *C. difficile*, which is particularly resistant. Without the other friendly bacteria to keep it in check, it breeds rapidly, producing toxins that cause serious illness.

C. difficile is very common in health care facilities. It is picked up on the hands, on bedpans, bedside commodes, toilets, sinks, countertops, bed rails, doorknobs, and other surfaces that have been contaminated by stool. It most commonly enters the body through the mouth by contact with unwashed hands.

Signs and Symptoms. Pseudomembranous colitis may occur several weeks or months after a course of antibiotic therapy is completed, so it can be difficult to diagnose. *C. difficile* produces a toxin that affects the lining of the intestine, causing inflammation. This results in sudden, severe, foul-smelling, watery diarrhea. Stopping the antibiotic will not stop the diarrhea. The diarrhea may be so frequent and severe that the patient becomes dehydrated rapidly and develops other serious imbalances within the body. Other signs and symptoms are:

- Cramping and pain in the lower abdomen; sometimes this begins several days before the diarrhea starts

- Fever
- Mucus, pus, or blood in the stool
- Abdomen very tender to touch
- In severe cases, low blood pressure and signs of shock

If the condition is not promptly treated, it can cause ruptured bowel and a condition in which the bowel becomes severely distended and retains stool.

Diagnosis and Treatment. If pseudomembranous colitis is suspected, the doctor will order laboratory analysis on one or more stool cultures. The laboratory will identify the bacteria that are causing the illness. The antibiotic suspected of causing the problem is stopped, if possible. Another antimicrobial drug is used to eliminate the harmful bacteria in the colon. The patient may be given yogurt to eat and several other medications to increase the balance of healthy flora in the bowel. Although drug therapy usually eliminates the condition, it sometimes recurs, making a second course of therapy necessary. The patient is placed in contact precautions (Unit 13) until 72 hours after the appearance and frequency of stools return to normal, or as ordered by the physician. Standard precautions must also be used.

INFECTIOUS DIARRHEA

Spores are microscopic reproductive bodies that are responsible for the spread of some diseases. They can survive in a dormant form until conditions are ideal for reproduction. The spores will then multiply and continue to spread infection. They are very difficult to eliminate.

Norovirus (Norwalk virus) is a highly contagious pathogen that causes infectious diarrhea. You may have heard of these viruses on the news, as they caused diarrhea outbreaks on many cruise ships. Very few particles are needed to transmit infection. The pathogen originates in the stool. *Rotavirus* is plentiful throughout environments in which many young children spend time (such as day care centers), especially during the winter months. Both viruses are highly resistant to disinfectants used for cleaning environmental surfaces. *Norovirus* is also highly resistant to alcohol-based hand cleaners. *Rotavirus* and *Norovirus* remain active on the hands for at least 4 hours, on hard dry surfaces for 10 days, and on wet surfaces for weeks.

Patients with infectious diarrhea will be placed on contact precautions. When caring for patients with infectious diarrhea, especially conditions known to be spread by spores, such as *C. difficile* or *Norovirus*, you must use good handwashing. The friction and running water will remove spores and viruses from your hands.

Environmental Cleanliness

When patients have infectious diarrhea or another condition spread by spores, special attention must be paid to environmental cleanliness. These pathogens have the following features in common:

- *C. difficile*, (Figure 12-10), *Rotavirus*, and *Norovirus* are usually plentiful in the environment (room or unit) of patients with infectious diarrhea.
- They have been found on the hands of health care workers providing care to affected patients or touching items and surfaces in the patient's room.
- They are capable of surviving for days to months in the environment.
- *C. difficile* and *Norovirus* are resistant to many chemical disinfectant products, including alcohol.
- They have caused outbreaks of infectious diarrhea in hospitals and long-term care facilities.
- They are transmitted through the digestive tract (usually entering through the mouth via the hands).
- *C. difficile* and *Norovirus* are spread by spores.
- Studies have shown that environmental surface contamination is a common source of infection.
- Good handwashing, with soap, water, and friction, is required to eliminate pathogens and spores from hands.
- Environmental cleaning is required, with friction and a disinfectant product known to kill the pathogen, such as those containing sodium hypochlorite (bleach).

VIRAL INFECTIONS

Several viral infections are listed in this section:

- Shingles (herpes zoster)
- Influenza

FIGURE 12-10 *C. difficile* is a spore-forming bacterium. It is a major cause of pseudomembranous colitis and diarrhea. People become infected if they touch items or surfaces that are contaminated with feces and then touch the mouth or mucous membranes. Health care workers can spread the bacteria to other patients or contaminate surfaces through hand contact. (Courtesy of Centers for Disease Control and Prevention)

- Hepatitis
- Acquired immune deficiency syndrome (AIDS)
- Hantavirus
- Smallpox
- Severe acute respiratory syndrome (SARS)

The viral infection genital herpes is covered in Unit 46.

Shingles

Shingles (herpes zoster) (Figure 12-11A) occurs in people who were infected by the virus that causes chickenpox. The organisms did not leave the body. They remained hidden in the nervous system in a nonactive (dormant) state.

Years later, when the person is in a weakened condition, the organisms become active. Painful blister-like lesions develop in the skin along the paths of sensitive nerves. The blisters contain infectious organisms. Workers who never had chickenpox, and those who have not been immunized against chickenpox should not care for a person with shingles. Workers who are pregnant should not enter the room because of the risk of complications from possible exposure. The patient is no longer infectious and will be removed from isolation when all the lesions have burst and have crusted over (Figure 12-11B).

Influenza

Influenza (flu) is caused by a family of viruses. The infection can have serious consequences for elderly or frail people. Each year new types of viruses spread rapidly from person to person by way of respiratory secretions, causing many to become ill. Vaccines offer some protection against influenza viruses and are often given to residents in long-term care.

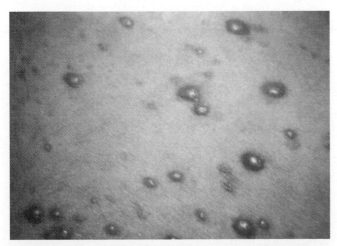

FIGURE 12-11A A rash in a patient with shingles. The blisters are intact, so the patient is infectious. Compare the blisters with the photo of chickenpox. (Courtesy of Centers for Disease Control and Prevention)

FIGURE 12-11B These shingles blisters have erupted and crusted over into scab-like areas. The patient is no longer infectious when all blisters have ruptured. (Courtesy of Centers for Disease Control and Prevention)

Someone with the flu may experience:

- Malaise (general unwell feeling)
- Chills
- Fever
- Muscle aches and pains
- Coldlike symptoms

In addition to making the person feel ill, the viruses may lower the patient's resistance to other infectious organisms. These other organisms can cause pneumonia and other life-threatening infections. Medicines may be given to limit the effects of the viruses and antibiotics are given to combat bacterial infections that may develop.

You can help protect the patients in your care by:

- Staying healthy
- Not reporting for duty when you are ill
- Carrying out standard precautions faithfully
- Following the facility's policies regarding special precautions when a patient has a respiratory infection
- Encouraging the patient to drink fluids
- Reporting to the charge nurse when a visitor seems to be ill

Hepatitis

Hepatitis is an inflammation of the liver caused by several viruses, including:

- Hepatitis A virus
- Hepatitis B virus
- Hepatitis C virus
- Hepatitis D virus
- Hepatitis E virus
- Hepatitis G virus

Characteristics of these viruses are:

- Hepatitis A virus (HAV)
  - Most common
  - Transmitted by feces, saliva, and contaminated food
  - Signs and symptoms are **jaundice**, a yellow color of the skin and sclera (Figure 12-12), fever, nausea, vomiting, diarrhea, fatigue, abdominal pain, dark urine, and appetite loss. Respiratory symptoms, rashes, and joint pain may also develop. Some people do not notice any signs of illness. As a rule, the symptoms are more severe in older patients.
  - Vaccine available
  - Rarely fatal
  - Treated with bedrest and avoidance of alcoholic beverages
- Hepatitis B virus (HBV)
  - Can cause liver cancer and death
  - Transmitted by blood, sexual secretions, feces, and saliva
  - Signs and symptoms may mimic the flu; they include fever, aches and pains, nausea, fatigue, and urine that may turn a dark color
  - Infectious for life, even after the patient recovers from acute illness
  - Some patients have no symptoms at all but are still infectious
  - Vaccine available for protection
- Hepatitis C virus (HCV)
  - 50% of people infected develop chronic hepatitis
  - Transmitted mainly through blood and blood products
  - May be mistaken for the flu
  - Common signs and symptoms are extreme fatigue, depression, fever, mood changes, weakness, pain, loss of appetite
  - May cause liver cancer and liver failure

  - Disease may be present for years before patient becomes aware of it; during this time it silently destroys the liver
  - Leading cause of need for liver transplants in the United States
  - Treated with alpha interferon; treatment is not always successful

Any infection of the liver is serious because the liver is a vital organ. Health care workers must take hepatitis very seriously because many individuals have no signs and symptoms of illness, yet are able to transmit the infection to others. You can best protect yourself by:

- Using standard precautions (Unit 13)
- Taking the vaccine, if available
- Practicing safe sex (using condoms)
- Not using illegal drugs
- Giving your full attention to the handling of sharps, such as needles or razors

Acquired Immune Deficiency Syndrome (AIDS)

Acquired immune deficiency syndrome (AIDS) is a viral disease. It is transmitted primarily through direct contact with the bodily secretions of an infected person. The virus that causes AIDS is the **human immunodeficiency virus (HIV)**.

The ways in which HIV is transmitted include:

- Blood to blood through:
  - Transfusion of infected blood. Note that federal regulations prohibit the use of untested and unregulated blood in the United States
  - Treatment of hemophilia with clotting factor from infected blood
  - Needle sharing among drug users
  - Prick from a contaminated needle or sharp
  - Unsterile instruments used for procedures such as ear piercing or tattooing
- Unprotected vaginal, oral, or anal intercourse when one partner is infected
- Infected mother to infant during:
  - Pregnancy
  - Birth process
  - Breast-feeding

The AIDS Virus. The AIDS virus (HIV):

- Has many variants
- Does not live long outside the body
- Is affected by common chemicals such as bleach
- Depresses the body's immune system
- Makes the infected person more susceptible to infections
- Makes the infected person more likely to experience complications such as:

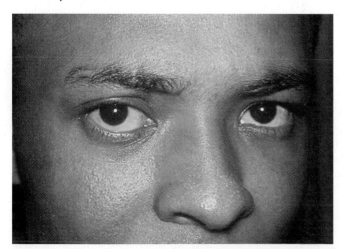

FIGURE 12-12 Jaundice is a yellowing of the skin and whites of the eyes caused by hepatitis and other conditions. (Courtesy of Centers for Disease Control and Prevention)

FIGURE 12-13 The Kaposi's sarcoma lesion is commonly seen in the mouth and lining the intestinal tract. It may also develop on the skin surface. (Courtesy of Centers for Disease Control and Prevention)

- *Pneumocystis carinii* pneumonia—a serious lung infection
- Kaposi's sarcoma (Figure 12-13)—a serious malignancy affecting many body organs
- Brain involvement leading to dementia
- Eye involvement leading to blindness
- Tuberculosis
- Other opportunistic infections

Incubation Period. Not everyone who comes in contact with the HIV virus becomes infected. For those who are infected, there is always a period of time between contact and the start of the signs and symptoms of infection.

- During this period the virus is in infected cells but is not active. The body does not make antibodies to the virus.
- Most people become **seropositive** or HIV positive (show antibodies to HIV in the bloodstream) approximately 3 to 6 months after infection. The person has HIV disease, which may progress to AIDS.
- The asymptomatic period (when no signs and symptoms are present) following infection may last months to years. AIDS does not always develop, but the person is an HIV carrier for life.

Disease Progression. Progression of the disease process is determined by the effect of the viruses on spe-

cial protective white blood cells known as CD4 cells (T cells). Over time, the number of these protective white blood cells drops. As a result, the immune system of the infected person becomes more suppressed (weaker) and less able to fight infection. When the number of CD4 cells drops to a critical level (below 200 cells/mm^3), the person is diagnosed with AIDS.

Symptoms of HIV infection, when they do appear, consist of:

- Acute flulike symptoms
- Fever
- Night sweats
- Fatigue
- Swollen lymph nodes
- Sore throat
- Gastrointestinal problems
- Headache

One-fourth to one-half of people exposed to HIV show evidence of disease within 5 to 10 years of antibody development (becoming seropositive).

Testing. Several tests have been developed to confirm the presence of antibodies to HIV (positive for HIV infection), to test the level of viral activity, and to confirm the presence of AIDS.

The test for antibodies is also used to check the national blood supply. When people donate blood, it is tested to be sure that it is free of HIV antibodies, to protect the people who receive blood transfusions and other blood products.

Treatment. No specific treatment is able to cure AIDS at the present time. A combination of drugs currently in use reduces both the symptoms and viral activity.

- No vaccine prevents the infection from developing. However, millions of dollars are being spent on research to develop a vaccine.

- Therapy is directed toward vigorously treating each infection as it appears.
- Nutritional and other forms of preventive therapy are aimed at maintaining a person with AIDS in the best health possible.
- The drug industry continues to develop drugs that slow down the disease process or reinforce the immune system. Patients treated with combinations of drugs show decreased viral loads and improved CD4 counts. Every dose must be taken properly. When patients fail to follow the protocol exactly, the disease state returns quickly and more strongly than before. These drugs, however, do not cure the disease.
- At present there is no evidence that AIDS is transmitted:
  - Through kissing, touching, or hugging an HIV-infected person
  - By eating at the same table with an infected person
  - By using the same toilet seat
  - Through insect bites

Hantavirus

In May 1993, a cluster of unexplained deaths occurred among young Native Americans in the southwestern United States. An investigation revealed a new virus that was previously unknown. This situation attracted a great deal of media attention. Several additional outbreaks have been reported since 1993. This strange disease is called **hantavirus**. It is spread by contact with rodents (rats and mice) or their excretions, including urine and stool. Once disturbed, viral particles in the excretions become airborne and are inhaled by the susceptible host. Signs and symptoms appear one to five weeks later and include high fever, chills, muscle aches, cough, nausea, vomiting, diarrhea, dizziness, and feeling very tired. As the disease progresses, the patient becomes very short of breath. When this occurs, the disease progresses rapidly, and the patient becomes seriously ill. Respiratory support may be necessary. Hantavirus is not transmitted from person to person. Spread of this condition can be reduced by taking steps to prevent rodents from entering the home or eliminating them if they are present.

Severe Acute Respiratory Syndrome

Severe acute respiratory syndrome (SARS) was first seen in China in late 2002. It has now spread throughout the world. SARS is a viral respiratory illness caused by a coronavirus. It is highly contagious. The virus is elusive, and much remains to be learned. SARS seems to spread by very close person to person contact. Scientists believe the virus is spread through respiratory droplets, which are inhaled by a susceptible host who is within three feet of the patient. However, the droplets are heavy, and they fall to environmental surfaces, causing contamination. They are picked up on the hands and introduced into the host's body. It appears that it may also be spread by the airborne method.

Signs and Symptoms of SARS. SARS begins with a fever that is higher than 100.4°F. Other signs and symptoms are:

- Headache
- Flu-like symptoms of malaise, discomfort, and body aches
- Some people have mild respiratory symptoms at the outset
- Some patients develop diarrhea

The patient develops a dry cough in 2 to 7 days. The cough usually progresses to pneumonia. As the oxygen level in the blood decreases, the patient experiences respiratory distress. Many SARS patients need mechanical ventilation.

Treatment. SARS is treated similarly to very serious pneumonia. Antiviral drugs are given and respirations are supported. Your facility will require frequent handwashing, and special isolation precautions (Unit 13).

OTHER IMPORTANT INFECTIONS

Infection Caused by Fungi

Coccidioidomycosis (valley fever) is caused by *Coccidioides immitis*. It occurs primarily as a respiratory infection. It is treated with antibiotics and is seldom fatal in otherwise healthy people. In people with immunosuppression, however, the death rate is high. It is treated with antibiotics.

Aspergillosis is a serious fungal infection that affects patients with weak immune systems, such as those with HIV and AIDS, cancer patients, and transplant patients. An infection in the bloodstream can be deadly, and few drugs are available to treat it. There are more than 150 species of the Aspergillus genus, but only a few are harmful. Most healthy people are immune to this fungus, which is spread by spores. Aspergillus produces many well-known toxins. Some strains have caused infections in humans who consumed peanuts and grains. One strain resulted in a dog-food recall in 2005. A number of dogs died after consuming food containing the toxins (called *aflatoxins*).

Infection Caused by Protozoa

Two diseases caused by protozoa are becoming more common in the general public and in health facilities. Giardiasis is caused by *Giardia lamblia*, which is found in the water supplies of many communities. It also causes severe diarrhea. Cryptosporidiosis is caused by the *Cryptosporidium* protozoan, which is found in the digestive tracts of domestic animals and is transferred by contact. It also causes diarrhea, especially in immunosuppressed

GUIDELINES *for*

Preventing Infection

- Assist patients to maintain adequate fluid intake. This helps prevent urinary tract and respiratory tract infections and keeps the skin healthier.

- Assist patients to maintain adequate nutritional intake. Report to the nurse when patients eat less or refuse food.

- Assist patients to carry out exercise programs established by the nurse or physical therapist. Follow positioning schedules and orders for range-of-motion exercises and ambulation. Exercise improves breathing and circulation.

- Toilet patients who need assistance. This keeps the bladder empty and also assures patients that they will receive help when they need to urinate.

- When cleaning the perineal area of patients, be sure to wipe women from front to back. This avoids contaminating the urethra (bladder opening) with stool or vaginal excretions.

- Perform catheter care as directed. Avoid opening the drainage system.

- Observe patients carefully and report any unusual signs or changes, such as:
  - Changes in frequency of urination or amount of urine voided
  - Complaints of pain or burning on urination
  - Changes in character of urine
  - Coughing or respiratory problems
  - Confusion or disorientation that was not present before or that has increased
  - Drainage or discharge from any body opening or skin wound
  - Changes in skin color
  - Complaints of pain, discomfort, or nausea
  - Elevated temperature
  - Red, swollen areas on body

- Keep patients clean.

- Staff members who have an infectious disease should not be on duty. Caring for your own health is vital in preventing illness in patients. Friends and family of patients should be advised not to visit when they do not feel well. If you notice a visitor coughing and sneezing, or otherwise obviously sick, inform the nurse.

- Follow your facility policies and procedures for prevention of infection and injury. If you identify health risks, take the proper precautions. It is your responsibility to learn and follow these practices. Cooperate with your infection control nurse or department during audits, education, investigation of outbreaks and exposure, and review of infection control practices. Sometimes recommendations to prevent infection change. It is your responsibility to learn new techniques and make changes in the way you practice.

---

people. Both pathogens are spread by spores. Avoid alcohol hand cleanser if these organisms are present.

BIOTERRORISM

Bioterrorism is the use of biological agents, such as pathogenic organisms or agricultural pests, for terrorist purposes. Since October 2001, state, local, and federal public health authorities have been investigating cases of bioterrorism-related illness. Specifically, some individuals died from inhalation anthrax, a condition that was spread by a powdery substance containing anthrax spores that was sent through the mail. A number of other individuals developed the cutaneous (skin) version of this disease. Cutaneous anthrax is not fatal. Anthrax cannot be passed from one person to the next. It is transmitted only through contact with spores. Fortunately, the number of

workplaces and individuals contaminated was small, but it raised concerns regarding future terrorist attacks. Many individuals could be infected by a biological weapon before the exposure is detected and diagnosed. Some of the diseases that can potentially be used as biological weapons have been considered eradicated for years, and today's health care professionals have never seen or treated them. Thus, bioterrorism is a significant threat.

Many health care facilities have developed disaster plans to address bioterrorism. The plans outline the steps necessary for responding to bioterrorism with the most common agents, including smallpox, botulism toxin, anthrax, and plague. The disaster plan includes information for patients, employees, and visitors, and specifies public health precautions and protocols to follow in the event of an emergency. Sadly, given the state of world affairs, health care facilities must be prepared for potential terrorist actions in the future.

Smallpox

Smallpox (Figure 12-14) is a serious viral infection that is sometimes fatal. The disease emerged thousands of years ago, but was eliminated during the 20th century. Unfortunately, laboratory stockpiles of the virus that causes smallpox still exist, and there is concern that these samples might be used for terrorist purposes.

Mode of Transmission. Smallpox is caused by the variola virus. It usually spreads through direct face-to-face contact with an infected person. It may also be spread by:

- Direct contact with infected bodily fluids
- Direct contact with contaminated objects, such as linen or clothing
- The air in buildings, buses, and trains, although this is less common

The virus does not live long in the air, and 90% of the virus dies within 24 hours after airborne release. Ultraviolet light (Unit 13) eliminates even more of the virus.

Signs and Symptoms. After exposure to the smallpox virus, the newly infected person goes through a 7- to 17-day incubation period in which there are no symptoms of illness. The first symptoms of smallpox include:

- High fever ranging from 101°F to 104°F
- Feeling very tired
- Headache
- Body aches
- Vomiting

Infected persons are usually too sick to carry on their normal activities. This phase lasts for about two to four days.

A rash emerges about four days after the onset of fever. At first, small red spots appear in the mouth and on the tongue. The spots become sores that break open, spreading large amounts of virus into the mouth and throat. The patient is extremely contagious during this time. A rash also develops on the skin, beginning on the face and spreading to the arms, legs, hands, and feet. Within 24 hours, the rash spreads to all parts of the body. When the rash appears, the fever drops and the person begins to feel better. By the third day of the rash, raised bumps appear. By day four, the bumps fill with a thick, cloudy fluid. The bumps develop a depression in the center. Their appearance has been compared to the appearance of a navel, and is a distinguishing feature of smallpox. During this time, the patient's fever rises again and remains high until scabs develop. The bumps become round and firm to the touch; they may feel like pellets from a BB gun. After approximately five days, the bumps develop scabs. The scabs fall off, leaving scars on the skin. This occurs about three weeks after the rash appears. The person is contagious until the last scab falls off.

Vaccination. A vaccine is available to prevent smallpox, but it has not been routinely given since the 1970s, when the disease was eradicated worldwide. Presently, there is no treatment for smallpox, although this is an area of current research. Receiving the vaccine within three days of exposure will completely prevent or significantly reduce the severity of the illness. Vaccination four to seven days after exposure likely offers some protection from disease or may modify the severity of disease.

In 2002, the United States began recommending that hospitals immunize certain key personnel against smallpox. In case of an outbreak, these individuals would be able to care for patients without contracting the disease. Not everyone can receive the vaccine. For example, health care workers who are HIV positive, pregnant, or have had certain skin and other health conditions should not receive the vaccine.

The smallpox vaccine contains a weakened live virus that stimulates the body into developing immunity. A normal reaction to the vaccine is to develop a blister, which fills with pus, drains, then crusts over (Figure 12-15). The crust falls off, leaving a scar. Because the vaccine contains a live virus, the injection site must be kept covered.

An individual who has just been immunized can work, but may be under work restrictions for some time after

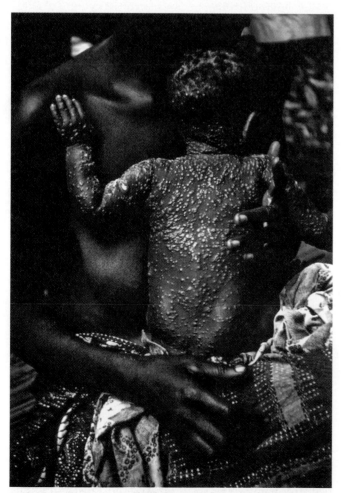

FIGURE 12-14 This photograph shows the back of a Nigerian child with smallpox. Compare this photo with the pictures of chickenpox and shingles. (Courtesy of Centers for Disease Control and Prevention)

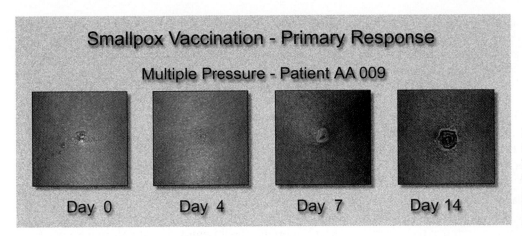

FIGURE 12-15 Photographs of normal smallpox vaccination site "takes" shot at different intervals over a two-week period. (Courtesy of Centers for Disease Control and Prevention)

the smallpox immunization. Personnel who have been immunized should not care for newborn infants or patients who are immunocompromised for at least three weeks. The virus is not transmitted in the air, but can be spread by contact with the injection site and dressings or clothing covering the area.

If your facility offers the smallpox vaccine, become familiar with the actions, use, conditions in which the vaccine is not given, and potential side effects and risks. The vaccine provides high-level immunity for three to five years, but then immunity progressively decreases. Individuals who were immunized previously may have longer immunity.

PARASITES

You have learned that yeast and mold are opportunistic parasites. Some insects are also parasites, because they survive by feeding off another human or animal. Fleas and ticks are common examples of parasites.

Head Lice

Head lice are parasites that spread primarily by direct contact with an infected person. They can also be spread by sharing personal belongings such as brushes, combs, ribbons, caps, clothing, and bedding with others. You cannot contract head lice from pets and animals. The lice (Figure 12-16A) do not hop, jump, or fly, but they can crawl very quickly. When performing hair care, check patients for **nits** (Figure 12-16B). Nits are tiny, oval-shaped eggs that are yellow-white in color. They look like dandruff, but are firmly attached to the hair and are very difficult to remove. Dandruff brushes off readily. It may be difficult to differentiate nits from other conditions of the scalp. The nits hatch into live lice. Lice are tiny brown insects about the size of a sesame seed. They run away from light quickly. Notify the nurse for further assessment if you notice nits or other abnormalities.

Treatment for Head Lice. If nits or lice are suspected, you will wear a gown and gloves for contact with

FIGURE 12-16A A magnified view of a head louse. Head lice are tiny, but can be seen with the unaided eye. (Courtesy of Centers for Disease Control and Prevention)

FIGURE 12-16B A head louse hatching from a nit. The empty nit case remains firmly attached to the hair shaft. (Courtesy of Centers for Disease Control and Prevention)

the patient until the patient has been treated. You must also wear gloves and a gown when handling the patient's clothing or linen. The physician will order a medicated shampoo to kill the parasites. Contact precautions will be used for 24 hours after the patient is treated. It is important to remove all of the nits, as the shampoo may not kill them. To be effective, all the nits must be removed from the scalp, or the nits will hatch, producing more lice. A special comb is used. This is a time-consuming task. You may be directed to check other patients for the presence of head lice.

As with other diseases, some head lice have become resistant to medicated shampoos. If the lice cannot be eliminated with a shampoo, the only way to remove them is by checking the head and eliminating them manually. Manual removal of lice and nits is done using a comb, tweezers, or double-sided tape. Two people may need to check the head simultaneously, because the lice run very fast. Shining a flashlight on the head may be helpful, as the lice will move away from the light source.

The patient's clothing must be bagged. Send it home with a family member, if possible. The linen and pillows in the room should be sent to the laundry. Furniture and personal items in the room must be vacuumed to eliminate lice in the environment. Vacuuming is safer and more effective than using pesticide sprays, which leave a toxic residue. After vacuuming, wipe environmental surfaces with a facility-approved disinfectant to eliminate microbes left from the outside of the vacuum cleaner. Previously, toxic sprays were used to eliminate lice from environmental surfaces and personal belongings, but this is no longer recommended.

Scabies

Scabies is a disease of the skin caused by a parasite called a **mite** (Figure 12-17A). A mite is a microscopic organism that cannot be seen with the eye. Scabies is highly contagious and is spread by direct and indirect contact. It causes a rash (Figure 12-17B) and severe itching of the

skin. The rash may be seen in the webs of the fingers, inside the wrists, outside the elbows, and in the underarm, waist, and nipple area. It is also sometimes seen in the genital area in men and around the knees and lower buttocks. One type of scabies causes scaling and crusts on the palms of hands and soles of feet. If you notice a rash, notify the nurse immediately. As with head lice, you will be directed to wear a gown and gloves for further patient contact.

Treatment for Scabies. Special medicated creams and lotions are used to kill the mite. Some strains of scabies have become resistant to this treatment. If new lesions erupt after a patient has been properly treated, another product will be ordered. When treating for head lice or scabies, use the products exactly as directed. Products for treating lice and scabies are pesticides and repeated use can cause toxicity and other complications.

The patient's nails should be clipped before beginning. Work the medicated product into and around the fingernail area with a cotton swab. You may be directed to apply the lotion to the patient's entire body, not just the rash area. Avoid the eyelids or lips. Wear a gown and gloves when applying this treatment. The lotion remains

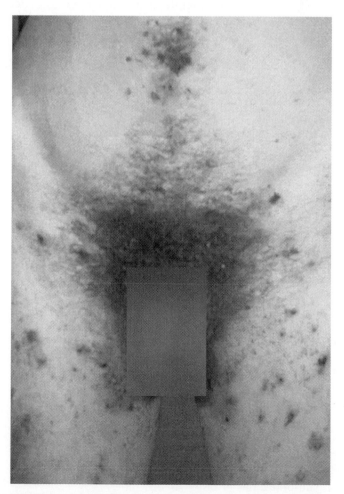

FIGURE 12-17B The scabies rash is often severe in the abdomen, groin, genital area, and knees. (Courtesy of Centers for Disease Control and Prevention)

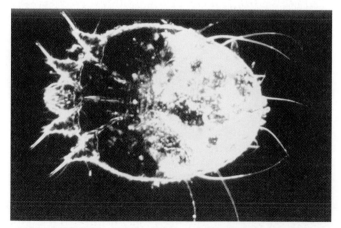

FIGURE 12-17A A microscopic view of the scabies mite, which cannot be seen with the unaided eye. (Courtesy of Centers for Disease Control and Prevention)

on the patient's skin for 12 to 24 hours, then is washed off in the tub or shower. If the patient's hands are washed during this period, reapply the lotion. Depending on the solution used, another treatment may be required several days to several weeks later. It takes about a month from the first treatment for the rash to disappear. The patient may experience itching even after the scabies are eliminated. You may be directed to check other patients for the appearance of a rash. Facility personnel may also be treated to prevent the spread of the mite.

The patient's room, clothing, and linen must also be cleaned. The room and furnishings should be vacuumed well to capture mites in the environment. Check the mattress and furniture for cracks, as the mite often crawls into the foam padding. If items cannot be vacuumed, they are bagged in a sealed plastic bag for 14 days. The mite cannot live beyond this time without food. Some facilities expose the bags to extreme heat or cold to kill the mite more quickly. The mattress is vacuumed and turned, then wiped with a facility-approved disinfectant to remove microbes left from the outside of the vacuum cleaner. Contact precautions are used for 24 hours after the patient is treated. If the patient requires a second treatment, the cleaning procedure is repeated for clothing, linen, and furnishings.

Bedbugs

Most people think **bedbugs** (Figure 12-18A) are imaginary pests from a nursery rhyme. In fact, bedbugs are real parasites that have been found throughout the world, with the exception of Antarctica. They have been found in hotels, hospitals, doctors' offices, and nursing homes in the United States. The bugs are usually seen at night, and are stealthy and fast-moving. They can survive in hot and cold environments. Although there is no recorded incidence of disease as a result of bedbugs, they are parasites that bite, causing a painful, rash-type area on the skin. Bedbugs have an anticoagulant in their saliva that prevents blood from clotting while they are eating. Some people are very sensitive to this substance, and have an allergic skin reaction. Others can live with bedbugs and not be aware of them. Some people develop welts that look like flea or mosquito bites. The tiny, red bumps itch. The bites may appear in lines, similar to scabies. Adult bedbugs can survive for up to a year without eating. Like lice and scabies, some bedbugs are resistant to over-the-counter insecticides, and setting off pesticide bombs may scatter them farther.

A bedbug is tiny, a little smaller than a pencil eraser. They are flat, and clear or white in appearance before feeding. After eating a blood meal, they develop a red-brown hue (Figure 12-18B). They leave little excretion droppings on the sheets and may give off a sickly sweet smell. Finding tiny bloodstains on the linen from crushed bugs, or dark spots from the droppings, is a strong indication that bedbugs are present. They hide in the seams of clothing and furnishings, so the patient may have brought them from home and may not be aware of it. Bedbugs can also live on bats, chickens, pigeons, other birds, laboratory animals, and some domestic pets. They run fast and multiply quickly. They may hide in cracks and crevices in mattresses, bed frames, behind headboards, inside nightstands, behind baseboards, and in window and door casings, pictures, and moldings. They have also been found hiding in furniture and clutter, such as piles of books, papers, and boxes, and items near sleeping areas. Shining a flashlight and aiming a hot hair dryer into crevices will help force the insects out.

If bedbugs are noted, a professional exterminator will be called to eliminate them. Everything in the room must be cleaned and washed. Items that cannot be washed should be sealed in plastic bags and exposed to very hot or freezing temperatures. The eggs must also be found and eliminated, or more bugs will hatch. If you suspect bedbugs in a patient's room, inform the nurse immediately.

FIGURE 12-18A The bedbug is tiny, but can be seen with the unaided eye. (Courtesy of Centers for Disease Control and Prevention)

FIGURE 12-18B The bedbug is clear in appearance until it ingests a blood meal, causing it to darken to a red-brown color. (Courtesy of Centers for Disease Control and Prevention)

OUTBREAK OF INFECTIOUS DISEASE IN A HEALTH CARE FACILITY

An outbreak of an infection in the facility can be serious. All patients, workers, volunteers, and visitors are at risk of exposure. Unless steps are taken immediately, the infection can spread rapidly. Examples of outbreaks include:

- Influenza
- Gastroenteritis, diarrhea
- Hepatitis
- MRSA
- Scabies

Most facilities have an action plan for responding to an outbreak of infection. Nursing assistants will receive instructions from the nurse.

SELF-CARE

You can take steps to stay healthy and free from infections:

- Eat a healthy diet.
- Get enough sleep each day.
- Keep your body clean.
- Live in a clean environment.
- Avoid unhealthy habits such as smoking and substance abuse.
- Learn how to cope with stress.

REVIEW

A. Matching.

Match Column I with Column II.

Column I

1. _____ spiral-shaped bacterium

2. _____ organism that causes ringworm

3. _____ bacteria that grow in pairs

4. _____ organism that causes AIDS

5. _____ bacteria that grow as clusters

Column II

a. staphylococci

b. protozoan

c. diplococci

d. streptococci

e. virus

f. fungus

g. spirillum

B. Word Choice.

Fill in the blanks for questions 6–10 with the correct word or phrase from the following list.

insects
method of transmission
portal of entry
portal of exit
reservoir

sexual contact
sneezing
susceptible host
water

6. Complete the chain of infection by naming the parts missing from the following figure.

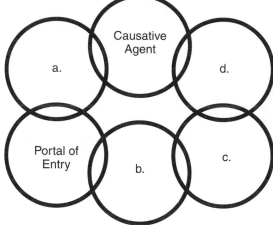

a. _____

b. _____

c. _____

d. _____

7. An example of transmission by direct contact is _____.

8. An example of transmission by indirect contact is _____.

9. A common vehicle for the transmission of microbes is _____.

10. Vectors, such as animals and _____ also transmit disease organisms.

C. True/False.

Mark the following true or false by circling T or F.

11. T F Normal body flora are the same in each part of the body.

12. T F The rectum is a common portal of exit for some infectious organisms.

13. T F The general health of an individual is an important factor in determining if infectious disease will occur.

14. T F Unbroken skin is a mechanical defense against infection.

15. T F A boil is an example of a generalized infection.

16. T F Allergies are sensitivity reactions.

17. T F The term *reservoir* may refer to a human body in which the organisms live.

18. T F An immunizing vaccine causes the body to produce antibodies that protect the person against certain infectious diseases.

19. T F MRSA infections are easy to control.

20. T F Bedpans and urinals can act as fomites.

D. Multiple Choice.

Select the one best answer for each of the following.

21. White blood cells that multiply and attempt to destroy pathogens are
   a. antigens.
   b. phagocytes.
   c. antibodies.
   d. red blood cells.

22. Which of the following is not a natural body defense?
   a. Antibiotic
   b. Hydrochloric acid in the stomach
   c. Hair in the nose
   d. Tears

23. Which is an example of a local infection?
   a. Pneumonia
   b. Septicemia
   c. Boil
   d. AIDS

24. One patient's visitor is coughing and looks flushed. Your best action is to
   a. ask the visitor to leave.
   b. put a mask on the visitor.
   c. put a mask on the patient.
   d. refer the matter to the nurse.

25. You woke up not feeling well this morning. You have an elevated temperature. Your best action is to
   a. call in sick.
   b. go to work.
   c. stay home without notifying the facility.
   d. call a friend to go to work for you.

26. Infection with *Escherichia coli O157:H7*
   a. is mildly uncomfortable.
   b. can cause renal failure and death.
   c. is caused by inhaling spores.
   d. is highly infectious to health care workers.

27. *Streptococcus A*
   a. is spread only by the droplet method.
   b. is easily treated and eliminated with antibiotics.
   c. causes pain out of proportion to the injury.
   d. is a common cause of infectious diarrhea.

28. Spores
   a. remain dormant until conditions are ideal for reproduction.
   b. can be eliminated by cleansing the environment with alcohol.
   c. are usually responsible for boils and skin abscesses.
   d. can be treated with antibiotics and increased fluids.

29. SARS
   a. can be treated and eliminated by antibiotics.
   b. is spread by more than one mode of transmission.
   c. is contagious only as long as the patient is coughing.
   d. requires no special precautions beyond standard precautions.

30. *Rotavirus* and *Norovirus*
   a. die quickly after leaving the body.
   b. can live up to an hour on environmental surfaces.
   c. are readily eliminated with alcohol-based hand cleaner.
   d. can remain on the hands for at least 4 hours.

31. Hantavirus is spread by
   a. rodent excretions.
   b. indirect contact with fomites.
   c. contact with an infected person.
   d. inhalation of droplets from an infected patient.

32. Bioterrorism is
   a. not a concern in the United States.
   b. the use of chemicals to cause illness.
   c. the use of biological agents for terrorist purposes.
   d. easily detected and treated.

33. Hepatitis B
   a. is spread by oral–fecal transmission.
   b. can be readily cured with antibiotics.
   c. causes visible signs of serious illness.
   d. can be prevented by vaccination.

E. Nursing Assistant Challenge.

34. Your patient, Mrs. Wallace, has a cold.
   a. What organism is responsible? _____
   b. Could Mrs. Wallace be immunized against this condition? _____
   c. How is the condition most likely transmitted? _____

35. Mr. Reynolds has a staphylococcal infection in his finger.
   a. What class of organisms are staphylococci? _____
   b. What shape are these organisms? _____
   c. How might Mr. Reynolds have acquired this infection? _____

UNIT 13

Infection Control

OBJECTIVES

After completing this unit, you will be able to:

- Spell and define terms.
- Explain the principles of medical asepsis.
- Explain the components of standard precautions.
- List the types of personal protective equipment.
- Describe nursing assistant actions related to standard precautions.
- Describe airborne precautions.
- Describe droplet precautions.
- Describe contact precautions.
- Demonstrate the following:
  - Procedure 1 Handwashing
  - Procedure 2 Putting on a Mask
  - Procedure 3 Putting on a Gown
  - Procedure 4 Putting on Gloves
  - Procedure 5 Removing Contaminated Gloves
  - Procedure 6 Removing Contaminated Gloves, Eye Protection, Gown, and Mask
  - Procedure 7 Serving a Meal in an Isolation Unit
  - Procedure 8 Measuring Vital Signs in an Isolation Unit
  - Procedure 9 Transferring Nondisposable Equipment Outside of the Isolation Unit
  - Procedure 10 Specimen Collection from a Patient in an Isolation Unit
  - Procedure 11 Caring for Linens in an Isolation Unit
  - Procedure 12 Transporting a Patient to and from the Isolation Unit
  - Procedure 13 Opening a Sterile Package

VOCABULARY

Learn the meaning and the correct spelling of the following words and phrases:

AII room (A2 room)
airborne precautions
airborne transmission
anteroom
asepsis
autoclave
biohazard
communicable disease
contact precautions
contact transmission
contagious disease
contaminated
dirty
disposable

disinfection
droplet precautions
droplet transmission
expanded precautions
exposure incident
face shield
goggles
high-efficiency particulate air (HEPA) filter mask
isolation
isolation technique
isolation unit
medical asepsis

N95 respirator
National Institute of Occupational Safety and Health (NIOSH)
negative air pressure room
nosocomial infection
occupational exposure
personal protective equipment (PPE)
PFR95 respirator
potentially infectious material
sharps

standard precautions
sterile
sterile field
sterilization
surgical mask
transmission-based precautions
ultraviolet germicidal irradiation (UVGI)
work practice controls

DISEASE PREVENTION

In the last unit you learned what infections are and some of their causes. In this unit, you will be introduced to actions and procedures that can help prevent the transmission (spread) of infection to protect yourself, your coworkers, and those in your care.

MEDICAL ASEPSIS

Asepsis is defined as the absence of disease-producing microorganisms. Two ways of achieving asepsis are by medical aseptic technique and surgical aseptic technique. **Medical asepsis** refers to medical practices that reduce the numbers of microorganisms or interrupt transmission

---

GUIDELINES *for*
Maintaining Medical Asepsis

To maintain medical asepsis, the nursing assistant should follow these guidelines:

- Wash hands thoroughly and at appropriate times. Protect the skin on the hands by using warm water, drying thoroughly, then applying lotion if needed.

- Treat breaks in the skin immediately by washing thoroughly, cleaning with an antiseptic, and covering. Report any breaks in the skin to your supervisor.

- Use gloves when required.

- Bathe or shower daily. Daily changes of clothing are necessary. Keep your hair clean and away from your face and shoulders. Avoid artificial nails. Keep fingernails short and clean. Do not wear rings, other than a plain wedding band.

- Assist patients with their personal hygiene.

- *Never* use one patient's items for another patient.

- Keep patient personal care items in the proper areas. In the top two drawers of the patient's bedside stand, place:
    - toothbrush and toothpaste
    - comb and hairbrush
    - denture cup if patient wears dentures

Items such as a toothbrush, denture cup, wash basin, and emesis basin should always be placed on a different shelf (or drawer) from items such as a bedpan and a urinal.

In the second drawer or on the shelf of the bedside stand, or in the bathroom, place:
    - emesis basin
    - wash basin
    - soap and soap dish

Store on the lower shelf:
    - bedpan
    - urinal for male patients

- Disinfect bathtubs and shower chairs after each use, according to facility policy.

- Disinfect equipment that is used by more than one health care provider or patient, such as a stethoscope, before and after each use.

- Disinfect personal care equipment, such as bedpans, urinals, and commodes, according to facility policy.

- Be careful when handling bedpans and urinals after use to prevent spills and splashes. Use a cover when transporting.

- Avoid contaminating environmental surfaces by touching them while wearing used gloves.

- Use the overbed table only for clean items, such as food trays, water pitcher, and clean supplies.

- The water pitcher should always be covered at the bedside.

- Keep food and water supplies clean. Food trays are to remain covered until they reach their destination. Remove food dishes immediately after use. Do not place used trays on a cart until all clean trays have been delivered to patients.

- Do not allow patients to keep puddings or custards from meal trays. Bacteria multiply rapidly in these foods when they are not refrigerated.

- Carry soiled equipment, supplies, and linens away from your uniform. Dispose of items according to facility policy.

- Do not use anything that has touched the floor without recleaning or sterilizing it first. If you are in doubt about whether an item is clean, do not use it. Any personal items that touch the floor should be disinfected before use. The floor is heavily contaminated with pathogens.

- Avoid raising dust.

continues

- Do not shake linens. This scatters contaminated dust and lint. Gather or fold linens inward with the dirtiest area toward the center. Keep soiled linen hampers covered. Keep linens (even if soiled) off the floor.

- The soiled linen hamper and housekeeping cart must be separated from the clean linen cart and food cart by at least one room's width.

- Clean from least soiled areas toward the most soiled.

- Keep work areas such as utility rooms clean. Return clean equipment to the proper storage areas after use.

from one person to another person or from person to place or object. These practices are often referred to as *medical aseptic technique (clean technique).*

You will hear the terms *clean* and *dirty* applied to equipment and supplies used in the facility. For example, the linen you take from the linen cart is "clean." After it is carried into the patient's room, it is considered "dirty." If it is not used, it cannot be returned to the clean linen cart; it must be placed in the laundry hamper. Once linen is in the patient's room, it is exposed to the patient's pathogens. To prevent the spread of these pathogens to other patients, the linen must be laundered. Keeping each patient's equipment and supplies separate from those for other patients is part of medical aseptic technique. Articles that have come into contact with known pathogens or have been exposed to potential pathogens are called **dirty** or **contaminated**. Articles that are free of pathogens are considered clean or uncontaminated.

It is not possible to eliminate all microorganisms from our bodies or the environment. However, microbes can be reduced by always using the essential practices of medical aseptic technique:

- Handwashing
- Using nonsterile gloves when contact with blood, moist body fluids (except sweat), mucous membranes, or nonintact skin is likely
- Cleaning and/or disinfecting equipment

For additional information on medical asepsis, see the online Appendix at the Online Companion for this textbook.

HANDWASHING

Handwashing is the single most important health procedure any individual can perform to prevent the spread of microbes. Handwashing is a vigorous, short rubbing together of all the surfaces of soap-lathered hands. It is followed by rinsing under a stream of running warm water. Warm water is used because it makes a good lather. It is also less damaging to the skin than hot water. In health care facilities,

soap is provided in a dispenser. Bar soap is easily contaminated because microbes can grow in the wet soap dish and on the surface of the soap.

Sinks in health care facilities vary in design. In most, you turn the water on by using faucets. Most people wash their hands when their hands are soiled or contaminated, so it stands to reason that the faucets are a potential source of contamination. Although not a requirement in most facilities, holding a paper towel under your hand when turning the faucet on is a good idea. The water flow in some sinks is controlled by using a knee pedal or foot pedal, reducing the risk of inadvertent contamination. These are operated by stepping on the foot pedal or pushing the knee lever to the right to turn the water on. Push the knee lever to the left to turn the water off.

When washing your hands, always keep your fingertips pointed down. Never lean against the sink with your uniform or touch the inside of the sink with your hands.

The most important aspect of handwashing is the friction created by rubbing the hands together. This friction mechanically removes microbes from the hands. Routine handwashing with soap, running water, and friction by all health care providers:

- Is the most significant control measure for the prevention of a **nosocomial infection** (infection acquired by a patient while being cared for in a health care facility)
- Is the single most important control measure to break the chain of infection

The recommended handwashing technique depends on the purpose of the handwashing. Hands can usually be washed effectively in 15 to 20 seconds. More time will be needed, however, if hands are visibly soiled (refer to Procedure 1).

Handwashing should be done:

- At the beginning of your shift
- After picking up any item from the floor
- Before handling food
- After personal use of the bathroom
- After using a tissue
- After you cough or sneeze
- Before handling a patient's food and drink

PROCEDURE

HANDWASHING

1. Check that there is an adequate supply of soap and paper towels. A waste container lined with a plastic bag should be in the area near you.

2. Remove rings, if possible, or be sure to lather soap underneath.

3. Remove watch, or push up over wrist.

4. Turn on the faucet.

5. Adjust water to a warm temperature. Once used, drop the paper towel in the waste container.

Stand back from the sink so you do not contaminate your uniform. Wet your hands, keeping your fingertips pointed downward (Figure 13-1).

6. Apply soap and lather over your hands and wrists, between fingers, and under rings. Use friction and interlace your fingers (Figure 13-2). Work lather over every part of your hands and wrists. Clean your fingernails by rubbing them against the palm of the other hand to force soap under the nails for 15 to 20 seconds (Figure 13-3).

7. Rinse hands with your fingertips pointed down. Do not shake water from hands.

8. Dry hands thoroughly with a clean paper towel.

9. Turn off the faucet with a paper towel (Figure 13-4); drop the towel in the waste container.

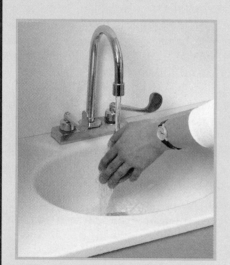

FIGURE 13-1 Keep your fingertips pointed down when washing hands.

FIGURE 13-2 Interlace the fingers to clean between them.

FIGURE 13-3 Rub nails against the palms of the hands to clean under the nails.

FIGURE 13-4 Use a clean, dry paper towel to turn faucets off.

- After handling a patient's belongings
- After touching any item or environmental surface that is soiled or in the immediate vicinity of patients
- Before handling any supply considered clean
- Immediately before touching mucous membranes or nonintact skin; if you are already wearing gloves, change them
- Immediately after accidental contact with blood, moist body fluids, mucous membranes, or nonintact skin
- Before and after any contact with your mouth or mucous membranes, such as touching, eating, drinking, smoking, using lip balm, or manipulating contact lenses
- Before and after every patient contact
- Before applying and after removing gloves
- Whenever your hands are visibly soiled
- Any time your gloves become torn
- At the end of your shift before going home

Most health care facilities do not permit caregivers to wear artificial fingernails of any type, including nail tips, overlays, silk wraps, gels, sculptured, or acrylic nails. Long nails (beyond the fingertips) are also not usually permitted. This is because the long and artificial nails have been proven to harbor bacteria and increase the risk of infection to both the patient and the worker. They are difficult to clean properly and increase the risk of tearing gloves. Facilities may also have restrictions on the types of rings worn when on duty. Rings with many stones and elaborate settings can also hold harmful bacteria, and are difficult to clean. Rings may also tear gloves. Rings other than flat bands are better left at home when you are on duty.

Hand Lotion and Cream

Maintaining the integrity of the skin on your hands is very important to prevent injury and exposure to microbes. However, you must be careful when selecting and using hand care products. Several episodes of infection have been reported in hospitals as a result of workers using community containers of hand care products. The skin and fingernails are a good reservoir for growth and multiplication of bacteria and viruses. Lotions and creams from jars or squeeze bottles in which hands touch the dispenser opening become a source of contamination to everyone who uses them. Another concern is that the petroleum in some hand care products can damage your gloves, causing holes and tears and increasing your risk of exposure to pathogens. If you prefer to use hand lotion, select a light, non-oily product. A personal-size bottle that you do not share is best. Avoid any product that comes in a jar. You may use bottles with pump dispensers and squeeze bottles, but avoid touching the dispensing spout.

Waterless Hand Cleaners

Many facilities provide dispensers containing waterless hand cleaners in various locations in the facility. The hand cleaners contain an alcohol-based gel, lotion, or foam that is dispensed in small dime- to quarter-sized portions (approximately 2 to 3 mL). In addition to the alcohol, most solutions contain moisturizers that prevent drying of the skin. Each facility has directions for using the product and policies and procedures for when waterless hand cleaners may be used. In many, the waterless cleaner may be used instead of handwashing during routine patient care. However, washing at the sink may still be required in certain areas, such as the nursery, operating room, and others. Washing at the sink should also be done any time the hands are visibly soiled. To use the waterless cleaning product, dispense the proper amount into the palm of your hand. Rub the product into the hands until it dries, making sure to rub all areas and surfaces, including the nail beds and between the fingers. This takes about 15 seconds. Become familiar with the products used by your facility and their applications. They are very effective in reducing infection and eliminating pathogens from the hands.

Infection Control ALERT

Always wash your hands with soap and water if a patient has infectious diarrhea or another condition spread by spores. *Alcohol-based cleaners will not eliminate spores.* The mechanical action of soap, water, and friction used during handwashing will remove spores from your hands and wash them down the drain. ■

PROTECTING YOURSELF

As you perform your duties, you may contact **potentially infectious material** such as blood or other body fluids that may contain pathogens. This is called **occupational exposure.**

OSHA ALERT

Health care facilities are required to have an *exposure control plan* that describes what to do if you contact blood or body fluid. Immediately wash the area well. Report accidental contact with blood or body fluid to the nurse immediately. You will be treated according to the established plan, have blood samples taken, and may begin drug therapy to prevent a bloodborne disease. Medical care and monitoring may continue over a long period of time. ■

Using proper medical asepsis technique and following standard precautions according to facility policy are the best ways to limit the potential for being infected.

An **exposure incident** means that your eyes, nose, mouth, mucous membranes, or nonintact skin had contact with blood or other potentially infectious material. Rinse your eyes, nose, or mouth immediately with clear water. Wash exposed skin and nonintact areas on your skin well with soap and water. Report this at once to your supervisor and follow facility procedure.

STANDARD PRECAUTIONS

Standard precautions (Figure 13-5) are the infection control actions used for all people receiving care, regardless of their condition or diagnosis. Standard precautions apply to situations in which care providers may contact:

- Blood, body fluids (except sweat), secretions, and excretions
- Mucous membranes

Culture/Infection Control ALERT

Alcohol-based hand cleaners are usually mounted throughout the facility and are available to anyone who wants to use them. Patients sometimes use alcohol preparations in the dispensers in their rooms. Persons of the Muslim faith often do not use alcohol hand cleaners because the use of alcohol violates Islamic law. The Koran states that alcohol is permitted for medicinal purposes, but some individuals are not aware of this provision or are simply not comfortable with the practice. Make sure that patients who are practicing Muslims have another, acceptable means of handwashing available to them. ■

STANDARD PRECAUTIONS FOR INFECTION CONTROL

Wash Hands (Plain soap)
Wash after touching blood, body fluids, secretions, excretions, and contaminated items. Wash immediately after gloves are removed and between patient contacts. Avoid transfer of microorganisms to other patients or environments.

Wear Gloves
Wear when touching blood, body fluids, secretions, excretions, and contaminated items. Put on clean gloves just before touching mucous membranes and nonintact skin. Change gloves between tasks and procedures on the same patient after contact with material that may contain high concentrations of microorganisms. Remove gloves promptly after use, before touching noncontaminated items and environmental surfaces, and before going to another patient, and wash hands immediately to avoid transfer of microorganisms to other patients or environments.

Wear Mask and Eye Protection or Face Shield
Protect mucous membranes of the eyes, nose and mouth during procedures and patient-care activities that are likely to generate splashes or sprays of blood, body fluids, secretions, or excretions.

Wear Gown
Protect skin and prevent soiling of clothing during procedures that are likely to generate splashes or sprays of blood, body fluids, secretions, or excretions. Remove a soiled gown as promptly as possible and wash hands to avoid transfer of microorganisms to other patients or environments.

Patient-Care Equipment
Handle used patient-care equipment soiled with blood, body fluids, secretions, or excretions in a manner that prevents skin and mucous membrane exposures, contamination of clothing, and transfer of microorganisms to other patients and environments. Ensure that reusable equipment is not used for the care of another patient until it has been appropriately cleaned and reprocessed. Ensure that single-use items are properly discarded.

Environmental Control
Follow hospital procedures for routine care, cleaning, and disinfection of environmental surfaces, beds, bed rails, bedside equipment, and other frequently touched surfaces.

Linen
Handle, transport, and process used linen soiled with blood, body fluids, secretions, or excretions in a manner that prevents exposure and contamination of clothing, and avoids transfer of microorganisms to other patients and environments.

Occupational Health and Bloodborne Pathogens
Prevent injuries when using needles, scalpels, and other sharp instruments or devices; when handling sharp instruments after procedures; when cleaning used instruments; and when disposing of used needles.

Never recap used needles using both hands or any other technique that involves directing the point of a needle towards any part of the body; rather, use either a one-handed "scoop" technique or a mechanical device designed for holding the needle sheath.

Do not remove used needles from disposable syringes by hand, and do not bend, break, or otherwise manipulate used needles by hand. Place used disposable syringes and needles, scalpels, blades, and other sharp items in puncture-resistant sharps containers located as close as practical to the area in which the items were used, and place reusable syringes and needles in a puncture-resistant container for transport to the reprocessing area.

Use resuscitation devices as an alternative to mouth-to-mouth resuscitation.

Patient Placement
Use a private room for a patient who contaminates the environment or who does not (or cannot be expected to) assist in maintaining appropriate hygiene or environmental control. Consult Infection Control if a private room is not available.

FIGURE 13-5 Standard precautions (Courtesy of BREVIS Corporation, Salt Lake City, UT)

- Nonintact skin

Some examples of secretions and excretions are:

- Respiratory mucus (phlegm)
- Cerebrospinal fluid
- Urine
- Feces
- Vaginal secretions
- Semen
- Vomitus

This means that all health care workers follow specific procedures, called **work practice controls**, to prevent the spread of infections.

Standard precautions stress handwashing and the use of **personal protective equipment (PPE)**: gloves, gown, mask, and goggles or face shield.

OSHA ALERT

Regular eyeglasses do not provide the same level of protection as goggles or a face shield. If you wear glasses, remove them to wear goggles. Most face shields fit comfortably over eyeglasses, making removal unnecessary. ∎

GUIDELINES *for*

Standard Precautions

1. Wash hands in the situations listed under "Handwashing."

2. Wear gloves for any contact with blood, body fluids, mucous membranes, or nonintact skin, such as when:
   - Hands are cut, scratched, chapped, or have a rash
   - Cleaning up body fluid spills
   - Cleaning potentially contaminated equipment

3. Gloves are provided in patient rooms on supply carts, or in wall-mounted dispensers.

4. Carry gloves with you so they will always be available as you need them.

5. If you have a sensitivity to latex gloves, follow your physician's advice. Three possible options are:
   - Change to nonlatex gloves (facilities must supply them because latex allergies are common).
   - Apply a skin barrier cream to your hands before putting on latex gloves; the cream protects hands against most irritants, including latex.
   - Put on glove liners that prevent direct contact between the skin of the hands and the latex gloves.

6. Change gloves:
   - After contacting each patient
   - Before touching noncontaminated articles or environmental surfaces
   - Between tasks with the same patient if there is contact with infectious materials

7. Dispose of gloves according to facility policy.

8. Wear a waterproof gown for procedures likely to produce splashes of blood or other body fluids.
   - Remove a soiled gown as soon as possible and dispose of it properly according to facility policy.
   - Wash your hands.

9. Wear a mask and protective eyewear or face shield for procedures likely to produce splashes of blood or other moist body fluids. This is to prevent contact between pathogens and your mucous membranes.

   The surgical mask covers both the nose and the mouth. The mask is used once and discarded. When a mask is required, a new one is put on for each patient receiving care. If the mask becomes wet, a new one must be put on because the mask loses its effectiveness when moist.

10. Goggles or a face shield help protect the mucous membranes of the eyes from splashes or sprays of blood and other body fluids. A surgical mask must be worn with goggles and with a face shield to protect the nose and mouth.

11. When using PPE, you should:
    - Know where to obtain these items in your work area.
    - Always remove the items before leaving the work area, whether the patient's room, an isolation unit, or the utility room.
    - Place used PPE items in the proper container for laundering, decontamination, or disposal, according to facility policy.

GUIDELINES *for*
Environmental Procedures

1. Handle all patient care items so that infectious organisms will not be transferred to skin, mucous membranes, clothing, or the environment. Reusable equipment must be cleaned and decontaminated according to facility policy before it can be used with another patient. Dispose of single-use items according to facility policy.

2. Follow facility procedures for routine care and cleaning of environmental surfaces, such as beds, bedside equipment, and other frequently touched surfaces.

3. Dispose of **sharps**—needles, razors, and other sharp items—in a puncture-resistant, leakproof container near the point of use (Figure 13-6). The container should be labeled with the **biohazard** symbol (Figure 13-7) and color-coded red. Biohazardous waste contains items contaminated with blood or body fluids. Items discarded here must be labeled. Special precautions are taken to dispose of these waste containers.

4. Do not recap or handle needles before disposal.

5. Mouthpieces or resuscitator bags should be available to eliminate the need for mouth-to-mouth resuscitation. Remember that you must be taught how to use them.

6. Waste and soiled linen should be placed in plastic bags and handled according to facility policy. There are separate containers for regular waste and for biohazardous waste. Containers for biohazardous waste should have the biohazard symbol, or be color-coded in red (Figure 13-8). Learn your facility policy for what is biohazardous waste and follow the guidelines.

7. Wipe up blood spills immediately. Disinfect the floor according to facility policy.
   - Use disposable gloves.
   - For small spills, use 1:10 or 1:100 dilution of bleach or facility-approved disinfectant.
   - For larger spills, use a commercial blood cleanup kit. Begin by sprinkling absorbent powder on the blood to absorb the spill. The blood and powder are cleaned up with the scoop provided in the kit. Discard the material and scoop in a biohazard bag (Figure 13-9).
   - Wipe with disinfectant and disposable cleaning cloths.

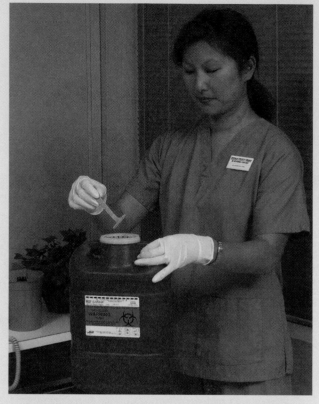

FIGURE 13-6 Carefully discard sharps in a safety container specifically designated for this use.

FIGURE 13-7 Containers for contaminated items are identified with the biohazard label. The symbol is black with a red or orange background.

   - Discard gloves and cleaning cloths in biohazard waste.

8. Dispose of body fluids and contaminated articles according to facility policy. This includes the contents of:
   - Urinary drainage bags
   - Bedpans

continues

GUIDELINES *continued*

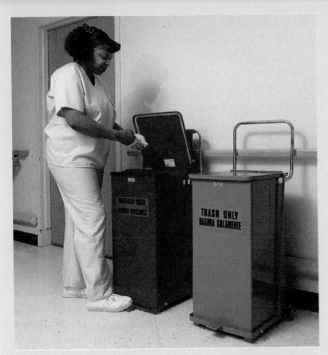

FIGURE 13-8 Discard all potentially infectious materials in the proper container.

- Urinals
- Emesis basins
- Drainage receptacles from tracheal and gastric suction
- Solutions returned from vaginal douches, enemas, and bladder irrigations
- Soiled dressings
- Incontinence pads, Chux, underpads, linen savers, blue pads
- Vaginal pads
- Incontinent briefs

9. Eating, drinking, chewing gum, smoking, applying cosmetics or lip balm, and handling contact lenses are prohibited in work areas where there may be exposure to infectious material.

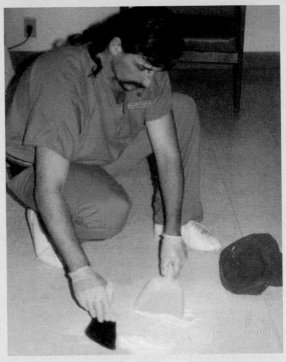

FIGURE 13-9 Clean blood spills immediately and then disinfect, using a 1:10 or 1:100 bleach solution (according to facility policy) or facility-approved disinfectant. For larger spills, a blood spill kit can be used. The powder in the kit solidifies the blood so it can be easily scooped into a plastic biohazard bag.

10. Food and drink should not be kept in refrigerators, freezers, shelves, cabinets, or on countertops or benchtops where they may be exposed to blood or other potentially contaminated items.

11. Do not pick up broken glassware with your bare hands. Use a brush and dust pan, tongs, or forceps. Clean and disinfect properly. Discard according to facility policy.

12. Consider laboratory specimens and specimen containers to be potentially infectious materials.

TRANSMISSION-BASED PRECAUTIONS

Standard precautions do not eliminate the need for other isolation precautions. A second set of precautions is used with certain highly transmissible diseases. This second tier of precautions is called **transmission-based precautions**. Transmission-based precautions are designed to interrupt the mode of transmission so that the disease cannot spread to others. *Standard precautions are always used in addition to transmission-based precautions.*

Diseases may be transferred from one person to another either directly or indirectly. Such diseases are called **communicable** or **contagious diseases**. Some diseases are transmitted more easily than others. Specific precautions must be taken to control their spread.

Communicable diseases may be spread:

Infection Control ALERT

Items that have contacted blood or body fluids are biohazardous waste. Dispose of linen and trash contaminated with blood or body fluids according to facility policy. These items must always be disposed of in leakproof, tightly closed containers. Biohazardous waste is stored in special areas until it is removed, and requires special handling during removal. This type of handling is very expensive, and storage space is often limited, so do not place non-biohazardous materials in the biohazard disposal containers. ■

- Through upper respiratory secretions by **airborne transmission** and **droplet transmission**
- By **contact transmission** (direct contact or indirect contact) with feces or other body secretions and excretions
- Through draining wounds or infective material such as blood on needles

Each mode of transmission requires special precautions to interrupt the movement of microbes from the infected person to others.

If a disease is transmitted by more than one mode, all methods of transmission must be considered when selecting precautions for a specific patient. Table 13-1 lists transmission-based precautions and common diseases in each category.

TABLE 13-1 TRANSMISSION-BASED PRECAUTIONS FOR COMMON DISEASES

Transmission-Based Precautions Category	Disease or Condition
Airborne	Tuberculosis Measles
Airborne and Contact	Chickenpox Widespread shingles
Droplet	German measles Mumps; Influenza
Contact	Head or body lice, scabies Impetigo Infected pressure ulcer with with heavy drainage

Isolation

Isolation means being separated or set apart. The purpose of isolation is to separate the patient who has a communicable or contagious disease, to help prevent the spread of the infectious pathogens.

When a patient is in isolation precautions, a private room is used. Two patients with the same disease may share a room. (This practice is called *cohorting*.) For patients in isolation, the proper use of precautions requires extra effort by all care providers, but especially nursing assistants, and is more time-consuming. The fear of infection also makes working with these precautions more stressful for the care providers. Patients in isolation and their families and other visitors also feel stress.

Psychological Aspects of Isolation

The patient in isolation fears both the disease that makes the isolation precautions necessary and the practices that must be followed for these precautions to be effective. These include:

- PPE worn by all who enter the isolation unit, including visitors
- Special procedures for handling waste, specimens, food, linens, and personal effects of the patient
- Restrictions on the patient's movement in the facility
- Procedures to be followed when patient is moved outside of the isolation unit
- Possible restrictions on visiting hours or number of visitors
- Likelihood that close personal contact, such as kissing of family members, will not be permitted

The patient may be afraid of passing the infection to family and friends. If the patient does not understand the infectious process, this fear is increased. If the patient is confused, he or she may be very fearful of the PPE.

Because of the patient's fears and the need for decreased contact with other patients, family, and friends, the patient in isolation requires more emotional support and care. The extra time required to follow the isolation precautions, such as putting on PPE, could easily lessen the time the care providers spend with the patient at a time when emotional attention is most needed. Nursing assistants should be mindful of the patient's needs and plan their schedules to spend the necessary time with a patient in isolation.

Transmission-Based Isolation Precautions

Standard precautions are used with all patients regardless of their condition. When patients are known to have or are suspected of having an infectious disease, isolation precautions are used *in addition to* standard precautions.

The isolation precautions used depend on the way in which the infectious pathogens are transmitted. Guidelines from the Centers for Disease Control and Prevention (CDC) indicate the specific precautions and personal protective equipment to be used based on how the disease is transmitted. The three transmission precautions are:

- Airborne precautions
- Droplet precautions
- Contact precautions

Airborne Precautions. **Airborne precautions** are used for diseases that are transmitted by air currents. The pathogens are small and light and are suspended in the air or on dust particles in the air. They can travel a long distance from the source by natural air currents and through ventilation systems. Tuberculosis is a disease that requires airborne precautions. Figure 13-10 shows the required precautions.

The patient must be in a private room with special air handling. Hospitals use many different methods of handling the air to reduce the risk that pathogens will escape into the ventilation system. A **negative air pressure room** is commonly used. Your facility may call this an **AII** (A2) **room** because of the type of air handling used. This means that air is drawn into the room and leaves the room through a special exhaust system to the outside. Air from the isolation room does not circulate directly into the facility.

Some isolation rooms have special **ultraviolet germicidal irradiation** (UVGI) lights in the room, air ducts, or suspended from the ceiling in the room and anteroom. In some facilities, these lights are in the hallway outside the room. UVGI uses ultraviolet-C light in the room air or air duct. It is not used for lighting the room. Rather, these lights are a secondary measure to kill or inactivate

AIRBORNE PRECAUTIONS
(in addition to Standard Precautions)
VISITORS: Report to nurse before entering.

Patient Placement
Use **private room** that has:
Monitored negative air pressure,
6 to 12 air changes per hour,
Discharge of air outdoors or HEPA filtration if recirculated.
Keep room door closed and patient in room.

Respiratory Protection
Wear an N95 respirator when entering the room of a patient with known or suspected infectious pulmonary **tuberculosis.**
Susceptible persons should not enter the room of patients known or suspected to have **measles** (rubeola) or **varicella** (chickenpox) if other immune caregivers are available. If susceptible persons must enter, they should wear an **N95 respirator.** (Respirator or surgical mask not required if immune to measles and varicella.)

Patient Transport
Limit transport of patient from room to essential purposes only. Use **surgical mask** on patient during transport.

FIGURE 13-10 Airborne precautions (Courtesy of BREVIS Corporation, Salt Lake City, UT)

pathogens in the upper portion of the room or passing through the air duct. When the air is irradiated, droplets containing pathogens are inactivated so that they no longer pose a risk for infection. The lights are not on all the time, and their use is regularly monitored to ensure that the radiation is not a threat to the patient or health care workers.

Most facilities have an **anteroom** adjoining an AII room (Figure 13-11). An anteroom is a small room just inside the entrance to the patient room. It typically has a sink

FIGURE 13-11 The floor plan for an isolation room. Note the anteroom, which is an entrance room that is often used in rooms with negative pressure ventilation for respiratory (airborne) precautions.

and containers for trash disposal. Having an anteroom reduces the possible escape of infectious organisms when the door is opened and closed. It also serves as a buffer between the changes in air pressure in the patient room and the hallway. When caring for a patient in airborne precautions:

- The door to the room is kept closed.
- All care providers who enter the room must wear a **high-efficiency particulate air (HEPA) filter mask** or other specially filtered mask (Figure 13-12). The filters in the mask protect the care provider from the very small disease-causing pathogens. A surgical mask does

FIGURE 13-12 The HEPA respirator filter is individually fitted to the worker. The respirator is reusable. Store it according to facility policy.

not provide this level of protection. Each care provider must be fitted with a HEPA or other filter mask. This ensures that air entering the mask comes through the filters only with no air leaks. Follow all facility policies for the use of filter masks.

The HEPA mask may be disposable or reusable. Men with facial hair cannot wear a HEPA mask because the hair prevents an airtight seal. In this case, a special filter hood can be worn. The filter mask is the only mask that can be used in an airborne isolation room. Masks that are worn in an airborne precautions room must be approved by the **National Institute of Occupational Safety and Health (NIOSH)**. This agency is part of the CDC, and is responsible for conducting research and making recommendations for the prevention of work-related disease and injury. The **PFR95 respirator** (Figure 13-13) and the **N95 respirator** (Figure 13-14) are approved alternatives. Some workers prefer these masks because they are lighter in weight and more comfortable to wear. The employee must self-test the respirator each time it is applied to be sure there are no air leaks. Figure 13-15 shows the procedure for fit-testing the N95 respirator.

Before beginning work in airborne precautions rooms, employees must:

- Attend a comprehensive class about respirator use, fit, storage, cleaning, and maintenance
  - workers must attend an annual educational update
- Have a medical examination to ensure that working in the mask will not harm the worker's personal health
  - the medical examination must be repeated annually and upon request if the worker believes the mask may be causing health problems

FIGURE 13-13 The PFR95 respirator filter is preferred by many health care workers because it is lightweight and comfortable.

FIGURE 13-14 The N95 respirator is disposable. Some facilities store it for one shift, then discard it. (Courtesy of 3M Health Care, St. Paul, MN)

Donning instructions (to be followed each time product is worn):

1 Cup the respirator in your hand with the nosepiece at fingertips, allowing the headbands to hang freely below hands.

2 Position the respirator under your chin with the nosepiece up.

3 Pull the top strap over your head so it rests high on the back of head.

4 Pull the bottom strap over your head and position it around neck below ears.

5 Using two hands, mold the nosepiece to the shape of your nose by pushing inward while moving fingertips down both sides of the nosepiece. Pinching the nosepiece using one hand may result in less effective respirator performance.

6 FACE FIT CHECK
The respirator seal should be checked before each use. To check fit, place both hands completely over the respirator and exhale. If air leaks around your nose, adjust the nosepiece as described in step 5. If air leaks at respirator edges, adjust the straps back along the sides of your head. Recheck.

NOTE: If you cannot achieve proper fit, do not enter the isolation or treatment area. See your supervisor.

Removal instructions:

1 Cup the respirator in your hand to maintain position on face. Pull bottom strap over head.

2 Still holding respirator in position, pull top strap over head.

3 Remove respirator from face and discard or store according to your facility's policy.

FIGURE 13-15 Fit-test the respirator each time you wear it. (Courtesy of 3M Health Care, St. Paul, MN)

- Be fitted for the mask by a qualified professional
  - the fit test involves performing several different activities while wearing the mask, then demonstrating application and removal several times
  - after the professional fit test, workers must wear only the type and size mask approved by the fit tester
- Learn how to store the mask in a properly labeled container that prevents damage and deformation of the facepiece and exhalation valve
- Learn how to protect the respirator from damage, contamination, dust, sunlight, extreme temperatures, excessive moisture, and damaging chemicals, and how they must be packed or stored

When working with patients who are in airborne precautions rooms:

- People who are not immune to measles (rubeola) or chickenpox (varicella) should not enter the room of a patient known or suspected to have either of these infections. People who have not had chickenpox should not enter the room of a patient in isolation for shingles.
- If transport from the room is necessary, the patient must wear a surgical mask.
- Remember: standard precautions must be used in addition to airborns precautions.
- Some facilities do not have the special ventilation required for airborne precautions rooms. These facilities use portable units that are placed in the room to filter the air, creating a negative pressure environment. They are slightly noisier than a ventilation system, but are effective in eliminating pathogens.

Droplet Precautions. **Droplet precautions** are used for diseases that can be spread by means of large droplets in the air. A person can spread droplets containing infectious pathogens by sneezing, coughing, talking, singing, or laughing. The droplets generally do not travel more than three feet from the source. Influenza is an example of a disease spread by droplets.

Figure 13-16 shows the requirements for droplet precautions.

- If a patient cannot be placed in a private room, then patients with the same infection may be placed together.

- Caregivers should wear surgical masks if they expect to be working within three feet of the patient. The door can be open if the bed is more than three feet from the door.

- If transport from the room is necessary, the patient must wear a surgical mask.

- Remember that droplet precautions are used in addition to standard precautions.

Contact Precautions. Contact precautions are used when the infectious pathogen is spread by direct or indirect contact. *Direct contact* occurs when the caregiver touches a contaminated area on the patient's skin or blood or body fluids containing the infectious pathogen. *Indirect contact* occurs when the caregiver touches items contaminated with the infectious material, such as the patient's personal belongings, equipment or supplies used in the care of the patient, contaminated linens, and so on. Examples of infections requiring contact precautions are scabies, infected pressure ulcers, and gastroenteritis.

Figure 13-17 shows the requirements for contact precautions.

- The patient should be in a private room. If this is not possible, then patients requiring the same type of infection can be placed in the same room. The door can be open.

- Gloves are put on before the caregiver enters the patient's room. Gloves are changed whenever there is contact with highly contaminated matter in the room.

After removing gloves, always wash your hands before putting on a new pair of gloves. After care is completed, remove gloves and wash hands. Use a paper towel to open the door to leave the room and discard the towel in the trash container inside the room.

- Wear a gown when entering the patient's room if your uniform may contact the patient, blood or body fluids, environmental surfaces, or other items in the room. Remove the gown before leaving the room and dispose of it according to facility policy for biohazardous waste. Be careful not to touch environmental surfaces or other items with your uniform as you leave the room.

- Transport the patient from the room only when necessary. Continue precautions to minimize contamination of environmental surfaces, other patients, and health care personnel.

- Disposable equipment and supplies should be used whenever possible. Noncritical, nondisposable equipment should be used for one patient only. If equipment must be used for more than one patient, it must be cleaned and disinfected between patients.

- Remember that contact precautions are used in addition to standard precautions.

New Precautions and Screening. Some health care workers contracted SARS as a result of exposure incidents that occurred during patient care. It is believed that these exposures occurred before the patients had been diagnosed with the disease. This makes a case for taking precautions when the patient is highly symptomatic, even before a diagnosis has been made. Because SARS is highly contagious, and all methods of transmission may not be known, special precautions were developed to care for patients. These precautions may also be necessary in the care of patients with other highly contagious infections. In fact, as a result of the 2003 SARS outbreaks, the CDC identified weaknesses in the way infection control precautions are implemented when patients with signs of respiratory disease first present themselves at the hospital for treatment. As a result, CDC is recommending that facilities implement measures to prevent the spread of *all respiratory infections*, beginning at the first point of contact with a potentially infected person. The new recommendations are considered to be part of standard precautions.

As part of the new guidelines, hospitals and other health care facilities are posting signs at the entrance to outpatient facilities, in the emergency room, admissions office, and other areas of initial contact. The signs instruct the patients and persons who accompany them to:

- Notify facility personnel if symptoms of a respiratory infection are present when they first register for care

- Practice respiratory hygiene/cough etiquette, such as:
  - containing all respiratory secretions
  - covering the nose and mouth when coughing or sneezing
  - using tissues to contain respiratory secretions
  - discarding tissues in the nearest trash can after use

DROPLET PRECAUTIONS
(in addition to Standard Precautions)

VISITORS: Report to nurse before entering.

Patient Placement
Private room, if possible. Cohort or maintain spatial separation of **3 feet** from other patients or visitors if private room is not available.

Mask
Wear mask when working within **3 feet** of patient (or upon entering room).

Patient Transport
Limit transport of patient from room to essential purposes only. Use **surgical mask** on patient during transport.

FIGURE 13-16 Droplet precautions (Courtesy of BREVIS Corporation, Salt Lake City, UT)

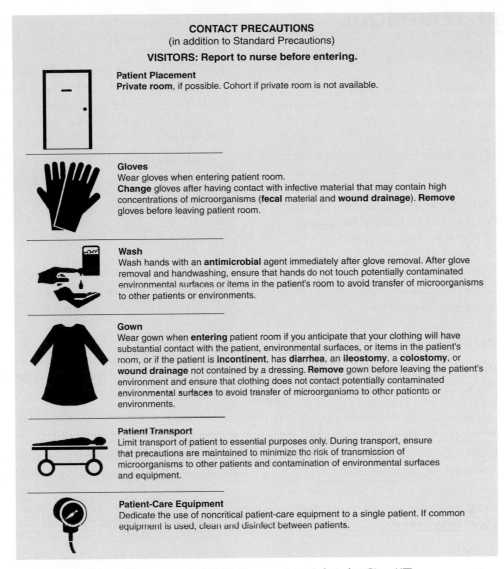

CONTACT PRECAUTIONS
(in addition to Standard Precautions)
VISITORS: Report to nurse before entering.

Patient Placement
Private room, if possible. Cohort if private room is not available.

Gloves
Wear gloves when entering patient room.
Change gloves after having contact with infective material that may contain high concentrations of microorganisms (**fecal** material and **wound drainage**). **Remove** gloves before leaving patient room.

Wash
Wash hands with an **antimicrobial** agent immediately after glove removal. After glove removal and handwashing, ensure that hands do not touch potentially contaminated environmental surfaces or items in the patient's room to avoid transfer of microorganisms to other patients or environments.

Gown
Wear gown when **entering** patient room if you anticipate that your clothing will have substantial contact with the patient, environmental surfaces, or items in the patient's room, or if the patient is **incontinent**, has **diarrhea**, an **ileostomy**, a **colostomy**, or **wound drainage** not contained by a dressing. **Remove** gown before leaving the patient's environment and ensure that clothing does not contact potentially contaminated environmental surfaces to avoid transfer of microorganisms to other patients or environments.

Patient Transport
Limit transport of patient to essential purposes only. During transport, ensure that precautions are maintained to minimize the risk of transmission of microorganisms to other patients and contamination of environmental surfaces and equipment.

Patient-Care Equipment
Dedicate the use of noncritical patient-care equipment to a single patient. If common equipment is used, clean and disinfect between patients.

FIGURE 13-17 Contact precautions (Courtesy of BREVIS Corporation, Salt Lake City, UT)

– performing hand hygiene after contact with respiratory secretions and/or contaminated objects and/or materials

Many facilities are also mounting dispensers of alcohol-based hand cleaner in public areas, lobbies, and areas in which patients first encounter facility staff.

Expanded Precautions. **Expanded precautions** is a term that has been used in the draft guidelines, but has not been formally adopted. Initially, CDC proposed using this title instead of transmission-based precautions. The term is introduced here in consideration of future policy changes. Remember it, but continue using the transmission-based precautions terminology until your employer notifies you that the name has been officially changed. Some of CDC's print materials use this term instead of transmission-based precautions, so this can be confusing. There is little difference between expanded precautions and transmission-based precautions. However, expanded precautions focus more on proper application and removal of PPE. You will use transmission-based precautions in patient care, and be conscientious when applying

and removing PPE. If a patient with pneumonia has been diagnosed with SARS, when SARS is strongly suspected, or the patient has one or more risk factors for the condition, attention to PPE is important. However, standard, contact, and airborne precautions are all used in patient care.

A patient with SARS will be in an AII (A2) room. Apply a gown, gloves, and disposable NIOSH-approved respirator when entering. Discard the respirator when leaving the room. It is not reused. When caring for a SARS patient, you will also wear eye protection (goggles or face shield) when working within three feet of the patient.

OSHA ALERT

When wearing gloves:

- Avoid touching your face with contaminated gloves.

- Avoid unnecessary touching of surfaces and objects with contaminated gloves. ■

ISOLATION TECHNIQUE

There are four key points to be remembered at all times for isolation technique:

1. **Isolation technique** is the name given to the method of caring for patients with easily transmitted diseases.
2. It is essential that every person knows how to select the correct PPE and takes responsibility for using the proper isolation techniques to prevent the spread of disease to others.
3. All items that come into contact with the patient's excretions, secretions, blood, body fluids, mucous membranes, or nonintact skin are considered contaminated. This potentially infective material must be treated in a special way.
4. Standard precautions are always used in addition to transmission-based precautions.

Isolation Unit

The **isolation unit** may be an area or a private room. Patients with the same disease may share a room. A room with handwashing facilities and an adjoining room with bathing and toilet facilities is best. A private room is indicated for patients who:

- Are highly infectious
- Have poor personal hygiene
- Require special air control procedures within the room

Preparing for Isolation

To prepare a patient room for isolation, do the following:

1. Place a card indicating the type of isolation precaution on the door to the patient's room. Hospitals have become very creative in alerting their personnel to the need for special precautions while observing the privacy and confidentiality rules. Some place colored dots on the door frame or signs on the door. The key to the color code is known only by personnel. Some place patient care information on the backs of door signs. Others place a precautions sticker on the chart cover or care plan. Information about the organism and special precautions are found inside. Follow your facility procedures for posting signs and other information.
2. Place an isolation cart outside the room, next to the door. Place in it quantities of personal protective equipment as needed:
   - Gowns
   - Masks
   - Gloves
   - Goggles or face shields
   - Plastic bags marked for biohazardous waste
   - Plastic bags for soiled linen

3. Line the wastepaper basket inside the room with a plastic bag labeled or color-coded for infectious waste.
4. Place a laundry hamper in the room and line it with a color-coded biohazard laundry bag.
5. At the sink, check the supply of paper towels and soap. Soap should be in a wall dispenser or foot-operated dispenser.

OSHA ALERT

You are responsible for selecting your own PPE. For maximum protection, you must consider three key things:

- *The type of anticipated exposure,* such as touch, or whether splashes, sprays, or large volumes of blood or body fluids, secretions, or excretions may be present.
- *The durability and appropriateness of the PPE* for the task. For example, some facilities may make aprons available to cover your clothing, instead of gowns. You must consider whether your arms will be exposed to an infectious substance. Also, you must consider the fabric of the item. Is it fluid-resistant, fluid-proof, or neither? Select the item based on the type of exposure you expect and degree of protection provided by the item.
- *How well the PPE fits you.* PPE that is too small or large will not provide optimal protection. Select items that fit you. The employer must ensure that PPE are available in sizes that will fit the workers to be protected. ■

PERSONAL PROTECTIVE EQUIPMENT

Personal protective equipment includes gloves, gown, mask, and goggles or face shield. The following sections describe the correct use of this equipment (see Procedures 2 through 6).

Cover Gown

A gown made of a moisture-resistant material is used when soiling or splashing with blood, body fluids, secretions, or excretions is likely (Figure 13-18). The gown prevents contamination of the health care provider's uniform. Discard gowns according to facility policy after use.

Gloves

The use of gloves prevents the spread of disease. Usually the nursing assistant will wear nonsterile latex or vinyl disposable gloves, but there are also times when other types of gloves are worn. Gloves should be worn for most

FIGURE 13-18 Put on a gown if your uniform may have contact with blood or body fluids.

health care procedures, and they are always worn when contact with blood, body fluids (except sweat), secretions, excretions, mucous membranes, or nonintact skin is expected. You should also wear gloves if you have cuts or open sores on your hands. Gloves are also used during many routine cleaning procedures that the nursing assistant performs. In this case, utility gloves may be worn. The use of gloves does not replace the need for handwashing. Always wash your hands before and after glove use. If you accidentally touch a potentially contaminated environmental surface after removing your gloves, wash your hands again.

Gloves are used for three main purposes:

1. To prevent the health care provider from picking up a pathogen from the patient
2. To avoid giving the patient a pathogen that the health care provider has picked up on the hands
3. To avoid picking up a pathogen on a patient or the environment and carrying it to another patient on the hands

For gloves to be effective, they must be intact and have no visible cuts, tears, or cracks. They must fit your hands well. Gloves come in different sizes. Select the size that most comfortably fits your hand. If the glove is too large or too small, a measure of protection is lost. Do not wash your hands while wearing gloves. Handwashing damages the pores of the gloves and may allow microbes to enter. If your hands need to be washed, remove the gloves, wash your hands, then reapply new gloves. Table 13-2 lists times when gloves should be changed. Remember to wash your hands every time you remove gloves. Table 13-3 lists common nursing assistant tasks and the correct personal protective equipment to use for each job.

Gloves are for single patient use only. Do not wear them to care for more than one patient. Take care that you do not contaminate environmental surfaces with your gloves. Some facilities use the "one-glove technique" (Figure 13-19). This involves carrying a contaminated item in a gloved hand. The glove on the other hand is removed to open doors, turn on faucets, and touch other environmental surfaces and supplies.

FIGURE 13-19 The one-glove technique is used to carry contaminated items.

TABLE 13-2 SUGGESTED TIMES
TO CHANGE GLOVES

Remember to wash your hands before applying and after removing gloves. Never touch environmental surfaces with a contaminated glove.

Change gloves:

- Before giving any patient care

- After giving patient care

- Immediately before touching mucous membranes

- Immediately before touching nonintact skin

- Immediately after touching secretions or excretions

- Immediately after touching blood or body fluids

- After touching equipment or environmental surfaces that are potentially contaminated

- Any time your gloves are torn

- If your gloves become visibly soiled

Health care facilities have many different policies regarding how and where gloves are discarded. Many facilities require the staff to discard gloves in sealed or covered containers and prohibit you from discarding gloves in open wastebaskets in the room. Know and follow your facility policy.

Communication HIGHLIGHT

Remember that one way to communicate is through touch. Do not carry glove use to the extreme. Use gloves when necessary, but avoid using them for all patient contact. Using gloves at all times sends a negative message. It says that the patient is untouchable. Touching is very important to all human beings. Use gloves only when contact with blood, body fluids, secretions, excretions, mucous membranes, or nonintact skin is likely. Also, wear gloves if the skin on your hands is cut, cracked, or chapped. Be very careful not to contaminate clean equipment, supplies, or environmental surfaces with used gloves. ■

Face Mask

Surgical masks should be worn when exposure to droplet secretions may occur. The mask should cover the nursing assistant's nose and mouth. For example, a mask would be worn when caring for a patient with influenza who is coughing and releasing droplets containing the flu pathogen into the environment. The mask protects you when you are working within three feet of the patient. It is also used whenever protective eyewear is worn. When a surgical mask is needed, it is:

- Used only once and discarded
- Changed if it becomes moist
- Handled only by the ties
- Never left secured around the neck, because it can contaminate the uniform and the environment

OSHA ALERT

Becoming familiar with the principles of standard precautions is one of the most important things you will learn. You need not fear contracting an infection from the patient if you apply precautions correctly. There are many variables in patient care situations, so there are no absolute guidelines for the use of PPE. Think about the situation and use good judgment. You are responsibile for applying the principles of standard precautions and selecting the personal protective equipment according to the task to be done. ■

OSHA ALERT

In some patient care situations, a mask is worn to prevent contamination of a sterile field or an exposed area of the body. A mask may be worn without eye protection, but in most situations eye protection (face shield or goggles) should not be worn without a mask. Some vendors produce extra-large face shields. These may be worn without a mask only if the design is such that there is no risk of exposure from a splash or spray of fluid at the sides or bottom of the mask. Wearing a mask with all types of eye protection offers the highest level of defense to the nursing assistant. ■

TABLE 13-3 PERSONAL PROTECTIVE EQUIPMENT IN COMMON NURSING ASSISTANT TASKS

Note: Use this chart as a general guideline only. Add protective equipment if special circumstances exist. Know and follow your facility policies for using personal protective equipment.

Nursing Assistant Task	Gloves	Gown	Goggles/ Face Shield	Surgical Mask
Washing/rinsing utensils in the soiled utility room	Yes	Yes, if splashing is likely	Yes, if splashing is likely	Yes, if splashing is likely
Holding pressure on a bleeding wound	Yes	Yes	Yes	Yes
Wiping the shower chair with disinfectant	Yes	No	No	No
Emptying a catheter bag	Yes	Yes, if facility policy	Yes, if facility policy	Yes, if facility policy
Passing meal trays	No	No	No	No
Passing ice	No	No	No	No
Giving a backrub to a patient with a rash	Yes	No	No	No
Giving special mouth care to an unconscious patient	Yes	Yes, if facility policy	Yes, if facility policy	Yes, if facility policy
Assisting with a dental procedure	Yes	Yes	Yes	Yes
Changing the bed after an incontinent patient has an episode of diarrhea	Yes	Yes	No	No
Taking an oral temperature with a glass thermometer (gloves are not necessary with an electronic thermometer unless this is your facility policy)	Yes	No	No	No
Taking a rectal temperature	Yes	No	No	No
Taking an axillary temperature	No	No	No	No
Taking a blood pressure	No	No	No	No
Assisting an alert patient to brush teeth	Yes	Yes, if facility policy	Yes, if facility policy	Yes, if facility policy
Washing a patient's eyes	Yes	No	No	No
Giving perineal care	Yes	No	No	No
Washing the patient's abdomen when the skin is not broken	No	No	No	No
Washing the patient's arms when skin tears are present	Yes	No	No	No
Brushing a patient's dentures	Yes	No	No	No
Assisting the nurse while he or she suctions an unconscious patient with a tracheostomy	Yes	Yes	Yes	Yes

continues

TABLE 13-3 *CONTINUED*

Nursing Assistant Task	Gloves	Gown	Goggles/ Face Shield	Surgical Mask
Turning an incontinent patient who weighs 85 pounds	Yes, if linen is soiled	Yes, if your uniform will have substantial contact with the linen	No	No
Shaving a patient with a disposable razor	Yes, because this is a high-risk procedure	No	No	No
Shaving a patient with an electric razor	No	No	No	No
Cleaning the soiled utility room at the end of your shift	Yes	No	No	No

Protective Eyewear

A full **face shield** (Figure 13-20), or **goggles** (Figure 13-21), are worn any time splashing of blood, body fluids, secretions, or excretions may occur. The eyewear does not protect the mucous membranes of the nose and mouth, so a surgical mask is always worn with eyewear. A good rule to follow is that a surgical mask may be worn without protective eyewear, but protective eyewear is never worn without a surgical mask. Some masks have a protective eyeshield attached to them. The mask is put on before the protective eyewear. When removing the mask and eyewear, wash your hands, remove the eyewear, then the mask.

Sequence for Applying Personal Protective Equipment

1. Wash hands
2. Gown
3. Mask

FIGURE 13-20 A surgical mask is always worn under a face shield.

FIGURE 13-21 Always protect your nose and mouth with a mask when wearing goggles.

OSHA ALERT

Remember four key points about using PPE:

- Apply PPE before having contact with the patient.
- Use the PPE carefully to prevent spreading contamination.
- When you have finished, remove PPE carefully and discard it properly.
- After removing PPE, wash your hands or use alcohol-based hand cleaner before doing anything else. ■

4. Goggles or face shield
5. Gloves

Sequence for Removing Personal Protective Equipment

1. Gloves
2. Wash hands
3. Goggles or face shield
4. Gown
5. Mask
6. Wash hands

Figure 13-22 shows the CDC recommendations for application and removal of PPE. Once applied, certain parts of the PPE are considered clean, and other areas contaminated. Clean areas are those that will be touched when you remove the apparel. Note that the CDC recommends removing PPE at the doorway to the patient room, or in the anteroom, if there is one. If a respirator is worn, remove it after leaving the patient's room and closing the door. Always wash your hands well or use alcohol hand cleaner immediately after removing PPE.

Equipment

Disposable (used once and discarded) patient care equipment is used by many facilities. It is ideal for patients on isolation precautions. Frequently used equipment remains in the patient's unit. Most articles will not require special handling unless they are contaminated (or likely to be contaminated) with infective material.

Containment of Contaminated Articles

Contaminated articles leaving the patient's room must be handled so that pathogens will not be spread. It is important that contaminated equipment be bagged, labeled, and disposed of according to the health care facility's policy for

OSHA ALERT

If a mask has elastic head bands, separate the two bands. Hold the mask in one hand with the bands in the other. Position the mask over your nose, mouth, and chin, then stretch the bands over your head. Secure them comfortably, with one on the upper back of your head and the other below the ears at the base of the neck. You cannot touch the mask during use, so take the time to adjust it to fit comfortably. It should be secure, but not too tight. Make sure it fits snugly around your face, with no gaps. Position the straps so they do not slip. ■

the disposal of infectious waste. Used articles are placed in an impenetrable bag (such as plastic) before they are removed from the room or unit of the patient. A single bag may be used if it is waterproof and sturdy enough to confine and contain the article without contaminating the outside of the bag. (Refer to Procedures 7 through 10.)

OSHA ALERT

Always select a gown that fits you correctly. The opening should be in the back and fit securely at the neck and waist. If the gown is too small, it will not cover your body completely. If necessary, put on two gowns. Put the first one on with the opening in the front. Put the second gown on over the first with the opening in the back. ■

PROCEDURE

2

PUTTING ON A MASK

1. Assemble equipment:
   • Mask

2. Tie top strings of mask first, then bottom strings.

3. Adjust mask over nose and mouth by fitting the flexible bridge to the nose.

4. Adjust the mask so it fits snugly around the face and chin.

5. Replace your mask if it becomes moist during procedures.

6. Do not reuse a mask and do not let the mask hang around your neck.

SEQUENCE FOR DONNING PERSONAL PROTECTIVE EQUIPMENT (PPE)

The type of PPE used will vary based on the level of precautions required; e.g., Standard and Contact, Droplet or Airborne Infection Isolation.

1. GOWN
- Fully cover torso from neck to knees, arms to end of wrists, and wrap around the back
- Fasten in back of neck and waist

2. MASK OR RESPIRATOR
- Secure ties or elastic bands at middle of head and neck
- Fit flexible band to nose bridge
- Fit snug to face and below chin
- Fit-check respirator

3. GOGGLES OR FACE SHIELD
- Place over face and eyes and adjust to fit

4. GLOVES
- Extend to cover wrist of isolation gown

USE SAFE WORK PRACTICES TO PROTECT YOURSELF AND LIMIT THE SPREAD OF CONTAMINATION

- Keep hands away from face
- Limit surfaces touched
- Change gloves when torn or heavily contaminated
- Perform hand hygiene

SECUENCIA PARA PONERSE EL EQUIPO DE PROTECCIÓN PERSONAL (PPE)

El tipo de PPE que se debe utilizar depende del nivel de precaución que sea necesario; por ejemplo, equipo Estándar y de Contacto o de Aislamiento de infecciones transportadas por gotas o por aire.

1. BATA
- Cubra con la bata todo el torso desde el cuello hasta las rodillas, los brazos hasta la muñeca y dóblela alrededor de la espalda
- Átesela por detrás a la altura del cuello y la cintura

2. MÁSCARA O RESPIRADOR
- Asegúrese los cordones o la banda elástica en la mitad de la cabeza y en el cuello
- Ajústese la banda flexible en el puente de la nariz
- Acomódesela en la cara y por debajo del mentón
- Verifique el ajuste del respirador

3. GAFAS PROTECTORAS O CARETAS
- Colóquesela sobre la cara y los ojos y ajústela

4. GUANTES
- Extienda los guantes para que cubran la parte del puño en la bata de aislamiento

UTILICE PRÁCTICAS DE TRABAJO SEGURAS PARA PROTEGERSE USTED MISMO Y LIMITAR LA PROPAGACIÓN DE LA CONTAMINACIÓN

- Mantenga las manos alejadas de la cara
- Limite el contacto con superficies
- Cambie los guantes si se rompen o están demasiado contaminados
- Realice la higiene de las manos

SEQUENCE FOR REMOVING PERSONAL PROTECTIVE EQUIPMENT (PPE)

Except for respirator, remove PPE at doorway or in anteroom. Remove respirator after leaving patient room and closing door.

1. GLOVES
- Outside of gloves is contaminated!
- Grasp outside of glove with opposite gloved hand; peel off
- Hold removed glove in gloved hand
- Slide fingers of ungloved hand under remaining glove at wrist
- Peel glove off over first glove
- Discard gloves in waste container

2. GOGGLES OR FACE SHIELD
- Outside of goggles or face shield is contaminated!
- To remove, handle by head band or ear pieces
- Place in designated receptacle for reprocessing or in waste container

3. GOWN
- Gown front and sleeves are contaminated!
- Unfasten ties
- Pull away from neck and shoulders, touching inside of gown only
- Turn gown inside out
- Fold or roll into a bundle and discard

4. MASK OR RESPIRATOR
- Front of mask/respirator is contaminated — DO NOT TOUCH!
- Grasp bottom, then top ties or elastics and remove
- Discard in waste container

SECUENCIA PARA QUITARSE EL EQUIPO DE PROTECCIÓN PERSONAL (PPE)

Con la excepción del respirador, quítese el PPE en la entrada de la puerta o en la antesala. Quítese el respirador después de salir de la habitación del paciente y de cerrar la puerta.

1. GUANTES
- ¡El exterior de los guantes está contaminado!
- Agarre la parte exterior del guante con la mano opuesta en la que todavía tiene puesto el guante y quíteselo
- Sostenga el guante que se quitó con la mano enguantada
- Deslice los dedos de la mano sin guante por debajo del otro guante que no se ha quitado todavía a la altura de la muñeca
- Quítese el guante de manera que acabe cubriendo el primer guante
- Arroje los guantes en el recipiente de deshechos

2. GAFAS PROTECTORAS O CARETA
- ¡El exterior de las gafas protectoras o de la careta está contaminado!
- Para quitárselas, tómelas por la parte de la banda de la cabeza o de las piezas de las orejas
- Colóquelas en el recipiente designado para reprocesar materiales o de materiales de deshecho

3. BATA
- ¡La parte delantera de la bata y las mangas están contaminadas!
- Desate los cordones
- Tocando solamente el interior de la bata, pásela por encima del cuello y de los hombros
- Voltee la bata al revés
- Dóblela o enróllela y deséchela

4. MÁSCARA O RESPIRADOR
- La parte delantera de la máscara o respirador está contaminada — ¡NO LA TOQUE!
- Primero agarre la parte de abajo, luego los cordones o banda elástica de arriba y por último quítese la máscara o respirador
- Arrójela en el recipiente de deshechos

PERFORM HAND HYGIENE IMMEDIATELY AFTER REMOVING ALL PPE

EFECTÚE LA HIGIENE DE LAS MANOS INMEDIATAMENTE DESPUÉS DE QUITARSE CUALQUIER EQUIPO DE PROTECCIÓN PERSONAL

FIGURE 13-22 Sequence for applying and removing personal protective equipment (Courtesy of Centers for Disease Control and Prevention)

PROCEDURE

3

PUTTING ON A GOWN

To be effective, a gown should have long sleeves, be long enough to cover the uniform, and be big enough to overlap in the back. Gowns should be waterproof.

1. Assemble equipment:
   - Clean gown
   - Paper towel
2. Remove wristwatch; place it on a paper towel.
3. Wash hands.
4. Put on the gown outside the patient's room. Put on gown by slipping your arms into the sleeves (Figure 13-23A).

5. Slip the fingers of both hands under the inside neckband and grasp the ties in back. Secure the neckband (Figure 13-23B).
6. Reach behind and overlap the edges of the gown. Secure the waist ties.
7. Take your watch into the isolation unit, leaving it on the paper towel.

Remember when using gowns:
- A disposable gown is worn only once and then is discarded as infectious waste.
- A reusable cloth gown is worn only once and then is handled as contaminated linen.
- Carry out all procedures in the unit at one time, to avoid unnecessary waste of gowns.

FIGURE 13-23A Select a cover gown that is the right size for you. Unfold the gown, then slip your arms in and pull it up to your shoulders. (Courtesy of Centers for Disease Control and Prevention)

FIGURE 13-23B Slip your hands inside, under the neckband and adust it to fit. Tie the neck ties. Then reach behind, overlapping the edges of the gown so your uniform is completely covered, and tie waist ties. (Courtesy of Centers for Disease Control and Prevention)

Soiled linen is a source of pathogens and should be handled with care. (Refer to Procedure 11.) Some facilities place dirty linen in water-soluble bags that melt in the washer. If these bags are used, they must be placed inside a second plastic bag, because the water-soluble bag will begin to melt if it touches wet linen.

- Handle linen as little as possible.
- Fold the dirtiest side inward.
- Do not shake.
- Do not place soiled linen on the floor or tabletop.

- Bag linen before leaving the room.
- Keep soiled linen separate from general linen.
- Transport soiled, wet linen in a leakproof bag.

Transporting the Patient in Isolation

Sometimes a patient in isolation has to be transported to another area of the health care facility for treatment or testing. Notify the receiving unit of your intention to

PROCEDURE

PUTTING ON GLOVES

1. Assemble equipment:
   - Disposable gloves in correct size

2. Wash your hands.

3. If a gown is required, put gloves on after the gown is put on.

4. Pick up a glove by the cuff and place it on the other hand.

5. Repeat with a glove for the other hand.

6. Interlace fingers to adjust the gloves on your hands.

7. If wearing a gown, pull cuffs of gloves up over the gown sleeves (Figure 13-24).

8. Remember when using gloves:
   - Wash hands before and after using gloves.
   - Remove gloves if they tear or become heavily soiled. Wash hands and put on a new pair.
   - Gloves are used whenever there is the possibility of contacting body fluids, blood, secretions, excretions, mucous membranes, or nonintact skin.

- Change gloves between patients and wash hands.

- Discard gloves immediately after removing them. Put them in a biohazardous waste receptacle.

- Avoid touching your face, exposed skin, or environmental surfaces with used gloves.

FIGURE 13-24 If you are wearing a gown, pull the cuffs of the gloves up to cover the gown sleeves. (Courtesy of Centers for Disease Control and Prevention)

OSHA ALERT

To remove PPE safely, you must be able to identify what parts are clean and what are contaminated.

- These areas are contaminated:
  - The outside front and sleeves of the gown
  - The outside front of the goggles, mask, respirator, and face shield
  - The outside of the gloves
  - Any area with visible blood, body fluids, or soiling

Touch only clean areas when removing PPE.

- These areas are clean:
  - Inside the gloves
  - The inside and back of the gown, including the ties
  - The ties, elastic, or earpieces of the mask, goggles, and face shield ∎

transport the patient and describe the type of transmission-based precautions being used. If the patient is on airborne or droplet precautions, the patient should wear a surgical mask while out of the isolation room. (HEPA masks are not used on patients.) If the patient is on contact precautions, the infectious area of the skin should be covered while the patient is out of the room. The nursing assistant wears personal protective equipment when picking up and returning the patient to the isolation room, but does not wear the PPE while transporting the patient in the hallway. (Refer to Procedure 12.)

You may remove your PPE after you have finished all tasks in the patient's room. Follow the instructions in Procedures 5 and 6.

PROCEDURE

5

REMOVING CONTAMINATED GLOVES

1. Grasp the cuff of one glove on the outside with the fingers of the other hand (Figure 13-25A).

2. Pull the cuff of the glove down, drawing it over the glove (Figure 13-25B). Pull that glove off your hand.

3. Hold the glove with the still-gloved hand.

4. Insert the fingers of the ungloved hand under the cuff of the glove on the other hand (Figure 13-25C).

5. Pull the glove off inside out, drawing it over the first glove.

6. Drop both gloves together into the biohazardous waste receptacle (Figure 13-25D).

7. Wash your hands. Dry with a paper towel and discard the towel in the proper container. Use a dry towel to turn off the water faucet. Discard the towel.

FIGURE 13-25B Pull the cuff of the glove down over the hand and fingers and remove it.

FIGURE 13-25A With the fingers of one glove, grasp the cuff or palm of glove on the other hand.

FIGURE 13-25C Hold the glove just removed in the gloved hand. Insert fingers of the ungloved hand inside the cuff of the other glove.

FIGURE 13-25D Pull the glove down over the hand and then pull both gloves off, holding the inside (clean side of glove). Discard the gloves in the proper container.

PROCEDURE

6

REMOVING CONTAMINATED GLOVES, EYE PROTECTION, GOWN, AND MASK

1. Assemble equipment:
   - Biohazardous waste receptacle for disposable items
   - Waste receptacle for gown if it is not disposable
   - Paper towels

2. Undo waist ties of gown, if they are in the front. Follow Procedure 5 for removing contaminated gloves.

3. Grasp the earpieces or head strap of goggles or face shield and lift the eye protection outward, away from the face and up (Figure 13-26A). Discard or reprocess according to facility policy.

4. Undo waist ties of gown, if they are in the back (Figure 13-26B).

5. Undo the neck ties and loosen gown at shoulders.

6. Slip the fingers of your dominant hand inside the cuff of the other hand without touching the outside of the gown (Figure 13-26C).

7. Using the gown-covered hand, pull the gown down over the other hand (Figure 13-26D) and then off both arms.

8. As the gown is removed, fold it away from the body with the contaminated side inward and then roll it up (Figure 13-26E). Dispose of the contaminated gown in the appropriate receptacle.

9. Turn faucets on with a clean paper towel. Discard the towel.

10. Wash your hands and dry them with a clean paper towel.

11. Use a clean, dry paper towel to turn off the faucet.

FIGURE 13-26A With ungloved hands, grasp the clean elastric strap or earpiece and lift the eye protection away from the face. (Courtesy of Centers for Disease Control and Prevention)

FIGURE 13-26C Slip the fingers of one hand inside the cuff of the other hand. Pull the gown down over the hand. Do not touch the outside of the gown with either hand.

FIGURE 13-26B Untie the gown waist ties.

FIGURE 13-26D Using the gown-covered hand, pull the gown down over the other hand.

continues

PROCEDURE 6 CONTINUED

FIGURE 13-26E Pull the gown down off the arms, being careful not to touch the outside of the gown. Hold the gown away from your uniform and roll it with the contaminated side in.

12. If you brought a watch into the area (see Procedure 3), remove the watch from the paper towel. Hold the clean side of the paper towel and dispose of the towel in a wastepaper receptacle.

13. Use a paper towel to grasp the door handle as you leave the patient's room. Discard the paper towel in an appropriate receptacle before you leave the unit.

14. Remove mask:
    • Undo the bottom ties first, then the top ties.
    • Holding the top ties, dispose of mask in appropriate waste receptacle.

15. Wash your hands.

PROCEDURE

SERVING A MEAL IN AN ISOLATION UNIT

1. Before entering the isolation unit:
   • Wash your hands.
   • Obtain the meal tray for the patient. Check the meal card on the tray and check that the correct menu was provided.
   • Ask for the assistance of another member of the team.
   • Place the tray on the isolation cart.
   • Put on PPE as required by the type of isolation precautions used.

2. Enter the isolation room and identify the patient.

3. Explain what you plan to do.

4. Provide privacy.

5. Allow the patient to help as much as possible.

6. Raise the bed to a comfortable working height.

7. Pick up the meal tray that remains in the room. Make sure the tray is clean.

8. Return to the door and open it. The team member assisting holds the meal tray while you carefully transfer items to the isolation tray.

9. Place the isolation meal tray on the overbed table. Prepare the patient for the meal.

10. Check the patient's identification band against the meal tray card.

11. Assist the patient with food preparation and feeding as needed.

12. When the patient finishes, note how much food and liquid have been eaten. Uneaten food (except bones) is flushed down the toilet.

continues

PROCEDURE 7 CONTINUED

13. All disposable items (bones, dishes, eating utensils, covers, plastic wrap, foil, napkins, cups, cartons) are placed in the appropriate waste receptacle.

14. Reusable dishes may be handled as follows:
    - Use a paper towel to open the door to the isolation unit.
    - Prop the door open with your foot. Transfer dishes to a tray held by another assistant outside the door.
    - Assistant outside the room covers the dishes and returns the tray to the food cart.

    Note: CDC does not require the use of disposable dishes for patients in transmission-based precautions. Either disposable or reusable dishes and utensils can be used for patients on isolation precautions, according to facility policy. Personnel in the dish room routinely wear gloves when handling used (soiled) dishes. The combination of hot water and detergents used in hospital dishwashers is sufficient to decontaminate dishes, glasses, cups, and eating utensils.

15. Clean the isolation meal tray and store it in the isolation unit.

16. Carry out all ending procedure actions (see Unit 15).

17. Remove PPE and discard in the appropriate receptacle.

18. Wash your hands.

19. Use a paper towel to open the door to leave the isolation unit. Discard the towel before leaving the unit.

PROCEDURE

8

MEASURING VITAL SIGNS IN AN ISOLATION UNIT

Note: Equipment to measure vital signs in isolation should be dedicated to the patient. (This means that the equipment will remain in the room with the patient.) It must be cleaned and disinfected before use with another patient.

1. Before entering the isolation unit:
   - Wash your hands.
   - Remove your wristwatch and place it on a clean paper towel.
   - Put on PPE as required by the type of transmission-based precautions used.

2. Pick up the paper towel with the watch. Enter the isolation unit.

3. With the watch still on the paper towel, place it where you can see it during the procedures.

4. Identify the patient and explain what you plan to do.

5. Provide privacy.

6. Allow the patient to help as much as possible.

7. Raise the bed to a comfortable working height.

8. Using the equipment dedicated to the patient, measure vital signs.

9. Note the readings so you do not forget them.

10. Clean and store the equipment used according to facility policy.

11. Carry out all ending procedure actions (see Unit 15).

12. Remove and discard PPE according to facility policy.

13. Wash your hands, dry them, and pick up your watch.

14. Handling only the clean side of the paper towel, discard it in the appropriate receptacle.

15. Pick up your notes. Use a clean paper towel to open the door and leave the isolation unit. Discard the paper towel before you leave the unit.

PROCEDURE

9

TRANSFERRING NONDISPOSABLE EQUIPMENT OUTSIDE OF THE ISOLATION UNIT

1. Nondisposable equipment used with a patient in transmission-based precautions may be dedicated to that patient. This means that the equipment remains in the isolation unit and is used only by that patient. Cleaning as required is done in the room by the nursing assistant or the housekeeping staff according to facility policy.

2. If the equipment must be used for other patients, it must be removed from the isolation unit and disinfected or sterilized before use with another patient.

3. Before leaving the isolation unit, clean the equipment with a disinfectant.

4. Place the equipment in a biohazard plastic bag. In some facilities, a second person opens a large plastic bag and folds the top over into a cuff to cover his or her hands. The second person stands outside the door and holds the bag open. The person inside the room places the disinfected item into the open bag. The second worker fastens the top of the bag. This is done to prevent possible contamination of the outside of the plastic bag in the isolation room.

5. Follow Procedures 5 and 6 for removing contaminated PPE.

6. Pick up the bag containing the equipment and leave the isolation unit.

7. Once outside the unit, follow facility policy for disinfecting or sterilizing the equipment.

8. Some equipment may be terminally (finally and completely) cleaned with disinfectant in the patient's unit when isolation is discontinued.

PROCEDURE

10

SPECIMEN COLLECTION FROM A PATIENT IN AN ISOLATION UNIT

1. Outside the isolation unit, assemble equipment:
   - Clean specimen container and cover
   - Paper towel
   - Biohazard bag for specimen container (Figure 13-27)
   - Two completed labels, one for the specimen container and one for the specimen bag

 Note: The specimen bag may have a preprinted block on the bag that can be completed with the required information. In this case, a second label is not needed.

2. Place the equipment on the isolation cart while you put on PPE.

3. The biohazard bag for specimen transport remains outside the isolation unit.

4. Carry the specimen equipment into the isolation unit. Place the container and cover on a paper towel.

5. Identify the patient and explain what you plan to do.

6. Provide privacy.

7. Allow the patient to help as much as possible.

8. Raise the bed to comfortable working height.

9. Obtain the specimen. Place it into the container without touching the outside of the container.

continues

PROCEDURE 10 CONTINUED

10. Cover the container and apply a label.

11. Clean the equipment used to obtain the specimen according to facility policy.

12. Carry out all ending procedure actions (see Unit 15).

13. Remove personal protective equipment as described in Procedures 5 and 6.

14. Wash your hands.

15. Use a paper towel to pick up the specimen container. Use another paper towel to open the door to leave the isolation unit.

16. Outside the unit, gather the towel in your hands so the edges do not hang loosely. Place the specimen container in the biohazard transport bag, being careful not to allow the paper towel to touch the outside of the transport bag.

17. Discard the paper towels in the appropriate receptacle.

18. Follow facility policy for transporting the specimen.

19. Wash your hands.

1) Insert Specimen in Longer Pouch.

2) Pull Off Liner, Press to Close.

3) Insert Requisition into Outside Pocket.

4) Tuck Top of Requisition Under Flap.

SPECI-GARD®
PAT.#4,932,791

FIGURE 13-27 Transport specimens in the sealed, labeled transport bag.

PROCEDURE

CARING FOR LINENS IN AN ISOLATION UNIT

1. Assemble any linen required and place on a chair or stand outside the isolation unit.

2. Wash and dry your hands.

3. Outside the isolation unit, put on PPE as required by type of transmission-based precautions.

4. Once inside the isolation unit, place the clean linen on a chair.

5. Identify the patient and explain what you plan to do.

6. Provide privacy.

continues

PROCEDURE **11** CONTINUED

7. Allow the patient to help as much as possible.

8. Raise the bed to a comfortable working height.

9. Remove the soiled linen from the bed by starting at the edges and working toward the center. Roll the linen toward the center with the soiled side inside.

10. Handle soiled linen as little as possible. Pick up the linen from the bed and hold it away from your uniform and gown (if used).

11. Place soiled linen in a meltaway laundry bag (a bag that dissolves in the wash water in the laundry), if used, or follow facility policy.

12. Place the meltaway bag in a laundry hamper lined with a biohazard plastic bag, or follow facility policy. Bag should be labeled as biohazardous material for laundry.

13. Secure the bag and route soiled linen to the laundry according to facility policy.

14. If gloves are heavily contaminated from the soiled linens, remove gloves and dispose of them in the appropriate receptacle. Wash your hands, dry them, and put on a clean pair of gloves. Then remake the patient's bed with the clean linens.

15. Carry out all ending procedure actions (see Unit 15).

PROCEDURE

12

TRANSPORTING A PATIENT TO AND FROM THE ISOLATION UNIT

1. Wash your hands.

2. Assemble equipment:
   - Transport vehicle (wheelchair or stretcher)
   - Clean sheet
   - Mask for patient, if isolation precautions require it

3. Notify the department to which the patient is to be transported that a patient from an isolation unit is being transported.

4. If the patient is to be transported by stretcher, ask for assistance in moving the patient to the stretcher. Two other care providers will be needed.

5. Cover the transport vehicle with a clean sheet. Do not let the sheet touch the floor.

6. Wash your hands.

7. Put on PPE as required by type of precautions being used. If other care providers are needed to move the patient onto a stretcher, they also must put on PPE.

8. Wheel the transport vehicle into the isolation unit.

9. Identify the patient. Explain what you plan to do.

10. Provide privacy.

11. Allow the patient to help as much as possible.

12. If the patient is to be transported by wheelchair, the bed must be in the lowest horizontal position. For transport by stretcher, raise the bed to the same height as the stretcher.

13. Assist the patient into the wheelchair or onto the stretcher.

14. Put a mask on the patient, if required.

15. Wrap the patient in a sheet, if required. Make sure the sheet does not touch the floor.

16. Remove PPE and wash your hands. Open the door and take the patient out of the isolation unit (Figure 13-28).

17. To return a patient to an isolation unit, place the wheelchair or stretcher near the wall of the room as you put on PPE.

continues

PROCEDURE 12 CONTINUED

18. Enter the isolation unit, unwrap the patient from the sheet, and remove the patient's mask, if used.

19. Assist the patient from the wheelchair or stretcher (with help of other caregivers) and return the patient to bed.

20. Carry out ending procedure actions (see Unit 15).

21. Place the sheet in the laundry hamper for contaminated linens and discard the patient's mask in the biohazardous trash receptacle.

22. Remove PPE and wash your hands.

23. Remove the transport vehicle from the isolation unit. Follow facility procedure for cleaning and storing the vehicle used for the patient in isolation.

24. Report completion of procedure: transport of patient in isolation to another department and back to isolation unit.

FIGURE 13-28 This patient is leaving her room, where contact precautions are in effect. The receiving area has been notified of her arrival.

Table 13-4 summarizes some rules for nursing assistants in the practice of infection control.

TABLE 13-4 RULES OF INFECTION CONTROL

Do
• Observe standard precautions and use barrier equipment (PPE) any time contact with blood, body fluids, secretions, excretions, mucous membranes, or nonintact skin is likely. Contact may be with a patient or an environmental surface.
• Clean up dishes immediately after use.
• Damp-dust daily and be conscientious about cleaning while you carry out a task.
• Provide a bag for the disposal of used tissues.
• Turn the face to one side so that the assistant and the patient are not breathing directly on each other.

continues

TABLE 13-4 *CONTINUED*

Do, *continued*

- Cover your nose and mouth when coughing or sneezing.

- Protect the skin on your hands by using warm water for washing, drying thoroughly, and applying lotion if needed.

- Treat breaks in the skin immediately by washing thoroughly, cleaning with an antiseptic, and covering. Report any breaks in the skin to the nurse.

- Disinfect equipment that is used by more than one staff member or patient, such as a stethoscope, before and after each use.

- Gather or fold linen inward, with the dirtiest area toward the center.

- Clean reusable equipment immediately after use.

- Handle and dispose of soiled material according to facility policy.

- Practice good personal hygiene.

- Wash your hands frequently.

- Keep clean and dirty items separate in patient rooms and storage areas.

- Bring only needed items into the patient's room.

- Keep soiled linen and trash covered in closed containers.

- Perform procedures in the manner in which you were taught.

- Empty wastebaskets frequently, if this is your responsibility.

Do Not

- Shake bed linens, because any microbes present could be released into the air.

- Allow dirty linen to touch your uniform.

- Eat or share food from a patient's tray.

- Borrow personal care items from another patient or employee, or use such items for another patient.

- Permit the contents of bedpans or urinals to splash when being emptied.

- Report for duty if you have an infectious disease.

- Permit linen to touch the floor, which is always considered dirty.

- Carry clean linen against your uniform or bring more linen than necessary into the patient's room.

- Store lab specimens in the refrigerator with food.

DISINFECTION AND STERILIZATION

Disinfection is the process of eliminating harmful pathogens from equipment and instruments. A chemical called a *disinfectant* is used for this procedure. You may be required to disinfect personal care items such as wash basins, bedpans, and urinals. You may also use disinfectants to clean wheelchairs and other furniture items. Items are usually washed before they are disinfected. The procedure for disinfection depends on the chemicals used. Follow the directions of your facility for use of disinfectants. Wear gloves and a gown for completing these procedures. You may also need a face shield. Wear PPE that is appropriate to the procedure.

Sterilization removes all microorganisms from an item. This process can be completed in an **autoclave**, which uses steam and pressure to kill organisms. Gas sterilization is also used in some health care facilities. Sterilization procedures are used for all nondisposable equipment that is exposed to potentially infectious materials. Equipment to be sterilized is wrapped in special material. Tape on the packaging material changes color when the package is sterilized (Figure 13-29). Do not use the package if the tape has not changed color. Do not use a sterilized package that has been accidentally opened.

STERILE PROCEDURES

Surgical asepsis is the means by which the environment is kept free of all microbes, both pathogens and non-pathogens. In procedures where surgical asepsis is used,

FIGURE 13-29 Before sterilization, the stripes on the tape are not visible. The stripes appear in the autoclave when the tape is exposed to heat and steam. This indicates the package has been sterilized.

equipment and supplies must be **sterile**. In other words, items used in the procedure must go through a sterilization process.

In most facilities, you will not be expected to use sterile technique. If you are responsible for sterile procedures, you should first be given thorough education. Your responsibilities may include opening sterile packages. (See Procedure 13.) Also see Unit 51.

Sterile Field

The term **sterile field** refers to an area of sterile equipment and materials. When working with a sterile field and sterile equipment, keep the following points in mind:

- The sterile field may be a table covered with a sterilized sheet or a sterile towel placed on an overbed table.
- Only the center of the towel is actually used.
- Equipment is kept two inches in from the edges all around, as an added precaution.
- Never reach for or pass anything that is unsterile over a sterile field. You might drop the unsterile article onto the field or touch the field. Instead, carry the unsterile object around the sterile field or hold it away from the sterile field.
- If there is even a suspicion that anything unsterile has touched any part of the sterile field, the field must be considered contaminated. The entire setup must be discarded.
- Coughing or sneezing while preparing a sterile field, or after the field has been set up, contaminates the field.
- Moisture means contamination. If a sterile towel is placed on an unsterile surface, any wetness on the towel means that the towel is contaminated. The towel and anything on the towel must be replaced.

PROCEDURE

OPENING A STERILE PACKAGE

1. Wash your hands.
2. Assemble equipment:
   - Sterile package
3. If color code has not changed, or seal does not look intact, do not consider article sterile. *If you have any doubt about sterility, consider the item unsterile and inform the nurse.*
4. Touch only the outside of the package. Only sterile surfaces contact other sterile surfaces. Never reach over a sterile field.

5. Commercially prepared products will be sealed. If the package is in poor condition or discolored, do not consider the item sterile. Discard the item.
6. Place the package with the fold side up on a flat, clean surface.
7. Remove the tape.
8. Unfold the flap farthest away from you by grasping the outer surface only between your thumb and forefinger (Figure 13-30A).

continues

PROCEDURE **13** CONTINUED

9. Open the right flap with your right hand using the same technique.

10. Open the left flap with your left hand using the same technique (Figure 13-30B).

11. Open the final flap (nearest you) (Figure 13-30C). Touch only the outside of the flap. Be careful not

to stand too close. Do not allow your uniform to touch the flap as it is lifted free. Be sure the flaps are pulled open completely to prevent them from folding back over sterile items.

FIGURE 13-30A Touching only the corner, open the distal (top) flap away from your body.

FIGURE 13-30B Carefully grasp the wrapper, opening the left side of the package.

FIGURE 13-30C Open the proximal (closest) flap toward you. Avoid touching the flap or inside of the package with your hands or clothing.

REVIEW

A. True/False.

Mark the following true or false by circling T or F.

1. T F When working in the droplet precautions room, always wear a HEPA mask.

2. T F Surgical masks may be reused.

3. T F It is permitted for two patients in the same room to share equipment.

4. T F Food and drink should not be kept where they may be exposed to contaminated materials.

5. T F When a patient is placed in transmission-based precautions, only licensed nurses are responsible for carrying out proper isolation technique.

6. T F Disposable patient care equipment is preferred when caring for a patient in isolation.

7. T F Droplet precautions do not require the use of a covering gown.

8. T F Handwashing should be done in cold water to prevent skin damage.

9. T F Always hold fingertips up when rinsing hands during handwashing.

10. T F Handling sterile equipment is a routine procedure for the nursing assistant.

11. T F A mask need not be worn if protective eye equipment is in place.

12. T F Asepsis is the absence of pathogens.

13. T F If an article is "clean," that means it is sterile.

B. Completion.

Complete the statements by writing in the correct word(s).

14. The single most important health procedure a nursing assistant can carry out is _____.

15. Accidental contact with infectious or potentially infectious materials is known as a/an _____.

16. Gloves, gown, masks, goggles, and face masks are part of_____.

17. Small blood spills may be cleaned up by using ____.

18. Sharps and needles should be disposed of by placing them in the _____.

C. Complete the Chart.

In addition to standard precautions, indicate the transmission-based precautions required by each disease or condition. Place an x to make your choice.

Disease	Airborne	Droplet	Contact
19. Draining infected pressure ulcer			
20. Tuberculosis			
21. Mumps			
22. Infected surgical wound			
23. Influenza			

D. Multiple Choice.

Select the one best answer for each of the following.

24. Housing and caring for a person with an infection is known as
   a. segregation.
   b. isolation.
   c. sequestration.
   d. separation.

25. To remove PPE after caring for a patient on isolation precautions, you should
   a. remove the gown first.
   b. remove the gloves first.
   c. remove the mask first.
   d. remove PPE in any order.

26. If a nursing assistant is sensitive to latex gloves, he or she
   a. need not wear gloves.
   b. should wear the latex gloves anyway.
   c. should ask for nonlatex gloves.
   d. should put powder in the gloves.

27. The basic foundation of medical asepsis is
   a. handwashing.
   b. wearing goggles.
   c. wearing a mask.
   d. wearing a gown.

28. If there is an exposure incident, you should
   a. ignore the situation.
   b. report it at once to the supervisor.
   c. call the doctor.
   d. tell other nursing assistants.

29. An AII (A2) isolation room
   a. must have the air conditioner on at all times.
   b. has the window cracked open 12 hours a day.
   c. is connected to the facility ventilation system.
   d. uses a negative pressure ventilation system.

30. When a patient is suspected of having SARS, workers will use
   a. standard, contact, and airborne precautions.
   b. standard and contact precautions.
   c. standard, contact, and droplet precautions.
   d. standard and airborne precautions.

31. If a patient has signs of respiratory infection upon initial facility contact, he or she is
   a. instructed to apply a surgical mask.
   b. asked to use respiratory hygiene and cough etiquette.
   c. placed in airborne or droplet precautions promptly.
   d. instructed to leave and return when symptom-free.

E. Nursing Assistant Challenge.

32. Mrs. Minion has just been placed on isolation. Your assignment is to set up the room.

   a. What equipment should be assembled and where is each item placed? _____

   b. What effect might being placed on isolation have on Mrs. Minion? _____

   c. What might you do to make her adjustment easier? _____

   d. How might her visitors feel? _____

33. You are reporting on duty. Some of your responsibilities will be handling food trays, making beds, straightening out your patients' overbed tables, and helping to change a patient who is wet with urine. During your shift you will use a facial tissue and visit the rest room.

List six times you will need to wash your hands.

   a. _____

   b. _____

   c. _____

   d. _____

   e. _____

   f. _____

Safety and Mobility

UNIT 14

Environmental and Nursing Assistant Safety

OBJECTIVES

After completing this unit, you will be able to:
- Spell and define terms.
- Describe the health care facility environment.
- Identify measures to promote environmental safety.
- List situations when equipment must be repaired.
- Describe the elements required for fire.
- List five measures to prevent fire.

- Describe the procedure to follow if a fire occurs.
- Demonstrate the use of a fire extinguisher.
- List at least 10 guidelines for dealing with a violent individual.
- List techniques for using ergonomics on the job.
- Demonstrate appropriate body mechanics.
- Describe the types of information contained in Material Safety Data Sheets (MSDS).

VOCABULARY

Learn the meaning and the correct spelling of the following words and phrases:

concurrent cleaning	incident report	private room	ward
environmental safety	Material Safety Data	RACE	workplace violence
ergonomics	Sheet (MSDS)	semiprivate room	
incident	PASS	side rails	

INTRODUCTION

The hospital room is the patient's home while he or she is hospitalized (Figure 14-1). The room becomes the patient's world. Cheerful and pleasant surroundings give the patient a better sense of well-being. Attention to safety helps foster feelings of security in this strange environment. *Both* help speed recovery.

The nursing assistant helps keep the patient's unit safe and clean. All health care providers share the task of keeping the entire nursing unit safe and clean.

Environmental safety refers to the condition of an entire facility—patient rooms, hallways, and all departments. The environment includes:

- Temperature (heating and air conditioning)
- Air circulation
- Light
- Cleanliness
- Noise control
- Walls, ceilings, and floors
- Plumbing
- Electricity
- Equipment and furniture

Prevention of injuries to patients, visitors, volunteers, and staff members is of primary concern.

FIGURE 14-1 The patient's unit is home during the hospital stay.

FIGURE 14-2 All hospital beds are equipped with side rails. These are split rails that can be raised and lowered in any combination.

Infection Control ALERT

Some hospitals do not permit flowers in certain areas, such as the burn unit, intensive care unit, or rooms of patients with weakened immune systems. This is because flowers increase the risk for the spread of infection, especially *Pseudomonas*. Plants and flowers should be cared for by staff who are not involved in patient care, or by the patient or a family member. If you must touch flowers or plants, wear gloves. Perform thorough hand hygiene with soap and water or an alcohol preparation when finished. ■

THE PATIENT ENVIRONMENT

In a health care facility, the basic patient unit consists of a/an:

- Hospital bed with rails (Figure 14-2)
- Bedside table
- Chair
- Reading lamp
- Waste basket
- Overbed table
- Signal cord

This equipment may be located in a single-, double-, or multiple-bed room. A **private room** contains only one bed. **Semiprivate rooms** contain two beds. **Wards** are multiple-bed rooms, usually with 3 or 4 beds.

Each room is numbered. The beds are marked by letters or numbers. For example, Room 871 in a large medical center may be a four-unit ward. The beds are labeled A,

B, C, D (or 1, 2, 3, 4). The patient in the fourth bed is in Unit 871–D or Unit 871–4.

The equipment from one unit should not be used by other patients. For home care, the same unit elements will be present, but they will be modified. For example, there may not be an adjustable hospital bed or an overbed table.

Hospital Beds

Hospital beds mostly have the same features, but there may be some differences. Hospital beds:

- Differ in the ways in which they operate. Some are controlled electrically (Figure 14-3). Others are operated by the turning of cranks or gatch handles (Figure 14-4).

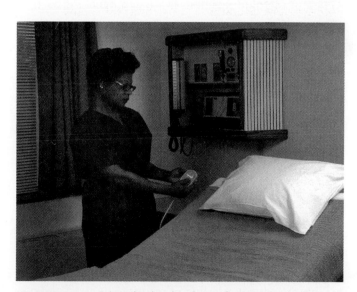

FIGURE 14-3 Some beds also have foot controls that are used to change the angle of the bed. The manual switch controls the head and knee elevation.

Raises and lowers height of bed

Raises and lowers head of bed

Raises and lowers knee portion or foot of bed

FIGURE 14-4 Gatch handles are used to change the position of nonelectric beds. Some stretchers also use handles similar to these.

- May be raised to a high horizontal position. In this position, there is less strain for those giving care. Beds must be returned to the lowest horizontal position when you leave the room.
- Are on wheels, to make it easy to move beds from one place to another. The wheels should always be locked unless the bed is being moved.
- Break in the middle so that the head may be raised.
- Break behind the knees to increase physical comfort for the bedridden patient.

Side rails are attached to the hospital bed. They protect the patient from falling. Side rails are considered to be restraints in some circumstances. Most health care facilities have policies, procedures, and guidelines describing their use. Potential benefits of side rails are that they:

- Provide support and a "handle" for the patient to use for turning and repositioning in bed.
- Provide a "handle" for getting into and out of bed.
- Give the patient a feeling of security.
- Reduce the risk of the patient falling out of bed when he or she is being transported in the bed.

- Provide access to bed and television controls that are part of the bed rail design.

The potential risks of side rails include:

- Strangulation, suffocation, bodily injury, or death when the patient or part of the patient's body becomes entrapped between the bars of the side rails or between the side rails and the mattress
- Serious injuries if the patient climbs over the rails and falls from this height
- Skin tears, bruises, cuts, scrapes
- Agitation caused by a feeling of being trapped or caged in
- Feelings of isolation or restriction
- Sadness because of loss of independence and having to call for help
- Actual loss of independence, such as the ability to get up to use the bathroom or to retrieve an item dropped on the floor

Several types of side rails are used on hospital beds. One type is a single rail that runs the length of the bed. Split rails are more common in acute care hospitals. Each side of the bed has two half-rails. One or both can be raised, depending on the patient's needs and plan of care. When side rails are used, they:

- Should be checked and attached securely before you leave the bedside, unless ordered otherwise.
- Should be down only when beds are in the lowest horizontal position, or if a release form has been signed by the patient.
- Should never be used for the attachment of tubes such as IV lines or catheters. Raising and lowering the side rails could put undue stress on such tubes and even pull them out.
- Should never be used for the attachment of restraints.

The use of side rails may upset some patients. Sometimes it may be necessary to reassure the patient that her condition is not becoming worse. The patient should be told that the raising of side rails is hospital policy or is being done as a reminder of a new environment.

Temperature, Air Circulation, and Light

As you adjust and maintain the temperature, light, and ventilation, keep in mind the patient's condition, the patient's personal preference, and the needs of the other patients in the room.

- The best temperature is about 71 to 81°F, according to patient comfort and facility policy. Lower temperatures may cause chilling and higher ones may make the patients uncomfortable.
- Movement of air and the temperature may be controlled by opening windows at the top and bottom if air conditioning is not being used. (In some facilities the windows are sealed shut.)
- Patients can be shielded from drafts by screens or curtains.

In most hospitals and health facilities, rooms are automatically air-conditioned. The thermostat may be set from a central location, or set individually in each patient's room.

Lighting comes from several sources. There will be times when less light is desired. At other times, more light will be needed (Figure 14-5). Use as much light as needed to safely carry out your job. Be careful to shield other patients as much as possible.

Patients often find it difficult to sleep if lights are too bright. There should be only enough light at night to enable staff to work safely.

- Rooms are equipped with lights above each bed. These illuminate a single patient bed.
- There may also be a ceiling light.
- Additional spotlights can be brought from the utility room when needed to provide extra light for delicate procedures.
- The best lighting is indirect; glare causes fatigue.
- Be sure to return extra lights as soon as you are finished, because clutter in a room is hazardous.

FIGURE 14-5 The overbed light can be adjusted to several different lighting levels.

- Be sure to turn ceiling lights off when leaving the room.
- Night lights are often left on for very ill or elderly patients.

Infection Control ALERT

Make sure clean and soiled items are separated in patient rooms and storage areas. Keep the lids tightly closed on trash cans and linen hampers. Avoid putting biohazard contaminated trash into open wastebaskets. Discard soiled items in a plastic bag or a covered trash can. ■

Cleanliness and Noise Reduction

You are responsible for the cleanliness, quiet, and order of the patient units to which you are assigned. To contribute to the comfort of the patient:

- Speak quietly.
- Report squeaky equipment wheels that should be oiled.
- Avoid banging equipment and trays against other surfaces.
- Keep the area neat as you work. Check its overall appearance before you leave.
- Return equipment to its proper location after completing patient care.
- Do not turn the TV on or up while giving care to patients unless the patient asks you to do so.

You are responsible for keeping the patient supplied with fresh water, ice, disposable drinking cups, tissues, and straws. Make sure that all necessary pieces of equipment, such as the wash basin, emesis basin, bedpan, urinal, soap, and towels, are always available, clean, and in good condition (Figure 14-6). These items should always be stored in the bedside table.

Infection Control ALERT

When two or more patients share a room, make sure that all personal care items are labeled with each patient's name. Keep personal care items in the appropriate area. Store grooming supplies in a clean area. Avoid storing personal care equipment and supplies in community areas, such as bathrooms; storage in these areas increases the risk that personal care items will be used for the wrong patient(s). ■

FIGURE 14-6 Personal care supplies are stored in the bedside stand. Items considered clean and dirty are stored in separate shelves or drawers.

SAFETY MEASURES

Safety is the responsibility of everyone. A safe environment is essential for both patients and staff. Safety must be a part of everything you do. This concern extends to the safety of the unit and the entire environment. The number of accidents involving patients and staff can be greatly reduced if simple measures are followed.

When an accident occurs in the health care facility, it is referred to as an **incident**. An incident is any unexpected occurrence or event that interrupts normal procedures or causes a crisis. Incidents can cause harm to a patient, employee, or any other person. If you see an incident or are involved in one, you need to report it to the nurse. The nurse fills out an **incident report** (Figure 14-7) after obtaining information from the persons involved and witnesses. Prevention of incidents depends on employees:

- Knowing their jobs and following all safety policies and procedures
- Maintaining a safe environment
- Knowing the patients and implementing safety measures to decrease their risk of injury

Environmental Safety Conditions

Incidents can be prevented by keeping hallways and other walkways free of equipment and clutter. Most facilities require that equipment and carts be kept on the same side of the hallway. This leaves the opposite side free so patients and visitors can use the hand rail, if needed. Keeping equipment on the same side reduces the risk of falls, and means that no one has to navigate through a maze of equipment to walk down the hallway. Report these situations promptly:

- Burnt-out light bulbs and light switches or electric plugs that do not work
- Water leaks from faucets or pipes
- Faucets or water fountains that do not flow properly
- Loose or missing floor tiles
- Windows that do not close tightly or are cracked or broken
- Temperatures that are too hot or too cold and cannot be controlled within the room
- Loose or missing ceiling tiles or leaks from the ceiling
- Toilets that do not flush properly

INCIDENT REPORT

Family Name	First Name	M.I.	Room No.	Hosp. No.

Address	City	State	Zip Code	Age	Sex M F

Date of Incident	Time a.m. p.m.	Place	Attending Physician

Status of person involved: Patient _____   Employee _____ Visitor _____   Other _____

Diagnosis: _____

_____

Describe condition before incident: Disoriented _____ Senile ___ Sedated ___ Normal ___ Other ___

_____

Was height of bed adjustable? Yes ___ No ___   Was bed up? Yes ___ No ___ Was bed down? Yes ___ No ___
Were bed rails ordered? Yes ___ No ___ Were they present? Yes ___ No ___   Were they up? Yes ___ No ___
Were they down? Yes ___ No ___ Other _____

Describe incident entirely, include part of body injured and treatment:

_____

_____

_____

_____

_____

_____

_____

_____

_____

_____

Vital Signs: Temp _____   Pulse _____   Resp _____   Blood Pressure _____

Indicate on diagram location of injury

– over –

FIGURE 14-7 A special report is completed any time an incident occurs.

Was physician called? Yes _____ No _____ Time _____ a.m. p.m.

Who responded? _____ Time _____ a.m. p.m.
              Attending physician _____ On-call physician _____

Statement of physician _____

_____

_____

_____

_____

Was family called? Yes _____ No _____ Time _____ a.m. p.m. Who: _____

Give names, addresses, and phone numbers of any who witnessed incident _____

_____

_____

_____

A copy of this report will be sent to Patient's physician.

Date of Report _____ Signed _____
                                                Signature and title of person preparing report

Nursing Office Review of Incident: Date _____ Signed _____

Comments: _____

_____

_____

_____

_____

_____

FIGURE 14-7 *CONTINUED*

Equipment and Its Care

The daily or **concurrent cleaning** of equipment is an important part of your job. It contributes to the safety of your patient. The housekeeping department maintains environmental cleanliness. However, spills must be mopped up immediately to avoid falls.

In most health care facilities, equipment is tagged when it needs repair (Figure 14-8). That equipment is not to be used again until the tag is removed. Facility policy differs as to who is responsible for applying and removing the tag. Reporting broken or nonfunctioning equipment is the responsibility of everyone.

You can prevent accidents related to equipment by:

1. Reporting needed repairs promptly. Possible hazards include:
   - lost screws
   - frayed straps
   - loose wheels
   - broken control knobs
   - latches that do not hook
   - side rails that do not fasten correctly
   - faulty brakes on wheelchairs and stretchers
   - frayed electrical cords

2. Reporting immediately if call lights (signal cords) are not working.

3. Disposing of equipment in proper containers. Facilities must dispose of sharps, such as needles and blades, in special puncture-resistant containers.

4. Never handling broken bits of glass with your hands. Put on gloves. Large pieces can be picked up with forceps. Broken glass can also be cleaned up using a brush or broom and a dustpan (Figure 14-9).

5. Always knowing what you are handling and the proper method for its disposal.

6. Inspecting mechanical lifts (Figure 14-10) carefully before using. Check:
   - Handle, to make sure legs open and close safely

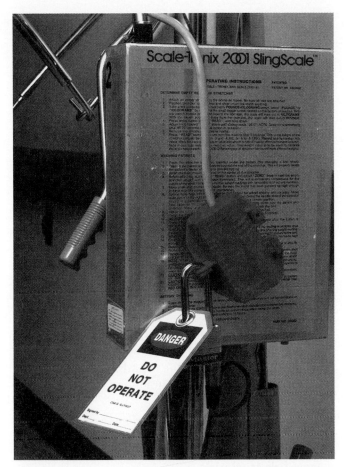

FIGURE 14-8 Unsafe electrical equipment is tagged and locked until it can be repaired.

FIGURE 14-10 Carefully examine the mechanical lift before using it.

– Release mechanism for raising and lowering lift
– All straps and chains for frayed areas or clasps that do not close correctly
– Sling, to be sure it is the right sling to use with that lift and that there are no frays or tears
– For hydraulic fluid on the floor—do not use the lift if fluid is present

7. Making sure that equipment and supplies are stored properly. Never block a doorway with equipment. Items in boxes should not be stored on the floor.

FIGURE 14-9 When cleaning up broken glass, wear gloves to protect your hands. Always use an instrument, broom, or dustpan. Resist the temptation to pick it up with your fingers. Discard the broken glass in the sharps container or other designated location.

OSHA ALERT

Handle needles, razors, and other sharp objects with care. Needles are never cut, bent, broken, or recapped by hand. After using a sharp object, dispose of it in a puncture-resistant "sharps" container. Avoid overfilling the sharps container. Seal the cap when it is three-quarters full. The cap is designed so it cannot be snapped back off after it is closed. The sealed sharps container is stored until it can be picked up with the biohazardous waste. The biohazardous waste disposal area is used for discarding items contaminated with blood or body fluids. Special precautions are taken to contain waste in this area. ■

FIRE SAFETY

It is a scientific fact that if three elements are present in the right proportions (Figure 14-11), there will be a fire. The three elements are heat, fuel, and oxygen.

It is the responsibility of every staff member to know and regularly practice the fire and evacuation plans for the facility.

- Role-play the emergency procedures until you are completely secure. Remember that in any emergency the welfare and safety of the patients are most important.
- Learn the location of escape routes and the location and operation of all fire control equipment (Figure 14-12), such as:

    Fire alarms
    Extinguishers
    Sprinklers
    Fire doors
    Fire escapes

- Know and practice fire drill procedures. These are conducted on a regular basis by each facility. Many

FIGURE 14-12 All personnel must be familiar with the evacuation plan, and must know the location of fire alarms and extinguishers and how to use them.

patients could be injured during a fire because of the confusion and their inability to help themselves.

- Keep alert to all possible fire hazards. Report them immediately to the proper authorities.

Fire Hazards

Some possible fire hazards include:
- Frayed electrical wires
- Overloaded circuits
- Plugs that are not properly grounded
- Accumulated clutter such as papers and rags
- Improper protection during oxygen therapy
- Uncontrolled smoking; most health care facilities prohibit smoking throughout the facility
- Matches left where children or others have unauthorized access to them
- Smoking in rooms where oxygen is in use

Fire Prevention

You and every staff member can do a great deal to prevent the disaster of fire. In general:
- Check for frayed electrical wires.
- Do not overload circuits with too many electrical cords.
- Do not use a lightweight electrical cord with equipment that draws a heavy power load.
- Use three-prong grounded plugs.
- Do not allow clutter to accumulate in doorways or traffic lanes.
- Empty wastepaper cans in proper receptacles.
- Do not store oily rags or paint rags.
- Report any possible hazards right away.
- Report smoke and/or burning smells.

FIGURE 14-11 The fire triangle displays the elements needed to start a fire.

- Keep all fire exits clear of equipment and debris.
- Know and practice fire drill safety.
- Do not let visitors give cigarettes to patients.

Safety ALERT

Avoid stacking linen and supplies on upper shelves closer than 18 inches to the ceiling. If supplies are stacked close to the ceiling, the sprinkler system will not be effective during a fire. ∎

Smoking

Smoking in bed should never be permitted. Smoking should be strictly limited to specific areas, if it is permitted at all. Most health care facilities do not permit smoking by anyone in any area.

This applies to patients, visitors, and staff alike. The use of matches should be watched. Smoking materials are usually stored at the nurse's station. Patients who do not have smoking privileges should not have smoking materials. Some patients may need direct supervision whenever they smoke.

Oxygen Precautions

The use of oxygen presents a specific hazard. When oxygen is in use:

- Never permit smoking, lighted matches, or open flames in the area.
- Do not use flammable liquids such as oils, alcohol, nail polish, aftershave, lotions, perfume, or hair spray.
- Do not use electrical equipment such as radios, hair dryers, electric razors, heating pads, or toys.
- Post a sign indicating that oxygen is in use.
- Use cotton blankets and gowns for the patient.
- In some facilities, the call signal is replaced with a hand bell.
- Wear cotton uniforms and nonwool sweaters when providing care.

Safety ALERT

Oxygen is a prescription item, like a medication. Using oxygen is safe as long as you follow facility policies and safety guidelines. Never change the fittings from one type of oxygen bottle to another. Make sure you use the correct adaptor and plug for the unit. Make sure the oxygen cylinder is secure in an upright position. If it is accidentally knocked over, it has the potential to turn into a missile and cause great damage. If you have reason to believe that an oxygen tank or liquid oxygen canister is leaking, remove the patient from the room and close the door. Report the problem to the proper person. Never attempt to carry or move an oxygen cylinder or canister if it is leaking. ∎

Safety ALERT

Bed linen can absorb oxygen. Any time oxygen is in use, avoid sparks. Static electricity can start a fire. ∎

- Be certain there are no cigarettes, matches, or lighters in the room.
- Do not adjust the liter flow of oxygen.

RACE System

You must be familiar with the fire policies and procedures for your facility. In case of fire, keep calm. Be sure those in immediate danger are moved to safety, then sound the alarm according to facility policy. Follow the evacuation plan as you have practiced. The patients may be confused and frightened. Therefore, the staff must be calm and in control. In a fire emergency, remember **RACE** as defined here (Figure 14-13):

Remove   Activate   Contain or   Extinguish or   Evacuate

FIGURE 14-13 Remember the sequence of critical actions in case of fire.

- **R** = Remove patients. Move patients to safety. Patients who can walk can be escorted. In some cases, they may be called upon to assist others to escape routes. Patients may need to be moved in their beds out of the danger areas. If a person is unable to walk and the bed cannot be moved, bed sheets may be used as cradles and the patient pulled to safety.
- **A** = Alarm. Sound the alarm. Use the intercom, emergency signal bell, telephone, or fire alarm as directed by facility policy. Give the location and type of fire.
- **C** = Contain fire. Close windows and doors to prevent drafts, which cause the fire to spread more rapidly. Before entering a closed door, touch the surface with the back of your hand (Figure 14-14). If the door is hot, do not open it. A fire in the room will quickly (and explosively) spread into the hallway when the door is opened.
- **E** = Extinguish fire or evacuate the area.

Follow the fire emergency plan for your facility:

- Keep calm. Be prepared to follow directions when a person in authority takes charge.
- Shut off air conditioning and other electrical equipment.
- Shut off oxygen.
- Do not use elevators.
- Close all doors into the hallway.
- Remove carts and equipment from the hallway. Get anything that may burn behind a door.

FIGURE 14-14 When you suspect a fire, touch the door with the back of your hand, which is more sensitive to heat than the palm. If the door feels hot, do not open it.

Safety ALERT

Health care facilities are built with safety features that prevent fires from spreading. These features include doors that close automatically when the fire alarm sounds, an automatic sprinkler system, smoke detectors, and fire exits. Many materials used on the floors, doors, walls, and furnishings are fire-rated. This means that they will take longer to burn. Nevertheless, fire prevention is an important responsibility. Despite the built-in safety features, health care facilities can catch fire. Many lives can be lost. ■

Safety ALERT

When a fire occurs, patients are removed from immediate danger. After the alarm is sounded, the fire is contained by closing doors and windows. Patients are moved behind closed doors to keep them safe. Closing doors and windows slows the spread of fire. The hallways are cleared of patients and pieces of equipment that will burn. If the fire is large and spreading rapidly, patients may be evacuated from the building. ■

Use of a Fire Extinguisher

If you have been taught how to use a fire extinguisher, you may use it on small fires.

- Fire extinguishers should be carried upright.
- Remove the safety pin.
- Push the top handle down.
- Direct the hose at the base of the fire.

Remember the letters **PASS**.

 P—PULL the pin.

 A—AIM the nozzle at the base of the fire.

 S—SQUEEZE the handle.

 S—SWEEP back and forth along the base of the fire.

OTHER EMERGENCIES

There may be other disasters for which you and your facility must be prepared. Tornadoes, hurricanes, floods, earthquakes, and bomb threats are examples of such disasters. Each facility has its own policies. Be sure you are familiar with them.

In all emergency situations, get patients to safety, follow your facility's policy, and keep calm.

VIOLENCE IN THE WORKPLACE

Episodes of violence in the workplace are increasing in our society. Hospitals and other health care facilities are not exempt from violence. Serious violence has occurred in both rural and urban communities. Many facilities have violence prevention education programs to eliminate or reduce worker exposure to conditions that can lead to injury. OSHA has developed guidelines for preventing violence in the health care facility and many employers use these guidelines.

Workplace violence is any physical assault, threatening behavior, or verbal abuse that occurs in the workplace. The workplace includes, but is not limited to, the facility buildings and the surrounding perimeters, including parking lots, field locations, clients' homes, and traveling to and from work assignments. Workplace violence includes:

- Beatings
- Stabbings
- Suicides and attempted suicides
- Shootings
- Rapes
- Psychological traumas
- Threats or obscene telephone calls
- Intimidation
- Verbal or physical harassment

- Being followed, sworn at, or shouted at
- Drug holdups

Violence in the workplace can be committed by strangers, patients, coworkers, or personal acquaintances. Some of the potential causes of health care facility violence are:

- The prevalence of handguns and other weapons
- Use of hospitals by the criminal justice system for criminal holds and the care of disturbed, violent individuals
- Acute and chronically mentally ill patients
- Poor judgment and loss of inhibition due to abuse of alcohol, street drugs (Figure 14-15), or illicit use of prescription drugs
- The availability of controlled substances in the facility, making it a likely target of robbery
- The increasing number of gangs and gang members in many communities
- Unrestricted movement of the public in health care facilities
- Distraught family members and other individuals who become angry and frustrated

FIGURE 14-15 Crack cocaine and similar drugs are stimulants that may perpetuate violence. The user may have increased energy, euphoria, and delusions of grandeur. Speech may be incoherent, and the drug user may hallucinate and become paranoid. He or she may become violent suddenly and without warning. (Courtesy of UPI/Corbis)

- Low staffing levels, particularly during meals and at other times when staff is busy caring for patients and unable to observe activity in the hallways
- Poorly lit parking lots, garages, and ramps
- Lack of staff awareness of risk factors
- Failure to use safety precautions, such as locking doors and reporting suspicious individuals

NURSING ASSISTANT SAFETY

The work performed by nursing assistants requires a great deal of lifting and moving of patients, objects, and equipment. It is important that you use your body correctly to avoid injury.

Ergonomics

The word **ergonomics** means adapting the environment and using techniques and equipment to prevent injury to the body. If certain risk factors are present, it is more

---

GUIDELINES *for*

Violence Prevention

Follow all facility policies and procedures involving safety and security. Other things you can do to prevent potential incidents are:

- Participate in continuing education programs to learn how to recognize and manage escalating agitation, assaultive behavior, or criminal intent.

- Attend classes on cultural diversity that offer sensitivity training on racial and ethnic issues and differences.

- If you are responsible for a secured area, control access to the area and keep it locked. Avoid propping locked doors and windows open. Never disable a door alarm.

- Do not leave keys unattended. Never share security alarm codes with unauthorized persons.

- Close shades or curtains at night.

- Report assaults or threats of assaults to the nurse immediately.

- Avoid wearing scarves, necklaces, earrings, and other jewelry that could cause injury if a patient or other individual attacks you.

- Do not carry valuables or large sums of cash to work.

- Avoid remote, dark areas when you are alone.

- Report lights that are burned out and locks that are not working.

- Exercise caution in elevators, stairwells, and unfamiliar areas. Immediately leave the area if you believe that a hazard exists.

- Use the "buddy system" if personal safety may be threatened.

- If a patient or other person is "acting out," or you believe you may be assaulted, do not let the person come between you and the exit.

- Keep your head up, look ahead, and be aware of your surroundings.

- If your facility has security personnel, request that they escort you in dark or potentially dangerous areas. If no security personnel are on duty, ask other staff members to accompany you.

- Park in well-lighted areas. Always lock your car after parking. Look in the car before getting in, then lock the doors after you get in. Do not roll windows down to speak with individuals approaching your car.

- Report suspicious individuals or other potential safety hazards to the proper person. Never approach a suspicious person by yourself.

GUIDELINES *for*
Dealing with a Violent Individual

- Remain calm and avoid raising your voice, which may further agitate the person.
- Speak slowly, softly, and clearly.
- Call for help, if possible, or send someone to get help.
- Move away from heavy or sharp objects that may be used as weapons.
- Monitor your body language and avoid movements that could be challenging, such as placing your hands on your hips, moving toward the person, pointing your finger, or staring directly at the person. However, focus your attention on the person so you know what he or she is doing at all times.
- Position yourself at right angles to the person. Avoid standing directly in front of him or her. Maintain a distance of 3 to 6 feet.
- Position yourself so that an exit is accessible. Never let the person come between you and the exit.
- Avoid making sudden movements.

- Listen to what the person is saying. Encourage the person to talk, and communicate that you genuinely care and will try to help. Acknowledge that you understand that he or she is upset. Break big problems into smaller, manageable ones.
- Avoid arguing and defensive statements. Accept criticism in a positive way. Ask clarifying questions.
- Ask the person to leave and return when he or she is calmer.
- Ask questions to help regain control of the conversation.
- Avoid challenging, bargaining, or making promises you cannot keep.
- Describe the consequences of abusive behavior.
- Avoid touching an angry person.
- If a weapon is involved, ask the person to place it in a neutral location while you continue talking. Avoid trying to disarm the person, which may put you in danger.

likely that an ergonomic (work-related) problem will occur. These risk factors include:

1. Performing the same motion or motion pattern every few seconds for more than two to four hours at a time.
2. Being in a fixed or awkward posture for more than a total of two to four hours.
3. Using forceful hand exertions for more than two to four hours at a time.
4. Doing heavy lifting, unassisted, for more than one to two hours.

Here are several ergonomic techniques you can use to reduce the risk of having an incident:

1. Use correct body mechanics at all times, both at work and when you are off duty.
2. Raise beds to a comfortable working height (remember to lower the bed when you finish your task).
3. Use mechanical lifts when you need to transfer very heavy and/or dependent patients from a bed or chair.
4. Use back supports if your employer requires them or if this is your preference. The use of back supports is controversial, but many nursing assistants find them helpful (Figure 14-16).

FIGURE 14-16 The back support belt reminds you to use your muscles correctly when lifting and moving patients and heavy objects. Fasten the belt before lifting and moving. Release it when you have finished.

5. Get another person to help when you need to transfer a patient who cannot bear his own weight fully.
6. Use a cart to move heavy items.

OSHA ALERT

The back support belt works by keeping your spine in good alignment. You are less likely to be injured if your spine is straight and you are using good body mechanics. Do not lift more than you would if you were not wearing the belt. Using a back support belt does not make you stronger. ∎

If you follow these eight commandments for lifting, you will greatly decrease the risk of injuring yourself.

1. Plan your lift and test the load (Figure 14-17A).
2. Ask for help (Figure 14-17B).
3. Get a firm footing (Figure 14-17C).
4. Bend your knees (Figure 14-17D).
5. Tighten your abdominal muscles (Figure 14-17E).
6. Lift with your legs (Figure 14-17F).
7. Keep the load close (Figure 14-17G).
8. Keep your back upright (Figure 14-17H).

Warming up before working is another way to maintain a healthy body. Exercises can be performed before each work shift. Check with your physician before beginning any exercise program.

Remember that you can avoid many problems if you also:

- Exercise every day.
- Eat a nourishing, well-balanced diet.
- Get adequate sleep.
- Avoid alcohol, cigarettes, drug use, and too much caffeine.
- Wear comfortable shoes with good support.

Hazards in the Work Environment

All health care facilities have hazards in the work environment that can potentially cause injury to employees.

A. Plan your lift and test the load.
Before you lift, think about the item you are going to move and ask yourself: "Can I lift this alone?" "Is it too awkward for one person?" "Is the path clear?" Also, test the load to see approximately how heavy it is before lifting.

B. Ask for help.
If the load is too heavy or too awkward for you to lift, ask for assistance.

C. Get a firm footing.
Keep your feet apart for a stable base and point your toes out.

D. Bend your knees.
Don't bend at the waist. Keep the principles of leverage in mind at all times. Don't do more work than you have to.

E. Tighten your stomach muscles.
Use intra-abdominal pressure to support your spine when you lift, offsetting the force of the load. Train your muscles to work together.

F. Lift with your legs.
Let your leg muscles do the work of lifting. Don't rely on your weaker back muscles.

G. Keep the load close.
Don't hold the load away from your body. The closer it is to your spine, the less force it exerts on your back.

H. Keep your back upright.
Whether lifting or putting down the load, don't add the weight of your body to the load. Avoid twisting.

FIGURE 14-17 Eight rules for lifting and moving. (Reprinted with permission from Ergodyne Corporation, St. Paul, MN)

Safety ALERT

Have you ever heard the expression, "When your feet hurt, you hurt all over"? Most experienced health care workers will tell you this old adage is true. Buying a sturdy pair of athletic shoes or duty shoes is one of the best investments you will make in your uniform. Make sure that the shoe soles are appropriate for the floor surface in your facility. In most cases, this means having a nonslip sole. Having proper footwear will make you feel better and reduce your risk of falls and injuries. ∎

OSHA ALERT

Many chemicals can be hazardous to both patients and nursing assistants. Always use chemicals according to the directions on the label. Make sure they are properly diluted and that containers and surfaces are properly rinsed. Never repackage chemicals into unmarked containers. Use only the original container or special, small containers provided by the manufacturer. Chemicals should always be under your visual control, meaning you can see them. If you cannot see a chemical, it should be stored in a locked area. Wear utility gloves when using chemicals for cleaning procedures. Many chemicals will cause defects in the examination gloves used for patient care. This can irritate your hands, and the chemicals may be absorbed through your skin. Wear eye protection if there is a possibility of splashing or spraying chemicals during a cleaning procedure. Learn the locations of your facility's MSDS sheets, eye wash station, and body wash station. ∎

Many of these items are chemicals that you may have in your own home (chlorine bleach, for example). On a nursing unit you might find cleaning supplies, disinfectants, and other products that are considered hazardous. Injuries can be prevented if you know what the hazards are and how to protect yourself and others. The Occupational Safety and Health Administration (OSHA) is a section of the Department of Labor under the federal government. OSHA is responsible for employee safety. OSHA requires that all manufacturers of these items supply **Material Safety Data Sheets (MSDS)** with any hazardous products they sell. The MSDS provide hazard communications that explain:

- What precautions to take in the presence of a hazard (for example, wearing personal protective equipment)
- Instructions for safe use of the potentially dangerous substance
- How to clean up and dispose of the hazardous product
- First aid measures to use if exposure occurs

OSHA has also established other rules for a safe environment. Employers are required to inform employees of:

- The location of the MSDS
- The hazards that exist in the work environment and where they are in the building

- The location of information related to the hazards
- How to read and understand chemical labels and hazard signs
- What type of personal protective equipment should be worn while working with these chemicals, and where the PPE is stored
- How to manage spills and where cleaning equipment is stored

All hazardous products must be kept in their original containers with the original labels intact and legible. Health care facilities must keep all chemicals in locked cupboards.

REVIEW

A. Multiple Choice.

Select the one best answer for each of the following.

1. The patient's name is Phe Quan. She is in Room 116–D. From this information, you know that she is occupying a bed in a
   a. private room.
   b. rehabilitation department.
   c. semiprivate room.
   d. ward.

2. Side rails should be up and secure when
   a. the bed is at the lowest horizontal height.
   b. the patient has a catheter.
   c. you must leave the bedside with the bed in the high position.
   d. the patient does not have an order for restraints.

3. The best room temperature is approximately
   a. 45°F.
   b. 65°F.
   c. 72°F.
   d. 88°F.

4. Which of the following represents a fire hazard?
   a. Frayed electrical wire
   b. Using three-prong plugs
   c. Supervised smoking
   d. Using UL-approved items

5. The elements needed to start a fire are
   a. cigarettes, matches, and call signal.
   b. heat, fuel, and oxygen.
   c. electricity, oxygen, and matches.
   d. oxygen, linen, and electricity.

6. Which of the following contributes to unsafe conditions in the facility?
   a. Equipment in the halls
   b. Chemicals in locked cupboards
   c. Allowing patients to smoke with supervision
   d. Teaching patients how to use assistive devices

7. When oxygen is in use, you should not
   a. use cotton blankets on the patient's bed.
   b. remove cigarettes from the room.
   c. adjust the liter flow.
   d. post a sign on the door.

8. Every staff member should know
   a. how to open sealed windows in case of fire.
   b. the RACE procedure.
   c. the distance from the fire department to the facility.
   d. how to extinguish a fire by aiming the extinguisher at the top of the flames.

9. The word that means adapting the environment to prevent body injury is
   a. body mechanics.
   b. incident.
   c. ergonomics.
   d. RACE.

10. One principle of good body mechanics is to
    a. bend from the waist when lifting.
    b. keep your feet close together when lifting.
    c. use the strong muscles of your legs for lifting.
    d. keep the load as far from your body as possible.

11. Material Safety Data Sheets (MSDS) are required to include information that
    a. describes how to repackage the product.
    b. explains first aid measures to use if exposure occurs.
    c. describes how to use the product.
    d. lists other approved uses of the product.

12. When dealing with a potentially violent individual, the nursing assistant should
    a. speak loudly and clearly.
    b. maintain a distance of 2 feet.
    c. listen to what the person is saying.
    d. attempt to touch the person gently.

B. Completion.

Choose the correct word from the following list to complete each statement in questions 13–20.

body mechanics	mechanical lift
call light	Material Safety Data Sheets
ergonomics	(MSDS)
hips and knees	OSHA
incident	RACE

13. Using your body correctly while you are working is called _____.

14. Basic rules for lifting include bending from the _____ and not from the waist.

15. An unexpected situation that can cause harm to an employee, a patient, or a visitor is called (a, an) _____.

16. Adapting the environment and using techniques and equipment to prevent body injury is called _____.

17. You should use a _____ when you need to transfer very heavy or dependent patients.

18. All patients must have access to a _____ because it may be the only way they have to summon help.

19. All manufacturers must supply _____ with the hazardous products they sell.

20. The section of the federal government that oversees employee safety is called _____.

21. The acronym used to remember the sequence of critical actions in case of fire is _____.

C. True/False.

Mark the following true or false by circling T or F.

22. T F The bed should be left in the lowest horizontal position when the patient is sleeping.

23. T F Side rails are restraints in certain circumstances.

24. T F There should always be enough light to enable staff to work safely.

25. T F Noise and clutter are very disturbing to most people.

26. T F Needed repairs should be reported immediately.

27. T F The signal cord is the patient's way of letting the staff know that he is in need.

28. T F It is all right to play while at work as long as no one gets hurt.

29. T F You are responsible for knowing and practicing fire drill procedures.

30. T F In case of a fire, follow your own plan of action.

31. T F It is wise to use an elevator during a fire emergency.

D. Nursing Assistant Challenge.

Mary Hernandez is a new nursing assistant at Community Memorial Hospital. She has just completed her CNA course. Consider the information she needs to receive in orientation in order to be a safe and efficient worker.

32. What information does Mary need to learn about the facility to prevent fires and to follow correct procedures in the event of a fire?

33. Mary will need information on equipment she will be working with. What items of equipment is she likely to be using on her job?

34. Discuss everything Mary can do to prevent work-related injuries.

35. What chemicals is she likely to be using?

UNIT 15

Patient Safety and Positioning

OBJECTIVES

After completing this unit, you will be able to:
- Spell and define terms.
- Identify patients who are at risk for having incidents.
- List alternatives to the use of physical restraints.
- Describe the guidelines for the use of restraints.
- Demonstrate the correct application of restraints.
- Describe two measures for preventing accidental poisoning, thermal injuries, skin injuries, and choking.
- List the elements that are common to all procedures.
- Describe correct body alignment for the patient.

- List the purposes of repositioning patients.
- Demonstrate these positions using the correct supportive devices: supine, semisupine, prone, semiprone, lateral, Fowler's, and orthopneic.
- Demonstrate the following procedures:
  - Procedure 14 Turning the Patient Toward You
  - Procedure 15 Turning the Patient Away from You
  - Procedure 16 Moving a Patient to the Head of the Bed
  - Procedure 17 Logrolling the Patient

VOCABULARY

Learn the meaning and the correct spelling of the following words and phrases:

ambulate	high Fowler's	physical restraint	Sims' position
aspiration	laceration	postural support	spasticity
body alignment	lateral	pressure ulcer	splint
chemical restraint	mobility	procedure	supine
contracture	90-90-90 position	prone	supportive device
draw sheet	orthopneic position	semi-Fowler's	transfer
enabler	orthotic devices	semiprone	trochanter roll
Fowler's position	(orthoses)	semisupine	turning (moving) sheet

PATIENT SAFETY

In Unit 14, you learned how to maintain a safe environment and how to avoid personal injuries. The prevention of patient injuries is another very important part of your job as a nursing assistant. Patients in health care facilities are at risk for incidents, because they may:

- Have impaired **mobility** (ability to move about) due to an injury, disease, or surgery

- Be receiving medications that affect mental status, balance, and coordination
- Be disoriented because of the change in environment or because of a medical disorder
- Have impaired hearing or impaired vision

Because of these risk factors, most incidents involving patients in any health care setting are falls. Falls may occur because the patient:

- Misjudges the distance from the bed to the floor
- Feels weak or dizzy when trying to get up
- Changes position too rapidly and loses balance when trying to stand up
- Encounters hazards when walking
- Is walking in a poorly lit area
- Is in denial about his or her ability and does not call for help

USE OF PHYSICAL RESTRAINTS

In the past, restraints were often used routinely as a preventive measure to avoid falls. Research has shown that side rails and restraints do not necessarily accomplish this purpose. In fact, many falls occur with side rails up and restraints intact. This can result in serious injury and even death. There are two types of restraints: physical restraints and chemical restraints. **Chemical restraints** are medications that affect the patient's mood and behavior. As a nursing assistant, you will be more concerned with the use of physical restraints. **Physical restraints** are defined as any technique or device that is attached or next to the patient's body that the patient cannot easily remove and that restricts freedom of movement and normal access to the body. OBRA (1987) clearly states when and how chemical and physical restraints may be used in a long-term care facility. The Residents' Rights state that "residents have the right to be free from physical and chemical restraints." According to this definition, many devices qualify as restraints if the patient does not have the physical or mental ability to remove the device readily. These guidelines have been implemented in acute care facilities as well. Physical restraints are to be used only when the safety of the patient or other persons is at risk. Before a restraint is used, the staff must:

- Document all patient behavior indicating the need for a restraint.
- Document all actions that were taken as an alternative to restraints.
- Consult with the patient and the family or legal guardian when alternatives are unsuccessful and obtain their approval and consent to apply a restraint (Figure 15-2).

GUIDELINES *for*

Preventing Patient Falls

- Always leave the bed in its lowest horizontal position when you have finished giving care.
- Keep brakes locked on bed wheels at all times except when the bed is being moved.
- Check to see whether the side rails are to be raised. Make sure they are attached securely.
- Check and adjust protruding objects such as bed wheels or gatch handles.
- Do not block or clutter open areas with supplies and equipment.
- Wipe up spills immediately.
- Encourage patients to use the rails along corridor walls when walking (Figure 15-1).
- Monitor patients for signs of weakness, fatigue, dizziness, and loss of balance.
- Monitor patients for safe practice if they independently:

  - propel their wheelchairs
  - **transfer** (get out of bed)
  - **ambulate** (walk)

- Provide adequate lighting.
- Eliminate noise and other distractions that may increase confusion and create anxiety.

- Avoid leaving patients alone in the tub or shower unless you are given specific permission to do so.
- Check patients' clothing for fit and safety. Loose shoes and laces, long robes, and slacks increase the risk of falling. Footwear should be appropriate for the floor surface. In general, this means using nonskid shoes on

FIGURE 15-1 Encourage patients to hold rails on corridor walls when walking.

continues

GUIDELINES *continued*

tile floor surfaces. For carpeted floors, consult the physical therapist if there is a question about appropriate footwear for the patient. Nonskid shoes may stick to the carpeting, causing falls. A leather or synthetic shoe sole may be more appropriate for a carpeted surface.

- Care for the patient's physical needs promptly. Many incidents occur when patients attempt to get out of bed to go to the bathroom.

- Always use the correct techniques for transferring and walking patients.

- Use a gait belt when assisting patients to transfer or ambulate.

- Follow the care plan when assisting patients with transfers and ambulation.

Examples of physical restraints include:

- Wrist/arm (Figure 15-3) and ankle/leg restraints
- Vests (Figure 15-4)
- Jackets (Figure 15-5)
- Hand mitts (Figure 15-6)
- Geriatric and cardiac chairs (Figure 15-7)
- Wheelchair safety belts, bars, and tables (Figure 15-8)

TABLE 15-1 COMPLICATIONS OF RESTRAINTS

Potential Physical Problems	Potential Psychosocial Problems
Decreased independence	Worsening of behavior problems
Pressure ulcers	
Weakness	Withdrawal, loss of social contact
Decreased range of motion	
Muscle wasting	Depression
Contractures (frozen, deformed joints)	Forgetfulness
	Fear
Loss of ability to ambulate	Anger
Edema of ankles, lower legs, feet, fingers	Shame
	Agitation
Decreased appetite, weight loss	Mental confusion
	Combativeness
Dehydration	Restlessness
Acute mental confusion	Sense of abandonment
Distended abdomen	Frustration
Urge to void frequently, dribbling	Loss of self-esteem
	Depression
Incontinence	Screaming, yelling, calling out
Urinary tract infection	
Constipation	
Fecal impaction	
Lethargy	
Shortness of breath	
Pneumonia	
Bruising, redness, cuts, skin tears	
Falls	
Impaired circulation	
Blood clots	
Choking	
Death	

- Bed rails (if they meet the definition of a restraint)

Restraints are medical devices. They should never be used as a form of punishment, or for the convenience of the nursing staff. Patients have been seriously injured and died as a result of restraint use, so restraint application must be considered very seriously and avoided whenever possible. Other potential complications of restraints are listed in Table 15-1.

Another important concern is restraint size. Manufacturers provide literature, teaching aids, and guidelines for restraint size, based on patient weight. The color of the trim on the vest, jacket, and poncho restraints is often a key to its size (see Table 15-2). Belts are usually one size fits all. A restraint that does not fit correctly will not hold the patient securely and increases the risk for injury.

Before restraints are used, the staff must assess the patient's capabilities and the reasons for use of the restraint. If the cause of the patient's problem can be identified and corrected, the need for a restraint may be eliminated. For example, if restraints are being considered to prevent falls, the patient's individual risk factors associated with falls are assessed. If some risk factors can be eliminated or modified, this reduces the risk of falls, and restraints may not be necessary. For example, an unsteady male patient gets up

TABLE 15-2 EXAMPLE COLOR CODES AND WEIGHTS

Size	Approximate Weight	Trim Color
Small	90 to 115 pounds	Red
Medium	115 to 145 pounds	Green
Large	145 to 185 pounds	Yellow
Extra Large	Over 185 pounds	Blue or gray

The guidelines are used for the restraints pictured in Figures 15-4 and 15-5. *Follow the manufacturer's directions for the device you are using.*

Physical Restraint Informed Consent

Patient's name _____

Method of physical restraint used _____

The reason the physical restraint is needed _____

_____

Times when restraint will be applied _____

Alternatives tried _____

In compliance with federal and state regulations, this facility is committed to limiting of the use of physical restraints only to situations necessary to maximize a patient's physical, mental, and psychological well-being. It is the policy of this facility that, if physical restraints are deemed necessary, the least restrictive method will be applied for the shortest amount of time possible.

Physical restraints will be used by this facility only when it has been determined that they are required to treat a patient's medical symptoms or a therapeutic intervention, as ordered by a physician, and based on (1) a documented assessment, by an appropriate health professional, of the patient's capabilities; the physical condition or mental treatment that requires the use of physical restraints; the less restrictive measures or therapeutic interventions that have proved ineffective; and the specific physical restraint most effective for the patient's condition; and (2) demonstration by the care planning process that using a physical restraint as a therapeutic intervention will promote the care and services necessary for the patient to attain or maintain the highest practicable physical, mental, or psychosocial well-being.

This patient has been assessed regarding his or her need for appropriate physical restraint. He or she will be reassessed at least quarterly or as his or her needs change throughout the stay at this facility. A report will be made each quarter as to the effectiveness of the physical restraint in maximizing the patient's physical, mental, or psychosocial well-being. Ongoing assessments help to further this goal. The duration of consent for the use of this physical restraint is good only until the next annual assessment of the patient's needs, or if there is a need for more restrictive physical restraints. At those times, a new informed consent will be required.

The benefits of physical restraints include the prevention of injuries to oneself or to others, enhancement of functional abilities, reduced potential for falling, and continued provision of medically necessary procedures. Potential complications associated with physical restraints include incontinence, decreased range of motion, decreased ability to ambulate, symptoms of withdrawal or depression, or reduced social contact. This facility will monitor the use of physical restraints daily and respond to any developing complications to physical restraint use.

By virtue of my signature, I state that I received, read, and had an opportunity to discuss any questions I may have regarding the application of physical restraints in this facility. I give consent for the use of physical restraints when the benefits outweigh the identified risks in accordance with this informed consent. I understand that I can revoke consent for this physical restraint at any time. I further consent to physical restraint reduction as soon as feasible.

_____

(Signature of Patient or Authorized Individual)   (Date)

_____

(Signature of Witness)   (Date)

[   ] Patient unable to sign.

FIGURE 15-2 Most facilities obtain written consent from the patient or responsible party before applying a restraint.

FIGURE 15-3 Wrist restraints may be used to prevent the patient from pulling on IVs and other tubes. (Courtesy of J.T. Posey Co., Inc., Arcadia, CA)

FIGURE 15-4 Vest restraints must be applied as pictured here, with the straps crossed over in front of the patient. Look closely at the strap placement, which is the key to keeping the hips down. The straps are threaded between the seat and the armrests, not through the armrests. (Courtesy of J.T. Posey Co., Inc., Arcadia, CA)

FIGURE 15-5 A jacket restraint has sleeves, whereas a vest does not. However, the straps for both restraints are tied in exactly the same manner. Note the position of the straps. They are threaded through the seat and the armrests, then go around the outside of the side posts. Once the straps are threaded through to the back of the chair, you may loop one strap over the other in the center, if desired. This makes it a little more secure. Then tie each strap in a slip knot on the kickspur on the opposite side. (Courtesy of J.T. Posey Co., Inc., Arcadia, CA)

FIGURE 15-6 Hand mitts may be applied to keep the patient from injuring himself (such as by scratching) or pulling on tubes. (Courtesy of J.T. Posey Co., Inc., Arcadia, CA)

FIGURE 15-7 Geriatric chairs are restraints in some circumstances.

FIGURE 15-8 Most wheelchair safety belts are designed to go over the patient's lap, not around the waist. Check the manufacturer's information if you are unsure. This belt is applied over the lap, then threaded between the seat and armrest. Finish tying it exactly like the vest restraint. Once the straps are threaded through to the back of the chair, you may loop one strap over the other in the center, then tie each strap in a slip knot on the kickspur on the opposite side. (Courtesy of J.T. Posey Co., Inc., Arcadia, CA)

Safety ALERT

The vest is a very secure restraint used for patients at high risk of injury. It looks like a vest and crosses over in the front. Other similar restraints are pulled over the head. These are called by different names, such as *jacket* or *poncho*, but the principles of application are the same for all three devices. Years ago, health care providers were taught to cross the vest restraint over the patient's back. Some personnel still apply vests in this manner, but doing so is not safe. Crossing the vest in the back can cause choking and other serious injury. A vest restraint that fits properly, and is crossed in front according to manufacturer's directions, will safely and securely hold the patient. ■

Safety ALERT

The wheelchair is an important piece of equipment in all health care facilities. Patients come in many shapes and sizes. Because of this, wheelchairs come in many sizes, and various accessories are available to support the user's body and meet the user's medical needs. Attention to wheelchair size and patient positioning are important for patient comfort and safety. Restraints are sometimes used because the wheelchair does not fit the patient! Using a proper-fitting chair eliminates the need for restraints. You will find information about wheelchair size and safety in Unit 17. Always consider the type and size of the wheelchair you are using when determining whether to apply a restraint! ■

to use the bathroom at night, but does not call for help. His risk of falls can be modified by making sure a urinal is within reach and emptied regularly.

If a patient is a danger to himself or others, or requires emergency medical treatment, restraints may be appropriate. However, less restrictive alternatives to restraints must be considered first. Many alternative devices are available to use instead of restraints. If a restraint is determined to be the best approach, it is applied. However, an ongoing assessment of the factors creating the need for restraints is necessary, and personnel must work to reduce or eliminate the need for the restraint.

If restraints are indicated, the least restrictive restraint required to keep the patient safe should be selected. The restraint should be used as infrequently as possible. Using restraints requires careful assessment, planning, and monitoring. Studies have proven that it takes more time to care for patients in restraints than to care for patients who are not restrained. The physician must agree to the use of restraints and write an order before they can be used. The care plan will provide information about the type of restraint to use, the time the restraint is to be applied, and other special information and instructions.

Enablers. Enablers are devices that empower patients and assist them to function at their highest possible level. For example, a patient in a wheelchair is unable to sit up straight to feed herself, so she is fed by staff. If a supportive device is applied to correct her posture and allow her to feed herself, the device is an enabler. Devices used as enablers that maintain body position and alignment are commonly called **postural supports**. Used correctly, they give patients a higher degree of independence and enable them to perform tasks they were previously unable to do. In this case, using the restraint improves the patient's self-esteem.

The wheelchair lap tray (Figure 15-9) is a restraint alternative that is also used as an enabler. The tray is simple to use: it is attached to the back of the wheelchair with Velcro straps. Patients can lean on it, and its surface can hold personal items or reading and writing supplies. A tray may enable the patient to feed himself by moving the food closer so he can reach it. The tray also reminds the patient not to stand up. If the tray allows the patient to perform a task, it is an enabler. If it is used strictly to keep the patient in the chair, and he does not have the physical or mental ability to remove the tray, it is considered a restraint. If the tray can be removed by the patient, it is a restraint alternative.

FIGURE 15-9 The lap tray is an enabler if it improves function, permitting the patient to eat independently. This tray is lined with gripper, a nonslip surface, to hold the dishes in place. The tray is a restraint if it is used to keep the patient in the chair and he cannot remove it by himself. (Courtesy of Skil-Care Corporation, Yonkers, NY, (800) 431-2972)

Side Rails as Restraints. By definition, side rails are restraints. They can also be an enabler. Many facilities consider the use of three half-rails an enabler, and four rails a restraint. Many patients pull on rails to position and turn themselves in bed. Some patients feel more secure if the rails are up. Side rails must always be up for patients who are restrained in vests, belts, or extremity restraints in bed.

Serious injuries can occur if patients attempt to climb over side rails and fall. This is a common cause of hip fractures in confused elderly patients. Leaving the rails down may be a much safer alternative. Alarms are available that sound if the patient attempts to get up. If side rails are used, monitor the patient frequently.

When side rails are used, it is important to check the space between the rail and the mattress. Hospital beds are permanent pieces of equipment that are used for years. Mattresses wear out and are replaced. There have been cases of injury and death in which patients became trapped between the mattress and side rails because the replacement mattress was not the same size as the original. Patients at high risk for entrapment include those with conditions such as confusion, restlessness, lack of muscle control, or a combination of these factors. Make sure that the gap between the mattress and the side rail is not large enough to cause injury. Figures 15-10A and 15-10B show areas of potential entrapment.

Gaps between the mattress and bed frame or rails can be caused by movement or compression of the mattress due to patient weight, movement, or bed position. If you observe a gap that is wide enough to entrap a patient's head or body part, inform the nurse promptly. Another bed can be used or the mattress modified (Figure 15-11A) to prevent injury.

The nursing orders often specify the use of padded side rails for patients with seizure disorder and those who are taking high doses of blood-thinning medication. In addi-

tion, patients who are at risk for climbing through the side rails may also have orders for side rail padding. Bath blankets may be wrapped around the rails as a temporary measure, but these often worsen the patients' agitation because they cannot see through the bars. Leaving a space at the top of the padding for the patient to look through may be perceived by the patient as like being in jail. Using a commercial side rail pad (Figure 15-11B) is the best solution to the problem, if they are available in your facility. The pad is thicker than a bath blanket, but the patient can look through the space.

Facilities and commercial manufacturers have developed many excellent alternatives to the use of side rails. Each patient's care plan or critical pathway will provide instructions regarding use of restraints, side rails, or alternative devices. Before applying restraints or raising the rails, ask yourself if the risks associated with their use presents less danger than other available options, including making the environment as safe and user-friendly as possible. Other possible alternatives to the use of side rails are:

- Keeping the bed in the lowest possible position with the wheels locked.
- Beds that can be raised and lowered close to the floor.
- Placing mats on the floor next to the bed, so that if a fall occurs, the patient will fall on a padded surface instead of the hard floor.

FIGURE 15-10B Seven additional zones of entrapment have been identified:

Zone 1: within the rail
Zone 2: between the top of the compressed mattress and the bottom of the rail, between the rail supports
Zone 3: between the rail and the mattress
Zone 4: between the top of the compressed mattress and the bottom of the rail, at the end of the rail
Zone 5: between the split bed rails
Zone 6: between the end of the rail and the side edge of the headboard or footboard
Zone 7: between the headboard or footboard and the mattress end
(Courtesy of U.S. Food & Drug Administration)

FIGURE 15-10A Entrapment between the mattress and side rails may occur: (1) through the bars of an individual side rail; (2) through the space between split side rails; (3) between the side rail and mattress; or (4) between the headboard or footboard, side rail, and mattress. (Courtesy of U.S. Food and Drug Administration)

FIGURE 15-11A The mattress can be modified to fit the bed and decrease the risk of injury. (Courtesy of Skil-Care Corporation, Yonkers, NY, (800) 431-2972)

FIGURE 15-11B Padded side rails are a good safety precaution for patients with seizure disorder, as well as patients who might climb through the rail to get out of bed. (Courtesy of Skil-Care Corporation, Yonkers, NY, (800) 431-2972)

FIGURE 15-12 Bed control bolsters are a good option to use in place of side rails. (Courtesy of Skil-Care Corporation, Yonkers, NY, (800) 431-2972)

- Anticipate reasons why the patient might get up, including need to use the bathroom, hunger, thirst, restlessness, and pain. Meet these needs promptly and provide calm interventions when you are in the room.
- Using side rail bolster cushions (Figure 15-12).
- Pressure-sensitive bed and chair alarms that sound when a patient attempts to get up (Figures 15-13A, 15-13B, 15-13C).

FIGURE 15-13A The pressure-sensitive pad is placed under the sheet. When the patient attempts to stand, an alarm sounds. (Courtesy of RN⁺ Systems, Boulder, CO)

FIGURE 15-13B This pressure-sensitive pad is placed under the sheet beneath the patient's shoulders. When he lifts his upper body off the pad, the alarm will sound. (Courtesy of RN⁺ Systems, Boulder, CO)

Signal Unit

Receiver

Sensor

FIGURE 15-13C The pressure-sensitive pad is placed under the sheet. The sensor box is placed in the room. When the patient removes pressure from the pad, a distinctive alarm sounds at the desk. The alarm does not sound in the room. (Courtesy of RN⁺ Systems, Boulder, CO)

- Some self-release belts sound an alarm immediately when the closure is released (Figure 15-13D), so staff have time to respond before the patient gets out of the chair.
- Some pressure-sensitive mats can be placed on the floor next to the bed to sound an alarm if the patient's feet touch the surface (Figure 15-13E).

FIGURE 15-13D This self-release belt is a restraint alternative because the patient can remove it. This type of belt is designed to sound an alarm when the patient begins to open the closure, providing time for staff to respond before the patient gets up. (Courtesy of Skil-Care Corporation, Yonkers, NY, (800) 431-2972)

FIGURE 15-13E This battery-operated mat can be placed on one or both sides of the bed. An alarm will sound as soon as the patient's foot touches the mat. (Courtesy of Skil-Care Corporation, Yonkers, NY, (800) 431-2972)

Each health care facility has policies addressing when side rails may be used. Know and follow your facility policies.

Applying Restraints in Bed

When applying wrist, vest, poncho, jacket, or belt restraints to a patient in bed:

- Center the patient's hips in the middle of the bed. This is where the bed bends when the head is elevated.
- Make sure the straps are not at an angle when extended over the edge of the mattress. If the straps are angled even slightly, they will loosen if the patient moves up or down in bed.
- Wrap the strap around the frame deck (the movable part of the frame that supports the mattress) once or twice (Figure 15-14A).
- Never wrap the strap around the lower frame, or the restraint will tighten and inhibit respiration when the head of the bed is elevated. Never tie the end of the strap to the outside of the frame. This enables the patient to reach down and untie it.
- Thread the strap through the bed springs at least 6 to 8 inches in from the side of the bed and 6 to 8 inches toward the head of the bed (Figure 15-14B).
- Loop the end of the strap around the spring (Figure 15-14C).

FIGURE 15-14 Tie the straps to the inner springs, where the patient cannot reach them. (A) Wrap the strap around the frame deck once or twice. (B) Thread the strap through the bed springs at least 6 to 8 inches in from the side of the bed and 6 to 8 inches toward the head of the bed. (C) Loop the end of the strap around the spring. (D) Loop the strap around itself again and tighten to form a slip knot. If the bed has a solid frame, a modification for fastening the straps and/or alternate instructions for fastening the straps are available from the restraint manufacturer.

- Loop the strap around itself again and tighten to form a slip knot (Figure 15-14D).
- Always raise the side rails when the patient is restrained in bed. Never fasten the straps to the side rails or loop or wrap the straps around the side rails.

Alternatives to the Use of Restraints

Alternatives to restraints should be tried before restraints are applied. Restraints are used only as a last resort in situations where the patient may harm himself or others. Nursing assistants can take a number of actions to help reduce the need to use restraints.

1. Care for patients' personal needs promptly.
   - Take patients to the bathroom regularly.
   - Provide adequate food and fluids to prevent hunger and thirst.
   - Report signs and symptoms of pain or illness promptly.
   - Follow all instructions for positioning and for assisting patients with exercise.
   - Be sure that patients have their eyeglasses and hearing aids if they need them.
   - Answer call signals promptly.
   - Check patients often to see if they need anything.
   - Provide appropriate exercise and activities.
2. Know which patients are at risk for falling. Monitor these patients regularly during your shift.
3. Observe patients who walk and transfer independently. Sometimes falls occur because patients use incorrect and unsafe methods. Report these situations and learn how to teach patients the correct way.
4. Report immediately any physical or mental change that could increase the risk of an incident, such as:
   - Disorientation (patient does not know time, place, or self)
   - Complaints of dizziness
   - Problems with balance and coordination
5. Maintain a safe, quiet, calm environment.
6. Provide comfortable chairs. Use supportive devices as necessary.
7. A number of security devices are available that are designed to prevent falls and eliminate the need for restraints. These devices include:
   - Special sensors attached to a patient's wrist, leg, or wheelchair. The sensor will set off an alarm if the patient tries to leave the unit or building.
   - Special sensors (a pad) placed in the patient's bed or chair that will set off an alarm if the patient attempts to rise.

Safety ALERT

When applying restraints to a patient in a chair, make sure the patient's hips are all the way back on the seat. Most restraints are designed to keep the hips down, so they must be applied in a manner that accomplishes this. The straps are usually inserted between the seat and the armrest. A common mistake is threading the straps through the armrest. Patients in wheelchairs frequently try to stand or slide their hips toward the front of the seat while restrained, causing injury. Threading the straps through the armrest places the restraint straps around the abdomen and fails to keep the hips down. If the patient attempts to stand or slides forward, the chair may tip, or another injury may occur. Attention to the manufacturer's directions for strap placement in the wheelchair is very important for preventing injuries. ■

Legal ALERT

The law is very clear regarding the use of restraints. It specifies that restraints must be applied according to manufacturers' directions. Each manufacturer determines the best way to apply its restraints. The directions for restraint application are sent to the government, which approves the instructions. There are many restraint manufacturers, so you must become familiar with the directions for applying the type of restraints used in your facility. You must also consider the size of the restraint. Restraints come in different sizes. Each manufacturer lists weight and size guidelines for its restraints. Some restraints are color-coded so you can tell the size at a glance. Using a restraint that does not fit the patient correctly is dangerous. Applying the correct size is very important. ■

Many commercial devices are available to use in place of restraints. Sometimes clothing or other items can be used as restraint alternatives. For example, a male patient who pulls at his urinary catheter can be fitted with boxer shorts. A patient with a feeding tube in the abdomen can

GUIDELINES *for*
The Use of Restraints

There are a few situations in which a patient may need a restraint, no matter how many alternatives are tried. When restraints are necessary, these guidelines must be followed:

1. A physician's order must be obtained by the nurse before restraints may be used. The order must indicate the type of restraint to use and the reason for its use. Try the least restrictive device first.

2. Use the right type and size of restraint. All restraints must be applied according to manufacturer's directions.

   Check the device before use—do not use if it is frayed, torn, has parts missing, or is soiled. Restraints are put on over clothing, never next to bare skin. When applying a restraint to a female patient, make sure the breasts are not under the strap to the restraint.

3. Even if the patient does not seem to understand, always explain what you are doing. After application, check the fit of the device. You should be able to slip the width of three fingers between the restraint and the patient's body. The device should never restrict breathing.

4. The straps should be positioned so the patient is unable to reach them. The restraint straps should be smooth. Avoid twisting. Pad the restraint if necessary to prevent irritation to the skin.

5. Tie restraint straps with slip knots for quick release in an emergency.

6. The patient should always have access to the signal light. Check every 15 minutes for the patient's comfort and safety. Make changes as needed.

7. When the patient is restrained in a wheelchair, the brakes should be locked when the chair is parked. The large part of the small front wheels of the chair should face forward. This changes the center of gravity of the chair, making the chair more stable and preventing tipping.

8. Release the restraint at least every 2 hours for at least 10 minutes to:
   - Check for irritation or poor circulation
   - Change the patient's position
   - Exercise—ambulate the patient or do passive range-of-motion exercises
   - Take the patient to the bathroom
   - Change incontinent patients and cleanse their skin
   - Provide fluid or nourishment
   - Attend to any other needs
     Document each of these actions.

9. Maintain good body alignment whether the patient is in bed or a chair.

10. When restraints are used in bed:
    - There must be full side rails on the bed, and they must be raised
    - The patient should always be positioned in the middle of the mattress
    - Always secure the restraint to the movable part of the bed frame

11. Do not use restraints in moving vehicles or on toilets unless you are sure the device is intended for that use by the manufacturer. (This does not apply to safety restraints that are part of the vehicle. Follow state laws.)

be covered with a T-shirt or abdominal binder. A patient with an intravenous infusion in the arm can wear a long-sleeved shirt. Covering the medical device may be all that is necessary to keep the patient from pulling on it. Previously, wrist restraints would have been used to keep the patient from dislodging tubes. Giving the patient something to hold, such as a Nerf ball, will occupy the hands and serve as a distraction.

Nursing Assistant Observations

The nursing assistant plays an important role in knowing the patients' needs and making recommendations for restraint alternatives. Making sure the patient is in touch with his or her environment reduces agitation and confusion. Simply ensuring that she can see or hear well may improve mental orientation. Other observations that will help eliminate the need for restraints are:

- Does the patient see and hear well? Does the patient normally wear glasses? Is she wearing them now? Are they clean? Does the hearing aid work? Are the patient's ears plugged with wax? Sometimes behavior problems, balance problems, and other safety concerns arise because the patient is out of touch with the environment. Applying these simple corrections may eliminate the need for a restraint.

- Is the patient able to make her needs known? Sometimes unsafe behavior is caused by an unmet need, such as hunger, thirst, or need to use the bathroom. Discovering the unmet need and meeting it may help you avoid using a restraint.
- Does noise or confusion in the environment cause the patient to become agitated? Noise can be caused by other patients or staff, the public address system, radios, or television. Eliminating or reducing the noise may stop the behavior.
- Does the behavior occur during a certain time of day, during a certain activity, or when a specific person is providing care?
- Does the patient seem uncomfortable? Physical pain, hunger, thirst, or need to use the bathroom can cause unsafe behavior.
- Does the patient seem lonely or isolated? Bored? Boredom, loneliness, or looking for a misplaced item can cause unsafe behavior.
- Does the patient try to get out of bed or chair without help? Is the patient steady on her feet? Does she normally use a cane or walker? Is she using it now? Is the call signal available, and does the patient know how to use it? Would the patient benefit from use of an alarm that sounds when she stands up? Would use of an alarm remind the patient to sit down, alert the staff, and eliminate the need for a restraint?

If you observe a condition that causes confusion or agitation, or discover an approach that is effective in eliminating or reducing the need for restraints, inform your nurse manager. Other common restraint alternatives are pictured in Figure 15-15 through Figure 15-21.

PREVENTION OF OTHER INCIDENTS

Many situations can result in an incident that may harm the patient. Incidents can be prevented when all staff members are aware of appropriate preventive measures.

Accidental Poisoning

Many common items, such as household chemicals, shaving lotion, plants, and cologne, are poisonous if ingested. Food kept in a bedside table may spoil and also cause illness. Patients who are disoriented may eat or drink any of these items. To prevent accidental poisonings:

- Keep all chemicals and cleaning solutions in locked cupboards.
- Store patients' personal food items in the refrigerator in dated labeled containers.

Thermal Injuries

Thermal injuries are those caused by heat or cold and result in burns. To prevent thermal injuries:

- Follow procedures accurately when administering warm or cold treatments.

FIGURE 15-15 The self-release belt serves as a reminder to call for help before rising. It is not a restraint if the patient has the physical and mental ability to release the Velcro fastener. (Courtesy of Skil-Care Corporation, Yonkers, NY, (800) 431-2972)

FIGURE 15-16 Some patients lean to the side, necessitating restraint to keep them upright in the chair. The lateral armrest supports and keeps the patient upright, making restraints unnecessary. (Courtesy of Skil-Care Corporation, Yonkers, NY, (800) 431-2972)

FIGURE 15-17 Some patients slide forward to the edge of the chair, and must be restrained to keep their hips back. The wedge cushion prevents sliding. A piece of gripper can be placed under or on top of the wedge for additional security. (Courtesy of Skil-Care Corporation, Yonkers, NY, (800) 431-2972)

FIGURE 15-18 The lap buddy is foam covered with vinyl. It is lightweight and comfortable and may be used in place of a heavier tray. It is a restraint if the patient cannot remove it. (Courtesy of Skil-Care Corporation, Yonkers, NY, (800) 431-2972)

FIGURE 15-19 Proper foot support is essential to good positioning. The feet and legs should never dangle. Unsupported legs are at increased risk for injuries and blood clots. The footrest elevator keeps the patient's legs from dangling and prevents sliding in the chair. (Courtesy of Skil-Care Corporation, Yonkers, NY, (800) 431-2972)

FIGURE 15-20 The geriatric chair can be used as a recliner for patient comfort. If the patient cannot stand, the chair is a restraint when in the reclining position. The tray is locked across the lap to prevent rising. It cannot be removed independently, so it is considered a restraint. (Courtesy of Hill-Rom® Long-Term Care Division)

FIGURE 15-21 The magnetic sensor bracelet is placed on the wrist of the patient's dominant hand. It enables cognitively impaired patients to wander freely within the unit. The door alarm will sound if the patient tries to exit. (©1996, RF Technologies. Used with permission)

- Check water temperatures before helping a patient into the bathtub or shower. Turn the hot water on last and turn it off first.
- Check food temperatures before feeding patients. Using a microwave oven to reheat food can be dangerous because of the uneven temperatures the oven produces.
- Store smoking materials in a safe place and supervise patients while they smoke. (Most health care facilities do not allow smoking by anyone.)

Skin Injuries

Skin injuries include **lacerations** (cuts or breaks in the skin) and punctures. To prevent these injuries:

- Store knives, scissors, razors, and tools in locked cupboards.
- Store syringes and needles in locked cupboards. These should not be recapped and must be disposed of in a sharps container immediately after use.
- Clean up broken glass immediately.

Choking

Aspiration is the accidental entry of food or a foreign object into the trachea (windpipe). This causes choking. Because swallowing becomes less efficient as people age, choking occurs more often in the elderly. Persons who are disoriented or who have impaired consciousness are also at risk. To prevent choking or aspiration:

1. Be aware of which patients have problems with swallowing. Follow all instructions when helping with feeding:
   - Cut food into small pieces.
   - Feed slowly.
   - Offer fluids carefully between solid foods.
   - If the patient has had a stroke, place the food in the unaffected side of the mouth.
   - Use thickeners for liquids if ordered.

Opening or Beginning Procedure Actions

2. Place patients upright in good body alignment before meals. Have them remain in this position for at least 30 minutes after eating.

3. At the end of the meal, give oral care to patients who are known to keep food in their mouths. Food may remain in the mouth for several minutes after a meal and be accidentally aspirated if the patient coughs or goes to sleep.

4. Know the procedure to clear an obstructed airway. (See Unit 52.)

INTRODUCTION TO PROCEDURES

Caring for patients safely means that you must faithfully and carefully carry out specific routines. The normal manner of carrying out a task is called a **procedure**. *Procedures* are the practices and processes used when following facility policies in patient care. The procedure prioritizes and orders your responsibilities when doing the task.

As you progress in your studies, you will learn the procedures for many nursing assistant tasks. You have already been introduced to the procedures for washing your hands and using PPE. The procedures that follow give you step-by-step directions for carrying out tasks that involve patients.

Certain things must be done before you begin patient care procedures. These actions are called preprocedure or initial procedure actions. At the end of each patient care procedure, you will carry out a standard series of ending procedure (procedure completion) actions.

COMMON STEPS IN ALL PROCEDURES

Certain steps are performed at the beginning and end of all nursing procedures. These are important and should not be omitted. Perform the steps in order, as appropriate to the patient and the procedure. This book calls these steps "initial procedure actions" and "ending procedure actions."

Initial Procedure Actions

Perform these steps, in order, at the beginning of every procedure.

Initial Procedure Action	Rationale
1. Wash your hands or use an alcohol-based hand cleaner.	Applies the principles of standard precautions. Prevents the spread of microbes and reduces the risk of cross-contamination.
2. Assemble supplies and equipment and bring to patient's room.	Improves efficiency, organizes your time, and ensures that you do not have to leave the room.
3. Knock on the door and identify yourself (Figure 15-22A).	Respects the patient's right to privacy. Informs the patient who is giving care.
4. Identify the patient according to facility policy (Figure 15-22B).	Ensures that you are caring for the correct patient.

FIGURE 15-22A If the door is closed or the privacy curtains are drawn, knock or speak before entering. Allow enough time for the patient to respond.

FIGURE 15-22B Identify the patient.

Initial Procedure Action	Rationale
5. Ask visitors to leave the room and advise where they may wait (as desired by patient).	Respects the patient's right to privacy. Shows respect and courtesy to visitors.
6. Explain what you are going to do and what is expected of the patient. Answer questions. (Maintain a dialogue with the patient during the procedure, and repeat explanations and instructions as needed.)	Informs the patient of what is going to be done and what to expect. Provides information about the procedure and shows respect.
7. Provide privacy by closing the door, privacy curtain, and window curtain (Figure 15-22C). (All three should be closed even if the patient is alone in the room.)	Respects the patient's right to privacy.
8. Wash your hands or use an alcohol-based hand cleaner.	Applies the principles of standard precautions. Prevents the spread of microbes and reduces the risk of cross-contamination.
9. Set up supplies and equipment at the bedside. (Use an overbed table, if possible, or other clean area. Cover with a clean underpad, according to nursing judgment, to provide a clean work surface.) Open packages. Position items for convenient reach. Position a container for soiled items so that you do not have to cross over clean items to access it.	Prepares for the procedure and helps organize time. Ensures that equipment and supplies are conveniently positioned and readily available. Reduces the risk of cross-contamination.
10. Wash your hands or use an alcohol-based hand cleaner.	Applies the principles of standard precautions. Prevents the spread of microbes and reduces the risk of cross-contamination.
11. Position the patient for the procedure. Support with pillows and props as needed. Place a clean underpad under the area, as needed. Make sure the patient is comfortable and able to maintain the position throughout the procedure.	Ensures that the patient is in the correct anatomic position for the procedure. Ensures that the patient is supported, comfortable, and can maintain the position for the duration of the procedure.
12. Cover the patient with a bath blanket and drape for modesty. Fold the bath blanket back to expose only the area on which you will be working.	Respects the patient's modesty and dignity. Ensures that the patient is warm and comfortable. (This step is essential even if the door, window, and cubicle curtains are closed.)
13. Raise the bed to a comfortable working height.	Prevents back strain and injury caused by bending at the waist.
14. Apply gloves if contact with blood, moist body fluids (except sweat), secretions, excretions, or nonintact skin is likely.	Applies the principles of standard precautions. Protects the worker and patient from transfer of pathogens.

FIGURE 15-22C Draw the curtains for privacy. If the bed is near a window, also close the window curtains.

Closing Procedure

Initial Procedure Action	Rationale
15. Apply a gown if your uniform will have substantial contact with linen or other articles contaminated with blood, moist body fluids (except sweat), secretions, or excretions.	Applies the principles of standard precautions. Protects your uniform and skin from contamination with bloodborne pathogens.
16. Apply a mask and eye protection if splashing of blood or moist body fluids is likely.	Applies the principles of standard precautions. Protects the worker's skin, mucous membranes, and uniform from accidental splashing of bloodborne pathogens.
17. Lower the side rail on the side where you will be working.	Provides an obstacle-free area in which to work.

Ending Procedure Actions

Perform these steps, in order, upon completion of each procedure.

Ending Procedure Action	Rationale
1. Remove gloves.	Prevents contamination of the patient, the environment, and clean supplies from used gloves.
2. Reposition the patient to ensure that he or she is comfortable and in good body alignment.	All body systems function better when the body is correctly aligned. The patient is more comfortable when the body is in good alignment.
3. Replace the bed covers, then remove any drapes used. Place used drapes in plastic bag to discard in trash or soiled linen.	Provides warmth and security. Contains linen and drapes that have been contaminated during the procedure.
4. Elevate the side rails, if used, before leaving the bedside.	Prevents contamination of the side rail from gloves. Ensures patient safety. Prevents falls, accidents, and injuries.
5. Remove other personal protective equipment, if worn, and discard in plastic bag or according to facility policy.	Prevents contamination of the patient, the environment, and clean supplies from used PPE.
6. Wash your hands or use an alcohol-based hand cleaner.	Applies the principles of standard precautions. Prevents the spread of microbes and reduces the risk of cross-contamination.
7. Return the bed to the lowest horizontal position.	Respects patient's right to a safe environment. Ensures patient safety. Prevents falls, accidents, and injuries.
8. Open the privacy and window curtains.	Privacy is no longer necessary unless preferred by the patient.
9. Position the call signal and needed personal items within reach (Figure 15-23A).	Prevents accidents and injuries. Gives the patient a sense of security by ensuring that help is available. Provides for patient convenience. Eliminates the need to call out or reach for needed personal items (which could result in a fall).
10. Wash your hands or use an alcohol-based hand cleaner.	Applies the principles of standard precautions. Prevents the spread of microbes and reduces the risk of cross-contamination. (Although the hands were washed previously, they have contacted the patient and other items in the room. Washing them again before leaving prevents potential transfer of microbes to other patients, equipment, and surfaces outside the patient's unit.)

Ending Procedure Action	Rationale
11. Remove procedural trash and contaminated linen when you leave the room. Discard in appropriate container or location, according to facility policy.	Applies the principles of standard precautions. Prevents the spread of microbes and reduces the risk of cross-contamination.
12. Inform visitors that they may return to the room (Figure 15-23B).	Shows respect, courtesy, and hospitality to visitors and patient.
13. Document the procedure, your observations, and the patient's response (Figure 15-23C).	Provides a legal record of ongoing progress and care. Provides a record of what has been done and observations of the patient's condition. Serves as a vehicle for communication for other members of the interdisciplinary team.

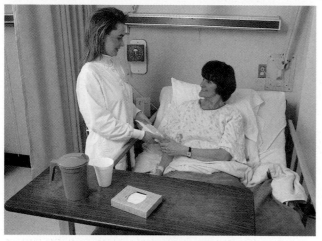

FIGURE 15-23A Lower the bed and place the signal cord within the patient's reach.

FIGURE 15-23B Let visitors know when they may reenter the room.

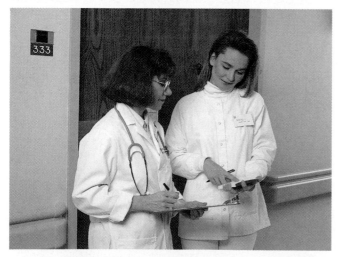

FIGURE 15-23C Report and document your actions and the patient's response.

Communication HIGHLIGHT

Communicate with the patient throughout the procedure. Whenever possible, use age-appropriate terms and explanations. Talk to the patient even if he or she is young, confused, may not understand, or cannot communicate verbally. Use gestures and body language to demonstrate, whenever possible. Continue to talk and smile throughout the procedure, regardless of the patient's age or level of understanding. This is important for the patient's well-being, and shows that you care. Remember that you also communicate with touch. Handle the patient gently to prevent injury and communicate caring. ■

So much handwashing may seem unnecessary, because of the short length of time that you are with the patient. Just remember that your hands can transmit germs. Patients already weakened by disease have a much lower resistance to germs.

Because the initial procedure and ending procedure actions are the same for each patient care procedure, they are not restated in this book as individual steps with each procedure. Rather, a general reference is made to these steps at the beginning and end of each procedure. You must, however, learn and faithfully complete each of these steps for each patient care procedure you perform.

BODY MECHANICS FOR THE PATIENT

Body mechanics for the patient are very similar to those for the health care team. Although the patient probably is not doing any lifting, good posture habits should not be neglected. Good posture for the patient means that moving in bed, getting out of bed, standing, and walking are done safely.

Bed patients sometimes find it hard to stay in a position; they tend to slide toward the foot of the bed when the head of the bed is elevated (Figure 15-24). Patients who are dependent are not able to change their position. These patients need extra help to gain and maintain proper alignment. Remember to:

- Get help
- Use turning or lifting sheets
- Change the patient's position frequently, at least every two hours
- Avoid creating friction by dragging the patient's heels across the sheets

Body Alignment and Positioning

Body alignment means a position in which the body can properly function. Patients who are weak, have impaired consciousness, are disoriented, or are in pain have problems keeping good alignment. Body alignment is maintained by moving, turning, and positioning the patient in a manner that:

FIGURE 15-24 Patients frequently slide down in bed, causing poor body alignment and increasing the risk for injuries to the skin caused by friction and shearing.

- Helps the patient feel more comfortable
- Relieves strain
- Helps the body function more efficiently
- Prevents complications like contractures and pressure ulcers

Complications of Incorrect Positioning

Complications can occur when body alignment is not maintained or when the patient's position is not changed often enough. The two most common complications are pressure ulcers and contractures. **Pressure ulcers** (bedsores) result when unrelieved pressure on a bony prominence interferes with blood flow to the area. Pressure ulcers are dangerous and expensive to treat. (These are discussed in Unit 39.) **Contractures** occur when a joint is allowed to remain in the same position for too long (Figure 15-25). The muscles stiffen and shorten (atrophy), preventing the joint from moving fully. The joint becomes fixed in a bent position (position of flexion). Contractures are painful, permanent, and can interfere with mobility.

Contractures can begin to develop within as little as four days of immobility and inactivity. After approximately 15 days, the patient loses the ability to move the joint freely. Contractures interfere with the patient's ability to move, complicate all nursing care, and interfere with proper positioning of the patient. Contractures promote the development of pressure ulcers and make treatment of existing pressure ulcers difficult. The contractures cause bony prominences to suffer reduced blood flow, increasing the risk for development of pressure ulcers. Contractures are a serious complication of immobility, making movement and activity painful and difficult. Voluntary movement of the contracted joint becomes impossible as the contracture worsens. Contractures can be prevented, and some can be reversed, with proper care. (Additional preventive measures for contractures are discussed in Unit 41.)

FIGURE 15-25 Contractures occur when joints are allowed to remain in the same position for too long.

Supportive Devices

Supportive devices are used to maintain proper body alignment and position in bed or in a chair. Supportive devices include:

- Pillows and/or folded sheets, bath blankets, or mattress pads to support the trunk and extremities.
- Splints and other specially designed **orthotic devices (orthoses)**. Orthoses restore or improve function and prevent deformity.
- Special boots or shoes that are worn in bed to keep the feet in alignment (Figure 15-26A).
- Bed cradles, which prevent pressure on the feet from the bed covers (Figure 15-26B).
- Footboards to maintain foot alignment.

FIGURE 15-26A Special boots will maintain the ankles and feet in good alignment. The boot prevents contractures of the feet and reduces friction and shearing of the skin upon movement. (Courtesy of Skil-Care Corporation, Yonkers, NY, (800) 431-2972)

FIGURE 15-26B The weight of the bedding pushes the toes downward, causing discomfort and increasing the risk for contractures. Patients with certain skin conditions also need to keep the bedding off the skin. Bed cradles prevent pressure and elevate the bedding so it does not contact the patient's body.

A folded pillow placed between the soles of the feet and the foot of the bed, or a pillow resting against the footboard (Figure 15-27), can take the place of a footboard alone. In some cases, a footboard may be harmful. For example, a footboard against the soles of the feet can stimulate **spasticity** (involuntary muscle contraction) in the legs and possibly cause skin breakdown from the rubbing of the feet against the footboard. Special shoes are sometimes worn in bed to maintain the feet in correct alignment. In most cases, ankle contractures can be avoided by doing passive range-of-motion exercises consistently (Unit 41).

Many other commercial products can be used as supportive devices. Remember that a supportive device is also a restraint if it is attached or next to the patient's body, if the patient cannot easily remove it, and if it restricts freedom of movement and normal access to the patient's body.

Basic Body Positions

There are four basic positions, with variations for each one. These are:

- **Prone** (on the abdomen), with a variation of **semiprone**
- **Supine** (on the back), with a variation of **semisupine**
- **Lateral** (on either side), with a variation of **Sims' position**
- **Fowler's position**, with variations of **high Fowler's**, **semi-Fowler's**, and **orthopneic position**

Changing a patient's position involves these steps:

1. Moving the patient into proper body alignment. You may need to move the patient up in bed or to one side of the bed. If the patient will be positioned on his left side, move him to the right side of the bed. If the patient will be positioned on his right side, move him to the left side of the bed. That way he will not be too close to the edge of the bed after he is turned.

2. Turning the patient onto the back, onto the abdomen, or to the side.

3. Placing the patient's trunk and extremities in proper position and maintaining alignment with the use of supportive devices.

FIGURE 15-27 Supporting the feet maintains good alignment and prevents contractures. (Courtesy of Skil-Care Corporation, Yonkers, NY, (800) 431-2972)

MOVING AND LIFTING PATIENTS

Lifting, moving, and transporting patients is a major responsibility of the nursing assistant. Using proper body mechanics and following safety rules will protect both you and your patients from injury. *Always* find out whether help is needed to lift or move a patient before proceeding with your assignment. Never be afraid to ask for help. By exercising caution, you are also preventing potentially serious injuries. Always check the care plan to see if there are special positioning instructions.

Safety ALERT

Using a lifting or turning sheet is better for the patient because it prevents injury to the skin. It prevents pain that sometimes occurs when you pull on the patient's body. It also reduces the risk of back injury in nursing assistants. When moving a patient on a sheet, make sure you have enough help. Two or three assistants may be necessary. Usually, two assistants are needed to reposition the patient's torso. A third may also be needed to prevent friction and shearing on the feet if the patient is being pulled up in bed. ■

OSHA ALERT

Your spine is one of the most important parts of your body, enabling you to maintain an upright position, move freely, stand, and walk. The vertebrae protect your spinal cord, a column of nerves connecting your brain with the rest of your body. Your organs would not function without it. Keeping your spine healthy is a vital concern for nursing assistants. Unfortunately, back injuries from improper lifting and moving are common in health care workers. Other contributing factors are rushing to get things done and not asking for help from others. Pay attention to your body and your position. Your back must last a lifetime. ■

A **turning sheet** or **draw sheet** (folded large sheet or half-sheet) may be placed under a heavy or helpless patient to make moving easier. The sheet must extend from above the shoulders to below the hips to be effective.

Procedures 14 to 17 should be followed when you are lifting or moving patients. As you practice these procedures, keep in mind the basic rules of good body mechanics that were discussed in Unit 14.

PROCEDURE

OBRA DVD

14

TURNING THE PATIENT TOWARD YOU

1. Carry out each initial procedure action.

2. Lower the side rail nearest to you. Cross the patient's far leg over the leg that is nearest to you.

3. Cross the far arm over the patient's chest. Bend the near arm at the elbow, bringing the hand toward the head of the bed.

4. Place your hand nearest the head of the bed on the patient's far shoulder. Place your other hand on the patient's hips on the far side. Brace your thighs against the side of the bed.

5. Roll the patient toward you (Figure 15-28A). Do it slowly, gently, and smoothly. Help the patient bring the upper leg toward you and bend it comfortably.

6. Put up the side rail. Be sure it is secure.

7. Go to the opposite side of the bed.

8. Place your hands under the patient's shoulders and then the hips. Pull toward the center of the bed (Figure 15-28B). This helps the patient maintain the side-lying position. Make sure the patient is not lying directly on the lower arm. The lower shoulder should be tipped slightly, so pressure is not centered directly over the joint.

9. Make sure the patient's body is properly aligned and safely positioned.

10. A pillow may be placed behind the patient's back. Secure it by pushing the near side under the patient to form a roll.

continues

PROCEDURE **14** CONTINUED

FIGURE 15-28A Place one hand on the patient's far shoulder and hip, then turn the patient toward you.

FIGURE 15-28B Move the patient to the center of the bed, keeping your back straight.

FIGURE 15-28C Place pillows to support the patient's body and maintain good alignment.

11. If the patient is unable to move independently, position the arms and legs. Support them with pillows between the shoulders, hands and knees, and ankles to prevent friction and contractures (Figure 15-28C). If the patient has an indwelling catheter, make sure the tubing is not between the legs, to prevent undue stress on the catheter and to prevent pressure ulcers.

12. Carry out each ending procedure action.

PROCEDURE

15

OBRA

TURNING THE PATIENT AWAY FROM YOU

1. Carry out each initial procedure action.

2. Lower the near side rail. Be sure the side rail on the opposite side of the bed is up and secure.

3. Have the patient bend his knees, if able. Cross the arms on the chest.

4. Place your arm nearest the head of the bed under the patient's head and shoulders. Place the other hand and forearm under the small of his back. Bend your body at the hips and knees. Keep your back straight. Pull the patient toward the edge of the bed.

5. Place your forearms under the patient's hips and pull them toward you.

6. Move the ankles and knees toward you by placing one hand under the ankles and one under the knees.

7. Cross the near leg over the other leg at the ankles.

8. Roll the patient slowly and carefully away from you (Figure 15-29) by placing one hand under the shoulder and one hand under the hips.

9. Place your hands under the head and shoulders. Draw them back toward the center of the bed.

continues

PROCEDURE **15** CONTINUED

FIGURE 15-29 Roll the patient away from you.

10. Move the hips to the center of the bed, as in step 5.

11. Place a pillow for support behind the back.

12. Make sure that the patient's body is in good position alignment. Support the upper leg with a pillow. Place the lower arm in a flexed position. Support the upper arm with a pillow.

13. Replace the side rail on near side of the bed. Return the bed to the lowest position.

14. Carry out each ending procedure action.

PROCEDURE **16**

MOVING A PATIENT TO THE HEAD OF THE BED

1. Carry out each initial procedure action.

2. Ask a coworker to assist from the opposite side of the bed.

3. Lock the wheels of the bed. Raise the bed to a comfortable horizontal working height. Lower side rails.

4. Lower the head of the bed if the patient can tolerate this position. Remove the pillow. Place it at the head of the bed, on its edge, for safety.

5. Lift top bedding and expose the draw sheet. Loosen both sides of the draw sheet.

6. Roll the draw sheet edges close to both sides of the patient's body (Figure 15-30).

7. Face the head of the bed. Grasp the draw sheet with the hand closest to the foot of the bed.

8. Position your feet 12 inches apart, with the foot that is farthest from the bed edge forward.

9. Place your free hand and arm under the neck and shoulders, cradling the head from both sides.

10. Bend your hips slightly.

11. Together, on a count of three, raise the patient's hips and back with the draw sheet, while supporting the head and shoulders. Move the patient smoothly toward the head of the bed.

12. Replace the pillow under the patient's head.

13. Tighten and tuck in the draw sheet. Adjust the top bedding.

14. Carry out each ending procedure action.

FIGURE 15-30 Using an overhand grasp, roll both edges of the turning (moving) sheet close to the patient's sides.

PROCEDURE

LOGROLLING THE PATIENT

Note: This procedure is performed when the patient's spinal column must be kept straight, such as following spinal surgery or spinal cord or vertebral column injury. It is a good procedure to use with any dependent patient.

1. Carry out each initial procedure action.

2. Get help from another nursing assistant.

3. Raise the bed to waist-high horizontal position. Lock the wheels.

4. Lower the side rail on the side opposite to which the patient will be turned. Both assistants should be on the same side of the bed.

5. One assistant places hands under the patient's head and shoulders. The second person places hands under the hips and legs. Then move the patient as a unit toward you.

6. Place a pillow lengthwise between the legs. Fold the patient's arm over the chest.

7. Raise the side rail. Check for security.

8. Go to the opposite side of the bed and lower the side rail.

9. Turning the patient to the side may be done by:

   a. Using a turning sheet that was previously placed under the patient.

   - Reach over the patient, grasping and rolling the turning sheet toward the patient (Figure 15-31A).

   - One nursing assistant should be positioned beside the patient to keep the shoulders and hips straight.

   - A second assistant should be positioned to keep the thighs and lower legs straight.

   b. If a turning sheet is not in position, the first assistant should position hands on the patient's far shoulder and hips.

   - Second assistant positions hands on the patient's far thigh and lower leg.

10. At a specified signal, roll the patient toward both assistants in a single movement, keeping the spine, head, and legs straight. If a turning sheet

is used, grasp the sheet and move the patient as a unit, onto her side (Figure 15-31B).

11. Place additional pillows behind the back to maintain the patient's position. A small pillow or folded bath blanket may be permitted under the patient's head and neck. Leave a pillow between the legs. Position small pillows or folded towels to support the arms.

12. Carry out each ending procedure action.

FIGURE 15-31A Roll the turning sheet against the patient.

FIGURE 15-31B Pulling together, turn the patient to the side in one smooth motion.

Positioning the Patient

After you have turned and moved the patient into proper body alignment, you can place pillows and other supportive devices to help the patient maintain the position. Directions are given here for the basic four positions and their variations.

Supine Position. (Figure 15-32A)

1. Start with the bed flat and the patient lying on the back. The patient's head should be about 2 to 3 inches from the head of the bed.
2. Place a pillow under the patient's head. It should extend about 2 inches below the patient's shoulders, with the head in the middle of the pillow.
3. Place a **trochanter roll** along the affected hip or along both hips if the patient has little control over the legs. A trochanter roll is devised by rolling a bath blanket into a shape about 12 inches long. The roll should be just long enough to reach from above the hip to above the knee (Figure 15-32B). The trochanter roll prevents external rotation (Figure 15-32C) of the hip.
4. Place pillows under the legs to reach from above the back of the knee to the ankle so that the ankles and heels do not rub on the sheets.
5. Lying flat on the back is very uncomfortable for some people. This is especially true for persons with low back pain. Elevating the knees with a foam bolster (Figure 15-32D) or one or more pillows will relieve pressure on the back and reduce discomfort.
6. If the care plan so indicates, position a footboard or place a folded pillow to support the patient's feet. The ankles should be at 90° angles.
7. Extend the patient's arms and place small pillows to reach from the elbow to below the wrist. The hand should be in alignment with the wrist and the palm should be down (Figure 15-32E).

Semisupine Position.

The semisupine position (Figure 15-33) is also called the *tilt position*. It should not be confused with the lateral position. The patient in this position is not lying directly on the side. When correctly used, semisupine position relieves pressure from the hip, sacrum, coccyx, and buttocks. The spine is straight and the patient is positioned so he is leaning against a pillow for support. Both legs are straight. The top leg is slightly behind the bottom leg. A pillow is placed under the top leg to keep it even with the hip joint. The lower shoulder is pulled slightly forward so that pressure is distributed over the back rather than the shoulder joint. The arms can be at the sides or folded across the abdomen. Begin the procedure with the patient in the supine position. It

FIGURE 15-32A Supine position

← 12" to 14" →
Partially rolled
trochanter roll

FIGURE 15-32B The trochanter roll should extend from the hip to just above the knee.

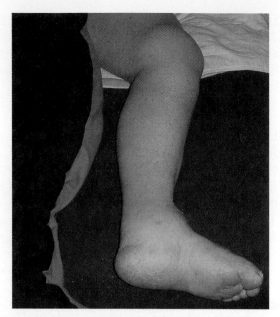

FIGURE 15-32C External rotation of the hip.

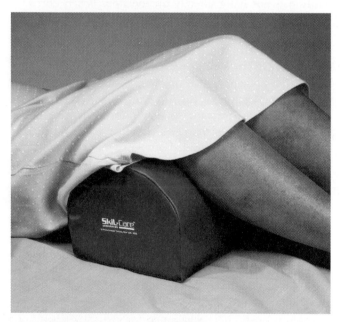

FIGURE 15-32D Supporting the knees relieves pressure and discomfort in the lower back. (Courtesy of Skil-Care Corporation, Yonkers, NY, (800) 431-2972)

will be easiest if you move him to the side of the bed that will be behind his back when you have finished positioning.

1. Turn the patient on the side, facing away from you. Leave about a 45° angle between the patient's back and the bed.
2. Position a pillow behind the patient's back. Push the patient slightly back against the pillow, then roll and tuck it under to support the back and relieve pressure on the arm or shoulder.
3. Pull the bottom shoulder slightly forward to prevent pressure on the joint.

FIGURE 15-32E Pillows support the wrist and arm in good alignment and are more comfortable for the patient.

4. Position another pillow under the patient's top leg, level with the hip joint.
5. Straighten both legs, positioning the top leg slightly behind the bottom leg and supported by a pillow.
6. Position the patient's upper arm in a position of comfort. The wrist may rest on a pillow or the abdomen, according to patient preference.

Prone Position. (Figure 15-34A) Start with the bed flat and the patient lying on the abdomen with the head turned to either side, spine straight and legs extended.

1. Place a small pillow under the head so that it extends to the patient's shoulders and 5 to 6 inches beyond the face.
2. Place a small pillow under the abdomen. This relieves pressure on the back and reduces pressure against a female patient's breasts. An alternate method is to roll a towel and place it under the shoulders.

FIGURE 15-33 The semisupine position is a variation of supine that is very comfortable and prevents pressure on the major pressure points.

FIGURE 15-34A Prone position

FIGURE 15-34B Position the arms in the way most comfortable for the patient.

FIGURE 15-34C The patient may be moved down in bed so that the feet hang over the end of the mattress.

3. Place a pillow under the arms to reach from the elbow to below the wrists. The shoulders and elbows may be flexed or extended, whichever is more comfortable for the patient (Figure 15-34B).

4. Place a pillow under the lower legs to prevent pressure on the toes. The patient may be moved down in bed before starting the procedure, so that the feet extend over the end of the mattress. This allows the foot to assume a normal standing position (Figure 15-34C).

Semiprone Position. The semiprone position (Figure 15-35) is the opposite of the semisupine position. It is usually a very comfortable position for the patient. Like the semisupine position, it eliminates pressure on the major areas at risk for pressure ulcer formation. Breathing is easier in this position than it is in the full prone position.

Begin the procedure by placing the patient prone. Lift the patient's chest and shoulder closest to you and place a pillow under them. The opposite arm is positioned behind the patient. A second pillow is folded in half and placed under the top leg. The legs and spine are straight. The

patient's head is turned to either side and a small pillow is used. Follow your facility policy for use of the semiprone position. Like the prone position, some facilities require a doctor's order, because lying on the abdomen may make breathing more difficult for some patients. When this position is used, check the patient every 15 minutes to be sure he can tolerate the position.

Sheepskin

FIGURE 15-35 The semiprone position is a very comfortable variation of the prone position.

1. Turn the patient into the prone position as described earlier.

2. Turn the patient's head to the side facing you, or according to patient preference.

3. Gently lift the patient's near shoulder. Position a pillow under the chest and shoulder, with the patient's arm resting on the pillow. Position the other arm behind (but not underneath) the patient.

4. Fold a second pillow in half and place it under the top leg.

5. Straighten and extend both legs for comfort.

6. Monitor the patient frequently for signs of respiratory distress.

Safety ALERT

The semiprone and semisupine positions may be a source of confusion for some health care workers. These positions are not the same as the lateral positions. Patients in semiprone and semisupine positions are tilted at an angle so that pressure is not applied to the bony prominences, whereas the lateral position places pressure on many vital areas. The semiprone and semisupine positions are very comfortable and relieve pressure from all major pressure points on the patient's body. ■

Right Lateral Position. (Figure 15-36) Reverse directions for left lateral position.

1. Start with the bed flat and the patient turned to the left side, with spine straight. Remember before turning to move the patient to the right side of the bed.

2. Place a pillow under the head so it extends 5 to 6 inches beyond the patient's face and down to the shoulders.

3. Position the right arm so the shoulder and elbow are flexed and the palm of the hand is facing up.

4. Place the left arm so it is extended or only slightly flexed and rest it on the hip or bring it forward and place it on a pillow. The patient's shoulder, elbow, and wrist should be at approximately the same height.

5. Place a pillow between the patient's legs, extending from above the knee to below the ankle. The patient's hip, knee, and ankle should be at approximately the same height.

6. A pillow may be placed behind the patient to help maintain the position.

Sims' Position. (Figure 15-37). This is a variation of the lateral position with the patient on the left side, left leg extended and right leg flexed. This position is often used for rectal examinations and treatments and enemas.

1. Place a pillow under the patient's head as for lateral position.

2. Start with the bed flat and the patient moved and turned onto the left side.

3. Extend the patient's left arm and position it behind the patient's back.

4. Flex the right arm and bring it forward. Support the arm with a pillow.

Fowler's Position. This position, or a variation of it, is used for feeding patients in bed, for certain treatments and procedures, for the patient's comfort while visiting or watching television, and for those who have trouble breathing. This position increases pressure on the buttocks and increases the risk of skin breakdown and pressure ulcers. Because of this, patients should not be left in Fowler's position for prolonged periods. Check the care plan for instructions.

1. Start with the patient on the back, in the middle of the bed and in good alignment. The patient's hips should be at the place where the bed bends when the bed head is rolled up. Place the head of the bed at 30° for semi-Fowler's (Figure 15-38A), 45° to 60° for Fowler's, and 90° for high Fowler's (Figure 15-38B).

2. Place one or two pillows behind the patient's head to extend 4 to 5 inches below the patient's shoulders.

3. Flex elbows and place a pillow under each arm to prevent pull on the shoulders.

4. Place a pillow under each leg to extend from above the knee and to the ankle, to prevent pressure on heels.

FIGURE 15-36 Right lateral position

FIGURE 15-37 Sims' position

FIGURE 15-38A Semi-Fowler's position

FIGURE 15-38B High Fowler's position

5. Place a footboard or folded pillow to keep the feet in position, if necessary.

Orthopneic Position. (Figure 15-39) This is a variation of high Fowler's position and is used for patients who have difficulty breathing. Like Fowler's position, the orthopneic position increases the risk of pressure ulcers. Special skin care may be necessary. Check the care plan or ask the nurse for further instructions.

1. The position of the bed remains the same as for high Fowler's.

2. Assist the patient to sit as upright as possible.

3. Have the patient lean slightly forward, supporting himself with the forearms. Placing the overbed table in front of the patient and extending the arms over it provides a good means of support and helps ease respirations. This makes the thorax larger, enabling the patient to inhale more air.

4. Place another pillow low behind the patient's back for support.

Sitting Position. Patients should be positioned in a comfortable, well-constructed chair, so that the head and spine are erect (Figure 15-40A). The back and buttocks should be up against the chair back. Stabilizing the patient's feet on the floor or wheelchair footrests is the first step in good positioning. Solid foot support also prevents forward sliding in the wheelchair. For good posture and even weight distribution, the feet should be at a 90° angle to the lower legs. The lower legs should be at a 90° angle to the thighs. The thighs should be at a 90° angle to the torso. This is called the **90-90-90 position** (Figure 15-40B).

FIGURE 15-40A Maintaining good body alignment is important when patients are sitting in chairs.

FIGURE 15-39
Orthopneic position

FIGURE 15-40B Remember the 90-90-90 position when positioning patients in chairs. The feet must be well supported at a 90° angle to the lower legs. The lower legs should be at a 90° angle to the thighs. The thighs should be at a 90° angle to the torso.

1. Pillows or postural supports may be needed to maintain the position.
2. A small pillow may be folded and placed at the small of the back to add comfort and support.
3. Do not permit the back of the patient's knees to rest against the chair.

FIGURE 15-41 Various orthoses are used to maintain good alignment and prevent contractures of the hand, wrist, and fingers.

GUIDELINES *for*

The Use of Splints

- The splint must be applied correctly. Follow the manufacturer's directions for each splint.
- Follow the care plan for the patient's wearing schedule.
- Keep the extremity under the splint clean and dry.
- If the splint becomes soiled, check with the nurse to see how it should be cleaned.
- Check the skin under the splint regularly for signs of redness, irritation, and skin breakdown.

Positioning Devices. Several types of devices, called orthoses, are used to maintain the position of an extremity. The correct use of these devices prevents contracture formation. Orthoses are also called **splints**. Figure 15-41 shows examples of orthoses for the upper extremities.

The physician may also order splints or orthoses for the lower extremities. A common type is called the *ankle foot orthosis (AFO)*. The AFO provides support for an unstable ankle and helps reduce extensor spasticity. The AFO is applied to the lower leg before the shoe is put on.

REVIEW

A. Multiple Choice.

Select the one best answer for each of the following.

1. Patients may be at risk for incidents because they
   a. ambulate in the hallway.
   b. use a wheelchair for long distances.
   c. keep one side rail up for turning independently when in bed.
   d. receive medications affecting balance, coordination, and mental status.

2. Patient falls can be prevented by
   a. encouraging patients to remain in bed.
   b. using restraints when the patient is up.

c. keeping the side rails up at all times.

d. meeting the patient's physical needs promptly.

3. Alternatives to restraints include

  a. taking patients to the bathroom regularly.

  b. giving medications to sedate the patient.

  c. playing music throughout the day to distract the patient.

  d. using side rails when in bed.

4. When restraints are used, they must be released

  a. every 2 hours.

  b. once each shift.

  c. every hour.

  d. every 4 hours.

5. When restraints are used on patients in bed,

  a. there must be full side rails on the bed, in the raised position.

  b. the bed should be elevated to the high position.

  c. the restraints should be secured to the stationary part of the bed frame.

  d. the electric bed adjustment switch should be removed to reduce the risk of injury.

6. Injuries caused by heat or cold are called

  a. lacerations.

  b. bruises.

  c. thermal injuries.

  d. aspiration.

7. Choking may be prevented by

  a. giving the patient only fluids.

  b. giving the patient finger foods.

  c. using thickeners for liquids.

  d. allowing only blended foods.

8. Initial procedure actions include

  a. handwashing.

  b. raising side rails.

  c. placing the call signal within reach.

  d. opening the door.

9. Correct body alignment will

  a. heal disease.

  b. prevent infection.

  c. help the body function more efficiently.

  d. be harmful in certain circumstances.

10. Examples of supportive devices include

  a. belts.

  b. pillows.

  c. side rails.

  d. vests.

11. Supine position is

  a. lying on the back.

  b. lying on the abdomen.

  c. lying on the side.

  d. sitting in the chair.

12. A position used for patients who have trouble breathing is

  a. orthopneic.

  b. semiprone.

  c. lateral.

  d. supine.

13. Logrolling is a procedure performed for

  a. persons who have had both legs amputated.

  b. ambulatory patients.

  c. all conscious patients.

  d. patients who have had spinal surgery or spinal cord injury.

14. A trochanter roll is used to

  a. maintain the hip in alignment.

  b. maintain the feet in alignment.

  c. support the patient's back.

  d. prevent contractures of the hand.

15. Splints may be used to

  a. maintain position of an extremity.

  b. provide support for a fractured femur.

  c. restrain the wrists.

  d. prevent pressure ulcers.

B. True/False.

Mark the following true or false by circling T or F.

16. T F Restraints are attached to the side rails for security.

17. T F Restraints may be needed for some patients.

18. T F A physician's order is not necessary before applying restraints.

19. T F The position of bed patients should be changed at least every 2 hours.

20. T F The left Sims' position is often used for rectal treatments and enemas.

21. T F When turning a patient toward you, cross the patient's near leg over the leg that is farthest from you.

22. T F You must wash your hands before beginning and after completing every nursing assistant task.

23. T F After patient care, the bed should be left in the highest horizontal position.

24. T F Turning sheets make moving heavy patients an easier task.

25. T F You should always explain what you plan to do even if the patient seems not to hear or understand.

C. Matching.

Complete the following by matching Column I with Column II.

Column I

26. _____ supine

27. _____ prone

28. _____ orthopneic

29. _____ trochanter roll

30. _____ splint

31. _____ contracture

32. _____ supportive devices

33. _____ physical restraints

Column II

a. prevents external rotation of hip

b. joint deformity caused by shortening of the muscles

c. devices used to maintain patient's position

d. device used to maintain position of an extremity

e. position for patients with difficult breathing

f. lying on the back

g. lying on the abdomen

h. devices that inhibit movement

D. Nursing Assistant Challenge.

Sara Abrams is 76 years old, has Parkinson's disease, and is a resident in a long-term care facility. She is ambulatory, with a shuffling walk, and has tremors of her hands related to the Parkinson's. She is disoriented and frequently walks into other patients' rooms.

34. Discuss safety issues related to Ms. Abrams's condition. _____

35. Which of the Residents' Rights may be a special issue in this situation? _____

36. What steps can you take to meet Ms. Abrams's physical needs? Will doing so lower her risk of falling? _____

37. How can you incorporate exercise into her daily routine? _____

38. What types of activities might interest Ms. Abrams? _____

39. Are there actions that can be taken to avoid restraints and falls? _____

UNIT 16

The Patient's Mobility: Transfer Skills

OBJECTIVES

After completing this unit, you will be able to:

- Spell and define terms.
- List at least seven factors to consider, before lifting or moving a patient, to determine whether additional equipment or assistance is necessary.
- Apply the principles of good body mechanics and ergonomics to moving and transferring patients.
- List the guidelines for safe transfers.
- Describe the difference between a standing transfer and a sitting transfer.
- Demonstrate correct application of a transfer belt.
- Demonstrate the following procedures:
  - Procedure 18 Applying a Transfer Belt
  - Procedure 19 Transferring the Patient from Bed to Chair—One Assistant
  - Procedure 20 Transferring the Patient from Bed to Chair—Two Assistants
  - Procedure 21 Sliding-Board Transfer from Bed to Wheelchair
  - Procedure 22 Transferring the Patient from Chair to Bed—One Assistant
  - Procedure 23 Transferring the Patient from Chair to Bed—Two Assistants
  - Procedure 24 Independent Transfer, Standby Assist
  - Procedure 25 Transferring the Patient from Bed to Stretcher
  - Procedure 26 Transferring the Patient from Stretcher to Bed
  - Procedure 27 Transferring the Patient with a Mechanical Lift
  - Procedure 28 Transferring the Patient onto and off the Toilet

VOCABULARY

Learn the meaning and the correct spelling of the following words and phrases:

contraindication	mechanical lift	partial weight-bearing	standing transfer
full weight-bearing	nonweight-bearing	pivot	transfer belt
gait belt	paralysis	sitting (lateral) transfer	weight-bearing
manual patient handling	paresis	sliding board	

INTRODUCTION

As a nursing assistant, you will work with many patients who have impaired mobility. In Unit 15 you learned how to move and position patients in bed. In this unit you will learn how to transfer patients (to move them from one place to another). Patients transfer:

- Out of bed into a chair and back to bed from the chair
- Out of bed onto a stretcher and back to bed from the stretcher

- Onto and off of a toilet
- Into and out of a car
- Into and out of a bathtub or shower

Refer to Procedures 19 through 28 later in this unit.

NURSING ASSISTANT SAFETY

Nursing work is always listed as one of the top 10 occupations for work-related musculoskeletal injuries. Having a previous history of back injury was identified as the biggest risk factor for either a new back injury or back pain. The rate of back injury in workers with a history of injury is about twice as high as the rate among workers with no history of back problems.

In 2005, the state of Texas passed the first state law requiring hospitals and long-term care facilities to implement safe patient handling and movement programs. Since then, several other states have passed or are working on passing laws that protect health care workers against injury from patient lifting. The American Nurses' Association (ANA) is working hard to get such legislation passed in all states.

Patient lifts and transfers are the tasks with the highest risk of injury. This is partly because workers often find themselves in awkward positions and confined spaces, and must bend or reach while the back is flexed. High-risk patient handling tasks vary by clinical setting. Other factors that increase the risk of injury are:

- Patient weight
- Transfer distance
- Confined workspace
- Lateral patient transfers
- Unpredictable patient behavior
- Stooping, bending, and reaching

need to remember

To reduce the risk of worker injury, facilities have implemented various programs, such as lift teams. These are specially trained personnel who do all patient moving in the facility. Some facilities have "no-lift" policies. This does not mean that workers should never lift a patient, heavy box, or equipment. Instead, this term usually means that no manual lifting should be done. Facilities with no-lift or "zero lift" policies usually depend on mechanical aids to reduce friction when moving patients. Some have a combination of mechanical, electrical, and ceiling-mounted lifts for moving patients vertically. Many require workers to use gait belts and mechanical aids for lifting and moving patients and heavy items. A no-lift policy is more of a pledge from management that equipment and/or personnel will be available to help with the task and reduce the risk of injury associated with manual patient handling. **Manual patient handling** is moving a patient by hand or bodily force, including pushing, pulling, carrying, holding, or supporting the patient or a patient's body part. When moving a patient from one surface to another:

- Use an assistive device whenever possible
- Know your limits
- Get assistance from another worker whenever possible

The procedures in this chapter are an overview of the basic methods for lifting, moving, and transferring patients. You must learn these before you can safely use a mechanical or friction-reducing device to assist with patient movement. Many new devices are available for lifting, moving, and repositioning patients to reduce the risk of worker injury. However, these vary widely from one facility to the next. You must adapt the procedures in this book to the policies, procedures, and equipment available in your facility for moving patients and protecting your back. When learning to use this equipment, your facility will teach you how to match the equipment and type of transfer to the patient's size and needs. Still, the basic procedures you will use are the ones in this book. In addition, practicing and using proper body mechanics is key to injury prevention. Before performing the procedures in this chapter, make sure you review and master the information on ergonomics, body mechanics, and safe patient handling in Unit 14. Also, OSHA and ANA have additional ergonomic and patient handling information to reduce the risk of injury.

Safety ALERT

Remember that having the right equipment is only one part of an ergonomics program. Using good body mechanics, reporting potential hazards, following facility policies and procedures, avoiding shortcuts, and using good judgment are all important to patient and nursing assistant safety. ■

TYPES OF TRANSFERS

There are basically two types of transfers. A **standing transfer** means the patient stands during the transfer with the help of one or two nursing assistants. A **sitting (lateral) transfer** means the patient sits throughout the transfer, such as when a sliding board is used (see Procedure 21). A **sliding board** is a plastic or wooden board about 2 feet long that has a slippery surface. It is used for a sitting, *lateral* transfer. A mechanical lift may also be used for sitting transfers, but this device is for *vertical* movement. The **mechanical lift** may be a manually operated hydraulic lift, an electrically (or battery) operated lift, or a ceiling-mounted lift. The mechanical lift is used to transfer dependent or heavy patients from one surface to another.

The nurse or the physical therapist determines which method is used to transfer a patient (Figure 16-1). It is important to follow instructions carefully to avoid injury. The method selected depends on:

FIGURE 16-1 The nurse or physical therapist determines the method of transfer, but you must also use good judgment, such as deciding that more help will be needed in the current situation.

• Absence of an extremity due to amputation
• Recent hip surgery

1. The patient's physical condition. This takes into consideration:
   • **Paralysis** (inability to move) of any extremity
   • **Paresis**, which is weakness of an extremity

2. The patient's strength, endurance, and balance. These abilities may be affected by:
   • Respiratory (lung) disease
   • Cardiac (heart) disease
   • Neurological disease, such as multiple sclerosis or a stroke
   • The ability to stand on one or both legs. This is called **weight-bearing**. For example, a patient may not be able to place full weight on a paralyzed leg. The physician may order the patient to be **non-weight-bearing** or only **partial weight-bearing** if the patient has had hip surgery. The ability to stand on both legs is called **full weight-bearing**. For a standing transfer, the patient must be able to stand and have at least partial weight-bearing on one leg.

3. The patient's mental condition. Can the patient understand and follow instructions?

GUIDELINES *for*
Safe Patient Transfers

Moving dependent patients can result in injury to you or the patient unless all safety measures are followed.

• Know the method of transfer that has been ordered by the nurse or physical therapist.
• Know the patient's capabilities.
• Use correct body mechanics.
• Place the bed in the lowest position before starting a standing transfer. Make sure the wheels on the bed and the transfer vehicle (wheelchair, stretcher) are locked before the move. It is helpful to elevate the head of the bed for bed-to-chair transfers.
• *Never allow patients to place their hands on your body during a transfer.* This is a dangerous practice. A patient who is disoriented or frightened can cause you to lose your balance. If this happens, the patient can pull you down, possibly injuring both of you.
• *Never place your hands under a patient's arms or shoulders.* This practice can cause severe shoulder injury to the patient.
• Use a transfer belt for standing transfers unless contraindicated.
• Make sure the patient is wearing shoes with sturdy, nonslip soles and that clothing is not too loose or dragging on the floor.

• Be aware of any tubes, orthoses, or other items that must be dealt with during the transfer.
• Transfer the patient toward the strongest side, if possible.
• Always explain to the patient what you are doing and how he can help.
• Test the patient's understanding and make sure she knows what you expect her to do during the transfer.
• Allow the patient to see the surface to which he is being transferred. Encourage the patient to keep his head up.
• Stand close to the patient during the transfer.
• If the patient has a weak or paralyzed leg, brace the knee of that leg with your knee or leg. If the patient has a paralyzed arm, be sure it is supported during the transfer to avoid dangling and pulling on the patient's shoulder.
• Give the patient only the assistance that she needs.
• Never have the patient use a footstool for transfers.
• During the transfer and when the wheelchair is parked, always position the large part of the small, front caster wheels facing forward and lock the brakes (Figure 16-2). Make sure the patient's legs are comfortably positioned on the footrests or the floor.

FIGURE 16-2 The large part of the small, front caster wheels must face forward during transfers and when the chair is parked. Changing the position of the front wheels changes the center of gravity of the chair and makes the chair more stable. Tipping is less likely when the large part of the wheels faces forward and the brakes are locked.

4. The patient's size. For example, transfer of a very tall or large person who cannot bear full weight would require two assistants or a mechanical lift.

Although the nurse or therapist selects the method of transfer, you will have to determine if you need another person or piece of equipment to assist you. When using the procedures in this chapter with the equipment available in your facility, key elements for you to consider first are:

- Patient's ability to assist with the procedure.
- Patient's ability to bear weight.
- Patient's upper-extremity strength, if a sliding board or certain other transfers are used.
- Patient's ability to cooperate and follow directions.
- Patient's size (height and weight) compared with your size; in general, if the patient is larger than you are, you will need help from another assistant or a mechanical device. Even if the patient is smaller than you are, you may need help if the patient is dependent or cannot cooperate.
- Special circumstances, such as presence of wounds, surgical sites, catheters, IVs, tubes, contractures, or other factors that restrict or interfere with mobility; always get help if there is danger of pulling on or displacing a tube during the transfer.
- Special physician orders or therapy recommendations for transfers and positioning, such as you would see for a patient who has had hip surgery.

Use the information in Figure 16-3 to help you to determine the safest method of making the transfer. You will

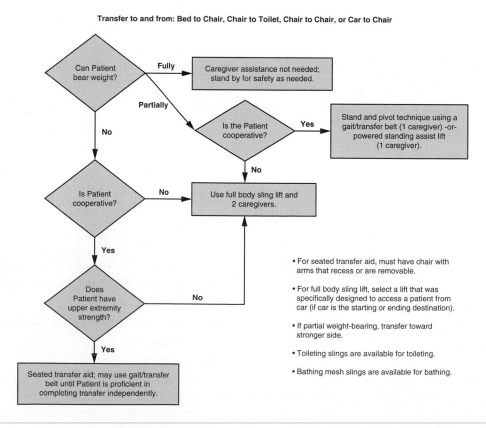

FIGURE 16-3 This algorithm helps you decide when extra help or a lifting device are needed during transfers onto a chair or toilet. Source: The Patient Safety Center of Inquiry (Tampa, FL), Veterans Health Administration & Department of Defense (October 2001).

find additional information in the online Appendix at the Online Companion for this textbook.

In some situations you may be instructed to take the patient's pulse before and after she gets out of bed. If the patient has been inactive for a long time, the heart muscle may be deconditioned. Checking the pulse when the patient is active provides an evaluation of the heart's condition.

TRANSFER BELTS

A **transfer belt** is a webbed belt $1^{1}/_{2}$ to 2 inches wide and about 54 to 60 inches long. It is an assistive and safety device used to transfer or ambulate patients who need help. (Refer to Procedure 18.) When it is used to assist a patient with ambulation, it is called a **gait belt**. Using a transfer belt avoids the need to grasp the patient around the ribcage or under the shoulders. Either of these methods can cause serious injury. It also allows you to have more control in directing the transfer. A transfer belt is not used to "lift" a patient. If the patient has no ability to bear weight, another method should be used for transfers.

Contraindications (situations in which something is not indicated, inappropriate, or potentially dangerous) for use of the transfer belt include:

- Abdominal, back, or rib injuries, fractures, or recent surgery
- Abdominal pacemakers

OSHA ALERT

Each year more than 12.8 million Americans consult their doctors about back problems. In fact, as many as 8 out of 10 individuals will suffer back pain during their lifetime. A transfer belt is an inexpensive item that helps protect you from injury and makes transfers safer and more secure for patients. Make the transfer belt a permanent part of your uniform. Wear it when you are on duty so it is readily available when needed to move a patient. ∎

- Advanced heart or lung disease
- Abdominal aneurysms
- Pregnancy
- Colostomy
- Gastrostomy tube or feeding tube

Medication pumps may be implanted under the skin of the abdomen in some patients. If the surgical site is well healed, it is probably safe to use the transfer belt. However, always follow the care plan or check with the nurse before using a transfer belt to move a patient with any type of implantable device.

PROCEDURE

18

APPLYING A TRANSFER BELT

1. Carry out initial procedure actions.

2. Assemble equipment:
   - Transfer belt

3. Explain the procedure. Tell the patient that the belt is a safety device that will be removed as soon as the transfer is completed.

4. Apply the belt over the patient's clothing (Figure 16-4A). If the patient is undressed and being transferred from wheelchair to tub or shower chair, either leave the patient's shirt on, put the patient's robe on, or place a towel around the patient's waist and then apply the belt over the towel.

5. If the patient is going to transfer from bed to chair, the belt may be applied after the patient comes to a sitting position on the edge of the bed. If the patient has inadequate balance, the belt can be applied while the patient is still lying down in bed. You may need to readjust the belt after the patient sits up.

6. Keep the belt at the patient's waist level. Avoid placing it too high. Make sure the belt is right side out and is not twisted.

7. Buckle the belt in front by threading the belt end through the teeth side of the buckle first and then through both openings (Figure 16-4B). The buckle must be in front.

8. Check female patients to be sure the breasts are not under the belt.

9. The belt should be snug, so that it does not slide up, but not tight (Figure 16-4C). Check the fit of the belt by placing three fingers under it. There should be just enough space for your fingers to fit comfortably.

continues

PROCEDURE 18 CONTINUED

FIGURE 16-4A Always apply the transfer belt over clothing.

FIGURE 16-4B Thread the belt through the teeth side of the buckle first.

FIGURE 16-4C The belt should be snug but not tight.

10. Before attempting to move the patient, be sure her feet are flat on the floor. If they are not, use the belt to assist the patient to the edge of the bed until her feet are resting firmly on the floor.

11. If you are transferring a patient into or out of a wheelchair, lock the brakes and keep the footrests out of the way during the transfer. After the patient is seated, her legs should not dangle. The feet are supported on the floor or on the wheelchair footrests.

12. Teach the patient to assist by pushing off the bed or arms of the chair with her hands when you count to three.

13. Use an underhand grasp when holding the belt. For transfers, one hand should be on each side of the buckle in front.

14. Do not overuse the belt by pulling the patient up with force.

15. When the patient is standing, **pivot** (turn the entire body as one unit) to transfer.

16. The chair should be close enough so the patient can feel it with her hands after you pivot.

17. Remove the belt after the patient is safely moved.

18. Carry out ending procedure actions.

PROCEDURE

19

TRANSFERRING THE PATIENT FROM BED TO CHAIR—ONE ASSISTANT

1. Carry out initial procedure actions.

2. Assemble equipment:
   - Transfer belt
   - Chair for patient

   - Bath blanket
   - Robe or clothing
   - Shoes and socks

continues

PROCEDURE 19 CONTINUED

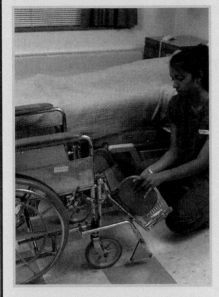

FIGURE 16-5A Lock the wheelchair and lift or remove the footrests before the patient transfers.

FIGURE 16-5B Instruct the patient to use her hands to push to the sitting position.

FIGURE 16-5C Place one arm under the patient's shoulders and one arm over and around the knees.

3. Place chair so the patient moves toward her strongest side. Set the chair parallel with the bed. Position the large part of the small front wheels facing forward. Lock the wheelchair and raise or remove the footrests (Figure 16-5A). Cover the chair with a bath blanket, unless the patient is fully clothed.

4. Lower the bed to the lowest horizontal position and lock the bed wheels.

These instructions are for getting out of the right side (patient's right side) of the bed.

5. Stand against the right side of the bed with the side rail down. Ask the patient to slide toward the right side of the bed.

6. Have the patient roll over onto her right side, flexing the knees and bending the right arm so it can be used for propping the upper body. Bend the elbow of the left arm so this hand can be used to push off from the bed.

7. Instruct the patient to use the elbow of her right arm to raise the upper body and to push with the hand of the right arm so she comes to an upright position (Figure 16-5B).

8. Instruct the patient to let her legs slide off the bed at the same time.

9. If assistance is needed, place one arm under the shoulders (not the neck) and one arm over and around the knees (Figure 16-5C). Raise the patient's upper body at the same time you move the legs off the bed.

10. Give the patient time to adjust to sitting up and then apply the transfer belt. Assist to put on shoes and socks. (If the patient has problems with balance, the shoes and socks can be put on while the patient is lying down in bed.)

11. If the patient has a weak or paralyzed arm, do not let it hang or dangle during the transfer. Put that hand in her pocket, or have her cradle that arm with her strong arm, or carefully tuck her weaker hand in the transfer belt or waist of the pants until she is again seated.

12. When the patient is ready to transfer:
   - Instruct her to move forward or closer to the edge of the mattress, to spread her knees, lean forward from the waist, and place her feet slightly back.
   - If one leg is weaker or should not bear weight, place this leg out in front with the strong leg slightly back.
   - Remember to spread your feet apart and bend your knees and hips, keeping your back straight.

continues

PROCEDURE **19** CONTINUED

- Hold the belt with an underhand grasp, one hand on each side of the front of the belt.
- If the patient has a weaker leg, press your knee against her knee, or block the patient's foot with yours to prevent the weaker leg from sliding out from under her.
- Tell the patient on the count of three to use her hands (if able) to press into the mattress, to straighten her elbows and knees, and to come to a standing position (Figure 16-5D).

13. If patient cannot walk, have her pivot around to the front of the chair until the chair is touching the backs of her legs.

14. Instruct the patient to place her hands on the arms of the chair (if able), to bend her knees, and to gently lower herself into the chair as you ease her downward (Figure 16-5E). Replace the footrests.

15. Position the patient comfortably. Place the signal light within easy reach.

16. Straighten the bed and prepare it for the patient's return.

17. Carry out ending procedure actions.

FIGURE 16-5D Tell the patient to straighten her elbows and knees to come to a standing position.

FIGURE 16-5E Tell the patient to bend her knees and lower herself into the chair.

PROCEDURE

TRANSFERRING THE PATIENT FROM BED TO CHAIR—TWO ASSISTANTS

Two people may be needed to transfer patients who are weak, disoriented, have limited weight-bearing ability, or are very large. Directions are given for transferring toward the patient's right side.

continues

PROCEDURE 20 CONTINUED

1. Follow steps 1 through 11 in Procedure 19.

2. The nursing assistants stand one on each side, facing the patient.

3. Each one places the hand closest to the patient through the belt, with an underhand grasp toward the front of the patient. The other hand of each assistant grasps the belt toward the back. Coordination of movement is necessary (Figure 16-6A).

4. The nursing assistant closest to the chair (on the patient's right side) stands in a position to step or pivot around smoothly to allow the patient access to the chair. This person stands with the left leg further back than the right leg.

5. The other nursing assistant uses the left knee to brace the patient's weaker left leg. This assistant's left leg is further back than the right leg.

6. Instruct the patient to bend forward and place the palms of the hands on the edge of the mattress to push off.

7. The patient's knees should be spread apart, with both feet back and the stronger foot slightly in back of the weaker foot.

8. The nursing assistants bend their knees and give a broad base of support.

9. On the count of three, the patient stands. Allow him to stand for a moment and bear weight. Tell him to keep the head up. Both nursing assistants help the patient pivot by slowly and smoothly pivoting their feet, legs, and hips to their left.

10. To sit, have the patient bend forward slightly, bend the knees, and lower onto the chair. At the same time, have him reach for the arms of the chair with both hands (Figure 16-6B).

11. Complete the procedure as described for a one-assistant transfer (Procedure 19).

FIGURE 16-6A Coordination of movement is necessary.

FIGURE 16-6B Instruct the patient to reach for the arms of the chair with both hands.

FIGURE 16-7 The sliding board is used when the wheelchair has removable arms and swing-away leg rests. Some fabrics tend to stick to the board. Make sure the patient is wearing pants that will slide across the board easily. (Photo courtesy of Briggs Corporation)

SLIDING-BOARD TRANSFERS

A sliding-board (Figure 16-7) transfer is used for patients with good upper body strength and sitting balance. This type of transfer is commonly used for patients with paraplegia, or weakness in both legs, such as those with post polio syndrome and other neuromuscular diseases. The procedure is performed by doing a series of push-ups. The patient locks the elbows and pushes with the hands. To transfer, the patient must be able to lift the buttocks off the bed. After lifting the buttocks, he or she lowers onto the sliding board, then lifts and slides until the transfer is complete. Some patients perform this transfer independently, whereas others need help. If you will be assisting, always use a transfer belt.

To use a sliding board for transfers, a wheelchair with removable armrests must be used. The chair must also have removable or swing-away leg rests. The patient must have clothing on the lower half of the body. Bare skin will stick to the board, creating friction and shearing and making the transfer very difficult or impossible. Blue jeans do not slide well on the board. Cotton or synthetic slacks are best. If the patient has difficulty sliding on the board, draping a pillowcase across the board may be helpful. (Do not encase the board in the pillowcase as you would a pillow.) If a wooden board is used, it can be waxed to maintain a slippery surface.

Two assistants can move dependent patients by using a sliding board. However, this transfers works best when the patient can understand and cooperate with your instructions. For a two-person transfer, one assistant stands in front of and the other behind the patient. At the count of three, both assistants hold the belt and slide the patient across the board.

PROCEDURE

SLIDING-BOARD TRANSFER FROM BED TO WHEELCHAIR

1. Carry out initial procedure actions.

2. Position the wheelchair parallel to the bed, or at a slight (about 35°) angle. Position the large part of the small front wheels facing forward. Lock the brakes.

3. Remove the arm of the wheelchair closest to the bed. Remove the leg rests or fold them back.

4. Apply a transfer belt. Check the fit with two or three fingers.

5. Assist the patient to move close to the edge of the bed.

6. Tell the patient to lean away from the wheelchair. Place the sliding board well under the buttocks, with the beveled side of the board facing up. Avoid pinching the patient's skin between the board and the bed.

7. Place the opposite end of the board well onto the seat of the wheelchair.

8. Instruct the patient to push up with the hands, lock the elbows, and move across the board. Repeat until the patient is seated in the chair with one buttock on the board. You will assist by

continues

PROCEDURE 21 CONTINUED

grasping the transfer belt with an underhand grasp and sliding laterally when the patient pushes down on the bed.

- The patient may push on the opposite armrest of the wheelchair with one hand when she has moved closely enough to reach it. This will help achieve greater height in the push-ups. The patient may also push on the board. Caution the patient to avoid placing the fingers under the edges of the board.

9. Be prepared to assist by lifting the patient's buttocks during the sitting push-up. If the patient is having trouble balancing, place your hands on the shoulders for support. Stop and allow the patient to balance before proceeding.

10. Support and move the patient's legs with your hands, if necessary.

11. Instruct the patient to lean away from the bed. Remove the board.

12. Remove the transfer belt.

13. Replace the arm of the wheelchair. Position the legs on the leg rests, or as instructed.

14. Assist the patient with positioning in good body alignment, as needed.

15. Perform ending procedure actions.

16. Reverse the procedure to return the patient to bed.

PROCEDURE

TRANSFERRING THE PATIENT FROM CHAIR TO BED—ONE ASSISTANT

1. Carry out initial procedure actions.
2. Assemble equipment:
   - Transfer belt
3. Place chair so the patient moves toward his strongest side. Set chair parallel with bed.
4. Move the bed to the lowest horizontal position and lock the wheels. Fanfold top covers to foot of bed if necessary and raise the opposite side rail.
5. Lock the wheelchair and raise or remove the footrests. Position the large part of the small, front caster wheels facing forward.
6. Have the patient place both feet flat on the floor.
7. Place the transfer belt around the patient's waist.
8. Instruct the patient to move forward in the chair, to bend forward, and to spread his knees apart. Both feet should be back, with the stronger foot slightly in back of the weaker foot. Both of the patient's hands should be on the arms of the chair (Figure 16-8).

FIGURE 16-8 Instruct the patient to assist by holding the arms of the chair with both hands.

continues

PROCEDURE 22 CONTINUED

9. Hold the transfer belt with an underhand grasp. Brace the patient's weaker leg with your knee or leg, as instructed in Procedure 19. Ask the patient to push off the chair on the count of three and to stand up as you provide the necessary assistance.

10. Allow the patient to remain standing for a time to stabilize position. Keep your grasp on the transfer belt and continue to brace the weak leg if necessary.

11. To complete the transfer, instruct the patient to step or pivot around to stand in front of the bed, facing away from it. Tell the patient to sit when the edge of the mattress is touching the back of

his legs. To sit, have the patient bend forward slightly, bend his knees, and lower himself onto the mattress.

12. When the patient is safely in bed, remove the transfer belt.

13. Remove the patient's slippers and robe. Assist the patient to lie down. Position the patient as necessary. Draw top bedding over the patient. Fold the bath blanket (if used) from the wheelchair and return it to the bedside stand. Make sure the signal light is within reach.

14. Move the wheelchair out of the way.

15. Carry out ending procedure actions.

PROCEDURE

TRANSFERRING THE PATIENT FROM CHAIR TO BED—TWO ASSISTANTS

The directions given here are for moving the patient toward his left side.

1. Follow instructions 1 through 8 in Procedure 22.

2. Each nursing assistant places the hand closest to the patient through the belt with an underhand grasp in front of the patient; the other hand goes toward the back.

3. The nursing assistant closest to the bed (on the patient's left side) stands in a position to step or pivot around smoothly to allow the patient access to the bed. This person stands with the right leg further back than the left leg.

4. The other nursing assistant uses the left knee to brace the patient's weaker right leg. This person's right leg is further back than the left one (Figure 16-9A).

5. Ask the patient to push off the chair on the count of three and to stand up as you provide the necessary assistance.

6. Allow the patient to remain standing for a time to stabilize position. Keep your hands on the

FIGURE 19–9A The nursing assistant uses the knee to support the patient's weaker right leg.

continues

PROCEDURE 23 CONTINUED

transfer belt and continue to brace the weak leg, if necessary.

7. To complete the transfer, instruct the patient to step or pivot around to stand in front of the bed, facing away from it. Tell the patient to sit when the edge of the mattress is touching the back of his legs. To sit, have the patient bend forward slightly, bend his knees, and lower himself onto the mattress (Figure 16-9B).

8. When the patient is safely in bed, remove the transfer belt.

9. Remove the patient's slippers and robe. Assist the patient to lie down and position as necessary. Raise side rails if ordered. Draw top bedding over the patient. Fold the bath blanket (if used) from the wheelchair and return it to the bedside stand. Make sure the signal light is within reach.

10. Move the wheelchair out of the way.

11. Carry out ending procedure actions.

FIGURE 16-9B Tell the patient to bend forward, bend the knees, and lower himself onto the mattress.

PROCEDURE

24

INDEPENDENT TRANSFER, STANDBY ASSIST

This method is appropriate for the patient who has good balance and strength and can understand instructions. Put a transfer belt on the patient the first time this is attempted.

1. Follow the instructions for getting the patient to a sitting position on the side of the bed. (See Procedure 19.) For an independent transfer, the patient should be able to do this without help.

2. Have the patient place the strongest foot slightly in back of the other foot. The patient's knees should be spread slightly apart.

3. Instruct the patient to place the palms of the hands at the edge of the bed and to lean slightly forward.

4. Tell the patient to press the hands into the bed to push off, at the same time the legs straighten, to assume a standing position.

5. Once standing, have the patient reach for the far arm of the chair and then step or pivot to stand in front of the chair. Instruct the patient to sit when the edge of the seat is felt against the back of the legs.

6. Carry out ending procedure actions.

Reverse these directions when transferring from chair to bed.

STRETCHER TRANSFERS

This procedure is used to move a patient from her room to another room for surgery, treatments, or diagnostic tests. The procedure may be very frightening to the patient. Assure the patient that the procedure is safe.

Note: Procedures 25 and 26 are for moving an unconscious or semiconscious patient. For alert, fully awake patients, two people may be able to perform this procedure with one person against the stretcher and the other person on the opposite side of the bed. Instruct the patient how to help you.

PROCEDURE   **OBRA**

25

TRANSFERRING THE PATIENT FROM BED TO STRETCHER

1. Carry out initial procedure actions.

2. Assemble equipment:
   - Stretcher
   - Bath blanket

3. You will need three to four people for transferring an unconscious or comatose patient from bed to stretcher.

4. Lock the wheels of the bed. Raise the bed to a horizontal position equal to the height of the stretcher. Lower the side rails.

5. Place a bath blanket over the patient and fanfold top covers to the foot of the bed, out of the way.

6. Roll the turning sheet up against the patient on both sides. The sheet should be long enough to support the patient's head and shoulders during the move.

7. Position the stretcher close to the bed. Lock stretcher wheels.

8. Two or three people stand along the open side of the stretcher. The other person stands on the open side of the bed. This assistant may need to get on the bed, on her knees, to avoid overstretching her back.

   Note: Use an overhand grasp on the moving sheet to avoid wrist strain. Using a friction-reducing sheet, roller, lifting pad (Figure 16-10A), or air-transfer device (Unit 31) will make this task much easier and reduce the risk of personal injury.

   - The assistant at the end of the bed grasps the moving sheet by placing one hand by the patient's legs and the other hand by the patient's hips.

FIGURE 16-10A The surface of the lifting pad slides readily and makes the transfer easier for the staff and more comfortable for the patient. (Courtesy of Skil-Care Corporation, Yonkers, NY, (800) 431-2972)

- The middle assistant grasps the moving sheet by placing one hand by the patient's hips and the other hand by the patient's shoulders.

- The assistant at the head of the bed grasps the turning sheet by the patient's shoulder and head.

- On the count of three, all persons slide the moving sheet from bed to stretcher (Figure 16-10B).

continues

PROCEDURE 25 CONTINUED

9. Center the patient on the stretcher in good body alignment. Secure the stretcher safety belt. Raise the side rails of the stretcher.

10. Transport the patient as directed.

11. Prepare the bed for the patient's return.

12. Carry out ending procedure actions.

Safety ALERT

Patients on stretchers are not left alone. ▪

FIGURE 16-10B All persons slide the lifting sheet from bed to stretcher.

PROCEDURE

26

OBRA

TRANSFERRING THE PATIENT FROM STRETCHER TO BED

1. Carry out initial procedure actions.

2. Assemble equipment:
   - Stretcher
   - Bath blanket (patient should already be covered with one on the stretcher)

3. You will need three or four people to transfer an unconscious or comatose patient from stretcher to bed.

4. Lock the wheels of the bed. Raise the bed to a horizontal position equal to the height of the stretcher. Lower the side rails. Fanfold top covers to the foot of the bed, out of the way.

5. Place a bath blanket over the patient, if necessary.

6. Roll the turning sheet up against the patient on both sides. The sheet should be long enough to support the patient's head and shoulders during the move.

7. Position the stretcher close to the bed. Lock the wheels and lower the side rails.

8. One person stands along the open side of the stretcher. The other two or three people stand on the open side of the bed. These assistants may need to get on the bed, on their knees, to avoid overstretching their backs.

Note: Use an overhand grasp on the moving sheet to avoid wrist strain. Using a friction-reducing sheet, roller, lifting pad, or air-transfer device will make this task much easier and reduce the risk of personal injury.

- The assistant at the end of the bed grasps the moving sheet by placing one hand by the patient's legs and the other hand by the patient's hips.

continues

PROCEDURE 26 CONTINUED

- The middle assistant grasps the moving sheet by placing one hand by the patient's hips and the other hand by the patient's shoulders.
- The assistant at the head of the bed grasps the turning sheet by the patient's shoulder and head.
- On the count of three, all persons slide the moving sheet from stretcher to bed (Figure 16-11).

9. Center the patient on the bed in good body alignment. Position the patient properly. Raise the side rails of the bed if ordered.

10. Carry out ending procedure actions.

FIGURE 16-11 All persons slide the lifting sheet from stretcher to bed.

MOVING THE PATIENT WITH A MECHANICAL LIFT

The mechanical lift is used for moving heavy patients who have little or no ability to assist. Using a mechanical lift for transfers is safer for both the patient and the nursing assistant. Various types of seats are available so the patient can be moved in the sitting or supine position. Some mechanical lifts may be used to weigh bedfast patients.

Safety ALERT

Some portable lifts are wheeled to the bedside. Some operate by using a ceiling-mounted hoist (Figure 16-12). However, the hydraulic lift is still in widespread use. The principles of use are the same for all lifts, and showing instructions for every lift available on the market is impossible. The principles of patient safety and movement given here for use of the hydraulic lift also apply to other lifts with a sling seat. Follow your facility policies and procedures for the lift you are using. Never use a mechanical lift until you have been instructed how to use it and are approved to use it independently. ∎

FIGURE 16-12 Some facilities permanently mount a ceiling hoist in certain rooms. These rooms are reserved for patients who are dependent for transfers, such as those with paralysis.

Several types of mechanical lifts are available. Some are manually operated, others are electric. The most commonly used lift is the hydraulic lift. It is used when a patient is heavy, unable to assist, unbalanced, or has an amputation or other condition that makes transfer with a belt difficult or impossible. For safety reasons, the manual hydraulic lift should be operated by two or more nursing assistants. Never attempt to operate it alone. Some electric and battery-operated lifts can safely be used by one person. Know and follow your facility policy for use of the mechanical lift.

PROCEDURE

27

TRANSFERRING THE PATIENT WITH A MECHANICAL LIFT

This procedure is used for heavy patients who have little or no weight-bearing ability.

> **Note:** Check slings, chains, and straps for frayed areas or clasps that do not close properly. Check the hydraulic lift and the leg spreader to make sure they are both working. Do not use if there is oil on the floor or if equipment is defective. Report need for repair and obtain safe equipment.

1. Carry out initial procedure actions.

2. Assemble equipment:
   - Mechanical lift
   - Sling
   - Chair

3. Place a wheelchair or other chair parallel to the foot of the bed, facing the head. Lock the wheelchair.

4. Elevate the bed to a comfortable working height. Lock the bed wheels. Lower the nearest side rail. Roll the patient toward you.

5. Position the sling beneath the patient's body behind shoulder, thighs, and buttocks. Be sure the sling is smooth (Figure 16-13A).

6. Roll the patient back onto the sling and position properly (Figure 16-13B). If the sling has inserts for metal bars, insert them now.

7. Position the lift frame over the bed with base legs in the maximum open position, and lock the lift legs (Figure 16-13C).

FIGURE 16-13B Roll the patient back onto the sling.

FIGURE 16-13A Position the sling under the patient.

FIGURE 16-13C Position the lift frame over the bed.

continues

PROCEDURE 27 CONTINUED

8. Attach suspension straps or chains to the sling (Figure 16-13D). Check fasteners for security.

   Note: Be sure that the correct end of the strap or chain is hooked to the correct place on the sling. Always hook straps or chains from inside to outside so the open part of the hook faces away from the patient.

9. Position the patient's crossed arms inside the straps.

10. Secure straps or chains if necessary.

11. One assistant operates the lift and the other assistant guides the movement of the patient. Lock the hydraulic mechanism, and slowly raise the boom of the lift until the patient is suspended over the bed. Talk to the patient while slowly lifting him free of the bed.

12. Guide the lift away from the bed.

13. Position the patient and lift over the chair or wheelchair (Figure 16-13E). Make sure that the wheels of the wheelchair are locked.

14. Slowly lower the patient into the chair or wheelchair. Pay attention to the position of the patient's feet and hands. One assistant stands behind the chair to pull and guide the patient's hips back into position.

15. Unhook the suspension straps or chains and remove the lift.

16. Position the footrests to support the feet.

   Note: Directions are reversed for moving patient from chair to bed. When raising the patient from the chair, monitor the position of the "S" hooks, which sometimes catch under the chair arms.

17. If the patient is in a chair, the sling can remain underneath the patient so it is in position for transfer back to bed. If the sling has metal bars, remove them and make sure the sling is smooth and wrinkle-free. Make sure the signal light is within reach.

18. If the patient has returned to bed, remove the sling. Pull top covers up and position the patient. Raise both side rails if necessary. Make sure the signal light is within reach.

   Note: The method for raising and lowering the lift and for moving the base legs varies for different types of equipment. Read the manufacturer's directions and practice using equipment before using it with patients.

19. Carry out ending procedure actions.

Safety ALERT

Two people should carry out these procedures to ensure patient and nursing assistant safety. ■

FIGURE 16-13D Attach the straps or chains to the sling.

FIGURE 16-13E Position the lift frame over the chair.

OSHA ALERT

Many health care facility bathrooms meet the OSHA criteria for confined spaces. Confined spaces cause health care workers to work in awkward positions and use forceful movements because the spaces are small, crowded, or have obstructions. Lifting and moving in a confined space increases your risk of injury. If you are in a confined space, you may need to use a creative method of doing toilet transfers, such as using a ceiling-mounted lift or by transferring the patient to a commode chair or shower chair outside the bathroom, then wheeling the chair in and positioning it over the toilet. Two or more workers will probably be necessary for this procedure. ■

TOILET TRANSFERS

The bladder is emptied much more efficiently if patients can use the toilet or commode rather than a urinal or bedpan. To use the toilet, the patient must possess transfer skills. Unless the patient has full weight-bearing on both legs and good balance, a wall rail is needed for support while transferring. (Refer to Procedure 28.) Towel racks are not safe for this purpose. Male patients may find it easier and safer to sit rather than stand while urinating.

Safety ALERT

Many falls occur going to and from the bathroom, as well as in the bathroom. Assist patients with toileting regularly. Respond to call signals promptly. Do not leave the patient alone if you think doing so is unsafe. ■

PROCEDURE

28

OBRA

TRANSFERRING THE PATIENT ONTO AND OFF THE TOILET

1. Carry out initial procedure actions.

2. Assemble equipment:
   - Toilet tissue
   - Transfer belt
   - Disposable gloves
   - Commode if toilet is not available

3. Position the wheelchair at a right angle to the toilet or commode to face the wall rail. Position the large part of the front caster wheels facing forward, and lock the wheels. Raise or remove footrests.

4. Place a transfer belt around the patient's waist. Use an underhand grasp with one hand toward the patient's back and the other hand toward the patient's front.

5. Tell the patient to lean forward slightly, to place the strongest foot slightly behind the other foot, to bring herself to a standing position by pushing off from the wheelchair, and to grasp the wall rail with both hands (Figure 16-14A).

6. Have the patient pivot or step around until she feels the toilet against the back of her legs.

7. Slide the pants and underwear down over the patient's knees. You may need to keep one hand in the transfer belt and use the other hand to manipulate the patient's clothing (Figure 16-14B).

8. Assist the patient to a sitting position on the toilet and allow her time to eliminate.

9. When the patient is finished, put on the disposable gloves. Instruct the patient to stand and to reach for the wall rail. Use the toilet tissue to clean the patient if she was unable to do this herself. If the patient is steady, remove and dispose of your gloves. Then pull the patient's pants or underwear up.

10. If the sink is close enough, the patient can pivot or step to the sink to wash her hands before sitting down in the wheelchair. Otherwise, unlock the wheelchair, replace the footrests, and move the wheelchair to the sink so this step can be completed while the patient is seated.

continues

PROCEDURE 28 CONTINUED

FIGURE 16-14A Tell the patient to grasp the wall rail with both hands.

FIGURE 16-14B Keep one hand on the transfer belt and adjust the patient's clothing.

11. Wash your hands.

12. Assist the patient to leave the bathroom. Make sure she is comfortable and has a signal light within reach.

13. Carry out ending procedure actions.

TUB TRANSFERS

In the institutional setting, a shower with chair or tub with hydraulic lift is available. If the patient is at home, a tub chair, rail on the wall beside the tub, and slip-proof mats in the tub are needed for safety. Add water to the tub after the patient has safely transferred, with cold water turned on first and off last. A hand-held shower attached to the faucet of the tub is safer and easier for self-bathing.

CAR TRANSFERS

You may need to assist a patient to transfer into a car when he is discharged from the facility. If you are working in the patient's home, you may need to help the patient into and out of the car. A two-door car makes the transfer easier because the door is wider and gives more room for moving in and out of the car. With either a two-door or four-door car, the patient should always transfer

Safety ALERT

Patient transfers into and out of personal vehicles are considered high-risk tasks, especially if the patient is very weak, confused, or acutely ill. Another concern is having to transfer a patient with one-sided weakness or paralysis toward the weaker side. (For most transfers, the stronger side is the leading side.) Make sure you have enough help and supplies, such as a transfer belt, friction-reducing sheet, or other special items, before transferring the patient. ■

onto the front seat. The front door is usually wider and opens wider.

REVIEW

A. Multiple Choice.

Select the one best answer for each of the following.

1. The method used for transferring a patient depends on
   a. the availability of two nursing assistants.
   b. the patient's personal preference.
   c. the patient's size, strength, endurance, and balance.
   d. where the patient is going.

2. A transfer belt should never be used on patients who
   a. have a long-term medication pump.
   b. have a colostomy.
   c. can stand on their feet.
   d. have an IV or catheter.

3. During a transfer, the patient should never
   a. be allowed to help in the move.
   b. place his hands on your body.
   c. wear shoes.
   d. be allowed to stand.

4. When transferring a patient, you should never place your hands under a patient's arms because the
   a. patient may not want you to stand so close.
   b. patient cannot see where she is going.
   c. patient's joints are fragile.
   d. patient may be ticklish.

5. Using a manual mechanical lift requires that
   a. two or more persons do the procedure.
   b. the patient be able to assist in the move.
   c. the patient be mentally alert.
   d. the patient weigh at least 300 pounds.

B. True/False.

Mark the following true or false by circling T or F.

6. T F During a transfer, the patient should place his or her hands on the nursing assistant's shoulders.

7. T F A transfer belt should always be used for standing transfers unless contraindicated.

8. T F Always transfer toward the patient's strongest side.

9. T F During a transfer, the nursing assistant should place his or her hands around the patient's trunk.

10. T F During a transfer, always explain to the patient how he or she can help.

11. T F Towel bars are not safe to use as grab bars.

12. T F Before using a mechanical lift, always check the slings and straps for damaged areas.

13. T F One person can safely transfer an unconscious patient from a stretcher to a bed.

14. T F When transferring a patient from a bed to a stretcher, raise the bed to the same horizontal height as the stretcher.

15. T F The unconscious patient should be secured with a safety belt during stretcher transport.

C. Nursing Assistant Challenge.

You are assigned to Mrs. McNeely, who is scheduled for surgery. She is alert and able to follow your directions. You know that when she returns from surgery she will be semiconscious from the medications and anesthesia. Consider the differences in procedures when she goes to surgery and when she returns to her room.

16. What instructions will you give Mrs. McNeely when she transfers from her bed to the surgical stretcher? _____

17. What will you need to do to transfer her back to bed after the surgery? _____

UNIT 17

The Patient's Mobility: Ambulation

OBJECTIVES

After completing this unit, you will be able to:
- Spell and define terms.
- Describe the purpose of assistive devices used in ambulation.
- List safety measures for using assistive devices.
- Describe safety measures for using a wheelchair.
- Describe nursing assistant actions for:
  - Ambulating a patient using a gait belt.
  - Propelling a patient in a wheelchair.

- Positioning a patient in a wheelchair.
- Transporting a patient on a stretcher
- Demonstrate the following procedures:
  - Procedure 29 Assisting the Patient to Walk with a Cane and Three-Point Gait
  - Procedure 30 Assisting the Patient to Walk with a Walker and Three-Point Gait
  - Procedure 31 Assisting the Falling Patient

VOCABULARY

Learn the meaning and the correct spelling of the following words and phrases:

ambulate	**gait**	**orthopedic**
assistive device	**gait training**	**prosthesis**

AMBULATION

The term **ambulate** means to walk. Some patients may not be able to walk because of a disease or injury. Patients who cannot walk may be able to self-propel their wheelchairs to increase their independence.

The term **gait** refers to the way in which a person walks. Many disorders can affect a person's gait, such as:
- A stroke—one side of the body is paralyzed (hemiplegia).
- Multiple sclerosis—one or both legs are weakened and balance may be disturbed.

- Huntington's disease—the patient has involuntary movements that disturb balance.
- Parkinson's disease—the patient has stiffness, tremors, and slowness of movements, causing shuffling.
- Arthritis—the patient has pain and stiffness of joints.
- Amputation—the patient has a **prosthesis** (artificial limb).
- **Orthopedic**—the patient has injuries or disorders of the musculoskeletal system and related structures.

Evaluation for Ambulation

Before initiating an ambulation program, the nurse or physical therapist (Figure 17-1) will evaluate the patient's:

- Tolerance to movement in bed
- Ability to participate in active (as opposed to passive) exercise
- Ability to safely transfer with minimal assistance
- Ability to stand and bear weight
- Strength, endurance, and balance
- Mental state, to determine if the patient can follow directions
- Ability to walk alone (whether the assistance of a person or equipment is needed)

Normal Gait Pattern

There are two phases to a normal gait (walking). The leg is on the floor during the first phase and the leg is brought forward during the second phase. Walking begins with the ankle in *dorsiflexion* (toes pulled toward shin) and the heel striking the floor first (Figure 17-2), rolling onto the ball of the foot. The patient must be able to stand straight on this leg while bringing the other leg forward. The arms normally swing slightly during walking. Each arm moves in the same direction as the opposite leg. To walk safely, the patient must have adequate joint motion in the hips and knees and strength in the muscles of the hips, buttocks, and legs. The physical therapist may work with the patient on exercises to promote movement and strength before the patient starts walking.

Gait Training

The physical therapist may work with the patient on **gait training** (teaching the patient to walk). The therapist will teach the patient how to:

- Walk correctly
- Walk on different surfaces, such as linoleum floors, carpet, grass, gravel, etc.
- Go up and down stairs
- Get in and out of a chair
- Use an assistive device if one is ordered

The therapist also teaches the staff measures to assist the patient and special safety precautions to follow during nursing care, if needed.

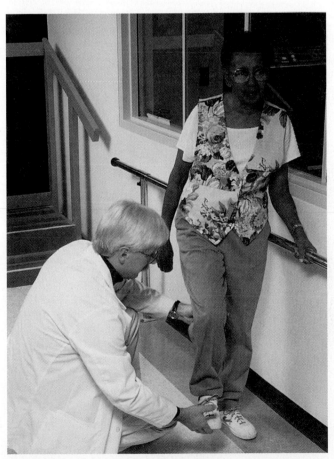

FIGURE 17-1 The physical therapist evaluates the patient's ability to ambulate and need for assistive devices.

FIGURE 17-2 Walking begins with the ankle in dorsiflexion and the heel striking the floor first.

GUIDELINES *for*
Safe Ambulation

- Encourage independent patients to use the hand rail when walking.
- Always stand on the patient's affected side when walking with her.
- Always use a gait belt (transfer belt) if the patient needs assistance with ambulation. Grasp the belt in the back with an underhand grip (Figure 17-3). Place your other hand on the patient's shoulder if balance is unsteady.
- Make sure the patient is wearing sturdy shoes with nonslip soles and that laces are tied. Clothing should not be too loose or drag on the floor.
- Check floor for clutter or puddles that could cause a fall.
- If you are unsure of the patient's endurance or balance, ask another nursing assistant to follow behind you with the wheelchair. If the patient becomes weak, dizzy, or tired, she can sit in the wheelchair.
- Check rubber tips on bottoms of canes, crutches, and walkers, and also check the rubber handgrips. These should be replaced if the ridges are cracked, loose, or worn down. If the ridges are filled with debris, use alcohol and cotton swabs to clean them. Replace the handgrip if it is loose or cracked.
- Check screws, nuts, and bolts for tightness. Do not use any device that appears unsafe. Report the problem to the proper person.
- Practice good body mechanics for both yourself and the patient.
- Teach the patient to practice safety.
- Position your body so it moves with the patient's body. You should not interfere with the patient's movement. Match the patient's stride.
- Encourage the patient to stand upright and erect when walking.
- Encourage the patient to take large, even steps. Teach her to maintain a wide base of support. The

distance between the feet should be equal to the patient's shoulder width.
- Allow adequate time for ambulation. Avoid making the patient feel rushed.
- Allow the patient time to rest, if necessary.
- Provide only the amount of assistance needed.
- If the patient is not motivated, place a chair ahead of her. Tell the patient the goal is to walk to the chair.
- Stop ambulation immediately if the patient shows signs of illness, pain, extreme fatigue, shortness of breath, dizziness, sweating, or anxiety. Notify the nurse.
- Never leave the patient standing unattended. When you are through, leave the patient safely sitting in a chair.

FIGURE 17-3
Hold the gait belt in back, using an underhand grip.

ASSISTIVE DEVICES

An **assistive device** is often prescribed. These devices include:

- Crutches
- Canes
- Walkers

An assistive device can help compensate for problems the patient has with walking. A walker or crutches may be ordered if the patient has only partial weight-bearing on one leg. Canes are usually ordered for persons who have problems with balance. There are several types of crutches, canes, and walkers. Each device is selected according to the needs of the patient and the cause of the problem. The nurse or physical therapist will adjust the device to fit the patient. The gait used with the device is determined by the patient's abilities, the cause of the impairment, and the type of assistive device being used. The nurse or physical therapist will select the appropriate gait. You should know the gaits that have been chosen. When you walk with the patient, you can then help make sure the patient is using the device correctly.

Use of Crutches

Standard crutches (Figure 17-4) are seldom recommended for older adults. They can be cumbersome to handle and require considerable balance and two strong arms. Metal forearm crutches may be used by patients who have weakness of both legs. These crutches are also called Lofstrand crutches or Canadian crutches. The cuff of the crutch encloses the forearm so the patient can release that hand without dropping the crutch (Figure 17-5).

Forearm crutches with platforms permit weight-bearing on the forearms, providing stability. During use, the elbows are at a constant 90° angle to the shoulder (Figure

17-6). The patient may need assistance in attaching the arm straps of the platforms. If you care for patients who use crutches, you will be taught the gaits the patients are to use.

FIGURE 17-4 Standard crutches are usually not appropriate for elderly patients.

FIGURE 17-5 Forearm crutches can be released to free the hand without dropping the crutch.

FIGURE 17-6 Forearm crutches with platforms permit weight-bearing on the forearms to provide stability.

Use of Canes

Quad canes and tripod canes provide a wide base of support. Pyramid canes are four-pronged devices with a broad base, and are narrower at the top. Single-prong canes with T-handles or J-handles have straight handles with a handgrip and are easier to hold than half-circle handled canes. For proper fit, the elbow is flexed 30° when the hands are on the handgrip, and the patient's wrist is even with the hip joint. Canes are recommended for aiding balance rather than for providing support. (Refer to Procedure 29.) The cane is always held by the arm on the *strong* side of the body. The patient will be taught to use either a two-point gait or a three-point gait with a cane.

PROCEDURE

29

ASSISTING THE PATIENT TO WALK WITH A CANE AND THREE-POINT GAIT

1. Carry out initial procedure actions.

2. Assemble equipment:
   - Cane as ordered
   - Gait belt

3. Make sure the patient has on sturdy shoes with nonslip soles. Check clothing to be sure it does not hang down over shoes.

4. Place the bed in the lowest horizontal position with brakes locked. Assist the patient to sit on the edge of the bed. Place a gait belt on the patient and assist the patient to a standing position. Stand on the patient's affected side. Place your closest hand in the gait belt, using an underhand grip.

5. Instruct the patient to hold the cane on her stronger side, with the tip about 4 inches to the side of the stronger foot. Her weight should be distributed evenly between her feet and the cane (Figure 17-7A).

6. Tell the patient to shift her body weight to the strong leg and advance the cane about 4 inches so she is supporting her weight on the strong leg and the cane. Move the weak leg forward so it is even with the cane (Figure 17-7B).

7. The patient then shifts her weight to the weak leg and the cane, moving the strong leg forward, ahead of the cane. This pattern is repeated while the patient is walking.

FIGURE 17-7A The patient holds the cane on the strong side of the body. The patient's weight should be distributed evenly between her feet and the cane before she starts to walk.

continues

PROCEDURE **29** CONTINUED

8. Note the patient's endurance, balance, and strength while walking. Stop immediately if the patient has trouble and help her to the closest chair. Call the nurse.

9. Assist the patient to sit in the chair or to lie down in bed. Remove the gait belt. Store the cane in an appropriate area.

10. Document the distance the patient ambulated and her tolerance of the procedure.

11. Carry out ending procedure actions.

FIGURE 17-7B Three-point gait

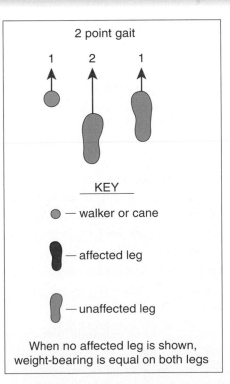

FIGURE 17-8
Two-point gait

Two-Point Gait with Cane. The steps for this procedure are as follows:

1. Follow steps 1 through 5 in Procedure 29.

2. Tell the patient to move the cane and weaker leg forward at the same time, while his weight is on the stronger leg (Figure 17-8).

3. He then shifts his weight to the weak leg and cane, and moves the stronger leg forward.

4. This pattern is repeated while the patient is walking.

5. Repeat steps 8 through 11 in Procedure 29.

Use of Walkers

Walkers also come in a variety of styles. Walkers are recommended for individuals who have general weakness of both legs, partial weight-bearing on one leg, or mild balance problems. The patient needs strength in both arms to pick up the walker. The walker should be wide enough to allow the patient to walk into it. For proper fit, the elbow is flexed 30° when the hands are on the handgrip, and the top of the walker reaches the hip joint. Most walkers are adjustable. The nurse or physical therapist will make any necessary changes. There are many additional features available from most manufacturers.

PROCEDURE

ASSISTING THE PATIENT TO WALK WITH A WALKER AND THREE-POINT GAIT

1. Carry out beginning procedure actions.

2. Assemble equipment:
    *   Walker as ordered
    *   Gait belt

3. Make sure the patient has on sturdy shoes with nonslip soles. Check clothing to be sure it does not hang down over shoes.

4. Place a gait belt on the patient and assist the patient to a standing position. Place the walker in front of the patient and have her grasp the walker with both hands. Stand on the patient's affected side. Place your closest hand in the gait belt, using an underhand grip (Figure 17-9).

    Note: The walker is not a transfer device and should not be used to help the patient stand up. The patient grasps the walker after she is standing. To sit, the patient releases her grip on the walker while still standing, and then places her hands on the arms of the chair before sitting.

5. Instruct the patient to stand with her weight evenly distributed between the walker and both legs, with the walker in front of her.

6. Have the patient shift her weight to the strong leg as she lifts and moves the walker 6 to 8 inches ahead. All four legs of the walker should strike the floor at the same time.

7. The patient then brings her weak foot forward into the walker.

8. Now have her bring her strong foot forward even with the weak foot.

9. This process is repeated while the patient is walking.

FIGURE 17-9 Stand on the patient's affected side while she grasps the walker with both hands.

10. Note the patient's endurance, balance, and strength while walking. Stop immediately if the patient has trouble and help her to the closest chair. Call the nurse.

continues

PROCEDURE 30 CONTINUED

11. Assist the patient to sit in the chair or to lie down in bed. Remove the gait belt. Store the walker in an appropriate area.

12. Document the distance the patient ambulated and her tolerance of the procedure.

13. Carry out ending procedure actions.

Two-Point Gait with Walker. The steps for this procedure are as follows:

1. Complete steps 1 through 5 in Procedure 30.
2. Have the patient shift his weight to the strong leg as he lifts and moves the walker and the weak leg 6 to 8 inches ahead.
3. Now have him shift his weight to the weaker leg and the walker (with most of the weight on the walker).
4. He then moves his strong leg 6 to 8 inches ahead.
5. This process is repeated while the patient is walking.
6. Note the patient's endurance, balance, and strength while walking. Stop immediately if the patient has trouble and help him to the closest chair. Call the nurse.
7. Assist the patient to sit in the chair or to lie down in bed. Remove the gait belt. Store the cane in an appropriate area.
8. Document the distance the patient ambulated and his tolerance of the procedure.
9. Carry out ending procedure actions.

THE FALLING PATIENT

If a patient starts to fall, you must protect both yourself and the patient. If the patient has started to fall, do not try to hold her upright. This will strain your back and

Safety ALERT

If you find a patient on the floor, remain in the room and call for help. Leave the patient on the floor. Provide any emergency measures that you are qualified to provide. If the nurse suspects a fracture, she will instruct you on how to return the patient to bed. Rolling the patient onto a sheet or blanket will make the transfer less traumatic. After emergency treatment and positioning on the sheet, the patient is lifted back to bed. ∎

Safety ALERT

Fall prevention is a major concern in health care facilities. Patients with a previous history of falls are always at higher risk than other patients. Other risk factors include advancing age, muscle weakness, gait and balance problems, neurological and musculoskeletal disorders, use of psychoactive medication, dementia, lower extremity disability or foot problems, and visual impairment. Environmental risk factors include slippery surfaces, uneven floors, loose rugs, poor lighting, unstable furniture, and objects on the floor.

Some elderly individuals have basic trust issues, particularly if the caregiver is young. They have their own way of doing things and believe they know best. The caregiver's way may be safest, but to gain cooperation, avoid telling the individual that he is wrong. Rather, try to incorporate the patient's method into a safer way of doing the task. ∎

may injure the patient. *If a patient does fall, call the nurse to assess the patient for injuries before she is moved.*

WHEELCHAIR MOBILITY

The wheelchair is an important piece of equipment in the health care facility. Many patients use wheelchairs for mobility. Some will progress to ambulation. Others will always use the wheelchair to move about. Whenever possible, the facility will restore the patient's ability to ambulate. Because patients spend so much time in wheelchairs, careful attention to fitting the chair to the patient is very important for comfort, pressure ulcer prevention, and restraint elimination. Sometimes wheelchairs are ordered or modified to meet special patient needs. For example, some patients with paralysis on one side of the body can

PROCEDURE

ASSISTING THE FALLING PATIENT

1. Keep your back straight, bend from the hips and knees, and maintain a broad base of support as you assist the falling patient. Maintain your grasp on the transfer belt.

2. Ease the patient to the floor, protecting her head.

3. As you ease the patient to the floor, bend your knees and go down with the patient (Figure 17-10).

4. Call for help.

5. Assist in returning the patient to bed or chair.

6. Carry out ending procedure actions.

FIGURE 17-10 Ease the falling patient to the floor; bend your knees and go down with the patient.

propel the wheelchair independently by using their strong arm on the wheel and pushing the strong leg on the floor. The leg rest is removed on this side.

The wheelchair is a mobility device, not a transportation device. Propelling the wheelchair independently is good exercise. It promotes communication, independence, confidence, and self-esteem. Wheelchair mobility provides opportunities for patients to make choices and decisions. They can decide where they will go, or what activities to attend. However, a facility emphasis on efficiency may create problems with wheelchair mobility. Pushing the chairs is faster for staff, but it deprives patients of much-needed exercise and independence. Some patients do not propel their wheelchairs because of physical problems, or because the chair does not fit correctly. However, adaptations may allow them to move independently. The therapy and restorative nursing departments will work with patients to fit the chair correctly and teach patients to move the wheelchair independently. Assist and encourage patients with independence whenever possible.

Wheelchair Size and Fit

A wheelchair should fit the person who is using it. Correct fit and body alignment (Figure 17-11) will prevent contractures and reduce the need for restraints, position-

ing aids, and body supports. A chair that fits correctly is also more comfortable, and reduces the risk of skin breakdown. If the chair fits correctly, there will be:

- About 4 inches between the top of the back upholstery and the patient's axillae (armpits).
- Armrests that support the arms without pushing the shoulders up or forcing them to hang.
- Two to three inches clearance between the front edge of the seat and the back of the patient's knee.

FIGURE 17-11 The wheelchair must fit the patient.

- Enough space between the patient's hip and the chair to slide your hand between the patient's hips on each side and the side of the wheelchair; the right amount of space avoids internal or external rotation of hips.
- Two inches between the bottom of the footrests and the floor.
- 90° angles between the feet and the legs, whether they are on the footrests or on the floor (when the footrests have been removed).

If the wheelchair does not fit the patient, check with the nurse or physical therapist to see how you can use pads or other devices to adapt the chair to the patient.

POSITIONING THE DEPENDENT PATIENT IN A WHEELCHAIR

The dependent person may slide down in the wheelchair, requiring assistance to regain body alignment. Several

Safety ALERT

There is no "one size fits all" wheelchair. Patients may have difficulty propelling a wheelchair that does not fit properly. A chair that does not fit correctly increases discomfort. Positioning problems are common. Patients may lean to the side, slide forward, or sit slumped in the chair. The risk of skin breakdown is increased. Positioning aids may be necessary. Sometimes unnecessary restraints are used to correct positioning problems. For many patients, a properly fit wheelchair solves the problem! If you suspect that the patient's problems are due to a wheelchair of the wrong size, inform the nurse. ■

GUIDELINES *for*
Wheelchair Safety

- Check the wheelchair to see that the brakes are working and wheels are securely attached. If the patient needs footrests, make sure they are in place. Replace the arm of wheelchair if it was removed during transfer.
- The small, front caster wheels of the chair provide the ability to move in all directions. The large part of the wheel faces back when the chair is moving. When the chair is parked, position the large part of the front wheel facing forward. This changes the center of gravity in the chair. Positioning the wheels to face forward prevents tipping if the patient leans forward. It helps stabilize the chair if the patient picks up an item from the floor. To reposition the wheels, back the chair up, then move it forward.
- The patient should be positioned in the 90-90-90 position, with the feet properly supported and the knees lower than the hips. Use pillows, props, adaptive devices, or restraint alternatives to ensure that the patient maintains an upright position.
- Apply brakes and lift footrests out of the way when the patient is getting in or out of the wheelchair.
- Instruct the patient not to try to pick up an object off the floor. If there is satisfactory trunk stability and balance, the patient may be taught to do so, but instruct the patient to:

  - avoid shifting weight in the direction of the reach
  - not move forward in the seat
  - not reach down between the knees

The safest method is to position the chair alongside the object with casters in forward position, lock the chair, and reach only as far as the arm will extend.

- Check the patient's body alignment while in the wheelchair and reposition the patient when necessary.
- Prevent bath blankets, lap robes, or clothing from getting caught in wheels.
- If the patient has a paralyzed arm, be sure is does not fall over the side of the wheelchair and become caught in the wheel.
- Guide the wheelchair from behind, grasping both handgrips (Figure 17-12).
- Approach corners slowly and look before you go around them.
- Take care when approaching swinging doors. Prop the door open to propel the chair through the door. If this is not possible, back through swinging doors.
- Back the wheelchair over the threshold in a doorway.

continues

GUIDELINES *continued*

- Always back into doorways and elevators when transporting a patient by wheelchair (Figure 17-13).
- When leaving an elevator, push the stop button and ask others to step out. Turn the wheelchair around and back it out the door.
- When transporting a patient in a wheelchair down a ramp or incline, walk backward, slowly pulling the chair. Periodically look over your shoulder, as you would when backing up in a car, to make sure that the path is clear.
- When parking a wheelchair, avoid blocking a doorway. Apply the brakes.

FIGURE 17-12 Guide the wheelchair from behind, grasping both hand grips.

FIGURE 17-13 Always back over the threshold when entering doorways and elevators.

procedures can be used to correct the dependent patient's position in the wheelchair. Lock the drive wheels and position the caster wheels in the forward position before repositioning the patient.

1. Stand in front of the patient; make sure that the feet are in alignment and the arms are on the armrests. Help the patient lean forward and push with the hands and legs as you push against the patient's knees (Figure 17-14).

2. For an alternate method, place a soft towel or small sheet under the patient's buttocks and use this as a pull sheet to move the patient up in the chair. This requires two people (Figure 17-15).

3. Another method involves using a manual lifting device, such as the TLC pad (Figure 17-16). The number of persons needed to lift is determined by patient size and the device you are using. One person can usually move an average-size patient by using the pad. Do not substitute a sheet for a manual lifting pad. The handles are necessary to coordinate the move and pull the patient safely. If the patient is uncooperative or heavy, two or more caregivers will be necessary. The TLC pad may also be used to turn a patient to the side or pull her up in bed. The pad is left in place when the patient is in a chair. Whether it is left in place when the patient is in bed is left to your discretion. The pad is soft and will not injure the skin, and the fabric is quite absorbent in the event of incontinence.

4. This method also requires two people. Place the transfer belt around the patient's waist. One assistant stands in back of the wheelchair and grasps the transfer belt with one hand on each side of the patient.

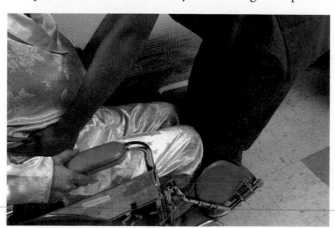

FIGURE 17-14 Push against the patient's knees as she pushes with her hands and legs.

FIGURE 17-15 A draw sheet or lifting pad may be used to correct the patient's body alignment.

FIGURE 17-16 One worker can move a small or average-size patient up in the geriatric chair by pulling the handles of the TLC pad up and out. If you are unsure about your ability to move the patient, always have help on standby. It is better to ask for help than to injure your back. (Courtesy of Skil-Care Corporation, Yonkers, NY, (800) 431-2972)

The other one stands in front of the patient and places her hands and arms under the patient's knees. On the count of three, this assistant supports the lower extremities while the other one moves the patient back in the chair (Figure 17-17). This is not recommended for a heavy patient.

5. This method also requires two people. Stand in back of the wheelchair and have another assistant in front of the patient. Both assistants work with knees and hips bent and backs straight. Lean forward with your head over the patient's shoulder. Instruct the patient to fold the arms. Place your arms around the patient's trunk. Grasp the patient's right wrist with your left hand and grasp the patient's left wrist with your right hand. The other assistant encircles the patient's knees with hands and arms. On the count of three, both assistants lift and move the patient up (Figure 17-18).

6. One person can do this procedure. The patient needs to be oriented and able to follow directions. Stand in front of the patient. Flex your knees and hips and keep your back straight. Position your feet, one on each side of the patient's feet. Brace your knees against the patient's knees. Have the patient lean forward. Lean forward over the patient's right shoulder with the patient's head under your right arm. Encircle your arms around the patient's trunk. The patient's arms are folded together (Figure 17-19). Rock the patient forward and on the count of three,

FIGURE 17-18 One assistant encircles the patient's legs with her hands and arms.

FIGURE 17-17 One assistant supports the lower extremities while the other uses the transfer belt to move the patient back in the chair.

FIGURE 17-19 Put your arms around the patient's torso.

when the patient's weight is over the legs, push against the patient's knees to move back in the chair.

If the patient can bear weight, it is easier and more beneficial to assist the patient to stand and then sit back down, getting the hips to the back of the chair. Wedge cushions placed in the wheelchair will prevent the patient from sliding forward.

WHEELCHAIR ACTIVITY

Pressure on the buttocks is dramatically increased when the patient is sitting. Teach the patient (and provide assistance if necessary) to periodically relieve the pressure by shifting weight every 15 minutes. *Be sure the wheelchair is locked,* *with the caster wheels in the forward position, before beginning any activities involving patient movement in the chair.*

Wheelchair Push-ups

1. Position the caster wheels in the forward position, and lock the brakes. (This may already have been done if the chair is parked.)
2. Teach the patient to place one hand on each armrest, keeping both elbows bent.
3. Then have the patient lean forward slightly, pushing on the armrests and straightening the elbows while lifting the buttocks off the seat of the wheelchair. Have the patient hold this position to the count of five if possible (Figure 17-20A).

GUIDELINES *for*

Chair and Wheelchair Positioning

- The patient's head should be upright and erect (or supported), and facing forward.
- If the patient leans to the side, make sure the chair fits correctly. Provide support with pillows, foam, or other props to support the patient upright.
- Position the arms on the armrests if this does not push the shoulders up. If the shoulders are elevated, adding a seat cushion will boost the patient, preventing shoulder strain.
- If the patient's shoulders are hanging, support the arms on pillows, foam, or other props.
- Position the hands on the armrests, or folded over the patient's lap. Place a small pillow for support and comfort, if needed.
- The upper back of the wheelchair is at the bottom of the shoulder blades.
  - If the chair back is too low, find another chair or ask the nurse about an extension.
  - If the chair back is too high, elevate the patient on a cushion.
- Place a folded bath blanket in the seat of the chair if the patient is wearing a hospital gown so the skin does not contact the vinyl. A reusable underpad may also be used to line the seat if the patient is wearing a hospital gown or is incontinent.
- Use a pressure-relieving pad in the seat if the patient plans to be up for a long time. The pressure-relieving cushion does more than make the patient comfortable. It has many hidden benefits:
  - The sling seat of the wheelchair tends to hammock (sag) in the center when a patient

sits on it. The sagging causes rotation of the inner thighs, which increases pressure on the coccyx and buttocks, two common sites of pressure ulcers.
  - Hammocking of the seat promotes sliding; the leveling pad at the bottom of many cushions corrects the sagging, distributing weight more evenly and reducing pressure.
  - Although foam is comfortable and reduces pressure, it also traps heat. Heat increases the potential for skin damage. To counteract this, use a cushion with a gel layer on top, which will provide a cooling effect on the skin (Figure 17-20B).
  - The gel also moves with the patient, which reduces the effects of friction and shearing.
- The hips are positioned at a 90° angle, at the back of the chair.
  - If the patient's hips slide forward, check the depth of the chair to make sure it fits. If the depth is correct, consult the nurse for postural supports, a wedge cushion, or restraint alternatives. A gripper or wedge cushion (Unit 15) may be placed on the seat to keep the patient from sliding.
  - The patient's weight should be supported by the legs and buttocks. Weight should be equally distributed on both sides.
  - When positioning the male patient, make sure the scrotum is in front of the body, not underneath the patient.

continues

- Avoid pressure on the backs of the knees. There should be at least three to four finger widths between the back of the knee and the seat of the chair.
- Support the feet on the floor or the footrests. If the patient's legs dangle:
  - Elevate the feet on a stool.
  - Use a commercial foot elevator.

- Check with the nurse to see if the leg rests can be shortened to fit.
- When the wheelchair is parked, make sure the large part of the small front wheels faces forward. Lock the brakes.

FIGURE 17-20A Wheelchair push-ups relieve pressure on the buttocks, preventing pressure ulcers. If the patient cannot lift up enough to relieve the pressure every 15 minutes, the care plan will list instructions and times for staff to move the patient to alleviate pressure.

Leaning

If the patient cannot do push-ups, teach her to place the hands on the armrests or thighs and lean forward slightly, and then to each side to relieve pressure on the buttocks. As for the other procedures, the caster wheels must be in the forward position, with the brakes locked. The patient's feet should be on the floor to prevent falling forward or chair tipping. Monitor patients who have balance problems.

Use pillows, pads, or other props to maintain the patient in good body alignment. Patients should always sit upright, without leaning to either side. Side leaning increases the risk for falls and other injuries, pain, discomfort, and other deformities. Patients who lean to the side are often restrained to prevent injury. Remember that good positioning begins with the feet. Make sure the feet are well supported on the footrests. Position the feet at a 90° angle to the lower legs. The lower legs must be at a 90° angle to the thighs. The patient's knees should not be higher than the hips. The thighs must be at a 90° angle to the torso. If the

FIGURE 17-20B A pressure-relieving gel and foam pad is very comfortable and is important for preventing breakdown and maintaining skin integrity. (Courtesy of Skil-Care Corporation, Yonkers, NY, (800) 431-2972).

Gel layer
Foam
Leveling pad

FIGURE 17-21 Padded side wings can be used on one or both sides. This semi-rigid, padded device provides additional support for patients with deformities and those who are difficult to maintain in an upright position. (Courtesy of Skil-Care Corporation, Yonkers, NY, (800) 431-2972)

patient is positioned in this manner and continues to lean, an additional postural support is needed.

Leaning to one side or the other (lateral leaning) alters weight distribution, increasing pressure on the hips and buttocks. Many types of restraint alternatives may be used to keep the patient upright, avoid the use of restraints, and maintain the patient's dignity and self-esteem. Devices such as lateral stabilizer bolsters are used on one or both arms to prevent patients with upper-torso weakness, paralysis, or deformities from leaning to the side and over the arm of the chair. The bolsters help maintain an upright position, use the arms to stabilize the torso, and provide armrest cushioning.

Some patients require more support than pillows or foam bolsters can provide. Padded side wings (Figure 17-21) can be used on one or both sides of the body, in a wheelchair or geriatric chair. A side wing is a semi-rigid device that provides additional support for patients with deformities and those who are difficult to maintain in an upright position. The side wings extend upward under the arms to provide stability to the torso. The padding prevents discomfort. The wings should extend to a few inches below the axilla on both sides. This maintains the patient in an erect, comfortable position and eliminates the needs for straps, harnesses, and restraints, which are often used for patients with positioning problems of the upper torso.

TRANSPORTING A PATIENT BY STRETCHER

Before moving a patient on a stretcher, make sure that the side rails are up and all safety belts are fastened. Push the stretcher by standing at the patient's head. Moving the stretcher in this manner enables you to use good body mechanics and see potential hazards. Approach corners slowly and look before you go around them. Take care when approaching swinging doors. Prop the door open to propel the stretcher through the door. If this is not possible, back through swinging doors.

When entering an elevator, push the stop button to lock the doors open. Back the stretcher into the elevator by walking backward and pulling the head end of the stretcher. Stand by the patient's head while the elevator is in motion. When the elevator stops, push the stop button to lock the door open. Push the stretcher out so the feet exit the elevator first. If the threshold is uneven, go to the foot end of the stretcher and pull it out of the elevator. After the stretcher is safely out of the elevator, unlock the door mechanism.

When transporting a stretcher down a ramp or incline, walk backward, slowly guiding the stretcher from the head end. Periodically look over your shoulder to make sure that the path is clear.

When parking a stretcher, avoid blocking a doorway. Never leave a patient who is on a stretcher unattended or unsupervised.

REVIEW

A. Multiple Choice.

Select the one best answer for each of the following.

1. When ambulating a patient who has a weak right side, you should stand
   a. in back of the patient.
   b. on the patient's right side.
   c. on the patient's left side.
   d. in front of the patient.

2. When ambulating a patient, you should hold the gait belt with
   a. an overhand grasp in back of the patient.
   b. an underhand grasp in back of the patient.
   c. one hand on each side of the patient.
   d. one hand in front of the patient.

3. Before helping a patient to walk with a cane or walker, you should check the
   a. distance between the patient's feet.
   b. screws and bolts for tightness.
   c. height of the wheelchair.
   d. length of each step.

4. The cane is always held
   a. on the patient's weaker side.
   b. on the patient's stronger side.
   c. in the dominant hand.
   d. in the nondominant hand.

5. When using a two-point gait with a cane, the patient will
   a. place the strong foot forward, then the cane, then the weaker foot.
   b. place the strong foot and cane forward at the same time and then the weaker foot.
   c. place the weaker foot and cane forward at the same time and then the stronger foot.
   d. place the weaker foot forward, then the stronger foot, and then the cane.

6. If a patient starts to fall, you should
   a. try to hold the patient upright to prevent a fall.
   b. let go of the patient immediately, to avoid back strain.
   c. ease the patient to the floor.
   d. leave the patient and go for help.

7. When using a walker, the walker is set down so that
   a. the front legs strike the floor first and then the back legs.
   b. the back legs strike the floor first and then the front legs.
   c. all four legs strike the floor at the same time.
   d. how the walker is set down depends on the patient's problem.

8. When transporting a patient in a wheelchair, always
   a. stay to the right in corridors.
   b. guide the wheelchair from the front going down ramps.
   c. push the patient into an elevator frontwards.
   d. position the patient's feet at a 45° angle.

9. Conditions that can affect a patient's gait include
   a. diseases such as Parkinson's disease.
   b. having a catheter.
   c. having hand surgery.
   d. transferring independently.

10. Assistive devices are usually selected by the
    a. nursing assistant.
    b. physician.
    c. physical therapist.
    d. family.

B. True/False.

Mark the following true or false by circling T or F.

11. T F Always back in as you move a patient in a wheelchair into an elevator.

12. T F When transporting a patient in a wheelchair, always walk on the left of the corridor.

13. T F A wheelchair should always be locked unless the patient is being moved.

14. T F A cane is held in the patient's weaker hand.

15. T F When using a walker, the front two legs of the walker should strike the floor first and then the back two legs should strike the floor.

16. T F When assisting a patient to ambulate, you need to use a gait belt only if the patient is using an assistive device.

17. T F To relieve pressure on the buttocks, the patient should be taught how to do wheelchair push-ups or how to lean to relieve pressure.

18. T F To pick an article up from the floor, the patient should lean forward and reach down between the knees.

19. T F A cane is used for patients who are unable to bear weight on one leg.

20. T F The patient needs to be able to use both hands to manipulate a walker.

C. Nursing Assistant Challenge.

Mr. Santozi is 76 years old and has had right hip surgery. His physician does not want him to bear full weight on the affected leg. He uses a walker to assist his ambulation. He has been taught to use a three-point gait. When you help him out of bed, he reaches for the walker to help pull himself up from the bed. As you watch him walk down the hall, you note that he is setting the walker down by the front legs first and then the back legs. When he walks, he moves the walker and his strong leg ahead at the same time.

21. What errors is Mr. Santozi making, and how can you help him? _____

Measuring and Recording Vital Signs, Height, and Weight

UNIT 18

Body Temperature

OBJECTIVES

After completing this unit, you will be able to:
- Spell and define terms.
- Name and identify the three types of clinical thermometers and tell their uses.
- Read a thermometer.
- Identify the range of normal values.
- Demonstrate the following procedures:
  - Procedure 32 Measuring Temperature Using a Sheath-Covered Thermometer
  - Procedure 33 Measuring an Oral Temperature (Electronic Thermometer)
  - Procedure 34 Measuring a Rectal Temperature (Electronic Thermometer)
  - Procedure 35 Measuring an Axillary Temperature (Electronic Thermometer)
  - Procedure 36 Measuring a Tympanic Temperature

VOCABULARY

Learn the meaning and the correct spelling of the following words and phrases:

body core	clinical thermometer	Fahrenheit scale	probe
body shell	digital thermometer	flagged	tympanic thermometer
Celsius scale	electronic thermometer	metabolism	vital signs

INTRODUCTION

Measurement of body temperature is a common nursing assistant task. Body temperature is one of the **vital** (living) **signs**. The patient's other vital signs include pulse, respiration, and blood pressure. Although they are not part of the vital signs, the height and weight of the patient are also commonly measured.

Specific equipment is used to determine or measure these values. Vital signs must be accurately measured because they tell us a great deal about the patient's condition. Do not tell the patient the results. This is not your responsibility. Tell the patient you will ask the nurse to discuss the results with him. Although they are usually determined as a combined procedure, each vital sign is discussed in a separate unit. Measurement of height and weight is discussed in Unit 21.

Many facilities use electronic equipment that automatically registers the four vital signs simultaneously.

TEMPERATURE VALUES

Temperature values may be expressed in either of two scales:
- **Fahrenheit scale**, which is indicated by an *F*.
- **Celsius scale** (centigrade scale), which is indicated by a *C*.

A small ° before either capital letter indicates degrees or levels of temperature.

A formula can be used to convert temperature readings from Celsius to Fahrenheit and from Fahrenheit to Celsius. See Table 18-1 for some important equivalents. Figure 18-1 compares the markings of the Fahrenheit and Celsius thermometers.

DEFINITION OF BODY TEMPERATURE

Temperature is the measurement of body heat. It is the balance between heat produced and heat lost.

Body temperature is:

- Fairly constant. There is a daily variation of 1 to 3°F. Body temperature is lowest in the morning. It is higher in the afternoon and evening.
- Lower the closer to the body surface it is measured. The temperature at the center of the body (**body core**) is much higher than the temperature at the surface of the body.
- Different in the same person when determined from different body areas (Table 18-2). It is important to know the "normal" temperature for an individual, because the normal may vary from person to person.
- Less stable in children. Table 18-3 shows average temperatures in infants and children.
- Affected by
  - illness
  - external temperature/environment
  - medication
  - age
  - infection
  - time of day
  - exercise
  - emotions
  - pregnancy
  - menstrual cycle
  - crying
  - hydration

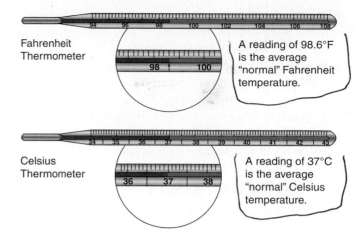

FIGURE 18-1 Fahrenheit and Celsius thermometers

Excessive body temperature puts stress on vital body organs.

TEMPERATURE CONTROL

Activities to control and regulate body temperature are managed by special cells in the brain.

TABLE 18-2 TEMPERATURE VARIATIONS IN THE SAME PERSON

	Oral	Axillary	Rectal
Average Temperature	98.6°F	97.6°F	99.6°F
Range	97.6–99.6°F (36.5–37.5°C)	96.6–98.6°F (36–37°C)	98.6°F–100.6°F (37–38.1°C)

TABLE 18-3 AVERAGE TEMPERATURES IN INFANTS AND CHILDREN

Age	Temperature
3 months	99.4°F
6 months	99.5°F
1 year	99.7°F
3 years	99.0°F
5 years	98.6°F
7 years	98.3°F
9 years	98.1°F
11 years	98.0°F
13 years	97.8°F

TABLE 18-1 COMPARISON OF FAHRENHEIT AND CELSIUS TEMPERATURE SCALES

	Celsius (C)	Fahrenheit (F)
Freezing	0°	32°
Body temperature	37°	98.6°
Pasteurization	63°	145°
Boiling	100°	212°
Sterilizing (Autoclave)	121°	250°

- Heat is produced by chemical reactions (**metabolism**) in the body core and muscular contractions. For this reason, rectal temperature is highest.
- Blood carries the heat to the skin (**body shell**). The heat is lost from the skin to the outside.
- Heat loss is largely controlled by regulating the amount of blood reaching the skin and through perspiration.
- Average oral temperature range is 96.8°F (36°C) to 100.4°F (38°C). Average temperature is 98.6°F (37°C).

MEASURING BODY TEMPERATURE

Temperature is usually measured in one of four body areas:
- Mouth (oral)—most common.
- Ear (aural or tympanic)—takes the least amount of time.
- Rectal—believed to be the most accurate of commonly used sites (mouth, rectal, axillary); rectal temperature registers 1°F higher than oral.
- Axillary or groin—least accurate; measures temperature under the arm or at the groin. (This method is used only when the patient's condition does not permit the use of oral, tympanic, or rectal sites.) An axillary or groin temperature registers 1°F (or 0.6°C) lower than oral temperature.

The patient's condition determines which is the best site for measuring the temperature. The site used most often is the mouth. It is not, however, always the best or safest site. In some situations, it is wiser to use the rectal site.

For example, if the patient is a child or irrational, a glass thermometer in the mouth could result in injury. Patients with respiratory problems, those who breathe through the mouth, or those who are very weak or unconscious may not be able to keep an oral thermometer in their mouths long enough to ensure an accurate recording. In these situations, the best choice is the tympanic site, because the care provider holds the thermometer in the ear. The reading registers within seconds, so the tympanic thermometer is a good choice for restless patients as well. If the tympanic thermometer is not available, the rectal site might be used. Use a rectal thermometer inserted in the anus for the proper time. Be sure to hold the rectal thermometer in place to avoid possible injury.

CLINICAL THERMOMETERS

A patient's temperature is determined by using a **clinical thermometer**. There are several types of clinical thermometers.

The Glass Clinical Thermometer

The glass clinical thermometer is a slender glass tube containing liquid; the liquid expands when exposed to heat and moves up or down the tube. Three types of glass clinical thermometers are in general use (Figure 18-2). They are the oral, security, and rectal thermometers. They differ mainly in the size and shape of the bulb. The bulb is the end that is inserted into the patient. When only the security or stubby type is in use, the rectal thermometers are marked with a red dot at the end of the stem.

Thermometers containing mercury have been used for many years. However, the trend in health care has been to avoid the use of products containing mercury, because mercury can be very toxic to humans and wildlife, if the product is broken. This is true even if mercury exposure occurs in very small amounts.

A mercury thermometer is a small glass tube containing liquid mercury, a silvery-white substance that registers body heat. Alternative products are now being used in many glass thermometers because of mercury's potential for toxicity. Some thermometers contain a red or blue liquid. These are alcohol thermometers and contain no mercury. Another thermometer contains galinstan, a substance similar to mercury in appearance. These thermometers are mercury-free, however, and are generally marked as such.

Mercury can be toxic in small amounts, particularly if it vaporizes and is inhaled. Even small mercury spills must be cleaned up properly to prevent contamination and illness. If you accidentally break a thermometer or other medical device containing mercury, follow your facility policies and procedures for cleaning the spill.

Electronic Thermometer

The **electronic thermometer** (Figure 18-3) is used in many hospitals. One unit can serve many patients because the nursing assistant simply changes the disposable sheath that fits over the probe.

- The electronic thermometer is battery-operated. It registers the temperature on the viewing screen in a few seconds.
- The portion called the **probe** is inserted into the patient.
- The probes are colored red for rectal use and blue for oral or axillary use.

FIGURE 18-2 Clinical thermometers (from top to bottom): oral, security, rectal

A   B   C   D   E
G   F

FIGURE 18-3 An electronic thermometer. The temperature is registered in large, easy-to-read numerals. The disposable protective sheath (probe cover) is placed over the probe tip. The probe is inserted in the patient's mouth in the usual manner. (A) Plastic cord goes around the nursing assistant's neck when carrying the thermometer. (B) Thermometer. (C) Box of disposable probe covers. (D) Probe (blue = oral, red = rectal). (E) Charging unit. (F) Probe cord. (G) Disposable probe cover.

- The probe is covered by a plastic sheath before use. The plastic sheath stays on during use. It is discarded after one use.

Digital Thermometer

Digital thermometers are hand-held and have a probe that is inserted into the patient's mouth or rectum (Figure 18-4). Sheaths are used to cover the oral or rectal probe

FIGURE 18-4 (A) Carrying case. (B) Digital thermometer. (C) Probe cover without backing. (D) Probe cover with backing.

before use and are discarded after use. The unit is battery-operated. After the sheath-covered probe is inserted, the temperature can be read within 20 to 60 seconds. The temperature is shown as a digital (number) display.

Disposable Oral Thermometers

Plastic or paper thermometers (Figure 18-5) are used for oral temperatures in some facilities. They are used once and discarded. They have dots on them. The dots change color from brown to blue, according to the patient's temperature.

> ## Safety ALERT
>
> The disposable thermometer is made of rigid plastic. Remove the thermometer from the patient's mouth slowly. Pulling the thermometer out rapidly from between closed lips can cause tears of the lips and mucous membranes in the mouth. ■

Tympanic Thermometer

The **tympanic thermometer** is an instrument that measures the temperature from blood vessels in the tympanic membrane (ear drum) in the ear (Figure 18-6). The temperature reading obtained is close to the core body temperature. To obtain an accurate reading, the probe must be placed solidly into the ear canal. The instrument has a built-in converter that provides the equivalent temperature in rectal or oral values (in both the Fahrenheit and Celsius systems). The type of temperature reading (mode) is selected by the user. The disposable speculum is inserted into the ear canal, gently sealing the canal. The instrument is activated, usually by pressing a button, and within a few seconds it registers the temperature of the blood flowing through the vessels in the eardrum.

Using the Glass Thermometer

The glass thermometer is a long, cylindrical, calibrated tube that contains a column of heat-sensitive liquid (Figure 18-7).

FIGURE 18-5 The chemical dot thermometer is used only for oral temperatures. It is used once, then discarded.

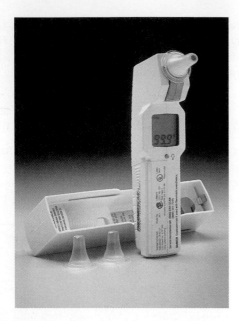

FIGURE 18-6 Cordless, hand-held tympanic thermometer that measures the temperature of the tympanic membrane in the ear. The window on the handset indicates the digital temperature reading. The thermometer can be set to provide an oral, rectal, Fahrenheit, or Celsius equivalent reading. (Courtesy of Thermoscan® Inc., San Diego, CA)

- Starting with 94°F (34°C), each long line indicates a one-degree elevation in temperature.
- Only every other degree is marked with a number.
- In between each long line are four shorter lines.
- Each shorter line equals two-tenths (2/10 or 0.2) of 1 degree.

The liquid (the solid color line shown in Figure 18-7) in the bulb of the thermometer rises in the hollow center of the stem as heat is registered. To read the thermometer:

- Hold it at eye level.
- Find the solid column in the center.
- Look along the sharper edge between the numbers and lines.
- Read at the point at which the liquid ends.
- If it falls between two lines, read it to the closest line.

Some glass thermometers come individually prepackaged for patient use. The patient receives it as part of the admission package.

Using the Electronic Thermometer

Battery-operated electronic thermometers are commonly used. The temperature registers in large numbers on the screen. The probe is placed into the patient. The probe stem is colored blue for oral or axillary use and red for rectal use. A new, disposable probe cover is used for each patient. Following use, the cover is discarded. The temperature registers in about 30 seconds.

FIGURE 18-7 Reading a thermometer. This thermometer reads 98.6°F. Most Fahrenheit thermometers have an arrow indicating 98.6°F.

Clinical Information ALERT

Each facility has policies and procedures about taking an oral temperature when the patient is using oxygen. In general, if the patient is using oxygen by mask, you should avoid taking an oral temperature. If the patient uses oxygen through a nasal cannula, the temperature reading may be slightly (approximately 0.3 degrees) lower because of the oxygen. Consult the nurse if you are unsure of the method to use for taking the temperature of a patient who is using oxygen. ■

Using the Tympanic Thermometer

Many facilities use tympanic thermometers. The temperature is taken by measuring the heat given off by the tympanic membrane (in the ear). This method has several advantages:

- Tympanic thermometers are accurate and easy to use.
- The temperature registers in a few seconds. Because of this, taking the temperature of an agitated patient is safer and faster.
- Temperatures that cannot be taken orally can be taken by the tympanic method, eliminating the need to take rectal or axillary temperatures.
- The tympanic thermometer allows you to select a core, oral, or rectal mode. This means the reading will correlate with the mode selected. Choose the mode according to your facility's policy.
- Wait for 15 minutes to take the temperature if the patient has been outdoors or if the patient has been lying on the ear you will use.

If you accidentally break a mercury thermometer, apply gloves and eye protection. Your facility may also require use of a mask to prevent inhalation. Pick up broken glass and other debris and place in a puncture-resistant container. Follow facility policies for picking up mercury. Use an index card to consolidate the droplets, then seal them in a plastic bag or covered container. Small droplets can be picked up with adhesive tape or wet paper towels. Seal the container and affix a label identifying the material as "mercury spill debris." ■

When a tympanic thermometer is used for children under age 3, pull the pinna down and back. In children over age 3, pull the pinna up and back. This straightens the ear canal, enabling the sensor to detect heat in the ear drum. When the probe is positioned correctly, the probe tip will point at the midpoint between the eyebrow and sideburn on the opposite side of the face. ■

The tympanic temperature is the fastest and most convenient method, but it can also give inaccurate readings if the user's technique is not precise. To ensure an accurate reading, insert the probe tip into the ear as far as it will go. Next, rotate the probe handle until it is aligned with the jaw, like speaking on the telephone. Quickly press the "scan" button. Using this method will help ensure accurate temperature readings.

Documentation

In many facilities, temperatures are recorded on a temperature clipboard. They are then transferred to the individual patient charts. Changes in readings may be **flagged** (specially noted) by placing a circle around the reading or a star beside it. Make sure to report any changes from previous temperature readings directly to the nurse. Your accurate observations, reporting, and documentation contribute to the nurses' evaluation and assessment of the patient.

GUIDELINES *for*
Using an Oral or Rectal Thermometer

Oral Thermometer

1. Do not use if the patient is:
   - uncooperative
   - restless
   - unconscious
   - chilled
   - confused or disoriented
   - coughing
   - an infant or child under the age of 6
   - unable to breathe through the nose
   - recovering from oral surgery
   - irrational
   - very weak
   - receiving oxygen (except nasal prongs)
   - on seizure precautions
2. An oral temperature reading could be inaccurate on denture wearers.

3. To measure an oral temperature accurately, wait 15 minutes if patients have been smoking, eating, or drinking, then take the temperature.

Rectal Thermometer

1. Do not use if the patient has:
   - diarrhea
   - fecal impaction
   - combative behavior
   - rectal bleeding
   - hemorrhoids
   - had rectal surgery or rectal or colonic disease
   - recently had a heart attack
   - recently had prostate surgery
   - a colostomy
2. Always hold a rectal thermometer in place the entire time.

GUIDELINES *for*

The Safe Use of a Glass Thermometer

- Make sure the thermometer is clean.
- Wear disposable gloves when measuring oral and rectal temperatures.
- Check glass thermometers for chips.
- Shake the thermometer down before use. Shake away from the patient and hard objects.
- Cover the thermometer with a disposable plastic sheath.
- Do not leave the patient alone with a thermometer in place.
- Allow a glass thermometer to register for at least 3 minutes for oral and rectal temperatures, and 10 minutes for axillary temperature.

- Hold rectal and axillary thermometers in place.
- When using a rectal thermometer, lubricate the bulb end of the thermometer before inserting it into the rectum. Some sheaths are prelubricated.
- After removing the thermometer and before reading it, wipe the thermometer from end to tip with an alcohol wipe or cotton ball.
- Do not touch a bulb end or disposable sheath that has been in patient's mouth (oral thermometer) or anus (rectal thermometer).
- Discard the sheath according to facility policy after use.
- Clean and disinfect the thermometer after use.

PROCEDURE

32

MEASURING TEMPERATURE USING A SHEATH-COVERED THERMOMETER

 Note: The guidelines for this procedure vary slightly from state to state, and from one facility to the next. Your instructor will inform you if the sequence in your state or facility differs from the procedure listed here. Know and follow the required sequence for your facility and state.

1. Carry out initial procedure actions.

2. Assemble equipment:
   - Gloves (standard precautions)
   - Clinical thermometer
   - Protective sheath (unopened package)
   - Pad and pencil

3. Have the patient rest in a comfortable position.

4. Ask the patient if he or she has had anything to eat or drink or has smoked within the last 15 minutes. Wait 15 minutes before taking an oral temperature if the answer is yes.

5. Apply gloves.

6. Shake the thermometer down to below 96°F.

7. Holding the thermometer in one hand, insert it into the marked end of a protective sheath wrapper (Figure 18-8A).

8. Holding onto the sheath tab on the stem end of the thermometer, peel back the paper cover to expose the plastic sheath (Figure 18-8B).

9. Hold the paper wrapper in one hand (Figure 18-8C). Twist the paper wrapper to break the seal with the tab and remove the paper wrapper,

FIGURE 18-8A Inserting a thermometer into a disposable thermometer sheath

continues

PROCEDURE 32 CONTINUED

leaving the plastic sheath on the thermometer (Figure 18-8D).

10. Keeping the protective sheath over the thermometer, insert the bulb end of the thermometer under the patient's tongue, toward the side of the mouth.

11. Tell the patient to hold the thermometer gently, with lips closed, for 3 minutes.

12. Remove the thermometer and discard the used sheath. Read and shake down. Record on notepad.

13. The thermometer can be stored in the patient's bedside stand for reuse with a new sheath.

14. Remove gloves and discard according to facility policy.

15. Carry out ending procedure actions.

FIGURE 18-8B To remove the sheath, peel back the outer paper wrapper to expose the inner plastic sheath.

16. Report any unusual variations to the nurse at once.

FIGURE 18-8C Grasp the outer paper wrapper.

FIGURE 18-8D Holding onto the paper tab with one hand, twist and remove the outer paper wrapper.

PROCEDURE

33

 DVD

MEASURING AN ORAL TEMPERATURE (ELECTRONIC THERMOMETER)

Note: The guidelines for this procedure vary slightly from state to state, and from one facility to the next. Your instructor will inform you if the sequence in your state or facility differs from the procedure listed here. Know and follow the required sequence for your facility and state.

1. Carry out initial procedure actions.

2. Obtain an electronic thermometer, disposable probe covers, and gloves, if this is your facility policy. (Gloves are not necessary with an *oral temperature* using this type of thermometer. Know and follow your facility policy.)

continues

PROCEDURE **33** CONTINUED

3. Ask the patient if he has had anything to eat or drink or has smoked within the last 15 minutes. Wait 15 minutes before taking an oral temperature if the answer is yes.

4. Cover the probe (blue) with a probe cover.

5. Insert the covered probe under the patient's tongue toward the side of the mouth (Figure 18-9A).

6. Hold the probe in position. Ask the patient to close the mouth and breathe through the nose.

7. When a buzzer signals that the temperature has been determined, remove the probe from the patient's mouth.

8. Discard the probe cover in the appropriate container (Figure 18-9B). Remove gloves, if used, and discard according to facility policy.

9. Return the probe to its proper position.

10. Record the temperature on your pad.

11. Return the thermometer unit to the charger.

12. Carry out ending procedure actions.

FIGURE 18-9A The thermometer probe is placed to one side of the patient's mouth and positioned under the tongue.

FIGURE 18-9B Discard the used probe cover according to facility policy.

PROCEDURE

34

MEASURING A RECTAL TEMPERATURE (ELECTRONIC THERMOMETER)

 Note: The guidelines for this procedure vary slightly from state to state, and from one facility to the next. Your instructor will inform you if the sequence in your state or facility differs from the procedure listed here. Know and follow the required sequence for your facility and state.

continues

PROCEDURE 34 CONTINUED

1. Carry out initial procedure actions.

2. Assemble equipment on a tray:
   - Gloves
   - Electronic thermometer with rectal (red) probe
   - Probe cover
   - Lubricant

3. Lower the backrest of the bed. Ask the patient to turn on his side. Assist if necessary.

4. Put on gloves. Place a small amount of lubricant on the tip of the probe cover (Figure 18-10).

5. Fold the top bedclothes back to expose the patient's anal area.

6. Separate the buttocks with one hand. Insert the covered probe about 1 inch into the rectum, or as recommended by the thermometer manufacturer. With many thermometers, the rectal probe is inserted approximately 1/4 inch. Hold in place. Replace the bedclothes for privacy as soon as the thermometer is inserted.

7. Read the temperature when registered on the digital display.

8. Remove the probe and discard the probe cover. Wipe lubricant from the patient. Discard tissue. Return the probe to its proper position.

FIGURE 18-10 Apply a small amount of lubricant to the tip of the sheath.

9. Remove and dispose of gloves according to facility policy.

10. Record the temperature on your pad.

11. Return the thermometer unit to the charger.

12. Carry out ending procedure actions.

PROCEDURE

35

OBRA DVD

MEASURING AN AXILLARY TEMPERATURE (ELECTRONIC THERMOMETER)

📝 **Note:** The guidelines for this procedure vary slightly from state to state, and from one facility to the next. Your instructor will inform you if the sequence in your state or facility differs from the procedure listed here. Know and follow the required sequence for your facility and state.

1. Carry out initial procedure actions.

📝 **Note:** Use disposable gloves if there may be contact with open lesions, wet linens, or body fluids.

2. Equipment needed: same as for oral temperature measurement using an electronic thermometer. (See Procedure 33.)

3. Wipe the axillary area dry and put the covered probe in place. Keep the patient's arm close to the body. Hold the probe in place until the temperature shows on the digital display and the buzzer signals that it has been recorded.

continues

PROCEDURE 35 CONTINUED

4. Remove the thermometer probe. Dispose of the probe cover. Return the probe to its proper position.

5. Record the temperature on your pad.

6. Return the thermometer unit to the charger.

7. Carry out ending procedure actions.

GUIDELINES *for*

Using a Tympanic (Ear) Thermometer

- Make sure the thermometer lens is clean and that there is no dirt or debris on the lens at the end of the probe tip.

- Use each probe cover only once. Make sure the cover is on snugly, without ripples.

- Store the thermometer out of the path of any cold air flow. If the thermometer is in a cold area, allow it to warm up before use, or it may read low.

- Make sure the patient is not directly in the path of cold air or being fanned. This action cools the ears, which can cause a low temperature reading.

- If the patient is or has been lying on one ear, use the opposite ear.

- If the patient has a hearing aid, use the opposite ear or remove the aid and wait 15 minutes.

- The tympanic thermometer can be set to oral, core, or rectal mode. In most cases, oral is appropriate. The mode will be shown in the readout screen. If the screen says "CAL," the thermometer is in the unadjusted mode, which is used only for calibration and other bench work.

- Insert the probe tip into the ear as far as possible, then rotate the handle to the correct position in alignment with the jaw.

Ear thermometers are similar to cameras. They provide the temperature of what you point them at. If the thermometer is not used correctly, you will get an inaccurate reading. Common causes of inaccurate tympanic temperatures are:

- Pressing the scan button before the probe is fully inserted

- Using a probe cover more than once

- Using a thermometer without a probe cover

- Improper cleaning of the thermometer lens

- Not following manufacturer's instructions for placing the probe tip into the ear; following instructions for the thermometer you are using is important

- Using a thermometer with a broken or missing lens (the lens is the shiny disc at the end of the probe tip through which the infrared energy must pass to be processed)

PROCEDURE

36

MEASURING A TYMPANIC TEMPERATURE

📝 **Note:** The guidelines for this procedure vary slightly from state to state, and from one facility to the next. Your instructor will inform you if the sequence in your state or facility differs from the procedure listed here. Know and follow the required sequence for your facility and state.

continues

PROCEDURE 36 CONTINUED

1. Carry out initial procedure actions.

2. Assemble equipment:
   - Disposable gloves if there may be contact with blood or body fluids, open lesions, or wet linens
   - Tympanic thermometer
   - Probe covers

3. Check the lens to make sure it is clean and intact (Figure 18-11A).

4. Select the appropriate mode on the thermometer.

5. Place a clean probe cover on the probe.

6. Put on disposable gloves if you may have contact with blood or body fluids, open lesions, or wet linens.

7. Position the patient so you have access to the ear you will be using.

8. Gently pull the ear pinna back and up (Figure 18-11B). This straightens the ear canal so the thermometer can be placed for an accurate reading.
   - If the patient is a child under age 3, pull the pinna down and back.
   - If the patient is a child over age 3, pull the pinna up and back.

9. Place the probe in the patient's ear, aiming it toward the tympanic membrane. Insert the probe until it seals the ear canal (Figure 18-11C). Do not apply pressure.
   - Check the position of the probe. The tip should be at an imaginary location inside the ear opposite the midpoint between the eyebrow and sideburn on the opposite side of the face.

10. Rotate the probe handle slightly until it is aligned with the jaw, as though the patient were speaking on the telephone.

11. Quickly press the activation button (Figure 18-11D). Leave the thermometer in the ear for the time recommended by the manufacturer.

12. When you have a reading, remove the probe from the patient's ear and dispose of the cover. See Table 18-4 for normal ranges of tympanic temperatures by age group.

FIGURE 18-11A Check the lens of the tympanic thermometer to make sure it is clean and intact.

FIGURE 18-11B Gently pull the ear pinna back and up.

continues

PROCEDURE 36 CONTINUED

FIGURE 18-11C Place the covered probe in the patient's ear, aiming it toward the tympanic membrane. Insert the probe until it seals in the ear canal, then rotate the handle until it is positioned like a telephone.

FIGURE 18-11D Press the activation button and leave the thermometer in the ear for the time recommended by the manufacturer.

13. Record the temperature on your pad.

14. Return the thermometer unit to the charger.

15. Carry out ending procedure actions.

TABLE 18-4 NORMAL RANGES FOR TYMPANIC TEMPERATURES

Years of Age	Fahrenheit	Celsius
0–2	97.5–100.4°F	36.4–38.0°C
3–10	97.0–100.0°F	36.1–37.8°C
11–65	96.6–99.7°F	35.9–37.6°C
>65	96.4–99.5°F	35.8–37.5°C

REVIEW

A. True/False.

Mark the following true or false by circling T or F.

1. T F When charting an axillary temperature, always print AX after the reading.

2. T F Readings taken with a plastic thermometer may not be entirely accurate.

3. T F Temperature is the measurement of body heat.

4. T F The most common method of measuring the temperature of a cooperative adult is by mouth.

5. T F To measure a rectal temperature, the patient is best positioned on her back.

6. T F 96.8°F is an average oral temperature.

7. T F Only temperature variations of more than 5°F should be reported to the nurse.

8. T F Clinical thermometers can be identified by the shapes of their bulbs.

9. T F The probe of an electronic thermometer is covered with a red sheath for rectal use.

10. T F The axillary temperature of a patient will register approximately one degree higher than his oral temperature.

11. T F The tympanic temperature reading is the most accurate.

12. T F A freezing temperature registered in Celsius readings would be 32°.

13. T F It would be unsafe to use a glass oral thermometer with a 2-year-old child.

14. T F If safely placed, rectal thermometers need not be held.

15. T F Wait 5 minutes after the patient has taken hot liquids to measure an oral temperature.

16. T F When washing used glass thermometers, use hot water.

17. T F Always wipe the axillary area before placing a thermometer.

18. T F When using an electronic thermometer, you should not allow your fingers to touch the tip of the probe sheath.

19. T F All rectal thermometers should be lubricated before insertion.

20. T F The oral thermometer should remain in place for 1 minute.

21. T F The liquid column in a glass oral thermometer should register below 96°F at the beginning of the procedure.

22. T F There may be times when a temperature has to be measured in the groin area.

23. T F Each long line on the stem of a clinical thermometer indicates a change of 2 degrees of temperature.

24. T F Each short line on the stem of the clinical thermometer indicates a 0.2-degree change in temperature.

25. T F Measuring the temperature in the groin area gives the most accurate indication of body temperature.

B. Completion.

Complete the statements by choosing the correct words from the following list.

Fahrenheit	less
higher	temperature
pulse	tympanic

26. Vital signs include _____, _____, respiration, and blood pressure.

27. A normal temperature reading of 98.6° would be in the _____ scale.

28. A _____ thermometer is used to measure the temperature in the ear.

29. A 3-month-old child might be expected to have a slightly _____ temperature normally than a child who is 9 years old.

30. Temperature is _____ stable in children than in adults.

C. Nursing Assistant Challenge.

31. Mrs. LeJune is having difficulty breathing and is very restless. The nurse instructs you to measure her temperature. What type of thermometer would you choose if all were available?

   a. Glass oral thermometer

   b. Glass rectal thermometer

   c. Electronic oral thermometer

   d. Tympanic thermometer

32. You are about to measure a rectal temperature with a glass thermometer. You find a small chip in the glass. What should you do?

   a. Use the thermometer, because it is just a small chip.

   b. Throw the thermometer in the wastepaper basket.

c. Break the thermometer in half so no one else will use it.

d. Discard the broken thermometer in the sharps container and replace it with another thermometer.

33. You are assigned to measure your patient's rectal temperature using a glass thermometer. How long should you hold the thermometer in place?

a. 3 minutes

b. 10 minutes

c. 15 minutes

d. 20 minutes

Pulse and Respiration

OBJECTIVES

60-90, Beat a mm (handwritten)

After completing this unit, you will be able to:
- Spell and define terms.
- Define pulse.
- Explain the importance of monitoring a pulse rate.
- Locate the pulse sites.
- Identify the range of normal pulse and respiratory rates.
- Measure the pulse at different locations.

- List the characteristics of the pulse and respiration.
- List eight guidelines for using the stethoscope.
- Demonstrate the following procedures:
  - Procedure 37 Counting the Radial Pulse
  - Procedure 38 Counting the Apical-Radial Pulse
  - Procedure 39 Counting Respirations

VOCABULARY

Learn the meaning and the correct spelling of the following words and phrases:

accelerated	cyanosis	radial pulse	stethoscope
apical pulse	dyspnea	rales	symmetry
apnea	expiration	rate	tachycardia
bradycardia	inspiration	respiration	tachypnea
Cheyne-Stokes respirations	pulse	rhythm	volume
	pulse deficit	stertorous	

INTRODUCTION

The pulse and respiration of the patient are usually counted during the same procedure. Because breathing is partly under voluntary control, a person is able to stop or alter breathing temporarily for a short period. For example, when a patient realizes that her breathing is being watched and counted, she alters her breathing pattern without meaning to do so. To avoid this, the respirations are counted immediately following the pulse count without telling the patient. The patient's hand is kept in the same position, and your fingers remain on the pulse point so that you seem to still be taking the pulse.

THE PULSE *test* (handwritten)

The **pulse** is:
- The pressure of the blood felt against the wall of an artery as the heart alternately contracts (beats) and relaxes (rests).
- More easily felt in arteries that come fairly close to the skin and can be gently pressed against a bone.
- The same in all arteries throughout the body.
- An indication of how the cardiovascular system is meeting the body's needs.

Radial Pulse

The **radial pulse** is the most commonly measured pulse. It is measured at the radial artery in the wrist. Figure 19-1 shows areas of the body where other large blood vessels come close enough to the surface to be used as sites for counting the pulse. Conscious patients can be checked at the radial artery. (See Procedure 37.) Unconscious patients should be checked at the carotid artery or apically (over the heart).

Pulse measurement includes determining the:

1. Rate or speed
   a. **Bradycardia**—an unusually slow pulse (below 60 beats per minute)
   b. **Tachycardia**—an unusually fast pulse (more than 100 beats per minute)
2. Character
   a. **Rhythm**—regularity
   b. Volume or fullness

Report:

- Pulse rates over 100 beats per minute (bpm) (tachycardia)
- Pulse rates under 60 bpm (bradycardia)
- Irregularities in character (rhythm and volume)

Pulse rates can be affected by:

- Illness
- Emotions
- Age
- Exercise
- Elevated temperature
- Gender
- Position
- Physical training
- Lowered temperature
- Drugs

Table 19-1 shows average pulse rates.

TABLE 19-1 AVERAGE PULSE RATES

Patient	Beats per Minute
Adult men	60–70
Adult women	65–80
Teenagers	60–90
Children over 7 years	75–100
Preschoolers	80–110
Toddlers	90–140
Infants	120–160

Using a Stethoscope

A **stethoscope** is a medical instrument used to listen to sounds inside the body. It intensifies sounds so they can be heard clearly. The parts of the stethoscope are seen in Figure 19-3. Many health care workers use stethoscopes on many patients. This creates the potential for infection to be passed to both workers and patients. Before and after using the stethoscope, wipe the earpieces and diaphragm with an alcohol sponge or other disinfectant. If the tubing of the stethoscope contacts the patient or bed linen, wipe the tubing as well.

You will use the stethoscope to take blood pressures. Your health care facility may teach you other procedures with the stethoscope, including taking an apical pulse.

The Apical Pulse

An **apical pulse** is measured by counting the heart contractions. The stethoscope is placed over the apex (tip) of the heart. Listen for the heart sounds that indicate closing

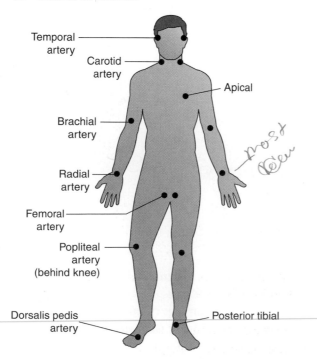

Temporal artery
Carotid artery
Apical
Brachial artery
Radial artery
Femoral artery
Popliteal artery (behind knee)
Dorsalis pedis artery
Posterior tibial

FIGURE 19-1 Common pulse sites of the body

PROCEDURE

OBRA DVD

37

COUNTING THE RADIAL PULSE

1. Carry out initial procedure actions.

2. Place the patient in a comfortable position. The palm of the hand should be down and the arm should rest on a flat surface.

3. Locate the pulse on the thumb side of the wrist with the tips of your first three fingers (Figure 19-2). Do not use your thumb—it contains a pulse that may be confused with the patient's pulse.

4. When the pulse is felt, exert slight pressure. Using the second hand of your watch, count for one minute. It is the practice in some hospitals to count for one-half minute and multiply by two and to record the rate for one minute. A one-minute count is preferred and must be done if the pulse is irregular.

5. Remember the reading when counting respirations. Record the reading on your pad as soon as possible.

6. Carry out ending procedure actions.

FIGURE 19-2 Locate the pulse on the thumb side of the wrist with the tips of your first three fingers.

FIGURE 19-3 The stethoscope is used to listen to sounds inside the body.

of the valves. These sounds occur as the heart pumps blood into the arteries. The sounds should occur at the same rate as the pulse that is felt as an expansion of the radial artery. The apex of the heart is found:

- On the left side of the front of the chest
- Between the fifth and sixth ribs
- Just below the left nipple
- In women, under the left breast

GUIDELINES *for*

Using a Stethoscope

- Clean the earpieces and diaphragm of the stethoscope before using it.
- Clean the stethoscope tubing if it contacts the patient or bed linen.
- Check the earpieces of the stethoscope for wax, and remove it if present.
- Check the stethoscope tubing. Do not use if it has cracks or holes in it.
- The earpieces of the stethoscope should face forward.

- The diaphragm of the stethoscope should not come in contact with the patient's clothing, blood pressure cuff, or other device.
- Place the diaphragm of the stethoscope flat against the patient's skin and hold it in place. If the diaphragm is at an angle, you will not be able to hear the sounds.
- Apply firm but gentle pressure when holding the diaphragm in place. If you press too hard, you may be unable to hear the sound.

Listen carefully for two sounds: lub dub. The louder sound (lub) corresponds to the contraction of the ventricles pushing the blood forward through the arteries, and the closing of the valves to prevent the backflow of blood. This is the sound to be counted. The softer sound (dub) corresponds to the relaxation of the ventricles as they fill with blood before the next contraction and the closing of the semilunar valves to prevent backflow from the arteries. When documenting an apical pulse reading, write "AP" after the value.

Apical-Radial Pulse Rate

The apical and radial pulse rate is a comparison of the apical rate and the radial rate. Usually they are the same.

Sometimes the contraction of the heart is so weak that it fails to send enough blood to the arteries to expand them. When this happens, no pulse is felt. In this case, the number of loud sounds does not correspond with the number of pulses felt in the radial artery.

The difference between the apical pulse (the loud sounds heard over the heart) and the radial pulse (the expansion felt over the radial pulse) is called a **pulse deficit**. Two people measure the heart rate and the radial pulse at the same time. (See Procedure 38.) The nurse measures the apical pulse while the second person counts the radial pulse for 1 minute. The rates are then compared.

Apical pulse rates are checked:

- Whenever a pulse deficit exists or is suspected
- Before the registered nurse administers drugs that alter the heart rate or rhythm
- In children whose rapid rates might be difficult to count at the radial artery
- For one full minute
- On any child 12 months of age or younger
- Whenever you are uncertain of the accuracy of the radial pulse or it is irregular

Pulse deficits are found in some forms of heart disease.

PROCEDURE

38

COUNTING THE APICAL-RADIAL PULSE

1. Carry out initial procedure actions.
2. Clean the stethoscope earpieces and bell or diaphragm with disinfectant.
3. Place the stethoscope earpieces in your ears with tips facing slightly forward for better fit.
4. Place the stethoscope diaphragm or bell over the apex of the patient's heart. If it is cold, warm the

diaphragm with your hands before placing it on the patient's chest.
5. Listen carefully for the heartbeat.
6. Count the louder-sounding beats for one minute.
7. Check the radial pulse for one minute. The best way to obtain these numbers is to have the nurse count the apical pulse while you take the radial pulse (Figure 19-4).

continues

PROCEDURE 38 CONTINUED

8. Note results on a pad for comparison.

9. Clean earpieces and bell of stethoscope with disinfectant.

10. Carry out ending procedure actions.

    Example: Apical pulse = 108

    Radial pulse = 82

    Pulse deficit = 26 (108 – 82 = 26)

FIGURE 19-4 The nurse takes the apical pulse while the nursing assistant takes the radial pulse.

RESPIRATION

The main function of **respiration** is to supply the cells in the body with oxygen and to rid the body of excess carbon dioxide. When respirations are inefficient, there is less oxygen in the blood available for body needs. In addition, carbon dioxide is released less efficiently. The skin takes on a bluish or dusky color and the patient develops a condition known as **cyanosis**.

There are two parts to each respiration: one **inspiration** (inhalation) followed by one **expiration** (exhalation). Special terms describe different breathing patterns:

- Normal—regular, 12 to 20 breaths per minute
- **Tachypnea**—rapid, shallow breathing
- **Dyspnea**—difficult or labored breathing
- Shallow—breaths that only partially fill the lungs
- **Apnea**—a period of no respirations
- **Cheyne-Stokes respirations**—a period of dyspnea followed by periods of apnea
- **Stertorous**—Snoring-like respirations

- **Rales** (crackles)—moist respirations. At times, fluid (mucus) will collect in the air passages. This causes a bubbling type of respiration. Crackles are common in the dying patient.
- Wheezing—difficult breathing accompanied by a whistling or sighing sound due to narrowing of bronchioles (as in asthma) or an increase of mucus in the bronchi.

Respirations should be checked for:

- **Rate**—number of respirations per minute
- Rhythm—regularity
- **Symmetry**—ability of the chest to expand equally as air enters each lung
- **Volume**—depth of respiration
- Character—terms used to describe the character of respirations include:
  - Regular
  - Irregular
  - Shallow
  - Deep
  - Labored (difficult)

The rate of respiration is determined by counting the rise or fall of the chest for one minute, using a watch equipped with a second hand. (See Procedure 39.)

- The average rate for adults is 12 to 20 respirations per minute.
- If the rate is more than 25 per minute, it is said to be **accelerated**. Accelerated respiration should be reported.
- If the rate is less than 12 per minute, it is too slow. It should be reported.

Remember that, if possible, respirations should be counted without the patient's knowing that you are doing so; the rate and volume may change if the patient knows they are being counted. You might count respirations

Clinical Information ALERT

When counting respirations, note whether the patient's breathing is normal (easy) or labored (dyspneic), shallow or deep, and quiet or noisy. Check the muscles of the neck and abdomen. If the patient is using these muscles for breathing, inform the nurse. ■

PROCEDURE

39

COUNTING RESPIRATIONS

1. When the pulse rate has been counted, you may leave your fingers on the radial pulse and start counting the number of times the chest rises and falls during one minute (Figure 19-5). Count one inhalation and one exhalation as one respiration.

2. Note the depth and regularity of respirations.

3. Record the time, rate, depth, and regularity of respirations.

FIGURE 19-5 Leave your fingers on the radial pulse while counting respirations.

before or after counting the radial pulse. Continue pressing on the pulse area while counting.

The factors affecting respiratory rates include:

- Illness
- Emotions
- Elevated temperature
- Gender
- Age
- Exercise

- Position
- Drugs

Average respiratory rates are listed in Table 19-2.

Temperature, pulse, and respiration (TPR) rates and character are recorded in a notebook or on a clipboard and then transferred to the patient's chart (Figure 19-6).

TABLE 19-2 AVERAGE RESPIRATORY RATES

Age	Normal Respiratory Rate per Minute
Infant	30–60
Toddler	24–40
Preschool child	22–34
School-age child	18–30
Teenager	12–24
Adult	12–20

GRAPHIC RECORD

DATE		10/5/xx						10/6/xx																																
HOSPITAL DAY		1						2																																	
POST OP DAY																																								

FIGURE 19-6 showing temperature, pulse, respiration, and blood pressure readings recorded over 10/5/xx (Hospital Day 1) and 10/6/xx (Hospital Day 2).

BLOOD PRESSURE readings:
AM 10/5: 12 112/66, 4 114/58, 8 126/76
AM 10/6: 12 118/64, 4 124/74, 8 130/82
PM 10/5: 12 116/68, 4 110/74, 8 142/78
PM 10/6: 12 122/72, 4 120/84, 8 126/88

WEIGHT/STOOL: 154 BM (10/5), 153.5 BM (10/6)

FIGURE 19-6 TPR readings are recorded in the patient's medical record.

REVIEW

A. True/False.

Mark the following true or false by circling T or F.

1. T F A pulse deficit results when there is a difference between the apical and radial pulses.

2. T F The pulse is the pressure of blood against the arterial wall.

3. T F Cheyne-Stokes respirations are deep and regular.

4. T F Pulses differ when counted at different pulse sites.

5. T F The pulse rate of an infant is 110 to 130 bpm.

6. T F An apical pulse should be counted in children.

7. T F The pulse site used most often is the carotid artery.

8. T F The respiratory system rids the body of excess carbon dioxide.

9. T F Mucus in the air passages causes crackles.

10. T F A pulse is best counted using the thumb placed over the artery.

B. Matching.

Choose the correct word from Column II to match the words and phrases in Column I.

Column I

11. _____ Snoring types of respiration

12. _____ Bluish discoloration to the skin

13. _____ Regularity

14. _____ Periods of no respiration

15. _____ Difficult breathing

16. _____ Rapid respirations

17. _____ Increased or speeded up

18. _____ Expiration

19. _____ Speed

20. _____ Slow pulse

Column II

a. accelerated

b. apnea

c. bradycardia

d. cyanosis

e. dyspnea

f. rate

g. rhythm

h. stertorous

i. tachypnea

j. inspiration

k. exhalation

C. Nursing Assistant Challenge.

21. Mrs. Morgan has a heart condition that makes her heart rate irregular and faster than normal. Her respirations are difficult or rapid, labored, and moist. She receives a medication that profoundly alters her heart action. Your orders are to assist in determining the pulse deficit. Answer the statements using the terms in the following list.

apical	rales
dyspnea	tachycardia
radial	tachypnea

   a. The faster heart rate is described as _____.

   b. The difficult respirations can be charted as _____.

   c. Moist respirations are best described as _____.

   d. Rapid respirations are also called _____.

   e. Which pulse rate will you count? _____.

   f. Which pulse rate will a second person count? _____.

22. List two reasons why a radial-apical pulse rate would be ordered.

   a. _____

   b. _____

UNIT 20

Blood Pressure

Skilled test

OBJECTIVES

After completing this unit, you will be able to:

- Spell and define terms.
- Describe the factors that influence blood pressure.
- Identify the range of normal blood pressure values.
- Identify the causes of inaccurate blood pressure readings.
- Select the proper size blood pressure cuff.

- List precautions associated with use of the sphygmomanometer.
- Demonstrate the following procedure:
  - Procedure 40 Taking Blood Pressure
  - Procedure 41 Taking Blood Pressure with an Electronic Blood Pressure Apparatus

VOCABULARY

Learn the meaning and the correct spelling of the following words and phrases:

aneroid gauge	depressant	fasting	sphygmomanometer
auscultatory gap	diastole	hypertension	stimulant
blood pressure	diastolic pressure	hypotension	systole
brachial artery	elasticity	pulse pressure	systolic pressure

INTRODUCTION

Blood pressure is the fourth vital sign. It is the measure of the force of the blood against the walls of the arteries. Blood pressure depends on the:

- Volume (amount of blood in the circulatory system).
- Force of the heartbeat.
- Condition of the arteries. Arteries that have lost their **elasticity** (stretch) give more resistance. The pressure is greater in these arteries.
- Distance from the heart. Blood pressure in the legs is lower than in the arms.

Pressure varies with contraction (**systole**) and relaxation (**diastole**) of the ventricles of the heart.

- Systolic blood pressure reading indicates the period when the pressure within the arteries is the greatest, during contraction of the ventricles. The systolic blood pressure is the working pressure.
- Diastolic reading indicates the lowest point of pressure between ventricular contractions. The diastolic blood pressure is the resting pressure.

Blood pressure is elevated by:

- Sex of the patient (males slightly higher than females before menopause)
- Exercise
- Eating
- **Stimulants** (substances that speed up body functions)
- Emotional stress, such as anger, fear, or sexual activity

Clinical Information ALERT

Taking accurate blood pressures and reporting and documenting abnormal values saves health care dollars and improves patients' health. For example, the physician will treat high blood pressure values leading to renal failure. High blood pressure causes 80% of all kidney failure. The annual cost of treating renal failure is approximately $20 billion. Controlling high blood pressure can delay the onset of renal failure by 4.5 years. Dialysis costs about $50,000 a year, so this control alone is a potential savings of $225,000. Even more important, being in good health and not using dialysis maintains the patient's quality of life. ∎

- Disease conditions, such as arteriosclerosis (hardening of the arteries), elevated cholesterol, or diabetes mellitus
- Hereditary factors
- Pain
- Obesity
- Age
- Condition of blood vessels
- Some drugs

Blood pressure is lowered by:

- **Fasting** (not eating)
- Rest
- **Depressants** (drugs that slow down body functions)
- Weight loss
- Emotions (such as grief)
- Abnormal conditions such as hemorrhage (loss of blood) or shock

- Dehydration and fluid loss
- Some drugs, such as antihypertensives (drugs that lower blood pressure in persons who have hypertension)
- Diuretics (drugs that lower the volume of body fluids)

Individual factors affecting blood pressure are:

- Age
- Sleep
- Weight
- Emotion
- Heredity
- Gender
- Viscosity of blood
- Condition of blood vessels

Average blood pressure values are listed in Table 20-1.

EQUIPMENT

The **sphygmomanometer** (blood pressure measuring apparatus) consists of:

- A cuff (different sizes are available) that fits around the patient's arm. There is a rubber bladder inside the cuff. A pressure control button is attached to the cuff. It is important to use the proper size cuff when measuring blood pressure. Cuffs that are too wide or too narrow will give inaccurate readings (Figure 20-1). To check the size of the cuff, compare the length of the rubber bladder inside the cuff (Figure 20-2) with the patient's arm circumference. The bladder should be at least 80% of the circumference of the arm. If it is larger or smaller, obtain a different size cuff.
- Two tubes. One tube is connected to the pressure control bulb and to the bladder inside the cuff. The other tube is connected to the pressure gauge.
- A pressure gauge, which may be a column of mercury (Figure 20-3A) or a round **aneroid gauge** (Figure 20-3B) dial. Both are marked with numbers.

The stethoscope magnifies sounds. It consists of:

TABLE 20-1 AVERAGE BLOOD PRESSURE VALUES

Age	Approximate Blood Pressure Value	
	Systolic	Diastolic
2–6 months	91	50 to 53
7–11 months	90	47 + age in months
1–5 years	90 + age in years	56
6–18 years	83 + (2 × age in years)	52 + age in years
Over age 18	120	80

FIGURE 20-1 The cuff must fit properly for accurate readings. A variety of cuff sizes are available.

- A bell or diaphragm.
- Tubing that carries sounds to the listener.
- Earpieces that direct the sounds into the listener's ears. The earpieces and diaphragm must be cleaned with antiseptic before and after each use to prevent transmission of disease.

Electronic sphygmomanometers with attached cuffs are used in some facilities. You do not have to use a stethoscope with these units, because they automatically register the readings on a digital display. Follow the manufacturer's directions for the type of unit you are using.

Some facilities use an instrument that measures pulse rate, temperature, and blood pressure (Figure 20-4).

FIGURE 20-2 The bladder inside the cuff should be 80% the circumference of the patient's arm.

FIGURE 20-3A A mercury gravity sphygmomanometer

MEASURING THE BLOOD PRESSURE

Blood pressure is usually measured in the upper arm over the brachial artery. Blood pressure readings taken anywhere else must be ordered by a doctor. The values are recorded in millimeters of mercury (mm Hg).

1. The cuff is smoothly applied directly over the **brachial artery** (1 inch above the antecubital area).
2. The stethoscope bell is placed over the brachial artery.

FIGURE 20-3B A dial (aneroid) sphygmomanometer

FIGURE 20-4 All vital signs may be checked with a single instrument. (Vital∎Check® patient monitor, photo courtesy of Alaris Medical Systems, Inc. San Diego, CA)

Clinical Information ALERT

Some facilities prefer measuring the blood pressure in the left arm, if possible, because it is closest to the heart. ∎

3. Pressure is then increased by inflating the rubber bladder in the cuff to stop the flow of blood through the artery.

4. The pressure is slowly released and the sounds of heart valves closing can be heard. The sounds correspond to pressure changes in the blood.

5. The blood pressure is measured:
   a. At its highest point as the **systolic pressure**. This will be the first regular sound you will hear. This is the sound of the bicuspid and tricuspid valves shutting.
   b. At its lowest point as the **diastolic pressure**. This will be the change or last sound you will hear. This is the sound of the semilunar valves shutting.
   c. The difference between systolic and diastolic pressure is called **pulse pressure**. The pulse pressure gives important information about the health of the arteries. The average pulse pressure in a healthy adult is about 40 millimeters (mm) of mercury (Hg) (range 30–50 mm Hg). However, factors in both health and disease can alter the pulse pressure. An increase in blood volume or heart rate or a decrease in the ability of the arteries to expand may result in an increased pulse pressure.

6. Blood pressure readings are recorded as an improper fraction; for example, systolic/diastolic or 130/92. This means the systolic pressure is 130 and the diastolic pressure is 92. Both numbers in the blood pressure are important, but for people who are 50 or older, systolic pressure gives the most accurate diagnosis of high blood pressure.

7. Blood pressure values:
   a. Average resting adult brachial artery pressure is less than 120 millimeters of mercury (mm Hg) systolic and less than 80 millimeters of mercury (mm Hg) diastolic.
   b. *Prehypertension* is a condition that means the person is likely to develop high blood pressure in the future. In this condition, blood pressure is between 120/80 mm Hg and 139/89 mm Hg. People with prehypertension can take steps to decrease their risk.
   c. **Hypertension** (high blood pressure) is when values are greater than 140 mm Hg systolic and 90 mm Hg diastolic.
   d. **Hypotension** (low blood pressure) is when values are less than 100 mm Hg systolic and 60 mm Hg diastolic. Excessive hypotension can lead to shock.
   e. For either hypertension or hypotension, unusual or changed readings must be recorded and reported. (See Procedure 40.)
   f. High blood pressure is a dangerous condition. There are no signs and symptoms. It increases the risk of several serious diseases (Unit 40). It can also cause complications of conditions such as diabetes. People with prehypertension and hypertension require regular blood pressure monitoring.
   g. Blood pressure classifications are listed in Table 20-2. When systolic and diastolic blood pressures fall into different categories, the higher category is used to classify blood pressure level. For example, 172/78 mm Hg would be stage 2 hypertension (high blood pressure).

Safety ALERT

For accurate blood pressure values, check the stethoscope tubing. Do not use if it has cracks or holes in it. The bell or diaphragm of the stethoscope should not come in contact with the patient's clothing, blood pressure cuff, or other device. Place the bell or diaphragm of the stethoscope flat against the patient's skin and hold it in place. If it is at an angle, you will not be able to hear the sounds. Apply firm but gentle pressure when holding the diaphragm in place. If you press too hard, you will be unable to hear the sound. ∎

GUIDELINES *for*

Preparing to Measure Blood Pressure

Before using the stethoscope:

1. Clean the earpieces with an alcohol wipe (Figure 20-5A) and clean the bell with a different alcohol wipe.

2. Point the earpieces forward when inserting them in your ears.

3. Use the diaphragm portion of the stethoscope.

4. Be sure the diaphragm portion is open so you will hear the beats.

Before using a sphygmomanometer:

1. If using a mercury manometer—if the mercury moves up the column very slowly (Figure 20-5B), it may have oxidized. Report this to the nurse and use another sphygmomanometer.

2. If using an aneroid manometer—make sure the needle is on zero before you inflate the cuff (Figure 20-5C). If it is not, report this to the nurse and use another sphygmomanometer.

Generally:

Turn off radio and television when taking blood pressure. Ask the patient not to talk. Do not take blood pressure on an arm that:

FIGURE 20-5A Clean the earpieces with an alcohol sponge before and after use.

- Has an intravenous feeding or other device inserted
- Is being treated for burns, fractures, or other injuries
- Has a dialysis access device
- Is on the same side as the patient's recent mastectomy (breast removal) or other surgical procedure
- Has a pulse oximeter

FIGURE 20-5B Do not use the sphygmomanometer if the mercury moves up the column slowly.

FIGURE 20-5C Make sure the needle is on zero before inflating the cuff on the aneroid sphygmomanometer.

TABLE 20-2 BLOOD PRESSURE CLASSIFICATIONS

Blood Pressure Level (mm Hg)		
Category	**Systolic**	**Diastolic**
Hypotension	<100 and	<60
Normal	<120 and	<80
Prehypertension	120-139 or	80–89
High Blood Pressure		
Stage I Hypertension	140–159 or	90–99
Stage II Hypertension	≥160 or	≥100

Legend: < means less than; ≥ means greater than or equal to

Inaccurate Blood Pressure Readings

Causes of inaccurate blood pressure readings include:

- Use of a wrong-size cuff
- An improperly wrapped cuff
- Incorrect positioning of arm
- Not using the same arm for all readings
- Not having the gauge at eye level
- Deflating the cuff too slowly
- Mistaking an **auscultatory gap** (sound fadeout for 10 to 15 mm Hg which then begins again) as the diastolic pressure

Safety ALERT

Do not attempt to measure blood pressure using an arm that is the site of an intravenous infusion, the site of a dialysis access device, paralyzed, injured, has edema present, is on the same side as a recent surgery, or has a pulse oximeter. ■

HOW TO READ THE GAUGE

The gauges on sphygmomanometers are marked with a series of lines. The large lines are at increments of 10 millimeters of mercury pressure. The shorter lines are at 2-mm intervals. For example, the first small line above 80 mm is 82 mm. The first small line below 80 mm is 78 mm (Figure 20-6).

To properly read the mercury gauge:

- It should be at eye level.

FIGURE 20-6 The aneroid gauge (left) and the mercury gauge (right). Take the reading at the closest line.

- It should not be tilted.
- The reading should be taken at the top of the column of mercury. It should not be taken at the "hump" in the middle of the mercury when you hear the first sound.

To properly read the aneroid gauge, observe the gauge at eye level. Do not read it at an angle.

Following completion of the blood pressure measurement, you will record and report the following:

- If you were unable to hear the reading
- If blood pressure is higher than in a previous reading
- If blood pressure is lower than in a previous reading
- If the site where you took the reading was other than the brachial artery

Infection Control ALERT

Clean the manual or electronic blood pressure cuff and tubing with a facility-approved disinfectant after each patient. Alternatives are to use a disposable cuff that is issued to each patient and used throughout the hospital stay or to cover the cuff with a disposable sleeve. ■

Pulse Oximeters

Some electronic vital signs monitors also measure the pulse oximeter value. A spring clip slips over the patient's fingertip, and the unit displays the value. If the unit you are using also measures the pulse oximeter, apply the spring finger clip to the hand on the opposite side from the blood pressure cuff. (Applying it to an arm with an inflated blood pressure cuff will cause inaccurate values.) The spring finger clip may be applied to an arm with an IV, dialysis access device, or the affected side of a stroke or mastectomy without causing injury. The unit will obtain

---

a reading quickly, usually within a few seconds. If you obtain a value below 95, have the patient take a few deep breaths, and check the reading again. You may remove the spring clip as soon as the reading is obtained. Review the information in Unit 36 on using the pulse oximeter so you are familiar with the reportable values.

PROCEDURE

40

TAKING BLOOD PRESSURE

📝 **Note:** This is the "two-step" procedure recommended by the American Heart Association (AHA) beginning in 1993. The AHA considers the two-step procedure the most reliable for normal blood pressure measurement. (The most accurate values are obtained by internal monitoring, in which a catheter is placed in an artery. The internal method is not practical for most clinical situations.) In some facilities and states, nursing assistants use a one-step procedure for measuring blood pressure. For more information, see the online Appendix at the Online Companion for this textbook.

1. Carry out initial procedure actions.

2. Assemble equipment:
   * Sphygmomanometer with appropriate size cuff
   * Stethoscope
   * Alcohol wipes

3. Remove the patient's arm from sleeve or roll sleeve 5 inches above the elbow; it should not be tight or binding.

4. Locate the brachial artery with your fingertips (Figure 20-7A).

5. Place the patient's arm palm upward, supported on bed or table, at heart level.

6. Wrap the cuff smoothly and snugly around the arm. Center the bladder over the brachial artery. The bottom of the cuff should be 1 inch above the antecubital space (inner elbow) (Figure 20-7B).

7. Place the bulb in your dominant hand and feel for the radial pulse with the fingers of your other hand (Figure 20-7C). To find out how high to pump the cuff:
   * Rapidly inflate the cuff until you no longer feel the radial pulse.
   * Add 30 mm to that reading. (If you no longer feel the pulse when the mercury or needle reaches 130, add 30 mm for a reading of 160.) Note that point.

FIGURE 20-7A Locate the brachial artery with your fingertips.

FIGURE 20-7B The bottom of the cuff should be at least 1 inch above the antecubital space (inner elbow).

8. Quickly and steadily deflate the cuff. Wait 15 to 30 seconds.

9. Place the stethoscope over the brachial artery (Figure 20-7D).

10. Reinflate the cuff quickly and steadily to the level you calculated (in the example in step 7, to 160).

11. Release the air at an even pace, about 2 to 3 mm per second. Keep your eyes on the needle or the mercury.

12. Listen for the onset of at least two consecutive beats. Note where the needle is on the sphygmomanometer when you first hear the sound. (Do not stop deflating the cuff.) This is your systolic reading.

13. Continue deflating the cuff. The last sound you hear is the diastolic reading. Continue to deflate and to listen for 10 to 20 mm more to make sure you have the correct diastolic reading.

continues

PROCEDURE 40 CONTINUED

FIGURE 20-7C Hold the bulb in your dominant hand and feel for the brachial pulse with the fingers of the other hand.

14. Record the reading (blood pressure is always recorded in even numbers, with the systolic on

FIGURE 20-7D Hold the stethoscope bell securely over the brachial artery.

top and the diastolic on the bottom, e.g., 128/82). Indicate the arm used and the position of the patient (sitting, lying down, or standing).

15. If you are not sure of the reading and need to retake the blood pressure, wait 1 to 2 minutes before repeating the procedure.

16. Clean the earpieces of the stethoscope with alcohol wipes. If the tubing has contacted the patient or linen, wipe it as well.

17. Return equipment to the appropriate area.

18. Carry out ending procedure actions.

GUIDELINES *for*

Electronic Blood Pressure Monitoring

Patient Selection (refer to Figure 20-8)

- This procedure can be done on patients of all ages and sizes, but appropriately sized cuffs must be used.
- At least one blood pressure reading should be taken using the auscultation method before an electronic blood pressure device is used. The auscultation reading is needed as a baseline with which to compare the values from the electronic device.

The procedure is contraindicated in patients with:

- Extreme hypertension or hypotension

- Very rapid heart rates
- Excessive body movement or tremors
- Irregular heart rhythms or atrial dysrhythmias

Patients for whom electronic blood pressure monitoring is not acceptable should be known to all caregivers and identified on the care plan or Kardex. If in doubt, check with the nurse for instructions for patients with very high blood pressure or rapid or irregular heart (pulse) rates.

Do not place the cuff on an arm that:

- Is paralyzed

continues

GUIDELINES *continued*

FIGURE 20-8 The electronic blood pressure monitoring unit takes the blood pressure automatically.

- Is the site of an intravenous infusion (IV)
- Has a pulse oximeter on it
- Has impaired circulation
- Is the site of a dialysis access device
- Is fractured
- Is burned
- Is on the same side as a recent mastectomy or other surgical procedure site

Application of the Cuff

- Select the proper cuff size. The length should be equal to 40% of the arm circumference.
- The upper arm is the preferred location for the monitoring cuff, but the forearm and ankle may also be used.

PROCEDURE

41

TAKING BLOOD PRESSURE WITH AN ELECTRONIC BLOOD PRESSURE APPARATUS

1. Carry out initial procedure actions.
2. Assemble equipment:
   - Electronic blood pressure device
   - Assortment of cuffs and tubes
3. Bring the electronic blood pressure unit to the bedside. Place it near the patient and plug it into a source of electricity.
4. Locate the on/off switch and turn the machine on.
5. Select the appropriate cuff for the machine and size for the patient's extremity.
6. Remove restrictive clothing.
7. Squeeze excess air out of the cuff.
8. Connect the cuff to the connector hose.
9. Wrap the cuff snugly around the patient's extremity, verifying that only one finger can fit between the cuff and the patient's skin. Make sure the "artery" arrow marked on the outside of

the cuff is correctly placed over the brachial artery.
10. Verify that the connector hose between the cuff and the machine is not kinked.
11. Set the frequency control for automatic or manual.
12. Press the start button.
13. If the cuff will take periodic, automatic measurements, set the designated frequency of blood pressure measurements.
14. Set upper and lower alarm limits for systolic, diastolic, and mean blood pressure readings.
15. Remove the cuff at least every 2 hours and rotate sites, if possible. Evaluate the skin for redness and irritation. Report abnormalities to the nurse.
16. Carry out ending procedure actions.

REVIEW

A. True/False.

Mark the following true or false by circling T or F.

1. T F The volume of blood in the circulatory system is a factor in the blood pressure.

2. T F Exercise decreases blood pressure.

3. T F To accurately measure blood pressure, you will need both a sphygmomanometer and a stethoscope.

4. T F Blood pressures taken over arteries closer to the heart will be lower than those taken over arteries farther from the heart.

5. T F A blood pressure below 100/60 suggests hypotension.

6. T F The large lines on the blood pressure gauge are in increments of 20 mm of Hg pressure.

7. T F Depressant drugs elevate the blood pressure.

8. T F Using a blood pressure cuff of the wrong size will give an inaccurate reading.

9. T F When measuring a blood pressure, always keep the gauge at eye level.

10. T F Stethoscope earpieces should be cleaned both before and after use.

B. Matching.

Choose the correct word from Column II to match each phrase in Column I.

Column I

11. _____ high blood pressure

12. _____ lowest blood pressure reading

13. _____ stretch

14. _____ most common artery used to determine blood pressure

15. _____ blood pressure apparatus

Column II

a. brachial

b. diastolic

c. stethoscope

d. femoral

e. sphygmomanometer

f. hypotension

g. hypertension

h. elasticity

i. systolic

C. Completion.

Complete the statements by choosing the correct word.

16. The closing of the heart valves is heard as the _____ sounds.
    (diastolic) (systolic)

17. High blood pressure is known as _____.
    hypotension) (hypertension)

18. Blood pressure is lowered when weight is _____.
    (gained) (lost)

19. Blood pressure is raised by _____.
    (rest) (exercise)

20. The earpieces of the stethoscope should be pointed _____ as they are placed in the ears.
    (forward) (backward)

D. Nursing Assistant Challenge.

You are assigned to take Mr. King's blood pressure at 12 noon. He is a very heavy man and has an IV inserted in his left arm. His blood pressure was 180/140 at 8 AM. Answer the following questions:

21. What effect will his size have on your selection of cuff? _____

22. On which arm will you apply the cuff? _____

23. Will you report your findings? _____

24. Why or why not? _____

UNIT 21

Measuring Height and Weight

OBJECTIVES

- Spell and define terms.
- Describe the proper use of an overbed scale.
- Demonstrate the following procedures:
  - Procedure 42 Weighing and Measuring the Patient Using an Upright Scale

- Procedure 43 Weighing the Patient on a Chair Scale
- Procedure 44 Measuring Weight with an Electronic Wheelchair Scale
- Procedure 45 Measuring and Weighing the Patient in Bed

VOCABULARY

Learn the meaning and the correct spelling of the following words and phrases:

balance bar
baseline

centimeter (cm)
increment

kilogram (kg)
pound (lb)

WEIGHT AND HEIGHT MEASUREMENTS

Changes in weight are frequently used as an indicator of the patient's condition.

- A **baseline** (original) measurement of height and weight is usually obtained on admission. These are usually noted on the Kardex.
- Weights are frequently measured when patients are given drugs (diuretics) to increase their urine output.
- Weight is an indicator of the patient's nutritional status.
- Measurements of weight and height must be accurately made and recorded according to facility policy because medications may be ordered according to the patient's size.
- Height measurements may be recorded in feet (') and inches (") or in **centimeters (cm)**.
- Weight measurements may be recorded in **pounds (lb)** or **kilograms (kg)**.

Note: Some facilities use the metric system, so you may be recording weight in kilograms. If your facility uses this measurement system, the scales will be calibrated for the metric system. You will not be required to convert measurements from the inch and pound system to the metric system.

- The upright scale is used for ambulatory patients who can stand unattended on the platform (Figure 21-1).
- A mechanical lift with scale can be used to weigh patients who cannot stand and a wheelchair scale is not available (Figure 21-2).
- Sling scales can be used to weigh patients whose conditions do not permit the use of a mechanical lift/scale (Figure 21-3).
- Chair scales are used to weigh patients in wheelchairs (Figure 21-4).

(See Procedures 42 to 45.)

FIGURE 21-1 An upright scale is used only for patients who can stand unaided on the platform.

FIGURE 21-2 The scale on the mechanical lift is used when patients cannot stand and a wheelchair is not available. (Photo courtesy Health O Meter®)

FIGURE 21-3 The sling scale is used for bedfast patients who are not ambulatory or are too heavy or difficult to move.

FIGURE 21-4 Electronic chair scales are used for patients who cannot stand on an upright scale.

Clinical Information ALERT

If the patient uses a lap tray on the wheelchair, remove the tray before weighing the patient. If the tray cannot be removed, weigh the empty wheelchair (with the tray), then subtract the combined weight from the total patient weight. Lap trays can add as much as 8 pounds to the total weight. (Refers to the type of scale pictured in Figure 21-4) ▪

Clinical Information ALERT

Some patients have orders for daily weight. Weigh the patient at the same time, with the same amount and type of clothing, using the same scale, if possible. A weight gain usually suggests fluid retention. A 2-pound gain in a short time indicates that the patient is retaining an extra liter of fluid. Weight loss means that excess fluid has left the body. ▪

GUIDELINES *for*
Obtaining Accurate Weight and Height Measurements

To obtain an accurate weight measurement, you must:

- Always balance the scale before using it.
- Have the patient empty his or her bladder.
- If the patient is wearing an incontinent brief, make sure it is dry before weighing.
- If the patient has an indwelling catheter, make sure the bag is empty before weighing.
- Weigh the patient at the same time of day each time.
- Have the patient wear the same type of garments each time.
- Use the same method and the same scale each time, if possible.
- If the patient has a cast, has recently had a cast removed, or has new onset edema, consult the nurse about possible weight discrepancies.

You must learn to read the scale correctly. There are two bars on the upright scale (see Figure 21-1). The **balance bar** should hang free to start.

- The lower bar indicates weights in 50-pound **increments** (amounts).
- The upper bar indicates one-quarter-pound increments (Figure 21-5).
- The even-numbered pounds are marked with numbers.
- The long line between each number indicates the odd-numbered pounds.
- Each small line indicates one-quarter pound, or 4 ounces.

The two figures are added and recorded as the person's total weight. The sum is recorded according to facility policy in either pounds or kilograms. For example:

>   Large bar = 100 pounds
>   Small bar = +22 pounds
>   Total = 122 pounds

- Height is measured with the ruler attached to an upright scale or with a tape measure when the patient is in bed.

Small Weight Indicator   Large Weight Indicator   Balance Bar

FIGURE 21-5 The upper bar indicates smaller pound weights. The weight shown on the lower bar is measured in 50-pound increments. This figure is added to the amount shown on the upper bar.

PROCEDURE

42

WEIGHING AND MEASURING THE PATIENT USING AN UPRIGHT SCALE

1. Carry out initial procedure actions.

 Note: Use disposable gloves if there may be contact with open lesions, wet linens, or body fluids.

2. Check notes or chart for previous weight as documented. Then escort the patient to the scales.

continues

PROCEDURE 42 CONTINUED

3. Place a paper towel on the platform of the scale.

4. Be sure the weights are to the extreme left and the balance bar (bar with weight markings) is hanging free.

5. Assist the patient to remove shoes and step up onto the scale platform, facing the balance bar. The balance bar will rise to the top of the bar guide. The patient should not hold the bar or other parts of the scale.

6. Move the large weight to the right to the closest estimated patient weight.

7. Move the small weight to the right until the balance bar hangs freely halfway between the upper and lower bar guides.

8. Add the two figures and record the total as the patient's weight in pounds or kilograms, according to the type of scale used.

9. Assist the patient to turn on the platform until facing away from the balance bar. Raise the height bar until it is level with the top of the patient's head.

10. The reading is made at the movable point of the ruler (Figure 21-6).

11. Note the number of inches (or centimeters) indicated. Record this information in inches ("), feet (') and inches ("), or centimeters (cm), according

to the type of scale. The height shown in Figure 21-6 is 62 inches. This may be recorded as 62 inches or 5 feet 2 inches (62 ÷ 12 = 5 feet 2 inches). Record the value on your notepad.

12. Assist the patient off the platform. Help the patient to put on shoes, if necessary, and return to the room.

13. Carry out ending procedure actions.

FIGURE 21-6 The height is read at the movable point of the ruler.

PROCEDURE

43

WEIGHING THE PATIENT ON A CHAIR SCALE

1. Carry out initial procedure actions.

2. Assemble equipment:
   - Chair scale

3. Take the patient in a wheelchair to the chair scale. Lock the brakes to the wheelchair. Check the brakes of the chair scale to make sure they are locked in place.

4. Apply a transfer belt to the patient and assist in a pivot transfer to the chair on the scale. Instruct

the patient to sit down when the chair is felt against the back of the legs. Be sure the patient's feet are on the footrest of the chair once seated.

5. Walk behind the scale to obtain the reading.

6. Transfer the patient back to the wheelchair.

7. Carry out ending procedure actions.

(This procedure refers to a scale with a permanently mounted chair.)

PROCEDURE

44

MEASURING WEIGHT WITH AN ELECTRONIC WHEELCHAIR SCALE

1. Carry out initial procedure actions.

2. Assemble equipment:
   - Wheelchair scale

3. Determine and record empty weight of a wheelchair by weighing it on the scale.

4. Take the wheelchair to the patient's room. Help the patient into the wheelchair and take the patient to the electronic wheelchair scale.

5. Open the metal ramp sides on the scale so that they rest on the floor. This allows wheelchair access to the scale.

6. Press the "on" button; the scale zeroes automatically (Figure 21-7).

7. Roll the wheelchair, with the patient in it, onto the platform of the scale (Refer to Figure 21-4). Lock wheelchair wheels.

8. The digital readout will show the weight.

9. Record weight of the patient and wheelchair. Subtract the wheelchair weight to obtain the patient's weight.

10. Unlock wheelchair wheels. Roll the wheelchair with patient off the scale.

11. Fold the scale ramps back into place.

12. Carry out ending procedure actions.

   (This procedure refers to the scale pictured in Figure 21-4.)

FIGURE 21-7 Press the "on" button to calibrate the scale. This will cause the reading to return to zero. (Courtesy of Scale-Tronix, White Plains, NY)

Clinical Information ALERT

To weigh a patient who is slightly unsteady or has a little trouble with balance, position a walker over the scale. Instruct the patient to hold the walker while stepping onto the scale. Hold the walker or assist as needed. If a balance scale is being used, move the weights to the approximate weight. When you are ready to obtain the weight, instruct the patient to let go for a moment. If he or she becomes unsteady, advise the patient to lean in and hold the walker. Keep one hand on the walker to stabilize it if necessary. ■

Clinical Information ALERT

Occasionally you will encounter a patient who is badly contracted in the fetal position. The easiest way to obtain the height for this patient is to use a tape measure when the patient is in the side-lying position. Measure the body in two or three segments, depending on the nature and location of contractures. Measure from the top of the head to the waist, and then write down the number. Next, measure the distance from the waist to behind the knees. Write down this number. Now measure from behind the knees to the bottom of the heels. Write down this number. Finally, add together all of the numbers you have recorded. This will give you the total height measurement. ■

PROCEDURE

45

MEASURING AND WEIGHING THE PATIENT IN BED

1. Carry out initial procedure actions.

2. Obtain assistance from a coworker.

3. Assemble equipment:
   - Overbed scale
   - Sheet
   - Tape measure
   - Pencil

4. Check scale sling and straps for frayed areas or straps that do not close properly.

5. Lower the side rail on your side. Make sure the side rail is up on the other side.

6. Fanfold the top linen to foot of the bed.

7. Position the patient flat on the back with arms and legs straight and body in good alignment. Make sure the sheet is straight and wrinkle-free.

8. Make a small pencil mark at the top of the patient's head on the sheet.

9. Make a second pencil mark even with the heels (Figure 21-8).

10. Roll the patient on the side. Using the tape measure, measure the distance between the two pencil marks.

11. Note the patient's height in feet and inches on a pad.

12. Cover the canvas sling with a sheet. Balance the scale according to the manufacturer's directions. The scale should be balanced with the sheet, canvas sling, chains, or straps attached.

13. Remove the scale sling from the suspension straps and position half of the sheet-covered sling under the patient.
    - Turn the patient away from you.
    - Place the sling, folded lengthwise, under the patient.
    - Return the patient to the supine position and place the sling so that the patient rests securely within it.
    - Attach the sling to the suspension straps. Check to be sure attachments are secure.

14. Position the lift frame over the bed with base legs in maximum open position, and lock the frame.

15. Elevate the head of the bed and bring the patient to a sitting position.

16. Attach the suspension straps to the frame. Position the patient's arms inside the straps.

17. Slowly raise the sling so the patient's body is off the bed. Be reassuring.

18. Guide the lift away from the bed so that no part of the patient touches the bed.

19. Take and note the reading.

20. Reposition the sling over the center of the bed.

21. Release the knob slowly, lowering the patient to the bed.

22. Remove the sling by reversing the process in step 13.

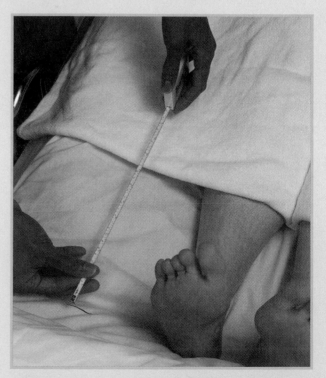

FIGURE 21-8 To find the height of the patient in bed, measure from the pencil line at the bottom of the feet to the pencil line at the top of the head.

continues

REVIEW

A. True/False.

Mark the following true or false by circling T or F.

1. T F The lower bar on the scale indicates pounds in increments of 25.

2. T F Always check the overbed scale for needed repairs before use.

3. T F To obtain a proper reading, the scale balance bar must hang freely.

4. T F The scale used most often to weigh ambulatory patients in care facilities is the upright scale.

5. T F A patient who cannot get out of bed cannot be measured.

6. T F When using an overbed scale, the patient's body must be free of the bed.

7. T F To measure a patient confined to bed, first help her assume the left Sims' position.

B. Short Answer.

Choose the correct word from the following list to complete each statement in questions 8–12.

ambulatory	inches
centimeters	kilograms
away	pounds

8. Weights may be measured in _____ or _____.

9. Height measurements may be recorded in feet and _____ or in _____.

10. The upright scale is used to weigh _____ patients.

11. A scale that is calibrated for the metric system will express weights in _____.

12. When a patient is measured on a balance scale, he should face _____ from the scale.

C. Nursing Assistant Challenge.

Mrs. Haughn is in bed recovering from a stroke. She is unable to walk or stand. She is receiving diuretics. Her doctor wants to order some new medication that is given according to the patient's size. You are assigned to weigh and measure the height of this patient. Answer each of the following by selecting the correct answer.

13. The best way to weigh this patient is with
   a. an upright scale.
   b. an overbed scale.
   c. a wheelchair scale.
   d. a chair scale.

14. The best way to measure this patient is
   a. with a height bar.
   b. with a tape measure.
   c. to ask the patient.
   d. to estimate the height.

15. One reason the physician might have asked for the patient's weight is because the patient
   a. is receiving diuretics.
   b. has had a stroke.
   c. cannot stand.
   d. cannot walk.

16. The patient measures 63 inches. This may be expressed as
   a. 5 feet 6 inches.
   b. 5 feet 8 inches.
   c. 5 feet 3 inches.
   d. 6 feet 3 inches.

Patient Care and Comfort Measures

UNIT 22

Admission, Transfer, and Discharge

OBJECTIVES

After completing this unit, you will be able to:
- Spell and define terms.
- List the ways the nursing assistant can help in the processes of admission, transfer, and discharge.
- Describe family dynamics and emotions that occur when a loved one is admitted to the hospital.
- List ways in which the nursing assistant can develop positive relationships with a patient's family members.
- Demonstrate the following procedures:
  - Procedure 46 Admitting the Patient
  - Procedure 47 Transferring the Patient
  - Procedure 48 Discharging the Patient

VOCABULARY

Learn the meaning and the correct spelling of the following words and phrases:

| admission | baseline assessment | discharge | transfer |

INTRODUCTION

The nurse is responsible for overseeing and carrying out hospital procedures and physician's orders regarding all admissions, transfers, and discharges. You will usually help the nurse by carrying out the routine procedures associated with these activities.

A nursing assistant, a volunteer, or someone from the admissions office accompanies the new patient to the unit. Someone must always escort the patient to the unit for admission. Also, someone must always escort the patient from the unit during transfer or discharge.

You can do much to make these activities easier for the patient, family, and the other staff members by:
- Having equipment and materials prepared for the activity.
- Being very observant during each activity.
- Documenting observations carefully and accurately. These make a valuable contribution to the nurse's initial **baseline assessment** of the patient's condition.
- Reporting observations directly to the nurse.
- Giving attention to the details of each procedure.
- Being aware of the emotional stress these activities cause patients and their families.
- Being courteous to everyone.

ADMISSION

When a person enters a health care facility for treatment of an illness or injury, the **admission** process often causes concern or stress to the patient, family, and friends. The first impression created is very important. You will be one of the first staff members the patient sees, so it is important that you be courteous, confident, and efficient. (See Procedure 46.)

Open the unit and prepare the bed as soon as you are notified of a new admission. If the patient will be admitted by ambulance or stretcher and put to bed, elevate the bed to the highest horizontal height, and open the bed. Move furnishings, if necessary, so the stretcher can be positioned next to the bed.

When a patient is ready for admission, ask the nurse if:

- The patient requires a stretcher or wheelchair to reach the unit.
- Any special equipment, such as oxygen or a fracture bed, is needed.
- There are any special instructions, such as withholding fluids or foods.

Introduce yourself and observe the patient carefully. Listen for complaints as you escort and assist the patient to the room and to bed. Initial observations are very important. They become the basis of comparison for future observations.

The nurse will assess the patient on admission and begin a care plan. Your observations, and vital sign, height, and weight measurements, contribute to this assessment. You should also note and report your observations about:

- Rashes
- Bruises
- Pressure ulcers
- Other skin problems
- Vision problems
- Hearing problems
- Communication problems, including ability to make needs known and call for help
- Ability to ambulate and transfer safely
- Ability to use the bathroom safely

Inform the nurse and document your findings on the admission record, or according to facility policy.

Offer to assist in unpacking and storing the patient's belongings. Complete the personal belongings inventory, if used by your facility, and ask the patient to sign it. Fill in all the forms for which you are responsible on admission, and make the patient and family as comfortable as possible.

If it is necessary to ask visitors to leave, do so in a kind and polite manner. They will be most anxious to remain and see the patient settled and comfortable, so

- Show them where they may wait.
- Let them know about how long they will have to wait.
- Tell them where they can get refreshments.
- Answer questions they may have about where to find a chapel and telephones, and visiting hours.
- After you have completed your part of the admission procedure, locate visitors and let them know they may return to the patient's room.

The nursing assistant is frequently the person who admits patients to the facility. This may be a difficult, stressful, frightening time for the patient. There is a common expression that "first impressions are usually lasting ones." The patient's perception of what is happening may be affected by illness, pain, and fear (Figure 22-1). Making a good first impression on the patient and family members is important. If the first impression of the nursing assistant is negative, this affects the patient's impression of all health care workers, and even the whole facility. Think about this and do your best to provide a positive, professional impression.

FAMILY DYNAMICS

The family is an extension of the patient. They must make many adjustments when the patient is admitted to the hospital. Admitting a loved one can be a very emotional time. Family members may feel relieved because the patient is getting help. They may also feel guilty for being unable to care for the loved one at home. Other common emotions family members experience are:

- Fear—Some family members will feel fearful and afraid to leave their relative in the facility.
- Anger—Some families become angry about the admission. This is usually because they feel a loss of control. However, occasionally they may take their anger out on the staff.
- Uncertainty—The family may feel uncertain about what will become of their loved one, causing them to feel afraid, worried, nervous, and tense (Figure 22-2).
- Sadness—The family may have difficulty coping with being separated from the patient.
- Guilt—The family may feel guilty for turning the care of the patient over to complete strangers. They may compensate by staying at the hospital most of the time to care for and protect the patient.

FIGURE 22-1 Treat patients and families with courtesy, respect, compassion, and understanding. Remember that admissions can be stressful for both the patient and family. First impressions are lasting ones, and you represent your facility to the patient.

FIGURE 22-2 Families experience a wide range of emotions when a loved one is admitted to the hospital. Use good communication skills and show that you care.

FIGURE 22-3 Families often worry about the patient's well-being and may fear a negative outcome.

- Helplessness—Family members may feel helpless because the patient's condition has worsened, and despite their best efforts, they cannot change the situation.
- Worry—Family members worry about their loved one's well-being (Figure 22-3). They may have other worries and demands on them, such as how to pay the bills, or what to do with the house or pets. They often feel overwhelmed with the decisions and responsibilities.

Understanding the emotions that families experience should give you an appreciation of why making a good first impression is so important. In addition, you must use good communication skills and show that you care. Greet each family member with warmth, courtesy, kindness, and respect. Introduce yourself and explain your responsibilities as a nursing assistant in the care of their loved one (Figure 22-4). Introduce the patient and family to roommates and other staff members. Make them feel welcome and show that you are sincerely interested in the patient.

FIGURE 22-4 Make it a point to speak to family members when they visit. Treat each family member with warmth, courtesy, kindness, and respect.

If appropriate, make comments such as, "I know this must be very difficult for you." Admission to the hospital does not have to be a negative experience. A competent, caring, professional staff will calm family members' fears and turn a potentially negative experience into a positive one.

Culture ALERT

The patient's religion may affect important issues, including admission to the hospital. In some cultures, patients are cared for at home. Other issues that may be affected by culture are consent to treatment, routines, schedules of care, bathing and toileting routines, food preferences, room arrangements (because of certain religious practices), and birth and death practices. Look for clues to the patient's practices and beliefs, such as making eye contact, wearing or displaying religious items, or maintaining a certain distance from others. ■

TRANSFER

It may be necessary for the patient to be moved to another unit. Preparations for the **transfer** will be handled by the nurse, but you may be asked to assist. (See Procedure 47.)

The transfer may be the patient's own preference, or may be done because a change in the patient's condition requires a different type of care. The transfer may be temporary or permanent. If it is permanent, the patient is discharged from one unit, then admitted to another. The patient may or may not fully understand the reasons for

GUIDELINES *for*

Family Dynamics

- Get to know family members. Greet them warmly when they visit.
- Wear a name badge. Introduce yourself by name and position.
- Work to build a positive and trusting relationship with family members.
- Be available to talk to the family. Tell them about the patient's activities, as appropriate. Listen carefully to what they have to say and respond appropriately.
- Let the family know that you respect and support their role as their loved one's caregivers.
- Familiarize the family with facility routines and services.
- Refer questions of a medical or personal nature to the nurse.
- Listen to family members' suggestions, complaints, and comments. Inform the nurse of family complaints or concerns, or refer the family to the nurse, as appropriate.
- If the family has been caring for the patient at home, they often know what works best. Listen closely to family members' advice about patient care. Pass the information on to the nurse.
- Inform the nurse if a visit is stressful or tiring to a patient.
- Avoid judging the family and decisions they make. Stay out of family disagreements.
- Avoid gossiping with the family, and do not discuss facility business with family members.
- Allow the family to participate in the patient's care, if the patient does not object. However, avoid making the family feel as if they must provide care for the patient.

Age-Appropriate Care ALERT

Pediatric patients may fear separation from the parents. Explain the unit policies for visiting or rooming in. Orient the child and family to the playroom, bathroom, and other areas as appropriate. Speak directly to the child. Show the child how to use the signal to call for help. Ask him or her questions about normal routines. Allow the child to respond before questioning the parents. A primary goal on admission is to make the child and parents as comfortable as possible, relieving anxiety about separation. ■

Safety ALERT

Never leave the room until the patient is safe, has the call signal in reach, and knows how to use it. ■

Communication HIGHLIGHT

Knowing when and how to ask a visitor to leave the room takes tact and diplomacy. Consult the nurse if you are unsure of how to handle a visitor situation. Try to schedule your care for when the patient is alone, if this is possible. If not, ask visitors to leave any time the patient's body will be exposed or a procedure will be performed. If the patient requests that the visitor be allowed to stay, honor the request. However, do not ask the patient if he would like the visitor to stay in the presence of others. For an infant or young child patient, parents are generally permitted to remain in the room during procedures. Some adolescent and teenage children will be uncomfortable if parents remain in the room during personal care. Ask the parents to leave the room unless the child asks that they be allowed to stay. ■

the transfer. Be positive and supportive. Recognize that the patient may be feeling very anxious. It would be helpful to know what the patient has been told about the reasons for the transfer. You may learn this from the nurse and by carefully listening to what your patient says.

PROCEDURE

46

ADMITTING THE PATIENT

1. Wash hands.

2. Assemble equipment:
   - Equipment for urine specimen collection
   - Equipment for taking temperature
   - Pad and pencil
   - Patient's chart or worksheet
   - Stethoscope
   - Admission kit
     - water pitcher
     - glass
     - liquid soap
     - washcloth
     - towel
     - basin
     - lotion
     - mouthwash
   - Scale
   - Blood pressure cuff and manometer
   - Watch with second hand
   - Disposable gloves (if urine specimen is required)

3. Prepare the unit for the patient by:
   a. Making sure that all necessary equipment and furniture are in their proper places and in good working order.

   b. Checking the unit for adequate lighting.
   c. Loosening the top linen at the foot of the bed. This is called a *toe pleat*.
   d. Opening the bed (Figure 22-5).

4. Identify the patient both by asking the name and checking the identification bracelet.
   a. Introduce yourself.
   b. Take the patient and the patient's family to the unit.
   c. Do not appear to rush the patient.
   d. Be courteous and helpful to the patient and the family.

5. Ask the patient to be seated, if ambulatory.
   a. Ask the family to go to the lounge or lobby while the patient is being admitted.
   b. Introduce the patient to the other patients in the room, unless it is a private room.
   c. As permitted, explain what will happen in the next hour.

6. Screen the unit to provide privacy (Figure 22-6).

7. Help the patient to undress and put on a hospital gown or night clothes from home. Care for clothing according to facility policy.

FIGURE 22-5 An open bed notifies everyone that a patient is expected.

FIGURE 22-6 Provide privacy so the patient can undress.

continues

PROCEDURE 46 CONTINUED

PATIENT PREFERS TO BE ADDRESSED AS:

_____

FROM: ☐ E.R.   ☐ E.C.F.   ☐ HOME   ☐ M.D.'S OFFICE

COMMUNICATES IN ENGLISH: ☐ WELL   ☐ MINIMAL

☐ INTERPRETER (NAME PERSON)   ☐ NONE

_____

MODE OF TRANSPORTATION:

☐ AMBULATORY   ☐ OTHER   **SMOKER:** ☐ Y ☐ N

☐ WHEELCHAIR   _____

☐ STRETCHER   _____

☐ NOT AT ALL   ☐ OTHER LANGUAGE (SPECIFY) _____

HOME TELEPHONE NO. (   ) _____

WORK TELEPHONE NO. (   ) _____

ORIENTATION TO ENVIRONMENT:

☐ ARMBAND CHECKED   ☐ CALL LIGHT

☐ BED CONTROL   ☐ PHONE

☐ TV CONTROL   ☐ SIDE RAIL POLICY

☐ BATH ROOM   ☐ VISITATION POLICY

☐ PERSONAL PROPERTY POLICY   ☐ SMOKING POLICY

PERSONAL BELONGINGS: (CHECK AND DESCRIBE)

☐ CLOTHING _____

☐ JEWELRY _____

☐ MONEY _____

☐ WALKER _____

☐ WHEELCHAIR _____

☐ CANE _____

☐ OTHER _____

DENTURES: **CONTACT LENSES:**

☐ UPPER   ☐ PARTIAL   ☐ HARD   ☐ LT   ☐ RT

☐ LOWER   ☐ NONE   ☐ SOFT

GLASSES: ☐ Y ☐ N   **HEARING AID:** ☐ Y ☐ N

PROSTHESIS: ☐ Y ☐ N

(DESCRIBE) _____

DISPOSITION OF VALUABLES:

☐ PATIENT

☐ HOME   GIVEN TO: _____

RELATIONSHIP: _____

☐ PLACED
IN SAFE _____

(CLAIM NO.)

IN CASE OF EMERGENCY NOTIFY:

NAME: _____

RELATIONSHIP: _____

HOME TELEPHONE NO. (   ) _____

WORK TELEPHONE NO. (   ) _____

VITAL SIGNS

TEMP: _____ ☐ ORAL   ☐ RECTAL   ☐ AXILLARY

PULSE: _____ ☐ RADIAL   ☐ APICAL   RESPIRATORY
RATE _____

☐ RT

B/P: _____ ☐ LT ☐ STANDING ☐ SITTING   ☐ LYING

HEIGHT: _____ WEIGHT: _____   ☐ BEDSIDE

☐ STANDING

ALLERGIES:

MEDICATIONS: ☐ NONE KNOWN   FOOD: ☐ NONE KNOWN

☐ PENICILLIN   ☐ TAPE   (SHELLFISH, EGGS, MILK, ETC.)

☐ SULFA   ☐ OTHER (LIST) _____

☐ IODINE   _____   _____

☐ ASPIRIN   _____   _____

☐ MORPHINE   _____   _____

☐ DEMEROL   _____   _____

(PRESCRIPTIVE & NON PRESCRIPTIVE)
MEDICATIONS: **DOSE/FREQUENCY**   (DATE/TIME)
LAST DOSE

1. _____   _____   _____
2. _____   _____   _____
3. _____   _____   _____
4. _____   _____   _____
5. _____   _____   _____
6. _____   _____   _____

DISPOSITION OF MEDICATIONS:

☐ NONE BROUGHT TO HOSPITAL

☐ SENT HOME _____

WITH _____

☐ TO PHARMACY: (LIST)

_____

_____

ADMITTING DIAGNOSIS: _____

NURSE'S SIGNATURE: _____ RN/LVN   DATE _____ TIME _____

CHARTER SUBURBAN HOSPITAL
16453 SOUTH COLORADO AVENUE
PARAMOUNT, CALIFORNIA 90723
NURSING ADMISSION ASSESSMENT PAGE 1 of 6

FIGURE 22-7 Recording accurate and complete admission information is an important contribution to the nursing assessment.

continues

PROCEDURE 46 CONTINUED

8. Check the patient's vital signs, weight, and height.

9. Help the patient get into bed. Adjust the side rails as needed.

10. If the patient is wearing any jewelry or has valuables:

    a. Make a list of them and ask the patient to sign it. This protects the facility and the patient.

    b. Ask the relatives also to sign the list and take the valuables home, or

    c. After checking and signing, give them to the nurse to put in the hospital safe.

11. Tell the patient if a urine specimen is necessary.

    a. Put on gloves and assist the patient as necessary.

    b. Allow the patient to use the bathroom, if ambulatory, or offer the bedpan or urinal.

12. Pour the patient's specimen from the bedpan or urinal into the specimen bottle. Apply the cap. Remove gloves and dispose of them according to facility policy. Be sure to label the specimen correctly (see Unit 45).

13. An admission form is usually completed at this time (Figure 22-7). Vital information includes:
    - Observations
    - Vital signs (TPR, BP, height, weight)
    - Known allergies
    - Medications being taken
    - Food preferences and dislikes

14. If admission is to a long-term care facility, label clothing and complete the personal belongings inventory form according to facility policy.

15. Orient the patient to the unit by explaining:
    - Visiting hours
    - How to use the telephone and/or television
    - How to use the call system for assistance
    - How to operate the bed and light switches, as appropriate
    - Standard hospital regulations
    - Television rental procedures, if applicable
    - Any questions about facility routines
    - When meals and refreshments are provided

16. Carry out ending procedure actions.

PROCEDURE

TRANSFERRING THE PATIENT

1. Find out which unit the patient will be transferred to. Check to see that it is ready.

2. Learn from the nurse in charge the method of transfer. Get the necessary vehicle (wheelchair, stretcher, or patient's own bed).

3. Check to see if any equipment is to be transferred with the patient.

4. Carry out initial procedure actions.

5. Explain to the patient what you are doing.

6. Gather all the patient's belongings together.

    a. Place disposables in a paper bag to transport with you.

    b. Check against clothes list.

7. Assist the patient to put on robe and slippers, if permitted. Assist the patient into wheelchair or stretcher, as directed. The entire bed is often used. Make sure the side rails are up during transport.

8. Obtain from the nurse:
    - Patient's chart
    - Nursing care plan
    - Medications
    - Paper bag

9. Transport the patient and his belongings to the new unit (Figure 22-8). Use all precautions related to safe transport.

continues

PROCEDURE 47 CONTINUED

10. Give any transferred medications, the nursing care plan, and the chart to the nurse in charge.

11. Introduce the patient to staff. Proceed to the patient's room.

12. Assist staff in helping the patient into bed. Assist in putting away the patient's belongings and helping the patient to get settled.

13. Before leaving the unit, carry out ending procedure actions.

FIGURE 22-8 Transfer the patient calmly and efficiently. Never leave the patient unattended.

All details must be taken care of according to facility policy. Following facility policy ensures that there is no interruption of health care services. Some facilities have transportation services for transferring patients.

After the new unit has been notified and prepared for the move, you will:

- Tell the patient what you are doing.
- Gather the patient's belongings. Explain to the patient what you are doing.
- If the patient is expected to return to the unit, you may be asked to gather only a few belongings, such as glasses, dentures, and toiletries.
- Get the patient's medicines, chart, and other personal data from the nurse.
- Assist in the physical transfer (Figure 22-9).
- Give the records and medication directly to the nurse on the new unit.
- Make sure the patient is safe and comfortable in the new environment before you return to your own unit.

Safety ALERT

Never leave the patient, the records, or medications unattended. ■

DISCHARGE

In recent years, the cost of health care has increased steadily. A government program known as *diagnosis-related groups* (*DRGs*) was introduced to control hospital costs. Hospitals are paid a specific amount of money for the care of an individual who has a particular condition or disease that is covered by a DRG.

FIGURE 22-9 Use a cart to transfer the patient's belongings, to avoid injury to your back.

If the hospital can provide the needed care and discharge the patient early, the hospital saves money and may keep the difference between the actual expenses and the DRG allotted payment. If the patient requires a longer hospital stay than is stated by the DRGs and the costs are higher, the hospital absorbs the additional cost. These standards do not apply to private patients. They apply to patients whose care is being paid for by the federal government, such as Medicare patients.

DRGs were developed for Medicare patients, but they are used today by all insurance companies to determine how many hospital days they will pay for. This has resulted in sicker patients being discharged from acute care facilities sooner.

Following hospitalization, many patients are discharged to subacute units or to long-term care facilities for further care, or to home to finish recuperation.

The discharge procedure is usually simple if the patient is going to another facility. The social worker and nurse relay information to the receiving facility. The patient and the patient's belongings are sent to the new facility. Discharge to the patient's home is more complicated and requires a number of actions called *discharge planning* (covered in Unit 34).

The Discharge Process

The **discharge**, or authorized release, of a patient requires a written order from the physician. If a patient indicates an intention to leave without an order, report it to the nurse immediately. He or she will make the necessary arrangements. Health care facilities have special policies that must be followed in these cases.

The patient should be spared any fatigue or unnecessary delay when being routinely discharged. (See Procedure 48.) You can help if you:

- Check with the nurse to make sure that the physician has written an order for discharge before preparing the patient.

PROCEDURE

48

DISCHARGING THE PATIENT

1. Check to be sure the physician has ordered the patient to be discharged. If a discharge order has not been written, check with the nurse before proceeding.

2. Carry out initial procedure actions.

3. Assemble equipment:
   - Wheelchair
   - Cart to transport items

4. Help the patient to dress, if necessary.

5. Collect the patient's personal belongings.
   a. Pack, if necessary.
   b. Check valuables against the admission list according to facility policy.
   c. Make sure that all of the patient's belongings have been removed from the closet and bedside stand.
   d. Check to see if medications or other equipment are to be sent home with the patient.
   e. Verify that the patient has received discharge instructions from the nurse, physician, or discharge coordinator.

6. Tell the patient or a member of the family how to collect valuables from the facility safe, if applicable.

7. Help the patient into a wheelchair.

8. Take the patient to the discharge entrance of the facility.
   a. Help the patient to transfer safely into the vehicle.
   b. Be gracious as you say goodbye.

9. Return the wheelchair.

10. Return to the patient unit.
    a. Strip the bed. Dispose of linen according to facility policy.
    b Clean and replace equipment used in patient care, according to facility policy.

11. Wash your hands.

12. Record the discharge in accordance with facility policy. Include:
    - Time
    - Method of transport
    - Patient's reaction
    - Signature

13. Report completion of task to the nurse.

- Gather all the patient's belongings and assist in packing, if necessary. Patients who are well enough usually prefer to assemble their own things. You will need to do this activity completely for other patients.
- Carefully check the closet and bedside table. Disposable equipment is often sent home with the patient. If this is the policy in your facility, be sure that the equipment is clean.
- After gathering all the patient's belongings, check them against the personal inventory record or clothing list, and have the patient sign the receipt.

- Check with the nurse for any medications or other treatment-related equipment that should be sent home with the patient.
- Verify that the patient has received discharge instructions from the nurse, physician, or discharge coordinator.
- Never allow a patient to leave the health care facility unassisted. The patient is the staff's responsibility until she has left the building.

REVIEW

A. True/False.

Mark the following true or false by circling T or F.

1. T F When transferring a patient, it is all right to leave the patient unattended and return immediately to your own unit.
2. T F Use all precautions related to safe transport when admitting or discharging a patient.
3. T F You do not need to waste time introducing a new patient to others, because facility stays are very short anyway.
4. T F It is all right to allow patients to leave a health care facility at any time.
5. T F After discharge, the patient's unit is stripped, cleaned, and restocked.
6. T F The patient's unit should be prepared as soon as you are notified that there will be an admission.
7. T F During a transfer, the patient's medications remain on the original unit.
8. T F Measuring the patient's height and weight is part of the admission procedure.
9. T F The discharge order is written by the physician.
10. T F You should observe the patient carefully during the admission procedure.

B. Multiple Choice.

Select the one best answer for each of the following.

11. The assistant can do much to help facilitate the admission procedure by
    a. preparing equipment after the patient arrives on the unit.
    b. letting the nurse make all the observations.
    c. giving attention to the details of the procedure.
    d. recognizing that admission to the facility causes more anxiety to the staff than to the patient.

12. When dealing with the newly admitted patient's family, you should
    a. treat them with courtesy and consideration.
    b. send them home.
    c. let the nurse deal with them.
    d. allow them to stay at the patient's bedside at all times.

13. Part of the admission procedure includes
    a. securing a stool specimen.
    b. obtaining a sputum specimen.
    c. working in a hurried manner so the patient knows you are efficient.
    d. measuring vital signs.

14. Valuables that accompany the patient to her unit should be
    a. taken away.
    b. listed and signed for.
    c. left in the bedside stand.
    d. tucked under the pillow for safety.

15. When a patient is transferred, you should always include his
    a. personal belongings.
    b. bed.
    c. pillow.
    d. blood pressure cuffs.

C. Nursing Assistant Challenge.

Mrs. Leon is being admitted because her emphysema is making it very difficult for her to breathe. She is accompanied by her husband and both are obviously nervous. The next morning, her condition worsens. She is moved to the intensive respiratory care unit. Answer the following questions yes or no.

16. _____ The anxiety of the patient and family is not natural.

17. _____ You should answer questions about facility routines during admission.

18. _____ When taking vital signs, you should use an oral thermometer.

19. _____ When Mrs. Leon is transferred, take all of her personal articles with her.

20. _____ One way to prepare the unit for admission might include checking for the need for oxygen.

21. _____ You should turn Mrs. Leon's oxygen up to at least 6 liters to assist with her breathing.

UNIT 23

Bedmaking

OBJECTIVES

After completing this unit, you will be able to:
- Spell and define terms.
- List the different types of beds and their uses.
- Operate each type of bed.
- Properly handle clean and soiled linens.

- Demonstrate the following procedures:
  - Procedure 49 Making a Closed Bed
  - Procedure 50 Opening the Closed Bed
  - Procedure 51 Making an Occupied Bed
  - Procedure 52 Making the Surgical Bed

VOCABULARY

Learn the meaning and the correct spelling of the following words and phrases:

box (square) corner	electric bed	low bed	open bed
closed bed	gatch bed	mitered corner	toepleat

INTRODUCTION

The room, especially the bed, is the patient's home while he or she is in the health care facility. A well-made bed offers both comfort and safety. It is an extremely important contribution to the well-being of the patient.

OPERATION AND USES OF BEDS IN HEALTH CARE FACILITIES

The types of beds and the methods used to operate them may vary in different health care facilities, but the basic principles of bedmaking are the same. The most common beds are the:

- **Gatch bed**—a stationary bed about 26 inches high. Modern facilities are equipped with beds that can be raised to the desired height for bedside nursing or low-ered to 13 inches to accommodate the out-of-bed patient. The position of the head and knee areas of the bed can be adjusted for comfort. This operation may be done manually by turning the cranks. Most hospitals have eliminated these beds. Some long-term care facilities continue to use them, although they are being phased out because they increase the risk of employee back injury.

- **Electric bed**—a bed similar to the gatch bed, in that it can be raised or lowered and the knee and head areas can be adjusted. It is operated electrically (Figure 23-1). You will be using this bed most often.

- **Low bed**—low beds (Figure 23-2) are commonly used in health care facilities for patients who are at risk of falls, for whom use of side rails is not desirable. The bed frame is 4 to 6 inches from the floor to the top of the frame deck. These beds reduce the risk of injury if the patient falls from the bed. Some facilities place pads on the floor next to the bed to further reduce the risk of injury.

FIGURE 23-1 The typical hospital bed is electronically operated. The head and foot can be adjusted for patient comfort. The height of the bed can be raised, making it easier to give care.

FIGURE 23-2 Low beds are often used for patients who are at high risk for falls. Organize the bedmaking procedure carefully to prevent back injury. (Courtesy of Skil-Care Corporation, Yonkers, NY, (800) 431-2972)

Low beds are wonderful tools for reducing patient injuries, but the nursing assistant must use good body mechanics and common sense to prevent back injuries when lifting, moving, and caring for patients, and when making beds. Some low beds have high/low features, but many are stationary, which increases workers' risk of back injury. If the bed you are using has a high/low feature, use it whenever caring for the bedfast patient, transferring the patient, or making the bed. A pad or mat on the floor reduces the risk of injury when a patient falls, but it can also be a trip hazard. Fold it and store it under the bed or according to facility policy when the patient is out of bed. Move slowly and carefully when working near a floor mat. Avoid entering the room in the dark. Leave a nightlight on, or turn the light on when entering. Squat or kneel on the floor mat when caring for the patient to reduce back strain caused by bending at the waist. Use good body mechanics, a transfer belt, or a ceiling or mechanical lift when assisting patients into and out of low beds, to prevent back injuries. The care plan will provide patient-specific instructions. Avoid bending at the waist when moving the patient.

Other types of beds are available for the treatment of patients with multiple or advanced pressure ulcers, flaps, grafts, burns, and intractable pain. For example, the Clinitron bed (Figure 23-3) is filled with a sand-like material. Warm, dry air circulates through the material to maintain an even temperature and support the body evenly.

A low air loss bed (Figure 23-4) provides pressure relief for patients who have pressure ulcers, those who are at risk of pressure ulcers, and some patients with burns. This mattress is designed to keep the patient cooler and drier than other types of beds. Low air loss beds reduce pressure on

FIGURE 23-3 Clinitron® therapy is used to provide comfort and faster healing of multiple pressure ulcers, flaps, grafts, burns, management of extensive skin disorders or fresh surgical wounds. The bed reduces the potential for friction and shear. It can be defluidized rapidly if CPR is necessary. (Courtesy of Hill-Rom, Charelston, S.C.)

FIGURE 23-4 The low air loss bed is used for pressure ulcer prevention and treatment. Although the specialty beds exert less presssure on the skin than a regular mattress, patients must be turned and repositioned frequently to prevent skin breakdown. (Courtesy of Hill-Rom, Charelston, S.C.)

Safety ALERT

Become familiar with the features of the low air loss beds used by your facility. Some have bed scales built in, making it possible to weigh the patient without moving her from the bed. CPR is not effective in a low air loss bed, even with a back board. The beds have an emergency switch that rapidly deflates the air pillows in the event CPR is necessary. This enables the users to do CPR by using the hard metal frame instead of a back board or CPR board. Become familiar with the location and operation of the features of the bed. ■

OSHA ALERT

Elevating the bed to a working height that is comfortable for you takes a minute, but it is one of the most important things you can do to protect your back. Stay on one side of the bed until it is completely made before moving to the other side. This helps organize your time and conserves energy. Avoid moving quickly. Studies have shown that rapid motion increases the risk of injury. To reduce stress on your low back, remove soiled linen a few pieces at a time, rather than in a large bundle all at once. Keep your spine straight and use good body mechanics. Make beds with a partner, if possible. ■

GUIDELINES *for*
Handling Linens and Making the Bed

Handling Linens

1. Wash hands and use gloves if necessary; other personal protective equipment may also be required.

2. Laundry hampers placed in the hallway should be placed at least one room away from clean linen carts, or according to facility policy.

3. The clean linen cart is always covered; replace the cover after removing required linen.

4. Take only the linens you need into the patient's room.

5. Unused linen is never returned to the clean linen cart; it is placed in the laundry hamper.

6. Linens that touch the floor are considered dirty and are placed in the laundry hamper; they are not used.

7. Avoid contact between the linens and your uniform (for both clean and soiled linens).

8. As soiled linen is removed from the bed, keep the soiled areas on the inside and fold or roll the linen toward the center.

9. Never shake bed linens, because microbes will be released into the air.

10. Soiled linen is never placed on environmental surfaces in the room, such as the overbed table, chair, or floor; soiled linens are placed in the appropriate laundry hamper (follow facility policy).

11. Fill laundry hampers no more than two-thirds full. Keep the lid of the hamper on tightly at all times.

12. Many facilities do not permit laundry hampers or barrels to be taken into the patient's room. Soiled linen may be placed in a plastic bag or a pillowcase in the room. Make a cuff at the top of the bag or open end of the pillowcase and place the cuff over the back of the chair. When the bag or case is two-thirds full, secure the top and place it in the hamper in the hallway.

13. Laundry hampers or barrels are returned to the utility room after use, or as directed by facility policy.

Making the Bed

1. Use proper body mechanics at all times to prevent back injury.

2. Work on one side of the bed at a time to complete removal of soiled linen and placement of clean linen.

3. Make sure the bottom sheet and draw sheet (if used) are smooth and unwrinkled (wrinkles in bed linens can lead to discomfort and skin breakdown, especially for patients who must remain in bed).

4. Follow the care plan for positioning the head and foot of the bed, the number of pillows to be used, and the use of pillows for positioning.

GUIDELINES *for*
Low Beds

Caring for and making the low bed is very similar to making a regular hospital bed. However, certain adaptations must be made to reduce your risk of injury. You should:

1. Mentally plan and prepare yourself for the procedure.
2. Use good body mechanics.
3. Organize your work well to reduce the total number of motions required to complete the task.
4. Make sure you have everything you need before entering the room.
5. Elevate the bed, if possible.
6. Place linen and needed items on the patient's chair or within close reach.

7. Maintain a neutral posture and bend from the legs, not the waist. Avoid twisting.
8. You may squat, sit, or kneel on the plastic mat next to the bed if doing so is easier for you and helps keep your spine straight.
9. Slowly remove the bed linen several pieces at a time. Avoid trying to remove all the linen in one bundle. The weight of the linen and your posture increase the risk of back injury.
10. Make one side of the bed at a time. This is faster, more efficient, and conserves energy.
11. Use a fitted bottom sheet to reduce the number of movements necessary for making the bed, thereby lowering the risk of back strain.

the patient's skin, and reduce friction and shearing, which contribute to skin breakdown. These beds use a system of air-filled pillows in which inflation pressure can be adjusted so the characteristics of the support surface are matched to those of the body being supported. The pillows can be inflated and deflated to adjust the level of pressure relief. The design of the bed allows slight air escape upon movement, which reduces pressure.

Patients using a low air loss bed must still be turned and positioned regularly to prevent skin breakdown, which can occur despite the pressure-reducing mattress. Avoid tucking the bottom sheet in tightly, as this increases pressure within the bed. Some facilities use these beds with special nylon covers only, without sheets. These are similar to fitted bottom sheets, but they are thicker and made of nylon. They require special handling and air drying in the laundry, so your facility will have several for each bed. Check to make sure an extra cover is available before routinely changing the bed. The nylon cover reduces friction and shearing. Follow the care plan and facility policies. Special underpads are used with the low air loss bed.

Correct operation of any bed or equipment is important for patient safety. Always seek help and instruction from the nurse or another health care professional when using any specialized beds. Never try to operate any bed or equipment with a patient in it without first practicing and gaining security and skill in the procedures. Although different types of hospital beds may be similar in design, the operating instructions vary. For safety, always follow the manufacturers' directions in operating the various therapeutic beds.

Bedmaking

Bed linen is always changed when soiled. It is routinely changed:

Safety ALERT

Be alert when removing bed linen. Look carefully for items that are a potential source of injury to yourself or the patient, such as lancets and needles. Make sure the patient's personal items are not accidentally sent to the laundry with the bed linen. It is not unusual to find a patient's glasses, hearing aid, or dentures in the bed linen. These items are expensive and will not survive a trip through the washer and dryer. ▪

- Daily in the acute care facility.
- Two or three times a week in long-term care facilities.

Residents in long-term care may prefer to use their own pillows, blankets, and spreads.

Supplies for Bedmaking

You will need to gather supplies when making a bed. The supplies needed will vary slightly, depending on your facility policies and the type of bedmaking procedure you will be using. Gather and stack them in the order of use, so that the item used first is on top and the item used last is on the bottom. Bring only needed linen to the room. If linen is not used, it must be washed before it is returned to the unit linen supply for use by another patient. To do a complete linen change, you will need:

- *Mattress pad*, if used by the facility. A mattress pad is a heavy, quilted cotton pad. Mattress pads may be either flat or fitted to the mattress. A flat pad may have diagonal pieces of elastic across the corners to slip over the mattress to hold the pad in place. The purpose is to protect the mattress from spills, secretions, and excretions. Some facilities do not use mattress pads because the bed mattresses are covered with plastic or rubber, which protects the mattress. However, some patients become very hot and sweat profusely when lying on a plastic mattress that is covered only with a thin sheet. The sheet stays damp, which is uncomfortable for the patient and promotes skin breakdown. If heat and sweating are a problem for a patient, you can cover the mattress with one or two folded, cotton bath blankets, then apply the sheet.

- Two sheets. In some facilities, two large flat sheets are used to make each bed. Many facilities use a flat sheet on top and a fitted sheet on bottom. This type of sheet makes it easier to make the bed, and the bottom sheet does not slip or wrinkle as much with patient movement. If you must use a flat sheet to cover the mattress, make sure to tuck it in tightly. Check the sheet frequently for bedfast patients, and straighten or tighten it as often as needed for patient comfort. The top sheet is always a regular twin-bed-size flat sheet.
- *Rubber or plastic draw sheet*, if used by the facility. This is a half-size sheet placed over the center of the bed to reduce the number of changes needed for the bottom sheet. It is used for patients who are incontinent, and those who use the bedpan or urinal in bed. When a rubber or plastic draw sheet is used, it must always be covered with a regular linen draw sheet. Both sheets are tucked securely under the mattress.
- *Linen draw sheet*, or half sheet, if used by the facility. This sheet may be used with or without a protective plastic or rubber draw sheet underneath. The draw sheet is placed on the mattress between the lower shoulders to the area just below the buttocks. The purpose of this sheet is to protect the patient's skin from the waterproof sheet underneath. If the patient is incontinent, or a bedpan or urinal spills, the linen draw sheet is usually the only sheet that has to be changed. The draw sheet may also be used or folded to form a *lift* (or *lifting*) *sheet*, which makes it easier for the patient and staff if it is necessary to move the patient in bed.
- *Incontinent pad, underpad*, or *bed protector*. These items are soft, absorbent paper pads with a plastic backing or heavy cotton pad. The pads may also be called by their brand name, such as Chux. These pads are large, usually about 30 to 36 inches square. They are used to protect the bed linen for patients who are incontinent, use the bedpan or urinal when in bed, or have heavy drainage from a wound or surgical site. The reusable cotton pads are sometimes used in place of a lifting sheet. The paper incontinent pads are not suitable for this purpose. The incontinent pad is usually used in place of the rubber draw sheet covered with a linen draw sheet. If a patient is incontinent, this is often the only item that has to be changed, which is more efficient for staff and economical for the facility.

- *Pillow and pillowcase*. Hospitals use various types of pillows. Many are disposable, and are sent home with the patient or discarded. Some are reusable. The reusable pillows are usually covered with a plastic pillow protector. The pillow is always covered with a linen pillowcase. Some patients with special positioning needs will need several pillows to prop and support various areas of the body for alignment and comfort.
- *Bath blanket*. A bath blanket is a soft flannel or cotton blanket that is used for modesty and warmth during procedures in which the patient's body is exposed. It is usually folded and stored in the closet or bedside stand when not in use.
- *Regular blanket*. A thermal cotton blanket is applied to the bed for patient comfort and warmth.
- *Bedspread*. A bedspread may be used for a decorative touch and to give the room a neat appearance.

Some facilities use other special items, such as foam *mattress overlays* and *pressure-reducing pads* or *mattresses*, which reduce friction and shearing and provide extra padding to decrease the risk of skin breakdown. These are issued only to high-risk patients. Many foam pads lose their fire-retardant protection if they are washed and dried, so facilities use incontinent pads to protect them. They are usually covered with a flat linen sheet. The mattress is covered with a separate sheet.

Occasionally, facilities use other items, such as *bed boards*, to meet special patient needs. Bed boards are placed between the mattress and bed frame to offer extra-firm support to the patient's back. Bed cradles (Unit 25) may be used to keep the weight of the linen off the patient's skin. A *footboard* (Unit 25) may also be applied to the foot of the

Infection Control ALERT

Some people associate bedbugs with unsanitary living conditions. However, bugs have been found in very clean hospitals and hotels. The bugs adapt well to any environment where they can obtain a blood meal. Always watch for signs of bedbugs, such as small red or black dots on the bed linen and clothing, egg cases, and tiny shed skins. Look in cracks and crevices near the mattress and bed frame. Pay close attention to the area under the mattress seams. Bedbugs can also hide behind headboards and behind the molding or baseboard of the walls. Although they tend to live around beds, they may also hide in furniture, such as sofas and upholstered chairs. ■

bed for patients who have special positioning needs or are at risk for contractures.

Closed Bed

The **closed bed** is made following discharge of a patient and after the unit is cleaned (terminal cleaning). It remains closed until a new patient is admitted. Details are impor-tant. The same procedure is followed when making an unoccupied bed, but the bed is opened as a final step when a patient is to occupy it shortly. (Refer to Procedure 49.)

The Unoccupied Bed

Beds are often made while patients are up in a shower or chair. Follow the procedure for making a

---

PROCEDURE

MAKING A CLOSED BED

1. Wash your hands and assemble equipment:
   - 2 pillowcases
   - Pillow
   - Spread
   - Blankets, as needed
   - 2 large sheets (90" × 108") (substitute one fit-ted sheet, if used)
   - Cotton draw sheet or half sheet (if used)
   - Plastic or rubber draw sheet (if used in your facility)
   - Mattress pad and cover, if mattress is not plastic-treated

   Note: Mattresses that are treated with plastic do not require a moisture-proof sheet or cotton half sheet (draw sheet). In some cases, the half sheet is used as a lifter to assist in moving the patient. It is sometimes used simply to keep the bottom sheet clean. Some facil-ities use fitted bottom sheets. If this is so, use a fitted sheet in place of one of the large sheets.

2. Elevate the bed to a comfortable working height in the horizontal position. Lock bed wheels so the bed will not roll. Place a chair at the side of the bed.

3. Arrange the linen on the chair in the order in which it is to be used.

4. Position the mattress to the head of the bed by grasping the mattress handles (or the edge of the mattress, if no handles are present).

5. If used, place a mattress cover on the mattress. Adjust it smoothly for corners. You will work entirely from one side of the bed until that side is completed. Then go to the other side of the bed. This conserves time and energy.

6. Place the mattress pad even with the top of the mattress and unfold it.

7. Place the bottom sheet on the bed and unfold it, seam side down and wide hem at the top. The small hem should be brought to the foot of the mattress (Figure 23-5). The center fold should be at the center of the bed. If a fitted bottom sheet is used, fit it smoothly around one corner (Figure 23-6).

8. Tuck 12 to 18 inches of sheet smoothly over the top of the mattress (Figures 23-7A to C).

FIGURE 23-5 Place the flat bottom sheet even with the end of the mat-tress at the foot of the bed.

FIGURE 23-6 If a fitted bottom sheet is used, pull and smooth it around the corner.

continues

PROCEDURE 49 CONTINUED

FIGURE 23-7A Gather about 12 to 18 inches of the top sheet at the bottom of the bed.

FIGURE 23-7B Face the foot of the bed and lift the mattress with your near hand.

FIGURE 23-7C Bring the sheet smoothly over the end of the mattress with your opposite hand.

9. Make a **mitered corner** (Figure 23-8). The square corner, preferred by some facilities, is made in a way similar to the mitered corner.

10. Tuck in the sheet on one side, keeping the sheet straight. Work from the head to the foot of the bed. If using a fitted sheet, adjust it over the head and bottom ends of the mattress.

11. If used, place the plastic draw sheet and half sheet with upper edge about 14 inches from the head of the mattress and tuck under one side. Be sure that the half sheet covers the plastic sheet. It should cover the area from above the patient's shoulders to below the hips.

12. Unfold and place the top sheet on the bed, seam up, top hem even with the upper edge of the mattress and the center fold in the center of the bed.

13. Spread the blanket over the top sheet and foot of the mattress. Keep the blanket centered.

14. Make a **toe pleat** by folding the top linen over two to three inches at the end of the bed (Figure 23-9). The toe pleat provides extra space and keeps the linen from pulling the feet downward. This is more comfortable for the patient and reduces the risk of contractures.

FIGURE 23-8 Making a mitered corner. A. The sheet is hanging loose at the side of the bed. B. Pick up the sheet about 12 inches from the head of the bed to form a triangle. C. Tuck the sheet in at the head of the bed. Pick up the triangle and place your other hand at the edge of the bed near the head to hold the edge of the sheet in place. Bring the triangle over the edge of the mattress and tuck it smoothly under the mattress. Tuck in the rest of the sheet along the side of the mattress. Make sure the sheet is wrinkle-free.

continues

PROCEDURE 49 CONTINUED

FIGURE 23-9 The toe pleat provides space for movement of the feet. For bedfast patients, the extra space reduces the risk of contractures and pressure ulcers. The extra space is much more comfortable for all patients.

15. Tuck the top sheet and blanket under the mattress at the foot of the bed as far as the center only. Make a **box (square) corner** (Figures 23-10A to 23-C).

16. Place the spread with its top hem even with the head of the mattress. Unfold the spread to the foot of the bed.

17. Tuck the spread under the mattress at the foot of the bed and miter the corner. Sometimes the spread may be placed directly on top of the sheet. Rather than tucking the sheet, blanket, and/or spread under the end of the mattress separately and forming separate corners, all of the covers may be tucked under at the same time and one corner formed (Figures 23-11A to 23-11E).

18. Go to the other side of the bed. Fanfold the top covers to the center of the bed so you can work with the lower sheets and pad.

19. Tuck the bottom sheet under the head of the mattress and miter the corner. Working from top to bottom, smooth out all wrinkles and tighten these sheets as much as possible to provide comfort. (Adjust a fitted bottom sheet smoothly and securely around the mattress corners.)

20. Grasp the protective draw sheet (if used) and cotton draw sheet in the center. Tuck these sheets tightly under the mattress.

21. Tuck in the top sheet and blanket at the foot of the bed and miter the corner.

22. Fold the top sheet back over the blanket, making an 8-inch cuff.

FIGURE 23-10A Make the square (box) corner following the steps shown in Figures 23-10A to 23-10C. Then, holding the corner with your left hand, grasp the bottom of the sheet and pull it straight down until the fold is even with the edge of the mattress.

FIGURE 23-10B Holding the square corner in place, tuck the remaining sheet under the mattress.

FIGURE 23-10C The finished square corner should look like this.

PROCEDURE 49 CONTINUED

FIGURE 23-11A Gather the top sheet and bedspread together. Smooth evenly over the end of the mattress.

FIGURE 23-11B Tuck the sheet and spread under the mattress together.

FIGURE 23-11C Continue as with the procedure for a mitered corner.

FIGURE 23-11D Slide your finger to the end to make a smooth edge.

FIGURE 23-11E The completed top bedding. Repeat the procedure on the other side of the bed.

23. Tuck in the spread at the foot of the bed and miter the corner. Bring the top of the spread to the head of the mattress.

24. Insert the pillow into a pillowcase:

    a. Place your hands in the clean case, freeing the corners.

    b. Grasp the center of the end seam with a hand outside the case and turn the case back over your hand (Figure 23-12A).

    c. Grasp the pillow through the case at the center of one end. Pull the case over the pillow with your free hand (Figures 23-B and 23-C). (Do not allow the pillow to touch your uniform.)

FIGURE 23-12A Grasp the pillowcase at the seam and fold it back and over your wrist, inside out.

FIGURE 23-12B Grab the end of the pillow in the center with your pillowcase-covered hand.

FIGURE 23-12C Unfold and smooth the pillowcase over the pillow.

continues

PROCEDURE 49 CONTINUED

   d. Adjust the corners of the pillow to fit in the corners of the case.

25. Place the pillow at the head of the bed with the open end away from the door.

26. Lower the bed to the lowest horizontal position.

27. Arrange the room as follows:

   a. Replace the bedside table parallel to the bed. Place the chair in its assigned location.

   b. Place the overbed table over the foot of the bed opposite the chair.

   c. Place the signal cord within easy reach of the patient.

   d. Leave the side rails down.

   e. Check for possible hazards, such as gatch handles that are out of place.

28. Leave the unit neat and tidy.

29. Wash your hands.

30. Report completion of the task to the nurse.

Infection Control ALERT

Wear gloves when removing bed linen that is wet or soiled. Place the soiled linen in a plastic bag or linen hamper. Avoid contaminating environmental surfaces with gloves that have handled soiled linen. Remove one glove, if necessary. Follow facility policy for disinfecting the mattress. Allow it to dry. Discard your gloves and wash your hands. It is not necessary to wear gloves when you are handling clean linen. Cracks in the mattress are a potential source of odors and contamination. Report cracks in the mattress to the proper person in your facility. ■

FIGURE 23-13 Open the closed bed by drawing the bedding to the foot of the bed and fanfolding it.

Safety ALERT

Never turn your back on the patient or leave the bedside when the bed is in the high position and the side rail is down. ■

closed bed but then fanfold the top bedding three-fourths of the way down. This "opens" the bed and makes it easier for the person to get into it.

The Open Bed

The **open bed** is like a sign saying "welcome" to the new patient (Figure 23-13). It indicates that the patient's arrival has been made known to the assistant. It also shows that the unit has been prepared. (See Procedure 50.) In long-term care facilities, the bed is not opened unless the resident is going to bed soon.

The Occupied Bed

Unless the patient is permitted out of bed by physician's order, the bed is made with the patient in it. (See Procedure 51.) Bedmaking usually follows the bed bath, while the patient is covered with a bath blanket. It may, however, be done any time it would add to the comfort of the patient.

Surgical Bed

The surgical bed provides a safe, warm environment to receive the postsurgical patient. It must be made in such a way that movement from stretcher to bed can be done with maximum safety and minimum effort. For this reason, the bed should be left open and at stretcher height. (See Procedure 52.)

All equipment needed to monitor vital signs and to supervise recovery should be in place and ready for use. You should also keep alert for the patient's return so you can help make a safe transfer from stretcher to bed.

Modern surgical techniques have shortened the time many patients stay in an acute care facility after surgery. Patients are often admitted on the morning of surgery to special units, have the surgery performed, return to these same units immediately after surgery, and are discharged the same day to recuperate at home. These units are called ambulatory, short-term, or day-care units. To prepare a postsurgical bed in one of these units:

- Tighten the bottom linen.

- Fanfold the top linen to the side or foot of bed.
- Raise the bed to stretcher height and lock the wheels.
- Place the equipment to check vital signs, emesis basin, and tissues by the recovery bed.

PROCEDURE   **OBRA**

50

OPENING THE CLOSED BED

1. Wash your hands.
2. Check assignment for bed location.
3. Raise the bed to a comfortable working height in the horizontal position. Move the overbed table to one side.
4. Lock the bed wheels.
5. Loosen the top bedding.
6. Facing the head of the bed, grasp the top sheet and spread and fanfold the top bedding to the foot of the bed.

7. Return the bed to the lowest horizontal position. Place the overbed table over the foot of the bed.
8. Place the call bell near the pillow or within easy reach. It should be visible and within reach of the patient at all times.
9. Leave the unit neat and tidy.
10. Wash your hands.
11. Report completion of the task to the nurse.

PROCEDURE   **OBRA**

51

MAKING AN OCCUPIED BED

1. Carry out initial procedure actions.
2. Assemble the equipment needed:
   - Disposable gloves (if linens are soiled with blood, body fluids, secretions, or excretions)
   - Cotton draw sheet or turning sheet for selected patients
   - 2 large flat sheets (or one large flat sheet and one fitted bottom sheet)
   - 2 pillowcases
   - Laundry hamper
3. Place the bedside chair at the foot of the bed.
4. Arrange the clean linen on the chair in the order in which it is to be used.
5. The bed should be flat, with wheels locked, unless otherwise indicated. Raise the bed to working horizontal height. Lower the side rail on your side of the bed.

FIGURE 23-14 The patient grasps the head of the bed and pushes in with the heels while two nursing assistants pull the mattress to the head of the bed.

6. If the bed linens are soiled with blood or other body fluids, wash your hands and put on disposable gloves.

continues

PROCEDURE 51 CONTINUED

7. Loosen the bedclothes on your side by lifting the edge of the mattress with one hand and drawing the bedclothes out with the other. Never shake the linen. This spreads germs.

8. Put the side rail up and go to the opposite side of the bed.

9. Adjust the mattress to the head of the bed (Figure 23-14). Get help, if necessary.

10. Remove the top covers except for the top sheet, one at a time. Fold to bottom. Pick up in the center. Place them over the back of chair if they are to be reused.

    Note: Carefully check each piece of linen for foreign articles (such as patient care equipment, eyeglasses, dentures, items of food, or eating utensils). Remove any such items.

11. Place the clean sheet or bath blanket over the top sheet. Have the patient hold the top edge of the clean sheet if able. If the patient is unable to help, tuck the sheet beneath the patient's shoulder.

12. Slide the soiled sheet out, from top to bottom. Put it in a hamper or plastic bag.

13. Ask the patient to move to the side of the bed toward you. Assist if necessary. Move one pillow with the patient and remove the other pillow. Pull up the side rail. (Alternatively, you may ask the patient to turn toward the opposite side of the bed, holding onto the raised side rail. You would then fanfold the sheet, as in step 15, but there would be no need to go to the other side of the bed.)

14. Go to the other side of the bed. Fanfold the soiled cotton draw sheet, if used, and bottom sheet close to the patient (Figure 23-15).

15. Straighten the mattress pad. If the bottom sheet is to be changed, place a clean sheet on the bed so that the narrow hem comes to the edge of the mattress at the foot. The seamed side of the hem is toward the bed. The lengthwise center fold of the sheet is at the center of the bed. Fanfold the opposite side of the sheet close to the patient.

16. Tuck the top of the sheet under the head of the mattress.

17. Make a mitered corner.

18. Tuck the side of the sheet under the mattress, working toward the foot of the bed.

FIGURE 23-15 Fanfold the soiled bottom sheet to the center of the bed as close to the patient as possible. Note that the bottom linen is flat and the patient is positioned to the far side of the bed with the rail up.

19. Position a fresh draw sheet, if used. Tuck it under the mattress.

20. Ask or assist the patient to roll toward you, over the fanfolded linen. Move the pillow with the patient.

21. Raise the side rails. Test for security.

22. Go to the other side of the bed. Lower the side rail. Remove the soiled linen by rolling the edges inward. *Keep soiled linen away from your uniform.* Placed soiled linen in the hamper or plastic bag. (Raise the side rail if leaving the bedside.)

23. Remove gloves, if worn, and discard according to facility policy.

24. Wash your hands.

25. Pull the clean bottom sheet into place. Tuck it under the mattress at the head of the bed. Make a mitered corner.

26. Pull gently to eliminate wrinkles. Then tuck the side of the sheet under the mattress, working from top to bottom.

27. Pull the draw sheet smoothly into place. Tuck it firmly under the mattress.

28. Place the top sheet over the patient. Remove the bath blanket.

29. Complete the bed as an unoccupied bed. To reduce pressure on toes, make a toe pleat or grasp the top bedding over the toes and pull straight up. Some patients prefer not to have the blanket and top sheet or spread tucked in.

continues

PROCEDURE 51 CONTINUED

30. Assist the patient to turn on his or her back. Place a clean pillowcase on the pillow that is not being used. Replace that pillow. Change the other pillowcase.

31. Carry out ending procedure actions.

PROCEDURE

52

MAKING THE SURGICAL BED

1. Wash your hands.

2. Check assignment for unit location.

3. Assemble the following equipment:
- Disposable gloves (if linens are soiled with blood or body fluids)
- Articles for basic bed
- One extra draw sheet
- Bath blanket for warmth
- One protective (rubber or plastic) draw sheet (if used in facility)
- Roll of one-inch gauze bandage

4. Lock the bed.

5. Apply gloves if linen is wet or soiled with blood or body fluids.

6. Strip and discard used linen.

7. Remove gloves and discard according to facility policy.

8. Wash your hands.

9. Make the bottom foundation bed (steps 1–11 in Procedure 49). Repeat on the opposite side of the bed.

10. Place a protective draw sheet over the head of the mattress sheet. Cover with a cotton draw sheet. Miter the corners and tuck them in on the sides.

11. Place the top sheet, blanket, and spread in the usual manner. Do not tuck them in.

12. Fold the linen back at the foot of the bed even with the edge of the mattress.

13. Fanfold the upper covers and top sheet to the far side of the bed (Figure 23-16).

14. Tie a waterproof pillow to the head of the bed with gauze bandaging, or place it according to facility policy.

15. Arrange the bed so there is adequate room to position a stretcher next to it. Leave the bed locked and at the same height as a stretcher.

16. Check the unit for obvious hazards.

17. Leave the room neat and tidy.

18. Wash your hands.

19. Report completion of the task to the nurse.

FIGURE 23-16 Prepare the surgical bed by fanfolding the covers to the far side of the bed. Raise the bed to stretcher height.

REVIEW

A. True/False.

Mark the following true or false by circling T or F.

1. T F The patient is most comfortable in a closed bed.

2. T F The low bed is used to avoid patient injury from falls.

3. T F You should not attempt to operate a bed until you have been thoroughly supervised.

4. T F The closed bed is made after terminal cleaning is finished.

5. T F Bottom bed linen can be loosely tucked as long as there are no wrinkles when you have finished.

6. T F A mitered corner is tucked in, forming a triangle.

7. T F Shaking linen as you change the bed spreads germs.

8. T F The open bed is like a sign saying "welcome."

9. T F Before making an occupied bed, adjust the mattress to the head of the bed.

10. T F The side rail opposite you must be up as you make an occupied bed.

B. Multiple Choice.

Select the one best answer for each of the following.

11. Loosening the top bedding at the foot of the bed is done
   a. to improve the appearance of the bed.
   b. in unoccupied beds.
   c. as folds in the bottom sheet.
   d. to reduce pressure on the toes.

12. When making an unoccupied bed, make the
   a. entire bottom first.
   b. far side of the bottom and top first.
   c. near side of the entire bed first.
   d. far side of the bottom first.

13. Before making an unoccupied bed,
   a. elevate it to a comfortable working height.
   b. keep the bed at the lowest horizontal height.
   c. raise the head portion.
   d. raise the side rails on the opposite side.

14. Before making any bed, always
   a. raise the side rails.
   b. lower the bed to the lowest horizontal height.
   c. lock the bed wheels.
   d. raise the head of the bed.

15. Sheets should be smoothly tucked in over the head of the mattress
   a. 5 to 7 inches.
   b. 12 to 18 inches.
   c. 20 to 24 inches.
   d. 26 to 30 inches.

16. If a draw sheet or lift sheet is used, it should be placed so that it covers the area under the patient's
   a. head and shoulders.
   b. heels and lower legs.
   c. buttocks only.
   d. shoulders to buttocks.

17. When placing the case on the pillow,
   a. tuck it under your chin.
   b. lay the pillow on the chair.
   c. pull the case over while grasping the pillow with the opposite hand.
   d. lay the pillow on the bedside stand.

18. When opening a closed bed,
   a. fanfold top bedding to the foot.
   b. loosen all top bedding.
   c. leave the bed at its highest horizontal height.
   d. raise the head of the bed.

19. The top bedding in a surgical bed is
   a. untucked and draped.
   b. tucked in on two sides.
   c. untucked and fanfolded.
   d. made without a blanket.

20. A common element in all bedmaking is
   a. fanfolding the linen.
   b. leaving the unit neat and tidy.
   c. leaving the bed in the high position.
   d. using the same linen and equipment.

C. Nursing Assistant Challenge.

21. You are assigned to make a closed bed. You have washed your hands and assembled the following equipment: pillow, blanket, spread, mattress pad, and mattress cover. What else will you need?

UNIT 24

Patient Bathing

OBJECTIVES

After completing this unit, you will be able to:
- Spell and define terms.
- Describe the safety precautions for patient bathing.
- List the purposes of bathing patients.
- State the value of whirlpool baths.
- Demonstrate the following procedures:
  - Procedure 53 Assisting with the Tub Bath or Shower
  - Procedure 54 Bed Bath
  - Procedure 55 Changing the Patient's Gown
  - Procedure 56 Waterless Bed Bath
  - Procedure 57 Partial Bath
  - Procedure 58 Female Perineal Care
  - Procedure 59 Male Perineal Care
  - Procedure 60 Hand and Fingernail Care
  - Procedure 61 Bed Shampoo
  - Procedure 62 Dressing and Undressing the Patient

VOCABULARY

Learn the meaning and the correct spelling of the following words and phrases:

axilla
cuticle

genitalia
perineal care

perineum
pubic

INTRODUCTION

A daily bath is as important for the patient as it is for you. Following the bath, the patient feels relaxed, clean, and refreshed. A bath with warm water and mild soap:
- Removes dirt and perspiration
- Increases circulation
- Provides the patient with mild exercise
- Provides an opportunity for close observation

You as the caregiver are able to see firsthand how the patient's condition is improving, declining, or changing in any way. Your observations are valuable aids to accurate nursing assessments.

With the physician's permission, the patient may be allowed to take regular tub baths or showers. Some patients will be bathed in bed.

Bathing may be performed as:
- Tub bath
- Shower bath
- Complete bed bath
- Partial bed bath
- Self-sponge bath or waterless bath
- Whirlpool bath
- Perineal care

During bathing, special attention should be given to skin areas that touch, including:
- Between the legs
- Under the arms
- Under the breasts
- Under the scrotum
- Between the buttocks

- Around the anus
- For obese people, under folds of skin or fat

Gently sponge and pat these areas dry. Follow facility policy for the use of talcum or corn starch.

A partial bath cleans the hands, face, back, axillae, buttocks, and genitals. It is very refreshing. Many patients will be able to help with bathing. Whenever possible, encourage patients to do so.

Culture ALERT

In the United States, we promote self-care in patient care and treatment. However, in some cultures, family members are expected to care for the patient. Some patients may expect certain people to be involved in their care. They may also expect certain people to be obligated to visit. ∎

Waterless Bath

Some facilities are taking a new approach to bathing called **waterless bathing**. It may also be called **bag bath**. The only equipment needed is a package of premoistened disposable washcloths (Figure 24-1). Each package contains washcloths moistened with a special cleansing solution that evaporates quickly after being applied so that drying is not necessary. Eight washcloths are supplied so that separate parts of the body (face, arms, legs, torso, and genitalia) can be washed. The washcloths can be warmed in the microwave or special product warmer (Figure 24-2). If the microwave is used, it may heat unevenly. Monitor for hot spots. This product can be used by the nursing assistant to administer a bath or by the patient to self-bathe.

FIGURE 24-1 Waterless bathing has become popular for its comfort and convenience. Although the product is more costly than more conventional methods of bathing, the time savings make it worthwhile. Bag bath contains a no-rinse cleanser and does not contain soap, so it is gentle on patients' skin. (Courtesy of Medline Industries, Inc. (800) MEDLINE)

FIGURE 24-2 The waterless bathing system may be used at room temperature, or warmed for comfort. Use the product warmer, if available, because heating the cloths in the microwave increases the risk for uneven heating and burns. (Courtesy of Medline Industries, Inc. (800) MEDLINE)

The procedure is similar to a bed bath, with cleansing done in the same order:

- Face and neck
- Far arm and hand
- Near arm and hand
- Chest and abdomen
- Far leg and foot
- Near leg and foot
- Back and buttocks
- Perineum

The waterless bathing system has several advantages:

Infection Control ALERT

Waterless bathing products are designed to be used for one bath. Smaller kits containing four cloths are also available for partial baths and perineal care. The package may be resealed if not all of the cloths are used. However, the open package should be dated and discarded in 48 to 72 hours, or according to facility infection control guidelines. Follow facility policy for discarding unused cloths after the bath is completed. Discard used cloths properly, according to facility policy. Avoid flushing them down the toilet. A plastic bag at the bedside works well for cloth disposal. ∎

- It is faster and more economical for the facility; each bath takes approximately 8 to 10 minutes.
- It is less fatiguing for the patient.
- It conserves moisture, reduces drying, and is gentler to skin than soaps.
- It creates less friction, because the cloths are softer than regular washcloths and towels, and drying is eliminated.

The following precautions are used when bathing patients with the waterless bathing system:

- The washcloths may be used at room temperature, but many facilities heat them for comfort.
- Peel the label back or open the package before heating to avoid bursting in the microwave.
- Follow manufacturers' directions for heating the package. One minute is usually sufficient to warm the contents to a comfortable temperature.
- The cloths in the package are for single use only.
- Discard unused cloths within 72 hours of opening the package, or immediately if they are dry.

Whirlpool Bath

The most stimulating form of bathing for patients is a therapeutic bath that is given in a whirlpool tub (Figure 24-3). The whirlpool bath benefits patients because:

- The temperature of the water can be regulated to a constant 97°F.
- The movement of the water stimulates circulation.
- Warm, circulating water is relaxing and invigorating.
- It provides the value of whirlpool activity with cleansing.

Care of the hair, teeth, and nails usually follows the bath procedure, but may be carried out as independent procedures. Range-of-motion exercises frequently follow bathing.

FIGURE 24-3 The water in the whirlpool circulates, maintaining a constant temperature and stimulating circulation. (Courtesy of Arjo-Century, Inc.)

Culture ALERT

A patient may prefer to receive personal care from someone of the same sex. Honor these requests, whenever possible, and do not be offended that the request was made. In some cultures, a male cannot even be in the same room with a female unless she is covered from head to foot. ■

Culture ALERT

Always learn ways to show respect in the patient's culture, such as how to address the patient and how to address privacy concerns, such as touching the body or wearing certain articles of clothing. Work on building a relationship of trust with each patient. ■

PATIENT BATHING

Nursing assistants are frequently assigned to bathe patients. It is important to follow the guidelines and the procedures for bathing carefully to ensure patient comfort and safety. (Refer to Procedures 53, 54, and 56 to 59.)

Safety ALERT

Make sure a chair is available next to the tub or shower in case the patient needs to sit quickly. Turn the hot water on last and off first to prevent injury. ■

Safety Measures for Special Treatments

Patients receiving special treatments can be bathed. They include, for example, the patient who is receiving an IV, has drainage tubes, or is receiving oxygen. These patients, however, need special care.

Be careful, as you bathe and move the patient, that you:

- Do not put stress on the tubes.
- Never lower the IV container below the level of the infusion site.
- Never raise the drainage tube above the drainage site.

GUIDELINES *for*
Giving a Whirlpool Bath

- Check with the nurse before giving a whirlpool to a patient with an infection, surgical incision, or pressure ulcer.

- If the patient is combative or disoriented, check with the nurse before giving the patient a whirlpool. The noise from the whirlpool may worsen agitation in some patients.

- Disinfect the whirlpool tub immediately before and after each use.

- The water temperature in the whirlpool tub is usually set at 97°F to 100°F because the temperature in the tub remains constant. (Use common sense; if the tub is steaming, the water is probably too hot. Use a thermometer to check the water temperature.) The constant movement of warm water stimulates the patient's circulation.

- Never leave a patient alone in the whirlpool tub, even for a minute.

- Always fasten the safety belt when moving a patient into or out of a whirlpool tub with a hydraulic lift seat. The safety belt should remain fastened throughout the procedure.

- The patient may be frightened when using the hydraulic lift. Explain the procedure and reassure the patient.

- Drape the patient's genital area with a bath towel for modesty during the whirlpool bath.

- Use low-suds or no-suds products that are designed specifically for whirlpool use.

- Never pour liquid soap or shampoo into the whirlpool tub. A tiny bit of liquid soap will result in an abundance of suds. If the patient accidentally creates a suds problem, rub a bar of soap against the walls of the tub to reduce the bubbles.

- The whirlpool activity provides a cleansing action. However, if you will be assisting the patient with bathing, apply the principles of standard precautions.

- Wrap the patient with a bath blanket for warmth and modesty immediately after removing him or her from the whirlpool tub.

- The jets in some whirlpool tubs have the potential to harbor dangerous pathogens. Follow facility policies for carefully cleaning the tub with the proper disinfectant solution. Make sure that you follow directions correctly and run the disinfectant through the tub for the correct length of time.

- When the bath is completed, raise the lift seat out of the soapy water and rinse with the hose using comfortably warm water.

Infection Control ALERT

Think about what precautions are necessary as you perform the procedures in this chapter. Apply the principles of standard precautions. However, avoid overkill. Patients need to be touched. Do not wear gloves for the entire bathing procedure unless there is a reason to do so. When bathing patients, remove the gloves and put on a clean pair immediately prior to contact with mucous membranes and nonintact skin. Do not cross-contaminate body sites by wearing the same pair of gloves for the entire procedure. Avoid contaminating the environment with your used gloves. Discard gloves properly. Wash your hands after removing gloves. ■

Age-Appropriate Care ALERT

Most patients, young and old, have some independence with activities of daily living when they are in the home. Sometimes they are able to continue to do all or part of these skills. If so, encourage them to continue, unless contraindicated. Provide the supplies needed and arrange them conveniently so the patient can use them. Supervise the patient and assist if needed. This may take longer, but you will reinforce the patient's feelings of self-worth by allowing her to do these things. Organize your work so that you can do something else while the patient is performing self-care skills, as appropriate. This makes good use of your time. If the patient is unable to complete the task, finish it promptly without complaint. ■

GUIDELINES *for*

Patient Bathing

- Wear disposable gloves if there may be contact with open lesions, blood, body fluids, secretions, or excretions.
- Make sure the shower or tub is cleaned before and after each use (Figure 24-4).
- Check that all safety aids, such as hand rails, shower chairs, and tub seats/benches are in good repair and proper working order.
- Protect patients from fatigue by transporting patients to and from the tub room and carrying out the bathing procedure as efficiently as possible.
- Make sure the patient's body is covered during transport.
- If a patient falls in the tub or shower room or feels faint during bathing, do not leave him alone. Signal for help, using the emergency call button in the bathroom. Do not lock the bathroom door.
- Use good body mechanics to protect yourself and the patient.
- Nonskid strips placed in the tub and on the floor of the shower prevent slipping.
- Hand rails secured to the walls help prevent falls as the patient transfers into and out of the tub.
- The patient should be assisted in all transfer activity related to the bath. Be sure to have enough help.
- The use of a shower chair will prevent patient stress and fatigue, but it must be secured so that it does not move as the patient transfers into and out of it.
- Wipe up all water spilled or dripped on the floor immediately, to prevent falls.
- The room should be comfortably warm (about 70°F) and free from drafts, to prevent chilling the patient.
- Cotton bath blankets should be used to cover the patient during a bed bath. They are also be used for added warmth following the tub bath or shower.
- Drape the patient's genital area with a bath towel for modesty during a tub bath or shower.
- The temperature of the water for a shower, tub bath, or bed bath should be maintained at about 105°F. Use a bath thermometer to check the temperature of the water.
- Observe the patient's skin for any changes or irregularities. Note any reddened areas. Do not disturb or injure warts or moles. Report anything unusual.

- If you will be using liquid soap from a dispenser mounted on the wall, avoid putting the soap directly into the bath water. Dispense some soap into a small cup and carry it to the tub or bedside. Pour the liquid soap onto the washcloth as needed.
- In some facilities, bar soap is not permitted. If refillable liquid soap bottles are used, each patient should have a bottle labeled with his or her name. The soap from that bottle is used for that patient only.
- Once a washcloth or towel has been used below the waist, avoid using it above the waist.
- The hand-held shower spray should be placed on the hook when not in use. Do not let it hang down or touch the floor, which is always considered dirty.

Safety ALERT

Never leave the patient alone in the tub or shower. A call signal in the bathing area is used to call for emergency help. ■

FIGURE 24-4 Clean the tub or shower chair before and after use. Wipe all areas, including the hand rails.

PROCEDURE

ASSISTING WITH THE TUB BATH OR SHOWER

1. Carry out initial procedure actions.

2. Assemble equipment:
   - Disposable gloves
   - Liquid soap
   - Washcloth
   - 2–3 bath towels
   - Bath blanket
   - Bath lotion
   - Deodorant
   - Chair or stool beside shower or tub
   - Bath or shower chair, as needed
   - Patient's gown, robe, and slippers
   - Bath mat

3. Take the supplies to the bathroom. Prepare the bathroom for the patient. Make sure the tub is clean.

4. Fill the tub half full of water at 105°F or adjust the shower flow. If a bath thermometer is available, check the water temperature. If a bath thermometer is not available, test the water with your wrist or elbow. The water should feel comfortably warm.

5. Help the patient put on a robe and slippers. Escort the patient to the bathroom. Completely cover the nonambulatory patient when going to or from the bath or shower.

6. Help the patient to undress. Give the patient a towel to wrap around the waist.

7. Position a shower chair in tub or shower, if needed (Figure 24-5).

8. Assist the patient into the tub or shower. For the patient's safety, the bottom of the tub and the shower floor are covered with a nonskid surface.

9. Put on disposable gloves if the patient has open skin lesions.

10. Encourage the patient to wash the rest of his or her body. Assist in washing as needed.

11. Wash the patient's back.

- Observe the skin for signs of redness or breaks. See Unit 38 for information on caring for pressure sores or other skin lesions.

12. The patient may wash the **genitalia** (external reproductive organs), if able.
    - If the patient is not able to wash the genitalia, then you will also perform this part of the bath. Apply disposable gloves before bathing the genital area.
    - After washing the genitalia, remove gloves, and discard according to facility policy.
    - Wash your hands.
    - After washing the genitalia, avoid using the same washcloth, towel, and gloves elsewhere on the body. If further bathing or touching is necessary, apply new gloves and use different linen.

13. If the patient shows any signs of weakness:
    - Get help. Use the call button.
    - Remove the plug and let the water drain.
    - Turn off the shower.
    - Allow the patient to rest until feeling better before making any attempt to assist the patient out of the tub or shower.
    - Keep the patient covered with a bath blanket to avoid chilling.

14. If the patient wants a shampoo and you have permission to do so:
    - Ask the patient to hold a washcloth over the eyes.
    - Pour a small amount of water on hair (enough to wet hair thoroughly).
    - Use a small amount of shampoo to lather hair.
    - Massage scalp gently.
    - Rinse hair with warm water.
    - Repeat lathering, massaging, and rinsing, if necessary.
    - Towel hair dry.

15. Hold the bath blanket around the patient as he or she steps out of the tub. The patient may choose

continues

PROCEDURE 5 3 CONTINUED

FIGURE 24-5 The shower chair is used to enable the patient to bathe safely. Lock the wheels during transfers.

to remove the wet towel from under the bath blanket.

16. Assist the patient to dry, apply deodorant, dress, and return to the unit.

17. Escort the patient back to his or her unit. Return supplies to the patient's unit.

18. Carry out ending procedure actions.

19. Return to the bath or shower room. Put on gloves and clean and disinfect the tub, shower chair, and hand rails.

20. Discard soiled linen.

21. Wash your hands.

Tips: It is important to use a bath blanket and towels to drape the patient during all bathing and personal care procedures, even if the room is completely private. Being exposed is uncomfortable for most people. Draping the patient properly provides a sense of dignity, reduces feelings of vulnerability, and protects the patient's modesty and self-esteem. Do not omit this important step for any patients, regardless of their age.

Clinical Information ALERT

Good personal hygiene provides comfort and a sense of well-being. Treat your patients with respect and be sensitive to their needs. Make sure to provide privacy when patients' bodies are exposed. The human body secretes substances that can cause unpleasant odors. Areas of greatest concern are the armpits and the perineum. Do not make the patient feel uncomfortable if he or she has an odor. Bathing will eliminate odors in these areas, and the patients will feel more comfortable and confident when they are clean. ■

Difficult SITUATIONS

Bathing can be very upsetting for patients with Alzheimer's disease and other types of dementia. Early signs of distress are increased motor activity and a change in tone of voice. The patient may perceive being disrobed and having the body handled as a form of sexual assault. As the patient becomes more distressed, he or she may scream, fight, and act out. Bathing becomes a source of stress for both the patient and nursing assistant. The patient's aggressive behavior tells you that this patient cannot tolerate the methods being used for bathing. He or she is asking you to find another, better way of doing it. Instead of using a tub bath, shower, or bed bath, consider another method of bathing, such as using a bag bath or towel bath, or doing a partial bath. Consult the nurse. Bathing should never be traumatic to a patient. Being flexibile and considerate of patients' needs improves their quality of life, reduces stress, and saves time for the nursing assistant. ■

PROCEDURE

54

BED BATH

> **Note:** Disposable gloves should be worn if the patient has draining wounds, nonintact skin, or if contact with blood, body fluids, mucous membranes, secretions, or excretions is likely.

1. Carry out initial procedure actions.

2. Assemble equipment:
   - Disposable gloves
   - Bed linen
   - Bath blanket
   - Laundry bag or hamper
   - Bath basin
   - Bath thermometer
   - Soap and soap dish, or liquid soap
   - Washcloths
   - Face towel
   - 2 bath towels
   - Hospital gown/patient's night clothes
   - Lotion
   - Equipment for oral hygiene
   - Nail brush, emery board, and orangewood stick (if needed)
   - Deodorant
   - Brush and comb
   - Bedpan and cover or urinal
   - Paper towel or protector

3. Close the windows and door to prevent chilling the patient.

4. Close the privacy curtain.

5. Put clean towels and linen on a chair in the order of use. Place a laundry hamper nearby.

6. Offer the bedpan or urinal. If the patient wants to use the bedpan or urinal, put on gloves. Empty and clean the bedpan or urinal before proceeding with the bath. Remove gloves and discard according to facility policy. Wash your hands.

7. Lower the head of the bed and the side rail on the side where you are working.

8. Loosen the top bedclothes. Remove and fold the blanket and spread and place them over the back of the chair.

9. Place a bath blanket over the top sheet (Figure 24-6) and remove the sheet by sliding it out from under the bath blanket. Place the sheet in a laundry hamper.

10. Leave one pillow under the patient's head. Place the other pillow on a chair.

11. Remove the patient's night wear and place it in a laundry hamper (assuming the patient has no IV).

12. Fill a bath basin two-thirds full with water at 105°F. Use a bath thermometer, if available, to be sure of the proper temperature.

13. Assist the patient to move to the side of the bed nearest you.

14. Fold a face towel over the upper edge of the bath blanket to keep the blanket dry. Put on gloves.

15. Form a mitt by folding a washcloth around your hand (Figure 24-7 shows a mitt being made on a gloved hand).
    a. Wet the washcloth.
    b. Wash eyes, using separate corners of the cloth for each eye.
    c. Wipe from inside to outside corner (Figure 24-8).
    d. Do not use soap near eyes.

FIGURE 24-6 Replace the top bedding with a bath blanket by covering the bedding with the bath blanket, then pulling the bedding out from underneath while the patient holds the blanket in place.

continues

PROCEDURE 54 CONTINUED

FIGURE 24-7 To make a mitt over a gloved hand, wrap the washcloth in thirds around one hand. Then bring the free end over the palm and tuck in the end. The thumb is free to hold the washcloth in place.

FIGURE 24-8 Avoid soap in the eye area. Wipe from the inner corner to the outer corner. Turn the washcloth before moving to the other eye.

FIGURE 24-9 Place the towel under the patient's arm. Support the arm as you wash it.

   e. After you have washed the eyes, remove gloves and discard according to facility policy.

   f. Do not use soap on the face unless the patient requests it.

16. Rinse the washcloth and apply soap if the patient desires. Squeeze out excess water. Do not leave soap in water.

17. Wash and rinse the patient's face, ears, and neck well. Use a towel to dry.

18. Expose the patient's far arm. Protect the bed with a bath towel placed underneath the arm.

   a. Wash, rinse, and pat dry arm and hand.

   b. Be sure **axilla** (armpit) is clean and dry.

   c. Repeat for other arm (Figure 24-9).

   d. Apply deodorant if the patient requests it.

19. Care for hands and nails as necessary. Check with the nurse first to see if there are any special instructions.

   a. Place the patient's hands in a basin of water. Wash each hand carefully. Rinse and dry. Push **cuticle** (base of fingernails) down gently with a towel while wiping the fingers. Be sure to dry between fingers.

   b. Clean under the nails with an orangewood stick. Shape the nails with an emery board. Be careful not to file nails too close. Do not

continues

PROCEDURE 54 CONTINUED

cut nails if the patient is diabetic. Inform the nurse if attention is needed.

20. Discard used bath water and refill the basin two-thirds full with water at 105°F.

21. Put a bath towel over the patient's chest. Then fold the blanket to the waist. Under the towel:

    a. Wash, rinse, and pat dry chest.

    b. Rinse and dry folds under the breasts of a female patient carefully to avoid irritating the skin.

22. Fold the bath blanket down to the **pubic** area (location of external genitalia). Wash, rinse, and pat dry abdomen. Fold the bath blanket up to cover the abdomen and chest. Slide the towel out from under the bath blanket.

23. Ask the patient to flex the far knee, if possible. Fold the bath blanket up to expose the thigh, leg, and foot. Protect the bed with a bath towel.

    a. Put the bath basin on the towel.

    b. Place the patient's foot in the basin.

    c. Wash and rinse the leg and foot (Figure 24-10).

    d. When moving the patient's leg, support it properly.

24. Lift the leg and move the basin to the other side of the bed. Dry the leg and foot. Dry well between toes.

25. Repeat for the other leg and foot. Take the basin off the bed before drying the leg and foot.

FIGURE 24-10   Support the leg and place the foot in the basin.

26. Care for toenails as necessary. Check with the nurse for any special instructions. Apply lotion to the feet of a patient with dry skin. Do not apply lotion between the toes, as this keeps the area moist and promotes fungal growth.

    • Do not attempt to cut thickened nails.

    • File nails straight across.

    • Do not round edges.

    • Do not push back the cuticle, because it is easily injured and infected.

    • If the patient is diabetic, inform the nurse if toenail care is required.

27. Change water and check for the correct temperature with a bath thermometer. It may be necessary to change the water before this point in the patient's bath if it becomes cold or too soapy.

28. Help the patient to turn on the side away from you. Help him to move toward the center of the bed. Place a bath towel lengthwise next to the patient's back.

    • Wash, rinse, and dry neck, back, and buttocks.

    • Use long, firm strokes when washing the back.

29. A back rub is usually given at this time (see Unit 25).

30. Help the patient to turn on the back.

31. Place a towel under the buttocks and upper legs. Change the water in the basin and check for the correct temperature. Place a washcloth, soap, basin, and bath towel within convenient reach of the patient. Have the patient complete the bath by washing the genitalia. Assist the patient if necessary. You must take responsibility for the procedure if the patient has difficulty. Many times patients are reluctant to acknowledge the need for help. If assisting a patient with genital washing, always put on disposable gloves.

    • For a female patient, wash from front to back, drying carefully.

    • For a male patient, carefully wash and dry the penis, scrotum, and groin area. If the patient is not circumcised, gently push the foreskin back and carefully wash and dry the penis. Then gently pull the foreskin down to its original position.

continues

PROCEDURE 54 CONTINUED

32. Remove gloves and discard according to facility policy.

33. Carry out range-of-motion exercises as ordered (see Unit 41 for Procedures 90 and 91).

34. Cover the pillow with a towel. Comb or brush the patient's hair. Oral hygiene is usually given at this time (see Unit 25).

35. Discard towels and washcloth in a laundry hamper.

36. Provide a clean gown.

37. Clean and replace equipment according to facility policy.

38. Put clean washcloth and towels in the bedside stand, or hang according to facility policy.

39. Change the bed linen, following the procedure for making an occupied bed. Replace and discard soiled linen in a laundry hamper.

40. Remove and discard disposable gloves according to facility policy. Wash your hands.

41. Raise the side rails, if required.

42. Carry out ending procedure actions.

PROCEDURE 55

OBRA

CHANGING THE PATIENT'S GOWN

Note: Wear disposable gloves if the patient has draining wounds, nonintact skin, or if contact with mucous membranes, blood, body fluids, secretions, or excretions is likely.

1. Carry out initial procedure actions.

2. Assemble equipment:
- Disposable gloves
- Bath blanket
- Clean gown
- Laundry bag or hamper

3. Place a bath blanket over the top sheet. Pull the sheet down by sliding it out from under the bath blanket.

4. Loosen the gown from the patient's neck.

5. Slip the gown down the arms.

6. Make sure the patient is covered by a bath blanket (Figure 24-11).

Note: This procedure is to be used only when the patient has an IV that is NOT run through an electric pump. When a pump is used, the patient may wear a gown that snaps at the shoulder. In this case, the gown can be removed without touching the IV bag or tubing. If the patient is wearing a nonsnap gown, call the nurse if the gown is to be changed. Never disconnect the tubing from the pump.

FIGURE 24-11 Keeping the patient covered with the bath blanket, remove the patient's gown.

7. For a patient wearing a regular gown (nonsnap):
- **a.** Remove the gown from the arm without the IV and bring the gown across the patient's chest to the other arm.
- **b.** Place a clean gown over the patient's chest to avoid exposure.
- **c.** On the arm with the IV, gather the gown material in one hand so there is no pull or pressure on the IV line (Figure 24-12A), and slowly draw the gown over the tips of the patient's fingers.

continues

PROCEDURE 55 CONTINUED

d. With your free hand, lift the IV off the standard and slip the gown over the bag of fluid (Figure 24-12B), removing the gown from the patient's body. *Never allow the bag of fluid to be lower than the patient's arm.*

e. Take the sleeve of a clean gown and slip it over the bag of fluid, over the tubing, and up the patient's arm.

f. Replace the bag of fluid on the IV standard.

g. Remove the soiled gown and place it at the end of the bed. Finish putting the clean gown on the patient's other arm. Secure the neck ties.

h. Place the soiled gown in a laundry hamper.

i. Make sure the IV is dripping at the required rate and that the tubing is not kinked or twisted.

8. If the patient has a weak or paralyzed arm, always undress the patient in the following manner:

a. Untie the gown and remove the back sides of the gown from underneath the patient.

b. Remove the gown from the stronger arm first.

c. Bring the gown across the patient's chest and slide the gown down over the weak arm.

d. Gently lift the patient's weak arm to finish removing the gown over the patient's hand.

e. Reverse the procedure to put a clean gown on the patient, by putting the gown over the weaker arm first.

9. Pull the sheet up over the bath blanket. Remove the bath blanket.

10. Carry out ending procedure actions.

FIGURE 24-12A Gather the gown material in one hand so there is no traction on the IV line. Slowly draw the gown over the tips of the patient's fingers.

FIGURE 24-12B With your free hand, lift the IV off the standard and slip the gown over the bag of fluid.

PROCEDURE

56

WATERLESS BED BATH

1. Carry out initial procedure actions.

2. Assemble equipment:

- Disposable gloves
- Bed linen

continues

PROCEDURE 56 CONTINUED

- Bath blanket
- Laundry bag or hamper
- Hospital gown/patient's night clothes
- Bath towel
- Lotion for backrub
- Waterless bathing product, heated according to facility policy or patient wishes
- Basin of warm water for soaking hands (optional)
- Comb, brush
- Bedpan or urinal with cover, as needed
- Supplies for oral hygiene, as needed
- Supplies for nail care, as needed
- Small plastic bag to discard used bathing cloths
- Large plastic bag or hamper for soiled linen

3. Close the windows and door to the room.

4. Pull the privacy curtain. Place clean supplies on the overbed table.

5. Offer the bedpan or urinal. Put on gloves if you will be assisting with this procedure.

6. Lower the head of the bed and the side rail on the side where you will be working.

7. Loosen the top bedclothes. Remove and fold the blanket and spread and place them over the back of the chair.

8. Place a bath blanket over the top sheet and remove the sheet by sliding it out from under the bath blanket. Place the sheet in the laundry hamper.

9. Leave one pillow under the patient's head. Place the other pillow on the chair.

10. Remove the gown (see Procedure 55) and place it in the laundry hamper.

11. Assist the patient to move to the side of the bed near you.

12. Warm the package according to facility policy and manufacturer's directions. Open the package. (If you used a microwave to heat the package, check the cloths for hot spots.) Remove one cloth and cleanse the patient's face and neck. (The solution on these cloths can safely be used around the eyes.)

13. Place a towel over the patient's chest. Fold the bath blanket down to the waist and cleanse the chest. Be sure the area under a female patient's breasts is carefully cleaned.

14. Fold the bath blanket down to the pubic area and wash the abdomen. Replace the bath blanket over the abdomen and chest. Remove the towel by sliding it out from under the bath blanket. Discard the used cloth in the plastic bag.

15. Uncover the far arm. Remove another cloth from the package and wash the arm and hand. It is nice to soak each of the patient's hands separately in a basin of warm water while you wash the opposite arm. This is refreshing for the patient who cannot be out of bed to bathe. Wash each axilla. Apply deodorant if the patient desires. Discard the used cloth in the plastic bag. Cover the arm with the bath blanket.

16. Uncover the near arm. Remove a new cloth from the package. Wash the arm, hand, and axilla. Apply deodorant. Discard the used cloth in the plastic bag. Cover the patient with the bath blanket.

17. Provide nail care as needed.

18. Ask the patient to flex the far leg, if possible. Fold the bath blanket up to expose the thigh, leg, and foot. Remove a new cloth from the package. Cleanse the thigh, leg, and foot. Be sure the area between the toes is left dry. Discard the used cloth in the plastic bag. Cover the leg and foot with the bath blanket.

19. Repeat step 18 with the near thigh, leg, and foot.

20. Make sure the side rail on the opposite side of the bed is up. Help the patient turn onto the side away from you. Place a bath towel lengthwise next to the patient's back.

21. Remove a new cloth from the package. Draw the bath blanket back to expose the back. Wash the back and buttocks. Discard the used cloth in the plastic bag. A backrub may be given at this time. Cover the patient with the bath blanket.

22. Assist the patient to turn onto the back. Position a towel under the buttocks by asking the patient to lift the hips, if possible. Remove a new cloth from the package. Hand the patient the cloth and

continues

PROCEDURE 56 CONTINUED

instruct the patient to wash the genitalia. Assist if necessary. (Wear gloves if you will be assisting.) Discard gloves and the used cloth in the plastic bag. Remove the towel.

23. Wash your hands.

24. Assist the patient to put on a clean gown.

25. Cover the pillow with a towel. Comb or brush the patient's hair. Assist with oral hygiene, if needed.

26. Change the bed linen, following the procedure for making an occupied bed (see Procedure 51). Put soiled linen in a plastic bag or linen hamper.

27. Carry out ending procedure actions.

Towel Bath

The towel bath procedure has become popular in long-term care facilities for bathing patients with dementia who become distressed and agitated with the tub or shower bath. The bathing environment is also considered, and the room may be darkened, with soothing music playing softly. Products that give off a pleasant aroma are used in the environment. The bath is done by using a no-rinse skin cleanser. Two washcloths, two hand towels, one large towel, and two bath blankets are usually needed. The patient is completely covered with a bath blanket, which is pre-warmed, if possible. The nursing assistant may use the call signal to ask another assistant to warm additional blankets, if necessary.

The nursing assistant usually prepares a bathing kit in advance, and brings it to the room in a large plastic bag so it is ready to use. The patient is covered with a bath blanket and gradually undressed. Warm, moist towels prepared with the skin cleanser are used, one at a time, over a large area of the patient's body. Rather than using an established sequence or routine, the bath begins in an area of the body that is least distressing to the patient, such as the feet and lower legs. The prepared towel is used to simultaneously massage and cleanse the skin. Because a no-rinse product is used, rinsing and drying are not necessary. The skin usual-ly dries quickly when the towel is removed. During the bath, the nursing assistant speaks with the patient in a calm, soothing manner. He or she avoids rushing, and uses warm bath blankets and towels to keep the patient comfortably warm.

The goal of this type of bath is to keep the patient clean and odor-free, while avoiding a situation that is potentially upsetting to the patient. A variety of techniques are used to personalize the procedure and make it as pleasurable as possible for the patient, while respecting his or her autonomy. This type of bath is more creative than normal bathing routines, but it is not more work and is not more time-consuming.

Difficult SITUATIONS

Bathing patients with dementia requires the use of many nursing assistant skills, including communication, problem solving, and creativity. Strive to make the bath pleasant and comforting, dignified, patient-centered, and based on the patient's individual needs instead of being a routine ritual of practice. ■

PROCEDURE

PARTIAL BATH

1. Carry out initial procedure actions.

2. Assemble equipment:

- Disposable gloves
- Bed linen
- Bath blanket

- Bath thermometer
- Soap and soap dish or liquid soap
- Washcloth
- Face towel

continues

PROCEDURE 57 CONTINUED

- Bath towel
- Gown and robe
- Laundry bag or hamper
- Bath basin
- Lotion
- Equipment for oral hygiene
- Nail brush, emery board, and orangewood stick
- Brush, comb, and deodorant
- Bedpan or urinal and cover
- Paper towels or protector

Note: A package of premoistened washcloths can be substituted for the basin of water, soap, washcloth, and towel if the facility has approved the use of the waterless bath. The nursing assistant or the patient (condition permitting) can use the premoistened washcloths for the partial bath.

3. Close windows and door and turn off fans to prevent chilling the patient.

4. Put the towels and linen on the chair in the order of use. Make sure a laundry hamper is available.

5. Put on disposable gloves.

6. Offer the bedpan or urinal (see Unit 25). Empty and clean it before proceeding with the bath. Remove gloves and discard according to facility policy. Wash your hands.

7. Elevate the head of the bed, if permitted, to a comfortable position.

8. Loosen the top bedclothes. Remove and fold the blanket and spread and place them over the back of the chair. Place a bath blanket over the top sheet. Remove the top sheet by sliding it out from under the bath blanket.

9. Leave one pillow under the patient's head. Place the other pillow on the chair.

10. Assist the patient to remove the gown. Place the gown in the laundry hamper. Make sure the patient is covered with a bath blanket.

11. Place paper towels or a bed protector on the overbed table.

12. Fill a bath basin two-thirds full with water at 105°F. Place the basin on the overbed table.

13. Push the overbed table comfortably close to the patient.

14. Place towels, washcloth, and soap on the overbed table within easy reach.

15. Instruct the patient to wash as much as she is able and tell her that you will return to complete the bath.

16. Place the call bell within easy reach. Ask the patient to signal when ready.

17. Wash hands and leave the unit.

18. Wash hands and return to the unit when the patient signals. Put on a new pair of gloves.

19. Change the bath water. Complete bathing those areas the patient could not reach. Make sure the face, hands, axillae, buttocks, back, and genitals are washed and dried.

20. Remove gloves and discard according to facility policy.

21. Wash your hands.

22. Give a backrub with lotion.

23. Assist the patient in applying deodorant and a fresh gown.

24. Cover the pillow with a towel. Comb or brush the patient's hair. Assist with oral hygiene, if needed (see Unit 25).

25. Clean and replace equipment according to facility policy.

26. Put a clean washcloth and towels in the bedside stand, or hang according to facility policy.

27. Change the bed linen, following the procedure for making an occupied bed. Put soiled linen in the laundry hamper.

28. Carry out ending procedure actions.

Perineal Care

The **perineum** is the area between the legs. In females, it is the area between the vagina and the anus. In males, it is the area between the scrotum and the anus.

Perineal care may be performed as part of general bathing or as a separate procedure, as needed. **Perineal care** means to wash the area including the genitals and anus (see Procedures 58 and 59). Always wear gloves and use standard precautions when caring for the perineal area.

Tips: If the patient has been incontinent, remove the wet pad or linen and replace with a dry pad before beginning perineal care. Clean excess stool off with toilet tissue before beginning.

Communication HIGHLIGHT

Patients who need assistance with perineal care and those who become incontinent may feel guilty and embarrassed. Avoid showing disgust. Be sensitive to the patient's feelings. Communicate with the patient tactfully. Use proper terms when referring to body parts and excretions. ■

Clinical Information ALERT

Urine and stool are very damaging to the skin. The effects of the excretions cause skin damage (similar to a rash or chemical burn) and skin breakdown. The damage to the skin worsens with the length of exposure to the substances. ■

Infection Control ALERT

Providing perineal care is one of the most important procedures you will perform as a nursing assistant. Always apply the principles of standard precautions. Remember that there are mucous membranes in the genital area. If you are wearing gloves, change them before beginning care. Using proper technique is critical because of the high risk of contamination and infection. Avoid scrubbing back and forth. Always wipe from clean to dirty with a single wipe, then turn or discard the cloth, according to facility policy. Guidelines for female perineal care vary with the institution. In some facilities, you will be instructed to clean the center first, then each side. In others, you will clean the sides of the genitalia first, then the center. Know and follow your facility policies. Discard your gloves properly and avoid contaminating environmental surfaces with your used gloves. ■

PROCEDURE

FEMALE PERINEAL CARE

Note: The guidelines and sequence for this procedure vary slightly from state to state, and from one facility to the next. Your instructor will inform you if the sequence in your state or facility differs from the procedure listed here. Know and follow the required sequence for your state and facility policies.

1. Carry out initial procedure actions.

2. Assemble equipment:
   - Disposable gloves
   - Bath blanket or top sheet
   - Bedpan and cover
   - Liquid soap
   - Basin
   - Bath thermometer
   - Bed protector
   - Washcloth and towel
   - Plastic bag(s), if needed to discard linen or trash
   - Laundry barrel or hamper

3. Lower the side rail on the side where you will be working. Be sure the opposite side rail is up and secure.

4. Remove the bedspread and blanket. Fold and place them on the back of the chair.

5. The patient is to be on her back. Cover the patient with a bath blanket and fanfold the sheet to the foot of the bed.

6. Put on disposable gloves. Fill a basin with water at 105°F.

continues

PROCEDURE 58 CONTINUED

7. Ask the patient to raise her hips while you place a bed protector underneath the patient.

8. Offer the bedpan to the patient.

   a. If used and the patient is on intake and output, record the amount.

   b. Empty and clean the bedpan before continuing with the procedure.

   c. Remove gloves and discard according to facility policy.

   d. Wash your hands and put on a new pair of gloves.

9. Position the bath blanket so that only the area between the legs is exposed.

10. Ask the patient to separate her legs and flex her knees.

     Note: If the patient is unable to spread her legs and flex her knees, turn the patient on her side with the legs flexed. This position provides easy access to the perineal area.

11. Wet the washcloth, make a mitt, and apply a small amount of liquid soap.

    Note: Heavy soap application may be difficult to rinse off completely. Soap residue is irritating.

Clinical Information ALERT

Be gentle when cleansing patients after incontinent episodes. Scrubbing produces extra friction. The excretions are irritating to the skin, and vigorous scrubbing is abrasive, furthering the risk of infection and skin breakdown. ■

12. Separate the labia with one gloved hand. When caring for the female patient, keep the labia separated as much as possible during the procedure. Avoid placing your fingers on an area after washing it. Turn the washcloth so you are using a clean section each time you move to a new area. Use a second washcloth, if necessary. You may need several washcloths to perform the procedure without contamination. (Some facilities require a second, clean washcloth for rinsing; the used cloth is not put back into the water basin). If a urinary catheter is present, hold the tubing securely to one side and support against the leg to avoid unnecessary movement or traction on the catheter. Keep the tubing and drainage bag below the level of the bladder.

    a. With the other gloved hand, wash the center of the labia, using a single downward stroke from top to bottom.

    b. Turn the washcloth to a clean area.

    c. Wash the far side of the labia, using a single downward stroke from top to bottom (Figure 24-13A).

    d. Turn the washcloth to a clean area.

    e. Wash the near labia, using a single downward stroke from top to bottom.

    f. Continue to alternate from side to side, working outward to thighs, using the same technique. Turn the washcloth or use a new washcloth, if necessary, so a fresh section is used to cleanse each area.

    g. If a urinary catheter is present, wash, rinse, and dry the perineal area surrounding the urinary meatus and catheter. Change the washcloth. Beginning at the urinary meatus, wash down the catheter approximately 3 to 4 inches. Use a single downward stroke. Do not rub back and forth. Rinse and dry in the same direction. Hold the catheter firmly to avoid pulling and traction. After washing the catheter, continue with perineal care.

    h. Rinse the area from top to bottom with the washcloth. Avoid rubbing back and forth. Rinse in the same sequence, beginning in the center and moving outward from side to side. Turn the washcloth so a clean surface is used for each downward stroke.

    i. Gently pat the area dry with a towel. Avoid rubbing back and forth. Dry in the same sequence, beginning in the center and moving outward from side to side. Position the towel so a clean surface is used for each downward stroke.

13. Turn the patient away from you. Flex the upper leg slightly, if permitted.

continues

PROCEDURE 58 CONTINUED

FIGURE 24-13A
Spread the vulva with one hand. With the washcloth in the other hand, start in the front and stroke downward along the outer labia.

FIGURE 24-13B
With one hand, lift up on the buttocks to expose the anal area. Wipe from the perineum back toward the anus.

14. Make a mitt, wet it, and apply soap lightly.

15. Expose the anal area. Wash the area, stroking from perineum to coccyx (front to back) (Figure 24-13B).

16. Rinse well in the same manner.

17. Dry carefully.

18. Return the patient to her back.

19. Remove and dispose of the bed protector according to facility policy.

20. Cover the patient with a sheet or bath blanket.

21. Remove and dispose of gloves according to facility policy. Wash your hands.

22. Remove, fold, and store the bath blanket according to facility policy.

23. Replace the top covers, tuck them under the mattress, and make mitered corners. (Some patients prefer that the top covers not be tucked in.)

24. Put up the side rail, if required.

25. Put on gloves. Empty the water. Clean equipment and dispose of or store it, according to facility policy.

26. Remove gloves and discard according to facility policy. Wash your hands.

27. Carry out ending procedure actions.

PROCEDURE

MALE PERINEAL CARE

Note: The guidelines and sequence for this procedure vary slightly from state to state, and from one facility to the next. Your instructor will inform you if the sequence in your state or facility differs from the procedure listed here. Know and follow the required sequence for your state and facility policies.

1. Carry out initial procedure actions.

2. Assemble equipment:
- Disposable gloves
- Bath blanket
- Bath thermometer
- Urinal and cover or bedpan and cover
- Soap, washcloth, and towel
- Plastic bag
- Bed protector or bath towel

continues

PROCEDURE **59** CONTINUED

- Ordered solution (if other than water)
- Basin
- Laundry hamper

3. Fill a basin with warm water at approximately 105°F.

4. Lower the side rail on the side where you will be working.

5. Fanfold the blanket and spread to the foot of the bed. Remove, fold, and place them on the back of the chair.

6. Cover the patient with a bath blanket and fanfold the sheet to the foot of the bed.

7. Put on disposable gloves.

8. Place a bed protector under the patient's buttocks.

9. Offer the bedpan or urinal.

   a. If used and the patient is on intake and output, record the amount.

   b. Empty and clean the bedpan or urinal before continuing with the procedure.

   c. Remove gloves and discard according to facility policy.

   d. Wash your hands and put on a new pair of gloves.

10. Have the patient flex and separate his knees.

 Note: If the patient is unable to spread his legs and flex the knees, the perineal area can be washed with the patient on his side with the legs flexed. This position provides easy access to the perineal area.

11. Draw the bath blanket upward to expose the perineal area only.

12. Make a mitt with a washcloth and apply a small amount of soap.

Note: Heavy soap application may be difficult to rinse off completely. Soap residue is irritating.

13. Grasp the penis gently with one hand and wash. Begin at the meatus and wash in a circular motion (Figure 24-14A). If a urinary catheter is present, hold the tubing securely to one side and support it against the leg to avoid unnecessary

FIGURE 24-14A Grasp the penis gently with one hand. With the other, wipe in a circular motion, beginning with the urinary meatus, working outward over the glans (head of the penis). Continue to wash down the penis and the rest of the perineal area, including the scrotum, using downward strokes and working outward to the thighs.

movement or traction on the catheter. Keep the tubing and drainage bag below the level of the bladder.

14. If the patient is not circumcised, draw the foreskin back (Figure 24-14B). Be sure the entire penis is washed. Rinse thoroughly.

15. Continue to wash down the penis and the rest of the perineal area, including the scrotum, using downward strokes and working outward to the thighs. Lift the scrotum and wash the perineum. If a urinary catheter is present, wash, rinse, and dry the perineal area surrounding the urinary meatus and catheter. Change the washcloth. Beginning at the urinary meatus, wash down the catheter approximately 3 to 4 inches. Use a single downward stroke. Do not rub back and forth. Rinse and dry in the same direction. Hold the catheter firmly to avoid pulling and traction. After washing the catheter, continue with perineal care.

16. Rinse the washcloth and remake a mitt. Rinse the urethral and perineal areas well, working in the

continues

PROCEDURE 59 CONTINUED

FIGURE 24-14B If the patient is not circumcised, gently push the foreskin back so the glans can be washed. Once the penis is washed and dried, return the foreskin to its normal position.

same direction until the entire area is clean and soap-free.

17. Dry the washed area with a towel. Reposition the foreskin if necessary.

18. Turn the patient away from you. Flex his upper leg slightly if permitted.

19. Make a mitt, wet it, and apply soap lightly.

20. Expose the anal area. Wash the area, stroking from perineum to coccyx.

21. Rinse well in the same manner.

22. Dry carefully.

23. Return the patient to his back.

24. Remove and dispose of the bed protector according to facility policy.

25. Cover the patient with a sheet.

26. Remove and dispose of gloves according to facility policy. Wash your hands.

27. Remove, fold, and store the bath blanket, according to facility policy.

28. Replace the top covers, tuck them under the mattress, and make mitered corners. (Some patients prefer that the top covers not be tucked in.)

29. Put up the side rail, if required.

30. Put on gloves. Empty the water. Clean equipment and dispose of or store it, according to facility policy.

31. Remove gloves and discard according to facility policy. Wash your hands.

32. Carry out ending procedure actions.

Infection Control ALERT

When giving perineal care, always wash from the most clean area to the least clean. Turn the cloth frequently and rinse well. After giving perineal care, avoid using the same washcloth, towel, and gloves elsewhere on the body. If further bathing or touching is necessary, apply new gloves and use different linen. Some patients may have orders for barrier cream or another product following perineal care. If you will be applying barrier cream, remove your gloves, wash your hands, and apply new gloves. Your gloves become contaminated during the perineal care procedure, and you must use new (clean) gloves to apply barrier cream. Avoid contaminating the jar or tube of cream with your used gloves. ■

Infection Control ALERT

In many facilities, nursing assistants are not permitted to use nail clippers. However, some facilities permit assistants to perform nail care on nondiabetic patients. Be aware that the clippers are a potential source of infection, especially *Streptococcus A.* Make sure you disinfect clippers and any other reusable items thoroughly after each use. ■

GUIDELINES *for*
Providing Hand, Foot, and Nail Care

- Know and follow your facility policy for who is allowed to clip and clean nails.

- Cleaning and trimming nails is easier immediately after they have been soaked or bathed.

- Avoid the use of nail files and other sharp objects for cleaning nails. An orange stick is a disposable, pointed, wooden stick that can be safely used.

- If your facility allows you to clip fingernails, use clippers, not scissors.

- When trimming nails, be very careful not to accidentally clip or damage the skin surrounding the nail.

- If you observe any abnormalities, such as redness, cracking, or signs of infection, by the finger or toenails, report it to the nurse.

- Fingernails are clipped straight across, then rounded at the edges with an emery board.

- Push the cuticles back with a washcloth or the dull end of the orange stick.

- After washing the feet, dry well between each toe and inspect for red or cracked areas. Moisture promotes fungal growth and skin breakdown, which can lead to more serious complications.

- Lotion may be applied to the hands or feet if the skin is dry. Do not apply lotion between the toes, as this may promote fungal growth.

- **Note:** In some facilities, nursing assistants are not permitted to perform this procedure. Know and follow your facility policies. Use clippers only if you are permitted to do so according to state law and facility policies.

PROCEDURE

60

HAND AND FINGERNAIL CARE

Note: Check with the nurse and nursing care plan to learn if this procedure is permitted for the patient or if it is to be modified because of the patient's condition.

This procedure can be carried out independently or can be modified and added to the bath procedure.

1. Carry out initial procedure actions.

2. Assemble equipment:
   - Basin
   - Bath thermometer
   - Soap
   - Bath towel and washcloth
   - Lotion
   - Plastic protector
   - Nail clippers
   - Emery board
   - Orangewood stick
   - Nail polish (optional)

3. Elevate the head of the bed, if permitted, and adjust the overbed table in front of the patient. If the patient is allowed out of bed, assist the patient to transfer to a chair and position the overbed table waist-high across the patient's lap.

4. Place a plastic protector on the overbed table.

5. Fill a basin with warm water at approximately 105°F, using the bath thermometer to test temperature. Place the basin on the overbed table.

6. Instruct the patient to put hands in the basin and soak for approximately 5 minutes. Place a towel over the basin to help retain heat. Add warm water if necessary. Remember to remove the patient's hands before adding water.

7. Wash the patient's hands. Push cuticles back gently with a washcloth or an orangewood stick (Figure 24-15A). (A cream may be used to soften the cuticles first.) Use a soft brush or orangewood stick to clean under nails. (Check with the

continues

PROCEDURE 60 CONTINUED

nurse before using an orangewood stick on a patient with diabetes.)

8. Dry the patient's hands with a towel. Remember to dry between the fingers.

9. Use nail clippers to cut fingernails straight across, if permitted by facility policy (Figure 24-15B).
   - Do not cut below the tips of the fingers.
   - Keep nail clippings on the protector to be discarded.

10. Shape and smooth the fingernails with an emery board (Figure 24-15C). Apply polish to nails if the patient desires.

11. Pour a small amount of lotion in your palms and gently smooth it on the patient's hands.

12. Empty the basin of water. Gather equipment. Clean and store it according to the facility policy.

13. Return the overbed table to the foot of the bed. If the patient has been sitting up for the procedure, assist the patient to get into bed.

14. Carry out ending procedure actions.

FIGURE 24-15A Gently push the cuticles back with a washcloth or orange stick, if permitted.

FIGURE 24-15B Clip the nails straight across.

FIGURE 24-15C Round the edges with an emery board. (Courtesy of Medline Industries, Inc. (800) MEDLINE.)

Clinical Information ALERT

In some facilities, a doctor's order is needed for a shampoo. If permitted, the hair can be washed in the tub or shower. Offer the patient a washcloth or towel to hold over the face while hair is being washed and rinsed. For patients on complete bedrest, this procedure must be done in bed. Some facilities use dry chemical shampoos that are brushed out. No-rinse shampoos are also available for bedfast patients. ■

Difficult SITUATIONS

Like bathing, washing a cognitively impaired patient's hair under running water can be a cause of great stress and distress. Consider washing the hair using a bed shampoo tray, an inflatable shampoo basin, or a shampoo cap or dry shampoo product. ■

PROCEDURE

61

BED SHAMPOO

1. Carry out initial procedure actions.

2. Assemble equipment needed:
   - Shampoo tray
   - Shampoo
   - Washcloths
   - 3 bath towels
   - Bath blanket
   - Pitcher of water (105°F)
   - Safety pin
   - 2 bed protectors
   - Waterproof covering for pillow
   - Large bucket to collect used water
   - Hair dryer, if available (portable)
   - Hairbrush and comb
   - Small empty pitcher or cup
   - Larger pitcher of water (105°F)—use if additional water is needed

3. Place a large, empty basin on the floor under the spout of the shampoo tray.

4. Arrange on the bedside stand, within easy reach (Figure 24-16A).
   - Large pitcher of water (105°F)
   - Washcloth
   - 2 bath towels
   - Shampoo
   - Small pitcher of water (105°F)

5. Replace the top bedding with a bath blanket.

6. Ask the patient to move to the side of the bed nearest you. Assist as needed.

7. Replace the pillowcase with a waterproof covering.

8. Cover the head of the bed with a bed protector. Be sure it goes well under the patient's shoulders.

9. Loosen neck ties of the gown.

10. Place a towel under the patient's head and shoulders. Brush hair free of tangles, working snarls out carefully.

11. Bring the towel down around the patient's neck and shoulders and pin it. Position the pillow under shoulders so that the patient's head is tilted slightly backward.

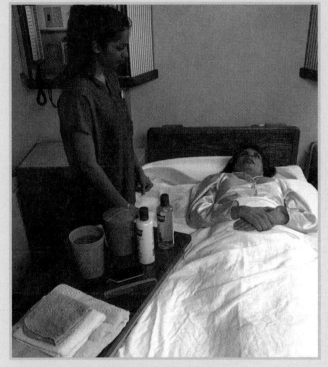

FIGURE 24-16A Assemble equipment.

12. Raise the bed to high horizontal position.

13. Raise the patient's head and position the shampoo tray (Figure 24-16B) so that the drain is over the edge of the bed directly above the basin.

14. Give the patient a washcloth to cover the eyes (Figure 24-16C).

15. Recheck the temperature of water in the basin.

16. Using the small pitcher (Figure 24-16D), pour a small amount of water over hair until thoroughly wet. Use one hand to help direct the flow away from the face and ears.

17. Apply a small amount of shampoo, working up a lather (Figure 24-16E). Work from scalp to hair ends.

18. Massage the scalp with your fingertips. Do not use your fingernails.

19. Rinse thoroughly, pouring from hairline to hair tips. Direct the flow into the drain. Use water from the pitcher if needed, but be sure to check the water temperature before use.

continues

PROCEDURE 61 CONTINUED

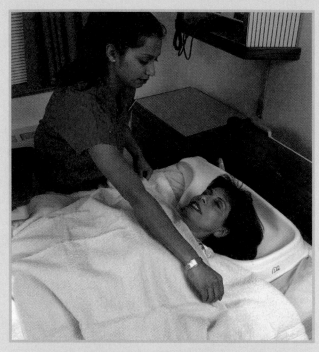

FIGURE 24-16B Position the patient with head on shampoo tray. Protect the patient with a towel and the bed with a protector.

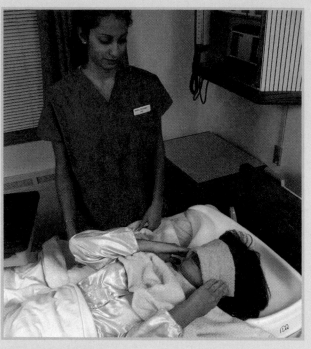

FIGURE 24-16C Give the patient a folded washcloth to protect her eyes.

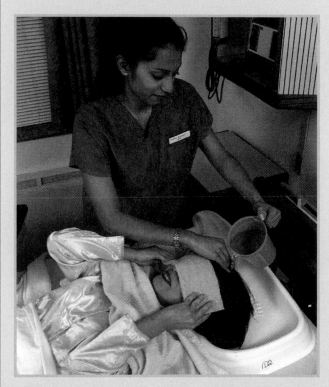

FIGURE 24-16D Wet the hair by slowly pouring warm water.

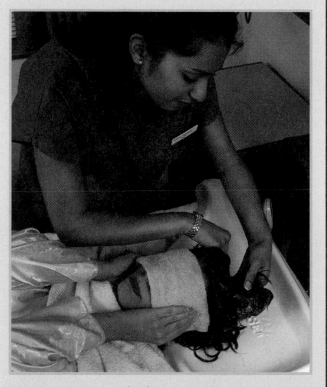

FIGURE 24-16E Apply shampoo and work it into a lather, using your fingertips.

continues

PROCEDURE 61 CONTINUED

20. Repeat lathering and rinsing (steps 16–19).

21. Lift the patient's head. Remove the tray and bed protector. Adjust the pillow and slip a dry bath towel underneath the head.

22. Place the tray on the basin. Wrap hair in a towel. Be sure to dry face, neck, and ears as needed.

23. Dry hair with the towel. If available and not otherwise contraindicated, a portable hair dryer may be used to complete the drying process. Brushing the hair as you blow-dry helps the hair to dry. Be sure to keep the dryer moving and not too close to the hair.

24. Comb hair appropriately. Remove the protective pillow cover. Replace with a cloth cover.

25. Lower the bed to a comfortable working position.

26. Replace the bedding and remove the bath blanket.

27. Help the patient assume a comfortable position. Lower the bed to the lowest horizontal position. Leave the call bell within reach.

28. Allow the patient to rest undisturbed. The length of this procedure may tire the patient.

29. Empty the water from the collection basin.

30. Carry out ending procedure actions.

The Waterless Shampoo

Various waterless preparations are available for washing the hair of patients whose hair cannot be shampooed by other methods. Shampoo caps (Figure 24-17) are a popular alternative for bathing bedfast patients. These are most comfortable for patients if they are warmed in a microwave for 30 seconds or less, or in the product warmer. If the microwave is used, feel the outside of the cap by pressing the various areas against your forearm to make sure there are no hot spots. Place the cap on the patient's head, then rub gently for 1 to 2 minutes for short hair and 4 to 5 minutes for long hair. After this time, remove the cap; towel-dry and comb the hair. Shampoo caps reduce tangling and do not leave residue like some dry chemical products.

FIGURE 24-17 Shampoo caps simplify the hair-washing procedure for bedfast patients, and require no rinsing. Conditioners in the product leave the hair soft and reduce the incidence of tangling. (Courtesy of Medline Industries, Inc. (800) MEDLINE)

DRESSING A PATIENT

Patients in hospitals generally wear hospital gowns because they are in bed most of the time. However, some patients may prefer to wear their own nightgowns or pajamas and will need assistance in dressing. Patients in the rehabilitation unit and those who participate in some special programs may be up and fully dressed each day. You may also need to assist patients to dress when they are discharged from the hospital. It is usually easier to help people dress while they are still in bed.

GUIDELINES *for*

Dressing and Undressing Patients

The patient who requires help in dressing may wish to sit in a chair with clothing placed nearby. You can help by:

- Allowing the patient to choose the clothing to be put on.

- Encouraging the patient to participate in the dressing or undressing procedure as much as he or she is able.

continues

GUIDELINES *continued*

- Being prepared to assist with shoes and stockings even for patients who can do much themselves. Bending over to adjust shoes and stockings can result in dizziness and loss of balance.

- Putting clothing on the affected or weakest side first if the patient has difficulty moving one side or is paralyzed.

- Removing clothing from the unaffected or strongest side first if the patient has difficulty moving one side or is paralyzed.

PROCEDURE

DRESSING AND UNDRESSING THE PATIENT

1. Carry out initial procedure actions.

2. Select appropriate clothing and arrange in order of application. Encourage the patient to participate in selection.

3. Cover the patient with a bath blanket and fanfold top bedclothes to the foot of the bed.

4. Elevate the head of the bed to sitting position.

5. Assist the patient to a comfortable sitting position.

6. Remove night clothing, keeping the patient covered with the bath blanket. Remove from strong side first and then from weaker side. Place night clothes in a laundry hamper or fold them to be taken home.

7. If the patient wears a bra, slip the straps over the patient's hands (weak side first), move the straps up her arms, and position them on her shoulders. Adjust the breasts in the bra cups. Then hook the bra in back (assist the patient to lean forward so the bra can be fastened).

8. For an undershirt, or any garment that slips on over the head:

   a. Gather the undershirt and place it over the patient's head (Figure 24-18A).

   b. Grasp the patient's hand and guide it through the armhole by reaching into the armhole from the outside.

   c. Repeat the procedure with the opposite arm.

   d. Assist the patient to lean forward, and adjust the undershirt so it is smooth over the upper body.

FIGURE 24-18A Gather the garment and pull it over the patient's head.

9. Alternate procedure for slipover garments:

    Note: A garment must be large enough or made of stretchy fabric for this procedure.

   a. Place the garment front side down on the patient's lap, with the bottom opening facing the patient.

   b. Put the patient's hands into the bottom of the garment and, one at a time, into the sleeve holes.

   c. Pull the sleeves up as far as possible on the patient's arms and pull the hands through at the wrist if it is a long-sleeved garment. The garment should now be high on the patient's chest.

continues

PROCEDURE 62 CONTINUED

   d. Gather up the back of the garment with your hand and slip the garment over the patient's head.

   e. Smooth the garment down and position it comfortably about the patient's body. Adjust sleeves and shoulders as needed.

10. Shirts or dresses that fasten in the front:

   a. Insert your hand through the sleeve of the garment and grasp the patient's hand. Draw the sleeve over your hand and the patient's.

   b. Adjust the sleeve at the shoulder.

   c. Assist the patient to sit forward. Arrange clothing across the patient's back.

   d. Gather the sleeve on the opposite side by slipping your hand in from the outside.

   e. Grasp the patient's wrist and pull the sleeve of the garment over your hand and the patient's hand. Draw the sleeve upward and adjust it at the shoulder.

   f. Button, zip, or snap the garment.

11. Underwear or pants:

   a. Facing the foot of the bed, gather the patient's garment from waist to leg hole.

   b. Slip the garment over one foot at a time (Figure 24-18B). Pull the garment up the legs as high as possible.

   c. Assist the patient to raise the hips. Draw the garment over the buttocks and up to the waist. If patient cannot raise the buttocks, assist the patient to roll first to one side, as

you pull up the garment, and then the other side (Figure 24-18C). Adjust the garment until comfortable.

   d. Fasten the garment, if required.

12. Socks or knee-high (or thigh-high) stockings:

   a. Roll a sock or stocking with heel in back and place it over the toes (Figure 24-18D).

   b. Draw the sock up over the foot and adjust until smooth. Pull stockings smoothly up to knee or thigh.

FIGURE 24-18C Have the patient roll onto the strong side first, then pull pants over hip. Then roll the patient to the other side and pull up pants. Adjust for comfort.

FIGURE 24-18D Adjust socks smoothly over toes. Leave about 1/4 inch of space between the ends of the toes and the toe of the stocking, to prevent pulling and pressure.

FIGURE 24-18B Slip pants over feet and lower legs.

PROCEDURE 62 CONTINUED

   c. Repeat for other foot.

13. Pantyhose:

   a. Gather pantyhose and adjust over toes and feet. Draw up legs as high as possible.

   b. Draw over hips as described in step 11c. Adjust until comfortable at waist.

14. Shoes:

   a. Slip shoe on, using a shoe horn if necessary. Open laces of shoes completely so the foot can easily slip into the shoe (Figure 24-18E).

   b. Be sure the shoe is fastened securely (Velcro tabs or ties). If the shoes tie, be sure that the ends of the shoelaces do not drag on the floor. The shoes should be fastened tight enough to prevent them from slipping off the patient's feet but not so tight that circulation is impaired.

   c. Shoes should be appropriate to the floor surface.

FIGURE 24-18E Open the shoelaces completely and slip the foot into the shoe.

15. To undress, reverse order of steps.

16. Carry out ending procedure actions

REVIEW

A. True/False.

Mark the following true or false by circling T or F.

1. T F The nursing assistant should carefully observe the patient during the bath procedure.

2. T F Perineal care is given with the patient positioned on a bedpan.

3. T F Range-of-motion exercises are often performed after the bath procedure begins.

4. T F The bath can be omitted if the patient is receiving an IV.

5. T F During the bed bath, only the part being bathed should be exposed.

6. T F Patients should be encouraged to use hand rails when getting in and out of the bathtub.

7. T F Traction may be placed on drainage tubes as long as they are not disconnected.

8. T F Because soap is used during the bathing procedure, the tub need not be cleaned between patient uses.

9. T F The bathing procedure can provide the patient with mild exercise.

10. T F Disposable gloves should be worn during bathing if the patient has draining wounds.

B. Matching.

Match the words in Column II with the statements in Column I.

Column I

11. _____ External reproductive organs

12. _____ Area at base of nails

13. _____ Area under the arms

Column II

  a. axillae

  b. midriff

  c. genitalia

  d. cuticle

  e. shampoo

C. Multiple Choice.

Select the one best answer for each of the following.

14. The room temperature during the bath procedure should be about
   a. 62°F.
   b. 68°F.
   c. 74°F.
   d. 86°F.

15. When providing perineal care to a female patient,
   a. wash from the front to the back.
   b. wash the genitals from side to side.
   c. wipe from back to front.
   d. scrub back and forth vigorously.

16. Bath water temperature should be approximately
   a. 105°F.
   b. 90°F.
   c. 80°F.
   d. 120°F.

17. When giving hand and nail care, the hands should be soaked approximately
   a. 1 hour.
   b. 1/2 hour.
   c. 20 minutes.
   d. 5 minutes.

18. When a patient takes a bath, the bathroom door should
   a. not be locked.
   b. be left wide open for easier access.
   c. be locked for privacy.
   d. be left partially open.

D. Nursing Assistant Challenge.

Mr. Rodriguez is taking a shower before going home. He had bowel surgery four days ago. Answer the following about his care by selecting the correct word.

19. The person responsible for the cleanliness of the shower is the _____.

   (patient) (nursing assistant)

20. The patient _____ be assisted into and out of the shower.

   (should not) (should)

21. You can protect the patient from fatigue by _____ to the shower.

   (walking slowly) (transporting him by wheelchair)

22. If Mr. Rodriguez feels faint during his shower, you should turn the water _____.

   (to cold) (off)

23. To prevent chilling if Mr. Rodriguez feels weak, you should _____.

   (turn on the warm water) (wrap him in a bath blanket)

General Comfort Measures

OBJECTIVES

After completing this unit, you will be able to:
- Spell and define terms.
- Discuss the reasons for early morning and bedtime care.
- Identify patients who require frequent oral hygiene.
- List the purposes of oral hygiene.
- Explain nursing assistant responsibilities for a patient's dentures.
- State the purpose of backrubs.
- Describe safety precautions when shaving a patient.
- Describe the importance of hair care.
- Explain the use of comfort devices.

- Demonstrate the following procedures:
  - Procedure 63 Assisting with Routine Oral Hygiene
  - Procedure 64 Assisting with Special Oral Hygiene
  - Procedure 65 Assisting the Patient to Floss and Brush Teeth
  - Procedure 66 Caring for Dentures
  - Procedure 67 Backrub
  - Procedure 68 Shaving a Male Patient
  - Procedure 69 Daily Hair Care
  - Procedure 70 Giving and Receiving the Bedpan
  - Procedure 71 Giving and Receiving the Urinal
  - Procedure 72 Assisting with Use of the Bedside Commode

VOCABULARY

Learn the meaning and the correct spelling of the following words and phrases:

AM care	caries	footboard	oral hygiene
anticoagulants	dentures	foot drop	PM care
bridging	feces	halitosis	

INTRODUCTION

You can do many things for your patients that will add to their general comfort and feeling of well-being. This includes:
- Providing AM and PM care
- Giving oral hygiene care
- Giving backrubs
- Brushing hair
- Shaving
- Using pillows and special equipment to maintain comfortable positions

AM CARE AND PM CARE

Early morning (AM) care prepares the patient for a day of activities and PM care prepares the patient for a night of rest. Each provides an opportunity for the patient to meet elimination needs and to be refreshed. The nursing assistant has an opportunity to closely observe the patient's condition and to interact supportively with the patient.

Early Morning (AM) Care

Early morning or AM care helps to set the tone for the entire day. If the patient is refreshed and comfortable before eating breakfast, the day is off to a good start. The nursing assistant provides AM care by:

- Awakening the patient gently—never abruptly—by saying the patient's name (Figure 25-1). If necessary, gently touch the arm.
- Awakening the patient before breakfast.
- Giving the patient the opportunity to use the bathroom, if permitted, or to use the bedpan or urinal.
- Helping the patient to wash hands and face.

The patient is not awakened early if he or she is:

- Going to surgery
- Having tests that prohibit eating

Bedtime (PM Care)

The care given to the patient just before bedtime is similar to that given in the early morning. Bedtime care is called PM care (or HS care). The nursing assistant gives PM care:

- In a quiet, unrushed manner that will help prepare the patient for sleep (Figure 25-2)
- Before medication for sleep is given by the nurse

Other routine procedures that may be carried out during AM and PM care include:

- Measuring vital signs
- Giving a backrub
- Providing mouth and hair care
- Giving the patient the opportunity to use the bathroom, if permitted, or to use the bedpan or urinal.

Infection Control ALERT

A clean mouth has about 100 million bacteria on the teeth, tongue, gums, and other surfaces. If the teeth are not regularly brushed, the bacteria can multiply quickly. They will move to other areas, including the pharynx, sinuses, larynx, and lungs. In patients with dysphagia (Unit 26), small amounts of oral fluid are aspirated frequently and rapidly. Even healthy adults occasionally aspirate small amounts of saliva during deep sleep, increasing the risk of pneumonia. However, they usually do not get sick because they brush their teeth daily and have healthy immune systems. ∎

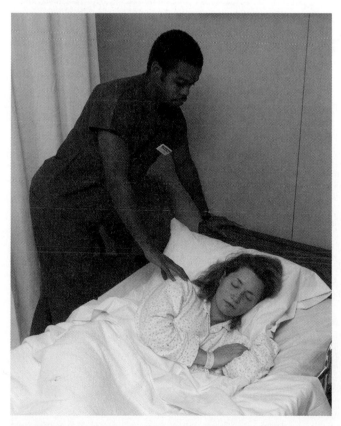

FIGURE 25-1 Early AM care. Wake the patient by saying the patient's name, then gently touching the arm, if necessary.

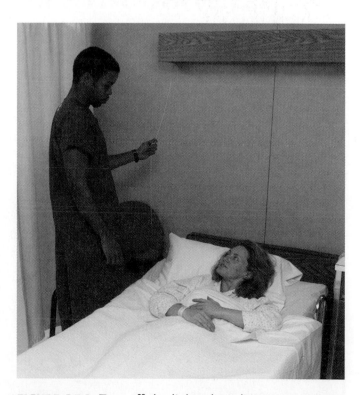

FIGURE 25-2 Turn off the light when the patient is settled and comfortable.

ORAL HYGIENE

Oral hygiene is care of the mouth and teeth. (Refer to Procedures 63 to 65.)

- Routine oral hygiene (including brushing and flossing the teeth) should be performed at least three times a day.
- Patients should be encouraged to do as much as possible for themselves.
- *Special oral hygiene* is the cleansing of the mouth of the helpless patient using commercially prepared lemon and glycerine swabs, Toothettes, and other preparations.

Patients requiring more frequent oral hygiene include those who are:

- Unconscious
- Vomiting
- Experiencing a high temperature
- Receiving certain medications
- Dehydrated
- Breathing through the mouth
- Receiving oxygen
- Receiving tube feeding
- Dying

Infection Control ALERT

Take care in storing the patient's toothbrush. Make sure it is covered or stored away from other items, such as the hairbrush. ▪

Infection Control ALERT

Apply the principles of standard precautions when selecting protective equipment for assisting with dental procedures. Always wear gloves. If there is a chance of spraying or splashing of oral secretions, you will need a gown, gloves, mask, and face shield. ▪

Proper cleansing of the teeth and mouth helps:

- Prevent tooth decay (**caries**)
- Eliminate bad breath (**halitosis**)
- Contribute to the patient's comfort

PROCEDURE

63

ASSISTING WITH ROUTINE ORAL HYGIENE

1. Carry out initial procedure actions.
2. Assemble equipment:
   - Disposable gloves and face mask
   - Toothbrush
   - Toothpaste
   - Dental floss
   - Mouthwash solution in cup
   - Emesis basin
   - Bath towel
   - Straw
   - Tissues
   - Cup of fresh water
   - Plastic bag
   - Bed protector
3. Raise the head of the bed so that the patient may sit up, if his condition permits.
4. Lower the side rails and position the overbed table across the patient's lap.

5. Cover the table with a protector and place equipment on the table.
6. Place a bath towel over the patient's gown and bedcovers.
7. Be prepared to help as the patient brushes and flosses teeth.
8. Pour water over the toothbrush and put toothpaste on the brush.
9. Put on disposable gloves. A face mask and eye protection may be used.
10. Brush teeth as follows (Figures 25-3A to 25-3E):
    a. Insert the toothbrush into the mouth with bristles pointing downward.
    b. Turn the toothbrush with bristles toward teeth.
    c. Brush all tooth surfaces with a back-and-forth motion using short strokes.

continues

PROCEDURE 63 CONTINUED

FIGURE 25-3A Place the head of the toothbrush beside the teeth, with the bristle tips at a 45° angle against the gumline. Move the brush back and forth in short strokes several times, using a gentle scrubbing motion. Brush the outer surfaces of each tooth, upper and lower, keeping the bristles angled against the gumline.

FIGURE 25-3B Use the same method on the inside surfaces of all the teeth, still using short back-and-forth strokes.

FIGURE 25-3C Scrub the chewing surfaces of the teeth.

FIGURE 25-3D To clean the inside surfaces of the front teeth, tilt the brush vertically and make several gentle up-and-down strokes with the "toe" (front part) of the brush.

FIGURE 25-3E Brushing the patient's tongue will help freshen breath and clean the mouth by removing bacteria.

FIGURE 25-3 Brush teeth in the direction they grow and across the chewing surfaces. (Toothbrushing photos and descriptions compliments of the American Dental Association.)

   d. Use the "toe" end of the brush to clean the inner surfaces of the front teeth, using a gentle up-and-down motion.

   e. Brush the front of the tongue gently, if tolerated by the patient. Avoid the back of the tongue, as touching this area may cause gagging and coughing.

11. Give the patient water in a cup to rinse the mouth. Use a straw, if necessary. Turn the patient's head to one side, with the emesis basin near the chin, for return of fluid.

12. Repeat steps 10 and 11 as necessary.

13. To floss the patient's teeth:

   a. Select a piece of dental floss about 12 inches long. Wrap the end of the floss around your middle fingers, leaving the center area free (Figure 25-4).

   b. Ask the patient to open her mouth. Gently insert the floss between each tooth down to, but not into, the gum line.

   c. Ask the patient to rinse her mouth using the emesis basin.

continues

PROCEDURE 63 CONTINUED

FIGURE 25-4 Floss is wrapped around the middle fingers (left). The proper method of using the floss to clean between the teeth (right).

14. Offer the patient mouthwash. Dilute the mouthwash if the patient wishes.

15. Remove the basin. Wipe the patient's mouth and chin with tissue. Discard the tissue in a paper bag.

16. Remove the towel.

17. Rinse the toothbrush with water.

18. Remove and dispose of gloves and mask according to facility policy.

19. Carry out ending procedure actions.

Culture ALERT

Many individuals have tongue piercings for fashion or cultural reasons. Many risks accompany this practice. Inform the nurse promptly if a patient with a tongue piercing has pain, bleeding, increased flow of saliva, swelling, or signs of infection in the mouth. Swelling of the tongue can become severe, closing off the airway. ■

Infection Control ALERT

Studies have shown that providing thorough, regular oral hygiene reduces the risk of infection in elderly persons and those with a weakened immune system. Avoid sponge swabs if there is a risk the patient may bite off or swallow the sponge. Lemon-glycerine swabs are drying, and should not be used frequently. The physician may order an artificial saliva product to increase patient comfort. ■

DENTURES

Some patients have full sets of dentures. Other patients have partial plates that are removable, but attach by small metal clips to existing teeth. Partial plates should be given the same care as full dentures. **Dentures** are artificial teeth that are removable. They must be cleaned. The patient may feel embarrassed about wearing dentures and may dislike being seen after the dentures have been removed.

Therefore, always provide privacy when dentures are to be removed and cleaned. (See Procedure 66.)

Denture Care

Denture care includes:

- Cleaning dentures daily under cool running water. Avoid hot water when caring for dentures.

PROCEDURE

ASSISTING WITH SPECIAL ORAL HYGIENE

 Note: Special oral hygiene is provided when the patient cannot participate actively in such care.

1. Carry out initial procedure actions.

2. Assemble equipment:
   - Disposable gloves
   - Toothettes or lemon-glycerine applicators
   - Emesis basin
   - 2 bath towels
   - Plastic bag
   - Premoistened applicators
   - Tissues
   - Tongue depressor
   - Water-based lubricant for lips
   - Laundry hamper

3. Put on gloves.

4. Cover pillow with a towel. If the patient is able to sit up, elevate the head of the bed. If the patient is unable or not permitted to sit up, turn the patient's head to one side and slightly forward so any excess fluid will not run down the throat. Cover the patient's upper chest with a towel. Place an emesis basin under the patient's chin.

5. Gently pull down on the chin to open the mouth, or open the mouth gently with a tongue depressor.

6. Using moistened Toothettes, wipe gums, teeth, tongue, and inside of mouth (Figure 25-5).

FIGURE 25-5 Using premoistened applicators, wipe gums, teeth, and tongue.

7. Discard used applicators in a plastic bag.

8. Using clean applicators, apply lubricant to the patient's lips. Place used applicators in a plastic bag.

9. Remove towels. Clean and replace equipment.

10. Remove and dispose of gloves properly. Wash your hands.

11. Carry out ending procedure actions.

PROCEDURE

ASSISTING THE PATIENT TO FLOSS AND BRUSH TEETH

1. Carry out initial procedure actions.

2. Assemble equipment:
   - Disposable gloves
   - Emesis basin
   - Toothbrush
   - Toothpaste
   - Dental floss
   - Glass of cool water

continues

PROCEDURE 6 5 CONTINUED

- Straw
- Mouthwash (if permitted)
- Hand towel
- Bed protector
- Plastic bag
- Laundry hamper

3. Elevate the head of the bed. Help the patient into a comfortable position.

4. Lower the side rails and position the overbed table across the patient's lap.

5. Cover the table with a plastic protector.

6. Place the emesis basin and a glass of water on the overbed table.

7. Place a towel across the patient's chest.

8. Be prepared to help as the patient flosses and brushes teeth. Remind the patient to clean the tongue and gums. Apply gloves and use standard precautions if you will be assisting with the procedure.

9. After the patient has flossed and brushed teeth:

    a. Push the overbed table to the foot of the bed.

    b. Remove the emesis basin, clean it, and replace it according to facility policy.

    c. Rinse toothbrush.

    d. Remove the towels and put them with the soiled linen.

    e. Remove gloves and discard according to facility policy. Wash your hands.

10. Carry out ending procedure actions.

Age-Appropriate Care ALERT

Elderly patients may experience dry mouth and reduced saliva production. This commonly occurs as a side effect of medications. Related complaints are burning or sore throat, difficulty in swallowing, hoarseness, and dry nasal passages. Saliva is needed to help break down food for digestion. It also neutralizes acids in the mouth caused by plaque. Artificial saliva products are available, as are medicated oral rinses. The dentist may recommend that the patient use sugar-free gum or candy to increase saliva production. Inform the nurse if the patient experiences problems with saliva production. ■

FIGURE 25-6 Dentures are stored in a cup labeled with the patient's name. The dentures are usually kept covered with water.

- Handling dentures carefully to prevent damage.
- Storing dentures in a safe place when they are out of the patient's mouth, such as in the drawer of the bedside stand in a container labeled with the patient's name (Figure 25-6).
- Brushing dentures daily. Soaking dentures in solution does not eliminate the need for daily brushing.
- Changing the soaking solution and washing the denture cup with soap and water daily. Rinse well.
- Rinsing dentures well before brushing under running water. Do not rinse them in standing water in the sink.
- Brushing the tissues and gums in the mouth daily, even if the patient has no teeth. Use a soft-bristled brush to clean the mouth. This improves circulation and removes oral debris.
- Cleaning and checking the patient's mouth for signs of irritation.
- Checking the patient's lips for cracking and dryness.
- Applying cream, petroleum jelly, or glycerin to lips to avoid excessive dryness.

If you must place items such as the toothbrush, toothpaste, or dentures on the counter, put them on a clean paper towel. Never place them in the sink or an unprotected countertop.

Safety ALERT

Remove dentures from a comatose patient to prevent accidental airway obstruction by the denture. Remove dentures from patients preoperatively to prevent potential damage to the dentures and accidental airway obstruction in surgery. ■

Age-Appropriate Care ALERT

Dentures are made to fit tightly in the patient's mouth. Natural aging changes in the bones and gums may cause the shape of the patient's mouth to change over time. If dentures are loose or ill-fitting, chances are that this is because of aging changes to the mouth. Loose dentures can cause sores in the mouth, and in the worst case can cause choking. Denture adhesives can be used temporarily to help keep dentures in place, but the patient will need to be referred to a dentist. Inform the nurse if the patient has problems with improperly fitting dentures. ■

PROCEDURE

66

CARING FOR DENTURES

1. Carry out Initial procedure actions.

2. Assemble equipment:
   - Disposable gloves
   - Tissues
   - Emesis basin
   - Tongue depressor
   - Toothbrush or denture brush (Figure 25-7)
   - Toothpaste or tooth powder
   - Mouthwash, if permitted
   - Cup of water
   - Straw
   - Gauze squares
   - Applicators
   - Denture cup

FIGURE 25-7 The denture brush has a smaller head than a toothbrush. The back side has a smaller tuft of bristles that works well for cleaning between teeth and in areas that are otherwise difficult to clean. (Courtesy of Medline Industries, Inc. (800) MEDLINE)

3. Apply disposable gloves.

4. Allow the patient to clean the dentures if she is able to do so. If the patient cannot, give a tissue to the patient and ask her to remove the dentures. Assist if necessary.

   a. To remove upper dentures, grasp the dentures firmly, ease them downward and then forward, and remove them from the mouth (Figure 25-8).

   b. To remove lower dentures, grasp the dentures firmly, ease them upward and then forward, and remove them from the mouth.

5. Place the dentures in a denture cup padded with gauze squares. Take them to the bathroom or utility room.

6. Place a paper towel or washcloth in the bottom of the basin to protect the dentures (Figure 25-9). Fill the sink half full with cool water. The combination of water and towel protect the dentures from chipping or breaking if they are accidentally dropped in the sink.

7. Dentures may be soaked in a solution with a cleansing tablet before brushing, if desired.

continues

PROCEDURE 66 CONTINUED

FIGURE 25-8 Grasp the upper dentures firmly with gauze-covered fingers to prevent slipping. Ease down and forward to remove.

FIGURE 25-9 Brush dentures until all surfaces are clean.

8. Wet the dentures by rinsing under cool water.

9. Put toothpaste or tooth powder on a brush. Hold the dentures and brush until all surfaces are clean.

10. Rinse the dentures thoroughly under cool running water. Never use hot water. Rinse the denture cup.

11. Place fresh gauze squares in the denture cup with clean, cool water unless instructed otherwise.

12. Place the dentures in the gauze-lined cup and take them to the bedside.

13. Assist the patient to rinse her mouth with mouthwash, if permitted. Otherwise, use water. Hold the mouth open gently with a wooden tongue depressor. Clean the gums and tongue with applicators moistened with mouthwash, or use foam Toothettes.

 Note: Carefully observe and report the condition of the teeth, mouth, tongue, lips, and dentures.

14. Use a paper towel or gauze to hand wet dentures to the patient. If the patient is able, she can remove the dentures from the cup. Insert if necessary, upper denture first.

15. Clean and replace equipment according to facility policy.

16. Remove and dispose of gloves according to facility policy.

17. Carry out ending procedure actions.

BACKRUBS

When properly given, backrubs can be:
- Stimulating to the patient's circulation
- A major aid in preventing skin breakdown (*pressure ulcers*)
- Soothing
- Refreshing

Keep your nails short to prevent injuring the patient. The backrub procedure provides a good opportunity for you to observe the condition of the patient's skin. Report all observations to the nurse. Look for:

Safety ALERT

Health care workers have known for years that denture cleaning tablets can cause serious injury to a confused or pediatric patient, if swallowed. The fizzing, foaming action of the tablet causes burns of the mucous membranes in the mouth, throat, esophagus, and stomach. In 2005, new information was published about the ingestion and systemic absorption of denture adhesive paste. Zinc is used in the paste as a bonding agent and odor blocker. It is not always listed on the label. Ingestion of denture paste poses a risk for zinc toxicity. Keep all denture cleaners and paste preparations out of the hands of confused and pediatric patients, as well as others (such as a suicidal patient) who may ingest them. ■

- Reddened areas that do not blanch (whiten) when pressed
- Raw areas of skin
- Condition of skin over bony prominences

Unless contraindicated, the backrub is given:

- Routinely as part of the bed bath or partial bath
- Following use of the bedpan
- When changing the position of the helpless patient
- At bedtime
- When it could be a comfort to the patient

Long, smooth strokes are relaxing. Short, circular strokes tend to be more stimulating. Avoid massaging red areas over bony prominences.

The backrub is given with warmed lotion.

OSHA ALERT

When giving a backrub, make sure the bed is elevated to a comfortable height for you. Stand with one foot slightly ahead of the other, with knees bent slightly. Use your arm and shoulder muscles to massage the back. Rock back and forth, using the strong muscles in your legs. Avoid bending from the waist. ■

Difficult SITUATIONS

For many years, backrubs were almost a sacred, routine part of nursing care. Over time, we have become much more dependent on technology. When we are busy or staffing is short, it seems as if there is no time to give backrubs. Yet, calming the agitated patient who cannot sleep is time-consuming; the pregnant mother with a backache may use the call signal frequently; the patient with spasticity just cannot get into a comfortable position.

You may find that taking a few minutes to give a backrub will save you a great deal of time in caring for your patients. A good backrub is comforting and relaxing. Agitated patients often calm down. Uncomfortable patients become more comfortable and demand less attention. Do not omit this important part of nursing care that pays such large dividends in patient comfort and satisfaction. In the long run, it may even make your job easier. ■

GUIDELINES *for*

Applying Lotion to the Patient's Skin

- Massaging the patient's skin is comforting and refreshing. It stimulates circulation and helps prevent skin breakdown.
- Warm the lotion in a basin of warm water or the palm of your hand.
- Refer to the care plan to see if massage is indicated.
- Applying lotion immediately after the bath helps hold moisture in the skin.
- Patients who are elderly and those with very dry, fragile skin will benefit from an application of lotion several times a day to keep skin supple and more resistant to injury.

- Each facility has a house lotion that is used for skin care. It is usually alcohol-free.
- Always use smooth, light strokes.
- Never rub red areas that may be stage I pressure ulcers.
- Avoid massaging the legs. If lotion is needed for dry skin, gently pat it on. Massage can cause complications related to blood clots. If the patient uses lotion on the legs, pat it on.
- Avoid putting lotion between the toes. The lotion keeps the area moist, which promotes fungal growth.

PROCEDURE

BACKRUB

1. Carry out initial procedure actions.

2. Assemble equipment:
   - Disposable gloves
   - Basin of water (105°F)
   - Washcloth
   - Bath towel
   - Soap and lotion

3. Put up the far side rail.

4. Place the lotion in a basin of water to warm (Figure 25-10).

5. Put on disposable gloves if the patient has open lesions.

6. Turn the patient on the side with the back toward you.

7. Expose and wash the back; dry carefully. This step is not necessary if the backrub is given after a bath.

8. Pour a small amount of lotion into one hand and warm it in the palm of your hand. Cold lotion may be very uncomfortable for the patient.

9. Apply the lotion to the patient's skin and rub with gentle but firm strokes. Give special attention to all bony prominences (Figure 25-11). Do not rub red areas. Report these to the nurse, if noted.

10. Begin at the base of the spine:
    - With long, soothing strokes, rub up the center of the back, around the shoulders, and down the sides of the back and buttocks (Figure 25-12A).
    - Repeat the previous step four times, using long, soothing upward strokes and a circular motion on the downstroke (Figure 25-12B).
    - Repeat, but on the downward stroke rub in small circular motions with the palm of your hand. Include areas over the coccyx (base of the spine) (Figure 25-12C).
    - Repeat long, soothing strokes on muscles for 3 to 5 minutes (Figure 25-12A).
    - Dry the area well.

FIGURE 25-10 Cool lotion causes an unpleasant sensation on the patient's back and may cause chilling. Warming the lotion in water for several minutes will make it more comfortable for the patient.

FIGURE 25-11 Use long, smooth, firm strokes to apply lotion.

- If redness on pressure areas is noted, report it to the nurse. Straighten and tighten the bottom sheet and draw sheet.

11. Change the patient's gown, if necessary.

continues

PROCEDURE 67 CONTINUED

12. Remove gloves if used. Discard according to facility policy and wash your hands.

13. Replace equipment.

14. Carry out ending procedure actions.

FIGURE 25-12 Strokes to be used during the backrub: A. soothing strokes B. circular movement C. passive movement

DAILY SHAVING

Daily shaving is part of the routine self-care of most men. It should not be neglected in a health care facility. When patients are unable to shave themselves and a barber is not available, it is your responsibility.

Older women have an increase in the growth and coarseness of hairs on the chin and upper lip. Many women find this distressing. Tweezers can be used to remove some of the hairs, but a more permanent method is to have the hairs removed professionally with an electric needle. Some women may require a shave. In some facilities nursing assistants are not permitted to shave female patients. Be sure to check the policy of your facility.

Infection Control ALERT

Shaving may be done with an electric razor that is the patient's personal property. Such a razor is used for one patient only and cleaned according to manufacturer's directions after each use. This usually involves brushing the heads with a small brush designed for this purpose. All hair should be removed from the head of the razor. Some electric razors must be recharged periodically. Electric razors are expensive. Handle the razor carefully and avoid dropping it. If the electrical cord is frayed or worn, report to the nurse and remove the razor from use. If an electric razor is not available, use a disposable safety razor. Wearing gloves is usually not necessary when an electric razor is used. ▪

Age-Appropriate Care ALERT

Elderly women may grow facial hair as a result of hormonal changes during aging. Coarse hair is common on the chin. Most women prefer to have facial hair removed. Many women also prefer to have hair removed from their legs and underarms. Honor the patient's preferences. Know your facility policy for removing facial hair from female patients. Some facilities use depilatories. Although some facilities shave women, check with the nurse before performing this procedure because shaving may worsen the problem, causing the hair to become thicker and coarser. ▪

OSHA ALERT

Always wear gloves when shaving patients with a nonelectric razor, because of the high risk of contact with blood. Discard the razor in a puncture-resistant (sharps) container. ▪

GUIDELINES *for*

Safety in Shaving

- Use the patient's own shaving equipment if possible. For safety, use an electric razor or rotary razor.

- If the patient is receiving **anticoagulants** (medications that thin the blood and increase the risk of bleeding), a special procedure may be required. For example, an electric razor provides the greatest safety. Check with the nurse for the proper procedure.

- If oxygen is being given, it may be possible to discontinue it during this procedure. Consult the nurse and follow hospital policy.

- The patient may use a preshave or aftershave product as desired. Keep these products out of the hands of patients who may swallow them.

PROCEDURE

SHAVING A MALE PATIENT

1. Carry out initial procedure actions.

2. Assemble equipment:
   - Disposable gloves
   - Electric shaver or safety razor
   - Shaving lather or preshave lotion for electric razor
   - Basin of water (105°F)
   - Face towels
   - Mirror
   - Washcloth
   - Aftershave lotion

3. Raise the head of the bed. Place equipment on the overbed table.

4. Put on gloves.

5. Place one face towel across the patient's chest and one under his head.

6. Moisten face and apply lather (or preshave lotion).

7. Starting in front of ear:
   a. Hold skin taut and bring razor down over cheek toward chin (Figure 25-13).
   b. Repeat until lather on cheek is removed and area has been shaved. Rinse frequently.
   c. Repeat on other cheek.
   d. Use firm, short strokes. Shave in direction of hair growth.
   e. Rinse razor frequently.

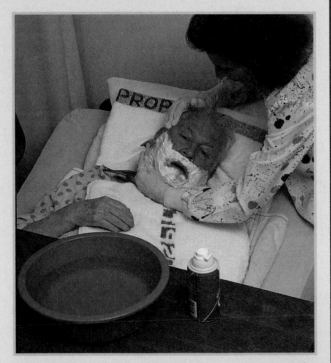

FIGURE 25-13 Shaving is part of the daily routine for most men.

8. Ask the patient to tighten his upper lip. Shave from the nose to the upper lip in short, downward strokes.

9. Ask the patient to tighten his chin. Shave the chin in downward strokes.

10. Assist the patient to tip his head back.

continues

PROCEDURE 68 CONTINUED

11. Lather the neck area and stroke up toward the chin. Rinse and repeat until all lather is removed.

12. Wash the patient's face and neck and dry thoroughly.

13. Apply aftershave lotion if desired.

14. If the skin is nicked, apply a small piece of tissue and hold pressure directly over the area. Then apply an antiseptic and bandage. Report the incident to the nurse.

15. Clean and replace equipment. Dispose of razor according to facility policy. Remove the head of an electric razor. Use a razor brush to remove clippings. Store the razor according to facility policy.

16. Remove and dispose of gloves according to facility policy.

17. Carry out ending procedure actions.

DAILY HAIR CARE

Daily care of the hair, for both male and female patients, is usually performed after the patient's bed bath.

The hair should be combed and brushed each morning. Tangles can be loosened by sectioning the hair with a comb or brush, working with one section at a time. Grasp the hair near the scalp to reduce pulling (Figure 25-14). Start combing or brushing tangles out starting at the ends and working toward the scalp. Braiding long hair after brushing can help reduce tangles. Tangles can be reduced in wiry, dry hair by using conditioner and keeping the hair short or in braids.

Tips: Avoid braiding a patient's hair tightly, because it can be uncomfortable. Secure the braids with hair ties. Avoid rubber bands, if possible. If the hair is very tangled, applying a small amount of alcohol or oil to the tangle will make it easier to remove.

Brushing the hair:

FIGURE 25-14 To remove tangles from long hair, divide the hair into sections. Work with one section at a time. Hold the hair near the scalp to reduce pulling and start combing at the end of the hair, working up toward the scalp.

- Stimulates circulation of the scalp
- Refreshes the patient
- Removes dust and lint
- Helps to keep the hair shiny and attractive

If additional care is needed, a fluid dry cleaner to shampoo the hair is available. It leaves the hair soft and manageable and the hairstyle intact. This procedure is so simple that it is often used instead of the regular shampoo for patients who must remain in bed.

Sometimes, however, a shampoo may be advisable for the patient in bed. Approval for the procedure must be obtained from the doctor. Bed shampoos should be given every two weeks when the patient is bedbound for an extended period. (See Unit 24, Procedure 61.)

Difficult SITUATIONS

Hair is important to everyone's self-esteem and appearance. Some diseases and medications cause hair loss. Some cause changes to the volume and texture of hair. Some medications cause hair to become dry and brittle. Patients who have problems with their hair may become anxious or angry because the appearance of the hair affects their self-esteem. If the patient is experiencing problems with hair, treat it gently. Use products such as baby shampoo and conditioner. Use tepid water. Pat the hair dry rather than rubbing it with a towel. Use a wide-toothed comb to style the hair gently. Avoid rubber bands, which may worsen the problem. Assist the patient to wear a scarf or turban, if desired. ■

PROCEDURE

69

DAILY HAIR CARE

1. Carry out initial procedure actions.

2. Assemble equipment:
   - Towel
   - Comb and brush

3. Ask the patient to move to the side of the bed nearest you; or the patient may sit in a chair if permitted. If the patient is sitting up, put a towel around her shoulders.

4. Cover the pillow with a towel.

5. Part or section the hair and comb with one hand between the scalp and the ends of the hair.

6. Brush carefully and thoroughly.

7. Have the patient turn so that you can comb and brush the hair on the back of her head. If the hair is tangled, work section by section to unsnarl it, beginning near the ends and working toward the scalp.

8. Complete brushing and arrange the hair attractively. Braid long hair to prevent repeated snarling. Allow the patient to choose the style, if able.

9. Clean and replace equipment according to facility policy.

10. Carry out ending procedure actions.

Procedure 69 assumes that the patient is a female. Hair care for a male is very similar, however, so the procedure can easily be adapted.

Care of African American Patients' Hair

African American patients have special hair-care needs. With these patients, hair texture can vary from soft and silky to coarse and thick. Patients with coarse hair need special care to prevent damage, tangling, and breaking. Asking the patient or family how to care for the hair is not offensive. In fact, it shows that you care about meeting the patient's needs. They have been caring for the hair for years, and are experts at it. They also know which products work and which do not.

In general, avoid using hair products designed for Caucasian persons. Most of these are designed to eliminate oil. Eliminating the oil from the hair is one of the worst things to do when caring for African Americans. Use a shampoo marketed specifically for black hair. In most cases, the patient or family will provide a product that works for them. Wash the hair once every week or two, as specified on the care plan, and according to the patient's preference. Washing more often than this dries the hair and causes breakage. If a special shampoo is not available, baby shampoo works best. Wash the hair using the guidelines in Procedure 61. Use a detangling conditioner according to product directions. After washing the hair, gently towel-dry. Cover the shoulders with a dry towel. Use a wide-toothed comb or pick to comb through the damp hair. Be gentle and patient. It may take time to work through the tangles.

African Americans need additional oil on the hair at all times. Some patients use products they refer to as hair "grease." If the patient does not have a product preference, apply baby oil *to the scalp, not the hair.* Then, using a soft brush, brush from the scalp to the ends of the hair until all the hairs are covered with oil. You may need to apply this heavily. If it is too oily, wipe the excess with a towel. If you use enough, the hair will appear shiny.

The patient's hair can be braided while damp. Run the wide-toothed comb through the hair to remove tangles, following the guidelines in Procedure 69. Gently twist the hair and apply a hair tie. Avoid using rubber bands, if possible. These cause breakage and damage hair. If a rubber band must be used, apply hair grease or baby oil liberally to your fingers. Roll the rubber band around in the hair grease until it is well coated, then apply it to the hair. Style the hair in a pony tail, then section and braid it. When you get to the end, apply more grease. Wrap the ends around a barrette and snap it shut, or use a hair tie or grease-coated rubber band.

COMFORT DEVICES

The physician, nurse, or physical therapist orders comfort devices such as bed cradles, footboards, and pillows. They are designed to relieve pressure on specific areas or to help maintain body position.

Bed Cradle

A bed cradle (Figures 25-15A and 25-15B) prevents the weight of the bedclothes from falling on some part of the

FIGURE 25-15A A bed cradle keeps the sheet and blanket from putting pressure on the feet.

FIGURE 25-15B A wide cradle is used for patients with skin conditions such as burns or widespread lesions. The wide cradle supports the weight of heavy bedding and relieves pressure from a larger area of skin surface.

body. It can be used therapeutically or as a comfort device. It is used:

- Over fractured limbs
- When there are burns
- To prevent skin lesions
- Over widespread skin conditions, such as psoriasis or eczema
- To prevent contractures of the feet
- Over a wet cast until it dries

Coverings that maintain some degree of warmth within the cradle may also be needed to keep the patient comfortable.

Care must be taken to position the limbs within the cradle. It may be necessary to pad the cradle edges.

Footboard or Footrest

The **footboard** or footrest is a device placed between the mattress and bed to keep the feet at right angles to the legs (natural standing position). A footboard is always padded. It is used to prevent a type of contracture called **foot drop**. In foot drop, the muscle in the calf of the leg tends to tighten, causing the toes to point downward. Foot drop may happen when the patient must remain in bed over a long period of time. Even a brief period in bed is sufficient to cause a degree of foot drop that makes walking difficult when the patient does get out of bed.

If a footboard is not available, a pillow folded lengthwise may be placed against the foot of the bed to serve the same purpose. Some facilities use special tennis shoes or soft boots to prevent foot drop in patients who are at risk because they are bedfast.

Pillows and Bath Blankets

Pillows can be used as comfort devices and to maintain alignment when properly arranged. For directions on properly altering the patient's position, refer to Unit 15.

The trochanter roll is used to prevent external rotation of the hip. Trochanter rolls should be used routinely for bedfast patients, to prevent deformities. Unless a specific medical condition, such as a hip fracture, is present, no special order is necessary.

A trochanter roll or support can be made as follows:

1. Fold a bath blanket lengthwise in thirds.
2. Position the patient in the center of the folded bath blanket. The blanket should extend from mid-thigh to above the waist.
3. Roll each side of the blanket under and toward the patient until the blanket roll is firmly against the patient. Then tuck the roll inward toward the bed and patient to maintain the patient's position.

Pillows are also used to relieve pressure in such a way that spaces are left for specific areas (Figure 25-16). This technique is called **bridging**. Bridging elevates an area of the body off the surface of the bed. It is useful for patients with healing pressure ulcers. Bridging is commonly used

FIGURE 25-16 The patient is positioned on her abdomen and pillows are used to form a bridge, preventing pressure on her breasts.

for the sacrum, hips, heels, and ankles. No special equipment is necessary. Facilities may use a combination of pillows, foam props, and bath blankets to support an area.

ELIMINATION NEEDS

Regular, periodic elimination of body wastes is essential for maintaining health. Patients who are confined to bed must rely on you to help them with this physical task. (See Procedures 70 to 72.) You should know that:

- The patient must regularly empty the bladder by urinating (voiding).
- A urinal (duct or bottle) is used by male patients when they need to urinate. A bedpan is used by female patients to void when they are confined to bed.
- A regular bowel movement (which is the discharge of solid waste from the body) is also important to a patient's health.
- The solid waste produced by the patient is called **feces** or *stool*.
- Both male and female patients use a bedpan for solid waste elimination when confined to bed.
- Many patients are somewhat sensitive about using a bedpan or urinal.
- Personal hygiene is exceedingly important in carrying out these procedures properly.
- Bedpans are very uncomfortable.

Four important points must be kept in mind. You must:

1. Wear disposable gloves.

Difficult **SITUATIONS**

Dusting the edges of the bedpan that contact the patient's skin lightly with powder will reduce friction, making the bedpan easier to insert and remove, especially if the patient is obese. ■

2. Wash your hands immediately before and after the procedure. This will help prevent the transmission of any disease to others and to yourself.
3. Provide privacy for the patient. Obtain the proper type of bedpan according to patient needs.
4. As soon as possible, answer the light indicating that the patient is finished.

One-Glove Technique

Some facilities require health care providers to use the one-glove technique when removing bedpans, urinals, and other contaminated items. Gloves are worn on both hands when the contaminated item is removed. The bedpan or contaminated item is covered if it is to be carried to the bathroom or into the hallway. A glove is then removed from one hand. Do not put the glove on an environmental surface. The gloved hand carries the glove that you removed and the contaminated item. The ungloved hand is used to open doors and turn on faucets. By using this method, you avoid contaminating the environment with your gloves.

PROCEDURE

GIVING AND RECEIVING THE BEDPAN

1. Carry out initial procedure actions.
2. Assemble equipment:
   - Disposable gloves
   - Bedpan and cover
   - Basin
   - Washcloth
   - Bath blanket
   - Paper towels/protector
   - Toilet tissue
   - Soap
   - Towel

3. Lower the head of the bed, if necessary.
4. Put on gloves.
5. Take the bedpan and toilet tissue from the bedside stand.
   - Place a protector on the chair. Place the bedpan (Figure 25-17) on it.
   - Never place a bedpan on the bedside stand or overbed table.
   - Put the remainder of the articles on the bedside table.

continues

PROCEDURE **70** CONTINUED

FIGURE 25-17 Orthopedic (fracture) bedpan (left) and regular bedpan (right).

FIGURE 25-18A Roll the patient away from you. Provide support by placing one hand on the hip. Position the bedpan with the other hand, then roll the patient back onto the bedpan.

6. Place the bedpan cover at the foot of the bed.
   - The bedpan may be warmed by running warm water into it and then emptying and drying it.
   - Plastic bedpans may be comfortable without warming.

   ✐ **Note:** Never carry or allow a used bedpan to sit uncovered. If a bedpan cover is not available, cover the bedpan with a towel, bed protector, pillowcase, or paper towels.

7. Cover the patient with a bath blanket. Fold the top bedcovers back at a right angle. Raise the patient's gown. If the patient is thin or has a pressure sore, consult the nurse for the appropriate action. The nursing care plan may have specific instructions for such cases. For example, it may be necessary to pad the bedpan with a folded towel or to take some other action.

8. Ask the patient to flex the knees and rest weight on the heels, if able.

9. Help the patient to raise the buttocks by:
   - Putting one hand under the small of the patient's back and lifting gently and slowly with that hand.
   - With the other hand, place the bedpan under the patient's hips.
   - The pan may also be placed by rolling the patient to one side, positioning the bedpan against the buttocks, and rolling the patient back onto the pan (Figure 25-18A). Check to be sure the bedpan is positioned properly.

   - Alternatively, if a trapeze is in place over the bed, place the bedpan under the patient as the patient lifts self using the trapeze (Figure 25-18B).
   - The patient's buttocks should rest on the rounded shelf of the regular bedpan.
   - The narrow end should face the foot of the bed. If a fracture pan is being used, the narrow end is positioned under the patient's buttocks, with the handle end facing the foot of the bed.

FIGURE 25-18B The patient assists by lifting with the trapeze as the nursing assistant places the bedpan. Support the small of the patient's back with one hand when he or she pulls up on the trapeze.

continues

PROCEDURE 70 CONTINUED

10. Replace the top bedcovers. Raise the head of the bed to a comfortable height. Remove gloves and dispose of properly.

11. Make sure the toilet paper and signal cord are within easy reach of the patient. Leave the patient alone unless contraindicated in the nursing care plan.

12. Wash your hands.

    📝 **Note:** If a specimen is to be taken, instruct the patient that toilet tissue is not to be placed in the bedpan. Provide a small plastic bag to discard tissue.

13. Watch for the patient's signal.

14. Answer the patient's call signal immediately. Wash your hands and put on disposable gloves. Fill the basin with warm water (105°F) and place it next to soap, washcloth, and towel on the overbed table.

15. Fold the top bedcovers back so that the patient remains covered only with the bath blanket.

16. Remove the bedpan from under the patient.

    • Ask the patient to flex the knees and rest weight on the heels. Place one hand under the small of the back and lift gently to help raise the buttocks off the bedpan. Take the bedpan with the other hand. Cover it and place it on the chair.

FIGURE 25-18C   Hold the bedpan securely while the patient turns to the side.

• If the patient is unable to raise the buttocks, roll the patient off the pan to the side and remove the pan. Lift and move carefully. Hold the pan firmly with one hand (Figure 25-18C).

• Many patients have difficulty cleaning adequately after using the bedpan. You may need to clean and dry the patient yourself.

17. If the underpad is wet, change it. Provide perineal care.

    • Discard used toilet tissue in the bedpan unless a specimen is to be collected.

    • Cover the bedpan again.

    • Cleanse the patient with warm water and soap, if necessary.

18. Replace the bedclothes, changing linen as necessary.

19. Cover the patient with top bedding and remove the bath blanket.

20. Assist the patient to wash hands and freshen up after the procedure. An antiseptic hand rub or alcohol product may be used, if desired.

21. Take the bedpan to the bathroom or utility room and observe its contents. Measure, if required. Always keep the soiled bedpan covered when carrying it in the patient's room or hallway. Some facilities use bedpans with self-fitting lids (Figure 25-18D). If no lid is available, use an underpad (Figure 25-18E), a plastic or paper bag, or a piece of newspaper. Wear a glove on the hand you use to carry the bedpan. Do not wear a soiled glove on the opposite hand if you will be using it to open doors or turn on faucets. Remove the soiled glove or hold a paper towel under your gloved hand to prevent contamination of the environment.

22. Empty the bedpan.

23. Turn on the faucet, using a paper towel. Rinse the bedpan with cold water and disinfectant. Rinse, dry, and return the bedpan to storage in the patient's bedside stand.

24. Remove gloves and dispose of them properly. Wash your hands.

25. Carry out ending procedure actions.

continues

PROCEDURE 70 CONTINUED

FIGURE 25-18D Always cover the full bedpan when carrying it. This bedpan has a lid that fits securely.

FIGURE 25-18E If a lid is not available, use a disposable underpad to cover the bedpan.

PROCEDURE

GIVING AND RECEIVING THE URINAL

1. Carry out initial procedure actions.

2. Assemble equipment:
   - Urinal (Figure 25-19)
   - Basin
   - Soap
   - Washcloth
   - Towel
   - Disposable gloves

3. Put on gloves. Lift the top bedcovers and place the urinal under the covers so the patient can grasp the handle. Instruct the patient to place his penis in the urinal opening. If he cannot do this, you must position the urinal and ensure that the penis is placed in the opening.

4. Remove gloves and dispose of them properly. Wash your hands. Make sure the signal cord is within easy reach of the patient. Leave the patient alone if possible. Watch for his signal.

FIGURE 25-19 A male urinal with a snap-on lid

continues

PROCEDURE 71 CONTINUED

5. Answer the patient's signal immediately. Wash your hands. Fill a basin with warm water (105°F), and place it next to soap, washcloth, and towel so the patient can wash and dry his hands.

6. Put on gloves. Ask the patient to hand the urinal to you. Cover it. Rearrange the bedclothes if necessary.

7. Take the urinal to the bathroom or utility room and observe the contents. Measure, if required. Do not empty the urinal if you observe anything unusual (such as blood). Rather, save the contents of the urinal for the nurse's inspection.

8. Empty the urinal. Rinse the urinal with cold water and clean it with warm soapy water. Rinse, dry, and cover the urinal. Remove gloves and dispose of them properly. Wash your hands.

9. Place the urinal inside the patient's bedside table. Clean and replace other articles.

10. Carry out ending procedure actions.

PROCEDURE 72

ASSISTING WITH USE OF THE BEDSIDE COMMODE

1. Carry out initial procedure actions.

2. Assemble equipment:
   - Disposable gloves
   - Portable commode
   - Toilet tissue
   - Basin
   - Washcloth
   - Soap
   - Towel
   - Bath blanket

3. Position the commode beside the bed, facing the head. Lock the commode wheels and open the lid. Be sure a receptacle is in place under the seat.

4. If the bed and side rails are elevated, lower the side rail nearest you and lower the bed to the lowest horizontal position. Lock bed wheels.

5. Put on gloves.

6. Assist the patient to a sitting position. Swing the patient's legs over the edge of the bed.

7. Assist the patient to put on a robe. Put slippers on the patient. Assist the patient to stand. If needed, use a transfer belt.

8. Support the patient with hands on either side of the chest. Remember to use proper body mechanics. Pivot the patient and lower her to the commode.

9. Cover the patient's legs with a bath blanket.

10. Leave the call bell and toilet tissue within reach.

11. Remove gloves and discard according to facility policy.

12. When the patient signals, return promptly. Wash your hands and put on gloves. Fill a basin with water at 105°F. Bring the basin to the bedside along with soap, a towel, and a washcloth.

13. Remove bath blanket. Assist the patient to stand.

14. Cleanse the anus or perineum if the patient is unable to do so.

15. Allow the patient to wash and dry her hands. Remove gloves and dispose of according to facility policy. Wash your hands.

16. Assist the patient to return to bed. Adjust bedding and pillows for comfort.

17. Leave the signal cord within easy reach.

18. Put on gloves.

continues

PROCEDURE 72 CONTINUED

19. Remove the receptacle from the commode and cover it. Close the commode lid.

20. Take the receptacle to the bathroom. Note its contents and measure if required.

21. Empty and clean the receptacle per facility policy. Replace it in the commode. Remove and dispose of gloves properly.

22. Put the commode in its proper place.

23. Carry out ending procedure actions.

Infection Control ALERT

Make sure that bedpans and urinals are labeled with the patients' names for patients in rooms with two or more beds. After cleaning the bedpan or urinal, store it properly in the bedside stand or according to facility policy. Do not leave uncovered bedpans and urinals on the floor or in the bathroom. ■

REVIEW

A. True/False.

Mark the following true or false by circling T or F.

1. T F Dentures should be stored in an antiseptic solution.

2. T F Backrubs are routinely given as part of the bath procedure.

3. T F A padded footboard is one method of preventing foot drop.

4. T F Routine oral hygiene should be carried out once daily.

5. T F Proper oral hygiene helps prevent tooth decay.

6. T F When not in the patient's mouth, dentures should be left on the back of the sink.

7. T F Patients who have no teeth and no dentures require regular oral hygiene.

8. T F When giving PM care, the bottom sheet should be tightened and the top linen straightened.

9. T F The nursing assistant should wear gloves when giving oral care.

10. T F The unconscious patient needs no oral care because he is not eating.

B. Matching.

Choose the correct word from Column II to match the phrases in Column I.

Column I

11. _____ bad breath

12. _____ mouth care

13. _____ tooth cavities

14. _____ means of relieving pressure

15. _____ artificial teeth

Column II

a. oral hygiene

b. caries

c. dentures

d. bridging

e. halitosis

f. foot drop

C. Completion.

Complete the statements in items 16–20 by writing in the correct word from the following list.

arm
breakfast
down
early AM care
hand

name
PM care
removed
surgery

16. After PM care, the bed should be left with the back-rest _____.

17. _____ should be completed before sleep medication is given.

18. The best way to awaken a patient is to place your _____ on the patient's arm and say his _____.

19. Patients are not wakened early if they are going to have _____.

20. Early morning care awakens the patient before _____.

D. Multiple Choice.

Select the one best answer for each of the following.

21. Which of the following patients should be given special mouth care?
   a. One who can brush her own teeth
   b. One who is drinking water ad lib
   c. One who has a broken leg
   d. One who has a nasogastric tube.

22. To warm lotion before giving a backrub,
   a. hold it under running water.
   b. soak it in a basin of warm water.
   c. let the patient hold the bottle for a few minutes.
   d. microwave the bottle for 15 seconds.

23. The best way to support a patient in a side-lying position is to
   a. use a footboard to keep the feet aligned.
   b. place a pillow doubled under the head.
   c. place two pillows lengthwise between the legs.
   d. double a pillow lengthwise behind the back.

24. When brushing a patient's teeth, the best technique includes
   a. inserting the toothbrush with the bristles down.
   b. scrubbing the outer surface well and avoiding the sensitive inner surface.
   c. inserting the toothbrush with bristles facing the teeth.
   d. brushing the teeth in a downward motion only.

25. Backrubs are given
   a. routinely as a comfort measure.
   b. before use of the bedpan.
   c. routinely every two hours.
   d. only for patients with red areas.

E. Nursing Assistant Challenge.

Your patient, Mrs. Ubanan, has a history of heavy smoking and breathes through her mouth. She has plastic dentures and her care plan indicates that she needs assistance with denture care. Complete the following statements regarding this patient.

26. State two reasons why special oral hygiene has been ordered for Mrs. Ubanan.
   a. _____
   b. _____

27. Where are the dentures stored when not in use? ____

28. Should the dentures be kept dry or wet? _____

29. Should you wear gloves when removing her dentures? _____

30. Will you clean the dentures in cool or hot water? _____

Principles of Nutrition and Fluid Balance

UNIT 26
Nutritional Needs and Diet Modifications

UNIT 26

Nutritional Needs and Diet Modifications

OBJECTIVES

After completing this unit, you will be able to:

- Spell and define terms.
- Define normal nutrition.
- List the essential nutrients.
- Name the food groups and list the foods included in each group.
- State the liquids/foods allowed on the basic facility diets.
- Describe the purposes of the following diets:
  - clear liquid
  - full liquid
  - soft
  - mechanically altered

- State the purpose of calorie counts and food intake studies.
- Define dysphagia and explain the risks of this condition.
- Describe general care for the patient with dysphagia and swallowing problems.
- State the purposes of therapeutic diets.
- List types of alternative nutrition.
- Describe the nursing assistant actions when patients are unable to drink fluids independently.
- Demonstrate the following procedures:
  - Procedure 73 Assisting the Patient Who Can Feed Self
  - Procedure 74 Feeding the Dependent Patient

VOCABULARY

Learn the meaning and the correct spelling of the following words and phrases:

amino acids	enteral feeding	intravenous infusion (IV)	percutaneous endoscopic gastrostomy (PEG)
aspiration	essential nutrients	jejunostomy tube (J-tube)	protein
carbohydrates	exchange list	mechanical soft	pureed diet
cellulose	excrete	mechanically altered	push fluids
clear liquid diet	fats	minerals	soft diet
defecation	fluid balance	nasogastric feeding (NG feeding)	supplement
dehydration	force fluids	nourishments	therapeutic diets
diaphoresis	full liquid diet	nutrients	total parenteral nutrition (TPN)
digestion	gastrostomy feeding	nutrition	vitamins
diuresis	graduate		
dysphagia	hyperalimentation		
edema	intake and output (I&O)		
emesis			

INTRODU

Nutrition is the e
food for growth a
The signs of good

- Shiny hair
- Clear skin and
- A well-develope
- An alert express
- A pleasant disp
- Healthy sleep p
- Appropriate ap
- Regular bowel
- Body weight a

NORMAL

Food is normally
The mouth is th
tion is the proc
substances that c
ment. These subs

ESSENTIA

To be well nouri

- Supply heat a
- Build and rep
- Regulate body

These foods are
tial to maintain

- Proteins
- Carbohydrate
- Fats
- Minerals
- Vitamins
- Water

Protein

Protein is an e
every body cell.
cells and rebuil
est amount of p

- Meat
- Poultry
- Eggs
- Milk
- Cheese

Proteins are m
acids. The bo
acids, but not

Vitamins and Minerals

Vitamins and minerals are present in a wi
foods. The best way to be sure that you
enough vitamins and minerals is to include
foods in your daily diet.

Vitamins are substances that regulate bo
They help to:

- Build strong teeth and bones
- Promote growth
- Aid normal body functioning
- Strengthen resistance to disease

You probably know the vitamins by their lett

- Vitamin A
- B-complex vitamins
- Vitamin C
- Vitamin D
- Vitamin E
- Vitamin K

Fat-soluble vitamins do not dissolve easily in that are liquid at room temperature; they
can be stored in the body. Vitamins A, D, E many different plants and fish. Some are
fat-soluble vitamins. as flavorings, such as walnut oil and

Vitamins B and C are water soluble. Water- oods such as nuts, olives, and avocados are
mins dissolve in water, so they can be lost in h in oil (Figure 26-5).
process. In general, these vitamins are not sto
amounts in the body. Deficiencies in water-s
mins are more common.

Fruits are healthy, good alternatives to
high in sugar.

Exercise

- Adults should be physically active for at least 30 minutes most days of the week, children for 60 minutes.
- Sixty to 90 minutes of daily physical activity may be needed to prevent weight gain or sustain weight loss.

CATEGORY	Grains	Vege
RECOMMENDATION	Half of all grains consumed should be whole grains.	Vary t of veg you
DAILY AMOUNT *Based on a 2,000 calorie diet.*	6 oz.	2.5

FIGURE 26-2 The USDA Food Guide Pyramid
pyramid to meet individual needs. This may be
Agriculture)

Mediterranean food is prepared with vari-
lives and oils.

- Free oils, such as mayonnaise, butter, margarine, lard, and shortening, should be used sparingly.
- Make the most of the fat sources in fish, nuts, and vegetable oils.
- If solid fat is used in cooking (such as frying chicken), the extra oil consumed is part of the discretionary calorie allowance.

Milk group

- Consume 3 cups each day (Figure 26-6).
- Use low-fat or fat-free products whenever possible.
- Cheese, yogurt, and milk-based desserts are included in this group.
- If you cannot consume milk because of lactose intolerance, choose lactose-free products and other sources that are rich in calcium.
- Foods such as cream, butter, and cream cheese are low in calcium and are not part of this group.

Meat and beans group

- Eat $5\frac{1}{2}$ ounces per day.
- This group includes meat, fish, poultry, and eggs.
- Dry beans and peas are part of this group as well as the vegetable group.
- Chose lean and low-fat meats and poultry.
- Meat may be baked, grilled, or broiled.
- Vary your choices with more fish, beans, peas, nuts, and seeds.
- Fish, nuts, and seeds contain healthy oils, so select these instead of meat and poultry when possible.
- If high-fat meats are used, the extra oil consumed is part of the discretionary calorie allowance.

Discretionary Calories. Each person needs a certain number of calories each day for proper body function and to provide energy for physical activities. The essential calories are the minimum calories required to meet your nutrient needs. By selecting food items that have low fat and low or no sugar content, you may be able to use more calories than the amount required to meet your nutrient needs. These are *discretionary calories*. A discretionary calorie is an extra calorie that can be used on solid fats, added sugars, alcohol, or extra food from any food group. For most people, the discretionary calorie allowance is very small (between 100 and 300 calories daily). Many people regularly use their discretionary calories by making unwise food choices, such as high-fat meats, cheeses, whole milk, or sweetened bakery products. You can use your discretionary calories to:

- Eat more foods from any food group than the food guide recommends.
- Eat higher-calorie forms of foods, such as those containing solid fats or added sugars, such as whole milk, cheese, sausage, biscuits, sweetened cereal, and sweetened yogurt.
- Add fats or sweeteners to foods, such as sauces, salad dressings, sugar, syrup, and butter.
- Eat or drink items that are mostly fats, caloric sweeteners, and/or alcohol, such as candy, soda, wine, and beer.

Water. Water is an essential nutrient that is necessary to life. A person can live only a few days without water. Water is necessary for all cellular functions in the body. An adequate intake of fluids is required to replace fluids lost through urine, stool, sweat, and evaporation through skin. The normal adult intake of fluids should be two to three quarts a day. Offering liquids to patients frequently is important for the following reasons:

- Some patients are not able to drink liquids without your help.
- Elderly patients have a decreased sense of thirst.
- Adequate fluid intake is necessary to prevent urinary problems and constipation.

BASIC FACILITY DIETS

The food you serve to patients in the health care facility will be prepared by the dietary department (Figure 26-7). It includes the essential nutrients. The way in which it is prepared and its consistency will depend on the individual patient's condition and needs. Sometimes very strict dietary control is needed.

The trays are usually delivered to the patient floors in large food containers. Each tray is labeled with the patient's name and type of diet. You will:

- Prepare the patient for the meal
- Check the tray card for the patient's name
- Check the tray card against the patient's armband
- Check the items on the tray to make sure they are allowed on the patient's diet
- Serve the tray to the patient
- Assist with feeding as necessary

FIGURE 26-6 Milk is an excellent source of calcium and phosphorus. These minerals are essential for growth and development of bones and teeth.

FIGURE 26-7 Patient diets are prepared in the dietary department and transported to the units in containers designed to maintain the temperature.

Health care facilities usually have many types of diets. Four common diets are:

- Regular or house, sometimes called a general diet
- Full liquid
- Clear liquid
- Soft

The progression of diets a patient is allowed following surgery is as follows:

1. Ice chips/sip of water
2. Clear liquids
3. Full liquids
4. Soft diet
5. Regular diet

In addition, the dietary department prepares special or **therapeutic** (treatment) **diets**. Therapeutic diets are discussed later in this unit.

Regular Diet

The regular or house diet is a normal or full diet based on the five food groups. The regular diet:

- Includes a great variety of foods
- Excludes only very rich foods: pastries, heavy cakes, fried foods, and highly seasoned foods, which might be difficult for inactive people to digest

- Has a lower caloric count, because an inactive person does not require as many calories as an active person

In many health care facilities, patients may select foods from a menu.

Liquid Diets

Clear Liquid Diet. A **clear liquid diet** (Figure 26-8) is a temporary diet because it is an inadequate diet. It is made up primarily of water and carbohydrates for energy. Feedings are given every two, three, or four hours as prescribed by the physician. It replaces fluids that may have been lost by vomiting or diarrhea. When a clear liquid food item is held up to the light, you can see through it. The clear liquid diet consists of liquids that do not irritate, cause gas formation, or encourage bowel movements (**defecation**).

Foods allowed on the clear liquid diet include:

- Tea, coffee with sugar but without cream
- Strained fruit or vegetable juice with gelatin (occasionally)
- Fat free meat broths
- Ginger ale (usually), 7Up, Coke, strained grape or apple juice
- Gelatin
- Popsicles

Full Liquid Diet. The **full liquid diet** does supply nourishment and may be used for longer periods of time than the clear liquid diet, but is also considered a temporary diet because it is not nutritionally complete. Six to eight ounces are usually given every two to three hours.

The full liquid diet is given to:

- Some patients with acute infections
- Patients with conditions involving the digestive tract

The diet includes all of the foods allowed on the clear liquid diet, in addition to the following:

- Strained cereal, such as cream of wheat or rice, blenderized soup, or potatoes pureed in soup
- Strained soups, milk-based soups

FIGURE 26-8 Items on a clear liquid diet include only liquids you can see through.

- Sherbet
- Gelatin
- Eggnog
- Malted milk
- Milk and cream
- Plain ice cream
- Strained vegetables and fruit juices
- Junket
- Solids that liquefy at room temperature
- Yogurt

Soft Diet

The **soft diet** usually follows the full liquid diet. Although this diet nourishes the body, between-meal feedings are sometimes given to increase the calorie count. Foods allowed on the soft diet are:

- Low-residue, which are almost completely used by the body
- Mildly flavored, slightly seasoned, or unseasoned
- Prepared in a form that is easy to digest

The diet includes liquids and semisolid foods that have a soft texture. It is given to patients who:

- Have infections and fevers
- Have minor difficulty swallowing
- Have conditions involving the digestive tract
- Are on a progressive postoperative dietary regime

The following foods are usually allowed on the soft diet:

- Soups
- Cream cheese and cottage cheese
- Crackers, toast
- Fish
- White meat of chicken or turkey (boiled or stewed)
- Fruit juices
- Cooked fruit (sieved)
- Tea, coffee
- Milk, cream, butter
- Cooked cereals
- Eggs (not fried)
- Beef and lamb (scraped or finely ground)
- Cooked vegetables (mashed or sieved)
- Angel food or sponge cake
- Small amounts of sugar
- Gelatin, custard
- Pudding
- Plain ice cream

Foods to be avoided include:

- Coarse cereals
- Spices
- Gas-forming foods (onions, cabbage, beans)
- Rich pastries and desserts
- Foods high in roughage/fiber
- Fried foods
- Raw fruits and vegetables
- Corn
- Pork (except bacon)

Clinical Information ALERT

Hospital food is the subject of many jokes. For example, after having a bad meal in a restaurant, a person may comment that he had better food at the hospital. Food is the issue most often complained about by hospital patients and their families. Some studies have shown that up to a third of the food served each day is not touched. Medical and nutritional professionals recognize that good-tasting, culturally appropriate food served at the correct temperature is well accepted by patients. Patients begin to feel better, and hospitals save money by wasting less food. Many facilities are now providing more diverse food. If you learn information about food choices that would benefit the patient, inform the nurse. ■

SPECIAL DIETS

Special diets are planned to meet specific patient needs. Patients may need special diets because of religious preferences or health needs.

Religious Restrictions

Religious practice requires changes in diet for some patients. For example, persons of the Orthodox Jewish faith follow strict food laws (Figure 26-9).

- There are strict prohibitions against shellfish and nonkosher meats such as pork.
- Certain fishes, such as tuna and salmon, are permitted.
- Foods may not be prepared with utensils that have been used for nonkosher food preparation.
- There are strict rules regarding the sequence in which milk products and meat may be consumed.

Some other faith restrictions are summarized in Table 26-1.

Therapeutic Diets

Standard diets can be changed to conform to special dietary requirements. For example, an order might be written for a low-sodium, mechanical soft diet when a patient has ill-fitting dentures and heart disease. These

TABLE 26-1 RELIGIOUS DIETARY PRACTICES

	Restricted Food						
Faith	Coffee	Tea	Alcohol	Pork/Pork Products	Caffeine-Containing Foods	Dairy Products	All Meats
Christian Science	▪	▪	▪				
Roman Catholic							1 hour before communion, Ash Wednesday, Good Friday
Latter Day Saints (Mormons)	▪	▪	▪		▪		
Seventh Day Adventist	▪	▪	▪	▪	▪		▪
Some Baptist	▪	▪	▪				
Greek Orthodox (on fast days)						▪	Fasting from meat and dairy products on Wed./Fri. during Lent and other holy days
Jewish Orthodox				▪ Also shellfish		Certain holy days	Forbids the serving of milk and milk products with meat; regulates food preparation; forbids cooking on the Sabbath
Muslim, Islamic			▪	▪			Fasting during Ramadan during day, feasting at night
Hindu							Some are vegetarians
Buddhist							Meat must be blessed and killed in special ways; some sects are vegetarians

FIGURE 26-9 Persons of the Orthodox Jewish faith eat only kosher foods, which require special preparation.

therapeutic diets are planned and prepared according to a patient's individual health problems. Commonly prescribed therapeutic diets include the diabetic diet, sodium-restricted diet, and low-fat diet.

The Diabetic Diet

Diet is an integral part of the therapy of the patient with diabetes mellitus. The diet is nutritionally adequate. It provides enough energy in the form of calories for a 24-hour period. Sometimes a proper diet is all that is needed to control the disease. Usually, however, the food intake is balanced by the administration of insulin or hypoglycemic drugs.

It is important for you to accurately evaluate and report the patient's intake. Foods and liquids have a major impact on diabetes management. Illness increases the need for insulin because the liver releases more glucose in response to the stress. Dehydration is a particularly serious

FIGURE 26-10 Many diabetics self-administer insulin injections one or more times each day for blood sugar control. Approximately 15.7 million people (5.9% of the U.S. population) have diabetes. An estimated 5.4 million people are not aware that they have the disease. Each day approximately 2,200 new cases of diabetes are diagnosed. Diabetes is a chronic disease that cannot be cured, but can be controlled through a combination of diet, exercise, and medications. The risk of complications is high if the condition is not diagnosed and medically managed.

problem for the diabetic. This can occur when not enough foods and fluids are taken in. Insulin administration may depend on your observations. Not all physicians prescribe dietary intake in the same way.

- Some physicians prescribe a very carefully balanced diet and insulin to maintain the level of blood sugar (glucose) within normal limits. All foods must be measured and repeated injections of insulin (Figure 26-10) may be required.
- Other physicians are much more liberal in their approach. They permit an unmeasured diet, limiting only sugar and high-sugar foods. This diet is known as a no-concentrated-sweets diet. It may be balanced by insulin or drugs that lower blood sugar.
- Many physicians treat diabetes with an approach that is midway between the preceding two methods. They prescribe the American Dietetic Association diets with

specific calorie levels, such as the 1,200-calorie diet or the 1,500-calorie diet. The dietitian teaches the patient about the diet and acts as a major resource for health care providers. The diet is balanced by insulin or hypoglycemic drugs.

The Exchange List. The **exchange list** method of balancing the diabetic diet:

- Is based on standard household measurements, to make it easier to measure
- Excludes sugar and high-sugar-content foods, to prevent rapid swings in blood sugar
- Divides foods into six groups
- Allows equivalent exchanges to be made within a group but not from group to group

The six groups are:

- Milk exchanges
- Vegetable exchange: Group A, Group B
- Fruit exchange
- Bread exchange
- Meat exchange
- Fat exchange

Sodium-Restricted Diet

Sodium-restricted diets may be ordered for patients with chronic renal failure and cardiovascular disease. Sodium-restricted diets are some of the most difficult diets to follow. The average American consumes 2 to 6 grams of sodium in food each day. Table salt is a major source of sodium in the diet.

TABLE 26-2 SODIUM-RESTRICTED DIETS

Type of Low-Sodium Diet	Amount of Sodium
No added salt (limited salt used in cooking, no salt added at meals)	3 to 4 grams daily
2 grams sodium	2 grams daily
1 gram sodium	1 gram daily
500-mg sodium	½ gram daily

Most Americans consume 2 to 6 grams of dietary sodium each day.

The physician may order several different levels of sodium restriction. These are listed in Table 26-2, in order of most to least salt content.

Processing may add significant amounts of sodium to foods. Food preservatives such as sodium citrate and sodium benzoate are added to many processed foods. This factor is considered in planning and selecting foods for the sodium-restricted diet. It is important to carefully read the labels for the contents of all commercially prepared foods.

Some foods naturally contain relatively large amounts of sodium. These foods may be restricted for this diet. They include:

- Meat
- Fish
- Poultry
- Milk and milk products
- Eggs

Avoid:

- Pork, ham, bacon
- Breads
- Potato chips, pretzels, and similar snacks
- Saltine crackers
- Pop (soda) containing sodium
- Pickles
- Processed meats
- Canned foods, such as vegetables and soups

Some foods are naturally low in sodium. They can be used more liberally. They are:

- Some cereals, such as shredded wheat
- Vegetables
- Fruits

Calorie-Restricted Diet

As long as activity remains constant, a person must take in approximately 500 calories a day less than usual (3,500 calories deficit per week) to lose one pound.

Calorie-restricted diets are prescribed for patients who are overweight. These diets are planned to meet general nutritional needs. They take into consideration the patient's energy output, general nutritional state, and weight goal.

In planning the calorie-restricted diet, the dietitian tries to create a realistic balance between fats, proteins, and carbohydrates. This type of diet encourages the patient to develop better, more consistent eating habits. Exact amounts of the three nutrients are not uniformly prescribed, but they may be balanced as follows:

- Proteins, 20%
- Fats, 25–35%
- Carbohydrates, 45–65%

Some physicians use a factor of 10 calories multiplied by the desired weight in calculating the daily calorie requirements. For example:

- Desired weight 120 lb. × 10 = 1,200 calories per day
- Desired weight 160 lb. × 10 = 1,600 calories per day

Low-Fat/Low-Cholesterol Diet

Low-fat/low-cholesterol diets are prescribed for patients who suffer from vascular, heart, liver, or gallbladder disease, and for those who have difficulty with fat metabolism. Fats are limited and calories are balanced by increasing proteins and carbohydrates. Foods are baked, roasted, or broiled, and the skin is removed from chicken. Low-fat foods include:

- Low fat cottage cheese (no other allowed)
- Skim milk, buttermilk, yogurt
- Lean meats, fish, chicken
- Vegetables and fruits
- Jams, jellies, ices
- Cereals, pasta, bread, potatoes, rice
- Carbonated beverages, tea, coffee

Mechanically Altered Diets

Any diet may be **mechanically altered**. This means that the consistency and texture are modified, making the food easier to chew and swallow. The **mechanical soft** diet (Figure 26-11) is commonly served to patients who have no teeth, or those with serious dental problems. Meats and hard foods are ground to the consistency of hamburger. Soft items, such as bread, are not ground. The **pureed diet** (Figure 26-12) is blended with gravy or liquid until it is the consistency of pudding. This diet is used for patients who have difficulty swallowing. Pureed foods should not be watery. Properly prepared food items will support a plastic spoon in the upright position.

FIGURE 26-11 The mechanical soft diet is blenderized so foods are the consistency of ground beef. Soft foods, such as bread and cooked carrots, are easily chewed and so are not blended.

FIGURE 26-12 The pureed diet is given to patients who have difficulty swallowing. Food should have a consistency firm enough to support a plastic spoon in an upright position. Attention is given to attractive appearance so food is not runny and does not resemble baby food.

SUPPLEMENTS AND NOURISHMENTS

Many patients receive a nutritional **supplement** or between-meal nourishments. Supplements are ordered by the physician and have a definite therapeutic value. Patients who have wounds may receive supplements high in protein to facilitate healing. Nutritional supplements are usually given to patients who have experienced weight loss and those who need additional calories to meet a medical need. Other special supplements are used to treat patients with specific medical needs, such as those with renal failure, diabetes, chronic obstructive pulmonary disease, HIV, and pediatric patients. These supplements may be liquid or in any form that is easy to eat and digest, such as pudding. It is essential that the patient consume the entire serving.

Nutritional supplements:

- Are ordered by the physician or dietitian. In some facilities, they are not given without an order.
- Are given for a specific therapeutic purpose. They are not nutritionally complete, and are not a replacement for meals. They are given to make up for a nutritional deficiency, strengthen the patient, or promote healing.
- Come in a variety of preparations and flavors to promote patient acceptance.
- Usually taste best when served cold.
- Contain approximately 250 calories per can.
- Are usually lactose-free, and higher in sodium and protein than most tube-feeding formulas.
- Are flavored and are used for oral nutrition. They are not recommended for tube feedings, and tube-feeding formulas are not recommended for nutritional supplementation.
- Are very filling, and should not be given with meals or immediately before mealtime.
- Are expensive and should not be wasted!

In most facilities, the nursing assistant must document the percentage of the product the patient consumed on a flow sheet.

Nourishments are substantial food items given to patients to increase nutrient intake. They are often planned and ordered by the facility dietitian and include foods such as:

- Sandwiches
- Instant breakfast
- Milkshakes
- Pudding
- Whole or chocolate milk
- Yogurt
- Cottage cheese
- Ice cream or sherbet
- Liquid milk-type products, such as Great Shake and Shake Up

Nourishments are usually given between meals to provide needed nutrients or prevent hunger. Serving snacks, nourishments, and supplements is an important nursing assistant responsibility. *Snacks* may be planned and regularly given, or unplanned upon patient request. They are given to patients to prevent or eliminate hunger between meals.

Between-meal nourishments are usually served:

- Midmorning—between 9:30 and 10:00 AM
- Midafternoon—between 2:30 and 3:00 PM
- At bedtime—between 8:00 and 10:00 PM

Snacks served include:

- Milk
- Juices
- Gelatin
- Custard
- Ice cream
- Sherbet
- High-protein drinks
- Fruits

Difficult SITUATIONS

Liquid nutritional supplements are very filling, which is why they are usually served between meals and not with meals. Most patients prefer them cold. If the beverage is warm, the patient may not accept it. Because some of these products are milk-based, serving them warm can also be an infection control hazard. When serving supplements and nourishments, make sure the patient is able to consume the beverage independently. Do not just set it on the table and walk out. Pour the beverage into a cup, if that is what the patient prefers. Provide a straw. If the patient cannot consume the product independently, assist him or her. Document the percentage consumed on the proper form. Record the amount if the patient is on intake and output. Inform the nurse if the patient expresses a preference or dislike for a certain product or flavor. ■

To serve nourishments:

- Wash your hands.
- Check the nourishment list for each patient for any limitations or special dietary instructions.
- Allow patients to choose from the available nourishments whenever possible.
- Assist those who are unable to take their nourishment alone.
- Remember to pick up used glasses and dishes after the patient has finished and return them to the proper area.
- Notice what the patient was or was not able to take.
- Record on intake and output (I&O) sheet if required.

CALORIE COUNTS AND FOOD INTAKE STUDIES

The physician or dietitian may order special food intake studies for patients with special nutritional needs. The patient's food intake is carefully recorded for a period of time, usually three days. The food intake is analyzed for nutritional adequacy and number of calories consumed. The dietitian uses this information to plan a diet to meet the patient's special medical needs.

If the physician orders a food intake study, nursing personnel will notify the dietary department. A special food documentation form (Figure 26-13) is prepared and placed on the medical record or other designated location. The food intake study usually begins with the breakfast meal on the day after the physician writes the order. Some facilities post a sign in the room or on the door to remind staff and visitors that a study is in progress. In some facilities, each food item is weighed or measured. At the end of each meal, you will accurately record the patient's food intake on the form. Facility policies vary on how food intake is documented, but this is usually done by recording an accurate percentage of each individual meal item consumed. You will also accurately document intake of all snacks, liquid nutritional beverages, and food items brought from home by visitors.

At the end of the study period, the form is returned to the dietitian or dietetic technician. He or she uses the information to calculate the amount of protein, carbohydrates, fat, and calories the patient consumed each day. In some facilities, nutrient, vitamin, and mineral intake are also calculated. The dietitian uses this information to adjust the patient's diet and nutritional plan of care. The results of the study and the dietitian's recommendations are communicated to the physician, who may order extra vitamin or mineral supplements necessary for the patient's medical condition. Completing a food intake or calorie count study requires a team effort, good communication, and accurate documentation.

DYSPHAGIA

Some patients have **dysphagia**, or difficulty swallowing food and liquids. This condition may occur in patients who have:

- Had a stroke
- Neurological diseases
- Cancer of the head, neck, or esophagus
- Undergone radiation therapy to the head or neck
- Dementia

People who take medications that cause sedation or reduce saliva production are also at risk of dysphagia. Signs and symptoms of dysphagia are:

- Taking a long time before beginning to swallow
- Swallowing three or four times with each bite of food
- Frequent throat clearing or coughing
- Lack of a gag reflex or weak cough
- Difficulty controlling liquids and secretions in the mouth
- Wet, gurgling voice
- Refusing to eat, spitting food out, or pocketing food in cheeks
- Unintentional weight loss
- Tightness in the throat or chest
- Feeling as if food is sticking in the esophagus or sternal area

If you observe any of these signs or symptoms, inform the nurse. Patients with dysphagia are at high risk of developing malnutrition, dehydration, aspiration, and pneumonia.

Diet _____

CALORIE/PROTEIN SUMMARY

PATIENT _____ ROOM # _____

	DAY 1					DAY 2					DAY 3			
	DATE ___/___/___					DATE ___/___/___					DATE ___/___/___			
	% 0–25	% 25–50	% 50–75	% 75–100		% 0–25	% 25–50	% 50–75	% 75–100		% 0–25	% 25–50	% 50–75	% 75–100
Breakfast					**Breakfast**					**Breakfast**				
Meat					Meat					Meat				
Milk					Milk					Milk				
Fruit					Fruit					Fruit				
Starch					Starch					Starch				
Fat					Fat					Fat				
Other					Other					Other				
AM Supp.					AM Supp.					AM Supp.				
Noon Meal					**Noon Meal**					**Noon Meal**				
Meat					Meat					Meat				
Milk					Milk					Milk				
Juice					Juice					Juice				
Starch					Starch					Starch				
Vegetable					Vegetable					Vegetable				
Bread					Bread					Bread				
Fat					Fat					Fat				
Dessert					Dessert					Dessert				
Other					Other					Other				
PM Supp.					PM Supp.					PM Supp.				
Evening Meal					**Evening Meal**					**Evening Meal**				
Meat					Meat					Meat				
Milk					Milk					Milk				
Juice					Juice					Juice				
Starch					Starch					Starch				
Vegetable					Vegetable					Vegetable				
Bread					Bread					Bread				
Fat					Fat					Fat				
Dessert					Dessert					Dessert				
Other					Other					Other				
PM Supp.					PM Supp.					PM Supp.				
Total Kcal					**Total Kcal**					**Total Kcal**				
Total Pro					**Total Pro**					**Total Pro**				

Avg. for 3 days Kcal: _____   **Avg. Protein for 3 days:** _____

PLEASE RETURN COMPLETED FORM TO NUTRITION CARE MANAGER

FIGURE 26-13 The calorie count provides an accurate picture of the patient's calorie and nutrient intake over a three-day period. The registered dietitian analyzes the information and uses it to make adjustments in the patient's diet and nutritional plan of care.

Consultation with a speech language pathologist and diagnostic tests for dysphagia may be necessary.

Dysphagia is treated with swallowing exercises, practice of proper swallowing techniques, and alteration of the consistency of food and beverages. The dietitian works closely with the speech language pathologist to ensure that the food is the proper consistency to meet the patient's needs and reduce the risk of aspiration. The goal is to keep the look, taste, and food consistency as close to normal as possible, considering the patient's safety needs. Extra gravies or sauces may be added to some foods. Adults may be resistant to eating pureed food because it resembles baby food. Molds and special methods of preparation are used to enhance the appearance of pureed foods, making them more acceptable to the patient. You may be instructed to monitor the patient's food and fluid intake accurately. Inform the nurse if the patient has special dietary requests. The physician may order frequent weight monitoring.

Patients with dysphagia will use special approaches to eating and drinking to prevent aspiration and ensure proper intake. The speech therapist works closely with these patients. Liquids are usually the most difficult to swallow. The speech professional may recommend using food thickeners (Figure 26-14) to slow the movement of fluid through the esophagus. Thickeners are nonprescription, powdered products that are mixed into beverages and some foods to make swallowing easier and prevent aspiration. The consistency of the liquid depends on the amount of powder added. It is important to add exactly the amount that has been ordered. Thickeners do not change the taste of food or liquids, but they may change the intensity, making it taste stronger. Prethickened liquids are also available.

The care plan will specify the type and amount of thickener to use to achieve the necessary texture. For example, the therapist may recommend that liquids be mixed to the consistency of peach juice, nectar, honey, or pudding.

Add the thickener immediately before serving the product. Follow the therapist's directions exactly. When adding thickeners:

- Use the correct product
- Use the correct amount
- Follow the manufacturer's directions
- Stir the thickener well
- Follow the speech therapist's instructions and plan of care for positioning and feeding

FLUID BALANCE

Fluid balance is the balance between liquid intake and liquid output. Because two-thirds of the body's weight is water, there must be a balance between the amount of fluid taken into the body and the amount lost under normal conditions. Generally, we do not need to concern ourselves about this balance. It usually takes care of itself.

The metric system is used for fluid measurements: milliliters (mL) or cubic centimeters (cc). A mL and a cc are the same amount. Table 26-3 compares U.S. customary and metric measurements.

Intake

Most adults take in approximately 2½ to 3 quarts (2,500 to 3,000 mL) of fluid daily:

- In liquids such as water, tea, and soft drinks
- In foods such as fruits and vegetables
- Artificially, such as by intravenous infusions or gavage

Most adult patients need to consume at least 600 to 800 mL of fluid during each eight-hour shift. Because patients may sleep during most of the night shift, additional fluids must be provided during waking hours to keep the body

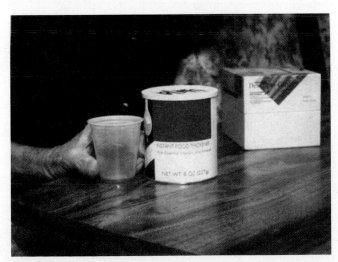

FIGURE 26-14 Food thickener is used to change the texture and consistency of liquids to prevent choking.

TABLE 26-3 COMPARISON OF U.S. CUSTOMARY AND METRIC MEASUREMENTS

U.S. Customary Units	Metric Units
1 minim	0.06 milliliter (mL)
16 minims	1 mL
1 ounce	30 mL
1 pint	500 mL
1 quart	1,000 mL (1 liter)
2.2 pounds	1 kilogram (kg)
1 inch	2.5 centimeters (cm)
1 foot	30 cm

in balance. Excessive fluid retention is called **edema**. Inadequate fluid intake results in **dehydration**, or the lack of sufficient fluid in body tissues. Some disease conditions may change the amounts of fluid the patient is allowed to have.

Output

Typical output equals about 2½ quarts daily in the form of:

- Urine, 1½ quarts (1,500 mL)
- Perspiration
- Moisture from the lungs
- Moisture from the bowel

Excessive fluid loss results in dehydration. This usually occurs through:

- Diarrhea
- Vomiting
- Excessive urine output (**diuresis**)
- Excessive perspiration (**diaphoresis**)
- Wound drainage or blood loss

Recording Intake and Output

An accurate recording of **intake and output (I&O)**, or fluid taken in and given off by the body, is basic to the care of many patients. Intake and output records are kept when specifically ordered by the physician and when patients:

- Are dehydrated or at high risk for dehydration
- Receive intravenous infusion
- Have recently had surgery
- Have a urinary catheter
- Are perspiring profusely or vomiting
- Have specific diagnoses, such as congestive heart failure or renal disease, that require accurate monitoring of I&O

Fluid intake may have to be encouraged in some patients. This is called **push fluids** or **force fluids**. In some situations (as in kidney disease), fluid intake may have to be restricted. Fluid restriction requires a physician order. You will find information regarding whether to push or restrict fluids on the patient's care plan.

Fluid intake and output is calculated by measuring and recording the fluids the patient takes in and the fluids the patient **excretes** (eliminates from the body) (Table 26-4). Because the fluids taken in by the patient cannot actually be measured, an estimate is made and recorded. This is done by:

- Knowing what the liquid container holds when full

📝 **Note:** Sizes of containers vary. Learn the fluid content of the containers used at your facility. Remember that there are 30 mL per ounce (240 mL ÷ 30 mL = 8 oz).

TABLE 26-4 COMPUTING INTAKE AND OUTPUT

Intake	
IV	1,500 mL
By mouth	2,000 mL
Total	3,500 mL
Output	
Urine	1,500 mL
Vomitus	500 mL
Drainage	600 mL
Total	2,600 mL

- Coffee/tea cup, 8 oz = 240 mL
- Water carafe, 16 oz = 480 mL
- Foam cup, 8 oz = 240 mL
- Water glass, 8 oz = 240 mL
- Soup bowl, 6 oz = 180 mL
- Jello, 1 serving = 130 mL
- Ice chips, full 4 oz glass = 120 mL

- Estimating how much is gone from the container (what the patient drank), such as one-third of a glass of juice or half of a cup of coffee
- Converting this to mL. *Example:* A water glass holds 240 mL when filled. The patient drinks ¾ of the glass of water. ¾ × 240 = 180 mL. Intake for the glass of water is recorded as 180 mL. Fluids that are calculated and recorded include all liquids, such as water, juices, soda, coffee, tea, milk, and soup. Also included are foods that melt at room temperature: ice cream, sherbet, and gelatin.

📝 **Note:** Containers may vary from one facility to the next. Each facility should have a chart available that tells you what each size of glass, cup, and bowl holds when full.

Fluids taken by mouth, through intravenous infusion, or through gastric feeding are all recorded separately (Figure 26-15). At the end of each 8-hour shift and the end of 24 hours, the figures are totaled.

Fluid output amount is obtained by measuring all fluids excreted from the body. This includes urine, **emesis** (vomitus), and drainage from body cavities, such as gastric drainage. A container called a **graduate** is marked in mL or cc. The substance is poured into the graduate to determine the amount of output. Urine and any other excretions are recorded separately.

Date Amount	Time	Method of Adm.	Solution	Intake Amounts Rec'd	Time	Output Urine Amount	Others	
							Kind	
7/16	0700	PO	water	120 mL		500 mL		
	0830	PO	coffee	240 mL				
			or. ju.	120 mL				
	1030	PO	cran.ju.	120 mL				
	1100					300 mL		
	1230	PO	tea	240 mL				
	1400	PO	water	150 mL				
Shift Totals	1500			990 mL		800 mL		
	1530	PO	gelatin	120 mL				
	1700	PO	tea	120 mL				
			soup	180 mL				
	2000					512 mL		
	2045						vomitus	500 mL
	2205						vomitus	90 mL
Shift Totals	2300			420 mL		512 mL		590 mL
	2345						vomitus	80 mL
	0130	IV	D/W	500 mL				
	0315					400 mL		
Shift Totals	0700			500 mL		400 mL		80 mL
24 Hour Totals				1910 mL		1712 mL		670 mL vomitus

FIGURE 26-15 Sample intake and output record

Note: Standard precautions must be followed when measuring any body excretion. Gloves are required for measuring all forms of output (Figure 26-16).

CHANGING WATER

It is important to provide fresh water for patients, because water is essential to life. In all cases, you should know whether a patient is allowed ice or tap water and if water is to be especially encouraged. Even without an order to force fluids, you must encourage patients to take 6 to 8 glasses of fluids every 24 hours, unless the patient is NPO (nothing by mouth) or on fluid restriction. Give special attention to confused patients, patients who may not be able to reach a source of water, and the elderly. The need for adequate water intake cannot be overstressed. Because patients often do not drink enough water, sometimes the physician will leave orders that fluids are to be forced to a specific number of mL per day.

FIGURE 26-16 The nursing assistant uses the principles of standard precautions to collect urinary drainage. The urinary output is accurately measured in the graduate pitcher, and the total amount is documented on the intake and output record.

Infection Control ALERT

Avoid contaminating the ice chest or ice scoop when filling pitchers and passing drinking water. Keep the ice scoop covered when not in use. Note that the handle is contaminated and should not touch the clean ice supply. Avoid filling the pitcher over the source of clean ice. (If ice hits the rim of the pitcher and drops back into the clean ice supply, the whole supply is contaminated.) Do not allow the scoop to touch the pitcher. Always keep water pitchers covered at the bedside. If more than one patient shares the room, make sure each pitcher and cup are labeled with a single patient's name. To reduce the potential for infection, some facilities are now giving patients a bottle of water each shift, and upon request, rather than filling a carafe. If ice is requested, staff provides it in a plastic bag or disposable cup with a lid. ■

Forcing fluids is an old term that is not quite accurate. Patients should never actually be forced to consume water or other beverages. When "force fluids" is ordered, encourage the patient to drink each time you are in the room. Offer to assist, if necessary. Some patients will not drink water. Find out what beverages the patient likes, and provide these, if possible.

Providing fresh water is one way to encourage the patient to increase intake of fluids. The procedure for providing fresh water varies greatly.

- In some hospitals, the water pitcher and glass are replaced with a new disposable set each time water is provided.
- In others, the pitcher and glass are washed, refilled, and returned to the patient's bedside table.

In all cases, be sure you know whether a patient is allowed ice or tap water. Some patients prefer no ice. Others have a specific doctor's order for no ice because of potential instabilities in their medical condition.

Clinical Information ALERT

An important nursing assistant responsibility is to accurately document each patient's meal intake. Accuracy is especially important for patients who are diabetic, on calorie counts, or on special diets. Many professionals depend on the accuracy of documented information. Make sure you record food intake accurately. If you have trouble understanding percentages, work with your instructor until you master the information. ■

FOOD ACCEPTANCE

Making mealtime special is an important responsibility. Having friendly staff who show sincere concern for patient welfare helps create a comfortable atmosphere at meals. If patients are satisfied with the quality of food and food service, they tend to view everything else in a positive light. Complaints do not necessarily reflect poor-quality food. They may reflect personal problems or dissatisfaction with care.

- Make the environment as pleasant as possible. Remove unpleasant sights and smells. Clear and wipe the overbed table before serving food trays.
- Provide supplies for patients to wash hands, if needed or desired.
- Be sure patients have dentures, glasses, and hearing aid, if used.
- Make sure that patients are positioned correctly. Ensure that they can reach the food. Make adjustments, if necessary.

The human sensory response to food is complicated. The brain coordinates signals of smell and taste with sight, temperature, and texture. Sensory disorders have many causes, including normal aging, various diseases, lack of certain vitamins and minerals, certain medications, cigarette smoking, and wearing dentures. Sensory problems are very difficult to overcome. Sensory problems may affect:

- Temperature
- Smell
- Taste
- Hearing and vision
- Touch
- Texture

The presentation and attractiveness of food are especially important for patients whose smell, taste, and texture sensations are impaired. They may not be able to smell the food. Taste and texture sensations may be altered. Always check food temperature. This is particularly important with hot foods. All patients are at risk of burns if food is too hot. Patients with abnormal temperature sensations are at greater risk than others. The facility dietitian and occupational, physical, and speech therapists will work with the patient to help resolve sensory problems.

Many patients look forward to meals. However, we know that certain common problems cause patient complaints and decreased food intake. Common complaints about food service are:

- Inability to make choices or select food
- Unappetizing appearance of food
- Lack of seasoning
- Dislike of food served
- Food temperatures not maintained
- Not getting enough to eat

PREVENTION OF FOODBORNE ILLNESS

Hot foods and beverages must be served hot and cold foods and beverages served cold. Food tastes best when it is served at the proper temperature. Imagine how a scrambled egg or cup of black coffee tastes when it is ice cold, or a popsicle or ice cream tastes when it is warm. Food acceptance is only one concern. The potential for foodborne infection is a much more serious problem. Many of the pathogens implicated in "food poisoning" (foodborne illness) have the potential to cause serious illness and death. Foodborne illness is often spread through the common-vehicle method of contamination (Unit 12).

In addition to proper sanitation and food preparation in the kitchen, nursing personnel have an important responsibility for ensuring that patients' trays are served and dependent patients are fed when food is the proper temperature. The temperature danger zone is fairly narrow (Figure 26-17). Foods served in the danger zone are potentially hazardous and have an increased risk for pathogen growth. Hot foods must be served at 140°F or above, and cold foods must be 40°F or below. You may be surprised to learn that hot foods are often 140°F to 150°F when they are delivered to your unit. Food trays must be served promptly because the food cools quickly.

FEEDING THE PATIENT

Eating should be an enjoyable experience. (See Procedures 73 and 74.) Prepare the patient for the meal tray before it arrives by:

- Offering the bedpan or helping the patient to the bathroom
- Assisting the patient to wash hands and face
- Assisting with oral hygiene, if needed
- Raising the head of the bed, if permitted, or assisting the patient out of bed and into a chair, if permitted
- Adjusting the in-bed patient's position with pillows
- Clearing away anything that is unpleasant, such as the emesis basin and bedpan
- Clearing the overbed table
- Encouraging the patient to do as much as possible

When you have served the tray and after you have washed your hands, assist the patient as needed by:

- Being unhurried and pleasant
- Opening prepackaged items
- Cutting meat
- Pouring liquids
- Buttering bread
- Explaining the arrangement of the tray as if items were on the face of a clock (Figure 26-18) if the patient cannot see

There are times when you will be responsible for the entire feeding procedure.

 Note: Carry some extra straws with you during mealtimes. It can save you steps.

Mealtime Assistance for Patients Who Have Swallowing Problems

Patients who have difficulty swallowing may require one-to-one assistance, prompting, or supervision at meals. The speech therapist will recommend special techniques and positions for improving swallowing and preventing aspiration. These will be listed on the care plan. The therapist may work closely with each staff member who may feed the patient. In general:

- Before serving food or beverages, make sure the patient is fully awake and alert.

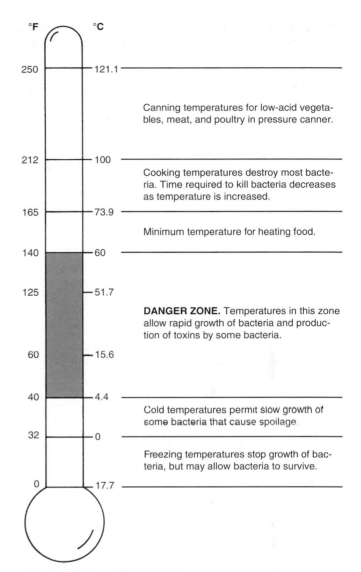

FIGURE 26-17 Temperatures of food for control of pathogens. The danger zone is very close to the average serving temperature, so the temperature of food trays must be carefully maintained. Food should be served promptly upon arrival on the unit.

FIGURE 26-18 Describe the location of each food item compared with the positions on the face of a clock.

PROCEDURE   **OBRA** **DVD**

73

ASSISTING THE PATIENT WHO CAN FEED SELF

1. Carry out initial procedure actions.

2. Assemble equipment:
   - Bedpan/urinal
   - Disposable gloves
   - Basin of warm water
   - Towel
   - Soap
   - Washcloth
   - Oral hygiene items
   - Tray of food

3. Offer bedpan/urinal. Use standard precautions if you anticipate contact with blood, body fluids, mucous membranes, or nonintact skin when assisting the patient with elimination or feeding.

4. If permitted, elevate the head of the bed or assist the patient out of bed.

5. Provide a washcloth to wash the patient's hands and face.

6. Assist with oral hygiene or assist with dentures.

7. Remove and discard personal protective equipment, if used, according to facility policy.

8. Clear the overbed table and position it in front of the patient. Remove unpleasant equipment from sight.

9. Wash your hands. Obtain the meal tray from the dietary tray conveyor.

10. Check the diet with the dietary card and with the patient's identification band (Figure 26-19A).

11. Place the tray on the overbed table and arrange food in a convenient manner.

12. Assist in food preparation as needed (Figure 26-19B). Encourage the patient to do as much as possible.

13. Remove the tray as soon as the patient is finished. Make sure to note what the patient has and has not eaten.

14. Record fluids on intake record, if necessary. Record food intake.

15. Push the overbed table out of the way.

16. Carry out ending procedure actions.

FIGURE 26-19A Check the patient's identification band against the tray card.

FIGURE 26-19B Assist with food preparation as needed.

74

FEEDING THE DEPENDENT PATIENT

1. Carry out initial procedure actions.

2. Assemble equipment:
   - Bedpan/urinal
   - Basin
   - Soap
   - Towel
   - Washcloth
   - Clothing protector
   - Oral hygiene items
   - Tray of food

3. Offer the bedpan or urinal. Follow standard precautions.

4. Provide oral hygiene, if desired.

5. Remove unnecessary articles from the overbed table.

6. Elevate the head of the bed with the patient's head bent slightly forward.

7. Place a towel or protector under the patient's chin (Figure 26-20A). Avoid calling this item a bib, which is demeaning to adults.

8. Obtain the meal tray. Check the diet against the patient's identification band and dietary card.

9. Place the tray on the overbed table (Figure 26-20B).

10. Butter bread and cut meat. Do not pour a hot beverage until the patient is ready for it.

11. Use different drinking straws to give each fluid, or use a cup. Thick fluids are more easily controlled by using a straw. Use adaptive devices as indicated on the care plan.

12. Sit down while you are feeding the patient, so that you are at eye level.

13. Holding the spoon at a right angle:
    - Give solid foods from the point of the spoon (Figure 25-20C).
    - Alternate solids and liquids.
    - Ask the patient in what order she would like the food.

FIGURE 26-20A Place a towel or garment protector over the patient. Avoid calling this item a bib.

FIGURE 26-20B Uncover the food and arrange it on the overbed table.

continues

PROCEDURE 74 CONTINUED

FIGURE 26-20C Give solid foods from the tip of the spoon.

- Describe or show the patient what kind of food you are giving.
- If the patient has had a stroke, direct food to the unaffected side and check for food stored in the affected side. Watch the patient's throat to check for swallowing.
- Test hot foods by dropping a small amount on the inside of your wrist before feeding them to the patient (Figure 26-20D).

FIGURE 26-20D Check the temperature of food and beverages by placing a drop on your wrist or forearm.

- Never blow on the patient's food to cool it.
- Never taste the patient's food.
- Do not hurry the meal.

14. Allow the patient to assist to the extent that she is able.

15. Use a napkin to wipe the patient's mouth as often as necessary.

16. Remove the tray as soon as the patient is finished. Record percentage of food eaten. Record fluid intake.

17. Carry out ending procedure actions.

- Position the patient as upright as possible.
- The head should face forward, with the neck flexed forward slightly.
- During the meal, reduce distractions.
- Limit conversation. The patient with dysphagia should not try to carry on a conversation while eating. Focus the patient on eating.
- Prompt or feed the patient slowly, offering small bites. Remind the patient to chew the food well.

The speech language pathologist may order other special positions and exercises, depending on the patient's medical condition and needs. The care plan will provide additional directions, such as reminding the patient to tuck the chin in when swallowing. In some types of dysphagia,

this changes the position of the airway, further reducing the risk of aspiration. In other types, this technique increases the risk. Because dysphagia care is highly individualized, many staff members must work as a team to ensure that the patient's nutritional needs are safely met.

DOCUMENTING MEAL INTAKE

Each facility has a policy and procedure for documenting and recording the amount of food patients consume at each meal. Every staff member should use the same method of calculation and documentation. The system may also be used for snacks, nourishments, and supplements. A clipboard is commonly used to record meal intake. The clipboard is usually on top of the cart where used trays are returned. After the meal, the information is later transferred to the patient's chart. Remember that documented information is confidential. Keep the information covered with a piece of paper when the clipboard is not in use.

Many different methods are used for documenting percentage of meals consumed. Wait until each patient has finished eating before calculating meal intake. Documenting appetite is more than eyeballing the food tray and estimating how much of the food was eaten. Instead, you must document the percentage of the significant food items on the tray. Some facilities use fractions to record the amount of the food consumed. Some write "good," "fair," or "poor." Some facilities record the percentage of each individual food item. Others estimate and document a percentage of the total meal (Figure 26-21). Know and follow your facility policy. Inform the nurse if a patient eats less than 75% of the meal, or according to facility policy. The nurse may instruct you to obtain a substitute meal. Follow the nurse's instructions.

Legal ALERT

Facility staff are responsible for documenting meal intake. One three-month study showed that facility staff overestimated meal intake 22% of the time. This was statistically significant, and exposes staff to great legal exposure if the patient has a negative outcome. Be sure your documentation of meal intake is accurate.[1] ∎

ALTERNATIVE NUTRITION

There may be situations in which the patient is unable to take in food in the usual way. This may occur if the patient:

- Is unconscious.
- Has a disease of the digestive tract.
- Has persistent vomiting and cannot hold down food.
- Is unable to swallow without **aspiration** (choking).

Aspiration is a very serious condition in which food, water, gastric contents, or other objects enter the trachea and lungs. It is usually accidental, such as when the

FIGURE 26-21 Accurate documentation of meal intake is an important nursing assistant responsibility. (Photo used with permission of Ross Products Division, Abbott Laboratories, Columbus, Ohio)

patient "swallows down the wrong tube" or accidentally inhales food or fluids. If you suspect a patient has aspirated, inform the nurse promptly.

To maintain life, the body must meet its requirements for daily essential nutrients. This may be done by:

- administration of **total parenteral nutrition** (**TPN**) (also called **hyperalimentation**), which is a form of **intravenous infusion** (**IV**), or by
- **enteral feedings** (tubes inserted into the digestive tract)

Total Parenteral Nutrition

TPN is a technique in which high-density (concentrated) nutrients are introduced into a large vein, such as the subclavian or the superior vena cava. This method of feeding is used for patients with diseases of the digestive tract. Caring for patients with TPN is discussed in Unit 36.

Enteral Feedings

Enteral feedings may be administered by a tube that is

- Inserted through the nose and into the stomach (**nasogastric** or **NG feeding**) (Figure 26-22A).

[1]Simmons, S. F., & Reuben, D. (2000). Nutritional intake monitoring for nursing home residents: A comparison of staff documentation, direct observation, and photography methods. *Journal of the American Geriatric Society, 48,* 209–213.

A. Nasogastric route

B. Gastrostomy route

C. Jejunostomy route

FIGURE 26-22 Common methods of enteral feeding: A. Nasogastric (NG) tube B. Gastrostomy (G) tube C. Jejunostomy (J) tube

- Inserted directly through the abdominal skin and into the stomach (**gastrostomy feeding**) (Figure 26-22B).

The **jejunostomy tube (J-tube)** (Figure 26-22C) is a long, small-bore tube that is threaded through the GI tract until the tip reaches the small intestine. Occasionally, you may see a J-tube that has been placed through the nose (nasojejunostomy), but these are less common. The most common J-tube is surgically inserted through an incision in the abdominal skin. This is considered to be a long-term tube. Jejunostomy tubes are used for patients who do not have a stomach, and those in whom recurrent formula aspiration is a problem.

Many different types of tubes may be used for these feedings. The nurse or physician inserts the feeding tube. Some tubes are placed surgically, such as the gastrostomy (Figure 26-23) and **percutaneous endoscopic gastro-** **stomy (PEG)** tube. The PEG tube is surgically inserted by the physician by threading the tube through the patient's mouth and into the stomach. The tube is pulled out through an incision in the patient's abdomen. Tubes that have been surgically placed are covered with a dressing for the first few weeks. Once the insertion site has healed, the area is usually left uncovered. Specially prepared solutions contain all the nutrients required by the body. The feeding may be administered intermittently or it may run continuously. In either case, the container of solution is hung from an IV (intravenous) pole and is usually attached to a device that automatically controls the administration (Figure 26-24).

FIGURE 26-23 Gastrostomy tubes are surgically inserted through the abdminal skin into the stomach. This type of tube is used when long-term tube feeding is anticipated.

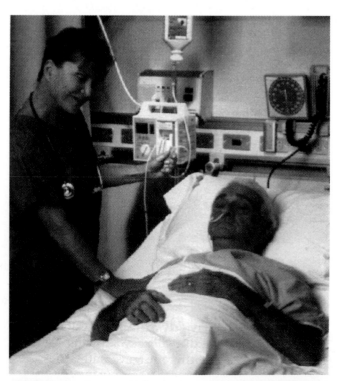

FIGURE 26-24 Enteral feedings are usually administered through a mechanical pump. (Photo used with permission of Ross Products Division, Abbott Laboratories, Columbus, Ohio)

Safety ALERT

Most patients receiving tube feedings are NPO, but some are also permitted to have food or liquids orally. Verify the orders for that patient before giving food or fluids. When a patient receives a continuous tube feeding with a pump, the head must be elevated at all times. Keeping the head of the bed elevated when the tube feeding is infusing is critical to prevent accidental aspiration of formula into the lungs. Monitor the patient for signs of respiratory distress. If formula is aspirated into the lungs, the patient will begin coughing, choking, or gurgling, or will become cyanotic. If any of these occur, call for the nurse immediately. Monitor the skin on the hips and buttocks frequently, as this position increases pressure and the risk of skin breakdown. Move the patient in bed with an assistant. Elevation of the head of the bed also increases the risk of skin damage from friction and shearing. ◼

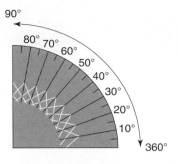

FIGURE 26-25 Elevate the head of the bed at least 30° to 45°, or as specified on the plan of care during feeding, and for at least an hour after the feeding is completed.

Safety ALERT

Know the location of the tube at all times and avoid pulling on it. Avoid pulling on the tube when moving and transferring the patient. Serious complications can result if a feeding tube is dislodged. The skin around the feeding tube must be kept clean and dry. Sometimes the skin around a gastrostomy tube is covered with gauze. After the incision has healed, no dressing is necessary. If the patient has a nasogastric tube, it may be clipped to the gown or clothing to prevent pulling. ◼

When caring for the patient with tube feedings, you need to:
- Keep the head of the bed elevated at least 30° to 45° (Figure 26-25) during feeding and for 60 minutes after feeding.
- Check the taping of tubes. If tape is loose, or pulls, or is causing skin irritation, inform the nurse.
- Report any retching, nausea, or vomiting immediately.
- Check the tubing for kinks. Be sure the patient is not lying on the tubing.

- Provide frequent mouth hygiene. Patients with an NG tube will also need nasal care.
- Notify the nurse if a controlling device alarm sounds.

Adjusting to tube-feeding formula can be difficult for the patient. The rate and strength of formula must be adjusted to meet the patient's needs. In some patients, the formula causes diarrhea. Inform the nurse if the patient's bowel activity increases, or if the patient experiences multiple loose or liquid stools. Keep the perineum clean and dry, and wash the patient well after each bowel activity.

REVIEW

A. True/False.

Mark the following true or false by circling T or F.

1. T F Vitamins are nutrients that help regulate body activities.
2. T F The exchange lists are used by patients on low-salt diets.
3. T F Fats are one of the six essential nutrients.
4. T F Ice cream would be served to a patient on a clear liquid diet.
5. T F Labels of canned foods must be checked when planning their use in low-sodium diets.
6. T F A gastrostomy tube introduces nutrients directly into the stomach.
7. T F Carbohydrate foods are used to make new body cells and build tissues.
8. T F Green leafy vegetables are a good source of calcium, iron, and B vitamins.
9. T F Complete protein foods like poultry contain all of the essential amino acids.

B. Matching.

Match the correct term from Column II with the words and phrases in Column I.

Column I

10. _____ difficulty swallowing

11. _____ roughage

12. _____ encourage liquid intake

13. _____ all the processes involved in taking in food and building and repairing the body

14. _____ treatment

15. _____ calcium

Column II

  a. therapeutic

  b. mineral

  c. dysphagia

  d. force fluids

  e. cellulose

  f. gastrostomy

  g. nutrition

C. Multiple Choice.

Select the one best answer for each of the following.

16. Feeding the patient through a nasogastric tube is known as a/an
  a. intravenous infusion.
  b. gastrostomy feeding.
  c. enteral feeding.
  d. hyperalimentation.

17. Which of the following is a water-soluble vitamin?
  a. Vitamin C
  b. Vitamin E
  c. Vitamin A
  d. Vitamin D

18. An example of a fat-soluble vitamin is
  a. vitamin C.
  b. vitamin B-complex.
  c. vitamin D.
  d. vitamin N.

19. Water is a/an
  a. vitamin.
  b. essential nutrient.
  c. mineral.
  d. discretionary calorie.

20. Which of the following is part of the meat group?
  a. whole grains
  b. rice

  c. fish
  d. butter

21. Foods naturally high in sodium include
  a. milk.
  b. cereals.
  c. vegetables.
  d. fruits.

22. Supplemental nourishments might include
  a. hot fudge sundaes.
  b. mashed potatoes.
  c. scrambled eggs.
  d. high-protein drinks.

23. Nutritional supplements are
  a. given for a specific therapeutic purpose.
  b. withheld if the patient has a fluid restriction.
  c. given on request when a patient is hungry.
  d. high in sugar, protein, and lactose.

24. It is especially important to report to the nurse that the patient only ate two-thirds of her meal when the patient is on a
  a. low-salt diet.
  b. calorie-restricted diet.
  c. diabetic diet.
  d. house diet.

D. Nursing Assistant Challenge.

Mrs. Gole is one of your assigned patients. She is 72 years old, is on a 1,500-calorie diabetic diet, and is a member of the Seventh Day Adventist Church. She also has Parkinson's disease with tremors of her hands, and occasionally has trouble swallowing. Mrs. Gole sometimes eats food brought in by family and friends that is not on the 1,500-calorie diet. Consider Mrs. Gole's care:

25. Discuss safety issues that you need to think about when Mrs. Gole is eating.

26. Are there conflicts between the ordered diet and the dietary restrictions of her church? If so, what are the conflicts and how might they be resolved?

27. Do you anticipate that Mrs. Gole will have any problems feeding herself? If so, what are those problems, and what can you do to help her eat independently?

28. Discuss the issues of residents' or patients' rights that may arise because of the conflict between the patient's desire to eat more food than ordered and foods different from what the physician has prescribed.

SECTION 9

Special Care Procedures

UNIT 27

Warm and Cold Applications

OBJECTIVES

After completing this unit, you will be able to:

- Spell and define terms.
- List the physical conditions requiring the use of heat and cold.
- Name types of heat and cold applications.
- Describe the effects of local cold applications.
- Describe the effects of local heat applications.
- List safety concerns related to application of heat and cold.

- Demonstrate the following procedures:
  - Procedure 75 Applying an Ice Bag
  - Procedure 76 Applying a Disposable Cold Pack
  - Procedure 77 Applying an Aquamatic K-Pad
  - Procedure 78 Giving a Sitz Bath
  - Procedure 79 Assisting with Application of a Hypothermia Blanket

VOCABULARY

Learn the meaning and the correct spelling of the following words and phrases:

Aquamatic K-Pad	hyperpyrexia	ice bag	warm soak
cold pack	hyperthermia	sitz bath	wet compress
core body temperature	hypothermia	thermal blanket	
diathermy	hypothermia-	vasoconstriction	
hemorrhage	hyperthermia blanket	vasodilation	

INTRODUCTION

Heat and cold applications are used only on written orders from the physician or nurse, and only for a specific length of time. Some facilities allow only professional personnel to apply heat and cold. *Some states have laws against nursing assistants applying heat or cold in a home health setting.* In other facilities, nursing assistants who have been specially trained are permitted to carry out these procedures under the supervision of the nurse. Be sure you know and follow the policy of your facility and are adequately prepared and *supervised*.

THERAPY WITH HEAT AND COLD

The physician orders the use of heat or cold applications to:

- Relieve pain
- Combat local infection, swelling, or inflammation
- Control bleeding (**hemorrhage**)
- Reduce body temperature

Local applications of heat and cold are made with:

- Ice bags.

- Electronically operated Aquamatic K-Pads. K-Pads come in many shapes and sizes. They can be used to apply dry heat. By using an attachment, they can also be used for cooling.
- Prepackaged, single-use units for the application of hot and cold. A single hit on the surface activates the contents, providing a controlled temperature.
- Gel packs that can be cooled or heated as needed.

General treatments of heat and cold consist of thermal mattresses known as **hypothermia-hyperthermia blankets**. These are widely used to:

- Lower body temperature when there is fever
- Elevate body temperature in cases of hypothermia

Applications of warm and cold may be either dry or moist. Moisture makes both heat and cold more penetrating. Therefore, moist heat or moist cold is more likely to cause injury. Extra care must be taken to protect the patient when moist treatments are used. Be sure you know:

- Exact method to be used
- Correct temperature and placement
- Proper length of time the warm or cold application is to be performed
- How often the area being treated is to be checked

Table 27-1 lists the average temperatures ordered for heat and cold applications.

Commercial Preparations

Easy-to-use commercial warm and cold packs are available for dry applications. For one type of pack, a single hit or

TABLE 27-1 AVERAGE ORDERED WATER TEMPERATURES FOR HYDROTHERAPY TREATMENTS AND PROCEDURES

Hot 100°F to 105°F
Warm 95°F to 100°F (this is the range that is used for bathing and most treatments)
Tepid 80°F to 95°F
Cool 65°F to 80°F
Cold 45°F to 65°F

- Never set the whirlpool for higher than 100°F without first checking with the nurse. (The whirlpool is preset to maintain a constant temperature of 97°F. Because it maintains a constant temperature, you should not have to adjust it.)

- These guidelines may also be appropriate for other heat treatments; follow facility policies.

Safety ALERT

Each state has laws governing the water temperature in patient care areas of the facility. These vary slightly from one state to the next, but in most, water temperature in patient care units and bathing areas should not exceed 120°F. The regulators sometimes fail, sending very hot water into the facility. However, water in bath and shower areas must be warm enough to bathe patients comfortably. Comfortable temperature for most people is 95°F to 105°F. Report water in bathing areas that does not warm up enough for comfortable bathing. Also report steaming water, or water that feels hot to touch at any faucet in a patient care area. Use bath thermometers to check water temperatures before patient care whenever possible. If a thermometer is unavailable, check the temperature on the inside of your forearm or wrist. ■

blow to the pack before application activates it. The pack is discarded after one use. Reusable packs are also available, but infection control issues make them less desirable.

USE OF COLD APPLICATIONS

Applications of cold are given only with a physician's order. The application of cold:

- Constricts or decreases the size of blood vessels (**vasoconstriction**) and reduces swelling
- Decreases sensitivity to pain
- Reduces temperature
- Slows inflammation
- Reduces itching

Cautions

Remember, moisture intensifies the effect of cold just as it does heat. Caution must be used in the application of moist cold.

- Excessive cold can damage body tissues.
- Report color changes such as *blanching* (turning white) or *cyanosis* (becoming bluish).
- Report feelings of numbness or discomfort experienced by the patient.
- Stop the cold treatment if the patient starts to shiver. Cover the patient with a blanket and report immediately to the nurse. (See Procedures 75 and 76.)

GUIDELINES *for*

Warm and Cold Treatments

You must be very watchful when applying cold or warm treatments. When assigned to this task, keep in mind the following:

- The age and condition of the patient. Give extra care to:
  - Young children
  - The aged
  - Patients with cognitive impairment
  - Patients who are uncooperative
  - Patients who are unconscious
  - Patients who are paralyzed
  - Patients with tissue damage
  - Patients with poor circulation
- Apply the principles of standard precautions if your hands will contact blood, moist body fluids (except sweat), secretions, excretions, nonintact skin, or mucous membranes.
- If the patient has a dressing covering the area to be treated, consult the nurse for directions.
- Check the temperature of the solution with a thermometer. You may need to add more liquid during the treatment to maintain the temperature. Avoid pouring hot or cold liquid directly over the patient.
- Remove all metal jewelry, buttons, or zippers that could conduct heat or cold and thereby injure the skin.
- Avoid using heat treatments with temperatures over 105°F. Temperatures greater than this can cause burns, particularly in infants and the elderly.
- Avoid using heat in the first 48 hours after an injury.
- Follow all safety rules to prevent spills and falls.
- An electric heating pad must not be used with moist dressings unless a rubber cover is placed over the pad. If the wires become damp, a short circuit may result. The patient must not lie on the pad, because severe burns can result. Sensitivity to heat varies, so patients receiving heat treatments must be checked frequently. Although heating pads are not used in health care facilities, they are used by individuals in homes.
- Heat is not applied to the head because it could make blood vessels in the area dilate, causing headache.
- Heat should not be applied to the abdomen if there is any chance that the patient has appendicitis, because it would increase the chance of the appendix rupturing.
- Check the skin under the application every 10 minutes, or according to facility policy. If the skin under a heat application appears red, or a dark area appears, stop the treatment. Notify the nurse immediately. Stop a cold application and notify the nurse if the patient's skin appears cyanotic, pale, white, or bright red; if the patient complains of numbness; or if the patient is shivering. Cover the patient with a blanket.
- Rubber or plastic should never touch the patient's skin. Be sure all appliances are covered with cloth.
- Heat and cold applications are usually not left in place longer than 20 minutes, according to the purpose and type of treatment. Follow the care plan and the nurse's instructions.
- After the treatment, pat the skin dry. Make the patient comfortable. Clean and store used equipment. Remove gloves, if worn, and dispose of them according to facility policy. Wash your hands. Inform the nurse that the procedure was completed and the patient's reaction to the treatment.

Dry Cold Applications

There are several methods for applying therapeutic cold. Careful attention to the application is needed to prevent injury.

- Disposable **cold pack**—This single-use commercial pack can be stored until needed. Reusable commercial packs are also available (for both warm and cold applications). The pack remains effective for approximately 15 to 30 minutes. If the cold pack must be activated,

follow the manufacturer's instructions exactly. When activating the pack, do not hold it in front of your face. If the pack leaks or bursts, the chemicals inside the pack may splash. Check the area being treated every 10 minutes. Discard the chemical cold pack after one use, or when the pack warms. Do not attempt to refreeze it.

- **Ice bag**—This reusable, waterproof, canvas or rubber container can be filled with ice to provide temporary local cold. An ice bag is never placed directly on the affected area because the weight of the bag will cause the patient discomfort.

- **Thermal blanket**—This is a large, fluid-filled blanket that is placed over or around the patient. The temperature of the fluid in the blanket may be raised or lowered. The blanket is used to lower or raise the patient's body temperature. However, it is most often used in care facilities to lower the body temperature. This process is called inducing **hypothermia**. A licensed professional usually monitors the use of this type of blanket.

Tips: Paper or styrofoam cups of ice are sometimes used to gently massage an injured area. To apply cold this way, hold the cup and make small, overlapping circles on the affected area for 20 minutes. An examination glove filled with ice and secured with a rubber band is also sometimes used as an alternate ice application.

Moist Cold Applications

- **Wet compresses** are moistened with a solution and placed on the affected area.

Clinical Information ALERT

A partially filled bottle or application is flexible and molds to the patient's body easily. The weight of a full bottle may cause pain to an injured area. A partially filled bottle with the air expelled stays warm longer. Extra air in the bottle cools the hot water. You can tie the application to the treatment area with roller gauze to hold it in place. Make sure the patient can tolerate the weight of the application without increasing or causing pain. ■

Safety ALERT

Cold therapy should not be used for patients with:

- Deep vein thrombosis
- Peripheral vascular disease
- Open wound(s)
- Skin sensation impairment
- Severe cognitive impairment
- Cold intolerance, cold allergy
- Some medical conditions such as rheumatoid arthritis and Reynaud's phenomenon.

If a patient has any of these conditions, check with the nurse before applying a cold application. ■

- A syringe may be used to add water to the compresses to keep them moist.
- Compresses can be kept cold by placing a covered ice bag against the affected area. Make sure the patient can tolerate the weight of the ice bag without increased pain.
- Each time the pad is removed and replaced, be careful to reposition the protective covering.

Follow facility policy for:

- Method of applying the treatment
- Length of time the treatment is to be applied
- How often the patient is to be checked for condition of the skin in the treatment area and general response to the treatment
- Signs that treatment should be discontinued

USE OF WARM APPLICATIONS

Warm applications are ordered to:

- Relieve muscle spasms
- Reduce pain
- Reduce inflammation
- Promote healing
- Combat local infection
- Increase circulation
- Improve mobility before exercise periods
- Soothe the patient

Safety ALERT

The heat application should feel comfortably warm to the patient, not uncomfortably hot. If you will be applying a pack or pad, touch the device to your forearm to check the temperature before applying it. If the patient complains of burning, remove the application and consult the nurse. ■

The value of heat treatments (**diathermy**) is that heat dilates or increases the size of blood vessels (**vasodilation**). This brings more blood to the area to promote healing. Warmth is very soothing when there is pain.

There must be a specific order for a warm application. Some groups of people require extra care when they receive warm applications.

Cautions

Follow these cautions when working with patients:

- Constant warmth must be carefully monitored.
- Moisture intensifies the effect of warmth. Use extra caution.

PROCEDURE

APPLYING AN ICE BAG

1. Assemble equipment:
   - Ice bag
   - Cover (usually cotton, such as a towel, or cover specified by your facility)
   - Paper towels
   - Spoon or similar utensil
   - Ice cubes or crushed ice

2. Prepare the ice bag as follows:
   a. Fill the ice bag with cold water and check for leaks.
   b. Empty the bag.
   c. If ice cubes are used, rinse them in water to remove sharp edges. The use of crushed ice makes the bag more flexible and is more comfortable for the patient.
   d. Fill the ice bag half full, using an ice scoop, paper cup, or large spoon (Figure 27-1).

   Avoid making ice bags too heavy. Do not allow the scoop to touch the ice bag.
   e. To remove air from the ice bag:
      - Rest the ice bag flat on a paper towel on a flat surface.
      - Put the top in place, but do not screw it on.
      - Press the bag until the air is removed (Figure 27-2).
   f. Fasten the top securely.
   g. Test for leakage.
   h. Wipe the ice bag dry with paper towels. Place it in a cloth cover.

   Notes: As an alternative, a gel pack stored in the freezer can be used for cold applications. These packs can be refrozen and reused if this is facility policy.

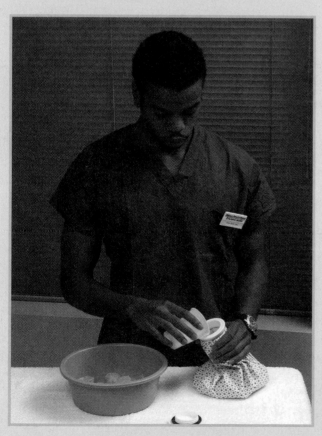

FIGURE 27-1 Fill the ice bag half full.

FIGURE 27-2 Place the ice bag on a flat surface, then press firmly to remove air.

continues

PROCEDURE 75 CONTINUED

3. Take the equipment to the bedside on a tray. Carry out initial procedure actions.

4. Apply the ice bag to the affected part.

5. Refill the ice bag before all the ice has melted.

6. Check the skin area under the ice bag every 10 minutes. Report to nurse immediately if skin is discolored or white or if the patient reports that the skin is numb.

7. Continue the cold application for the amount of time specified by the nurse. If the patient feels cold, cover with a blanket, but do not cover the area being treated.

8. Carry out ending procedure actions.

9. When the treatment is complete, wash the bag with soap and water. Rinse and dry it completely, and then screw the top on. Wipe the bag with a disinfectant if this is your facility policy. Leave air in the ice bag to prevent the sides from sticking together.

10. If a reusable cold pack is used, wash it thoroughly with soap and water or wipe with a disinfectant, according to facility policy. Return the pack to the refrigerator. Discard a disposable pack.

PROCEDURE 76

APPLYING A DISPOSABLE COLD PACK

1. Carry out initial procedure actions.

2. Assemble equipment:
   - Disposable commercial cold pack
   - Cloth covering (towel, warm water bag cover, or other cover specified by the facility)
   - Tape or rolls of gauze

3. Expose the area to be treated. Note the condition of the area.

4. Place the cold pack in a cloth covering (Figure 27-3).

5. Strike or squeeze the cold pack to activate chemicals. (Follow manufacturer's instructions.)

6. Place the covered cold pack on the proper area and cover it with a towel (Figure 27-4). Note time of application.

7. Secure the cover with tape or gauze, if necessary, to hold it in place.

8. Leave the patient in a comfortable position, with the signal cord within easy reach.

9. Return to the bedside every 10 minutes. Check the area being treated for discoloration or numb-

ness. If these signs and symptoms occur, discontinue treatment and report them to the nurse.

10. If no adverse symptoms occur, remove the pack after 30 minutes, or after the amount of time given in your instructions. Note the condition of

FIGURE 27-3 Cover the disposable cold pack with a flannel cover or towel before applying it to the patient.

continues

PROCEDURE 76 CONTINUED

FIGURE 27-4 After positioning the cold pack, cover the application with a towel.

the area. Continuous treatment requires application of a fresh pack.

11. Remove the pack from the cover and discard according to facility policy. Return unused gauze and tape.

12. Put the cover in a laundry hamper.

13. Carry out ending procedure actions.

- Hot packs are contraindicated for paralyzed areas or areas without sensation, acute edema or inflammation, infection, and hemophilia. They must be used with caution for patients with many medical conditions, including impaired circulation, sensory impairment, cancer, rashes, and open skin conditions. Take extra care with hot packs for very young and very old patients.
- Never allow a patient to lie on a constant heat unit, because heat may be trapped and build up to dangerous levels.
- Temperature of a constant heat unit should be between 95° and 100°F.
- Always use a bath thermometer to check solution temperatures.
- Always remove the body part being soaked before adding warm solution.
- Protect areas not being treated from excessive exposure.
- Warmth is not applied to the head because it could cause blood vessels in the area to dilate, resulting in headache.
- Rubber or plastic should never touch the patient's skin. Be sure all appliances are covered with cloth.

Dry Warm Applications

The **Aquamatic K-Pad** is commonly used to provide dry warmth. It consists of a plastic pad with fluid-filled coils

Safety ALERT

Heat therapy should not be used for patients with:

- Acute inflammation
- Dermatitis
- Deep vein thrombosis
- Peripheral vascular disease
- Open wound(s)
- Recent soft tissue injuries in which swelling or bleeding would be increased by heat
- Skin sensation impairment and paralysis
- Severe cognitive impairment

Some physicians also recommend avoiding heat use with children and women during pregnancy. If a patient has any of these conditions, check with the nurse before applying a heat application. ■

and a control unit that maintains a constant temperature of the fluid.

The fluid in the pad is distilled water that is supplied from a reservoir in the control unit. The control unit is placed on the bedside stand and is plugged into an electrical outlet. In most facilities, the temperature is preset by the central supply department. The temperature is usually set at 95° to 100°F.

Tips: When setting up the K-Pad for the first time, check the pad for leaks. Tip it back and forth several times to eliminate air pockets, which cause hot spots. Place the control unit on the bedside stand so it is higher than the patient, so that water will run into the pad by gravity. Make sure the tubing is free of kinks.

Safety ALERT

Moisture intensifies heat, so you must use extra care. ■

Moist Warm Applications

For each of the warm treatments, follow facility policy for:
- Method of applying the treatment
- Length of time the treatment is to be applied
- How often the patient is to be checked for condition of the skin in the treatment area and general response to the treatment

- Signs that treatment should be discontinued

Moist warm treatments include:
- **Warm soaks**—The patient, or the part of the patient's body that is being treated, is immersed in a tub filled with water at a specific temperature, usually 105°F.
- Wet compresses—The same cautions apply to warm compresses as to cold compresses. They may be kept wet with a syringe and warm by covering them with an Aquamatic K-Pad.

Sitz Bath

A **sitz bath** is a method of bathing in which only the pelvic area is immersed. This is a cleansing or therapeutic bath in a small tub that holds enough water for the patient to sit with the hips covered and the legs and torso above water. It is usually done to relieve discomfort following childbirth, perineal surgery, or rectal surgery. Immersing the perineum in warm water enhances healing by reducing inflammation, stimulating circulation, and promoting wound healing. It is also very relaxing. The water temperature must be constant for maximum effect.

Some older hospitals have permanent sitz bath tubs (Figure 27-6). Most newer facilities use a portable (disposable) sitz bath kit. The kit is issued to the patient, and sent home or discarded upon discharge. The kit holds a plastic

PROCEDURE

77

APPLYING AN AQUAMATIC K-PAD

1. Carry out initial procedure actions.

2. Assemble equipment:
   - K-Pad and control unit
   - Distilled water
   - Covering for pad

3. Check the cord for frayed or damaged insulation. Also check that the tubing between the control unit and the pad is intact.

4. Place the control unit on the bedside stand (Figure 27-5).

5. Remove the cover of the control unit and check the level of the distilled water. If it is low, fill the unit two-thirds full or to the fill line using distilled water. Tilt the unit back and forth gently to clear the tubing of air.

6. Screw the cover in place and loosen it one-quarter turn.

FIGURE 27-5 The control unit for the aquathermia pad maintains a constant temperature.

continues

PROCEDURE 77 CONTINUED

7. If the temperature was not preset, check with the nurse for the proper setting before turning on the unit. Remove the key after setting the temperature.

8. Plug in the unit.

9. Cover the pad with an appropriate cover, according to facility policy or as specified by the manufacturer of the unit. Do not use pins to hold the cover in place.

10. Expose the area on the patient to be treated. Place the covered pad on the patient and note the time.

   - Be sure the tubing between the control unit and the pad does not hang over the side of the bed. It should be coiled on the bed to promote the flow of liquid.

11. Following facility policy, periodically check the skin under the pad.

12. Check the level of the water in the control unit. Refill if necessary to the fill line.

13. Remove the pad after the prescribed amount of time.

14. Carry out ending procedure actions.

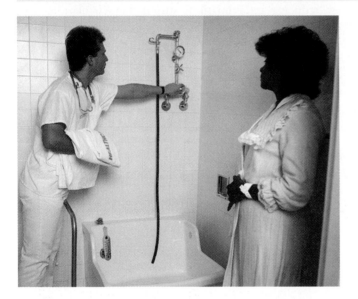

FIGURE 27-6 Some hospitals have stationary sitz bath tubs in areas of frequent use, such as obstetrics and surgical units.

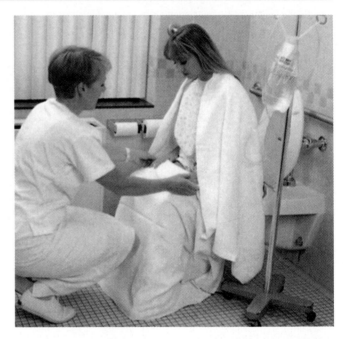

FIGURE 27-7 After the patient is seated, cover her with a bath blanket, if desired, to prevent chilling.

basin that fits over the toilet and an irrigation bag with tubing and clamp.

Drape the patient's lower body with a bath blanket during the bath (Figure 27-7), and keep him or her warm throughout the procedure. Dress the patient promptly after the sitz bath to maintain body heat.

ABNORMALITIES IN TEMPERATURE REGULATION

Human survival depends on the person's ability to maintain a stable body temperature between 97°F and 100°F. Normally, the nervous system controls the body response to heat and cold, and regulates temperature automatically to keep the body at normal operating temperature. This normal body response is disrupted in extreme environmental conditions and various medical problems.

Hypothermia

When heat loss exceeds heat production, the nervous system will trigger certain involuntary responses, such as shivering, to restore the balance. If the cold stress is great, and the person's system is overwhelmed, body temperature decreases. **Hypothermia** is a lowering of **core body temperature** to 95°F or below. Very young and very old persons are at high risk for this condition. Core body temperature is the normal operating temperature of the

PROCEDURE

78

GIVING A SITZ BATH

1. Carry out initial procedure actions.

2. Assemble equipment:
   - Disposable exam gloves
   - Permanent sitz tub, portable sitz tub, or bathtub
   - Bath towels (2–3)
   - Bath blanket (2)
   - Floor bath mat
   - Rubber bath mat
   - Bath thermometer
   - Gown
   - Footstool, if needed
   - Overbed table
   - Pitcher, if needed to refill irrigation bag
   - IV standard (if needed, to hold irrigation bag)
   - Dressings
   - Supplies to disinfect tub, as needed
   - Plastic bag for used supplies

3. Clean and disinfect the tub, if necessary.

4. Instruct the patient to void before beginning this procedure.

5. Remove dressings and/or peri pad, if used. If a dressing adheres to a wound, soak it off in the tub. Discard it in a plastic bag.

6. Fill the sitz tub (Figure 27-8) or bathtub one-third to one-half full, so that the water will cover the perineum, or will reach the patient's umbilicus if a permanent sitz tub is used. Use hot water, 105°F to 110°F, or as instructed by the nurse. (The water will cool before the patient uses it; if the patient will be using it immediately, temperature should not exceed 105°F.)

7. Check the water temperature with a bath thermometer.

8. If you are using a disposable kit, fill the basin to the designated line.

9. Place the basin under the commode seat.

10. Close the plastic clamp on the irrigation tubing.

11. Fill the irrigation bag with 105°F to 110°F water. (The water will cool before use.)

12. Hang the solution bag from the towel bar, hook, or an IV standard.

13. Insert the irrigation tubing through the entry hole near the front of the plastic bowl.

14. Pull the tubing inside the bowl.

15. Secure the tubing by snapping it into the channel in the center bottom of the bowl.

16. Make sure the small hole at the end of the tube faces up.

17. Assist the patient to sit on the seat. If the patient's legs do not reach the floor, support them on a footstool.

18. Cover the patient's shoulders and lap with a bath blanket.

19. Position a folded towel behind the lower back to reduce discomfort.

20. Offer to place the overbed table in front of the patient, if desired to provide additional support and comfort.

21. Open the clamp to begin the flow of solution. Show the patient how to regulate the flow.

22. Follow your facility policies for remaining in the room during the procedure.

23. Frequently monitor the patient's color and condition. If she becomes dizzy or weak, check the pulse and blood pressure promptly. Use the call signal to get help. Return the patient to bed using a wheelchair.

24. Refill the irrigation bag when necessary.

25. After the prescribed time (usually 15 to 20 minutes), clamp the tubing.

26. Assist the patient to stand. Encourage her to use the hand rails. Monitor closely for dizziness, weakness, faintness, or nausea.

27. Assist the patient to dry, if necessary.

28. Apply a clean dressing or peri pad, if necessary.

continues

PROCEDURE 78 CONTINUED

FIGURE 27-8 A portable sitz bath tub is placed under the base of the toilet after the seat is lifted. Some hospitals prefer this type of sitz bath because it is for single patient use and may be taken home for continued therapy after hospital discharge.

29. Assist the patient to dress and return to her room.

30. Disinfect the sitz tub.

31. Store the disposable tub for reuse.

32. Carry out ending procedure actions.

body center, or core. This temperature value reflects the temperature in deep structures of the body such as the liver. The severity of hypothermia is determined by the degree to which core temperature is lowered. Rectal temperatures are taken when hypothermia is suspected or diagnosed.

- Mild hypothermia: 93°F–95°F (R)
- Moderate hypothermia: 86°F–93°F (R)
- Severe hypothermia: less than 86°F (R)

Indications of hypothermia to report include:

- Drop in body temperature
- Poor coordination and confusion
- Slurred speech
- Decreased respiratory and heart rates

Nursing Assistant Actions

- Report observations to the nurse.
- Check the environmental temperature and adjust it.
- Provide external warmth with a sweater or blanket.
- Reduce drafts with screens or curtains.
- If permitted, give something warm to drink.
- Check vital signs.

Untreated, the patient's condition worsens, with dehydration, liver and kidney failure, and death. In the early stages of hypothermia, the pulse, respirations, and blood pressure may rise. If the body temperature drops below 90°F, these vital signs decrease markedly. If the temperature drops to 86°F, most people become comatose. If the temperature continues to drop to 82°F or below, serious heart problems will occur.

Heat-Related Illness

Abnormally high body temperature is called **hyperpyrexia** or **hyperthermia**. It occurs when the rectal temperature is 104°F or above. When environmental temperature exceeds body temperature or the humidity is high, the body retains heat, increasing body temperature. Certain medical problems can also cause severe temperature elevation. When the patient has a fever, the normal mechanisms causing thirst are reduced. The body sweats to cool off. Aging and many chronic diseases further reduce the effectiveness of sweating in cooling the body. Untreated, high body temperature is a very serious condition that leads to brain damage and death. Very high temperatures are treated aggressively by a variety of methods.

Indications of hyperthermia to report include:

- Elevated body temperature
- Hot, flushed skin
- Faintness
- Headache

- Nausea
- Convulsions

Fever (*pyrexia*) occurs when core body temperature rises to at least 101°F (rectally). Fever is often associated with infections, injury, surgery, and serious trauma. Indications of fever are the same as those for general hyperthermia.

Nursing Assistant Actions

- Report observations to the nurse.
- Check the environmental temperature and adjust it.
- Reduce external warmth. Cover the patient with only a gown or sheet.
- If permitted, give a cooling drink.
- Carry out cooling procedures as ordered. For example, give cooling baths or enemas.
- Check vital signs frequently.

TEMPERATURE CONTROL MEASURES

Excessively high or low body temperatures are treated in acute care facilities by placing hypothermia-hyperthermia blankets (Figure 27-9) over and under the patient. These blankets are units filled with water. The blankets may be called *aquathermia blankets.* "Aqua" is the Latin term for *water.* The temperature of the water can be adjusted higher or lower depending on whether the patient's body temperature is to be raised or lowered.

Using the Aquathermia Blanket

The aquathermia blanket is operated either manually or automatically. For manual operation, the licensed nurse will set the blanket to a predetermined temperature, which is ordered by the physician. The blanket maintains this temperature regardless of changes in the patient's body temperature. When the unit is set for automatic operation, it monitors the patient's temperature through a rectal, skin, or esophageal probe. The probe is secured to the body with tape to prevent injury. The blanket temperature changes according to the patient's temperature. The goal is to maintain the patient's body temperature. An alarm will sound for abnormal temperature variations. Before using the blanket, check it for cracks, tears, or leaks in the system. Do not use it if there are cracks or an electrical malfunction.

The patient should wear a hospital gown when the aquathermia blanket is used. Use a gown with tie closures. Snaps, pins, or other metal may cause injury to the skin. Before beginning the procedure, check and record the patient's baseline vital signs as a basis for comparison.

One or two aquathermia blankets may be used. The nurse may instruct you to place one under the patient, and to cover him or her with the other. The blankets must be

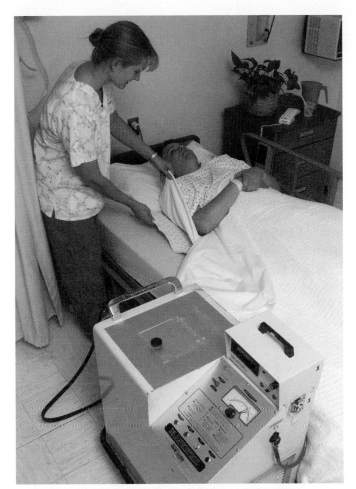

FIGURE 27-9 Hypothermia-hyperthermia blanket

Safety ALERT

Always read the instructions before using a hyper-thermia-hypothermia blanket. Some units are manually operated. This means that the blanket will maintain the preset temperature regardless of the patient's temperature. You will have to adjust the temperature setting manually. Make sure you are familiar with the directions for the unit you are using. ■

covered with a disposable cover, sheet, or bath blanket to absorb perspiration and prevent complications. Avoid using pins to cover the blanket. These can puncture the unit or injure the patient's skin by creating hot or cold spots. Use tape or Velcro fasteners, if necessary, to cover the unit.

The blanket should be set up and preheated or precooled before it is applied to the patient. Connect the blanket to the control unit by plugging in the tubing. The nurse will set the blanket for automatic or manual operation. He or she will also set the desired body temperature or blanket temperature and instruct you as to what temperature values are being used. Turn the device on, then add distilled water to the reservoir. Position the controls at the foot of the bed. After the blanket has reached the designated temperature, apply it to the patient. If the patient will be lying on a blanket, place a pillow or folded bath blanket under the patient's head.

The patient's head should not contact the blanket directly. The combination of heat or cold and the surface of the blanket promotes skin breakdown on the back of the head. The nurse may instruct you to apply lanolin or another designated product to the skin in exposed areas that contact the blanket directly. You may wrap the patient's hands and feet to prevent chilling, if desired.

Complications. Immediately notify the nurse if you observe any of these complications:

- Changes in skin color
- Cyanosis of the lips or nail beds
- Sudden changes in body temperature
- Marked changes in pulse, respirations, and blood pressure
- Respiratory distress
- Pain
- Changes in sensation
- Edema
- Shivering and chills
- Urinary output below 50 mL/hour

Discontinuing Blanket Use. The nurse will inform you when to discontinue use of the blanket. Follow the manufacturer's directions for the type of blanket you are using. Turn the unit off. (Some types must remain plugged in for 30 to 60 minutes to dry condensation inside the unit.) Dry the patient's skin and assist him or her into a dry gown. Position the patient in a comfortable

position. Remove the aquathermia blanket from the bed after the designated time. Continue checking vital signs and intake and output every 30 minutes for the first 2 hours, then hourly or as directed by the nurse.

Safety ALERT

The nurse will instruct you on how often to monitor vital signs when an aquathermia blanket is being used. The patient's temperature and the blanket temperature are usually monitored and documented every 15 to 30 minutes. Inform the nurse immediately if the patient's temperature drops more than 1° in 15 minutes. Continued temperature monitoring is necessary after the blanket is removed because the patient's temperature can continue to drop as much as 5° after the procedure ends. ■

Age-Appropriate Care ALERT

In children, temperatures tend to rise higher than in adults. This puts children at greater risk for seizures. ■

PROCEDURE

79

ASSISTING WITH APPLICATION OF A HYPOTHERMIA BLANKET

Applying a hypothermia blanket and monitoring a patient who is receiving a hypothermia treatment is a professional nursing responsibility. The nurse will supervise the procedure and monitor the patient throughout the treatment. The nurse will check the specific gravity of the patient's urine, and nervous system response. The nursing assistant may be asked to assist in setting up equipment, positioning

the patient and the thermal blanket, observing the patient during the treatment, and keeping the patient comfortable. In addition, the nursing assistant may be asked to transport equipment to and from the central supply service.

1. Wash your hands, collect equipment, and take equipment to the bedside.

continues

PROCEDURE 79 CONTINUED

2. Assemble equipment:
   - Disposable gloves
   - Hypothermia-hyperthermia control unit
   - Fluid for control unit
   - Thermometer probes (rectal or skin)
   - Adhesive tape
   - Sphygmomanometer
   - Stethoscope
   - Hypothermia-hyperthermia blanket (disposable or reusable), 1 or 2 as ordered
   - Bath blanket or sheet, 1 or 2 as ordered
   - Lanolin-based skin cream

3. Follow manufacturer's directions for setting up equipment. Check equipment for safety. Be sure the control unit is grounded.

4. Connect the blanket(s) to the control unit and set the control.

5. Turn on the control unit and add liquid.

6. Allow the blanket(s) to precool as you prepare the patient.

7. Carry out initial procedure actions.

8. Place the patient in a hospital-type gown with ties.

9. Measure vital signs and record.

10. Place the hypothermia-hyperthermia blanket on the bed and cover it with a sheet. Position the patient on the sheet-covered thermal blanket in the recumbent position, with the head on a pillow that does not touch the blanket.

11. Wash your hands. Put on gloves.

12. Insert a rectal thermometer probe into the patient's rectum (unless contraindicated) and tape it in place. (Alternatively, place a skin probe into an axilla and tape it in place.)

13. Plug the end of the probe into the proper jack on the control panel.

14. Place a second sheet over the patient and place a second thermal blanket over the sheet, if ordered.

15. Apply lanolin-based cream to the patient's skin where it contacts the blanket.

16. Remove gloves. Discard according to facility policy. Wash your hands.

17. Monitor vital signs, and intake and output every 5 minutes until the desired body temperature is reached, and then every 15 minutes, or as ordered.

18. Report color changes in skin or excessive shivering.

19. The blanket's texture increases the risk of skin breakdown. The patient should be repositioned every 30 minutes to 1 hour. Reapply skin cream as necessary. Change the gown and top sheet as often as necessary if the patient is actively perspiring. Put on gloves each time you care for patient. At the end of care, remove gloves, discard according to facility policy, and wash your hands.

20. At completion of the treatment, follow manufacturer's instructions for turning off the unit, disconnecting the blanket(s), and returning them to storage.

21. Put on gloves. Continue to monitor the patient as you remove the equipment.

22. Replace any damp bedding or garments and cover the patient. Continue to monitor the patient every 30 minutes until he or she has been stable for 2 hours.

23. Clean the thermometer probe and store it according to facility policy.

24. Remove gloves and discard according to facility policy.

25. Carry out ending procedure actions.

REVIEW

A. True/False.

Mark the following true or false by circling T or F.

1. T F Heat and cold treatments should be supervised by the nurse.

2. T F If a patient has a possible diagnosis of appendicitis, heat should not be applied to the abdomen.

3. T F The temperature of a warm soak solution should be approximately 100°F.

4. T F Special blankets used to alter the patient's temperature are called infrared blankets.

5. T F A patient who is unconscious must receive special attention during a heat treatment.

6. T F Hyperthermia is reducing core body temperature to below 95°F.

7. T F Heat is frequently applied to the head.

8. T F When charting an application of cold, always include the length of time of the application.

9. T F Aquamatic K-Pads are usually set at 115°F.

B. Multiple Choice.

Select the one best answer for each of the following.

10. Heat affects the body by
   a. causing constriction.
   b. increasing blood supply to the area.
   c. reducing oxygen in tissues.
   d. increasing white blood cells.

11. Special care with heat and cold treatments must be taken when the patient is
   a. alert and oriented.
   b. very young.
   c. cooperative.
   d. ambulatory.

12. Dry cold is provided by
   a. compresses.
   b. a sitz baths.
   c. ice caps.
   d. soaks.

13. Cold affects the body by
   a. reducing pain sensations.
   b. stimulating life processes.
   c. promoting inflammation.
   d. promoting healing.

14. Moist cold is applied with
   a. ice bags.
   b. ice caps.
   c. ice collars.
   d. soaks.

15. When applying heat and cold treatments, the nursing assistant should
   a. always remain in the room for the duration of the treatment.
   b. check the temperature of the solution with an elbow.
   c. monitor the skin under the application every 30 minutes.
   d. remove jewelry, buttons, or zippers that may conduct heat or cold.

16. When caring for a patient who is using an aquathermia blanket, the nursing assistant should
   a. regulate blanket temperature at least every 15 minutes.
   b. give the patient plenty of iced liquids to drink to reduce fever.
   c. monitor the patient for cyanosis or changes in vital signs.
   d. turn the patient at least every 2 hours.

C. Matching.

Choose the correct word from Column II to match each blank in Column I.

Column I

17. _____ excessive blood loss

18. _____ increase in size of blood vessel

19. _____ heat treatment

20. _____ decrease in size of blood vessel

21. _____ used to lower body temperature

Column II

   a. diathermy
   b. vasoconstriction
   c. vasodilation
   d. hypothermia blanket
   e. hemorrhage
   f. infrared

D. Nursing Assistant Challenge.

Peggy, 17 years of age, was admitted to your unit from the emergency room. She fractured an ankle and will require internal repair with screws and wire. You will care for her prior to surgery. The physician has ordered an ice bag for her ankle and her leg is to be elevated. Answer the following questions.

22. What are two reasons for applying the ice bag?

23. How full should the ice bag be filled?

24. Why should ice cubes be rinsed?

25. How should the metal cap be positioned when the ice bag is placed on the patient?

26. When should the ice bag be refilled?

27. How is the ice bag held in place?

28. What important observation should be reported immediately to the nurse?

UNIT 28

Assisting with the Physical Examination

OBJECTIVES

After completing this unit, you will be able to:
- Spell and define terms.
- Describe the responsibilities of the nursing assistant during the physical examination.
- Name the various positions for physical examinations.
- Drape patient for the various positions.
- Name the basic instruments necessary for physical examinations.

VOCABULARY

Learn the meaning and the correct spelling of the following words and phrases:

dorsal lithotomy
    position

dorsal recumbent
    position

knee-chest position
Trendelenburg position

INTRODUCTION

Physical examinations are done in the physician's office, in clinics, after the patient's admission to the facility, and in the patient's home. Remember to carry out each initial procedure action and ending procedure action as you assist.

The physical examination helps the primary care provider:
- Evaluate the patient's current status
- Establish a diagnosis
- Determine the patient's progress and response to therapy

Nursing physical assessments will be performed by the nurse in the facility after the patient is admitted. This information is used by the nurse to establish a nursing diagnosis.

Both of these procedures are carried out in a similar manner. The responsibilities of the nursing assistant include:
- Providing for the comfort and privacy of the patient
- Trying to anticipate the examiner's needs
- Draping and positioning patients
- Using proper body mechanics and exposing only the part of the patient being examined
- Preparing equipment that might be needed
- Reassuring the patient
- Caring for and labeling specimens
- Handing equipment as needed
- Cleaning equipment after use
- Adjusting lighting
- Remaining available during the examination
- Assisting the patient after the examination

The examination is typically done in a treatment room, examination room, or clinic setting that has the necessary equipment and supplies available. In this setting, disposable items are commonly used, such as disposable:
- Gown (Figure 28-1)
- Drapes or sheets
- Instruments and equipment

FIGURE 28-1 A disposable gown is commonly used for a physical examination. (Courtesy of Medline Industries, Inc. (800) MEDLINE)

The gowns are usually one size fits all, but may not fit larger patients. Regular cloth gowns are usually available. The disposable gown and drapes are paper. Caution the patient to handle them gently because they tear easily. They are discarded when the examination is complete.

Tips: Adjust the room temperature for comfort and make sure the room is free of drafts. Cover the examination table with a clean sheet or disposable paper. Instruct the patient to empty the bladder before beginning.

POSITIONING THE PATIENT

When the physical examination takes place on an examination table, extra attention must be given to safety. The examination table may be raised or lowered in sections and stirrups and shoulder braces applied to assist in positioning. Be sure you know how to properly operate the examination table before positioning a patient on it. In Figures 28-2 to 28-9, an examination table is shown.

Modifications

Some of the positions discussed here may be modified and used for other purposes. For example, they might be used to change the position of a patient who is confined to bed, or to perform specific procedures. Pillows must be used to support a patient who is to be kept in position for a period of time. Remember, the patient who "feels" covered and comfortable will be able to cooperate more fully. Providing privacy for the patient is one of your tasks.

Dorsal Recumbent Position

The **dorsal recumbent position** is the basic examination position.

- Assist the patient to be flat on the back, with knees flexed and slightly separated. The feet should be flat on the bed or table (Figure 28-2).
- Place a small pillow under the patient's head.
- Loosen the gown at the neck.
- Cover the patient with a sheet.

Supine or Horizontal Recumbent Position

- Assist the patient to lie flat on the back. The legs are extended and slightly separated (Figure 28-3).
- Place a pillow under the patient's head.
- Cover the patient with a sheet.
- Loosen the gown at the neck.

Knee-Chest Position

The **knee-chest position** may be used to examine the rectal or vaginal areas and to relieve pain following childbirth. This is a difficult position to maintain, so never leave the patient alone. Position the patient in a prone position until the examiner is ready.

- Draping may be done with one or two sheets.
- Place a small pillow under the patient's head.
- Assist the patient to turn and lie on the abdomen with head turned to one side.

FIGURE 28-2 Dorsal recumbent position. (Draping has been omitted for clarity.)

FIGURE 28-3 Supine or horizontal recumbent position

- Have the patient flex the arms and bring them up on either side of the head.
- Assist the patient to flex the knees and draw them up as far as possible toward the chest (Figure 28-4).

Prone Position

This position is used to examine the patient's back.

- Assist the patient to lie on the abdomen with head turned to one side.
- Place a small pillow under the patient's head.
- Arms may be extended at the patient's side or flexed and brought up on either side of the head (Figure 28-5).
- One sheet is used for draping.

Sims' Position

This position is used for vaginal and rectal procedures, including enema administration.

- Assist the patient to turn on the left side, with the head turned to the same side and resting on a small pillow.
- Position the left arm extended behind the body.
- Flex the right arm and position it in front of the patient.
- The left leg is slightly bent, while the right leg is sharply flexed (Figure 28-6).

- One drape is usually adequate.

Semi-Fowler's Position

This is a common position for head and neck examinations of the in-bed patient.

- Assist patient to a semi-sitting position with backrest elevated at a 45° angle to the bed.
- The knees are supported in a slightly flexed position (Figure 28-7).
- The arms rest at the sides.
- One drape is usually enough.

Trendelenburg Position

The **Trendelenburg position** encourages circulation to the patient's heart and brain. It is used when the patient is in shock.

- Assist the patient to lie flat on the back with the head lower than the rest of the body.
- If possible, the lower half of the bed or table is tilted so the legs are slightly flexed (Figure 28-8A). In an emergency, the entire bed frame may be supported on blocks, tilting the bed to a 45° angle. Some hospital beds, stretchers, and examination tables have a switch that enables the user to position the device in the Trendelenburg position quickly in emergencies.

FIGURE 28-4 Knee-chest position

FIGURE 28-6 Sims' position

FIGURE 28-5 Prone position

FIGURE 28-7 Semi-Fowler's position

FIGURE 28-8A The Trendelenburg position

FIGURE 28-8B A variation of the Trendelenburg position used for some treatments and procedures. Some professionals also use this position to treat patients who are in shock, but this use has fallen out of favor in recent years.

Clinical Information ALERT

A modification of the Trendelenburg position is taught as an initial treatment for hypotension, and to prevent shock in emergency situations. When you are instructed to use the Trendelenburg position for this purpose, you will elevate the patient's legs so they are higher than the heart. If possible, the feet are elevated so they are higher than the head, with the patient in a 30° to 45°, head-down angle. The underlying principle is that in an emergency, this position will help shunt blood and oxygen from the legs to the vital structures of the heart and the brain. However, despite being a time-honored ritual and an accepted treatment since World War I, evidence to date does not support the use of this position for the treatment of shock, and limited data suggests it may be harmful. This is an area of clinical practice in which much additional research is needed. ∎

- Beds that are electrically powered may be adjusted to this position.
- Shoulder braces may be needed to prevent the patient from slipping.
- One drape is usually sufficient.

There are several other variations of the Trendelenburg position. Of these, Figure 28-8B shows the most common. Another variation may be used for some emergencies and surgical procedures. You will need to know the

nature of the examination or procedure being done to know which Trendelenburg position to use. Never use the head-down Trendelenburg position for a patient with a known or suspected head injury.

Dorsal Lithotomy Position

The **dorsal lithotomy position** is frequently used for the pelvic examination of female patients. This is a difficult examination for most women, so make sure your draping makes the patient feel covered.

- Make sure the patient voids her bladder before the examination.
- The patient is positioned on her back.
- The knees are well separated and flexed.
- Usually this position is achieved by placing the feet in stirrups (Figure 28-9).
- One or two drapes may be used to cover the patient. The draping may be similar to draping for the knee-chest position.
- This position can be difficult and uncomfortable for the patient to maintain. Do not place the patient's legs in the stirrups until the physician is in the room and ready to begin the examination.

PHYSICAL EXAMINATION

Some health care facilities have examining instruments and equipment collected on trays. At other facilities, you will gather the necessary equipment and assemble it (Figure 28-10).

FIGURE 28-9 The patient's feet are placed in stirrups for the dorsal lithotomy position, with the knees flexed and separated.

FIGURE 28-10 Equipment and supplies for the physical examination

OSHA ALERT

Apply the principles of standard precautions when assisting with a physical examination. Anticipate the equipment that will be needed and make sure it is available to you and to the physician or nurse who is doing the examination. ■

REVIEW

A. True/False.

Mark the following true or false by circling T or F.

1. T F The physical examination helps the physician establish a nursing assessment.

2. T F A patient who feels covered is able to cooperate more fully.

3. T F Positions used for the physical examination can only be used for that purpose.

4. T F The nursing assistant performs the actual physical exam.

5. T F When a patient is placed in the Trendelenburg position, the feet must be at the same level as the knees.

6. T F When positioning a patient for a physical examination, you must maintain proper body mechanics.

7. T F Once you have the patient positioned for a physical examination, you should leave the room.

8. T F The nursing assistant assists in the physical assessment by draping and positioning the patient.

9. T F Lighting may have to be adjusted during the examination.

10. T F The semi-Fowler's position encourages blood flow to the head and heart.

B. Multiple Choice.

Select the one best answer for each of the following.

11. The basic examination position is
    a. Sims'.
    b. dorsal recumbent.
    c. dorsal lithotomy.
    d. Trendelenburg.

12. The patient is to have a pelvic examination. In what position should she be positioned?
    a. Sims'
    b. lithotomy
    c. Trendelenburg
    d. semi-Fowler's

13. The patient has vaginal bleeding and the physician orders you to place her in a position that will increase blood flow to the head. Which position would you prepare for?
    a. Sims'
    b. semi-Fowler's
    c. Trendelenburg
    d. Lithotomy

14. Stirrups are used in which position?
   a. dorsal lithotomy
   b. semi-Fowler's
   c. Sims'
   d. Trendelenburg

C. Matching.

Choose the correct word from Column II to match the word or phrase in Column I.

Column I

15. _____ variation in position

16. _____ how a patient is placed

17. _____ fearful

18. _____ covering

Column II

   a. apprehensive

   b. drape

   c. modification

   d. position

D. Nursing Assistant Challenge.

Robert Ubek is to have a physical examination in the doctor's office. He is 88 years of age and appears very nervous. He tells you that he is afraid he has prostate cancer. You are to assist the doctor. Complete the following statements using words from the following list.

anticipate	off
dorsal recumbent	on
drape	reassure

19. One of your responsibilities will be to _____ the patient.

20. Because of Mr. Ubek's age, you will be especially careful in assisting him to get _____ and _____ the table.

21. You can help him feel more comfortable if you _____ him properly.

22. You can help the examination go more smoothly if you _____ the examiner's needs.

23. You will position Mr. Ubek in the _____ position to begin the examination.

UNIT 29

The Surgical Patient

OBJECTIVES

After completing this unit, you will be able to:

- Spell and define terms.
- Describe the concerns of patients who are about to have surgery.
- List the various types of anesthesia.
- Shave the area to be operated on.
- Prepare the patient's unit for the patient's return from the operating room.
- Give routine postoperative care when the patient returns to the room.
- Assist the patient with deep breathing and coughing.

- Apply elasticized stockings or bandages and pneumatic hosiery.
- Demonstrate the following procedures:
  - Procedure 80 Assisting the Patient to Deep Breathe and Cough
  - Procedure 81 Performing Postoperative Leg Exercises
  - Procedure 82 Applying Elasticized Stockings
  - Procedure 83 Applying an Elastic Bandage
  - Procedure 84 Applying Pneumatic Compression Hosiery
  - Procedure 85 Assisting the Patient to Dangle

VOCABULARY

Learn the meaning and the correct spelling of the following words and phrases:

ambulation	disruption	NPO	pulmonary embolism
anesthesia	distention	operative	recovery room
anti-embolism hose	drainage	orifice	sequential compression therapy
aspirate	dressings	perioperative	singultus
atelectasis	embolus	perioperative hypothermia	spinal anesthesia
bandages	general anesthetic	postanesthesia care unit (PACU)	stable
binders	hypoallergenic tape	postoperative	surgical bed
dangling	hypoxia	preoperative	TED hose
deep vein thrombosis (DVT)	local anesthetic	prosthesis	thrombophlebitis
depilatory	Montgomery straps		vertigo
	nosocomial		

INTRODUCTION

Patients facing any surgical procedure tend to be fearful. Remember that these patients require great emotional as well as physical support (Figure 29-1). Such support should be given from the time the patient is admitted through the discharge.

Patients are concerned with:

- Disfigurement
- Pain

FIGURE 29-1 Patients and family members need support during the preoperative period.

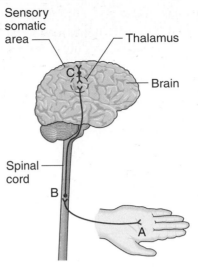

A Pain messages are picked up by free nerve endings in the skin. Local anesthetic blocks this.

B Message is carried into the spinal cord. Spinal anesthetic blocks this.

C Message is then carried to the cortex of the brain. General anesthetic blocks this.

FIGURE 29-2 Anesthetics will block pain impulses at points A, B, or C.

- Loss of control as they undergo anesthesia
- What serious conditions might be found
- Length and cost of recovery
- Possibility of death

Surgery is often associated with anxiety, pain, and discomfort. For this reason, medications are given before, during, and after surgery.

PAIN PERCEPTION

When a person feels pain sensations, the:

- Pain receptors record the sensation
- Sensation is sent by the spinal nerves to the spinal cord and then to the brain
- Sensation is received and interpreted in the brain

Before surgery, the patient is given medication to promote relaxation. During surgery, anesthetics are given to prevent pain (Figure 29-2). After surgery, medications are given to reduce discomfort.

ANESTHESIA

Anesthesia is given to prevent pain, to relax muscles, and to induce forgetfulness. The anesthetic agent (drug) and method of administration used are determined by the location and type of surgery to be performed, the length of time needed for surgery, and the patient's physical condition.

There are two main types of anesthetics:

1. **General anesthetics**—These induce the patient to become unconscious.
2. **Local anesthetics**—These induce loss of feeling in a specific area.

General Anesthetics

General anesthetics block reception of pain in the brain. They are usually given in one of two ways:

1. Inhalation—Some gases that are used as anesthetics include nitrous oxide and cyclopropane.
   - Inhaled anesthetics are apt to make the patient secrete more mucus and to experience nausea.
   - Special attention must be given after surgery to keep the respiratory tract clear.
   - There is a real danger that the patient may **aspirate** (inhale) vomitus into the respiratory tract.
2. Intravenous—Drugs are introduced directly into the veins.
   - These drugs, such as sodium pentathol, act rapidly.
   - The patient quickly loses consciousness.
   - IV anesthetics are often used with other types of anesthesia for short operations.

Local Anesthetics

Local anesthetics act by:

1. Blocking pain receptors in the operative area.
   - Drugs such as procaine hydrochloride may be injected into the patient around the operative area.
   - These drugs stop the sensation of pain only in that area.
   - The patient remains awake but free from pain during the operation.
2. Blocking transmission of the pain sensation at the level of the spinal cord.
   - A drug injected into the spinal canal prevents feeling in any point below the level of the injection.

– The patient remains awake.

– This type of anesthesia is commonly used for abdominal surgery because it produces good relaxation of the muscles.

– This technique is called **spinal anesthesia**.

After getting this type of anesthetic, the patient is unable to feel or move the legs for a period of time. If not prepared ahead of time, the patient may be frightened by this experience.

SURGICAL CARE

Care of the surgical patient (**perioperative**) can be divided into three parts:

- **Preoperative** (before surgery)
- **Operative** (in the operating room)
- **Postoperative** (after surgery)

PREOPERATIVE CARE

Preoperative care begins when surgery is planned by the physician with the patient. Your responsibilities begin when the patient is admitted to the facility. Remember that you may answer general questions that the patient asks, but you must refer specific questions about the surgery, its possible outcome, and anesthesia to the nurse. Although it is the responsibility of the physician and nurse to answer questions and give explanations, it is helpful if you are aware of the information that has been given.

Teaching

Time spent with the patient in the preoperative period is very helpful. Patients who are prepared are able to cooperate more successfully in their recovery. Ideally, this time is spent shortly after the patient's admission. Sometimes much of the information is given in the doctor's office or clinic.

During the preoperative period, the nurse will determine the patient's specific needs. The nurse also does preoperative teaching. The other staff members support this effort.

- Tests, medications, and preoperative procedures are explained.
- Questions regarding the postoperative period are answered.
- The patient is taught and given an opportunity to practice postoperative exercises, such as leg exercises and respiratory exercises.
- The patient and staff discuss the events of the preoperative period, and what the patient may experience while being taken to the operating room and being given anesthesia.

- The recovery period is outlined and the purpose of special procedures or equipment, such as tubes or intravenous fluid lines, that may be used after surgery is explained.
- Play therapy may be used to explain to children.
- Every effort is made to teach ways of decreasing discomfort and to assure the patient that pain relief will be available.
- Planning for the discharge period begins now.

Psychological Preparation

The nursing staff spends as much time as possible helping patients deal with their emotional stress.

All members of the health care team need to be sensitive and responsive to the psychological needs of the patient. Because you will be in frequent contact with the patient, you may be the first person to recognize signs of fear or concern. Listen to what the patient says and observe the patient's body language carefully. Report your observations to the nurse so that appropriate nursing intervention may be carried out.

Build patient confidence by:

- Performing your work in an efficient, calm manner.
- Being available to listen.
- Explaining what you plan to do before carrying out any procedure.
- Encouraging the patient to participate in his own care as much as possible. This helps the patient feel that he still has a measure of control over his life.
- Immediately transmitting requests for clergy visits.

Physical Preparation

The Evening Before Surgery. If the patient is in the facility the evening before surgery, part of the surgical preparation may be done then. It usually includes:

- Bath or shower with surgical soap
- Enema
- Surgical prep (shaving of the operative site)
- Special tests
- Medication to ensure a good night's rest, when indicated
- Insertion of special tubes for draining body cavities
- Being placed on **NPO** (nothing by mouth) orders after midnight
- Removal of the water pitcher from the bedside table and having the NPO notice posted over the bed, bedside stand, on the door, on the patient's chart, and on the Kardex.

Nosocomial infections are those acquired during the facility stay. It is known that such infections:

- Are more likely to occur the longer the patient is in the facility.

- Add days to the stay in the facility
- Increase the cost of hospitalization
- Can be life-threatening

To decrease costs and the potential for nosocomial infections, patients are often admitted on the morning of surgery and are sometimes discharged on the day of surgery or the day after. In this circumstance, much of the preoperative care must be done at home or immediately upon admission. This is called outpatient or "short-term" surgery.

Patients who remain at home until they are admitted for surgery usually have laboratory testing done on an outpatient basis before surgery. The patient is advised not to eat or drink anything after midnight on the evening before the scheduled surgery. He or she may be instructed to shower with a special antiseptic soap before coming to the hospital early in the morning, on the day of surgery. After admission, you may be assigned to complete the skin preparation. The patient then goes right to surgery. Many surgeries are performed on an outpatient basis. The patients go home, or return to a long-term care or subacute care facility, after they have recovered from the anesthesia. If the patient experiences complications, she will be admitted to the hospital. Many patients are first admitted to the nursing unit after surgery, so they are not familiar with the staff, and may need information about what to expect postoperatively.

When the patient is admitted before surgery, preoperative teaching is done on the nursing unit the evening before surgery. Because most patients are not admitted until after surgery, patient teaching may be done later. Patient teaching is also done in the physician's office before surgery. The office may mail instructions to the patient before hospital admission. Some physicians hold informational classes. Personnel in the operating room may also do some patient teaching, but you must reinforce it on the nursing unit. You will be assisting the nurse in teaching the patient how to move and turn, cough and deep breathe, do foot and leg exercises, manage pain, and other aspects of care.

The Surgical Prep Area. Skin preparation before surgery may or may not include hair removal. There is a trend away from removing the hair unless its thickness will interfere with the surgery. In fact, some studies have shown more infections among shaved patients compared with unshaved patients.

If shaving is ordered, it must be done according to facility procedure. It must be performed skillfully in a well-lighted area. Also, the area to be washed and shaved will be larger than the surgical incision area (Figure 29-3). In some cases, a **depilatory** (hair-removing) cream will be ordered for use the night before surgery. If a depilatory is to be used, check the skin for sensitivity. Apply a small amount to the skin of the forearm and wait 10 minutes. If redness occurs, do not continue, but report to the nurse.

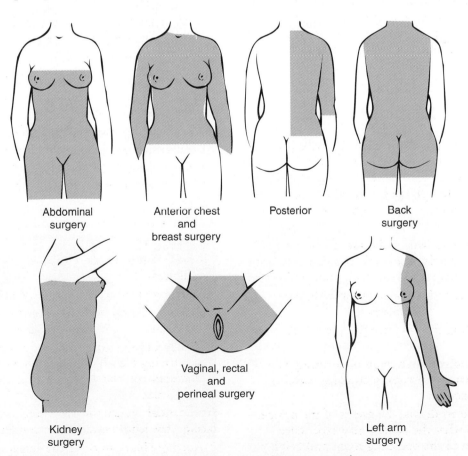

Abdominal surgery

Anterior chest and breast surgery

Posterior

Back surgery

Kidney surgery

Vaginal, rectal and perineal surgery

Left arm surgery

FIGURE 29-3 The shading indicates the areas that must be shaved preoperatively.

Skin preparation may be performed by:

- Special surgical prep team
- Operating room (OR) staff in the OR
- Nursing staff in the patient's unit just prior to surgery

Safety ALERT

All personnel involved in perioperative care of the patient must be alert to make sure that the correct surgical procedure is done on the correct patient, and that the surgery is done on the correct site. This often involves marking the site of the surgery. Various forms and checklists are used to verify the patient and surgical site. Take your responsibilities for identifying the patient and operative site seriously. There is no room for error in this area of nursing practice. ■

To prepare the surgical area by shaving:

- Make sure you know exactly what area is to be shaved. Most hospitals have routine prep areas.
- Do not shave the neck or face of a female patient. If in doubt, check with the nurse.
- Never shave the eyebrows.
- Be aware that the preparations for cranial surgery are usually performed after the patient has been medicated and taken to the operating suite. Doctors have special preferences in this regard.
- Remember that if a spinal anesthesia is to be given, the back may also be shaved.

Calm the patient's fears by explaining that the area prepared is much larger than the actual incision area. This is

Infection Control ALERT

Do the skin-prep procedure as close to the time of surgery as possible. This provides less time for microbes to proliferate on the skin. If the razor becomes dull, get another. The texture of some patients' body hair makes it difficult to remove, and a dull razor increases the risk of injury. If you observe a cut, rash, redness, irritation, or other break in the skin near the operative site, notify the nurse. In some facilities, hair is routinely removed with clippers unless a doctor's order specifies shaving. Know and follow your facility policies for hair removal. ■

to prevent contamination of the surgical site, which may lead to possible complications after surgery.

Immediate Preoperative Care. Approximately one hour before surgery, the patient will be given additional medication by the nurse. Your responsibilities regarding the patient must be completed before this time. You may be asked to do the following:

- Take and record vital signs (Figure 29-4) (see Section 6).
- Take care of valuables according to hospital policy. Remove dentures and any other **prosthesis** (artificial part), such as a hearing aid or glasses. See that they are safely marked with the patient's name and stored appropriately.
- Remove nail polish, makeup, hairpins, and jewelry. Long hair should be neatly braided or capped. Plain wedding bands may be taped in place.
- Dress the patient in a gown and cover the hair with a surgical cap.
- See that the patient voids and measure the urine. Drain the catheter, if present, and record.
- Make sure that the room is quiet and comfortable.

As soon as the nurse gives the preoperative medication:

- Be sure the side rails are in place for safety.
  - Always keep the side rails up after the patient receives the preoperative injection. Make sure the call signal is within reach. Never allow a patient to get up and go to the bathroom alone after the preoperative medication has been given. Assist with using the bedpan or urinal, if necessary.
- Remove all unnecessary equipment.
- Push the bedside table, overbed table, and chair out of the way to make room for the stretcher when it arrives from surgery.
- Complete the surgical checklist:
  1. Admission sheet
  2. Surgical consent
  3. Sterilization consent (if necessary)
  4. Consultation sheet (if necessary)

FIGURE 29-4 Taking vital signs is an important part of preoperative care.

5. History and physical
6. Lab reports (pregnancy test also if necessary)
7. Surgery prep done and charted, if required
8. Latest TPR and blood pressure charted
9. Preoperative medication given and charted (if required)
10. Identification band on patient
11. Fingernail polish and makeup removed
12. Metallic objects removed (wedding ring may be taped)
13. Dentures removed
14. Other prostheses removed (such as artificial limb or eye, wigs and hairpieces)
15. Glasses or contact lenses removed
16. Bath blanket and head cap in place
17. Bed in high position and side rails up after preop medication is given
18. Patient has voided
    - Check off those duties to which you were assigned.
    - Note the time your patient leaves for surgery.
- Follow facility policy regarding visitors. Sometimes they are allowed to wait quietly with the patient. Sometimes they should be directed to the visitors' waiting room.
- Elevate the bed to stretcher height when the transporter arrives to take the patient to surgery.

The nurse and surgical attendant will check the patient's identification and surgical checklist before the patient is moved. A staff member, and sometimes a family member, accompanies the patient to the doors of the operating room. You will probably be asked to assist in transferring the patient from the bed to the stretcher and, after surgery, from the stretcher to the bed. Review Procedures 25 and 26 in Unit 16.

DURING THE OPERATIVE PERIOD

While the patient is in the operating room, you will prepare the room for the patient's return.

- A special surgical bed will be prepared. This was described in Unit 23. The **surgical bed** is also called a postop bed or recovery bed.
- Everything should be removed from the top of the bedside stand except an emesis basin, tissue wipes, tongue depressors, and equipment to check vital signs.
- A pencil and small pad to record vital signs should also be available.
- Check with your team leader for any special equipment, such as oxygen, IV poles, suction, or drainage bags, that might be necessary for your patient.
- While carrying out your other assignments, watch for the return of your patient from surgery.

- Follow facility policy regarding the location of visitors and family during surgery. They are sometimes permitted to wait in the patient's room. In most cases they are directed to a special waiting area.

POSTOPERATIVE CARE

During the immediate postoperative period, the patient recovers from anesthesia. For this period, the patient is placed in a special area called the **recovery room** (Figure 29-5). The recovery room is located next to the operating room and is sometimes called the **postanesthesia care unit (PACU)**.

Safety ALERT

Remember that most patients receive many drugs when they are in surgery. Many of these drugs can alter the patient's mental status. The drugs are excreted from the body slowly. The patient may sleep soundly upon return to the unit. Keep the side rails up and follow all safety precautions until the patient is fully awake and the nurse instructs you that side rails are no longer necessary. Do not leave liquids at the bedside until the nurse instructs you that it is safe to do so. Check on the patient regularly. ■

When the patient's condition is stabilized, the patient is returned to the unit. Upon the patient's return from the recovery room, you should:

- Identify the patient
- Assist in the transfer from stretcher to bed (see Unit 16)

FIGURE 29-5 Postanesthesia care unit (PACU)—the unit where the patient wakes up from anesthesia after surgery. (Courtesy of Memorial Medical Center of Long Beach, CA)

- Never leave the unconscious patient alone at any time
- Check with the nurse for any special instructions
- Realize that the patient may be drowsy for several hours after return
- Notify the nurse if the patient's temperature is below 97°F.
- Have an extra blanket available—many patients complain of feeling cold upon return (Figure 29-6).

Safety ALERT

Anesthesia reduces body temperature. Keep the patient warm. If the patient's temperature is below 97°F, inform the nurse promptly. ■

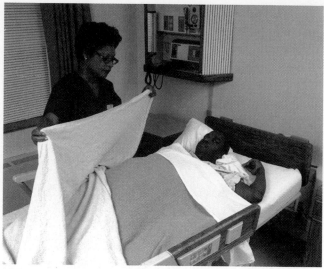

FIGURE 29-6 Patients may be cold after surgery. Cover them to prevent chilling. Use warmed blankets, if available.

GUIDELINES *for*
Postoperative Care

- Always wear gloves and follow standard precautions when contact with blood, body fluids, mucous membranes, or nonintact skin is likely.
- Take vital signs of the patient upon arrival on the unit (Figure 29-7) and every 15 minutes for four readings. The patient's temperature may not always be taken at this time.
- When taking postoperative vital signs, count pulse and respiration for one full minute. Most facilities have policies for postoperative vital signs at specified frequencies that decrease if the vital signs are **stable** (approximately the same), such as:
  - every 15 minutes for 1 hour
  - if stable, every 30 minutes for 1 hour
  - if stable, every hour for 2 hours
  - if stable, every 4 hours for 24 hours
- Always follow the protocol for vital signs used by your facility. The vital sign schedule may be altered by the nurse if the patient's condition warrants. The physician may also order vital signs at a specifically designated frequency. Monitor the patient's level of consciousness (drowsy, unresponsive, alert) each time you check the vital signs.
- Many facilities consider pain to be the fifth vital sign, so you should ask the patient if he or she is having pain each time you check the vital signs. Inform the nurse if pain is present.

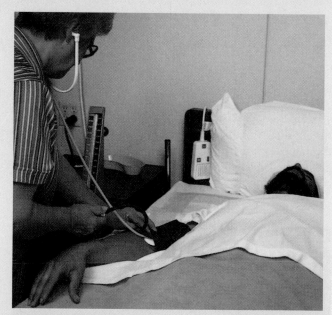

FIGURE 29-7 Check the vital signs regularly until they are stable.

- Check dressings for amount and type of any drainage. The nurse may reinforce them as necessary.
- Check IV solution for flow rate. Restrain the infusion site whenever ordered by the physician and report to the nurse. Remember that the flow rate is ordered by the physician.

continues

GUIDELINES *continued*

- Encourage the patient to breathe deeply, cough, and move in bed. Position should be changed every 2 hours.

- Turn the patient's head to one side and support if he is vomiting. Have an emesis basin ready, as well as tissues and wet cloth. If the patient is conscious, allow the patient to rinse the mouth with water after vomiting. Note the type and amount of vomitus and record on the output worksheet.

- Check the pulses distal to the operative site. Inform the nurse if the pulse is weak or cannot be felt.

- If the patient was given a spinal anesthetic:
  - Give extra care in turning frequently and maintaining proper alignment.
  - Remember that the patient will be unable to move independently until sensation and motor functions return. Make sure to calm the patient's fear about this.
  - Some physicians require that the patient remain flat on the back and without a pillow for 8 to 12 hours following spinal anesthesia, to avoid headaches.
  - Any complaints of a headache following spinal anesthesia should be reported promptly.
  - Provide extra blankets if the patient is cold.

- Be sure all drainage tubes have been connected (the nurse will usually attend to this). If you notice a tube clamped shut, check with the nurse.

- Measure and record the first postoperative voiding. Inform the nurse.

- Report any patient complaints of discomfort or pain to the nurse (Figure 29-8).

FIGURE 29-8 Report complaints of pain or discomfort to the nurse.

Safety ALERT

Some patients are very sensitive and will not let anyone see them unless their dentures are in the mouth. Monitor postoperative patients to be sure they have not inserted their dentures before they are fully awake. Remove dentures from an unconscious or comatose patient to prevent accidental airway obstruction by the denture. ■

Tubes

Patients often return from surgery with a variety of tubes and drains in place.

- Some tubes may deliver materials into the patient. Examples are oxygen tubes or intravenous tubes.
- Other tubes may have been placed in the patient to provide **drainage** from wounds or body cavities. Examples are drains in the incision or urinary catheters.

The following are some special precautions to be taken:

- Always wear gloves if contact with drainage from the tube is likely.
- Learn the type, purpose, and location of each tube.
- Check drainage for character and amount.
- Check for obstructions to the tube system.
- Check flow rate of infusions from intravenous lines.
- Keep **orifices** (body openings) clear of secretions and discharge.
- Never disconnect tubes or raise drainage bottles above the level of the drainage site.
- Never lower infusion bottles below the level of the infusion site.
- Never put stress on the tubes when moving the patient or giving care.
- Monitor levels of infusions and report to the nurse before they run out.
- Report any signs of leakage or disconnected tubes immediately.
- Report pain, discoloration, or swelling at sites or drainage and infusion.

Dressings and Bandages

Caring for surgical wounds, injuries, and ulcers is very important. **Dressings** are gauze, film, or other synthetic substances that cover a wound, ulcer, or injury. Some dressings have an adhesive backing. Some are affixed with tape. Many different types of tape are available in the health care facility. Some patients need special **hypoallergenic tape**, which reduces the incidence of a skin reaction in patients who are allergic to the adhesive backing. **Bandages** are sometimes used to hold dressings in place. These are fabric, gauze, net, or elasticized materials used to cover the dressing and keep it securely in place. Bandages are available in different sizes and shapes. Gauze bandages are commonly used to cover dressings. Elastic bandages are used to reduce edema and support injured body parts. When wrapping bandages, avoid wrapping them so tightly that they restrict circulation.

Occasionally, **Montgomery straps** (Figure 29-9) are used to hold dressings in place. These are long strips of adhesive attached to the skin on either side of the wound. They are less traumatic to the skin because the adhesive is not removed with each dressing change unless the straps are soiled. After the dressing is in place, the straps are tied to hold the dressing securely. **Binders** (Figure 29-10) may also be used to hold dressings in place.

FIGURE 29-9 Montgomery straps hold dressings securely in place so they can be observed, changed, and reinforced without tape. This is much less traumatic for the patient.

Drainage

When a body cavity is the operative site, it may be necessary to drain fluid such as blood, pus, serous drainage caused by tissue trauma, or gastric contents from it before or after surgery. Always wear gloves if contact with drainage is likely. The drainage outlet may be a:

- Catheter
- T-tube

FIGURE 29-10 Various surgical binders support the body part and hold dressings in place.

- Jackson-Pratt (J–P) or Hemovac drain
- Penrose drain
- Cigarette drain

Infection Control ALERT

Body sites with tubes, drains, and surgical dressings are managed using sterile technique. Never open a tube or drain or remove a dressing. The nurse will use sterile technique to manage these areas. ■

When such a drain is in place, the drainage accumulates on the dressing (Figure 29-11). You should:

- Note the amount and character of the drainage
- Inform the nurse when the dressing should be changed or reinforced

At times, the withdrawal of fluids is controlled by attaching the drainage tube to a connecting tube and then a suction apparatus. The drainage accumulates in a container. The container is emptied and the contents measured at the end of each shift. The Jackson-Pratt or Hemovac drains are closed drainage systems. The drains are placed directly in the wound, and drainage goes directly into an expandable container. A record of the amount and character of the drainage is entered in both the output chart and the nurses' notes.

It is your responsibility to:

- Report either heavy or light drainage
- Report a change in the character or amount of the drainage
- Make sure that the flow of drainage is not blocked by kinking of the tube (Figure 29-12)

Never assume responsibility for chest drainage or attempt to empty chest bottles. Chest bottles and irrigations require the nurse's or physician's attention.

Careful preoperative preparation and postoperative care can help limit the extent of postoperative discomfort and complication.

Clinical Information ALERT

A closed wound drain and vacuum system are placed when the surgeon anticipates substantial wound drainage. The tubing exit site is considered a surgical incision, and the drain is often sutured to the skin. Some patients will have more than one closed drain. Having a drain in place prevents swelling and promotes wound healing. It reduces the risk of infection and skin breakdown. Fewer dressing changes are necessary. Fasten the vacuum unit for the drain to the bed or the patient's gown if the patient is ambulatory. Make sure the vacuum unit remains below the level of the wound. Avoid traction on the tubing. The nurse is responsible for caring for the drain. He or she will empty the drain and record the output at the end of each shift, and more often if the drain is full. Inform the nurse if the drain is full. A full drain applies less suction to the wound, and the additional fluid accumulation under the skin will strain the suture line. ■

The patient must be carefully observed, especially during the first 24 hours, for possible complications. Possible postoperative discomfort and complications and appropriate nursing assistant actions are summarized in Table 29-1.

When the patient has responded sufficiently and vital signs are stable, the patient may be refreshed by:

- Washing the hands and face
- Changing the linen
- Being given a light backrub

The patient is now ready to participate more actively in recovery. Exercises taught in the preoperative period are practiced, including:

- Deep breathing and coughing
- Leg exercises

FIGURE 29-11 Check dressings regularly for drainage or bleeding.

FIGURE 29-12 Monitor drainage tubes to make sure they are not twisted, kinked, or obstructed.

TABLE 29-1 POSTOPERATIVE COMPLICATIONS AND NURSING ASSISTANT ACTIONS

Possible Discomfort	Report	What You Can Do*
Thirst	Patient complaints of dryness of lips, mouth, and skin	Carefully check I&O. Give ice chips or increase fluid intake by mouth with permission. Monitor IV if ordered. Give mouth care. Check BP and pulse. Watch for signs of shock and hemorrhage.
Singultus (hiccups)—intermittent spasms of the diaphragm	Incidence of hiccups	Allow the patient to rest; hiccups can be tiring. Support the incisional area. Assist the patient to breathe into a paper bag.
Pain	Location, intensity, type	Change position. Apply warmth if instructed. Monitor carefully for and report effects of medication given by nurse.
Distention (accumulation of gas in bowel)	Distention of abdomen, complaints of pain	Increase mobility. Insert a rectal tube if instructed and permitted.
Nausea, vomiting	Nausea, character of vomitus	Keep an emesis basin at the bedside. Monitor IV fluids, which are substituted for oral fluids. Give mouth care. Limit fluids by mouth. Encourage the patient to breathe deeply.
Urinary retention	Amount and time of first voiding. Distention, restlessness, imbalance between I&O	Monitor I&O carefully. Check for distention.
Hemorrhage (excessive blood loss)	Fall in blood pressure; cold, moist skin; weak, rapid pulse; restlessness; pallor/cyanosis; condition of dressing; thirst	Report immediately to nurse. Keep the patient quiet. Check vital signs.
Shock	Fall in blood pressure; weak, rapid pulse; cold, moist skin; pallor	Report immediately to nurse. Keep the patient quiet. Monitor ordered oxygen. Be prepared to follow additional instructions.
Hypoxia (lack of oxygen)	Restlessness, dyspnea, crowing sounds to respirations, pounding pulse, perspiring	Report immediately to nurse. Monitor oxygen, if ordered.
Atelectasis (decreased or absent air in all or part of a lung, resulting in loss of lung volume and inability to expand lung fully)	Dyspnea; cyanosis/pallor	Report immediately to nurse.
Wound infection	Increased pain in incisional area; fever; chills, anorexia, increased drainage on dressing	Be observant. Report findings promptly to nurse. Check dressing.
Wound **disruption** (separation of wound edges)	Pinkish drainage. Complaints by the patient that he "feels open," "broken," "given away"	Report immediately to nurse. Keep the patient quiet. Support incisional area.

continues

TABLE 29-1 *CONTINUED*

Possible Discomfort	Report	What You Can Do*
Pulmonary emboli	Anxiety, difficulty breathing; feelings of "heaviness in chest," cyanosis, chest pain	Keep the patient quiet. Report immediately to nurse. Elevate head of bed.

*In all cases, be prepared to follow the nurse's additional instructions.

Perioperative Hypothermia

During the perioperative period, many factors interfere with the patient's normal temperature-regulating mechanisms. Normally, we shiver when we are cold. The blood vessels constrict. **Perioperative hypothermia** develops in the operating room. Anesthesia and some sedatives disrupt the internal ability to regulate temperature. The drugs promote heat loss by reducing the shivering response and preventing blood vessel constriction. Underlying factors such as age, presence of chronic disease, and body size also affect temperature regulation.

The operating room is a very cool environment. This is done deliberately, because cooler temperature reduces oxygen requirements. Open body cavities and administration of blood and IV fluids further contribute to temperature loss. In the first 30 minutes after being given general anesthesia, body temperature usually decreases. The American Association of Nurse Anesthetists (AANA) recommends continuous temperature monitoring on pediatric patients receiving general anesthesia and, when indicated, on all other patients. Some experts recommend checking the temperature at 15- to 30-minute intervals while the patient is in the operating room.

The body cannot return the temperature to normal until the concentration of anesthetic in the brain decreases and the normal temperature-regulating responses are triggered and can take over. Pain further decreases the effectiveness of these responses. Because of these factors, return to normal temperature may take 2 to 5 hours, depending on the degree of hypothermia and the age of the patient. Perioperative outcomes are better if the patient does not become hypothermic.

To maintain patient temperature during and after surgery, the hyperthermia-hypothermia blanket may be used. The circulating water is known to be a very effective warming mechanism. The blankets may be used under or over the patient, but are most effective when positioned over the patient's body. If the patient is not hypothermic, wrapping him or her with several warm bath blankets is a good comfort measure that will help maintain body heat.

Deep Breathing and Coughing

Deep breathing and coughing clear the air passages. This helps to prevent postoperative respiratory complications

Safety ALERT

Although we routinely encourage postoperative patients to cough and deep breathe, there are a few exceptions you must be aware of. Avoid this procedure with patients who have had eye, nose, or neurologic surgery. Coughing and deep breathing will increase pressure, causing complications in these patients. Check with the nurse if you are unsure of what action to take. ■

such as pneumonia and atelectasis, which is the collapse of the alveolar air sacs. This may be an uncomfortable task when the patient has a new incision and feels fatigued. (See Procedure 80.) You can best assist the patient by:

- Explaining the value of the exercise and carrying out Procedure 80.
- Checking with the nurse to see if medication for pain is to be administered before the exercise. If so, wait for 45 minutes after the medication has been given before carrying out the exercise.
- Learning from the nurse how many deep breaths and coughs should be attempted. The usual number is 5 to 10 breaths and 2 to 3 coughs.
- Using a pillow or binder to support the incision during the procedure.

OSHA ALERT

Apply the principles of standard precautions when assisting with coughing and deep breathing procedures. If the patient is expelling loose secretions, select and wear appropriate protective equipment, including gloves, gown, mask, and face shield. Show the patient how to contain secretions in a tissue. Assist him or her with handwashing after the activity. ■

PROCEDURE

80

ASSISTING THE PATIENT TO DEEP BREATHE AND COUGH

1. Carry out initial procedure actions.

2. Assemble equipment:
   - Disposable gloves
   - A pillowcase-covered pillow or binder, if ordered
   - Tissues
   - Emesis basin

3. Elevate the head of the bed and assist the patient to assume a comfortable semi-Fowler's position.

4. Have the patient place his hands on either side of his rib cage or over the operative site (Figure 29-13). A pillow over the operative site can be used to support an incision during respiratory exercises.

5. Ask the patient to take as deep a breath as possible and hold it for 3 to 5 seconds; then exhale slowly through pursed lips.

6. Repeat this exercise about five times unless the patient seems too tired. If so, stop the procedure and report to the nurse.

7. Place the pillow across the incision line as a brace. Have the patient hold the pillow on either side or have the patient interlace fingers across the incision to act as a brace (Figure 29-14).

8. Pass tissues to the patient and instruct him to take a deep breath and cough forcefully twice with the mouth open, collecting any secretions that are brought up in tissues.

9. Put on disposable gloves to handle the tissues.

10. Dispose of tissues in an emesis basin.

11. Assist the patient to assume a new, comfortable position.

12. Clean the emesis basin.

13. Remove and dispose of gloves according to facility policy.

14. Carry out ending procedure actions.

15. Report to nurse on the number of times the patient performed each exercise, how the patient tolerated the exercise, and the type and amount of any sputum coughed up.
    - Be sure the patient does not become overly fatigued.
    - Encourage the patient to cough and clear the respiratory passages.
    - Report to your team leader if the patient seems overly fatigued during the procedure.
    - Carefully observe and report any unusual responses such as pain, dizziness, or throat and airway irritation.

FIGURE 29-13 Remind, encourage, and assist the patient to perform deep breathing exercises.

FIGURE 29-14 A pillow helps support the abdomen and splint the incision during coughing and deep breathing.

Leg Exercises

Leg exercises following surgery encourage steady circulation. This helps to prevent another serious complication of the postoperative period—the development of blood clots.

A blood clot or **deep vein thrombosis (DVT)** could develop in the venous system and block the essential blood flow. A small piece of thrombus broken off (**embolus**) could travel throughout the vascular system and block a vessel in the lungs.

A specific order must be written for leg exercises when there has been surgery on the legs themselves. Otherwise, leg exercises are routinely performed by the patient. If the patient is very weak, you may need to assist.

- Encourage leg exercises and be sure they have been performed.
- Each exercise should be performed 3 to 5 times at least every 1 or 2 hours, and at other times as well.
- Carry out leg exercises as you assist with position changes.
- Apply or reapply support hose after exercises if ordered.

Elasticized Stockings

Elasticized stockings, called **TED hose** or **anti-embolism hose**, extend from the ankle or foot to calf or mid-thigh. They may also be called *graduated compression stockings (GCS)*, which refers to the graduation of pressure.

PROCEDURE

81

PERFORMING POSTOPERATIVE LEG EXERCISES

1. Carry out initial procedure actions.

2. Explain how the exercise is to be performed. Have the patient:

   a. Brace the incisional area with laced hands.

   b. Dorsiflex (bring toes toward knee) and plantar flex (point toes and foot down) each ankle (Figure 29-15A).

   c. Rotate each ankle by drawing imaginary circles with the toes (Figure 29-15B).

   d. Flex and extend each knee (Figure 29-15C).

   e. Flex and extend each hip.

   f. Repeat each exercise 3 to 5 times. Assist as needed.

3. Lower the side rail.

4. Cover the patient with a bath blanket and draw the top bedding to the foot of the bed.

5. Supervise exercises or assist. Apply or reapply support hose as ordered after exercises.

6. Draw bedding up and remove the bath blanket.

7. Fold the bath blanket and place in the bedside stand for reuse.

8. Carry out ending procedure actions. Report to nurse on the number of exercises done and how they were tolerated by the patient.

A. Curl the toes down and up. Repeat 5 times.

B. Make circles with the feet clockwise 3 times and counterclockwise 3 times. Repeat 5 times.

C. Slide one leg up and down in bed. Do the same with the other leg. Repeat 5 times.

FIGURE 29-15 Help the patient perform leg exercises to encourage circulation.

Sometimes they are referred to by the brand name, such as TED or Jobst hose. The stockings are tightest at the ankle, and become looser as they move up the leg. They are often applied during the preoperative and postoperative periods to support the veins of the legs. This reduces the incidence of **thrombophlebitis**, which is inflammation of the veins that can lead to blood clots. The stockings must be applied smoothly and evenly before the patient gets out of bed. They should be removed and reapplied at least every 8 hours—more often if necessary or as ordered.

Several different types of anti-embolism hose are used. Some have closed toes, but most have an opening near the toe end. The hole is positioned on the top or the bottom of the foot, just proximal to the toes. Check the heel placement on the stocking. By using the heel as a landmark, you will see where to position the hole in the stocking.

Preventing Complications. A physician's order is needed to apply special hosiery. The ordering physician will specify if knee-high or thigh-high hose should be used. Anti-embolism hosiery is available in various grades of pressure, ranging from 8 mm Hg through 46 mm Hg. Become familiar with the criteria used by your facility to establish what constitutes light, medium, and firm compression. Make sure you apply the correct hosiery, according to the original order and facility policies.

The risk of complications from anti-embolism hosiery is low. However, they are not risk-free. The greatest risk is a reduction in blood flow from pressure. This leads to decreased oxygen in the tissues and potential for blood clots. Patients with diabetes and certain circulatory conditions are at high risk. Other reported complications are pressure ulcers, gangrene, and arterial occlusion. These often occurred when the patient sat for a prolonged period without moving. In another case, the tourniquet effect created by bunched-up layers of elastic hose, combined with swelling of the leg, caused serious skin breakdown, leading to amputation. The tourniquet effect of stockings that do not fit properly may also increase the risk of blood clots and occlusion of blood flow.

Follow your facility procedure manual and the product package for applying anti-embolism hosiery. Never guess at the size. Always use a tape measure to ensure that the size is accurate. Measuring and fitting the initial hosiery

are nursing responsibilities in some facilities. Ill-fitting hosiery is the most common cause of complications, so nursing personnel must:

- Measure legs with a tape measure to ensure correct hosiery fit. Compare the measurements with the size chart (Figure 29-16), then select the correct size.
- Follow the schedule for applying and removing the hosiery. Remove the hosiery for patient bathing each day. Evaluate the appearance of the feet and legs regularly, at least several times each day.
- Promptly inform the nurse of abnormalities or complications. Intervene early with the occurrence of complications.

FIGURE 29-16 Measure the patient's leg with the disposable paper tape measure, then compare the measurements to the manufacturer's chart to determine the correct size hosiery. Discard the tape measure.

GUIDELINES *for*
Applying Anti-Embolism Stockings

- The care plan will specify the wearing schedule for the stockings, according to physician orders and facility policies. For most patients, the hosiery is applied during the day and removed at bedtime.

- It is best to apply the stockings before the patient gets out of bed in the morning. Elevating the legs for 20 to 30 minutes before applying the hosiery will reduce swelling and make hose easier to apply.

GUIDELINES *continued*

- Make sure the legs are dry before attempting to apply the hosiery. An apparatus is used in some facilities to make them easier to apply. If this is not available, the nurse may permit you to dust the legs lightly with baby powder, making the hose easier to apply. Avoid using baby powder if the patient has respiratory difficulty, a rash, or dressings on the legs.

- Never apply the hosiery over open areas, fractures, or deformities. If the patient has an open or abnormal skin area, fracture, or deformity on the legs or feet, inform the nurse.

- Make sure the stockings are applied smoothly, with no wrinkles.

- Check the stockings every few hours to be sure the tops have not rolled or turned down. Keep the fabric straight.

- Monitor circulation in the patient's toes every 2 to 4 hours, or as specified on the care plan. Note color, sensation, swelling, temperature, and ability to move. Report abnormalities to the nurse. Document that you have done regular skin and circulation checks.

- Follow your facility policy for washing anti-embolism stockings. These must be hand-washed and drip-dried. The stockings are damaged by the commercial washers and dryers used in health care facilities. Because of this, your facility may issue two pairs to each patient.

- To preserve the life of the stockings, avoid contact with lotions, ointments, or oils containing lanolin or petroleum products. These products deteriorate the elastic.

PROCEDURE

82

APPLYING ELASTICIZED STOCKINGS

1. Carry out initial procedure actions.

2. Assemble equipment:
   - Elasticized stockings of proper length and size

3. Always apply stockings with the patient lying down. Expose one leg at a time.

4. Grasp the stocking with both hands at the top and roll it toward the toe end (Figure 29-17A).

5. Adjust over the patient's toes, positioning the opening at the base of the toes (unless the toes are to be covered) (Figure 29-17B). Remember that the raised seams should be on the outside.

6. Apply the stocking to the leg by rolling it upward toward the body (Figure 29-17C).

7. Check to be sure the stocking is applied evenly and smoothly and that there are no wrinkles (Figure 29-17D).

8. Repeat the procedure on the opposite leg.

9. Carry out ending procedure actions.

FIGURE 29-17A Gather the stocking and slip over the patient's toes.

continues

PROCEDURE 82 CONTINUED

FIGURE 29-17B Position the opening on the top of the foot, at the base of the toes.

FIGURE 29-17C Draw the stocking smoothly up to the knee.

FIGURE 29-17D Check to make sure the stocking is free from wrinkles.

Elastic Bandage

An elasticized bandage (Ace bandage) may be used to keep dressings in place, especially on an extremity or on the head. You may need to remove and reapply the bandage once or twice on your shift. Elastic bandages are also used on nonsurgical patients, to promote venous blood flow in the legs, and for injuries of the musculoskeletal system, to reduce swelling. Elastic bandages come in 2-inch to 6-inch widths and in 4-foot and 6-foot lengths (Figure 29-18). Check with the nurse for the appropriate size bandage.

FIGURE 29-18 Elastic bandages are available in a variety of widths.

PROCEDURE

83

APPLYING AN ELASTIC BANDAGE

1. Carry out initial procedure actions.

2. Assemble equipment:
   - Appropriate size bandage (check for cleanliness)
   - Tape, pins, or self-closures that come with bandage

3. Check the area to be bandaged.
   a. If there are lesions or signs of skin breakdown, report to the nurse before bandaging.
   b. If there are dressings underneath the bandage, the nurse may want to check them before you reapply the bandage.

   c. If an arm or leg is to be bandaged, elevate it for 15 to 30 minutes before application to promote venous blood flow.
   d. Apply the bandage so that two skin surfaces do not rub together (toes, fingers, under breasts and arms). Place cotton between the toes to prevent friction, if this is your facility policy.

4. Hold the bandage with the roll facing upward in one hand and the free end of the bandage in your other hand (Figure 29-19A).

continues

PROCEDURE 83 CONTINUED

a. Hold the roll close to the part being bandaged so that pressure is even.

b. When bandaging an extremity, always wrap from the distal (far) area to the proximal (near) area (Figure 29-19B).

c. Unroll the bandage as you wrap the body part. Never unroll the entire bandage at once.

5. Use appropriate bandaging technique (Figure 29-19C). Overlap each layer of bandage by one-half the width of the strip.

6. When finished rolling (Figure 29-19D), secure the bandage with pins, tape, or self-closures. Avoid using the clips that may come with the bandage, if possible. They tend to come loose and could

injure the patient's skin. The bandage should be smooth and wrinkle-free.

7. Check distal circulation just after the bandage has been applied and once or twice every 8 hours thereafter (check the skin under the bandage for color and temperature; note patient complaints of burning, tingling, or other discomfort).

8. Remove and reapply the bandage every shift, or more often if needed. The patient should have two bandages so that they can be laundered daily. Ask the nurse whether the bandage is to be worn continuously or only at specified times.

9. Carry out ending procedure actions.

A.	B.	C.	D.
Foot and ankle Use 3-inch width. Hold foot at right angle to leg. Start bandage on ridge of foot just back of the toes.	Pass bandage around foot from inside to outside. After two or three complete turns around foot, ascending toward the ankle on each turn, make a figure-eight turn by bringing bandage up	over the arch–to the inside of the ankle–around the ankle–down over the arch–and under the foot.	Repeat the figure-eight wrapping two to three times. Fasten end by pressing the last 4 to 6 inches of unstretched bandage to the preceding layer.

FIGURE 29-19A Bandage-wrapping technique (Courtesy Becton Dickinson, and Co., Rutherford, NJ)

Sequential Compression Therapy

Deep vein thrombosis and **pulmonary embolism** (blood clot in the lungs) are serious postoperative complications. Approximately 10% of all patients with DVT die from pulmonary embolism. Most have no symptoms until they develop the pulmonary embolus. The femoral vein, the large blood vessel in the groin, is particularly susceptible to clot formation. Because of the high risk and serious consequences associated with blood clots, the physician may order **sequential compression therapy** to reduce the risk. Sequential compression therapy massages the legs using a milking, wavelike motion.

Pneumatic hosiery (Figure 29-20) is also called *sequential compression hosiery*. This device prevents blood clots by massaging the legs mechanically. Pneumatic hosiery inflates and deflates rhythmically to produce a milking, wavelike massaging motion. The device should not be used on patients with lower leg ulcers, blood clots, massive edema, deformities, infected or broken skin, or arterial disease. Shiny, hairless skin is an indication of arterial

FIGURE 29-20 Pneumatic compression hosiery are used to prevent blood clots.

problems. If you observe any hard nodules, red areas, or warm areas on the patient's lower legs, inform the nurse before applying the hosiery.

Measuring and Connecting the Hosiery.
Before beginning this procedure, you must determine the proper size hosiery for the patient. Do this by measuring the circumference of the patient's upper thigh with a tape measure when she is in bed. Hold the measure snugly against the leg and note the circumference. Compare the measurement with the sizing chart, and select the proper size hosiery.

Familiarize yourself with the hosiery and compression controller if you have not used them before. Open the package and lay the hose on a flat surface. Open them completely, with the cotton lining facing up. Inside you will notice markings for the ankle and knee. When you apply the garment to the patient's leg, line it up exactly with these landmarks. Next, familiarize yourself with the compression controller. The device may have a cooling adjustment. This is used to cool the patient. It is turned off during routine use. Follow your facility policy and the nurse's instructions for activating this feature. The controller also has arrows to adjust the pressure inside the hose. It should be set at 35 mm Hg to 55 mm Hg. The unit may automatically set at 45 mm Hg, the midway point. The nurse will set the unit or instruct you on the setting to use.

Both hosiery must be connected to the controller for the unit to operate. Position the arrows on the hose opposite the arrows on the tubing. Push the ends together firmly until you hear a clicking sound. If the patient will be using only one sleeve, such as when she has a cast on one leg, leave the unused sleeve in the sealed plastic bag. Cut a small hole in the bag and connect the tubing.

Applying Pneumatic Hosiery. Before applying the hosiery, palpate the pedal (Figure 29-21A) and posterior tibial pulses (Figure 29-21B). In most facilities, staff mark the location of these pulses with a marker, making a small "X" on the patient's skin. Compare the movement, sensation, and color in both feet. If abnormalities are noted, consult the nurse before continuing. The nurse will assess the patient's legs and check for contraindications. Follow the nurse's instructions.

Pneumatic hosiery may be applied over anti-embolism hose, but both the sleeves and the anti-embolism hose must be smooth and wrinkle-free to reduce the risk of skin breakdown. The device is used 24 hours a day, when the patient is lying down, until the patient is completely ambulatory. It may be removed for bathing and ambulation, then reapplied immediately. The nurse may instruct the patient to perform certain leg exercises while the device is being used.

Caring for the Patient with Pneumatic Hosiery. The compression controller has a visual display that notes which chamber is inflated. When the chambers decompress, the unit will say "vent." Make sure the audible alarm is turned on, and check that the key has

FIGURE 29-21A The pedal (dorsalis pedis) pulse

FIGURE 29-21B The posterior tibial pulse

been removed. If the alarm sounds, the panel will display a message code. A card in a slot in the top of the unit will display the numerical message code with the nature of the problem. Follow the directions on the card to correct the problem, or notify the nurse, according to facility policy. The hose deflates automatically when the alarm sounds.

Turn the power off and remove the hose every 4 hours. Disconnect the sleeves from the tubing by releasing the latches on each side of the connectors, then pulling the connectors apart. Observe the skin under the device, and provide skin care as ordered. Avoid massaging the legs. Massage may dislodge a blood clot, which will quickly migrate to the lungs. Inform the nurse when you will be removing the device so that he or she can assess the patient's legs.

Use of the hose will be discontinued when the patient is fully ambulatory. The unit is not disposable. Clean and store the device according to facility policy after use, or return it to central supply.

PROCEDURE

84

APPLYING PNEUMATIC COMPRESSION HOSIERY

1. Carry out initial procedure actions.

2. Assemble equipment:
   - Hosiery of proper size
   - Compression controller

3. Open the hose, laying them flat on the bed with the markings opposite the knee and ankle.

4. Lift the patient's leg and slide the hose under it. Begin on the side of the leg opposite the plastic tubing. Wrap the sleeve smoothly around the leg with the opening in front, over the knee. Make sure there are no dents, folds, or creases in the garment.

5. Beginning at the ankle, fasten the Velcro fasteners securely. Next, secure the ankle and calf, then the thigh.

6. Check the fit by inserting two fingers between the sleeve and the patient's leg. The fit should feel snug and secure, but not tight.

7. Wrap the other leg in the same manner, beginning on the side opposite the plastic tubing. After wrapping the leg, check the fit.

8. Attach the plastic tubing on each leg to the compression controller by lining up the arrows on the tubing.

9. Plug the controller in and turn on the power.

10. Remain with the patient for one complete cycle (usually 60 to 90 seconds) to ensure that he tolerates the procedure.

11. Carry out ending procedure actions.

Documentation. Follow your facility policy for documenting use of the pneumatic compression device. You may be asked to document the procedure, pulse checks in the feet, skin color, the patient's response, and the settings, including use of the alarm and cooling settings.

Initial Ambulation

Some time after surgery, a patient is permitted to sit up with the legs over the edge of the bed. This position is called **dangling**.

- Watch carefully for signs of fatigue or dizziness (**vertigo**).

- Assist the patient to assume the position slowly.

The first **ambulation** (walk) is usually short. The patient usually dangles for a short time before ambulating. Dangling is an important part of postoperative care because it stimulates circulation and helps prevent the formation of blood clots (thrombi). (Refer to Procedure 85.)

The patient may need assistance the first few times he stands up to ambulate. The anesthesia and medications administered before, during, and after surgery may affect the patient's balance, endurance, and strength. There may be drainage tubes or an intravenous feeding that must be moved with the patient (Figure 29-22).

PROCEDURE

85

ASSISTING THE PATIENT TO DANGLE

1. Carry out initial procedure actions.

2. Assemble equipment:
   - Bath blanket
   - Pillow

3. Check the pulse.

4. Lower the side rail nearest to you. Lock the bed at the lowest position.

5. Drape the patient with a bath blanket and fanfold the top bedcovers to the foot of the bed.

6. Gradually elevate the head of the bed.

7. Help the patient to put on a bathrobe.

continues

PROCEDURE 85 CONTINUED

8. Place one arm around the patient's shoulders and the other arm under the knees.

9. Gently and slowly turn the patient toward you. Allow the patient's legs to hang over the side of the bed.

10. Roll a pillow and tuck it firmly against the patient's back for support.

11. After putting slippers on the patient, ask the patient to swing the legs.

12. Have the patient dangle as long as ordered.
    - If the patient becomes dizzy or faint, help him lie down.
    - Report to the supervising nurse immediately.

13. Check the patient's pulse.

14. Rearrange the pillow at the head of the bed. Remove the patient's bathrobe and slippers.

15. Place one arm around the patient's shoulders and the other arm under the knees. Gently and slowly swing the patient's legs onto the bed.

16. Check the patient's pulse. Lower the head of the bed and raise the side rails.

17. Carry out ending procedure actions. Remember to wash your hands, report completion of your task, and document the time dangled (duration), pulse, and the patient's reaction.

Safety ALERT

Remain next to the patient during the first dangling and ambulation. For patient safety, do not turn your back or leave the bedside. These precautions will probably not be necessary as the patient recovers and gains strength. Use common sense and follow the care plan and the nurse's instructions. ∎

FIGURE 29-22 Drainage tubes and IV lines may be in place after surgery. Carefully move these with the patient.

GUIDELINES *for*

Assisting the Patient in Initial Ambulation

- Check with the nurse to see if a transfer belt can be used.
- Assist the patient to sit on the edge of the bed with the bed in low position.
- Assist the patient to put on footwear appropriate to the floor surface. Never allow a patient to ambulate with bare feet or socks.

- Take the patient's pulse before and after standing. If there is more than 10 points difference, return the patient to bed and inform the nurse.
- If the patient becomes dizzy or faint, return the patient to bed and inform the nurse.
- Walk with the patient as instructed in Unit 17.

REVIEW

A. True/False.

Mark the following true or false by circling T or F.

1. T F Patients receiving local anesthetics lose consciousness during the surgery.

2. T F When spinal anesthetics are used, patients may lose feeling and movement in their legs.

3. T F Preoperative teaching has little effect on the patient's postoperative recovery.

4. T F You help build patient confidence when you explain what you plan to do when carrying out procedures.

5. T F Skin preparation involves shaving an area larger than the size of the incision.

6. T F The nursing assistant has no responsibilities related to the patient while the patient is in surgery.

7. T F Patients should be dangled without incident before initial ambulation.

8. T F Patients who are unconscious following surgery should not be left alone.

9. T F Nosocomial infections do not affect the cost or length of hospital stay.

10. T F Patients who are faced with surgery are often filled with apprehension and fears.

B. Matching.

Choose the correct word or phrase from Column II to match each item in Column I.

Column I

11. _____ inflammation of a vein leading to clot formation

12. _____ period before surgery

13. _____ medicine given to prevent pain

14. _____ hospital-acquired

15. _____ opening

16. _____ walking

17. _____ dizziness

18. _____ loss of lung volume; inability to expand lung fully

19. _____ blood clot

20. _____ area where immediate postoperative care is given

Column II

a. ambulation

b. orifice

c. nosocomial

d. PACU

e. umbilicus

f. vertigo

g. anesthesia

h. preoperative

i. aspiration

j. embolism

k. atelectasis

l. thrombophlebitis

C. Multiple Choice.

Select the one best answer for each of the following.

21. When assisting a patient with coughing and deep breathing exercises, teach him or her to
    a. inhale through the nose.
    b. inhale through the mouth.
    c. exhale through the nose.
    d. keep the hands behind the neck to expand the lungs fully.

22. The main purpose of coughing and deep breathing exercises is to prevent
    a. pneumonia.
    b. dizziness.
    c. pain.
    d. anxiety.

23. The main purpose of pneumatic compression hosiery is to prevent
    a. edema.
    b. pneumonia.
    c. blood clots.
    d. pain.

24. Pneumatic compression hosiery are contraindicated
    a. in patients who have had abdominal surgery.
    b. if the patient is using oxygen.
    c. if a rash or open areas are present.
    d. for patients with a cast on one leg.

25. Check the postoperative patient's vital signs every

    a. 5 minutes for the first hour, then every 15 minutes for 4 hours.

    b. 15 minutes for an hour, then every 30 minutes for an hour.

    c. 30 minutes for 4 hours, then every 8 hours for 72 hours.

    d. 60 minutes for 4 hours, then every 4 hours for 16 hours.

D. Nursing Assistant Challenge.

Mr. Dovetski is a 47-year-old patient on the surgical unit. He has had abdominal surgery. When he is returned to his room from surgery, you note that he has a Foley catheter, an intravenous feeding running, dressings on the abdominal incision, and elastic stockings. Think about what procedures you will include in your care of Mr. Dovetski.

26. How often will you take his vital signs? Which procedures are included in vital signs? What are the "normal" ranges for each vital sign for a person of this age? If there are changes in the vital signs, these changes may be indications of what complications?

27. What observations will you make regarding the Foley catheter? Why do you think he has the catheter in place?

28. What observations will you make regarding the intravenous feeding? Why do you think the physician ordered an IV?

29. You know you will need to have Mr. Dovetski perform deep breathing exercises and deep coughing. Why is this important? How can you help him do the exercises with the least discomfort?

30. Why do you think he has elastic stockings on? How often should you take the stockings off and reapply them? What do you need to remember when putting the stockings back on?

31. How will you report any complaints of pain?

32. How will you check for bleeding from the incision?

Caring for the Emotionally Stressed Patient

OBJECTIVES

After completing this unit, you will be able to:

- Spell and define terms.
- Define mental health.
- Define anxiety disorder, affective disorder, eating disorder, and substance abuse and give examples of each.
- Explain the interrelatedness of physical and mental health.
- Understand mental health as a process of adaptations.
- Identify commonly used defense mechanisms.

- Describe ways to help patients cope with stressful situations.
- Identify the signs and symptoms of maladaptive behaviors that should be documented and reported.
- List nursing assistant measures in providing care for patients with adaptive and maladaptive reactions.
- Identify professional boundaries in relationships with patients and families.

VOCABULARY

Learn the meaning and the correct spelling of the following words and phrases:

adaptation	coping	obsession	repression
affective disorders	defense mechanisms	obsessive-compulsive	schizoaffective disorder
agitation	delirium tremens (DTs)	disorder (OCD)	seasonal affective disor-
alcoholism	delusions	panic disorder	der (SAD)
anorexia nervosa	denial	paranoia	stressors
anxiety	depression	phobia	substance abuse
anxiety disorder	disorientation	posttraumatic stress dis-	suicide
bipolar affective disorder	eating disorders	order (PTSD)	suicide precautions
borderline personality	enabling	professional boundaries	suppression
disorder (BPD)	hypochondriasis	projection	
bulimia nervosa	maladaptive behavior	reaction formation	
compulsion	mental illness	reality orientation	

INTRODUCTION

There are varying degrees and differing aspects of health. A person who is in poor physical health may be mentally healthy. Because of good mental health, the person may be self-reliant, able to make decisions and to live an effective, productive life (Figure 30-1).

In contrast, a person with good physical health may not be able to cope with and adapt to changes. This inability limits the person's chances to participate successfully in society.

FIGURE 30-1 A mentally healthy person leads a productive life.

MENTAL HEALTH

Mental health means exhibiting behaviors that reflect a person's **adaptation** or adjustment to the multiple stresses of life, such as:

- Illness
- Hospitalization
- Loss of a loved one
- Loss of a job
- Loss of status

Stresses or **stressors** are situations, feelings, or conditions that cause a person to be anxious about his or her physical or emotional well-being. Good mental health leads to positive adaptations. Poor mental health is demonstrated by maladaptive behaviors (behaviors that harm the person or her adjustment).

Physical and mental health are interrelated. Physical illness is often preceded by stressful life situations. Ill health causes emotional stress. It is easy to understand that each of these factors contributes to the total health pattern of each person.

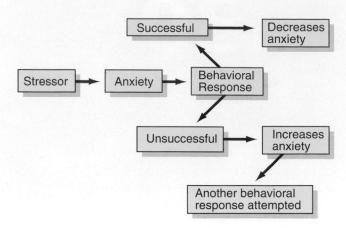

FIGURE 30-2 Each individual has ways of coping with stress.

Ways of **coping** with (handling) stressful situations (Figure 30-2) are learned early in life. As people grow, they find the behaviors that work best for them. They learn to use those behaviors to reduce stress and protect self-esteem. These coping patterns become part of the individual's habitual responses, becoming more and more obvious as the person ages.

ANXIETY DISORDERS

Anxiety is fear, apprehension, or a sense of impending danger. It is often marked by vague physical symptoms, such as tension, restlessness, and rapid heart rate. An **anxiety disorder** is one of a group of recognized mental illnesses involving anxiety reactions in response to stress. These include:

- Generalized anxiety (the most common condition)
- Panic disorder, in which a person has panic attacks
- Obsessive-compulsive disorder
- Posttraumatic stress disorder, which is most common in combat veterans or survivors of major trauma
- Phobias, which include various fears, such as fear of snakes, spiders, crowds, or other things

Agitation

Agitation is defined as inappropriate verbal, vocal, or motor activity due to causes other than disorientation or real need. It includes behavior such as:

- Aimless wandering
- Pacing
- Cursing
- Screaming
- Repeatedly asking the same question
- Spitting
- Biting
- Fighting or arguing constantly

- Demanding attention
- Restlessness
- Constant activity

Agitation is a significant problem for the elderly, their families, and the nursing staff. It is one of the foremost management problems in acute care hospitals, in home care, and in long-term care facilities.

The major factors contributing to agitation are:

- Noise
- Frustration at loss of control (Figure 30-3)
- Feelings that one's space has been invaded
- Loneliness and need for attention
- Boredom
- Depression
- Restraints
- Too much sensory stimulation

Study this list carefully, because your awareness can lead to early intervention. Early intervention can often prevent serious problems.

Panic Disorder

Panic disorder is characterized by unexpected, chronic *panic attacks*. These are bouts of overwhelming fear. The person usually feels that he is in danger, but has no specific cause or basis for the fear. The person may be so fearful that he is unable to function. Panic attacks tend to recur. Between attacks, the person may worry about when and where the next attack will occur.

Obsessive-Compulsive Disorder

Obsessive-compulsive disorder (OCD) is an anxiety disorder in which the patient has recurrent obsessions, fre-

FIGURE 30-3 This patient is very frustrated because she feels as if she is powerless and lacks control over her life.

quent thoughts, ideas, impulses, or compulsions. It results in repeated ritualistic activity over which the person has no control. He derives no pleasure from the ritualistic behavior. An **obsession** is a frequent idea, impulse, or thought that is usually unrelated to current conditions and does not make sense. However, the person cannot suppress or eliminate it. He usually has a sense of urgency to act on this thought. Resisting causes increased stress. A **compulsion** is a purposeful, repetitive behavior that is done many times each day and that is problematic enough to cause distress, be time-consuming, or interfere with the person's normal routine, occupation, social activities, or relationships. Examples of ritualistic behavior

GUIDELINES *for*

Managing the Patient Who Is Anxious or Agitated

- Do not argue with or confront the person.
- Make the environment safe (secure the windows and lock the doors, as appropriate).
- Make sure each patient wears an identification bracelet and that it is fastened securely.
- Keep a recent photo of the patient in case the patient wanders off.
- Notify the nurse promptly if the patient wanders away from his unit, facility, or home.
- Assign the patient brief tasks.
- Engage the patient in games, walks, swimming, and other activities. These should be activities that enhance the patient's self-esteem.

- Use bean-bag seats and rocking chairs in the nursing home or the patient's home.
- Care for the patient—watch for injuries.
- Engage the patient in conversations and in reality therapy or remotivation groups.
- Engage the patient in short-term activities. Realize that the patient's attention span is short. Thus, the patient needs rewards for short-term activities.
- Prevent the patient from becoming exhausted.
- Carefully monitor the patient's activities, because the agitated patient is at risk for falls and injuries.

caused by OCD is washing the hands many times each day for no reason, hoarding items, cleaning over and over, checking and rechecking something (such as ensuring that the stove is turned off or the door is locked), counting or sorting items, silently repeating words or phrases, or having many superstitions.

Posttraumatic Stress Disorder

Posttraumatic stress disorder (PTSD) is the development of unusual symptoms after a psychologically traumatic event. The person may relive the event, or have nightmares or flashbacks. He or she may have trouble with normal emotional responses or feel detached from others, feel anxious, and have difficulty sleeping, remembering, or concentrating. Persons with PTSD usually avoid anything that reminds them of the traumatic event, even though they may not remember everything that happened. The onset of symptoms may be delayed for months to years after the event.

Phobias

A **phobia** is an unfounded, recurring fear that causes the person to feel panic. The person with a phobia usually fears an object, insect, activity, or situation. The phobia is most often expressed as an unreasonable fear. The affected person regards the subject of the phobia in various ways, such as dislike, fear, hatred, disapproval, or hostility. The fear may be about an insect or pest, such as spiders or rats (Figure 30-4), or may be external, such as feeling afraid to leave home or being afraid to ride on a train or airplane. Reaction to the phobia can range from feeling dread to terror, or having outright panic that may include shaking or crying. Phobias can range in severity from being mildly annoying to severely disabling.

FIGURE 30-4 Patients with phobias have unfounded fears, such as of having a rat enter the house. The sight of a domestic rat in a pet store may be enough to trigger feelings of anxiety and panic. (Courtesy of Centers for Disease Control and Prevention)

AFFECTIVE DISORDERS

Affective disorders are a group of mental disorders characterized by a disturbance in mood. They may also be called *mood disorders*, and are usually marked by a profound and persistent sadness. Depression is the most common of these disorders. Other common affective disorders include:

- Bipolar affective disorder
- Schizoaffective disorder
- Seasonal affective disorder (SAD)
- Borderline personality disorder

Bipolar Affective Disorder

Bipolar affective disorder may also be called *manic depression* or *bipolar depression*. It is a mood disorder in which the person has marked mood swings beyond what most people experience. Moods will swing from elation (also called *mania*) to severe depression (Figure 30-5). Some people have only a few episodes of mania and depression, but most have many cycles of depression or mania. This is a serious condition, but it can be treated with drugs and psychotherapy.

Schizoaffective Disorder

Schizoaffective disorder is believed to be a combination of schizophrenia and a mood disorder. It is a chronic, disabling mental illness. The person will have symptoms of schizophrenia, such as delusions, hallucinations, disorganized speech, and disorganized behavior, along with a period of time when he also has symptoms of major depression or a manic episode. This condition can be difficult to diagnose. The mood symptoms are usually more prominent and longer-lasting than those experienced in schizophrenia. However, delusions and hallucinations

FIGURE 30-5 Withdrawal is common when patients are depressed.

(which are normally not present in a mood disorder) must also be present for a diagnosis of schizoaffective disorder.

Seasonal Affective Disorder (SAD)

Seasonal affective disorder (SAD) is a depression that recurs each year at the same time, usually starting in fall or winter and ending in spring or early summer. The cause is not known, but it is believed to be related to lack of exposure to sunlight or abnormal melatonin levels. The most common symptoms are sleepiness, craving for carbohydrates, weight gain, irritability, difficulty in getting along with others, and heaviness in the arms and legs. Some doctors report that SAD can be successfully treated with light therapy.

Borderline Personality Disorder

Borderline personality disorder (BPD) is sometimes a controversial diagnosis. There has been much speculation about the cause. People with this condition usually feel very unstable. They are often impulsive, fear abandonment, and are prone to self-injurious behavior. Some mutilate themselves or attempt suicide. They often feel empty or bored, and can be very manipulative of family, friends, and health care workers. They have difficulty maintaining stable relationships. Although their moods are often inconsistent, these people are never neutral. They usually have concrete opinions, difficulty with emotional reasoning, disrupted relationships, and difficulty functioning in a way that society accepts as normal.

Depression

Depression is the most common functional disorder in older people, but younger people also may experience depression (Figures 30-6 and 30-7).

Note: Figures 30-6 and 30-7 were a gift to the author. They were drawn by a severely depressed patient who chronicled her feelings through her art. Each caption reflects her feelings at the time the picture was drawn.

Depression may be shown in a variety of ways:

- Preoccupation
- Secretiveness
- Limited conversation
- Crying spells

FIGURE 30-6 It is so lonely here. I struggle to communicate but there are no words for what I feel. I withdraw further and feel that I am being watched. I know that they laugh at my plight.

FIGURE 30-7 Depression's cave. It smothers me with thoughts of death, of futility. I feel so low and imagine that everyone thinks that it is all I deserve. Their looks are heavy and weigh me down. Which side of me do they judge or can they see all of me? Do they know how weak I am? Do they laugh at my inability to cope with life? I, also, have judged myself . . . it is the verdict which weighs me down.

- Trouble sleeping (insomnia)
- Excessive sleep
- Loss of appetite or increased appetite
- Significant weight loss or weight gain
- Fatigue
- Headaches
- Apathy
- Impaired concentration
- Lethargy
- Agitation
- Poor personal hygiene
- Feeling of dejection

- Less interest in sex
- Depressed mood most of the day, nearly every day (irritability in children)
- Markedly diminished interest or pleasure in almost all activities, most of the day and nearly every day
- Psychomotor agitation or retardation
- Feelings of worthlessness or guilt
- Recurrent thoughts of death or suicide

Depression is often masked by symptoms that make it seem as though the patient is physically ill. Your observations are doubly important because a patient who is depressed may actually have minor or major illnesses. These infirmities may in turn cause depression. Remember, physical and mental health are interrelated. Also, some drugs that are used to treat actual physical illness in the elderly may cause depression.

Severely depressed patients may be treated with:

- Antidepressants
- Electroshock therapy (in severe cases)
- Talk therapy

A mental health clinical nurse specialist, psychologist, or psychiatrist will direct and support the staff efforts.

When depression is severe, suicidal thoughts and attempts are a real possibility. You must be sensitive to the possibility of such a situation and report and document your observations. The suicidal patient must be carefully protected. Watch for and report:

- Change in response such as deepening depression or sudden elevation of mood
- Evidence of withdrawal or secretiveness
- Sudden loss of a support system (such as the death of a family member)
- Repeated, prolonged, or sporadic refusal of food (oral or through gastric tubes), care, medications, or fluids
- Hoarding of medication (stockpiling of pills)
- Sudden decision to donate body parts to a medical school
- Changes in behavior, especially episodes of depression, screaming, hitting, throwing things, or a sudden failure to get along with family, friends, or peers
- Sudden interest or disinterest in religion
- Purchase of a gun
- Purchase of razor blades and hiding them

- Statements such as: "I just want out," "I want to end it all," "I'll never get well," "I'm going to kill myself," or "You would be better off without me."
- Increased use of alcohol and drugs
- Anger, hostility, belligerence, loss of interest, or inability to concentrate
- Inability to do simple tasks, confusion, slurred speech, or retarded motor skills
- Deep preoccupation with something that cannot be explained

Nursing Care of a Patient with the Potential for Suicide. Never assume that a suicide attempt is a means of getting the attention of staff or family. At least 15% of people who try to commit suicide do it again. Keep in mind the at-risk individuals. These include:

- White males over the age of 65 who live alone
- The very old (75 years and above)
- Persons with a recent diagnosis of a terminal illness
- Persons with unrelieved chronic pain
- Those suffering the sudden loss of a spouse
- The elderly with recent multiple losses

Be aware that the suicide rate is higher in acute medical units than it is on psychiatric units. Most of the suicides occur while the patient is under the supervision of a health provider, who frequently either misses or ignores the clues to suicide. Suicide attempts may occur either when the patient is successfully recovering or is getting worse. It is the responsibility of all staff members to observe patients carefully and immediately report any signs of depression and/or suicide. You should:

GUIDELINES *for*

Assisting the Patient Who Is Depressed

- Reinforce the person's self-concept by emphasizing her continued value to society and helping the patient to use the support systems that are available.
- Do not act in a pitying way. This only validates the person's depressed feelings.
- Make sure physical supports, such as eyeglasses and hearing aids, are in place. These help the person to focus on reality.
- Report all complaints so that actual physical problems may be identified and corrected rather than being attributed to the depression.
- Provide the person with activities within her limitations to help her think beyond herself. For exam-

ple, engage the person in some meaningful activity such as reading, making puzzles, or conversing with others.
- Avoid tiring activities.
- Use simple language and speak slowly when giving instructions.
- Monitor elimination carefully; constipation is common.
- Provide fluids frequently, because the depressed patient may be too preoccupied to drink.
- Be alert to the potential for **suicide** (the taking of one's own life).

- Implement **suicide precautions** according to your facility policies and procedures. These are checks and practices a facility follows if a patient states that she no longer wishes to live and intends to harm herself. In some situations, this may involve modifying the physical environment and securing the assistance of mental health professionals. The facility maintains these procedures until the patient is discharged or believed to be out of danger.
- Be observant for clues to suicide attempts, and report them to the appropriate person.
- Be consistent in approaches and care.
- Encourage the patient to review his life, emphasizing the positive aspects.
- Give the patient hope while being realistic (Figure 30-8).
- Work to restore the person's self-esteem, self-worth, and self-respect, to preserve positive self-concept.
- Help the patient find a support network within the family, religious groups, and self-help groups.
- Make the person feel accepted as a unique, valued person.
- Never ignore the person's statements or threats about suicide.

Hypochondriasis

The patient suffering from **hypochondriasis** imagines or magnifies each physical ailment. Some authorities feel that hypochondriasis is an expression of depression and is one way these individuals reduce stress. These patients need reassurance and understanding but should not be encouraged to focus on or believe in their supposed illnesses. However, the staff must be careful not to overlook real illness when it occurs, just because they have become used to hearing the patient complain. Nursing assistants should report all complaints and never make a judgment that a patient is a hypochondriac.

FIGURE 30-8 Be helpful but realistic with a depressed person who is at risk of suicide.

Paranoia

Paranoia is another extreme maladaptive response to stress. It is characterized by a heightened, false sense of self-importance and delusions of being persecuted. **Delusions** are false beliefs about oneself, other people, and events. People with paranoia believe that everyone is against them. When treating the paranoid patient, you should:

- Find ways to reduce the patient's feelings of insecurity and misunderstanding
- Keep the person as involved as possible in reality activities
- Report and document observed responses to medication and psychotherapy
- Monitor nutrition and fluid balance—these patients often refuse to eat or drink for fear of poisoning
- Observe sleep patterns—the person may be fearful of being harmed while sleeping
- Be direct and honest in all interactions
- Not support any misconceptions or delusions that the person exhibits
- Never argue with anyone who has delusions, it can trigger a serious confrontation

EATING DISORDERS

Eating disorders are a group of disorders characterized by disturbances in appetite or food intake. The two most common eating disorders are **anorexia nervosa** and **bulimia nervosa**. Anorexia is an eating disorder in which the patient has a disturbed body image. Despite appearing skeletal, he or she views the body as being fat. The patient cannot maintain even a minimal body weight. He or she is so fearful of obesity that the person limits food intake through diet, exercise, purging, and taking laxatives and diuretics. Sufferers are typically more than 15% below the average weight for their height, sex, and age. Over time, females stop having menstrual periods. Males lose interest in sex.

Patients with bulimia usually binge-eat huge amounts, then vomit (*purge*) to undo the binge. The binge eating causes feelings of guilt, depression, and self-condemnation. People with bulimia also use laxatives, diuretics, and vigorous exercise to lose weight. To be diagnosed with bulimia, a person must show this behavior at least twice a week for three months in a row.

Symptoms of eating disorders often overlap and may be difficult to identify. Bulimia and anorexia are common in patients with borderline personality disorder. Most people with an eating disorder are very secretive about it. Even family members may be unaware of the condition until weight loss is so profound that it cannot be ignored. Serious medical problems can occur, as well as depression, moodiness, and low self-esteem. The electrolyte imbalance and starvation caused by these conditions can lead to death.

SUBSTANCE ABUSE

Substance abuse is a disorder characterized by the use of one or more substances (such as alcohol or drugs) that alter mood or behavior, resulting in impairment. Increased substance use often causes impaired (bad) judgment. Use of the substance(s) results in a maladaptive pattern of behavior that strains finances, causes irresponsibility, and makes the user unable to fulfill social or occupational obligations. The substance abuser often uses when it is dangerous or illegal to do so. Drug abuse can be by use of illegal (street) drugs or misuse of prescription drugs without proper physician knowledge or oversight. Drugs of abuse (Figure 30-9A) are swallowed, inhaled, injected, or smoked (Figure 30-9B). Some definitions of substance abuse also include use of anabolic steroids (body building drugs), tobacco, and overeating, but the discussion in this book is confined to alcohol and drug use. Although narcotic pain medications can be abused, these are also not discussed here, as they pertain to acute and chronic pain management under physician supervision. Marijuana is discussed only as it applies to nontherapeutic use.

Drug Abuse

Many individual drugs can be abused. Abusers may use a single drug or combination of drugs.

FIGURE 30-9A Methamphetamine (meth) in powder form, wrapped in foil (Courtesy of U.S. Drug Enforcement Administration)

FIGURE 30-9B A pipe for smoking methamphetamine (Courtesy of U.S. Drug Enforcement Administration)

ALCOHOLISM

Some people use alcohol as a means of coping with stress. The National Institute for Alcohol Abuse reports that two-thirds of the senior population uses alcohol. Fifteen percent of them become alcoholics. **Alcoholism** is regarded as a disease.

Alcohol slows down brain activity. It impairs mental alertness, judgment, physical coordination, and reaction time—increasing the risk of falls and accidents.

Alcohol can affect the body in unusual ways. It can make it difficult to diagnose diseases and conditions of the cardiovascular system. It can mask pain that might otherwise serve as a warning sign of heart attack.

Alcohol is a drug. It mixes unfavorably with many other drugs (Table 30-1). The use of alcohol can cause some drugs to metabolize more rapidly, producing exaggerated responses.

Patients who are withdrawing from alcohol may have **delirium tremens (DTs)**. DTs are part of a serious withdrawal syndrome seen in persons who stop drinking alcohol

TABLE 30-1 COMMON ALCOHOL–DRUG INTERACTIONS

Drug Taken by Patient	Effects to Report
Narcotics	Increased central nervous system (CNS) depression with acute intoxication
Salicylates	Gastrointestinal bleeding
Sedatives and psychotropic drugs	Increased CNS depression with acute intoxication
Barbiturates	Decreased sedative effect after chronic alcohol abuse
Chloral hydrate	Prolonged hypnotic effects
Chlordiazepoxide (Librium, Librax)	Increased CNS depression
Chlorpromazine (Thorazine)	Increased CNS depression
Diazepam (Valium)	Increased CNS depression
Oxazepam (Serax)	Increased CNS depression
Antihistamines	Increased CNS depression
Antabuse	Flushing, vomiting, excessive sweating, hyperventilation, confusion, and drowsiness

following continuous and heavy consumption. The DTs commonly begin 48 to 96 hours after the person takes the last drink. Signs and symptoms of DTs are:

- Severe confusion
- Tremors
- Hallucinations
- Overactivity of the nervous system
- Seizures

DTs can become life-threatening, and require immediate treatment.

The alcoholic in withdrawal feels depressed and defensive. He needs to identify the stressors that bring on his need for alcohol and to find new ways of coping. This process takes professional skill, but you can:

- Not allow the alcoholic to manipulate you
- Listen with empathy (Figure 30-10)
- Reflect the person's ideas and thoughts
- Be sure alcohol is not available
- Be consistent in the limits that have been set

Care of the intoxicated patient includes:

- Caution during feeding to prevent choking or strangling
- Supervision of activities to prevent injury and falls
- Safety checks during bathing to prevent burns
- Close supervision if there is confusion or delirium

DEFENSE MECHANISMS

When any person feels unable to cope with stress and the situation threatens self-esteem, the person tends to act in protective ways. These ways are called **defense mechanisms**. A diagnosis of cancer, for instance, may be so overwhelming that a person must temporarily defend himself against acknowledging the truth. Everyone uses these defense-oriented behaviors from time to time to protect themselves. You use them. Patients use them. Your coworkers use them.

FIGURE 30-10
Listen with empathy. Try to understand how the patient is feeling.

You must recognize and understand the need to use defense mechanisms. Do not be critical of their occasional use. Most people do not use one mechanism all the time. They usually rely on a combination of defenses. They may not even be aware that they are behaving in a defensive way. Defensive behavior becomes harmful only when it is the major means of coping with stress. In such cases, the person continuously avoids recognizing and responding to reality with problem-solving methods. The person's stress is temporarily reduced, but the stressor (feeling or situation) is not resolved. Such a person needs counseling from a trained mental health provider.

Some of the commonly used defense mechanisms include:

- **Repression**—The involuntary exclusion from awareness of a painful or conflict-creating thought, memory, feeling, or impulse. For example, a woman has a lump in her breast, but refuses to go to a physician for examination and diagnosis. She has recently lost her husband, her house, and her job. She feels that she cannot "acknowledge" any other illness or crisis, so she unconsciously represses the knowledge of the lump in her breast. She is not going to take the chance that the lump may be cancer. She cannot face the possibility of a terminal disease.

- **Suppression**—This mechanism differs from repression because the person is aware of the unacceptable feelings and thoughts but deliberately refuses to acknowledge them. For example, a man becomes immobilized by the fear of rejection by his wife if he tells her he has a diagnosis of AIDS. Therefore, he consciously suppresses the knowledge of the AIDS diagnosis because he cannot handle the anxiety associated with telling his wife.

- **Projection**—A person's own unacceptable feelings and thoughts are attributed to others. The person blames others for his own shortcomings. For example, a person blames his wife or family for his alcoholism and loss of jobs. He projects his failings onto his wife and children.

- **Denial**—Blocking out painful or anxiety-producing events or feelings. This is one of the most common defenses against the stress of diagnosis and illness. For example, a patient with very high blood pressure refuses to stop smoking. She continues to eat a diet high in fats. She cannot deal with her fear of disability and unemployment, so she refuses to accept the seriousness of her condition.

- **Reaction formation**—A person using this defense mechanism represses the reality of a situation and then behaves in a manner that is the exact opposite of the real feelings. For example, a woman dislikes one nursing assistant but is fearful that if she expresses that feeling, the assistant will be less caring. This patient may be overly friendly and cooperative with that assistant.

Other adaptive behaviors include:

- Displacement—Substituting an object or person for another and behaving as if it were the original object or person. *Example:* Being angry with the nursing assistant because another patient is annoying.

- Identification—Behaving like another person whom one holds as an ideal. *Example:* Speaking to coworkers with the same tone the supervisor uses with you.
- Compensation—Excelling in one area to make up for feelings of failure in another. *Example:* The nursing assistant who overachieves in the skill area because her ability to read written directions is poor.
- Conversion—Offering a socially acceptable reason to avoid an unpleasant situation. *Example:* The nursing assistant who calls saying she cannot report for duty because she has the flu, when she is just tired from staying up too late.
- Fantasy—The use of imagination to solve problems. *Example:* The supervisor criticizes the nursing assistant, who then daydreams of a time when she is the head of nursing and can fire the supervisor.
- Undoing—A method of reversing something wrong that was done. *Example:* The person who used his hands to hurt another may wash his hands repeatedly to try to undo the deed.

ASSISTING PATIENTS TO COPE

Here are some ways to help patients become better able to cope and adapt:

- Be a good listener.
- Try to determine the source of stress so it can be removed and the stress reduced.
- Be sensitive to nonverbal messages (body language) that may give clues to the source of stress.
- Treat the person with respect, recognizing him as a unique individual.
- Understand the behavior in the same way the patient is viewing it, without labeling the behavior and passing judgment.
- Let the patient know that you are reliable and that you respect her privacy and feelings.
- Never argue, enter into a power struggle, or debate with a patient, even when you know the patient is wrong.
- Be supportive of the person's own attempts to overcome the stress (Figure 30-11).

Remember that illness, age, and separation from family and home are major stress factors.

THE DEMANDING PATIENT

In every nursing care situation, you will meet patients who are very demanding. This can be a difficult experience for everyone if it is not handled correctly.

FIGURE 30-11 Be supportive while the patient works through her problem.

Difficult SITUATIONS

Patients with coping and behavior problems usually have a behavior management care plan that lists steps to follow when certain problems are exhibited. Become familiar with the care plan. Implement the approaches in the order listed. Modify your behavior in response to the patient's behavior by monitoring how the patient responds to you, then adjusting your approach to achieve results. Vary routines and equipment, if necessary. Put yourself in the patient's shoes and try to understand what is happening. ■

Being demanding is another way in which patients show their frustration. It is a coping behavior. Patients who are very demanding are usually frustrated by their loss of control. To be successful in caring for these patients, the nursing assistant must:

- Try to learn and understand the factors that are causing the demanding behavior.
- Show that you care about the patient's situation, but keep control of your emotions.
- Maintain open communications by listening to the patient's words and by being sensitive to the patient's body language.
- Provide opportunities that allow the patient to regain some control by making choices.
- Be consistent in the manner of care. This builds the patient's sense of security.

- Do not take the patient's demands personally.
- Report observations to the nurse with suggestions for changes in the care plan.

MALADAPTIVE BEHAVIORS

Mental illness or **maladaptive behavior** occurs when behaviors and responses disrupt the person's ability to function smoothly within the family, environment, or community.

You must be careful about labeling anyone as mentally ill. Even when an official diagnosis of mental illness has been made, take care not to stereotype the patient.

Remember that stereotypes are often associated with *myths* (false beliefs). It is far better to view the person as an individual who is demonstrating poor behavioral responses.

As a nursing assistant, you need to be aware that sometimes signs and symptoms such as fatigue, loss of appetite, insomnia, and pain may reflect either physical or emotional stress. Note and report any unusual behavior or symptoms. Be careful, however, to be objective. Do not make judgments about your findings.

Remember also that confusion, disorientation, and aggressive behavior may only be temporary responses to a fever, drug interaction, or a full bladder. Continuation of such behavior may be the result of organic brain changes. Blaming and judging a patient is inappropriate and unhelpful.

Assessing the Patient's Behavior

An initial assessment of the patient's mental and emotional state will be made by the licensed care provider. Because you make frequent contact with the patient, you can make a valuable contribution to the nursing assessment process by making careful and sensitive objective observations.

Report observations regarding:

- Physical responses related to eating, personal hygiene, sleeping, participation in activities, or any strange or unusual behaviors
- Emotional responses related to interactions between the patient and yourself or between the patient and other patients, emotional outbursts, or inappropriate responses
- Patient behavior as it relates to judgment and affects memory, comprehension, and orientation

When working in long-term care, you will find many people whose coping ability has failed and so are demonstrating maladaptive behaviors. The many losses these people have suffered add to their inability to cope. Physical problems make dealing with reality more difficult.

Common maladaptive responses result in:

- Depression
- Disorientation or delirium
- Agitation
- Paranoia

Tips: Reward patients for positive behavior. Behavior that is rewarded is usually repeated. The goal is to show the patient a healthy way of directing energy. Verbal praise, positive feedback, and other signs of approval are rewards. Nonverbal rewards such as a hug, smile, or pat on the back may also be used, when appropriate. Snacks and privileges are sometimes used as rewards.

Disorientation (Disordered Consciousness)

Disorientation is a condition in which a person shows a lack of reality awareness with regard to time, person, or place (Figure 30-12). Disorientation may be mild or sometimes severe; sometimes temporary but at times prolonged. It is important to report patient behavior, actions, and responses. The disoriented person has impaired:

- Judgment
- Memory
- Comprehension
- Orientation

Physical ailments and stresses that can bring about a disoriented state (called *delirium*) include:

- Recovery from surgery
- Pneumonia
- Myocardial infarction
- Renal infection
- Head trauma
- Organic brain disease

FIGURE 30-12 Disorientation is lack of awareness of time, place, or person. The patient may be oriented in one sphere, such as who he is, but not know the day, date, or where he is.

- Fevers
- Dehydration
- Malnutrition
- Drug interaction

The signs and symptoms that identify the disoriented person are:

- Inability to think clearly
- Bewilderment
- Faulty memory
- Inability to follow directions
- Misinterpretation of stimuli
- Confusion about time
- Confusion about place
- Confusion about who he or she is

Nursing Assistant Responsibilities. The nursing assistant must realize that disoriented people cannot be responsible for their actions or for protecting themselves adequately. The patient's sensory misinterpretations (delusions or hallucinations) may put others at risk. The disorientation does not allow the patient to take action for self-protection. *Protection of the patient is the most important nursing responsibility.* In addition, you should:

- Be calm and gentle when approaching the patient. Disoriented patients are startled by even minor stimuli.
- Give instructions slowly, clearly, and in simple words.
- Give only one instruction at a time.
- Provide activities of short length that do not require much concentration.
- Build the patient's self-esteem with the reward of positive comments.
- Assist patients to participate in reality orientation activities (Figure 30-13). **Reality orientation** is making the disoriented patient aware of person, place, and time by visual reminders, activities, and verbal cues. See the guidelines for reality orientation activities.

FIGURE 30-13 Calendars, clocks, and current magazines and newspapers may help maintain orientation in some patients.

- Maintain a constant, limited routine.
- Use restraints only when absolutely necessary and only with a physician's order, making sure all safety practices are followed.
- Reduce disorientation by keeping rooms well lighted, cool, and quiet. Also, provide reality orientation according to the nursing care plan.
- Make sure patients wear glasses and hearing aids, if used.

To maintain a safe environment for disoriented patients:

- Keep all sharps, such as knives, out of reach.
- Remove and store valuable or breakable items. If the patient is at home, make sure the family knows where you put these items.
- Use sturdy chairs and couches.
- Put rails on windows that are close to the floor.
- Provide adequate lighting.
- Protect stairways with gates.
- Do not permit poisonous plants.
- Control matches and smoking materials.
- Supervise use of stoves and appliances.
- Keep all medications out of reach.

PROFESSIONAL BOUNDARIES

As a nursing assistant, you must stay within certain **professional boundaries** in the care of each patient. *Boundaries* are unspoken limits on the physical and emotional relationship with patients. They limit how a health care

GUIDELINES *for*

Reality Orientation

- Address the patient by name with each contact.
- Identify yourself to the patient at each contact.
- Avoid reinforcing illusions, delusions, or hallucinations.
- Keep glasses, dentures, and hearing aids in place.
- Speak often with the patient.
- Be patient and repeat instructions.
- Keep clock and calendar in view.
- Encourage the presence of and refer to familiar objects.
- Post an activity board and draw attention to it.
- Call attention to color-coding of facility areas.
- Introduce day, date, time, season, and weather into conversation.

worker acts with patients. They involve using your best behavior, ethical practices, and good judgment in patient care.

It takes good judgment and experience to identify boundaries and keep from crossing them. When driving down the road, you do not see the boundary lines when you cross from one city to the next. Professional boundaries are the same way. They exist, but you cannot see them. You must be aware of boundaries and take steps to avoid crossing them. You may cross them thinking that you are meeting a patient's need.

Being aware of boundaries is particularly important when caring for patients with emotional stress. Patients who are at risk of inappropriate relationships with health care workers usually have one or more of these risk factors:

- Mental or emotional problems
- Poor impulse control
- Marital problems
- Low self-esteem
- Loneliness and/or need for caring

Health care workers who are at greatest risk for inappropriate relationships and boundary problems usually have one or more of these risk factors:

- Family or marital problems
- Naïveté
- Low self-esteem
- Loneliness, feelings of isolation
- Addiction (chemical or sexual)
- Financial problems
- Stress, burnout

To avoid crossing boundaries, strive to act professionally, as you were taught in class. Avoid putting yourself in a position in which you think and act as a family member or friend. You must use good judgment and determine the amount of contact and assistance that are right for the patient. Too much or too little contact can be unhealthy for both the assistant and the patient. Treat all patients professionally. Consult the nurse if you are uncertain.

Ethical Behavior with Patients and Families

As a nursing assistant, patients expect you to act in their best interests and treat them with dignity. You do this by not taking advantage of a patient's situation and by avoiding inappropriate involvement in the patient's personal and family relationships. Some relationships with patients and families are not healthy for the patient or the nursing assistant. It is not always easy to recognize unhealthy relationships until it is too late. Once you have crossed over a boundary line, it is difficult to turn back. Strive to keep your relationships professional.

Actively work to find a balance in your relationships with patients and families. If any of the following occur, you are probably crossing professional boundaries and may be in a relationship danger zone:

- Discussing your personal problems with the patient or family members
- Being flirtatious with a patient, including making sexual innuendos, telling jokes that are sexual in nature, or using offensive language
- Discussing your feelings of sexual attraction with a patient
- Feeling that you may become involved in a sexual relationship with the patient
- Keeping secrets with a patient and becoming defensive when someone questions your relationship or involvement in the patient's personal life
- Thinking you are immune from having an unhealthy relationship with a patient
- Believing that you are the only nursing assistant who can meet the patient's needs
- Spending an inappropriate amount of time with the patient, including off-duty visits or trading assignments with others to be with the patient
- Reporting only partial information about the patient to the nurse, because you fear disclosing unfavorable information or secrets the patient has told you
- Feeling that you must protect the patient from other workers and always siding with the patient's position

Questions to ask yourself that will help you decide whether you are crossing a boundary line are listed in Table 30-2. If you have trouble staying objective, or think you may cross a boundary, seek help from the nurse, pastor, or another professional person whom you trust.

Consequences of Boundary Violations

Boundary violations lead to inappropriate relationships. These cloud your clinical judgment, and often carry over into your personal life. The improper relationship may cause you to do things that you would not ordinarily do (such as stealing from your employer). There are many serious personal, legal, and professional consequences to inappropriate relationships. For your own well-being, be aware that professional boundaries exist, and actively take steps to keep from crossing them.

Enabling

Enabling behavior is reacting to a patient in a manner that shields the person from experiencing the full impact or consequences of his or her actions or behavior. Enabling behavior differs from helping behavior in that it allows the person to be irresponsible. As a paraprofessional health care worker, the nursing assistant should be aware of enabling behavior and avoid it when caring for patients, particularly those with mental and emotional

TABLE 30-2 QUESTIONS TO ASK

- Is this in the patient's best interest?
- Whose needs are being served?
- Does this action benefit me rather than the patient?
- Will this affect the care I am delivering?
- Should I be concerned or consult with a colleague?
- How would the patient's family view this?
- How would I feel telling a colleague about this?
- Am I treating this patient differently from other patients?
- Does this patient mean something special to me?
- Am I taking advantage of the patient?
- Am I comfortable about documenting this in the medical record?
- Is this a violation of nursing assistant ethics?

problems. By learning and respecting professional boundaries, you will avoid helping others inappropriately. Likewise, you must learn to set limits for yourself and prevent patients from crossing into your own personal territory. Enabling behavior with patients creates dependency rather than moving the patient toward independence and good mental health. Methods of enabling patients that you should avoid include:

- Protecting the patient from the natural consequences of his or her behavior
- Keeping secrets about a patient's behavior from others
- Making excuses for a patient's behavior
- Taking steps to get a patient out of personal trouble
- Blaming others for the patient's behavior
- Seeing the patient's problems as a result of something else
- Giving money to patients
- Attempting to control patients' lives and activities
- Doing things for the patient that she should do herself

Strive to keep your behavior in the zone of helpfulness (Figure 30-14) to avoid crossing professional boundaries and enabling patients.

FIGURE 30-14 Keep your relationship with patients and families in the zone of helpfulness.

GUIDELINES *for*

Assisting Patients Who Have Behavior Problems

- Follow the care plan.
- Control your own responses and reactions.
- Be a good communicator.
- Avoid lying to the patient.
- Avoid making promises you cannot keep.
- Avoid discussing facility or staff problems with the patient. If the patient complains, inform the nurse or other appropriate person.
- Protect the safety of the patient and others.
- If the care plan tells you to respond to a specific behavior, apply the approaches when the behavior starts. Do not wait until the patient loses control.
- Use good communication and listening skills.

- Practice empathy.
- Attempt to learn the cause of the behavior. Communicate with other team members.
- Remove the cause (or trigger) of the behavior, if known.
- Let others know if you discover an approach that works.
- Modify your own behavior in response to the patient's behavior.
- Watch the patient's response to your approaches. Adjust your approach, equipment, routine, and other care, if necessary.

continues

GUIDELINES *continued*

- Discuss family, friends, or other pleasant information with patients. This provides a source of strength, comfort, and support.
- Meet the patient's physical needs.
- Give patients as much control as possible. Offer choices in care and routines. Encourage them to direct their own care.

- Be patient. Control your reaction to the patient. Make sure your body language does not send the wrong message.
- Be happy. Smile. Make sure your body language sends a positive message. Positive behavior is contagious.

REVIEW

A. True/False.

Mark the following true or false by circling T or F.

1. T F Mental health refers to the adaptations a person makes to the multiple stressors of life.

2. T F Stressors are the physical and emotional problems that a person encounters throughout life.

3. T F Defense mechanisms are used only by mentally unhealthy persons.

4. T F If you know that the patient is wrong about something she is saying, it is proper to debate the issue with the patient.

5. T F The best way to handle the demanding patient is by trying to determine the underlying factors causing the patient's distress.

6. T F Panic attacks are isolated events that seldom recur.

7. T F The use of alcohol impairs mental alertness, judgment, reaction time, and physical coordination.

8. T F It is dangerous for a person to drink alcohol when taking other medications.

9. T F Alcohol is a drug.

10. T F An intoxicated person could choke on food.

11. T F Alcoholics have a poor chance for recovery.

12. T F Maladaptive behaviors reflect the failure of usual defense mechanisms.

13. T F Depression is the least common of the functional disorders in older people.

14. T F Obsessive-compulsive disorder is an affective disorder.

15. T F The onset of symptoms in posttraumatic stress disorder may be delayed for months to years after the event.

16. T F Phobias are seldom serious or disabling.

17. T F Mania is a period of elation.

18. T F If a patient threatens suicide, you need not be concerned.

19. T F The white male who is over age 65 and living alone is at high risk for suicide.

20. T F It is the responsibility of only the licensed staff to guard against suicide attempts.

21. T F Suicides are attempted only by patients in psychiatric institutions.

22. T F The patient who is agitated may ask the same question repeatedly.

23. T F Agitation is a significant problem for the elderly, their families, and facility staff.

24. T F Paranoia is a maladaptive response that usually requires medication and psychotherapy.

25. T F Paranoid individuals believe that others are out to get them.

B. Matching.

Choose the correct word from Column II to match each phrase or statement in Column I.

Column I

26. _____ conscious refusal to recognize the reality of a situation

27. _____ shielding a patient from the consequences of behavior

28. _____ blocking out painful or anxiety-producing events or feelings

29. _____ involuntary exclusion of the awareness of reality

30. _____ lack of awareness of reality

31. _____ handling stressful situations

32. _____ attributing one's own failing to another

33. _____ invisible lines that define relationships with patients

Column II

a. repression

b. suppression

c. projection

d. denial

e. professional boundaries

f. enabling

g. coping

h. disorientation

C. Multiple Choice.

Select the one best answer for each of the following.

34. The patient tells you that her doctor says she has AIDS, but she knows that isn't possible. She most likely is using the defense mechanism of
    a. repression.
    b. displacement.
    c. projection.
    d. denial.

35. The best way to enhance the patient's capability to cope with an unpleasant situation that has developed with another patient is to
    a. tell him to ignore it.
    b. let him know he can talk to you safely.
    c. tell him everyone has problems, his aren't so important.
    d. suggest he discuss it with his clergyperson.

36. The patient who refuses to eat or drink because she is convinced that she is being poisoned is suffering from
    a. paranoia.
    b. depression.
    c. agitation.
    d. disorientation.

37. The patient is depressed. You can best help him by
    a. pitying him.
    b. keeping him from interacting with others.
    c. agreeing that he probably deserves the way he feels.
    d. stressing his continued value to society.

38. The best way to help the patient remain oriented to reality is to
    a. keep glasses in the bedside stand so they will not be broken.
    b. isolate the patient.
    c. place a clock and calendar nearby.
    d. explain things in detail.

39. The person holding a doll and acting as if it were a baby probably is experiencing
    a. repression.
    b. denial.
    c. projection.
    d. displacement.

40. Agitation may be demonstrated by
    a. talking a lot.
    b. boredom.
    c. smiling for no reason.
    d. repetitive questions.

41. Professional boundaries
    a. apply only to licensed nursing personnel.
    b. involve assisting patients with activities of daily living.
    c. are set out in the job description.
    d. are unspoken limits on relationships with patients.

42. Health care workers who are at risk of having inappropriate relationships with patients
    a. are usually friendly and happy.
    b. may have financial or marital problems.
    c. exercise regularly to relieve stress.
    d. occasionally drink alcoholic beverages.

43. Enabling behavior
    a. is used when caring for patients who require total care.
    b. involves orienting patients to person, place, and time.
    c. is used to help patients relieve stress.
    d. shields an individual from the consequences of his or her actions.

44. Conditions that are diagnosed as affective disorders include
    a. anxiety disorders.
    b. eating disorders.
    c. substance abuse disorders.
    d. mood disorders.

45. Purging behavior is
    a. self-induced vomiting.
    b. refusing to eat.
    c. exercising vigorously.
    d. a form of substance abuse.

46. Substance abusers use alcohol or drugs to
    a. relieve chronic pain.
    b. alter their mood, causing impairment.
    c. get back at family members.
    d. treat medical problems under physician supervision.

D. Nursing Assistant Challenge.

You are assigned to care for Mr. Simonson, who was recently diagnosed with diabetes. He is a top executive in a large corporation and has a wife and three adult children. He is learning how to administer his insulin, how to plan his diet, and how to test his blood sugar. He has been very quiet and keeps his eyes closed most of the time, although he is not sleeping. One day as you enter the room, he screams at you to get out and then picks up his water pitcher and throws it. Think about what you learned in this unit about human behavior as you consider these questions.

47. What examples of nonverbal communication is Mr. Simonson displaying?

48. Do you think he is using defense mechanisms to cope with his diagnosis? If so, which ones?

49. If Mr. Simonson displays this kind of behavior again, what would be an appropriate response from the nursing staff?

50. How would you document this episode?

51. How can the nursing staff show respect and concern for this patient?

UNIT 31

Caring for the Bariatric Patient

OBJECTIVES

After completing this unit, you will be able to:

- Spell and define terms.
- Define overweight, obesity, and morbid obesity, and explain how these conditions differ from each other.
- Explain why weight affects life span (longevity) and health.
- Define comorbidities and explain how they affect a person's health.
- Briefly state how obesity affects the cardiovascular and respiratory systems.
- Explain how stereotyping and discrimination affect persons with obesity.

- List some team members and their responsibilities in the care of the bariatric patient.
- Explain why environmental modifications are needed for bariatric patient care.
- Describe observations to make and methods of meeting bariatric patients' ADL needs.
- List precautions to take when moving and positioning bariatric patients.
- List at least five complications of immobility in bariatric patients.
- Describe nursing assistant responsibilities in the postoperative care of patients who have had bariatric surgery.

VOCABULARY

Learn the meaning and the correct spelling of the following words and phrases:

advocate	gastric bypass	morbid obesity	reflux
bariatric surgery	hyperventilation	obesity	stenosis
bariatrics	ideal body weight	overweight	stricture
body mass index (BMI)	minimally invasive	panniculus	trapeze
comorbidities	surgery	pannus	

INTRODUCTION

Being **overweight** (Figure 31-1) is a condition in which a person weighs more than he or she should, according to standards based on height and bone (frame) size. A person who is overweight has a body weight greater than is considered desirable or medically advisable.

The disease of obesity is very misunderstood. It is a complex condition with multiple causes. A popular myth is that obese people eat an enormous amount of food and

lack willpower. This is untrue. Genetics plays an important role in the distribution of body fat, metabolism, and regulation of the appetite. In fact, heredity may account for up to 70% of all weight problems. Some experts believe that the hormones used to fatten our meat supply are also affecting the humans who consume the meat. The definition of **obesity** varies, but it is usually considered being overweight by 20 to 30% of the ideal body weight. The varied definitions affect prevalence statistics and make it difficult to compare data. Environmental factors are also

Clinical Information ALERT

Obesity has become a serious, major health problem in the United States, accounting for thousands of deaths each year. Approximately 67% of adults in this country are overweight. About 31% are obese, and 1 in 20 is morbidly obese, according to the Centers for Disease Control and Prevention. Obesity is increasing very rapidly. It is believed that approximately 60 million adults are considered obese today; 9 million can be categorized as extremely or morbidly obese. In 2004, approximately 140,000 bariatric surgeries were done. This represents an increase of 125% in 2 years. ■

Age-Appropriate Care ALERT

Expressions such as "A fat baby is a healthy baby" are myths, with no basis in fact. The opposite is true. Childhood obesity is at epidemic proportions. In 2006, the *Journal of the American Medical Association* published an article noting that more than 12.5 million U.S. children and adolescents are overweight. The children are at risk for developing the same comorbidities as adults. Early nutrition and obesity prevention education are essential for families with young children. ■

FIGURE 31-1
Obesity is a very misunderstood condition, in which the person is 20 to 30% above ideal body weight. Heredity may account for up to 70% of all weight problems. (Courtesy of the Armed Forces Institute of Pathology)

very important. Obesity negatively affects every system of the body and increases patient risk for many other serious medical conditions and diseases. Untreated, it results in a shorter life span.

Obesity is a chronic condition that is a factor in 5 of the 10 leading causes of death. Besides the health risks, obese persons often experience emotional problems, including depression, low self-esteem, social isolation, and affective, anxiety, substance abuse, and eating disorders (see Unit 30). Experts believe that society's treatment of and response to obese persons increases their risk for emotional problems.

Persons with obesity experience discrimination and prejudice in social and employment situations. Activities of daily living are difficult. The obese person often has limited access to public facilities. It is not unusual for an obese person to experience difficulty in forming and maintaining personal relationships. Many are victims of physical and psychological abuse. When they are hospitalized, they know that their size makes it hard for staff to

care for them, and they may be admitted to your unit with feelings of shame, embarrassment, and fear.

Bariatrics is a relatively new field of medicine that focuses on the treatment and control of obesity and medical conditions and diseases associated with obesity. Bariatric patients have many highly specialized needs. Treatment may be medical, surgical, or both. Some hospitals and long-term care facilities have special bariatric treatment units. Others integrate bariatric patients into the general population. Regardless of the setting, as a nursing assistant you are likely to encounter bariatric patients, and must know how to care for them correctly.

Providing quality care for the bariatric patient presents many challenges and risks, both physical and emotional. Care that is routine for normal-size patients often cannot be done the same way for the bariatric population. This includes many activities of daily living (ADLs) and nursing assistant tasks, including bathing, transfers, mobility, and patient transport. Doing routine activities is often very difficult. Simple activities such as standing up, sitting down, and walking to the bathroom can be strenuous (Figure 31-2A) or painful (Figure 31-2B) for the patient. These patients share the challenges and frustrations of care with you. Certain aspects of care can be frustrating or humiliating for them. For example, the patient may not be able to put on shoes and socks. Many hospitals do not have scales to weigh patients who are more than 350 pounds. To obtain an accurate weight, some patients have been taken to the laundry, loading dock, or maintenance department, where a freight scale was available to weigh them. Think carefully about the patients' feelings before performing an action like this. Using a freight scale to weigh a patient is a tremendous assault on dignity and self-esteem.

WEIGHT AND BODY MASS INDEX

A person's **ideal body weight** is determined by a mathematical formula. Ideal weight is a concept developed from life insurance statistics related to life span (longevity) and health. The registered dietitian routinely calculates the ideal body weight (IBW) for each patient. The formula used takes the person's height, age, sex, build, activity, medical condition, and need for nutrients into consideration.

Body mass index (BMI) is also a consideration. The BMI is a mathematical calculation used to determine whether a person is at a healthy, normal weight, is overweight, or is obese. The BMI measures body weight relative to a person's height by dividing a person's weight (in kilograms) by his or her height (in meters, squared). Table 31-1 lists the BMI and categories of body mass. *Ideal weight* is considered as having a BMI that is less than 26. Obesity is a BMI of 30–39. **Morbid obesity** (Figure 31-3) usually qualifies for surgical treatment. Patients who are morbidly obese have a BMI of 40 or higher and are 100 pounds or more over their ideal body weight.

Calculating BMI

Conversion charts are available that make calculating BMI simple. However, using a chart as the sole indicator of weight or health status has limitations. The BMI measurement tool was designed for use by licensed health care providers who also consider many other factors. The BMI is only one part of the evaluation. People who are very muscular may fall into the overweight category when they are actually healthy and fit. People who have lost muscle mass, such as the elderly, may be in the BMI healthy-weight category, yet have nutritional deficiencies. Because of this, the BMI is considered a very general guideline to monitor trends in the population. It should not be used in isolation, and by itself is not diagnostic of an individual's health status. Further evaluation should be done by a licensed health care professional to determine each individual's weight category, comorbidities, and risk factors.

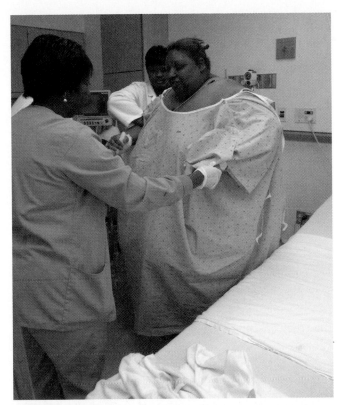

FIGURE 31-2A Many activities of daily living are difficult or painful for the patient.

FIGURE 31-2B The patient's large body is surrounding a normal-size frame. This causes wear on the musculoskeletal system and pain in the joints. Researchers theorize that each extra pound applies 4 to 5 pounds of pressure on the spine, making complaints of back pain common. Activities such as sitting in a chair can also be difficult and painful.

TABLE 31-1 CLASSIFICATION OF WEIGHT BODY MASS INDEX

BMI	Category
< 18.5	Underweight
18.5 to 24.9	Normal
25 to 26.9	Overweight
27 to 30	Mild obesity
31 to 35	Moderate obesity
36 to 40	Severe obesity
41 to 45	Morbid obesity
> 50	Super obesity

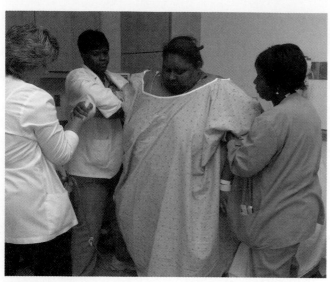

FIGURE 31-3 Patients who are morbidly obese qualify for bariatric surgery, but their medical problems must be stabilized first. Most have a BMI of 40 or higher and are 100 pounds or more over their ideal body weight.

Age-Appropriate Care ALERT

The rise in obesity has been rapid in children. Since 1971, the number of overweight children has more than doubled in the 6–11 age group. It has more than tripled for children ages 12–19. In the at-risk child population, 20% of all children ages 2–5 and 30% of children ages 6–19 are also at risk for being overweight and obese. Living with morbid obesity is extremely difficult for any individual, but especially so for children and adolescents. ■

Comorbidities

Being overweight or obese increases the risk for many health conditions, including chronic pain, arthritis and joint pain, sleep apnea, high cholesterol, hypertension, diabetes, heart disease, and stroke. These conditions are called comorbidities. **Comorbidities** are diseases and medical conditions that are either caused by or contributed to by morbid obesity. Comorbidities are listed and sorted by system in Table 31-2. Besides creating risk factors and medical management problems, comorbidities lower the weight threshold for surgical treatment. Medical problems are often compounded by mental health problems. Weight loss often improves or eliminates many comorbid conditions.

Some bariatric patients will be admitted for weight-loss surgery. They may also be admitted to your facility for management of complications of comorbidities. Because getting out of the house and to the hospital is very diffi-

Difficult SITUATIONS

The cardinal sign of sleep apnea is excessive daytime sleepiness. The patient may fall asleep at inappropriate times. Drowsiness interferes with the ability to concentrate and to perform complex tasks, such as operating machinery or driving. Other signs and symptoms include mood swings, personality changes, and irritability. If you observe patients with excessive sleepiness, snoring, or other signs of sleep apnea, inform the nurse, who will initiate screening for sleep apnea. ■

cult for these patients, they tend to wait a long time before going to the doctor or emergency room. Because of this, they are often very ill and unstable upon admission.

Patients with some comorbidities may need stabilization and management of comorbid conditions before bariatric surgery can safely be done. For example, patients may have severe sleep apnea, uncontrolled high blood pressure, or abnormally high blood sugar. The patient will be treated at home or admitted to the hospital with care targeted toward stabilizing the comorbid conditions, which will reduce the risk of perioperative complications. Once the comorbid conditions have been stabilized, weight-loss surgery will be done. Depending on the nature of the comorbid problem, this could take a long time. However, this initial management is essential to successful anesthesia and surgery, as well as stable postoperative recovery.

Malignancies. Persons with obesity are also at increased risk for cancer. Cancers believed to be related to obesity are:

- Breast cancer
- Colorectal cancer
- Endometrial cancer
- Gallbladder cancer
- Ovarian cancer
- Pancreatic cancer
- Prostate cancer
- Uterine cancer

EFFECTS OF OBESITY ON THE CARDIOVASCULAR AND RESPIRATORY SYSTEMS

Obesity places a great strain on the heart and lungs. The work of the heart is increased by the strain of supplying oxygenated blood to the tissues. Adipose (fat) tissue is poorly nourished and less resistant to injury than other tissues. Postoperatively, wound healing will depend on

TABLE 31-2 COMORBIDITIES RELATED TO OBESITY

Cardiovascular System	**Genitourinary System** *continued*
Atherosclerosis	Hirsutism
Congestive heart failure	Infertility
Hypertension	Polycystic ovarian disease
Varicose veins	Urinary stress incontinence
Venous insufficiency and stasis	Glomerulosclerosis and renal failure
Integumentary System	**Musculoskeletal System**
Cellulitis	Bone demineralization
Dermatitis	Carpal tunnel syndrome
Necrotizing skin infections	Low back pain
Panniculitis	Osteoarthritis
Endocrine System, Metabolic Disorders	**Neurological and Psychiatric Conditions**
Diabetes mellitus	Depression
Gout	Idiopathic intracranial hypertension
Hyperlipidemia	Stroke
Gastrointestinal System	**Ophthalmologic**
Abdominal wall hernia	Cataracts
Fatty liver	Glaucoma
Gallbladder disease	**Respiratory System**
Gastroesophageal reflux disease	Asthma
Irritable bowel syndrome	Obesity hypoventilation syndrome
Genitourinary System	Pulmonary hypertension
Dysmenorrhea	Sleep apnea

nutrients and oxygen, which are supplied by the circulatory system.

The respiratory system takes in oxygen and delivers it to body cells. Effective oxygen saturation of body parts depends on the volume of each ventilation, how well the oxygen is taken into the bloodstream, and how well saturated the blood is with oxygen when it moves through the system. Many obese patients hyperventilate because of the weight of the chest and the inability of the diaphragm to descend during inhalation. Normally, the descending

diaphragm provides space for the lungs to fill with air. In an obese person, the weight of the abdominal tissue prevents the diaphragm from descending fully. This inhibits chest expansion. **Hyperventilation** is breathing abnormally fast and deep, resulting in excessive amounts of oxygen in the lungs and reduced carbon dioxide levels in the bloodstream. The decrease in lung capacity and function results in inadequate oxygenation of the body and its tissues.

Wound healing is also affected by lack of oxygen. Some bariatric patients routinely use supplemental oxygen

(Unit 39). Others use BiPap and CPAP devices (Unit 39) for ventilatory assistance when in bed, because gravity plus the weight of the chest and abdomen further inhibit ventilation. Depending on the patient's size, a special mask may be needed. Monitor the fit of the mask when it is on the patient's face. If the mask is too tight, it may cause pain, redness, or skin breakdown on the nose. The patient may prefer to be in the semi-Fowler's position when the mask is being used. Wash the mask in soap and water each morning, or whenever the patient takes it off.

STEREOTYPING AND DISCRIMINATION

Being overweight brings many challenges. Overweight people often feel deep emotional pain caused by insensitivity and stereotyping by the public at large. Discrimination is a great obstacle for them. Making assumptions about others who are different from ourselves can be automatic, and assumptions about obese individuals are common. An online search using terms such as "fat" and "jokes" will bring up millions of hits. Negative comments and insensitive remarks are also common. Many people assume that overweight people lack self-discipline, overeat, and are unclean. These stereotypes are untrue. Finding flattering clothing that is affordable and fits correctly is difficult at best. As a health care worker, you must avoid passing judgment on patients. Be careful with remarks and body language that may be interpreted as insensitive, prejudicial, or discriminatory.

Bariatric patients may feel isolated or shunned by everyone. They may isolate themselves to protect against hurt

Difficult SITUATIONS

All patients have a right to considerate, respectful care. Patients do not choose to be overweight. Most bariatric surgery patients have tried every diet and exercise program available, without lasting success. The repeated diet failures negatively affect their self-esteem. These patients experience rejection and discrimination as part of everyday life. Imagine how that feels! Avoid passing judgment on patients because of their size and weight. Monitor your facial expressions and body language to avoid sending a negative message to the patient. Recognize that obesity is a chronic medical problem, like diabetes and other medical conditions. Always treat patients with consideration, dignity, and respect. ■

feelings. The care plan will list approaches to build trust and rapport with the patient. Show empathy. Try to put yourself in the patient's shoes and understand how he or she feels. Recognize that prejudices and stereotyping inflict great emotional pain. Be very compassionate in your dealings with these patients. If you regularly work with bariatric patients, your facility will provide classes on sensitivity, or you may wish to take a continuing education class on sensitivity training.

INTERDISCIPLINARY TEAM APPROACH TO CARE

A team effort is truly needed to provide care and ensure that bariatric patients' many needs are met. Here is an example of team members and their responsibilities for patients needing medical management or bariatric surgery:

- Licensed nurses—Assess the patient; plan, deliver, and supervise direct care; provide patient teaching
- Nursing assistants—Deliver direct personal care to meet the patient's ADL needs
- Social service and/or mental health workers—Care for emotional and psychosocial needs; coordinate services needed after discharge
- Pastoral workers—Care for spiritual and religious needs
- Attending physician and/or internal medicine specialist—Prescribes the medical plan of care
- Bariatric surgeon—Performs bariatric surgery, if planned for that patient
- Anesthesiologist—Delivers anesthesia; plans and supervises postoperative pain management
- Bariatric nurse (a nurse with additional education and experience in care of bariatric patients)—Oversees all nursing care and coordinates the care plan
- Infection control nurse—Addresses prevention and treatment of perioperative infection
- Wound, ostomy, and continence (WOC) nurse—Determines skin care plan for wound healing and prevention of new skin breakdown
- Respiratory therapist—Manages postoperative ventilation needs; cares for comorbid conditions, such as sleep apnea
- Dietitian—Writes dietary plan of care; supervises menu; addresses risk of malnutrition and dehydration and plans preventive care; provides patient teaching
- Physical therapist—Helps mobilize and exercise the patient
- Occupational therapist—Works to help the patient become independent in ADLs

Because the patient has so many special needs, other team members such as pharmacists and various physician specialists are also needed. Some facilities have additional specialists and advocates who work only with bariatric patients. An **advocate** is a person who speaks on behalf of the patient. A bariatrics advocate will have special knowledge and skill in this area of health care. Many of these workers have successfully been through bariatric surgery and massive weight loss themselves. They know better than anyone what it is like to walk in the patients' shoes. The advocate is responsible for looking at the patient as a whole to ensure that his or her needs are met. To be successful in treatment, the patient must also be a full partner in his or her own care. Those who are admitted for planned bariatric surgery often view the procedure with both fear and optimism. They often view this day as an important event, like a wedding anniversary; many consider it the first day of the rest of their lives.

Clinical Information ALERT

The care of medical and surgical bariatric patients differs in many ways from the care of adults with no weight problems. Avoid assuming that bariatric patients are just larger versions of the normal adult. Bariatric patients have many problems not seen in adults of normal weight, including internal fluid shifts and a change in the body's center of gravity. They have a higher risk of blood clots from immobility. Many have fragile skin and many skin-related problems. The increased weight of the chest may make it difficult to breathe, and the patient may need to use oxygen regularly (Figure 31-4). Breathing is even more difficult when the patient is lying down. The extra skin causes many to feel hot most of the time, and the patient may want to wear only lightweight clothing. Some have mental and emotional issues related to their weight. ■

FIGURE 31-4 The weight of the chest makes breathing difficult, so supplemental oxygen is often necessary.

ENVIRONMENTAL MODIFICATIONS

Many hospitals admit bariatric patients to private rooms that have been modified to meet their needs. The private room upholds the patient's dignity, and prevents potential infringement on the rights of other patients. The room must have a floor-mounted toilet. Wall-mounted toilets should not be used. Doorways must be wide enough to move beds and other special equipment in and out.

Bariatric patients often sweat profusely, and many feel as if they are chronically short of breath. The discomfort of these conditions is markedly relieved by using an electric fan. Most hospital rooms do not have fans, for a variety of reasons. A fan is an essential item in the bariatric patient's room. Some hospitals have ceiling fans. Many patients prefer portable, oscillating fans that they can position at will. They often position the fan to blow directly on the face or upper body. If a ceiling fan is used, the patient will appreciate having it mounted directly over the bed with an accessible control switch.

Specialized Equipment and Supplies

Some hospitals have bariatric units that are fully supplied with the equipment needed for patient care. If the hospital does not have dedicated bariatric beds, the nurse manager must anticipate patient needs and gather essential items promptly. Emergency or unplanned admissions can be challenging if the facility does not maintain a regular stock of basic items needed for bariatric care. Regular hospital furniture (including toilets) is designed to safely hold patients who weigh 350 pounds or less. Having a wall-mounted toilet break and fall off under a bariatric patient's weight would be emotionally traumatic and likely to cause a serious physical injury.

The obese patient may be unable to fit into a regular hospital bed or sit in a regular chair. If he or she is able to fit into the bed or chair, getting stuck is a real possibility. There is not enough space to turn the patient. In addition, regular furnishings may be unsafe and break under the patient's weight. Learning the weight limits of regular equipment and furniture is important. Many items that are marked "large size" may still be unsafe for a bariatric patient. Specially manufactured bariatric items are often necessary. Staff must learn the specific weight limits of equipment before using it. Many facilities mark this information directly on the back or underside of the equipment, where it is not visible to the public. Others use specially colored stickers, with abbreviations such as EC (expanded capacity), to denote bariatric-safe equipment. Bariatric furnishings reduce the risk of injury to patients and workers, and increase patient comfort.

The Bed

The bed is the most important piece of equipment in the hospital room. It is literally the center of the hospital patient's universe. From your class, you know that most daily activities are modified so they can be done when the patient is in bed. Because of concern for patient comfort and the risk of staff injury, special bariatric beds (Figure 31-5) have been developed that will safely support patients who are morbidly obese, and allow enough space for turning. Become familiar with the bed you are using. Most have an electronic high/low function, but the bed may not elevate as high as a regular hospital bed. The side rails on these beds have been strengthened so patients can safely pull on them for moving and positioning support. When a patient is in a regular hospital bed, he or she must go through a number of twists, turns, and pivots when getting out of bed to stand or transfer. These maneuvers can be awkward for the nursing assistant who is moving a bariatric patient, further increasing the risk of injury because of the positions and repetitive motions.

Special bariatric beds enable staff to move the bed from the flat position into the sitting position. After the patient is seated, the footboard to the bed can be removed so the patient can take a step and walk out of the bottom of the bed. Most beds of this type can also be used as a transport vehicle, so that the patient need not transfer to a stretcher or wheelchair. Keep the wheels locked when the bed is not in motion. An additional safeguard is to position the bed against the wall on one side, with the brakes locked, for staff-assisted transfers or for patients who are able to transfer at will. Bariatric wheelchairs (Figure 31-6) and walkers can be used when the patient is up, if needed.

FIGURE 31-6 A wide wheelchair is needed for bariatric patients. This chair also has a self-releasing tray that the patient leans on for upper body support. (Courtesy of Skil-Care Corporation, Yonkers, NY; (800) 431-2972)

Some hospitals use bottom sheets made of Gore-Tex or nylon, which have a surface that feels slippery. The fabric reduces friction and shear when moving the patient. Another benefit is that the fabric wicks moisture (perspiration) away from the skin. Some experts also recommend using these sheets to ease transfers, such as when moving the patient from the bed to a chair positioned against the bed. Various effective techniques have been developed in which caregivers pull on the sheet instead of the patient. This reduces the risk of discomfort and injury to the patient as well as the nursing assistant.

Depending on the type of bed used, an overbed or ceiling mounted **trapeze** (Figure 31-7) may also be used to assist the patient with independent bed mobility. The trapeze is also useful when bringing the patient to a standing position for ambulation. A *trapeze* is a triangular frame that hangs on a chain from the ceiling or base support attached to the bed. Several types of trapeze setups are usually available in every hospital. If you are instructed to obtain and set up a trapeze, select the *IV-Balkan type trapeze,* such as the one pictured. This trapeze is sturdy and will support a bariatric patient's weight without coming apart or causing injury. Special bariatric beds that convert to a chair position have a special trapeze that can be attached to the unit (Figure 31-8). A reg-

FIGURE 31-5 The Excel Care bed is manufactured for the care of bariatric patients. The trapeze is an accessory for the bed. (The Excel Care™ bed is a registered trademark of Hill-Rom Services, Inc. ©2007 Hill-Rom Services, Inc. Reprinted with permission. All rights reserved.)

FIGURE 31-7 The IV-type Balkan frame is sturdy enough to support the trapeze for a bariatric patient's bed.

FIGURE 31-8 The Total Care bariatric bed converts to a chair so the patient can step out of it rather than doing a standing transfer. (The Total Care® bariatric bed is a registered trademark of Hill-Rom Services, Inc. ©2007 Hill-Rom Services, Inc. Reprinted with permission. All rights reserved.)

FIGURE 31-10 The furniture in the patient's room is usually oversized to accommodate large-size family and friends. (Courtesy of Medline Industries, Inc. (800) MED-LINE)

ular trapeze defeats the purpose of the conversion bed, because the bed cannot be changed to the sitting position with the trapeze in place.

Low beds are also available for bariatric patients. These have a deck height of approximately 6 or 8 inches. Although they do have an electronic high/low feature, most cannot be elevated above 22 to 26 inches. If you are providing personal care for a patient in a low bed, follow the guidelines in Unit 23 to protect your back.

Your facility may also have pressure-reducing overlays for bariatric beds. Regular foam overlays are too thin to be of much benefit to the bariatric patient. Special bariatric low air loss beds and overlays are available (Figure 31-9) for bedfast bariatric patients and those with serious skin breakdown.

Bedside Chairs. Many of the bariatric patient's visitors will also be large. Chairs in the patient's room should have expanded capacity for the patient and visitors. Chairs the size of loveseats (Figure 31-10) and chairs without arms give the best fit, although the lack of arms will make standing difficult for some people.

Mechanical Lift. The mechanical lift you normally use may not support the bariatric patient's weight. The

hydraulic mechanical lift is normally safe for about 350 pounds. A special high-capacity lift (Figure 31-11A) is necessary to safely transfer bariatric patients. Some facilities mount a ceiling lift (Figure 31-11B) in each dedicated bariatric room. The lift moves on a track in the ceiling so you can safely slide the sling suspending the patient from bed to chair. After the patient is centered over the chair, the sling is lowered to seat the patient. The sling remains

FIGURE 31-11A This mechanical lift also has a digital scale feature. Its marking shows that it is safe to use to move patients weighing as much as 300 kilograms, or 660 pounds. It may also be used for normal-size adults, but the sling size is larger and may be more cumbersome for both staff and patient. (Photo courtesy of Alpha Modalities)

FIGURE 31-9 Low air loss beds are available for bariatric patients with pressure ulcers and other serious skin conditions. (Courtesy of Medline Industries, Inc. (800) MEDLINE)

FIGURE 31-11B This sling is suspended from a ceiling-mounted hoist that slides on a track to move from one location to another. A switch in the hoist releases a cord to lower the sling to seat the patient in the bed or chair. (Photo courtesy of Alpha Modalities)

in place. Some slings have a hole cut into the bottom so the lift can be used to lower the patient over the toilet or commode. Although these mechanical lifts are designed to be used by one person, having two or more caregivers is necessary for safety when moving a bariatric patient. When lowering the patient over a chair or commode, one person must hold the seat in place because there is a risk of tipping when the sling is lowered.

Gowns. Regular hospital gowns do not fit bariatric patients. Extra-large, or "ample" size gowns (Figure 31-12) are needed, and are stocked by most hospitals. If no large-size gown is available, use two regular gowns, with one on backward. However, this is an assault on the patient's dignity that should be avoided, if possible.

Toileting and Bathing. Double-size bedside commodes (Figure 31-13), shower chairs or benches, wheelchairs, and stretchers are also necessary. These devices normally cannot support more than 300 pounds. Many will not support even that much.

Scales. A number of scale options have become available for weighing bariatric patients without offending their dignity. Hospitals may purchase standing and chair or wheelchair scales that will accommodate patients who weigh less than 1,000 pounds. (Review the information in Unit 21 on obtaining weights using mechanical lifts.) Your facility may have a scale attachment for the regular

FIGURE 31-12 Oversize gowns are available for bariatric patients. These are much more comfortable than having to wear two regular-size gowns. (Courtesy of Medline Industries, Inc. (800) MEDLINE)

FIGURE 31-13 Oversize commodes often have drop arms so sliding transfers can be done. If the patient does sliding transfers, no lid is used. (The lid would be dislodged during sliding.) (Courtesy of Medline Industries, Inc. (800) MEDLINE)

mechanical lift. If so, check the weight limit. Some of these have only a 350-pound capacity. Some of the mechanical lifts used for bedfast patients also have a scale attachment. If your facility has a bed-size mechanical lift, check the weight limits for the scale attachment. Some older scales will weigh up to 400 pounds. Newer models will weigh 600-pound patients. Bed lifts that have scales with a capacity over 600 pounds are hard to find. Some bariatric beds have built-in scales, but this feature must be requested when the bed is ordered. The best option is use a scale that is built into the bed when it is manufactured.

ANTICIPATING PATIENT CARE NEEDS

When you are assigned to care for a bariatric patient, try to anticipate your needs in advance. You may have to request equipment from central supply. Make sure you have necessary supplies available, such as a hospital gown and a blood pressure cuff. Try to plan care, and inform the nurse if you will need additional items that are not routinely stocked on the unit. Because of the special nature of bariatric care, you should plan to spend more time doing tasks that you can do quickly for most adult patients. Expect bariatric patients to need more time than the average medical or surgical patient. On a bariatric unit, your assignment will be adjusted to allow enough time to provide conscientious patient care.

Patient Transport

When you must transport a patient to another area of the facility, conduct a dry run first. Evaluate the route you will take to make sure that doors, elevators, and other areas are wide enough, and that both the patient and extra equipment (such as an IV pole with a pump) will fit. If you will encounter ramps or inclines while transporting the patient, have another assistant accompany you to assist with pushing on inclines and prevent a runaway stretcher or wheelchair on a downward slope. Alert the receiving department of the patient's special needs, if necessary. They may also have to make special preparations and obtain extra help to care for the patient.

Taking Blood Pressure

Regular blood pressure cuffs are too small for bariatric patients, and will give inaccurate readings. A large, extra-large, or thigh-size cuff may be necessary. Occasionally, even these will not solve the problem. The upper arm is triangular in shape, with the wide part closest to the shoulder and the narrow part near the elbow. Because of this, sometimes no blood pressure cuffs will fit securely when wrapped, and will slip off. If this occurs, the care plan will identify how the blood pressure should be taken. Some facilities use a regular-size manual or electronic cuff on the forearm to take blood pressure. Occasionally, the lower leg is used.

For patients who need frequent or continuous blood pressure monitoring, some facilities use digital blood pressure units that register the blood pressure in an artery in the wrist or finger. The wrist blood pressure device (Figure 31-14) slips on like a bracelet. To obtain the reading, you just press a button. The finger blood pressure device clips on or slips over the finger. Pushing a button will enable you to obtain a digital reading. However, these devices are not always as accurate as a regular sphygmomanometer. Make sure to use them according to your facility's guidelines, which may indicate that they are to be used as a last resort.

FIGURE 31-14 The wrist blood pressure monitor is an excellent option for bariatric patients if frequent measurements are needed. (Courtesy of Medline Industries, Inc. (800) MEDLINE)

At least one blood pressure reading should be taken using the auscultation method before using the electronic wrist or finger device. The auscultation reading is used as a baseline with which to compare electronic values. Review the guidelines for electronic blood pressure monitoring in Unit 20. The electronic blood pressure device is contraindicated in patients with:

- Extreme hypertension or hypotension
- Very rapid heart rates
- Irregular heart rhythms, atrial dysrhythmias
- Excessive body movement, tremors

Patients for whom electronic blood pressure monitoring is not acceptable should be known to all caregivers and identified on the care plan or Kardex. If in doubt, check with the nurse for instructions for patients with very high blood pressure or rapid or irregular heart (pulse) rates.

Difficult SITUATIONS

The special care needed by bariatric patients is time-consuming. Plan your daily schedule and routines. Organize your work to allow enough time to meet patients' highly individual needs. ∎

ASSISTING WITH ADLS

Protect the patient's dignity at all costs. Avoid making insensitive comments about the patient's size. Some patients may refuse an offer of help with personal care because they are embarrassed by their inabilities or ashamed of their bodies. However, some patients are so large that they cannot complete their own personal hygiene. They may be unable to reach everywhere that needs washing, or lack the range of motion and flexibility required. Because of the excess skin and moisture, keeping patients' skin very clean and dry is essential. If the patient is perspiring heavily, he or she may need special skin care several times during your shift. Check the care plan for instructions.

When providing care, you will need to be very creative and modify some procedures to provide routine personal care. For example, when bathing the patient, you will find that he or she has so much extra skin that getting into some crevices and skin folds is very difficult. The umbilicus is often deep, making it difficult to clean. Use cotton swabs, if necessary, and be gentle. You must be very tactful and sensitive when providing personal hygiene, to avoid offending the patient. A second nursing assistant may need to assist, such as by holding skin folds back while you wash. An alternative may be to wrap an area with an abdominal binder or similar device to hold the skin back. If you cannot figure out how to solve a problem, ask the patient! He or she is usually an expert who knows what works, and asking the patient shows that you sincerely want to meet his or her needs. It also gives the patient a sense of control, which is often lost upon admission to the hospital.

Difficult SITUATIONS

Keeping the patient's skin clean is essential. However, if the skin is very sensitive, a washcloth and towel will be very irritating. Most facilities stock disposable washcloths that have a softer texture than terrycloth. Using a disposable washcloth and gently patting skin dry with a flannel bath blanket may be easier on the skin. Another alternative is to use a hair dryer on the cool setting to dry sensitive skin. A soft, clean, white cotton sock (such as a sweat sock) is also effective. You can put it over your hand to wash and rinse the skin, or use a dry sock for padding. The padding absorbs the moisture that further increases skin irritation. As you gain experience working with bariatric patients, improvising in this manner to complete tasks will become second nature to you. ■

Nutrition and Hydration

Obese patients often have nutritional problems. Surprisingly, many are malnourished, with a protein deficiency. For many, carbohydrates are dietary staples. This may be a financial issue. High-carbohydrate items stop hunger pangs and often cost less than foods with higher nutrient value. The dietitian will evaluate the patient and make dietary recommendations. The physician will write a diet order. Occasionally, a patient will have signs or symptoms

of an eating disorder, such as binging and purging. Bariatric patients are at risk for type 2 diabetes. Many patients' blood sugar must be controlled with insulin injections (Figure 31-15). Oral medications do not provide adequate control for all type 2 patients. Type 2 diabetes used to be considered an adult-onset condition, but we are now seeing young, obese teens with this condition. Nurses will monitor the patients' blood sugar. However, you should monitor for and report any signs and symptoms of thirst, fatigue, weakness, increased urination, or dehydration. Patients who are bedfast may have difficulty feeding themselves because of their size or position, or because they cannot use the overbed table. Assist the patient, if necessary (Figure 31-16).

You will probably be assigned to do intake and output (I&O) monitoring. The patient will need a large amount of fluid to support body needs. Many bariatric patients

FIGURE 31-15 Some patients have type 2 diabetes that cannot be controlled by oral drugs, making insulin injections necessary one to four times daily.

FIGURE 31-16 Assist the patient if her position prevents her from reaching the cup.

perspire excessively and eliminate a large amount of fluid through the skin. Be sure to inform the nurse if excessive perspiration is a problem. Fluids may be restricted if the patient has a comorbid condition, such as congestive heart failure. Tachycardia and decreased urinary output are early signs of dehydration. These are followed by a decrease in blood pressure. Inform the nurse promptly if the patient shows any of these signs.

Elimination

In many facilities, the bariatric patient is catheterized to monitor fluid balance. Because of the patient's size, you may wish to perform perineal care with the patient in the side-lying position instead of on the back. Usually, getting a condom catheter to stay in place on an obese male patient is difficult. An indwelling catheter may be a better option. Because of the patient's size, the catheter may appear short, and it may be difficult to attach to drainage tubing or secure to the thigh. Even more important, the catheter is at risk for being pulled out during patient movement. Attaching an extension tubing between the indwelling catheter and the drainage-bag tubing may be necessary. The patient is also at high risk for developing pressure ulcers in skin folds where a catheter or other device has burrowed into the skin surface. This may also be a problem if items, packaging, and supplies are accidentally dropped in the bed.

Patients may need assistance cleaning themselves after toileting. If the patient uses the bathroom or commode and is able to stand, one nursing assistant can stand in front of the patient to provide instruction and support while a second assistant cleans the perineum and rectum.

Skin Care

The skin is the largest organ of the body, and the bariatric patient has much extra skin. Usually, it has been stretched and is easily injured. You know that the skin is very sensitive to the effects of moisture, pressure, friction, and shear force. Pressure ulcers normally develop over bony prominences. The soft tissue is damaged by external pressure applied over the surface of the skeletal structure. Common areas of pressure ulcer development are the back of the ears and head, sacrum and coccyx, hips, heels, and any other area where high, prolonged external pressure exists. The buttocks are at high risk because patients tend to sit for long periods without moving or shifting their weight. A pressure-relieving cushion (Figure 31-17A) is much more comfortable to sit on and helps protect the skin (Figure 31-17B). The hips are also a high-risk area because of pressure from sitting for long periods in a chair or wheelchair that is too small or narrow. Bariatric patients have many skin folds (Figure 31-18). The patients' skin must be kept very clean and dry to reduce the risk of complications.

Each time you turn the patient to the side, check the skin folds carefully to make sure they are not red or "weeping"

FIGURE 31-17A The bariatric cushion comes with an internal leveling pad for sling-seat chairs or a contoured base for chairs with flat seats. The foam layer is comfortable to sit on. (Courtesy of Skil-Care Corporation, Yonkers, NY; (800) 431-2972)

FIGURE 31-17B The internal layer of visco foam provides excellent pressure relief. (Courtesy of Skil-Care Corporation, Yonkers, NY; (800) 431-2972)

FIGURE 31-18 Bariatric patients have many skin folds.

(overly moist). Wash and dry the skin folds frequently. Excessive moisture from perspiration in the warm, moist, dark environment of a skin fold carries a great risk for a painful yeast infection (Figure 31-19). Make sure the areas are kept dry. If necessary, a flannel bath blanket can be cut and folded to place in the skin folds. A better alternative to cutting a bath blanket is to obtain a supply of flannel receiving blankets, such as those used in the newborn nursery, and fold and place them between the skin folds. Avoid the temptation to use washcloths and towels in these fragile skin areas. The rough surface texture will further irritate tender skin.

If the patient is unconscious or using ventilator support, make sure to carefully check the skin folds behind the neck. These tend to become wet from sputum and saliva, and the patient's position produces constant pressure, placing him or her at risk of both yeast infection and pressure ulcers. The increased body weight promotes rapid ulcer development. Reposition the head manually each time the patient is turned. Otherwise, it tends to stay in the same position, and a pressure ulcer will develop quickly. Make sure that the various lines and tubes are not tunneled into, trapped between, or pressing on the patient's skin. Elevate the heels off the surface of the bed, or use a bariatric product that relieves pressure on the heel (Figure 31-20). The heels are also a very high-pressure, high-risk area. Remember, fleece and sock-type heel protectors prevent friction and shearing, but do not relieve pressure.

FIGURE 31-19 This painful condition is called candidiasis or intertrigo. It commonly develops in warm, moist skin folds, such as under the arms, breasts, abdominal apron, and groin. (Courtesy of Centers for Disease Control and Prevention)

FIGURE 31-20 The bariatric heel float eliminates all pressure from the heels. (Courtesy of Skil-Care Corporation, Yonkers, NY; (800) 431-2972)

Dressing the Patient

Because some bariatric patients feel warm and perspire, they may want to remain in a hospital gown or light pajamas all day. Some patients prefer to wear nothing and be covered only with a sheet. Make sure the patient is fully covered if he or she has visitors or must leave the room. Other clothing that is comfortable and easy to put on includes:

- Large T-shirts
- Loose, open-neck shirts that are not tucked into pants
- Caftans or ponchos for females instead of blouses
- Cotton house dresses or muu-muus
- Sweatshirts and sweatpants
- Boxer shorts and boxer briefs instead of brief-style underwear
- Sports bras instead of regular brassieres
- Overalls, coveralls
- Pants with an elastic waist instead of a button and zipper
- Slip-on shoes, shoes that have Velcro fasteners, bedroom slippers, or thong sandals
- Suspenders instead of belts

MOVING THE BARIATRIC PATIENT

Bariatric patients have many individual needs and many types of equipment are used in patient care. One staff person should never lift or move more than 35 pounds of body weight without extra help or a mechanical device. A variety of devices have been developed to make procedures as easy as possible for the patient and the nursing assistant (Figure 31-21).

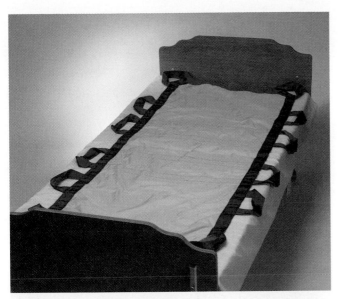

FIGURE 31-21 Many different devices are available to make moving the patient easier for staff and less traumatic for the patient. (Courtesy of Skil-Care Corporation, Yonkers, NY; (800) 431-2972).

FIGURE 31-22A The HoverMatt® Lateral Transfer and Repositioning System reduces friction, so it seems as if you are moving only about 10% of the patient's weight. (Courtesy of HoverTech International. (800-471-2776). http://www.hovermatt.com)

FIGURE 31-22B The edges of the HoverMatt® curve up and in, making the patient feel secure and less likely to roll off. Nevertheless, patients should not be left alone when the mat is inflated. (Courtesy of HoverTech International. (800-471-2776). http://www.hovermatt.com)

Another concern about equipment designed for lifting and moving is its ability to support the patient's weight adequately, to reduce the risk of injury for both the patient and the nursing assistant. Explaining positioning and moving techniques beyond the general principles of patient care is impossible. This is a subject for which an entire book is necessary. If you will be working with the bariatric population, your facility will teach you its policies and procedures and how to use its special equipment. Even when a device is used, two or more nursing assistants are often needed for procedures that involve moving the patient, as well as for personal hygiene.

The HoverMatt®

The HoverMatt® Lateral Transfer and Repositioning System (Figure 31-22A) is commonly used for lifting, moving, and transferring bariatric patients. The device improves patient comfort and helps reduce the risk of injury to nursing assistants. The HoverMatt® may be used on patients of any size. There is no weight limit. Larger mattresses are available for patients with greater body mass. The HoverMatt® transfer and repositioning device is inflated quickly (in about 5 seconds) by connecting a separate air supply unit. When the mattress is inflated, air escapes from tiny holes on the underside. The escape of air acts as a lubricant, reducing friction during transfers. Because the friction is reduced, nursing assistants are moving only about 10% of the patient's actual weight. A 400-pound patient seems to weigh only 40 pounds when the HoverMatt® is used. A two-person transfer is done for most bariatric patients, so each worker is moving about 20 pounds, thus reducing the risk of injury. When you

have finished the transfer, unplug the air supply. The mattress deflates on its own within 15 to 20 seconds.

The HoverMatt® cradles the patient when it is inflated (Figure 31-22B), so he or she feels secure and is less likely to roll off. Nevertheless, reassure the patient and never leave him or her alone when the mattress is inflated. Many facilities apply this mattress to the bed at the time of admission, so it is quickly available when the patient needs lifting and moving assistance. If the patient slides down in bed, the HoverMatt® slides as well. Inflating the mattress and using the handles on the sides is all that is necessary to move the patient up in bed.

Moving the Patient: Bed Mobility

Review the guidelines for moving patients in Units 15 through 17 of this book. Apply the principles of good body mechanics for yourself and the patient. Lifting and moving present a high risk of injury to the patient and the nursing assistant. Bedfast patients must be turned every 2 hours or more often, even if a special therapeutic, low air loss, rotational, or turning mattress is used. If the patient turns herself, check the position to ensure that she is turning often enough.

Bariatric patients who are able to move themselves tend to use their body weight to aid in movement. For example, when turning from side to side, they tug and pull on the side rail until they reach a point where only a little more effort will result in a comfortable position. In making this final turn, tubes such as the catheter, IV, or electrode monitoring wires may be pulled and the traction may result in tube removal. Make sure that all tubes are firmly secured, and monitor them for proper placement each time you are in the room.

Because the patient uses his arms for bed mobility, try to avoid devices that limit movement of the hands and arms. For example, having an IV in the left arm and an electronic blood pressure monitor on the right arm acts as a method of restraint and will restrict the patient's ability to move about in bed. Accessories such as the bed ladder (Figure 31-23) will help facilitate movement. The ladder is attached to the bed frame, and the patient pulls on it to rise to an upright position. If this device is not available, tying a sheet or rope to a secure spot on the frame at the end of the bed may help.

Manual Patient Handling Devices

Many bariatric patients prefer to keep the bed positioned in the high Fowler's position (Figure 31-24), which relieves pressure on the chest and helps maximize respiratory efficiency. However, this position promotes slipping down in bed. Elevating the knee of the bed slightly will reduce strain and help prevent downward sliding. If the patient complains of back pain when the head is elevated, elevating the knee of the bed will not provide sufficient relief. A commercial knee elevator (Figure 31-25) will relieve pressure on the back.

The TLC Pad (Figure 31-26A) and other similar patient-handling devices can be used for moving patients up in the bed or chair, and from side to side in bed. A regular-size patient can often be moved by a single caregiver (Figure 31-26B). Two to four workers may be necessary to move a bariatric patient up in bed or chair using this type of device. The handles make the job easier, and using a sturdy lifting device reduces the risk of injury.

FIGURE 31-24 Positioning the bed in the high Fowler's position makes breathing easier.

FIGURE 31-25 A knee elevator relieves pressure and pain on the back. (Courtesy of Skil-Care Corporation, Yonkers, NY; (800) 431-2972)

Some bariatric beds have an adjustable length feature at the foot end, which makes slipping down in bed less of a problem than it is in a regular bed. The nurse may instruct you to position the head slightly downward, in a modified Trendelenburg position, before turning and repositioning the bedfast patient. (This increases the risk of respiratory complications, so use the position only under the direction and supervision of the nurse.) A full Trendelenburg position places the head downward 60°. For this procedure, lowering the head 20 to 30° is sufficient. You should also use the modified Trendelenburg position when moving the patient up in bed because gravity will assist you, making the job easier and reducing the risk of injury. A Gore-Tex or nylon sheet or lifting device will also make this job easier.

FIGURE 31-23
The bed ladder fastens to the frame and enables the patient to sit up in the bed. (Courtesy of Skil-Care Corporation, Yonkers, NY; (800) 431-2972)

FIGURE 31-26A The TLC Pad is used for moving patients up in the bed or chair, and from side to side in bed. (Courtesy of Skil-Care Corporation, Yonkers, NY; (800) 431-2972)

FIGURE 31-26B A regular-size patient can be moved by a single caregiver. Two to four workers may be necessary to move the bariatric patient up in a bed or chair. (Courtesy of Skil-Care Corporation, Yonkers, NY; (800) 431-2972)

Note: Avoid leaving the patient in this position for more than a few minutes. Always check with the nurse before using the modified Trendelenburg position.

Return the bed to the flat position as soon as the move is done, then proceed with skin care and use pillows and props to support the body. Some bariatric beds have inflatable air bolsters on each side. These provide an adjunct for positioning and support, and can be inflated and deflated at will. This feature is also useful when moving the bed through narrow spaces and doorways.

Moving the patient by tugging on his or her body increases the risk of injury to patient and staff. If staff will be moving the patient in bed, use a lifting device made for this purpose. A draw sheet, two draw sheets, or a full-size sheet may also be used. Supporting the patient's body during positioning reduces the effects of gravity, making the move easier for both patient and staff. Four to six people may be needed to reposition a total-care patient safely. One person lifts the head. A second and third nursing assistant are positioned on each side, and a lift sheet or other device is also used. Another nursing assistant positioned at the foot of the bed lifts the patient's heels to eliminate friction and shearing.

When the patient is on the side, you may have to support the upper leg on pillows. The extra support reduces the risk of skin problems caused by the legs rubbing together, as well as preventing pressure on the bony prominence at the knee. However, supporting the upper leg also does much to relieve pain in the hip joint and lumbar-sacral area of the spine. Unsupported, the weight of the leg exerts a downward pull on both the hip and the spine, which can be very painful.

When moving and positioning the patient, remember that maintaining good body alignment is very important. The patient's skin and extremities are heavy and will not move on their own. You will have to move his or her body parts manually. Some hospitals have an arrangement of slings and pulleys for moving the arms and legs (Figure 31-27). The patient is encouraged to assist by pulling on the rope to which the sling is attached.

FIGURE 31-27 Various lifts, slings, and pulleys may be used to move the patient's extremities. This patient's legs are being elevated to relieve edema and pressure from the heels by using a ceiling-mounted hoist to hold them in place. (Photo courtesy of Alpha Modalities)

Moving the Patient: Transfers and Ambulation

Some bariatric patients can walk for short distances. Some will use a walker for support. Others use mobility scooters. Some will need help or use a mechanical device to come to a standing position (Figure 31-28), while others require assistance with transfers. The care plan will list instructions for mobilizing each patient. Some patients will be able to ambulate in their rooms with minimal assistance and support (Figure 31-29). The gait of an obese patient is usually wide-based. The legs are spread quite far apart. This helps the patient balance and the wide stance accommodates the width of the legs. The arms may be held out, slightly away from the body, and swing forward with each step to help propel the person forward. The patient may arch the back slightly to counterbalance the weight of the abdomen.

A gait/transfer belt may be used for transfers and ambulation if you have a long belt (Figure 31-30). A 72-inch belt will probably be necessary, in addition to two or three assistants to help. The transfer belt should not be used if the patient has recently had abdominal surgery or other contraindications are present (Unit 16). Check with the nurse if you are unsure. Avoid doubling a gait belt, if possible. If a long belt is not available and you must join two regular belts, make sure to lock the buckles down securely. Position both buckles close to your hands so you can see their position. If they begin to slip, even slowly, stop the procedure.

FIGURE 31-29 This patient can ambulate with minimum assistance. These nursing assistants are not pulling on the patient. Rather, they are providing encouragement, verbal instructions, and minor physical support to keep her balance and prevent falls.

FIGURE 31-30 A long belt may necessary for transferring and ambulating bariatric patients. A cloth belt holds more securely than a plastic belt. (Courtesy of Skil-Care Corporation, Yonkers, NY; (800) 431-2972)

FIGURE 31-28 Devices are available to assist patients in rising to their feet or to perform a standing transfer, such as for pivoting the patient to sit on a chair. (Photo courtesy of Alpha Modalities)

Some hospitals are using only plastic-type belts because of infection control issues. The buckles on these slip more readily, and they are not as gentle to the skin as cloth and canvas belts. Avoid connecting two plastic belts to make a single, long belt. The buckles may not hold. Your hospital may furnish a 72-inch cloth or canvas belt for each bariatric patient; often it is left in the room. (The patient takes the belt home or it is discarded upon discharge.)

When using any type of gait/transfer belt with an obese patient, avoid placing it over bare skin. Make sure the belt and buckle do not penetrate, rub, or cut into the skin folds, causing injury. Remember, the risk of this occurrence increases if plastic belts are used. The nurse may instruct you to apply an abdominal binder before moving the patient so that the abdomen does not interfere with safe patient handling and movement. The fatty apron of abdominal skin is called the **panniculus** or pannus. A **pannus** is a hanging flap of skin. It is usually seen in the abdomen of a person who has recently lost a significant amount of weight. Patients often like the feeling of support the binder provides.

Moving the patient is a high-risk procedure for the nursing assistant and patient alike. Whether moving the patient in bed or chair, you will need adequate help. Five or six caregivers may be needed. In addition to being at high risk for falls, patients are at risk of skin tears and abrasions. The nursing assistants are at risk for neck, shoulder, and back injuries, as well as other musculoskeletal injuries. Injury can occur even if a mechanical device is used. Instruct the patient to push herself to a standing position with the arms. Avoid straining or pulling on the patient to assist, especially under the arms. You will not be able to pull her up. Because of the highly individualized needs of the bariatric patient, the care plan will list instructions for moving. In many cases, a special mechanical lift is used to stand or transfer the patient.

Falls

If a standing patient starts to fall to the floor, you may instinctively try to hold her up or break the fall. Trying to do so will cause injury. Do all you can to prevent injury, but avoid trying to stabilize or brace the falling patient. For example, quickly push items out of the way that could cause injury to the patient. Try to protect the patient's head. When standing or ambulating the patient for the first time, have plenty of help. Monitor the patient for dizziness or weakness. If he or she experiences these problems, stop the procedure and return the patient to the supine position. It is best to have a walker, arm chair, or wheelchair turned backward in position in front of the patient. Have one assistant on each side to hold and stabilize the device. If the patient starts to fall, he or she may be able to stop the fall by using the arms and holding the walker or chair.

If the patient falls to the floor, a team will be required to get him up. Several methods are used, depending on how much assistance the patient can provide. The HoverJack® (Figure 31-31) operates in a manner similar to the Hover-Matt®. The HoverJack® is used to lift a patient in a supine position from the floor to bed or stretcher. By placing the HoverMatt® on top, the patient is easily lifted from the floor and transferred back to bed.

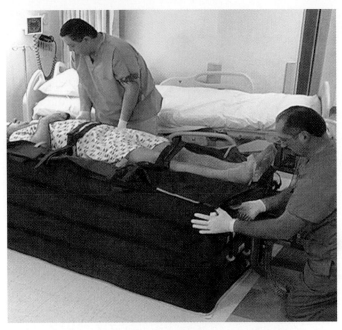

FGURE 31-31 The HoverJack® lifts the patient from the floor to a bed or stretcher. By placing the HoverMatt® on top, the patient is easily transferred back to bed. (Courtesy of HoverTech International. (800-471-2776). http://www.hovermatt.com)

A dependent patient may be rolled onto a bariatric sling made of nylon or canvas (Figure 31-32), or a heavy blanket. The patient is lifted only enough for a team member to slide a backboard or other solid lifting device underneath. The backboard (or other device) is used for moving the patient. If the patient is able to assist, a strong chair may be positioned against his back, then turned upright, or a team can lift the patient's arms and legs while another person slides a chair under him. These are potentially dangerous maneuvers for caregivers. Do not move an obese, dependent patient until you have proper instruction, supervision, adaptive mobility devices, and enough staff to accomplish the task.

COMPLICATIONS OF IMMOBILITY

Bariatric patients are at very high risk of complications when they are immobile. Even new postoperative patients are ambulated or gotten out of bed within 24 hours after

FIGURE 31-32 A dependent patient may be moved by rolling her onto a bariatric sling made of nylon or canvas. (Courtesy of Skil-Care Corporation, Yonkers, NY; (800) 431-2972)

Difficult SITUATIONS

The risk of aspiration is higher in obese patients than it is in adults of normal weight. Obese individuals have a greater volume of gastric fluid and increased intra-abdominal pressure. The incidence of reflux is higher. **Reflux** (also called *gastroesophageal reflux*) is the backflow of fluid, such as when stomach juices and food flow back from the stomach into the esophagus and mouth. This is typically the cause of heartburn. ■

surgery, whenever possible. Because of the risk of complications, some facilities strive to ambulate the patient within 2 hours after returning to the unit from surgery, then every 2 hours while awake. Patients who are unconscious or bedfast are at high risk of developing:

- Pneumonia
- Atelectasis
- Deep vein thrombosis (blood clots in the legs)
- Pulmonary embolism (a blood clot in the lungs)
- Pressure ulcers
- Yeast infections in the skin folds

BARIATRIC SURGERY

Bariatric surgery (Figure 31-33) is surgery on the stomach and/or intestines to help the patient with morbid or super obesity lose weight. Many different procedures may be done, depending on patient needs and doctor preference. Surgery is used as a treatment for weight loss for persons with a body mass index over 40. It is sometimes used as a treatment for people with a BMI between 35 and 40 who have health problems and potentially serious comorbidities, such as heart disease or type 2 diabetes.

Patients do not suddenly wake up one day, decide to have surgery, and schedule the procedure for the following day or week. The patient's BMI is only one of many considerations. The patient must have a thorough medical workup first. Medical instabilities and comorbidities may have to be treated and stabilized. The insurer, Medicare, or Medicaid must preapprove the procedure. It is never done on young children, and is seldom done on teenagers who are still growing. A few surgical centers will do bariatric surgery on teens as young as 15 or 16, if they meet the criteria established by the professionals at the facility. To be approved for bariatric surgery, most insurers require adult patients to:

- Be committed to making eating and lifestyle changes
- Have severe obesity (BMI over 35) with one or more comorbidities OR

Esophagus
Staples
Surgically strengthened outlet
Duodenum
Stomach
Jejunum
Large intestine

FIGURE 31-33 The gastric bypass and stomach banding are common bariatric surgeries.

GASTRIC BYPASS   STOMACH BANDING

- Have a BMI of 40 with or without comorbidities
- Have made numerous attempts at weight loss through diet and exercise

Goals and Objectives of Bariatric Surgery

Electing to have bariatric surgery is a major, life-altering decision. It is usually done after the patient has tried and failed at numerous diet and exercise programs. The physician has informed the patient that without weight loss, his or her life is at risk. Persons who elect to have bariatric surgery face many difficult problems and challenges. This surgery is much more than a painless, will-free approach to weight loss. As a full partner on the team, the patient makes a great investment in recovery and lifestyle changes. The surgery changes patients' lives completely. Their diet and manner of eating change forever. They must replace their clothing every few weeks as their body size decreases. When they reach their goal weight, they have an abundance of extra, stretched-out skin, which may require additional surgery. If the skin is not removed, the various fungal infection and skin problems related to friction will persist.

The goals of bariatric surgery are for the patient to achieve permanent weight loss and reduce the risk factors associated with the many comorbidities. The surgery is recognized as the only successful, permanent method for treating morbid obesity. Although some people lose weight by using nonsurgical methods, many regain the weight and often more. Few people have been able to successfully maintain the weight loss achieved with diet and exercise alone.

Surgical Procedure

Bariatric surgery has been evolving since the 1950s. Some procedures are minimally invasive. A **minimally invasive surgery** is any surgical procedure that does not require a large incision. It can be done by entering the body through a small cut or incision on the skin, or through a body cavity or other anatomical opening. Miniature scopes and instruments are used to visualize and repair the organs on the inside of the body. All of the accepted bariatric surgery techniques can be done by using a minimally invasive (also called *laparoscopic*) technique. There are both advantages and disadvantages to this method. Whether to use a minimally invasive or fully invasive procedure, in which the abdomen is opened, is determined by the surgeon, based on the patient's condition and needs. The minimally invasive technique is commonly used.

Patients who have minimally invasive bariatric surgery usually go home after the procedure, and can return to work and normal activities soon after surgery. However, certain risks are associated with this surgery. Some patients who anticipate immediate discharge must be admitted to the hospital because of complications. In fact, the rate of complications is higher than for other surgeries. However, living with morbid or super obesity is believed to be much more life-threatening than the potential for perioperative problems.

Patients who undergo bariatric surgery have an approximately 40% chance of developing complications within six months. In many surgical procedures, complications occur in the immediate postoperative period, while the patient is still in the hospital, or within a few weeks of surgery. The surgeon will continue to follow the postoperative bariatric patient closely for at least a year. Because this is somewhat different from the usual postoperative course, the surgeon will look for complications if a patient has a problem any time during the first year.

The most common complications (in 20% of patients) are vomiting, reflux, and diarrhea. About 10 to 12% of bariatric surgery patients develop problems from the surgical joining of the stomach and the intestine. Problems in this area usually involve leaking or strictures. A **stricture** is the narrowing of a passageway in the body, which is often caused by inflammation or scar tissue. This condition is also called **stenosis**. Approximately 7% of complications are abdominal hernias. A lower percentage of patients develop an infection or pneumonia after surgery.

Surgical Procedures

Three categories of surgical procedures are used for bariatric surgery. The category and specific type of surgical procedure selected are individualized to the patient's needs. The surgeon also makes the decision on whether to do an invasive or noninvasive procedure. The **gastric bypass** (Figure 31-33) is the most common of the six surgical techniques that are widely accepted. In this procedure, the surgeon creates a 2-inch-long pouch at the top of the patient's stomach. The surgeon attaches a portion of small intestine to the stomach pouch. After the surgery, patients can eat or drink only a small amount. The food will quickly pass through the stomach and digestive tract. Because of this, fewer calories are absorbed.

Postoperative Care

Gastric leaks are a very serious potential complication. Leaks often occur when a staple fails. This causes the stomach contents to leak internally, creating a serious or fatal infection. *Postoperative care is targeted to reduce pressure and strain on both the internal and external staples.* For example, splinting the abdomen with a pillow during deep breathing and coughing reduces pressure on the staples. The patient may use a nasogastric tube after surgery to reduce the strain on staples caused by vomiting. If an NG tube is present, the patient will be NPO (nothing by mouth) and will have an IV. A Foley catheter will be present that was placed during surgery. You will be expected to monitor intake and output. Each bariatric surgery has procedure-specific postoperative instructions. Other postoperative care includes:

- Using the incentive spirometer and coughing and deep breathing. The patient must be taught to firmly support the abdomen with pillows to reduce tension on the skin from coughing.
- Application of an abdominal binder (Unit 29). The binder should be fastened gently and released slowly. Make sure the tape over the incision does not stick to the binder. If it does, inform the nurse. Accidentally pulling the tape off when removing the binder will cause skin damage and potentially damage the operative site.
- Preventing constipation, which causes abdominal pressure. Inform the nurse if the patient complains of constipation or is straining to have a bowel movement.
- Draining the operative site to reduce fluid buildup and reduce the risk of infection and tension on the incision and operative area.
- Using nursing comfort measures to relieve pain and enhance the patient's comfort (Figure 31-34).

Other complications of bariatric surgery that may be seen in the immediate postoperative period are:

- Blood clots
- Hernias
- Cardiac abnormalities and rhythm disturbances

Potentially serious signs and symptoms of postoperative complications that should be reported to the nurse promptly are:

- Pulse/heart rate above 100
- Hypotension
- Patient feelings of anxiety, complaints of anxiety or a sense of impending doom
- Hypoxia, decreased oxygen saturation, signs of air hunger (Unit 39)

FIGURE 31-34 Use nursing comfort measures to relieve pain and enhance the patient's comfort.

- Fever above 102°F
- Abnormal changes in appearance or volume of gastric or wound drainage
- Signs or symptoms of wound infection
- Nausea, vomiting, or diarrhea
- Presence of blood in emesis or stool
- Persistent cough

Postoperative Care on the Night After Surgery.
Routine postoperative care given on the evening after surgery will probably include remote telemetry monitoring. The patient may be using oxygen through a cannula. Procedures the nursing assistant may be responsible for include:

- Vital sign monitoring according to postoperative routine, then hourly or as instructed by the nurse
- Application or care of an abdominal binder
- Application of ice packs to the incision
- Check dressing over the incision and drain hourly, or as instructed
- Using the incentive spirometer at least 10 times every hour
- Assisting with coughing and deep breathing
- Application of anti-embolism hosiery; circulation checks of feet every 2 to 4 hours
- Application of sequential compression devices, as ordered
- Getting the patient up in a chair with assistance one or more times
- Catheter care
- Intake and output monitoring and recording
- Monitoring the pulse oximeter for alarms (Unit 36)

The postsurgical patient will be NPO except for ice chips.

Postoperative Days 1 and 2. On the first postoperative day, the Foley catheter will be discontinued. The NPO status will be lifted, and the patient will be permitted measured amounts of clear liquids, such as 1 to 2 ounces every 30 to 60 minutes. Assist the patient with elimination. You will continue monitoring intake and output, and report the patient's first voiding to the nurse. If the patient does not urinate within 4 hours of catheter removal, inform the nurse. The patient will probably have dietary, physical, and occupational therapy evaluations on this day, so you must schedule care around these activities. Nursing assistant care from the evening after surgery will continue. Additionally, you will be assigned to ambulate the patient for longer distances, such as in the hallway. The patient should sit in a chair when not walking.

Postoperative Day 3. On the third postoperative day, IV fluids will be discontinued, but you will continue I&O monitoring. The patient's diet will advance to full liquid, low-carbohydrate items to see how she tolerates them. Stable patients are often discharged on Day 3 unless complications develop.

Discharge Instructions. The dietitian or registered nurse will teach the patient about the postoperative diet (Figure 31-35). The patient is instructed to advance food intake gradually every few days, as tolerated. In this case, "advancing" means adding new food items, not increasing portion size. The patient's stomach will hold only a few ounces, and overfilling it risks rupturing a staple and causing a leak. On the fifth and sixth postoperative days, the diet should advance to pureed foods, including baby foods, applesauce, blended soft foods, and potted meats. The patient needs to drink frequently to prevent dehydration.

On the sixth and seventh days, the diet progresses to soft foods, including all of the pureed items taken previously, all allowed liquids, and soft foods, such as baked white fish without bones, imitation crab meat, hot dogs, canned fruits, and overcooked vegetables. Hard meats, such as steak, pork, and chicken, are not allowed. During the second and third weeks, the patient begins a regular food trial. This trial includes all items eaten previously plus red meat, chicken, and well-cooked vegetables. The patient is permitted to try only one new item at a time. By adding one new regular food per day, 14 new items will have been added by the end of this period.

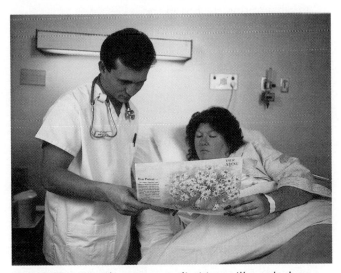

FIGURE 31-35 The nurse or dietitian will teach the patient about postoperative dietary restrictions.

ONGOING CARE AND SUPPORT

At home, the patient should be as active as possible, walking up to one mile a day by the appointment for the first postoperative office visit. The patient should continue wearing the abdominal binder when active. The patient must avoid heavy lifting until released by the physician. If a minimally invasive procedure was done, the patient should be able to return to work in a week. If an invasive procedure was done, he should plan to return to work after about six weeks. The patient must keep a food diary with exact amounts and portion sizes of everything he eats and drinks for the first month after surgery. The surgeon will evaluate this record to determine whether the patient's protein intake was adequate. This is very important to prevent malnutrition.

The commitment to the bariatric surgery patient does not end when the immediate perioperative period is complete. The surgeon and others continue to follow the patient's progress. Support groups are available for preoperative and postoperative patients. These are very important to patients' long-term weight-loss success. As you can see, an effective bariatric program encompasses many aspects besides the surgical intervention. Other key components are nutritional support, psychological support, and availability of health care professionals to help with any complications experienced by the patient.

The care of the bariatric patient is not technically or cognitively difficult. Nevertheless, it is physically demanding, and must be done according to directions to prevent injury to patients and staff. Paying close attention to detail and working as a member of a team are keys to successful care of bariatric patients. Bariatric surgery is a positive, health-promoting, life-sustaining intervention. Nursing assistants are essential members of the bariatric team. The care you give is vital to a quality outcome in the patients' care and quality of life. When a shapely, attractive patient returns to your unit to thank the staff, you will feel pride in yourself, your team, and your former patient that is well beyond expectation.

REVIEW

A. True/False.

Mark the following true or false by circling T or F.

1. T F Approximately 25% of adults in the United States are overweight.

2. T F Genetics and environment affect a person's weight.

3. T F Persons with mild to moderate obesity qualify for bariatric surgery if they have one comorbidity.

4. T F Comorbidities are genetic problems that cause or contribute to obesity.

5. T F Obesity places a great strain on the heart and lungs.

6. T F Bariatric patients are just larger versions of the normal-size adult.

7. T F When taking the blood pressure of a bariatric patient, a large, extra-large, or thigh-size cuff may be necessary.

8. T F Bariatric patients cannot develop an eating disorder.

9. T F Wall-mounted toilets should not be used for patients who weigh more than 500 pounds.

10. T F Obese patients do not develop malnutrition.

B. Matching.

Choose the correct phrase from Column II to match the words in Column I.

Column I

11. _____ minimally invasive surgery

12. _____ pannus

13. _____ ideal body weight

14. _____ advocate

15. _____ gastric bypass

16. _____ bariatrics

17. _____ overweight

18. _____ comorbidities

19. _____ reflux

20. _____ hyperventilation

Column II

a. most common bariatric surgery, in which the patient is left with a 2-inch-long stomach pouch

b. diseases and conditions that are caused by or contributed to by morbid obesity

c. a condition in which a person weighs more than he or she should, considering his or her height and bone size

d. breathing abnormally fast and deep

e. surgical procedure that is done through a scope and does not require a large incision

f. mathematical formula related to life span or longevity and health

g. backflow of stomach juices and food from the stomach into the esophagus and mouth

h. field of medicine that treats obesity and diseases associated with obesity

i. a large, hanging flap of abdominal skin

j. a person who speaks on behalf of the patient

C. Multiple Choice.

Select the one best answer for each of the following.

21. Early signs of dehydration in the bariatric patient include
    a. fever, high blood pressure, and edema.
    b. bradycardia and increased urination.

c. decreased urinary output and tachycardia.

d. diarrhea, edema, and tachycardia.

22. Bariatric patients who complain of feeling hot may obtain relief from
    a. removing the patient's clothes and top sheet, then closing the door.
    b. an electric fan that the patient can position and control.
    c. folding a newspaper to create a handheld fan.
    d. bathing the patient in ice water.

23. One staff person should never lift or move more than
    a. 5 pounds of body weight without extra help or a mechanical device.
    b. 35 pounds of body weight without extra help or a mechanical device.
    c. 65 pounds of body weight without extra help or a mechanical device.
    d. 90 pounds of body weight without extra help or a mechanical device.

24. When moving the bariatric patient up in bed, initially position the bed in the
    a. modified Trendelenburg position.
    b. semi-Fowler's position.
    c. lithotomy position.
    d. Sims' position.

25. If a standing bariatric patient starts to fall to the floor, you should
    a. protect the patient's head, if possible.
    b. grab the patient under the arms.
    c. hold the patient up however you can.
    d. run for extra help.

26. The goals of bariatric surgery include
    a. removing the large abdominal panniculus.
    b. temporarily reducing the size of the stomach until the patient loses at least 100 pounds.
    c. removing extra fat by using liposuction and cutting away massive areas of skin.
    d. helping the patient achieve permanent weight loss and reduce the risks of comorbidities.

27. A minimally invasive surgery is
    a. one in which the patient is under anesthesia for an hour or less.
    b. commonly done by using spinal anesthesia and IV sedation.
    c. done through a scope after making a small incision.
    d. done by making a large incision through which to enter the body cavity.

28. After bariatric surgery, the patient should be assisted or reminded to
    a. cough forcefully every 15 minutes.
    b. use the incentive spirometer 10 times every 4 hours.
    c. cough and deep breathe 10 times every shift.
    d. use the incentive spirometer 10 times every hour.

29. During the evening after bariatric surgery, the patient should be
    a. given 2 ounces of water every 4 hours.
    b. NPO except for ice chips.
    c. served a clear liquid diet.
    d. encouraged to eat to gain strength.

30. During the evening after bariatric surgery, the patient should be
    a. kept on bedrest for at least 12 hours.
    b. ambulated in the hall at least every 2 hours.
    c. gotten up in the chair one or more times.
    d. given a hot water bottle for incisional pain.

D. Nursing Assistant Challenge.

You are assigned to care for Mrs. Esmerelda Gonsalves, a 31-year-old female who has been admitted to room 306 on your unit. She is scheduled for bariatric surgery tomorrow. Mrs. Gonsalves tells you that she has gradually gained weight since she was a child. She tells you she has tried every diet she could find and nothing worked for her. She gets teary-eyed and tells you that surgery is her last hope for a normal life.

Her height on admission was 68 inches and her weight was 423 pounds. This calculates to a body mass index of 64.5. Her comorbidities include type 2 diabetes, sleep apnea, osteoarthritis of the lumbar spine and knees, and symptoms of depression.

31. The thigh blood pressure cuff slips down every time you apply it, so you have not finished taking Mrs. Gonsalves's admission vital signs. There is no electronic vital signs monitor on the unit. What action will you take?

32. You finally get the cuff to stay on the patient's arm, so you take a manual blood pressure. Your reading is 266/178. The patient has no history of hypertension. What action will you take?

33. The nurse informs you that the blood pressure cuff you used is broken. You cannot find another cuff that will stay on the patient's arm without slipping. What will you do?

34. After putting Mrs. Gonsalves to bed, you note that she has a large abdominal pannus. Under the pannus, the skin is bright red, with weeping and irritation. The patient tells you this is a chronic problem, which is painful for her. Is it necessary to notify the nurse? What else should you do to help this patient?

35. No special preoperative orders have been written. The nurse informs you to teach the patient about the routine care you will be giving after surgery. What will you tell this patient?

UNIT 32

Death and Dying

OBJECTIVES

After completing this unit, you will be able to:

- Spell and define terms.
- Describe how different people handle the process of death and dying.
- Describe the nursing assistant's responsibilities for providing supportive care.
- Describe the spiritual preparations for death practiced by various religious denominations.
- Describe the hospice philosophy and method of care.
- List the signs of approaching death.
- Demonstrate the following procedure:
  - Procedure 86 Giving Postmortem Care

VOCABULARY

Learn the meaning and the correct spelling of the following words and phrases:

acceptance	cardiopulmonary	durable power of attor-	no-code order
advance directive	resuscitation (CPR)	ney for health care	postmortem
anger	critical list	harvested	postmortem care
autopsy	denial	hospice care	rigor mortis
bargaining	depression	life-sustaining treatment	Sacrament of the Sick
cardiac arrest	DNR	living will	supportive care
		moribund	terminal

INTRODUCTION

Death is the final stage of life. It may come suddenly, without warning, or it may follow a long period of illness. It sometimes strikes the young but it always awaits the old. Death represents the final journey in the continuum of life. As a nursing assistant, you will be providing care throughout the period of dying and into the after-death (**postmortem**) period. Accepting the idea that death is the natural result of the life process may help you respond to your patient's needs more generously.

The concept of death and dying is handled differently by different people (Figure 32-1). There are many reactions to the diagnosis of a **terminal** (life-ending) illness:

- Some patients may have had time to prepare psychologically for their deaths. They may accept or be resigned to the inevitable.
- Some may actually look forward to relief from the pain and emotional burden of a long illness and await death calmly.
- Some may be fearful or angry and demonstrate moods that swing from outright denial to depression.
- Others may reach out, trying to verbalize feelings and thoughts of an uncertain future.
- In others, despair and anxiety may give way to moments of active hostility or periods of searching, groping questions.

FIGURE 32-1 Each person handles death differently.

None of the reaction states are predictable and no patient falls into one rigid pattern or another. You must accept the patient's behavior with understanding, interpret the patient's very real need for family support, and support the family in meeting their own needs during this adjustment period.

Communication HIGHLIGHT

Health care workers may feel helpless when caring for a dying patient. Remember that active listening is a means of therapeutic communication. Listening to a patient's concerns shows honest and caring regard for the patient. Using touch can also communicate caring and acceptance. When you are at a loss for words, consider these other means of showing the patient that you care. ■

FIVE STAGES OF GRIEF

Dr. Elisabeth Kübler-Ross identified five stages of grief that can occur in the dying patient. They are denial, anger, bargaining, depression, and acceptance (Table 32-1). If there is adequate time and support, some patients may be able to move psychologically through each stage to a point of acceptance of their illness and death.

- **Denial** begins when the person is made aware that he is going to die. He may not accept this information as truth, and may instead deny it. Making long-range plans that are not likely to be fulfilled may indicate that the patient is in the denial stage. Most people with a terminal illness must go through denial before they are able to eventually reach acceptance. This is a necessary and therapeutic stage. Other people should not try to convince the patient of his diagnosis or argue with the person. If denial begins to interfere with the person's adjustment, then professional counseling may be needed.

Clinical Information ALERT

The grieving process begins immediately when someone is diagnosed with a life-threatening or terminal illness. Mourning before someone dies is called *anticipatory grief*. Part of this process involves grieving for past, present, and future losses. Patients and families grieve for their former way of life, recognizing that returning to it will be impossible. Roles and responsibilities within the family change. Illness may change body image. Friends and family may begin to separate themselves from the dying person. This is one way they deal with loss, but it may make the patient feel isolated. Losses are many. Some are very private and personal. Each loss triggers the grieving process, causing feelings of isolation, abandonment, anger, and depression. ■

- **Anger** comes when the patient is no longer able to deny the fact that she is going to die. The patient may blame those around her, including those who are giving care, for her illness. Added stresses, however small, are likely to upset the patient who is in the anger stage (Figure 32-2). Statements such as, "It's all your fault. I should never have come to this hospital," are typical of a patient in the anger stage. Remember, if the patient expresses anger, that she is angry about her diagnosis, not with you personally. Remain calm and avoid saying anything that may make her angrier. If you think the patient is angry about something other than the diagnosis, report this to the nurse so the situation can be remedied.

- **Bargaining** is the stage in the grief process in which the patient attempts to bargain for more time to live. She may ask to be allowed to go home to finish a task before he dies. Trying to make private "deals" with God or her higher power is also common. For example, "If you will let me live another two months, I promise I will try to be a better person." Bargaining frequently involves an important event that the patient has been looking forward to, such as a child's wedding or the birth of a grandchild. The patient in this stage is basically saying, "I know I'm going to die and I'm ready to die, but not just yet." This may be done in private and not stated verbally.

- **Depression** is the fourth stage identified in the grief process. During this stage, the patient comes to a full realization that he will die soon (Figure 32-3). He is saddened by the thought that he will no longer be with family and friends, and by the fact that he may

TABLE 32-1 EMOTIONAL RESPONSES TO DYING

Stages of Grief	Response of the Nursing Assistant
Denial	Reflect patient's statements, but try not to confirm or deny the fact that the patient is dying. **Example:** *"The lab tests can't be right—I don't have cancer." "It must have been difficult for you to learn the results of your tests."*
Anger	Understand the source of the patient's anger. Provide understanding and support. Listen. Try to meet reasonable needs and demands quickly. **Example:** *"This food is terrible—not fit to eat." "Let me see if I can find something that would appeal to you more."*
Bargaining	If it is possible to meet the patient's requests, do so. Listen attentively. **Example:** *"If only God will spare me this, I'll go to church every week." "Would you like a visit from your clergyperson?"*
Depression	Avoid clichés that dismiss the patient's depression ("It could be worse—you could be in more pain"). Be caring and supportive. Let the patient know that it is all right to be depressed. **Example:** *"There just isn't any sense in going on." "I understand you are feeling very depressed."*
Acceptance	Do not assume that, because the patient has accepted death, she or he is unafraid, or that she or he does not need emotional support. Listen attentively and be supportive and caring. **Example:** *"I feel so alone." "I am here with you. Would you like to talk?"*

FIGURE 32-2 Patients may demonstrate feelings of frustration and anger.

FIGURE 32-3 Depression is a normal part of the grieving process.

not have accomplished some goals that he had set for himself. He may also express regrets about not having gone somewhere or done something: "I always promised my wife that we would go to Europe and now we'll never go."

- **Acceptance** is the stage during which a patient understands and accepts the fact that he is going to die (Figure 32-4). During this stage, he may try to complete unfinished business. Having accepted his eventual death, he may also try to help those around him to deal with it, especially family members.

Not all patients progress through these stages in sequential order. Nor does movement from one level to the next mean that the previous level will be completely left behind. Patients sometimes move back and forth between stages several times before completely resolving one stage and moving on to the next. The staff must be aware of

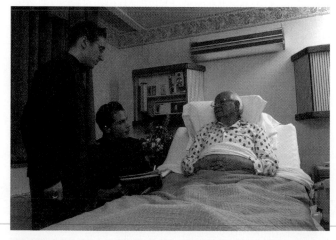

FIGURE 32-4 The patient may strive to complete unfinished business during the acceptance phase of the grieving process.

the possible psychological positions and be able to identify the patient's current reactions. For example, a patient who displays anger one day may be full of optimism and denial the next.

Denial frequently comes first, followed by anger and despair. Frustrated by feelings of helplessness, the person lashes out at those who are nearby. If each of these stages is expressed with some degree of success, the person is then able to move on to a level of grieving, for himself and for loved ones. When all five stages have been passed, it is believed that the patient is better able to accept the termination of life. If there is adequate time and support (Figure 32-5), many patients can be helped to reach a more accepting frame of mind.

The family and staff move through these same stages, but not necessarily at the same time. It is particularly difficult when the patient is in one stage and the family is at another stage.

Some experts believe that grief triggers the fight-or-flight mechanism, similar to when someone is chasing you. It causes the body to be in a state of alarm. These experts believe that some grieving people will not eat because the body is prioritizing for survival. This is one of the reasons that post-funeral meals are part of the death ritual in many cultures. Providing food for the surviving family is a means of offering emotional support. The belief is that survivors need nourishment to replace the nutrients that have been depleted by caregiving and bereavement.

PREPARATION FOR DEATH

The knowledge of impending death comes to the patient directly from the physician or indirectly from the staff. A diagnosis of terminal illness is very difficult to conceal from the patient. The staff may, without realizing it, reveal the information by:

FIGURE 32-5 The support of family and friends is very important to the dying patient.

- Exhibiting false cheerfulness
- Being evasive
- Making fewer visits to the patient's room
- Spending less time with the patient

You must realize that most terminally ill patients do eventually come to accept that death is part of their near future. Keep the following in mind:

- Each patient reacts to this understanding in a unique way.
- How many feelings the patient wishes to share and with whom are very personal decisions.
- You should be available to listen, but do not force the issue.

Upon being told of the terminal diagnosis, the patient may proceed through several stages of emotional adjustment. Initially, the

- Patient may react to the situation by denying the truth
- Patient may refuse all opportunities to discuss his illness with the staff or with family
- Patient's interpersonal relationships with family and staff may become greatly strained
- Patient may become defeated and full of despair, actively expressing a loss of hope

COMMON FEARS

Dying can be a lonely business. We experience various losses throughout life, but when a person is dying, he or she is losing everything—family, friends, pets, and belongings. It is natural to be afraid of the unknown, regardless of religious and spiritual beliefs. Some people do not feel good about how they lived their lives or things they have done. This causes feelings of guilt, grief, and remorse. Common fears associated with dying are:

- Fear of dying alone
- Fear of severe, unrelieved pain
- Fear of inability to finish personal business or manage affairs

Some people feel incomplete because they have failed to achieve all they wanted to do. They may also have a strong desire to do something that is no longer possible in light of their imminent death.

Reactions of Others

In a long-term care facility or other residential setting, other residents will also be upset about a terminal diagnosis or death of another resident. The age group in long-term care experiences many losses of friends and family to death. Each loss reminds residents that they are in the twilight years at the end of life. They must also cope with their own pain and grief. The nursing assistant will provide support and help others cope. In the residential care setting, others will:

- Be sad and grieve over the loss of a good friend
- Reminisce about the person who died
- Want to know how the person died (if they were alone, in pain, etc.)

Encourage others to express their feelings and talk about their sadness, loss, anger, and fear. This helps the grieving person come to grips with his or her own feelings. Be honest and answer questions as completely as possible, without violating confidentiality.

THE PATIENT SELF-DETERMINATION ACT

The Patient Self-Determination Act of 1990 requires health care providers to supply written information about state laws regarding **advance directives**. An advance directive is a document that is put into effect if the patient later becomes unable to make decisions. All health care providers, including hospitals, long-term care facilities, and home health care agencies, must have policies and procedures covering these issues. The patient must be informed of the right to execute an advance directive before or at the time of admission. The patient may choose to execute an advance directive at any time during his or her stay. Likewise, the patient may choose not to execute an advance directive.

Decisions often must be made when a patient is terminally or critically ill. These decisions involve provision of supportive care or life-sustaining treatment. The Patient Self-Determination Act was passed to assure patients and their families that their wishes will be followed. **Supportive care** means that the patient's life will not be artificially prolonged but that the patient will be kept comfortable physically, mentally, and emotionally. Supportive care includes:

- Oxygen to ease breathing if the patient needs it
- Food and fluids that the patient can consume by mouth
- Medications for pain, nausea, anxiety, or other physical or emotional discomforts
- The continuation of physical care such as grooming and hygiene, cleanliness, positioning, and range-of-motion exercises
- Caring and emotional support of staff

All patients deserve supportive care, but for terminally or critically ill patients, supportive care means the absence of life-sustaining treatment. **Life-sustaining treatment** means giving medications and treatments for the purpose of maintaining life. Life-sustaining treatments include all of the items listed under supportive care and may also include:

- Being placed on a ventilator to maintain breathing
- Receiving **cardiopulmonary resuscitation (CPR)** if **cardiac arrest** occurs (the heart and lungs stop functioning)
- Artificial nutrition through a feeding tube or hyperalimentation device

- Blood transfusions
- Surgery
- Radiation therapy
- Chemotherapy
- Other treatments that will maintain life

 Note: Radiation therapy and chemotherapy may also be given to relieve pain, not to extend life.

There are basically two types of advance directives: the living will and the durable power of attorney for health care. The **living will** is a request that death not be artificially postponed if the patient has an incurable, irreversible injury, disease, or illness that the physician judges to be a terminal condition. A living will must be witnessed by two other individuals who do not stand to benefit because of the person's death.

The **durable power of attorney for health care** is a directive that assigns someone else the responsibility for making medical decisions for the patient if the patient becomes unable to do so himself. In most states it must be signed by the *agent* (the person given the durable power of attorney) and by the *principal* (the person appointing the agent). The person designated as the agent may also be called the *proxy* or *health care proxy*. It also must be signed by an adult witness. The durable power of attorney may indicate whether the person:

- Does not want his life to be prolonged and does not want life-sustaining treatment
- Wants his life prolonged and wants life-sustaining treatment to be provided unless the physician believes he is in an irreversible coma
- Wants his life to be prolonged to the greatest extent possible without regard to his condition

The durable power of attorney is one way to ensure that the wishes and rights of an individual will be followed and protected when the person is no longer able to make personal decisions. The health care proxy must make decisions in keeping with the patient's wishes. As a nursing assistant, you must be aware of the patient's status for supportive care or life-sustaining treatment. The person on supportive care will have a **no-code order** or **DNR** (do not resuscitate) order. This means that no extraordinary means, such as CPR to resuscitate the person, will be used to prevent death. This allows a person to die peacefully with maximum dignity. A no-code decision is reached after discussion by the patient with her family and physician. Once made, the no-code decision is entered in the patient's chart. All staff members are made aware of the decision, but it is kept confidential. If the patient changes her mind, the order in the chart is changed.

Witnessing Advance Directives

The nursing assistant must become familiar with facility policies and state laws for witnessing advance directives. In many states, persons who care for the patient are not permitted to witness advance directives. In most states,

Legal ALERT

Health care workers sometimes become confused about the meaning of a living will in which the patient specifies that no heroic procedures are to be undertaken if the patient is in terminal, irreversible condition. If the patient is not known to be in terminal condition, resuscitation will be done (unless otherwise ordered). For example, a 32-year-old patient in good health enters the hospital for a diagnostic procedure that involves the injection of contrast material into the veins. The patient has an allergic reaction to the contrast material and suffers a cardiac arrest. In this case, *CPR would be done*, because the patient is not known to be in terminal condition.

In another instance, an elderly patient enters the hospital for insertion of a central intravenous catheter to be used for pain management as part of terminal care for cancer. The patient is known to have inoperable cancer, as documented by two or more physicians. The patient experiences a complication during the procedure and has a cardiac arrest. In this case, the provisions of the living will would be observed, and *CPR would not be done*.

The person designated as the agent in a durable power of attorney for health care should be familiar with the patient's wishes. The authority for making decisions takes effect only if the patient becomes physically or mentally unable to speak for herself. If the patient subsequently regains the ability to make decisions, the power of attorney and the agent's power are inactivated. Your facility will have a procedure for securing another person, usually a relative, to make decisions on the patient's behalf if she has not designated a durable power of attorney for health care. The durable power of attorney for health care covers only health care decisions, and only for the period of time during which the patient is unable to make decisions. It does not cover management of finances or other areas of the patient's life. ■

Legal ALERT

Your facility may have designations for different levels of emergency care, ranging from comfort care to full advanced life support. Become familiar with the criteria for these levels. Many facilities have ethics committees made up of professionals from many disciplines. The committee meets to review some difficult care situations. ■

caregivers cannot legally be appointed to be the agent (medical decision maker) for a patient unless they are related by blood or marriage.

Withdrawing or Modifying Advance Directives

Patients may withdraw or modify their advance directives at any time. For example, a patient's advance directive states that he wants full life support if his heart and breathing stop. The patient later finds out that he has cancer, and wants only supportive care at the end of life. If a patient informs you of changes that affect the advance directive, notify the nurse promptly.

THE ROLE OF THE NURSING ASSISTANT

As a nursing assistant, you spend much time with the patient. You have a unique opportunity to be a source of strength and comfort. You must behave in a way that instills confidence in both the patient and the patient's family. Developing the proper attitude and approach for this type of situation is not easy. It will come with experience. There are some things to keep in mind:

- Your response should be consistent. It should be guided by the patient's attitude and the care plan.
- You must be open and receptive, because the terminal patient's attitude may change from day to day.
- Make sure you inform the nurse of incidents related to the patient that reflect moods and needs.
- Remember that each person's idea of death and the hereafter differs. You must be open to patients' ideas and not force your own upon them.
- Your own feelings about death and dying influence your ability to care for the dying patient. Honestly explore your feelings by talking about them with others until you can resolve any conflicts you may have. Your acceptance of death as a natural occurrence will enable you to meet patient needs in a realistic manner.

Culture ALERT

The medical system and views about death and dying in the United States are based on Western values, which often differ greatly from those of other cultures. Cultural beliefs and values run deep and usually cannot be changed. People from other cultures have many views about care of the dying person. Many believe the family should care for the patient. Some cultures maintain that the patient should die at home, believing the spirit remains at the place of death and is comforted by the grieving of loved ones. Arab Americans may prefer not to die in a nursing home, whereas African Americans are comfortable using hospitals and nursing homes. Members of the Arab American culture often do not want lifesaving measures. They may not want the family told of the terminal nature of their illness, but want to be told themselves. With some, this is to ensure that their financial affairs are in order. Many Caucasians want the family close, but many prefer that someone other than family take care of them. Hispanics are often concerned with dying a dignified death. ■

- Give your best and most careful nursing care, with special attention to comfort measures such as mouth care and fluid intake.
- You should be quietly empathetic and carry out your duties in a calm, efficient way.

When a patient's condition is critical, the physician will place his name officially on the **critical list**. Then the family and the chaplain will be notified.

Providing for Spiritual Needs

Many people find spiritual faith to be a source of great comfort during difficult times.

- Some religions have specific rituals that are carried out when a person is very ill or dying (Table 32-2). Your role is to cooperate with the patient, family, and clergyperson so that these rituals may be performed in a dignified, caring manner.
- Other religions do not have specific practices, but patients of those religions may spend time in prayer. Allow the patient and family privacy, but let them know you are close by if you are needed.
- Some patients may have no formal religious affiliation. This does not mean they do not have spiritual needs. They may request the services of a clergyperson and not know who to call on. Relay this request to the nurse, because most health care facilities have chaplains to provide the services.

TABLE 32-2 BELIEFS AND PRACTICES RELATED TO DYING AND DEATH FOR MAJOR RELIGIONS

Religion	Autopsy	Organ Donation	Beliefs and Practices
Judaism (Orthodox)	Only in special circumstances	With consultation of rabbi	Visits to the dying are a religious duty.
			Witness must be present if death occurs, to protect family and commit soul to God.
			Torah and Psalms may be read and prayers recited.
			Conversation is kept to a minimum.
			Someone should be with the body after death until burial, usually within 24 hours.
			Body must not be touched 8 to 30 minutes after death.
			Medical personnel should not touch or wash body unless death occurs on Jewish Sabbath; then care may be given by staff wearing gloves.
			Water is removed from the room.
			Mirrors may be covered at family's request.
			Jewish practices and beliefs can be very different from family to family. Asking the patient or family members about their practices is probably best.
			Asking is not offensive, and shows that you care about and respect the patient's and family's wishes.

continues

TABLE 32-2 *CONTINUED*

Religion	Autopsy	Organ Donation	Beliefs and Practices
Hinduism	Permitted	Permitted	Priest ties thread around neck or wrist of deceased and pours water in the mouth. Only family and friends touch body.
Buddhism	Personal preference	Permitted	Buddhist priest is present at death. Last rites are chanted at the bedside.
Islam (Muslim)	Only for medical or legal reasons	Not permitted	Before death, read Koran and pray. Patient confesses sins and asks forgiveness of family. Only family touches or washes body. After death, turn the head towards the right shoulder.
Roman Catholic	Permitted	Permitted	Sacrament of the Sick administered to ill patients, to patients in imminent danger, or shortly after death.
Christian Scientist	Unlikely	Not permitted	No ritual is performed before or after death.
Church of Christ	Permitted	Permitted	No ritual is performed before or after death.
Jehovah's Witness	Only if required by law	Not permitted	No ritual is performed before or after death.
Baptist	Permitted	Permitted	Clergy ministers through counseling and prayers.
Episcopalian	Permitted	Permitted	Last rites are optional.
Lutheran	Permitted	Permitted	Last rites are optional.
Eastern Orthodox Christian	Not encouraged	Not encouraged	Last rites are mandatory and are given by ordained priest.

- Some patients do not believe in any higher spiritual being. This is their right and no one should try to change their feelings.
- Always respect the beliefs or nonbeliefs of any patient. Treat all religious items, such as holy books, medals, and rosaries, with respect.
- When a Catholic patient is ill, a priest may be called for the **Sacrament of the Sick** (Figure 32-6). It is preferable that the family be present and leave the room only while the confession is heard. The practicing Catholic and his family consider it a privilege to have the opportunity for confession. Many patients recover completely, but this hope should not prevent reception of this sacrament if this is the patient's wish.
- A Bible or spiritual reading of the patient's faith, if requested, may be of some spiritual help through this crisis. Be courteous and provide privacy when the patient's clergyperson visits.

Be aware that dying is a lonely business, a journey each person must finish alone. Until the final moment comes, privacy, but not total solitude, should be the guiding rule (Figure 32-7).

It is important to remember the family and other loved ones when a patient is dying. Check the policies of your health care facility and assist in the following actions:

- Allow the family to be with the patient as they desire.
- Allow the family to assist with some of the care, if they wish to do so and the patient does not object; for example, moistening the patient's lips or giving a backrub.
- Inform the family where they can get a cup of coffee or a meal.
- Show the family where they can use a telephone in private.
- If a family member stays during the night, offer a pillow and blanket. Some facilities provide recliners or cots for family members.

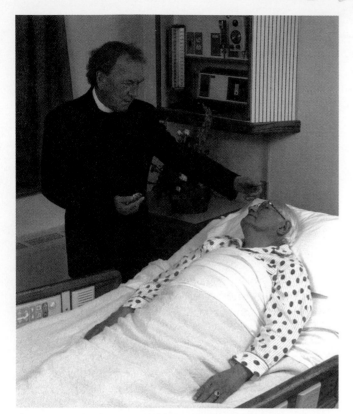

FIGURE 32-6 The Sacrament of the Sick may be administered to Roman Catholics who are gravely ill.

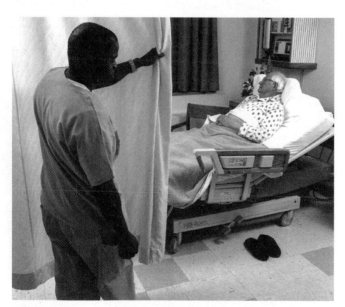

FIGURE 32-7 The dying patient needs privacy, but not total solitude.

• Avoid being judgmental of family members. Remember that each person grieves in his or her own way. The emotions that others see are not necessarily an accurate indication of what the individual is feeling.

HOSPICE CARE

Hospice care has evolved around the philosophy that death is a natural process that should neither be hastened nor delayed and that the dying person should be kept comfortable. **Hospice care** is:

• Provided to terminally ill people with a life expectancy of six months or less
• Involved with direct physical care when needed
• Supportive to both the family and the patient
• Provided in special hospice facilities, in other care facilities, and at home
• Largely carried out by a home health assistant or a nursing assistant under the direction of professional health care providers
• Follow-up bereavement counseling to help survivors accept the death of a loved one
• A program in which volunteers play an important role, making regular personal visits to the patient and family

Hospice care is provided by teams who work in conjunction with the terminally ill person and his family. The team usually consists of a physician, professional nurse, nursing assistant, and other professionals (such as social workers and clergy) as needed and desired.

The goals of hospice care include:

• Control of pain so the individual can remain an active participant in life until death
• Coordinating psychological, spiritual, and social support services for the patient and the family
• Making legal and financial counseling available to the patient and family

Because hospice care is a philosophy, it becomes part of the guide for your actions when caring for the terminally ill. Hospice care is provided as you give your usual care. Some things to keep in mind, however, are:

• Report pain immediately and give close attention to comfort measures.
• Encourage the person to carry out as much self-care as possible.
• Be readily available to listen. Spend as much time with the patient as possible and desired by the patient.
• Get to know the family and be supportive to them.
• Give the same care you would if a terminal diagnosis had not been made.
• Sometimes hospice care may seem to go against everything you have been taught. For example, a patient has bone cancer that is very painful. The patient is expected to die within a few days. Despite high doses of drugs, nurses are having trouble controlling the pain. Moving the patient worsens the pain, so the care plan instructs you to leave the patient on her back, rather than turning her every 2 hours. You know the patient has skin breakdown that will worsen if she is not turned. However, you must follow the care plan

and *not turn* the patient. This shows respect for the patient's needs and supports the quality of her final hours of life.

- Carry out all activities with dignity and respect.

PHYSICAL CHANGES AS DEATH APPROACHES

As death approaches, there are notable physical changes. As these changes occur, report them immediately to the nurse.

- The patient becomes less responsive (Figure 32-8).
- Body functions slow down.
- The patient loses general voluntary and involuntary muscle control.
- The patient may involuntarily void and defecate.
- The jaw tends to drop.
- Breathing becomes irregular and shallow.
- Circulation slows and the extremities become cold. The pulse becomes rapid and progressively weaker.
- Skin pales.
- The eyes stare and do not respond to light.
- Hearing seems to be the last sense to be lost. Do not assume that because death is approaching, the patient can no longer hear. You must be careful what you say.

In the period before death, the patient with a terminal diagnosis needs and receives the same care as the patient who is expected to recover. Attention is paid to physical as well as emotional needs.

As it becomes clear that death will occur very soon, you should call the nurse, who will supervise the care during the final moments of life.

Signs of Death

After death, changes continue to take place in the body. These changes are called **moribund** (dying) changes.

- Pupils become permanently dilated.

- There is no pulse or respiration.
- Heat is gradually lost from the body.
- The patient may urinate, defecate, or release flatus.
- Blood pools in the lowest areas of the body, giving a purplish discoloration to those areas.
- Within 2 to 4 hours, body rigidity, called **rigor mortis**, develops.
- Unless embalmed within 24 hours, there is indication of progressive protein breakdown.
- When circulation stops, the body begins to pull blood into the lowest areas of the body. This process can begin within 20 minutes of death. Over time, this will result in a stained appearance on the back of the body if the patient is in the supine position. To reduce the risk of staining about the head and neck, elevate the head of the bed 30°, in the semi-Fowler's position. Some facilities do not use ties in the morgue pack to position the body. Follow your facility policies. If used, tie them loosely. If the ties are too tight, they may also cause permanent marks on the body.

POSTMORTEM CARE

The patient's body should be treated with respect at all times. Before death occurs, the limbs should be straightened and the head elevated on a pillow. The body should be cleaned by gently washing it with warm water. Discharges must be washed off and wiped away.

Care of the body after death is called **postmortem care** (Figure 32-9). This may be your responsibility. You may find it easier if you ask a coworker to assist.

- Use gloves when giving postmortem care. The body may continue to be infectious following death.
- Treat the body with the same dignity you would a living person.
- Some facilities prefer to have the patient left alone until mortuary staff arrive. Your responsibility will be only to prepare the body for viewing by the family.

FIGURE 32-8 The patient becomes less responsive and body functions slow down as death approaches.

FIGURE 32-9 Postmortem care is given after death occurs.

FIGURE 32-10 Supplies needed for postmortem care

- Check the hospital procedure manual before proceeding with postmortem care.

The contents of morgue kits vary (Figure 32-10), but they usually include:

- A shroud of some kind (paper or cloth)
- A clean gown
- Tags used to identify the body
- Gauze squares for padding
- Safety pins

One procedure for postmortem care is described in Procedure 86. See also Figures 32-11A through 32-11E for instructions on using a shroud.

ORGAN DONATIONS

Some people desire to share their organs with others after death. They use an organ donor card that is part of the driver's license. The card specifies if particular organs or the whole body is being donated. At times, because of a special need, the patient's family is asked for permission so

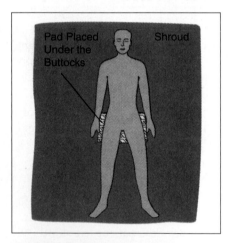

FIGURE 32-11A Position the shroud under the deceased with the pad under the buttocks.

FIGURE 32-11B Apply the chin strap as shown to keep the mouth closed.

FIGURE 32-11C Fasten the wrists and ankles together with the ties. Use gauze sponges under the ties so they do not make marks on the skin.

FIGURE 32-11D Fill out and attach four identification tags. Place one tag on the:
- right big toe or right ankle
- outside of the shroud
- patient's personal belongings (securely wrapped)
- compartment in the morgue

FIGURE 32-11E Fold the shroud around the body as shown. Use the long ties or tape to hold the shroud closed. Fasten another tag to the outside of the shroud.

PROCEDURE

86

GIVING POSTMORTEM CARE

1. Carry out initial procedure actions.

2. Assemble equipment:
   - Shroud or clean sheet
   - Basin with warm water
   - Washcloth
   - Towels
   - Disposable gloves
   - Identification tags
   - Cotton
   - Bandages
   - Pads as needed

3. Put on disposable gloves.

4. Remove all appliances, tubing, and used articles, if instructed to do so.

5. Work quickly and quietly; maintain an attitude of respect.

6. With the bed flat, place the body on the back, with head and shoulders elevated on a pillow.
   a. Close the eyes by grasping the eyelashes, gently pulling the eyelids down, and holding shut for a few seconds.
   b. Replace dentures in the patient's mouth, if used or clean the dentures and place them in a denture cup. Make sure they are sent to the funeral home with the body. Replace an artificial eye, if used.
   c. The jaw may have to be secured with light bandaging.
   d. Pad beneath the bandage. Handle the body gently, as tight bandaging or undue pressure from your hands may leave marks.
   e. Straighten the arms and legs and place the arms at the sides.

7. Bathe as necessary. Remove any soiled dressings and replace with clean ones. Groom hair.

8. Place a disposable pad underneath the buttocks. If the family is to view the body:
   a. Put a clean hospital gown on the patient.
   b. Cover the body to the shoulders with a sheet.
   c. Remove disposable gloves and wash your hands.
   d. Make sure the room is neat.
   e. Adjust the lights to a subdued level.
   f. Provide chairs for the family.
   g. Allow the family to visit in private.

9. Return to the patient's room after the family leaves. Wash your hands and put on disposable gloves.

10. Collect all belongings and make a list. Wrap properly and label. Valuables remain in the hospital safe until they are signed for by a relative.

11. Fill out the identification cards or tags in the morgue kit and attach them as follows:
    a. Place one card on the right ankle or right great toe.
    b. Attach one card to the bag with the patient's valuables.

12. Put the shroud on the patient and attach an identification card or tag to the outside.

13. Transport the body to the morgue.
    a. Call an elevator to the floor and keep it empty.
    b. Close patient corridor doors.
    c. Empty the corridor.
    d. With an assistant, place the body on a gurney.
    e. Keep the patient supine, with a rubber head elevator under the neck.
    f. Cover the body with a sheet.
    g. Remove disposable gloves and discard according to facility policy. Wash your hands.
    h. Take the body to the morgue.
    i. Attach one identification card or tag to the morgue compartment.

that certain body organs may be removed and saved or removed and **harvested** (reused). Such a request is made by the physician or the nurse, never by the nursing assistant.

If the patient or family make their wishes known to you without your asking, it is important to report this to the nurse.

POSTMORTEM EXAMINATION (AUTOPSY)

In certain situations, the law requires a medical postmortem examination or **autopsy** of the body. At other times, the family and physician may desire such an examination to understand the reasons for the patient's death.

It is possible that information learned from the examination can be used to protect other family members. As in the case of organ donations, however, requesting family permission for an autopsy is not part of the nursing assistant's responsibilities. The nursing assistant is responsible for being supportive of the family and the decision that has been made.

REVIEW

A. True/False.

Mark the following true or false by circling T or F.

1. T F All people respond to a terminal diagnosis in the same way.

2. T F Hearing is the first sense to be lost in the dying patient.

3. T F Death is the final stage of life.

4. T F The nursing assistant should call the physician when the patient dies.

5. T F Sometimes the staff, without realizing it, allow the patient to learn of a terminal diagnosis through their behavior.

6. T F The dying patient receives the same complete care that would be given to someone who is expected to recover.

7. T F Pain relief is one of the main goals of hospice care.

8. T F Permanent dilation of the pupils is a moribund sign.

9. T F Hospice-type care is only possible in the acute care facility.

10. T F The dying person needs a great deal of understanding and realistic support.

B. Matching.

Choose the correct word from Column II to match each phrase or statement in Column I.

Column I

11. _____ refusal to accept reality

12. _____ after death

13. _____ covering for the body after death

14. _____ stiffening of the body after death

15. _____ dying

Column II

a. moribund

b. rigor mortis

c. denial

d. hospice

e. postmortem

f. shroud

g. anger

C. Multiple Choice.

Select the one best answer for each of the following.

16. Organs from a dead person may be
    a. harvested without permission.
    b. obtained on an as-needed basis.
    c. donated with permission of the family at the time of death.
    d. donated only if listed in the patient's will.

17. Postmortem examinations
    a. are not done in hospitals.
    b. may provide valuable information.
    c. are arranged by the nursing assistant.
    d. are forbidden by law.

18. As death approaches, changes include
    a. constriction of the pupils.
    b. muscle spasm.
    c. slowing of circulation.
    d. skin developing yellow hue.

19. Moribund changes include
    a. permanent pupil constriction.
    b. increased body heat.
    c. pulse and respiration increase.
    d. blood pooling in the lower body.

20. A no-code order on a patient's chart means
    a. to start CPR immediately.
    b. do not resuscitate.
    c. begin postmortem care at once.
    d. to call the family if the patient seems in danger of dying.

D. Nursing Assistant Challenge.

Mrs. Goldstein is a patient in the hospital where you work. She was diagnosed with cancer of the ovaries two years ago. She has been at home but is admitted periodically for chemotherapy. You have taken care of her each time she has been in the hospital. The first time was right after Mrs. Goldstein was diagnosed. She seemed happy and made frequent comments like, "I'm glad I don't have cancer." The last time she was a patient, she refused to follow the suggestions of the nursing staff, but did allow her chemotherapy to be administered. When her family visited, she was irritated and hostile toward them. This time, she is agreeable with the staff on all matters and seems genuinely happy to see her family. She has told you that if she can live to see her granddaughter get married in two months, she will become a volunteer at the hospital so she can help other patients. She is not receiving chemotherapy anymore because the cancer is in an advanced stage. She is hospitalized for pain management now but plans to go home for hospice care. Consider these questions about Mrs. Goldstein:

21. Do you think she is preparing for her death?

22. How would you describe the stages of dying she has been experiencing?

23. What response is appropriate to her comments about the wedding?

24. Do you think hospice care will benefit Mrs. Goldstein? Give reasons for your answer.

25. Mrs. Goldstein is Jewish. What considerations must you give to her postmortem care?

Other Health Care Settings

UNIT 33

Care of the Elderly and Chronically Ill

OBJECTIVES

After completing this unit, you will be able to:
- Spell and define terms.
- List the federal requirements for nursing assistants working in long-term care facilities.
- Identify the expected changes of aging.
- Identify residents who are at risk of malnutrition and list measures to promote adequate food intake.
- Explain why elderly individuals are at risk of dehydration and list nursing assistant actions to prevent dehydration.

- List the actions a nursing assistant can take to prevent infections in the long-term care facility.
- Define delirium. List potential causes and signs and symptoms of delirium to report.
- Describe actions to use when working with residents who have dementia.
- Describe the management of wandering residents.

VOCABULARY

Learn the meaning and the correct spelling of the following words and phrases:

Alzheimer's disease	dementia	hand-over-hand	reminiscing
animal-assisted therapy	diverticula	technique	resident
assisted living	diverticulitis	intermediate care	sepsis
catastrophic reaction	diverticulosis	long-term care	skilled care
chronologic	eloping	music therapy	subacute care
debilitating	flatulence	pigmentation	sundowning
delirium		reality orientation (RO)	validation therapy

INTRODUCTION

Many individuals require continuing health care (Figure 33-1). These individuals are frequently elderly. This is because as people age, their risk of acquiring a chronic disease increases. A young person may also require continuing care for a chronic illness or severe injury. Persons of any age who are chronically ill or severely injured may require **long-term care**. This care is provided either in the patient's home or in a long-term care facility. This unit

provides information about caring for the elderly and working in a long-term care facility. Units 34 and 35 will teach you about home care.

Nursing assistants are valuable members of the health care team in these facilities (Figure 33-2). The skills you use in acute care facilities, such as hospitals, are also used in long-term care facilities. There are some changes in the application of these skills because of the differences between long-term and acute care.

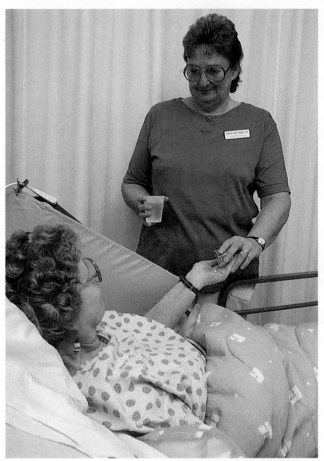

FIGURE 33-1 People of all ages need continuing health care.

FIGURE 33-2 Nursing assistants are valuable caregivers in long-term care facilities.

TYPES OF LONG-TERM CARE FACILITIES

Many types of facilities provide health care for persons with ongoing medical problems:

- **Assisted living** is designed for persons who need minimal assistance. The assisted living residence does not provide medical or nursing care. Residents receive daily supervision or assistance with activities of daily living and instrumental activities of daily living. The facility also coordinates services with outside agencies, and monitors the activities of the residents to ensure their health, safety, and well-being.

- **Intermediate care** is available for people who have health problems that are stable and who need assistance with activities of daily living. These facilities are designed for individuals with chronic conditions who are unable to live independently, but do not need constant care. Such a facility provides supportive care and nursing supervision under medical direction 24 hours per day, but not continuous nursing care.

- **Skilled care** facilities are licensed to provide care to persons with chronic health problems or who require specialized nursing care. Skilled nursing facilities provide the most intensive level of care on the residential care continuum. Residents of these facilities have complex medical care or rehabilitation demands. Some are chronically ill and can no longer live independently.

Some skilled care facilities have units called **subacute care**. The subacute care unit may provide services to persons who need rehabilitation, special cancer treatments, wound care, or pain management. Subacute care is discussed in Unit 36. Subacute care units may also be located in some hospitals.

Long-term care facilities used to be called *nursing homes*. The long-term care facilities of today bear little resemblance to those of the past. Employees must participate in staff development to maintain and update the knowledge and skills that are required to meet the needs of consumers.

Some long-term care facilities specialize in the care of people with a specific diagnosis or unusual care needs. Some are licensed to care only for children. The majority care for adults with various diagnoses and problems.

One important issue facing our country today is the financing of long-term health care. Few hospital insurance policies cover expenses of a resident in a long-term care facility. Insurance specifically for long-term care is now available. People who pay for care from private funds may find that their money is soon used up.

Medicaid is a government reimbursement system through which the federal government issues money to the states. The states determine how to distribute the money to health care facilities. These funds are used for the care of people who have no money of their own.

Medicare is another government program that partially pays for health care for persons over the age of 65 or who are permanently disabled. However, Medicare covers only limited long-term care expenses.

These funds are available only to facilities that participate in the Medicaid and Medicare programs.

LEGISLATION AFFECTING LONG-TERM CARE

Federal legislation has mandated improvements in the quality of long-term care. This legislation is called the Nursing Home Reform Act. It is the result of the Omnibus Budget Reconciliation Act of 1987 (OBRA). Each state is responsible for implementing this legislation.

The OBRA regulations require facilities to assist residents to attain and maintain the highest level of mental, physical, and psychosocial well-being possible in their individual circumstances. (People living in long-term care facilities are usually called **residents**.) Care must be provided in a home-like environment.

Much of the OBRA content affects nursing assistants directly or indirectly:

- OBRA requires all nursing assistants working in long-term care to complete a course of at least 75 clock hours. The course must be approved by the state agency appointed to oversee OBRA regulations. Many states require more than the minimum of 75 hours.
- After completing the course, written and manual (skills) competency tests must be passed. The tests may be taken three times.
- Nursing assistants must complete specific hours of in-service education (12 hours) per year (Figure 33-3). (Some states require more.)
- Nursing assistants who are not employed for 24 months must repeat the course or competency tests.

Federal regulations specify the content that must be included in a nursing assistant course:

- Residents' rights
- Communication and interpersonal skills
- Infection control

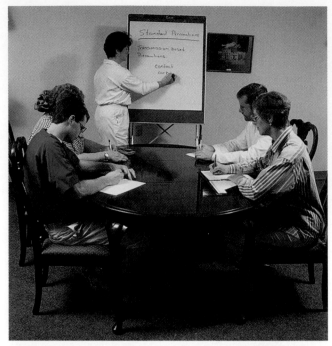

FIGURE 33-3 Nursing assistants working in long-term care facilities must complete at least 12 hours of in-service education each year.

- Safety and emergency procedures
- Basic nursing skills
- Personal care skills
- Mental health and social service needs
- Care of residents with Alzheimer's disease or other dementias
- Basic restorative services

These topics are covered in other units of this textbook. This unit provides specific information about long-term care and OBRA requirements.

ROLE OF THE NURSING ASSISTANT IN A SKILLED CARE FACILITY

As in the acute care facility, the nursing assistant carries out the procedures as taught, assisting in the health care of residents under the direct supervision of a nurse. Basic physical care as well as special procedures are done to help residents reach their maximum degree of well-being.

To be successful in this setting, you must:

- Be patient and caring
- Understand the character of the older age group
- Be able to care for persons who may be your own age and have chronic illnesses
- Be comfortable with the thought of your own aging
- Have the stamina to provide the assistance needed by residents

Legal ALERT

OBRA nursing assistant requirements apply only to long-term care facilities, including those in a hospital, such as the skilled nursing unit. The federal requirements do not apply to acute care hospitals, although many have voluntarily adopted the nursing assistant education as the minimum entry standard for employment. ∎

- Be able to derive satisfaction from being part of slow progress and small, if any, gains
- Have a sense of humor
- Be able to communicate effectively (Figure 33-4)

These attributes are important in any health setting, but in the long-term care facility they are essential.

FIGURE 33-4 Persons working in long-term care must have excellent communication skills.

Many residents will remain under your care for long periods of time, even for years. You will develop relationships that become important to both caregiver and care receiver. In those circumstances, communications take on greater importance. Greater significance may be attached to the attention to care or even the way thoughts are expressed in words. Thus, the long-term caregiver is a *very special person* who works in an important area of health care.

Nursing assistants provide approximately 75% to 80% of the care given in long-term care facilities. Because of this close contact, they come to know their assigned residents well. They know if a resident's condition or behavior is different from normal. When they are providing care, they are the eyes and ears of the nurses, who depend on them to report important changes, findings, and observations.

Nursing is both an art and a science. The science is doing tasks in the way you were taught. Each step of the procedures you do has a scientific rationale that is supported by nursing research. However, a robot could be programmed to be an efficient caregiver. This is why the art of nursing is so important. Being caring and compassionate in doing your assigned tasks is the art. Committed career nursing assistants are skilled in both. There are many demands on your time. Take a deep breath and avoid becoming overwhelmed. Never get so busy with technical tasks that you forget the caring and compassion. This is as important, or even more important, than the science, because it humanizes the care you give. As you gain experience, you will find ways to balance the art and science so you are organized and efficient, while also being caring and compassionate. This is the essence of nursing assistant care.

EFFECTS OF AGING

Many residents in the long-term facility are advanced in age and have one or more chronic, somewhat **debilitating** (weakening) conditions. Some are mentally alert. Others are confused and disoriented.

Some features of aging are characteristic of most elderly residents. Do not expect every resident to exhibit the same characteristics at the same **chronologic** (year) age. Remember that aging is a natural, progressive process that begins at birth and extends to death. Remember also that every resident is unique and must be treated with dignity and respect.

Physical Changes in Aging

Some investigators believe we are born with a biological time clock. This clock is programmed for a specific life span, barring accidents and disease. As we move toward old age, changes that have been taking place gradually become more evident. For example, the elderly person:

- May lose vitality.
- May sleep less at night.
- May benefit from rest periods during the day.

Age-Appropriate Care ALERT

Consider other factors that may affect care. For example:

- An older patient may assume that certain problems are a normal part of aging and not mention them.
- An older patient may not mention a change in his condition, such as an increase in pain, because he is afraid of what the change means, including loss of independence, worsening medical problems,

- Stores less fluid in body tissue and is apt to become dehydrated. This results in a loss of elasticity and resiliency in tissues.
- Has fibrous tissue changes. These decrease the tone, mass, and strength of skeletal and smooth muscle.
- Has secretory and endocrine cells that become less functional and reduced nerve sensitivity.

Certain changes occur in every body system. These are listed in Table 33-1. They do not necessarily occur at the same rate in each system.

SPIRITUAL NEEDS

Long-term care facility residents often have many spiritual needs. Finding a way to meet these needs is very important to residents' well-being. Many depend on spirituality

TABLE 33-1 PHYSICAL CHANGES OF AGING

Body System	Physical Changes
Integumentary	• Hair loses color and becomes thinner • Skin dries, becomes less elastic; wrinkles develop • Skin is fragile and tears easily • Bruises easily (senile purpura common) • Reduced blood flow in vessels that nourish the skin results in delayed healing • Fingernails and toenails thicken • Sweat glands do not excrete perspiration as readily • Oil glands do not secrete as much oil • There is increased sensitivity to cold • Skin discolorations (age spots) become more common • Blood supply to the feet and legs is reduced, increasing the risk of injury and ulcers, and sensations of cold
Nervous	• Tasks involving speed, balance, coordination, and fine motor activities take longer because of slowed transmission of nerve impulses • Balance and coordination problems result from deterioration in the nerve terminals that provide information to the brain about body movement and position • Temperature regulation is less effective • Deep sleep is shortened; the person awakens more during the night • Brain cells are lost, but intelligence remains intact unless disease is present • Decreased sensitivity of nerve receptors in skin (heat, cold, pain, pressure) • Risk of injury increases because of decreased ability to feel pressure and temperature changes • Decreased blood flow to the brain, which may result in mental confusion and memory loss
Sensory	• More difficult to see close objects • Night vision may decrease • Cataracts (clouding of the lens of the eye) are more common

continues

TABLE 33-1 *CONTINUED*

Body System	Physical Changes
Sensory, *continued*	• Dryness and itching of the eyes may result from decreased secretion of fluids • Side vision and depth perception diminish • Hearing diminishes in most elderly persons • Smell receptors and taste buds become less sensitive, so foods have less taste
Musculoskeletal	• Loss of elasticity of muscles and decrease in size of muscle mass result in reduced strength, flexibility, endurance, muscle tone, and delayed reaction time • Slower movements • Bones lose minerals, become brittle, and break more easily; arthritis and osteoporosis are common • Spine becomes less stable and flexible, increasing the risk of injury • Posture may become slumped because of weakness in back muscles • Degenerative changes in the joints result in limited movement, stiffness, and pain
Respiratory	• Lung capacity decreases as a result of muscular rigidity in the lungs • Coughing is less effective; this results in pooling of secretions and fluid in the lungs, increasing the risk of infection and choking • Shortness of breath on exertion, as a result of aging changes in the lungs • Gas exchange in the lungs is less effective, resulting in decreased oxygenation
Urinary	• Kidneys decrease in size • Urine production is less efficient • Bladder capacity decreases, increasing the frequency of urination • Kidney function increases at rest, causing increased urination at night • Bladder muscles weaken, causing leaking of urine or inability to empty the bladder completely; complete emptying of bladder becomes more difficult • Enlargement of the prostate gland in the male, causing frequency of urination, dribbling, urinary obstruction, and urinary retention
Digestive	• Saliva production in the mouth decreases, causing difficulty with swallowing and digestion of starches, and increasing risk of tooth decay • Tastebuds on the tongue decrease, beginning with sweet and salt; changes in tastebuds may result in appetite changes and increase in condiment use • Gag reflex is less effective, increasing the risk of choking and aspiration • Movement of food into the stomach through the esophagus is slower • Food in the stomach is digested slower, so food remains there longer before moving to the small intestine • Flatulence increases • Indigestion and slower absorption of fat result from a decrease in digestive enzymes • Food movement through the large intestine is slower, resulting in constipation
Cardiovascular	• Heart rate slows, causing a slower pulse and less efficient circulation. This results in decreased energy and a slower response, causing the individual to tire easily • Blood vessels lose elasticity and develop calcium deposits, causing vessels to narrow • Blood pressure increases because of changes to the blood vessel walls • Heart rate takes longer to return to normal after exercise • Veins enlarge, causing blood vessels close to the skin surface to become more prominent • Heart may not pump as efficiently, leading to decreased cardiac output and circulation

continues

TABLE 33-1 *CONTINUED*

Body System	Physical Changes
Endocrine	• Decrease in levels of estrogen, progesterone • Hot flashes, nervous feelings • Higher levels of parathormone and thyroid-stimulating hormone • Delayed release of insulin, increasing blood sugar level; incidence of diabetes increases greatly with age • Metabolism rate and body functions slow, reducing the amount of calories needed for the body to function normally. This increases the risk of overweight and obesity
Reproductive	*Females:* • Fewer female hormones are produced • Ovulation and menstrual cycle cease • Vaginal walls are thinner and drier • Vagina becomes shorter and narrower • Breast tissue decreases and the muscles supporting the breasts weaken *Males:* • Scrotum less firm • Prostate gland may enlarge • Male hormones (testosterone) begin to decrease at about age 50 at the rate of approximately 1% per year • As hormone production decreases, testes become smaller and sperm count is lower • More time required for an erection

Age-Appropriate Care ALERT

You may find that caring for elderly individuals is time-consuming. Aging changes may cause the person to move more slowly than she did previously. Do not complete tasks that residents can do themselves, just for the sake of saving time. Avoid assuming that the resident cannot do something because of physical or mental problems related to aging. Test her ability without making assumptions. Be patient and encourage independence, according to the care plan. ∎

and religion to help them cope with the many losses they experience. Losses common to long-term care facility residents are:

• Loss of home, belongings, and beloved pets
• Loss of independence
• Loss of those they love, such as friends and family members, through separation and death
• Loss of health and/or mental ability

The residents must cope with losses, find out what each loss means to them, and incorporate the loss into daily life. Residents have the spiritual need to:

• Love and be loved unconditionally
• Help or serve others
• Maintain and validate their relationship with their higher power
• Feel that they have a daily relationship with their higher power
• Engage in spiritual or religious behaviors and activities
• Have purpose, meaning, and hope in their daily lives
• Transcend their circumstances
• Have continuity in their lives
• Maintain personal dignity, a sense of worth, and self-esteem
• Have a support system or mechanism for dealing with loss or coping with problems
• Have a constructive way of managing and expressing anger and doubt
• Forgive others and be forgiven
• Be thankful for what they have
• Conduct a life review
• Prepare for their own death

NUTRITIONAL NEEDS

Malnutrition is a problem for the aged because the older person may develop an apathy toward food that becomes progressive. Malnutrition can and does occur in long-term care facility residents, despite the fact that a balanced diet is served and nutritional supplements are available. Factors that contribute to lack of appetite are:

- Decreased activity
- Inadequate teeth
- Bad dentures
- Decreased saliva
- Diminished smell and taste
- Poor oral hygiene
- Eating alone

The diet for the elderly person should:

- Be easy to chew and digest.
- Contain decreased amounts of refined sugars, fats, and cholesterol.
- Have adequate proteins and vitamins to provide for best bodily function and repair.
- Have many complex carbohydrates, found in fruits, vegetables, and grains (Figure 33-5). These foods are also good sources of vitamins and minerals, which tend to be deficient in the elderly diet.
- Be monitored for weight control. Obesity is a major nutritional problem among the elderly and those who are inactive. The excess weight increases the stress of existing conditions. Calories are generally limited to about 2,000 calories for the average woman and 2,400 to 2,500 calories for the average man.

Because of loss of muscle tone, three intestinal problems are commonly seen:

- Constipation—difficulty in eliminating solid waste
- **Flatulence**—gas production

- **Diverticulosis**—small pockets (**diverticula**) of weakened intestinal wall

Dietary adjustments can help reduce these problems.

- Soft bulk foods, such as whole-grain cereals and fruits and vegetables, are helpful in overcoming constipation.
- Skins and seeds should be avoided to prevent **diverticulitis**, which is an inflammation of the diverticula.

The presentation and service of food are important in stimulating appetites. Keep in mind the following:

- Several smaller meals seem to be more easily tolerated than three large meals.
- Residents should be allowed to feed themselves as much as possible. You may assist by cutting up the food into bite-sized pieces. Even if you must do most of the feeding, allow the resident to participate as much as possible.
- Fruit and vegetable juices, eggnogs, and soups can serve the dual purpose of providing both nourishment and fluids.

Nursing Assistant Actions

Mealtime is a very busy time in the long-term care facility, especially on the day shift, when two meals are served. Do not get so busy that you overlook residents who are having difficulty or who are not eating. Residents who are at greatest risk of malnutrition and unintentional weight loss are those who:

- Need help eating and drinking (Figure 33-6)
- Eat less than half their meals and/or planned snacks
- Have mouth pain
- Have no dentures, or have dentures that do not fit correctly
- Have difficulty chewing or swallowing
- Have difficulty getting utensils or glasses to the mouth
- Cough or choke while eating
- Are sad, have crying spells, or are withdrawn from others

FIGURE 33-5 Elderly people require complex carbohydrates for a healthy diet. (From "How to Eat for Good Health," courtesy of National Dairy Council)

FIGURE 33-6 Assisting residents with meals helps prevent weight loss and malnutrition.

- Are confused, wander, or pace
- Have diabetes, lung disease, cancer, HIV, or other chronic diseases

To increase food intake and prevent weight loss and malnutrition, create a pleasant, positive dining atmosphere for residents. Be aware of each resident's self-feeding ability and changes in eating patterns. Report your observations and changes in residents' conditions and appetite to the nurse. You should also:

- Provide oral care before meals.
- Position residents correctly for feeding.
- Honor food preferences, likes, and dislikes.
- Offer substitutes according to facility policy.
- Serve meals promptly so foods are at the proper temperature; check foods by dropping a small amount on your wrist (Figure 33-7).
- Offer a variety of foods and beverages.
- Help residents who are having trouble feeding themselves.
- Provide adaptive utensils and dishes, as ordered (Figure 33-8).
- Notify nursing staff if a resident has difficulty feeding himself, eating, or using utensils.
- Prompt and encourage residents to eat.

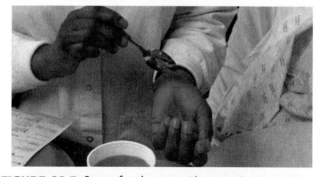

FIGURE 33-7 Serve foods promptly to maintain temperature. Check hot food temperature by dropping a small amount on your wrist.

FIGURE 33-8 Adaptive utensils enable residents with physical problems to feed themselves.

- Allow enough time for residents to finish eating; avoid rushing.
- Reheat cold food items, if necessary.
- Ask what's wrong if a resident's appetite decreases, or she seems sad.
- Accurately record the resident's intake at each meal.
- Assist and prompt residents to consume planned, ordered snacks and supplements.

Residents Receiving Tube Feedings

Tube feedings are common treatments in the long-term care facility. Residents receiving tube feedings are also at nutritional risk. Their medical needs sometimes change, and tube-feeding formula and fluid orders must be adjusted to keep up with their bodies' demands. Signs and symptoms that a resident is at risk for or experiencing tube-feeding complications are:

- Nausea
- Vomiting
- Diarrhea
- Swollen stomach
- Constipation
- Excessive flatus, cramping
- Pain, redness, heat, swelling, crusting, or fluid oozing from the site where the feeding tube enters the body
- Cough
- Wet breathing
- Feeling that something is caught in the throat

Infection Control ALERT

Reflux is the regurgitation of stomach contents back into the esophagus. When this occurs, the stomach contents can be aspirated into the trachea. If the patient is NPO, he or she will also have a dry mouth and fewer automatic swallows. This occurs in patients who are fed by tube, as well as those who do not eat regulary. People believe that those who do not eat frequently need less oral care. In fact, the reverse is true. The aspiration causes a burning pain, and the patient may complain of an acid taste. If the fluid enters the lungs, it can cause pneumonia. Patients receiving tube feeding are prone to reflux, which causes discomfort and the potential for aspiration. Because of this, proper positioning is very important. ■

FIGURE 33-9 Keep the head of the bed elevated at least 30° to 45° when the tube feeding is running, and for at least an hour after, to prevent reflux and choking.

- Complaints of dryness or discomfort in the mouth or throat
- Pulling at or removing the feeding tube

Nursing assistant actions to take when residents are at risk of tube-feeding complications are:

- Keep the head of the bed elevated 30° to 45° any time the tube feeding is running (Figure 33-9), and for one hour after feeding is completed.
- Provide frequent oral care.
- Follow the nurse's instructions and care plan for care of the skin around the feeding tube.
- Move the resident carefully and position him to avoid tension or traction on the tube.
- Make sure that the tube is not kinked or obstructed.
- Give the resident something to hold if she is pulling on the feeding tube; notify the nurse promptly.
- Turn the resident on the side if coughing or choking.
- Report observations and warning signs to the nurse promptly.

HYDRATION NEEDS

Like malnutrition, dehydration can and does occur in long-term care facility residents. This is partially due to decreased thirst in the elderly. Some residents deliberately avoid fluids because they fear incontinence. Some residents do not like to drink water, but willingly accept other liquids when provided. The majority of residents who become dehydrated do so because of medical illness and the physical or mental inability to ask for liquids; many cannot reach for or hold the cup, pour from the pitcher, or drink from a straw without assistance. Extra fluid is needed by all residents in very hot weather. Dehydration can be a very serious condition in the elderly, causing delirium and other complications. Residents who

are becoming dehydrated or are at high risk for dehydration are those who:

- Drink less than 6 cups of liquid a day
- Have dry mouth
- Have cracked lips
- Have sunken eyes
- Have dark urine
- Need help drinking from a glass
- Have trouble swallowing liquids
- Have diarrhea, vomiting, or fever
- Are mentally confused
- Are weak or tired
- Are lethargic and have difficulty staying awake

Nursing Assistant Actions

Nursing assistant actions to prevent dehydration are:

- Offer the resident a drink each time you enter the room; set a goal, such as 2 to 4 ounces of liquid each time.
- Drink with the resident, if permitted.
- Provide fluids the resident likes, as permitted on the diet.
- Make sure that fresh water is available (Figure 33-10), that the resident can reach it, and that the pitcher and cup are light enough to hold.
- Provide physical assistance to pour and consume fluids, as needed.
- Offer ice chips, if permitted.
- Follow all swallowing precautions listed on the care plan.

FIGURE 33-10
Provide fresh water frequently, and assist residents with cups and pitchers, if needed.

- Alternate liquids with solids when feeding meals.
- Encourage the resident to attend activities involving food and fluids.
- Accurately monitor and record intake and output, when ordered.
- Promptly notify the nurse of your observations.

PREVENTING INFECTIONS IN RESIDENTS

There are no additional or special infection control techniques in long-term facilities. Section 4 provides instruction on all infection control procedures performed in nursing homes. Effective and frequent handwashing is the best method of preventing the spread of disease from resident to resident, staff person to resident, or resident to staff person. Standard precautions should be implemented in the care of all persons when contact with blood, body fluids, secretions, excretions, mucous membranes, or non-intact skin is anticipated. Isolation techniques are used for residents with known infectious diseases.

It is important to follow these procedures because it is easy for elderly people to get infections. There are a number of reasons for this:

- Body changes due to aging make older people more susceptible to infection. The skin offers less protection because of its fragility. Any break in the skin, such as a pressure sore or skin tear, can quickly become infected.
- Changes in the urinary system cause the bladder to empty less efficiently. Urine left in the bladder contributes to urinary tract infections.
- The ability to cough and raise secretions is reduced. As a result, there is decreased ability to get rid of bacteria from the lungs.
- Elderly people do not always eat well and may be undernourished.
- Elderly people have less resistance to disease because the immune system becomes less effective with age.
- Resistance to disease is reduced when residents have several chronic health problems.
- The sense of thirst is diminished by aging, and elderly individuals frequently do not take in sufficient fluids.

The elderly do not readily show signs of infection. This means they may be sick for some time before you recognize the problem.

- The elderly do not always develop a fever with an infection. The average temperature for an older person may be one or two degrees less than that of a younger person. Therefore, average temperature may represent an increase or fever.
- The elderly do not readily develop signs of inflammatory response. A skin infection usually shows redness, swelling, heat, and pain. These signs may be missing or delayed in the elderly person.

- The elderly do not necessarily have an increase in the white blood cell count. This is usually a sign of infection but is often absent in the elderly.
- Elderly people do not cough as frequently when they have respiratory tract infections.
- Residents who are disoriented may not comprehend or be able to communicate feelings of pain or nausea.

The elderly are also more likely to develop serious complications from infections. A simple urinary tract infection can result in *bacteremia* (blood infection), causing the resident to become acutely ill. **Sepsis** (presence of pus-forming and other pathogens or their toxins in the blood) is also a serious complication of infection in the elderly. Rather than developing a fever, residents with sepsis often become hypothermic (Unit 27). Since elderly persons normally have a lower temperature than younger individuals, the definition of hypothermia (below 95°F) is probably not entirely accurate for this age group. A better definition may be that the elderly person *is cold relative to his or her baseline temperature*. Many elderly persons become hypothermic with sepsis and overwhelming infection, so monitor residents with abnormally low body temperature closely, and notify the nurse promptly of an abnormally low body temperature in an elderly person. Sepsis and some infections can be fatal to a person who has little ability to cope with additional health problems.

Prevention of infection in residents is an ongoing concern. There are some steps you can take to help in this process:

- Assist residents to maintain adequate fluid intake. This helps prevent urinary tract and respiratory tract infections and keeps the skin healthier.
- Assist residents to maintain adequate nutritional intake. Report to the nurse when residents eat less or refuse food.
- Assist residents to perform exercise programs established by the nurse or physical therapist. Follow positioning schedules and orders for range-of-motion exercises and ambulation. This increases circulation, thus lowering the risk of pressure ulcers (a frequent source of infection).

Age-Appropriate Care ALERT

Confusion often signals illness, infection, or a reaction to medication or anesthesia. Early mental changes may be subtle, and the nursing assistant is in the best position to detect them because of close patient contact. A change in mental status is a very important observation. Monitor patients carefully for signs of new and worsening confusion, and notify the nurse promptly. ■

Exercise also improves breathing, thereby decreasing the risk of respiratory tract infections.

- Attend to residents' personal hygiene and grooming needs. Regular bathing and oral care help prevent infection. Inspect the body and mouth when performing these procedures.
- Toilet residents regularly who need assistance. This keeps the bladder empty and also assures residents that they will receive help when they need to urinate. Some residents hesitate to drink fluids for fear they will become incontinent. When caring for incontinent residents, be sure to wipe female residents using strokes from front to back. This avoids contaminating the urethra with stool or vaginal excretions.
- Perform catheter care as directed. Avoid opening the closed drainage system. Use aseptic technique when emptying the catheter bag (Figure 33-11).
- Observe residents carefully and report any unusual signs or changes. Urinary tract infections may be discovered from changes in the urine or by incontinence. In some cases, the first sign of any infection is disorientation in people who are not usually disoriented. For persons with dementia, a change in behavior may indicate an infection. Incidents of falling often occur in residents with infections.
- You will be asked to collect urine specimens for culture and sensitivity. The specimen should be clean-catch (see Unit 45). You may need help when collecting the specimen. If it is contaminated because of inadequate cleaning or improper collection, the results will be altered.

Fighting infection in the long-term care facility is everyone's responsibility. As a nursing assistant, you can do your part by performing handwashing, standard precautions, isolation techniques, and all principles of medical

FIGURE 33-11 Use aseptic technique and avoid contamination when emptying the catheter drainage bag.

Age-Appropriate Care ALERT

Remember that incontinence is a medical problem. It is not a normal aging change. Loss of bladder control affects the resident's dignity and self-esteem. Make every effort to assist elderly residents with toileting and maintaining normal bowel and bladder function. ■

asepsis on a routine basis. Help new employees to acquire these skills, and assist residents to maintain good personal hygiene practices.

DELIRIUM

Mental confusion is not a normal aging change, and is often caused by reversible conditions. **Delirium** is an acute confusional state caused by reversible medical problems. It is common in the elderly, particularly those over age 75. Delirium is a nonspecific symptom of acute illness and dehydration in the elderly. It may also occur when elderly adults are given anesthesia or some other medications. Sensory losses, including uncorrected vision or hearing, may cause the resident to be unable to interpret the environment correctly. Changes in resident routines and the environment, as well as complications of many different medical conditions, can cause delirium. See Table 33-2 for common causes of delirium. These conditions can occur simultaneously, or can worsen problems in residents with dementia. Because so many factors contribute to delirium, it is often misunderstood, and may be confused with dementia.

Delirium is a very serious condition. Unrecognized and untreated, the mortality rate is high, particularly in residents with chronic disease, mental problems, or dementia. This is unfortunate, because delirium can be reversed if promptly identified and treated.

Signs and Symptoms of Delirium

Delirium develops rapidly. In most cases, the onset is within a few hours or days. Delirium may not be recognized until the resident is critically ill. Staff believe that the resident became ill suddenly, because of the rapid onset of mental changes, but a closer look often reveals subtle changes in the resident's physical or mental condition over the course of several days before the onset of delirium. *Any change in a resident's mental status is significant.*

Residents with acute delirium develop disorientation, behavioral changes, and decreased awareness of the environment (Figure 33-12). Other common signs and symptoms are:

TABLE 33-2 COMMON CAUSES OF DELIRIUM

- Unfamiliar environment, such as relocation to a new room or being new to the facility
- Vascular insufficiency
- Central nervous system infection
- Trauma
- Tumors or masses, malignancies
- Chemotherapy
- Seizures
- Migraine
- Decreased cardiac output, reduced blood flow, interrupted blood flow
- Urinary retention, urinary tract infection
- Pressure ulcers
- Hypotension
- Inadequate oxygenation
- Pneumonia or other lung infection
- Systemic infections, acute and chronic
- Metabolic disorders
- Anemias
- Decreased renal function
- Endocrine system disorders
- Nutritional deficiencies, malnutrition
- Emotional stress
- Pain
- Surgery, anesthesia
- Alteration in temperature regulation; hyperthermia, hypothermia
- Dehydration, fluid and electrolyte imbalances
- Depression
- Anxiety
- Grief/grieving
- Fatigue
- Sensory/perceptual deficiencies
- Sensory deprivation, isolation, confinement to a restricted area
- Sensory overload
- Immobility, bedrest
- Exposure to toxic substances
- Restraints
- Medication reactions
- Use of invasive equipment such as nasogastric tube or catheter
- Lack of prosthetic devices, including glasses, hearing aid, dentures
- Lack of items that complete body image, such as canes, purses, walkers
- Loss of family contact
- Loss of control over body processes

FIGURE 33-12 Residents with delirium develop confusion and decreased awareness of the environment.

- Reduced or fluctuating levels of consciousness
- Misinterpretating the environment, misunderstanding or misinterpeting conversations
- Hallucinations
- Illusions
- Delusions
- Insomnia and disturbance of sleep-wake cycle
- Change in motor activity
- Mental confusion and memory impairment

Nursing Assistant Responsibilities

Early identification and careful observation are essential to preventing more serious problems. As a nursing assistant, you work more closely with residents than other caregivers. This places you in an ideal position to notice subtle changes in mental status and other signs of dehydration, infection, or physical illness that may lead to delirium. You will become familiar with the resident's usual or normal condition. If something differs from the resident's usual condition, do not overlook it. Monitor changes in residents carefully, and report them to the nurse in charge promptly. Keep changes in resident routines and environment minimal. Monitor for and promptly report signs and symptoms of physical illness to the nurse.

GENERAL HYGIENE

Cleanliness of the skin is essential, but a full daily bath for the older person is neither necessary nor advisable. In fact, most elderly are reluctant to bathe daily. Hygiene also includes care of the hands and feet, hair, facial hair, mouth, and observations of the eyes, ears, and nose.

Partial Baths

Although a daily bath is unnecessary, frequent sponging of specific areas is necessary. The face, hands, underarms, perineum, and other body creases need regular cleaning and care. Use standard precautions when cleaning the eyes and genital area.

Skin areas that touch must be kept free from perspiration and should not be allowed to rub together. Whenever moisture, perspiration, urine, or feces are present, skin breakdown and infection are possible. Gently wash and dry local areas.

Total Baths

Bed baths clean the skin, but they are a rather passive activity for the resident. Therefore, a tub or shower bath is desirable two or three times a week to stimulate the resident.

Hand and Foot Care

As we age, fingernails and toenails become thickened and brittle. They split frequently because of decreased peripheral circulation. Fingernails can be cleaned during the morning care period. They should not be neglected.

- A soft brush and blunt-edged orangewood stick will clean the nails without causing injury.
- The hands can be soaked in warm water and the cuticles pushed back gently with a towel.
- Softening creams and olive-oil soaks help to soften the cuticles.
- Fingernails should be cut and filed, following the contour of the fingertips (check your facility policy).
- Care should be taken not to injure the corners; improper cutting of fingernails and toenails is the biggest single cause of infections.

Foot care should also be a routine part of morning care. This should include:

- Careful washing and drying of the foot (Figure 33-13).
- Close inspection for any abnormalities.
- Application of olive oil, lanolin, cocoa butter, hand cream, or lotion to dry, scaly skin.
- Application of a very light dusting of powder to perspiring feet.
- Cutting toenails straight across (check your facility policy). Thickened nails, which are difficult to cut, or nails of diabetic residents that must be cut should always be reported to the nurse.
- Providing slippers or shoes that fit well and are in good repair.

 Note: Check facility policy regarding nail and foot care for diabetic residents.

FIGURE 33-13 Foot care is an important part of personal hygiene.

GUIDELINES *for*
Bathing the Elderly

- Some soaps may be drying. Superfatted soaps and lotion soaps are less drying and less irritating.
- The skin of an elderly resident is easily damaged and takes a long time to heal because of inefficient general circulation, so care must be taken in handling the skin.
- Dry the skin by patting gently rather than by rubbing. All contact with the skin must be gentle. Even pulling a sheet from under a resident too rapidly can cause trauma.
- Lotions should be applied to dry areas to protect them. Bath oils lubricate the skin, but they are dangerous because they make the bath tub slippery. It is better to use spray-on dry oil or to apply lotions

directly to dry areas of skin. Make sure you cover the floor with a towel or bath blanket while spraying cosmetics. The spray tends to get on the unprotected floor, making it slippery.

- Applying lotion and skin moisturizer immediately after the bath helps to seal moisture into the skin.
- General safety factors and the resident's physical limitations should be considered before giving a tub or shower bath. Placement of hand rails, and availability of tub and shower seats or hydraulic lifts (Figure 33-14), should be checked. Be sure you know how to use the hydraulic lift before trying to use one with a resident.

continues

GUIDELINES *continued*

- Warm baths may decrease cerebral circulation. This can lead to confusion. Warm baths may be best just before the resident retires.
- Elderly people tend to be sensitive to deodorants, so care should be used when applying them.
- Inspect the resident's skin over bony prominences for signs of skin breakdown, including redness, warmth, and ischemic pallor.
- The skin should be carefully observed for abnormalities and care must be taken not to disturb them. Any change in color, size, or texture should be reported immediately. Cancer of the skin, often seen in the elderly, has an excellent cure rate (93%) when treated early. This is because skin cancer tends to grow slowly and the cells tend not to spread. These lesions are usually painless. All skin lesions are suspect. You must immediately report any changes noted in a resident's skin.

FIGURE 33-14 Check shower chairs and hydraulic lifts before using them. Always fasten the seat belt on the lift chair when moving the resident into and out of the tub.

Hair Care

Hair changes in amount and color as a person ages. These changes are part of the normal aging process. Graying or loss of **pigmentation** (color) is usual. Some graying may be evident as early as the second or third decade of life.

- Genetics probably plays an important role in the change rate. As more and more pigment is lost, the hair becomes white.
- Decreased oil makes the hair dull and lifeless.
- The amount of hair may be reduced in both males and females, and the texture becomes coarser in other areas such as the eyebrows and face.
- Balding is an aging characteristic that first appears at widely varying ages. Again, genetics has a strong influence.

Hair care is important in maintaining the resident's overall personal appearance.

- Hair should be styled and neatly arranged (Figure 33-15).
- Hair is commonly washed when the resident is showered. Check the care plan for specific instructions.
- Dry and no-rinse shampoos are also available. They simplify shampoos for residents confined to bed.

- A mild conditioning shampoo is best.
  - A dryer will dry the hair quickly, decreasing the chance of chilling.
  - The resident must be kept out of drafts while the hair is being washed and dried.
- Hair care may be provided by a beautician or barber, if available, or by a family member or nursing assistant.

Age-Appropriate Care ALERT

Style residents' hair in age-appropriate styles. Avoid juvenile hairstyles and accessories, which can be demeaning to elderly individuals. ■

Facial Hair

Elderly women tend to have an increase in the growth and coarseness of the hair on their chins and upper lips. These can be removed:

- With tweezers
- By electric needles used by a professional
- By shaving

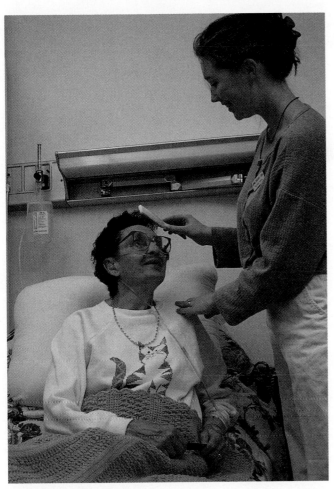

FIGURE 33-15 An attractive hairstyle is important for resident self-esteem.

- With a depilatory

Facial hair may also be lightened by mildly bleaching it. Elderly men need to be shaved regularly, usually daily. You may need to:

- Only provide the equipment
- Use a safety razor or electric razor to shave the resident yourself
- Assist the person to obtain barbering services

Mouth Care

The condition of the teeth affects the aged person's total health. Hygienic routines and observations are your responsibility when an individual is no longer able to do these things for himself. See Unit 25 for specific care procedures.

Natural Teeth. Poor oral hygiene can result in loss of appetite and weight, and may be the focus of any infection. Even if teeth are missing, the remaining teeth should be cleaned regularly. Dental checkups should be done as often as in younger years.

Dentures. False teeth, called *dentures*, must be cleaned daily (see Procedure 66 in Unit 25).

- Check the mouth and gums routinely for signs of irritation. Use a soft brush to clean mouth and gums.
- Teeth should be checked and polished during periodic dental examinations.

Mouth care is especially important for the resident who has lost teeth and is no longer able to keep dentures in the mouth. Check the mouth and gums for irritation. Dentures should be inspected for cracks, rough edges, and broken parts.

- A commercial mouthwash, a warm wash of saline solution, or baking soda should be used before and after meals.
- Wiping with moistened sponge-tip applicators, between meals, is very refreshing.
- Lips should be inspected for excessive dryness or fissures.
- Creams, petroleum jelly, or lip balm applied to the lips can prevent fissures from developing into deep sores and infections.

Eyes, Ears, and Nose

Eyes, ears, and nose should also be observed daily for any signs of irritation, redness, drainage, or excessive dryness of the skin that could lead to breaks and fissures. Observations of this nature by staff members should be part of routine care.

MENTAL CHANGES

Mental deterioration is not a normal part of aging. However, as people age, the risk of mental deterioration increases. Mental deterioration may stem from physical (organic) or emotional causes. A combination of both may occur in the residents in your care. Periods of mental confusion are often temporary. They may be due to unusual stress, such as an infection; sudden injury, such as a fracture; or transfer to an unfamiliar environment. In some situations, the changes may signify a progressive deterioration of mental abilities. The term **dementia** refers to any disorder of the brain that causes deficits in thinking, memory, and judgment.

CARING FOR RESIDENTS WITH DEMENTIA

You will care for many residents with dementia in the long-term care facility. Dementia is not a disease in itself, but is a group of symptoms seen in a number of different diseases. You will recall that delirium is a temporary condition, caused by medical illness. Dementia is a permanent condition that is not related to acute physical problems. Residents who have dementia may also develop delirium when they become acutely ill. In such cases, their confusion worsens. It returns to baseline when the medical problem is resolved.

Alzheimer's disease is the most common form of dementia. Other types of dementias are related to cardiovascular disease, Parkinson's disease, and Huntington's disease and are listed in Table 33-3. The term *dementia* is used here when referring to symptoms, behavior, and nursing actions that are appropriate for people with any dementia. Alzheimer's is used when the information is specific to that dementia.

Alzheimer's Disease

Alzheimer's disease can begin during middle age, but is more common in older persons. The disease affects people of all races, levels of intelligence, education, and financial status. It is progressive and cannot be cured. It has been called a "slow death of the mind." In the past, the term *senility* was used to describe these symptoms. We know now that it is a disease of the brain cells and is not normal aging. The cause of Alzheimer's is unknown. There is no diagnostic test. When symptoms appear, the person should have a medical workup to rule out other diseases. Nutritional problems, depression, medications, and metabolic diseases can all cause similar symptoms. However, these conditions can be reversed with treatment.

In Alzheimer's, changes occur in both the structure and function of the brain. The brain shrinks and becomes smaller. If an autopsy of the brain is performed after death, changes are noted in the brain cells. These changes are called *neuritic plaques* and *neurofibrillary tangles*.

Clinical Information ALERT

Approximately 40% of patients with severe Alzheimer's disease experience a significant weight loss. Several promising studies have shown that patients with advanced Alzheimer's disease eat and drink more when food is served on brightly colored dishes, such as the bright colors of some disposable plastic plates and cups. ■

Individuals with Alzheimer's often live as long as 20 years after the onset of the disease. Their bodies can be surprisingly healthy. Families and friends have difficulty believing that the person is ill. Much is unknown about this disease. Caregivers can increase the quality of life for those who have the illness.

The disease generally has three stages, with symptoms becoming progressively worse. The best-learned skills tend to remain the longest. An English teacher, for example, may maintain verbal skills longer than usual. However, once a skill is lost, it is lost forever.

Stage I: Mild Dementia. During the first stage, most people remain at home if they have a supportive family to provide assistance. They are usually physically capable and can attend to the activities of daily living with supervision.

TABLE 33-3 DESCRIPTION OF MAJOR FORMS OF DEMENTIA

Disease	Features	Course
Alzheimer's disease	Lack of chemical in brain causing neurofibrillary tangles, neuritic plaques	Onset age: 60–80 Slowly progressive
Multi-infarct dementia	Interference with blood circulation in brain cells due to arteriosclerosis or atherosclerosis	Onset age: 55–70 Outcome depends on rate of damage to brain cells
Huntington's disease	Inherited from either parent who has gene for the disease	Onset age: 25–45 Average duration 15 years
Parkinson's disease	Deficiency of chemical in brain (dopamine)	Onset age: 55–60 Several years duration
Creutzfeldt-Jakob disease	Noninflammatory virus causes changes in brain	Onset age: 50–60 Rapidly progressive
Syphilis	Spirochete (bacteria) causes brain damage	Occurs 15–20 years after primary infection
AIDS dementia	HIV-1 infection	Symptoms sometimes precede diagnosis of AIDS

Characteristics of Stage I include:

- Short-term memory loss
- Personality changes with loss of spontaneity and indifference (Figure 33-16)
- Decreased ability to concentrate and shortened attention span
- Disorientation to time and space
- Poor judgment
- Lack of safety awareness
- Carelessness in actions and appearance
- Anxiety, depression, and agitation
- Delusions of persecution—the person thinks that others are conspiring to do him harm
- Enough alertness to recognize that the person has a memory problem; may fabricate stories and make excuses to cover for memory loss

Stage II: Moderate Dementia. Symptoms of this stage are:

- Increased short-term memory loss and deterioration of memory for remote events.
- Complete disorientation.
- Wandering and pacing.
- **Sundowning**, which is confusion and restlessness that occur during the late afternoon, evening, or night.
- Sensory/perceptual changes. The person is unable to recognize and use common objects, such as eating utensils, combs, and pencils. Also, the person is unable to distinguish between right and left, up and down, hot and cold.
- Perseveration phenomena. This refers to repeating an action. Examples are repeating the same word or phrase, lip-licking, chewing, or finger-tapping.
- Problems with walking.
- Problems with speech, reading, writing.
- Good eating habits continue.

- Incontinent of bowel and bladder.
- Catastrophic reactions, hallucinations, delusions. A **catastrophic reaction** is the response of a person with dementia to overwhelming stimuli (Figure 33-17).

Most people with Alzheimer's are admitted to long-term care facilities during the second stage. Although they may still be healthy physically, they require constant care. Most families do not have the emotional resources and physical energy to cope. Admission may be traumatic to families. Families are vital members of the interdisciplinary team. They can provide staff with valuable information about the resident and how to deal with the problems.

Stage III: Severe Dementia. The person in Stage III:

- Is totally dependent
- Is verbally unresponsive
- May have seizures

Work with residents who have Alzheimer's disease or any dementia is challenging, rewarding, and gratifying. Caregivers must be compassionate, patient, calm, and have a sense of humor. When you are caring for residents with dementia, remember to:

FIGURE 33-17 Catastrophic reactions can occur when the person with dementia feels overwhelmed.

FIGURE 33-16 People with dementia exhibit indifference and loss of spontaneity.

- Protect residents from physical injury
- Allow residents to maintain independence as long as possible
- Provide physical and mental activities within residents' abilities
- Support residents' dignity and self-esteem

To meet these goals, the care must be:

- Consistent
- Provided with a structured but flexible routine
- Given in a peaceful, quiet environment that is simple, uncluttered, and unchanged

It is helpful to:

- Make eye contact with residents.
- Use appropriate body language. Residents with dementia can "read" the staff. Therefore, residents' behavior will reflect the mood of the staff (Figure 33-18).
- Be able to "tune" into and accept residents without being judgmental or critical.
- Use touch appropriately. This can be soothing. If a resident is surprised by the body contact, though, it can result in a catastrophic reaction.
- Avoid using logic, reasoning, or lengthy explanations.
- Remember that when the ability to use speech is lost, communication occurs through nonverbal means.
  - Biting, scratching, and kicking may be the only way the resident can express displeasure.
  - Watch for facial expressions and body language for clues to feelings and moods.
  - Learn what triggers agitation or anger. Work on preventing those situations.
- Use techniques of diversion and distraction. For example, calmly take the resident by the hand and walk together or direct the resident's attention to another activity. These techniques work well because of the shortened attention span.

FIGURE 33-18 Residents with dementia are in tune with the body language of the caregiver.

- Realize that people with dementia are not responsible for what they do or say.
  - Their behavior is not intentional, and they cannot change.
  - They are not aware of what they are doing.
  - They lose the ability to control their impulses.
  - Avoid confrontations and always allow them to "save face"—that is, keep their dignity.
  - No one really knows what is happening in the minds of people with dementia.

GUIDELINES *for*

Activities of Daily Living for Residents with Dementia

- Allow the resident to do as much as possible.
  - Use the hand-over-hand technique for personal care and eating. The **hand-over-hand technique** means that the resident's hand is placed around an object, such as a glass. The caregiver then places a hand over the resident's hand and guides the object to the resident's mouth.
  - Give only one short, simple direction at a time.
- Observe the resident's physical condition. People with dementia are usually unaware of signs of illness.

- Assist residents to maintain a dignified, attractive appearance by helping them with grooming and dressing.
- Monitor food and fluid intake.
  - Encourage and provide sufficient fluids to prevent dehydration.
  - Offer the resident a drink each time you enter the room.
  - Some residents do not like water, but will drink fruit juice, soda, or sugarless beverages. Provide

GUIDELINES *continued*

fluids that the resident likes and will consume readily.

— Too many foods at once are confusing.

— Place one food at a time in front of the resident.

— Do not use plastic utensils that can break in the resident's mouth.

— Provide nutritious finger foods when the resident is unable to use utensils.

— Avoid pureed foods as long as possible.

— Check food temperatures.

— Prepare foods for eating by buttering bread, cutting meat, and opening cartons.

— Check the resident's mouth after eating for food. "Squirreling" food (hoarding food in the cheeks) can cause aspiration.

— Weigh residents regularly to detect patterns of weight gain or loss.

— The dining area should be quiet and calm.

• Persons with dementia eventually lose bowel and bladder continence. Taking residents to the bathroom every 2 hours keeps residents dry and prevents skin breakdown.

• Residents with dementia need activities geared to their abilities.

— Avoid large groups or competitive activities.

FIGURE 33-19
Daily exercise is important to maintain physical health and well-being.

— In later stages, use sensory stimulation with quiet music, soft touching, and calm talk.

— Holding puppies or kittens (pet therapy) brings pleasure to severely impaired residents.

• Daily exercise should be planned according to residents' habits and abilities (Figure 33-19). The resident who wanders throughout the day may only need range-of-motion exercises.

SPECIAL PROBLEMS

Problems with Bathing

Resistance to bathing is common in residents with Alzheimer's disease. The resident may have forgotten the purpose of bathing. Residents may be uncomfortable and resist removing their clothing in front of you. They may misinterpret your assistance as a sexual assault. Staff may label this behavior "uncooperative" or "aggressive" when in fact the resident is just using normal defense mechanisms. The behavior may worsen if the resident's requests to stop bathing are ignored. Try to view the procedure from the resident's perspective. Observe and listen to the resident's verbal and nonverbal behavior.

If a resident steadfastly refuses a bath, consider whether it is really necessary to bathe the resident in this way at this time. Return and try again later, or consult the nurse. Try to avoid agitating the resident further. Consider a different method of bathing, such as using a towel bath or bag bath. Individualize your approach to the resident. Modify the environment so it is comfortable and pleasurable, and be flexible in your approach to and communication with the resident.

Before bringing the resident to the tub or shower room, make sure the room is warm and private. Noises from running water, the whirlpool tub, and heaters in the shower room may frighten the resident. Sound tends to echo in some shower and tub rooms, making the problem worse. Encouraging the resident to sing an old song or playing pleasant music may help. (You may also use a special battery-operated shower radio, or keep the radio plug away from sources of water.)

Wrapping a towel or bath blanket around the shoulders and pinning it securely may help with modesty problems. Leave it in place during the bath. Some residents appear to be fearful of water or afraid of washing. Alzheimer's disease causes problems with sensation, so bathing may be uncomfortable. The resident may not be able to feel the water temperature. Bathing is a complex task involving many steps. Taking a bath may simply be too overwhelming for the resident. Residents in the early stages of Alzheimer's disease may also be sensitive with an unfamiliar nursing assistant.

Before beginning, ask the resident to feel the water. Say something like, "This feels good." Explain what you are going to do and what you want the resident to do, one step at a time. Giving too many directions at once may overwhelm the resident and trigger a catastrophic reaction. If you will be giving a complete bath, giving the resident something to hold, to occupy the hands, may be helpful. Squeezing a sponge or washcloth may distract the resident. Washing the hair may also be frightening. Use the resident's responses to guide your actions. Washing the hair in the sink or with a no-rinse product may be less traumatic to both the resident and the nursing assistant.

Modify your behavior and care according to the resident's responses to the procedure. Be slow, calm, patient, and reassuring. If you are successful in bathing the resident, share the approaches you used with the nurse and other team members so they can be added to the care plan.

Dressing Problems

Some residents are resistant to dressing. Like bathing, they may view changing the clothes as a form of sexual assault. Others remove their clothing after they are dressed. Keep the morning routine consistent and familiar. Once you start, avoid interruptions, which cause the resident to forget what she is supposed to be doing. Make sure the room is warm and private. Ask the resident to select the clothing, if this is not too overwhelming. The clothing should be color-coordinated and appropriate for the resident's age and the season. Lay out clothing in the order in which it will be put on. Break the task down into simple, manageable steps and give the resident easy instructions, one step at a time. Assist with dressing, if needed. Allow the resident to do as much for herself as possible, but do not let her become overwhelmed or frustrated. Understand the resident's need for privacy and unwillingness to completely disrobe in front of you. Be sensitive to grooming issues and encourage residents to comb hair, shave, or wear cosmetics and jewelry. Praise the resident and compliment her appearance.

Sexual Behavior

Sexuality is a basic need in all humans, according to Maslow. Sexuality does not diminish with age. Sexual expression may be physical or psychological. Always knock before entering a resident's room and wait for a response before entering.

Many health care workers feel that masturbation is inappropriate behavior. Masturbation is satisfying to the resident and is not harmful. It is an acceptable behavior as long as it is done in a private area. If you enter a resident's room and find the resident masturbating, provide privacy and leave the room.

If you enter a room and find two consenting adults engaged in a sexual act, provide privacy and leave. Adults have a legal right to do whatever is pleasing to them, as long as it is not medically contraindicated and both partners are mentally capable of consent. Do not pass judgment on the resident's choice of partner or methods of sexual expression.

Facility staff is responsible for protecting residents who are physically or mentally vulnerable to unwanted sexual contact. Sexual contact with unwilling, alert residents who are physically unable to defend themselves, or with confused residents who cannot give full informed consent, is sexual abuse. Sexual abuse is a violation of resident rights and is illegal. No health care worker, visitor, or other resident may sexually abuse others. If sexual abuse occurs, the police are notified. Anyone who sexually harasses or abuses a resident or care provider should be reported to the nurse, manager, or other appropriate person according to facility policy.

Sometimes residents may make unwanted sexual advances toward the nursing assistant. The resident's desire for sexuality is normal, but the choice of person is not. If a resident makes sexual advances, do not ridicule or belittle him or her. Be patient and understanding, and speak to the resident in a matter-of-fact manner. Tactfully inform the resident that the behavior is not acceptable. Follow your facility policy for reporting sexual advances.

Disrobing

Sometimes mentally confused residents disrobe in public areas. Residents who are bedfast may remove the covers many times each day, exposing their bodies to anyone who looks in the door. This sight can be traumatic to a young child who is visiting. It is your responsibility to keep residents covered. This may be a difficult task. As with all other behavior problems, look for a cause. Frequently residents disrobe because they need to use the bathroom. Other causes are uncomfortable clothing and very warm environmental temperatures. The resident may be bored or tired and ready for bed. Evaluate the situation and common triggers of the problem. Sometimes there is no apparent cause.

You are not permitted to put the resident's clothing on backward to keep him or her from disrobing. Ask the nurse to contact the appropriate person in your facility to obtain clothing that fastens in back and is difficult for the resident to remove. Consult the care plan and nurse about approaches to use. Find out whether tying the sheet to the side rails of the bed constitutes a restraint. Tying a sheet to the bed or chair is usually a restraint, but wrapping it around the resident's body only, then tying it in back, may be effective. If the sheet does not limit the resident's movement or access to his own body, it is not a restraint. Monitor the resident who disrobes frequently and do your best to keep him or her covered.

Wandering and Pacing

Persons with Alzheimer's may wander or pace for hours at a time. No one knows why this occurs. Some reasons may be:

- They are looking for companionship, security, or loved ones.
- It is a way to handle stress.

The resident may not know where he is, but knows he does not want to be there. He is seeking a state of mind, not a physical location. Ask the resident his intended destination. A man may tell you he is going to work. A woman may say she is going home to cook dinner for the children. Avoid arguing or providing reality orientation. These techniques will probably agitate the resident. Instead, use reminiscence (Figure 33-20). Talk about the resident's activities, work, meal preparation, or cooking. Make appropriate comments, such as, "That must be very interesting work," or "You must have been a very good cook." Ask the resident about his former work routines. This approach restores the state of mind the resident seeks, reducing stress and the risk of **eloping** (wandering away from the facility).

Many different things trigger wandering behavior. The facility may keep a log to help identify the resident's wandering triggers. You will record information such as the resident's behavior, staff on duty, and temperature and noise in the environment on the log. The nurse uses this information to develop a plan of care. Several studies have shown that noise increases wandering. Health care facilities can be very noisy at times. Loud talking, using the intercom, loud televisions, and residents calling out for help can be very upsetting to wanderers. Hot or cold environmental temperature may also be a problem. If the resident is uncomfortable, he may wander to escape. Other common wandering triggers are:

- Boredom
- Unmet physical needs
- Feeling stressed
- Pain
- Hunger

- Thirst
- Needing to use the bathroom

Other, less common wandering triggers are dehydration, illness, inadequate coping mechanisms, medications, and an unfamiliar environment.

Nursing Assistant Approaches. Allow the resident to wander. Using restraints increases anxiety and frustration, worsening the problem. Walk with the resident whenever possible. Adapt the environment to the wandering resident, to ensure that it is safe and secure. Keeping the resident's stress as low as possible is important because if he feels overwhelmed, he may wander to elope. If the resident's stress is not relieved, he may have a catastrophic reaction. As a rule, try to meet the resident's needs for hunger, thirst, and elimination. If you meet the need, the wandering will cease.

Thinking is a very complex process. If someone tells you *not to think* of a purple dog, you will think of it, then have to unthink it. "Unthinking" is a complex process for a cognitively impaired resident. Avoid saying, "Don't go outside," or "Don't go in that room," because that will cause the resident to think about doing exactly what you told him not to. A better approach is to say, "Stay inside," or "Stay here." Communication is best if it is concrete and does not require abstract thinking.

Remember that nonverbal communication can have a powerful effect on residents. Confused residents are very sensitive to the moods and body language of staff members. Send the right message through facial expressions and body language. Approach the resident in a calm, nonthreatening manner (Figure 33-21). Avoid forcing your own agenda on the resident, which will cause agitation and worsen the behavior. Instead, use gentle persuasion. Avoid making too many demands on the resident during ADLs and direct care. Keep instructions simple and brief. As the resident completes one task, give him another. Be

FIGURE 33-20
Some residents with Alzheimer's disease wander continually. They must be reminded to rest, to eat, and to drink.

FIGURE 33-21
Your demeanor has a powerful effect on residents. Approach the resident slowly, calmly, and in a nonthreatening manner.

patient, calm, and reassuring. Tell him that he is in the right place, safe, and you will help him. Compliment him for his successes, even if they are small. The resident will probably not remember the compliment, but will feel good about himself. He will be more cooperative and less likely to act out or wander.

Seeing items associated with going outdoors may trigger wandering. Remove purses, hats, coats, shoes, or other outerwear from sight. There is no single effective approach for all wandering behavior. Use the approaches listed here and see if they work. If you discover an effective approach, inform the nurse so he or she can add it to the care plan. Remember that identifying and modifying the resident's agenda, feelings, and unmet needs will usually modify or stop the behavior. Effective management is individualized to the resident. It is often the result of trial and error. Other approaches that may be listed on the care plan are:

- Taking the resident to the bathroom frequently.
- Adjusting room temperature and ensuring that the resident is wearing appropriate clothing for the temperature and season.
- Reducing environmental noise and stimulation; check residents yelling, television, intercom announcements, and other sources of noise in the facility.
- Providing something to eat or drink.
- Informing the nurse if the the resident complains of pain; he or she may not admit to having "pain," but may admit to having pressure, discomfort, or another unpleasant sensation.
- Providing a magazine, newspaper, book, or picture album (Figure 33-22).
- Visiting with the resident.
- Escorting the resident to activities.
- Having the resident fold towels and washcloths, perform a repetitive task, or sort other harmless items.
- Providing a stereo with earphones and playing soft, soothing music, or the resident's favorite type of music, if known. This approach is often effective when others fail.
- Placing an identifying object, such as a bow, hat, or gender-appropriate decoration on the door of the resident's room and directing him to it.
- Making sure the resident wears glasses and hearing aids, as appropriate. Wandering may worsen if the resident misinterprets environmental signals.
- Avoiding clutter and safety hazards in the environment.
- Ensuring that chemicals and potential hazards are stored properly.
- Providing a nightlight at night, or leaving the bathroom light on.
- If nighttime wandering is a problem, avoid letting the resident nap during the day. Limit caffeinated food and beverages after the evening meal.

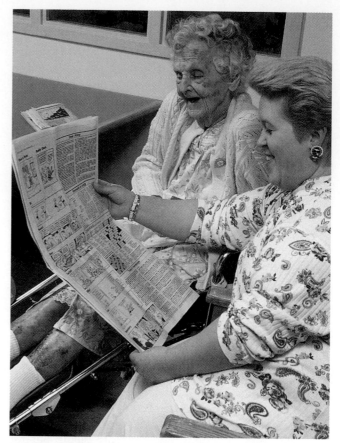

FIGURE 33-22 Some residents with Alzheimer's wander in their wheelchairs. Distracting the resident with a newspaper will provide an opportunity to rest.

- Avoiding the use of side rails. This resident may climb the rails and suffer a serious fall.
- Attaching the call signal cord to the back of resident's clothing so the cord will pull from the wall and turn the signal on when he rises. Other types of tab signals or magnetic sensor systems may be used to alert staff if the resident rises or attempts to leave the facility through an exit door.
- Responding promptly to door alarms, bed, or other alarms that alert you to a problem with a wandering resident.
- Covering elevator buttons with soft fabric or duct tape to disguise them. The soft material permits staff and visitors to push the buttons, but wandering residents will usually not recognize them.
- Avoiding restraints, which often worsen agitation.
- Always knowing what the resident is wearing. Write this information down at the beginning or end of each shift. Wanderers are often discovered missing at mealtime, when staff cannot find the resident to deliver the tray. This is commonly a problem for second-shift staff. Day shift dresses the resident. Staff on second shift may not know what she is wearing.
- Checking on the resident frequently to note her whereabouts. If you will be with another resident for a pro-

longed period of time, inform the nurse so that another worker can be assigned to monitor the wandering resident in your absence.

Remember that residents who wander will burn extra calories and are at risk for weight loss. Some are so busy wandering they will not sit long enough to eat a meal. Give them finger foods and walk with them, if necessary. Follow the plan of care to ensure that the resident takes in enough nutrients.

Residents who wander may become physically exhausted. They have forgotten how to sit down and may need reminders. Special reclining chairs (Figure 33-23) and beanbag-type chairs may be used to allow residents to rest. Again, the care plan will specify the method to use.

Agitation, Anxiety, and Catastrophic Reactions

Agitation and anxiety are shown by an increase in physical activity, such as pacing, or the perseveration behaviors described for Stage II. If appropriate interventions are not implemented in time, a catastrophic reaction will likely occur. You may note any or all of the following.

- Increased physical activity
- Increased talking or mumbling
- Explosive behavior with physical violence

To avoid catastrophic reactions:

- Monitor behavior closely.
- Watch for signs of increasing agitation.
- Check to see if the resident:
  - Is hungry
  - Needs to go to the bathroom
  - Is too hot or too cold
  - Is overtired or in pain
  - Has signs of physical illness
- Check the environment for:
  - Too much noise.
  - Too many people.
  - Staff anxiety.
  - Television programs. People with dementia cannot distinguish fiction from reality.
- People with dementia cannot make decisions. For example, the question "What do you want to wear today?" may be more than they can handle.

When agitation or catastrophic reactions occur:

- Do not use physical restraints or force in any attempt to subdue the resident. This increases agitation and can result in injury to the resident or staff.
- Avoid having several staff persons approach the resident at the same time. This is frightening to the resident.
- Use a soft, calm voice. Do not try to reason with the resident. Using touch may or may not be appropriate. Some residents respond to smooth stroking of the arms or back with lotion. Others may react violently if they are already agitated.

Sundowning

Sundowning is increased confusion and restlessness during the late afternoon, evening, or night. It is sometimes prevented by avoiding too much activity before bedtime and by establishing a consistent bedtime routine.

- Overfatigue can cause sundowning. Encourage the resident to nap or rest in the early afternoon.
- Try to prevent the resident from sleeping too much during the day.
- The evening meal should be eaten at least 2 hours before bedtime. Eliminate or limit caffeine in the resident's diet.
- Involve the resident in quiet evening activities, listening to soft music, or interactions with a caregiver or family member.
- Provide a light bedtime snack that is easily chewed and digested.
- Take the resident to the bathroom. Allow sufficient time for bladder and bowel elimination.
- Give a slow back massage.
- Check with family members and continue the resident's established habits, such as wearing socks to bed, using two pillows, or having a nightlight.
- Check the lighting of the room. Shadows and reflections are disturbing.
- If the resident awakens during the night, repeat the bedtime routine. If this is ineffective and the resident does not remain in bed, try a recliner or Alzheimer's chair.

Pillaging and Hoarding

These events do not present a major problem unless residents collect items from other residents' rooms or they

FIGURE 33-23 Some residents wander until they are physically exhausted. Seating the resident in a recliner enables him to rest.

hide things that are difficult to find. This resident usually believes he is in his own home, and he can explore and take whatever he wants because everything in the "house" belongs to him. The resident has very poor safety awareness and is at high risk of injury from entering housekeeping closets and service areas and ingesting chemicals or becoming injured by sharp objects. Other residents may harm the resident, such as by hitting him, because they believe the resident is stealing their belongings.

- Label all residents' belongings.
- If a missing item is located, note where it was found. The resident probably will choose the same hiding place the next time.
- Check the room daily for stale food and items belonging to other residents.
- Keep the resident's hands busy. Activities like folding washcloths or "fiddling" with keys on a ring may help.

- Provide a dresser, nightstand, suitcase, or box in the hallway with items that he can safely rummage through.
- Give the resident junk mail, linen, or other items to sort, coupons to clip, or some other activity.
- Post paper streamers across doorways.
- Post signs that say "stop," "do not enter," or "construction zone."
- Listening to a radio with headphones may calm the resident.
- Provide reassurance that the resident is safe.

Reality Orientation

Reality orientation (RO) is used to help disoriented residents regain connections to the environment, to time, and to themselves. When used appropriately, it decreases anxiety in the resident. RO may be effective in

GUIDELINES *for*

Reality Orientation

- Always treat residents as adults, with respect and dignity, no matter how confused they are.
- Speak clearly and directly. Avoid the temptation to speak louder when the resident does not understand you.
- Give simple, brief instructions and responses.
- Establish and maintain a structured routine.
- Be polite and sincere.
- Give residents adequate time to respond.
- Allow residents to be independent as long as possible.
- Set residents' watches to the correct time.
- Make sure residents have clean eyeglasses and effective hearing aids if they need them.
- Place large numbered calendars in rooms and cross off the days as they pass.
- There should be clocks with large numbers around the facility.
- Signs with large letters and color codes on walls, floors, and equipment help residents find their way around the facility.
- Call residents by name. Disoriented residents usually respond to the first name more quickly.
- Tell residents your name—do not expect them to remember you.

- Use RO in conversation with the residents, for example, "It's only March 5 today but it is warm outside."

When using RO:

- Do not put residents on the spot. For example, do not ask, "Do you remember who I am?" or "Do you know what day this is?" If you need to verify orientation, ask "What are your plans for today?"
- Answer questions honestly but avoid confronting residents with information they are unable to handle. If a resident whose husband is deceased asks, "Is my husband coming today?" it is cruel to answer by saying, "Remember, your husband died two years ago." This response will likely trigger a catastrophic reaction. It is better to answer by asking another question, such as, "Tell me about your husband, Emma." She will receive pleasure from reminiscing and will probably work up to present time on her own.
- Never argue with a resident's reality. When a resident has a delusion, arguing increases the individual's anxiety and agitation. Many delusions are based on past experiences. Because the resident is disoriented, the experience seems to be happening now.
- Do not reinforce the resident's disorientation.
- Remember that a pleasant facial expression, relaxed body language, and a caring touch are the most important aspects of caring for confused residents.

the first stage and the early part of the second stage of Alzheimer's disease. In later stages it is meaningless and increases agitation.

Reminiscing

Reminiscing (remembering past experiences) is a natural activity for people of all ages. We tend to reminisce when we see old friends or get together with families.

- Past experiences are remembered and enjoyed as we think of pleasant times from the past.
- As people age, the tendency to reminisce increases, and the activity becomes more important.
- It is an appropriate activity for residents with dementia if long-term memory is still intact (Figure 33-24).
- Reminiscing may serve as a life review. Elderly people often review the past experiences of their lives. This can bring back unpleasant memories. If these experiences are resolved, peace of mind can be found.
- Reminiscing can help people adapt to old age. It helps to maintain self-esteem. It allows them to work through personal losses.
- When we listen to residents reminisce, we understand them better.
- Reminiscing therapy can be a group activity if done with a leader who is skillful and sensitive to the feelings of the members.

Validation Therapy

Validation therapy was developed by Naomi Feil. **Validation therapy** is a technique that tries to maintain the disoriented person's dignity by acknowledging the person's memories and feelings. It is based on these ideas:

- Maintain the identity and dignity of residents.
- Help disoriented people with dementia feel good about themselves.

FIGURE 33-24 Residents with dementia retain long-term memory even though short-term memory is lost. Looking at family pictures is an excellent way to reminisce.

Difficult SITUATIONS

The Velveteen Rabbit is a children's story that was copyrighted in 1922. This is a conversation between two stuffed animals:

"What is REAL?" asked the Rabbit one day, when they were lying side by side near the nursery fender, before Nana came to tidy the room. "Does it mean having things that buzz inside you and a stick-out handle?"

"REAL isn't how you are made," said the Skin Horse. "It's a thing that happens to you. When a child loves you for a long, long time, not just to play with, but REALLY loves you, then you become REAL."

"Does it hurt?" asked the Rabbit.

"Sometimes," said the Skin Horse, for he was always truthful. "When you are REAL you don't mind being hurt."

"Does it happen all at once, like being wound up," he asked, "or bit by bit?"

"It doesn't happen all at once, like being wound up," said the Skin Horse. "You become. It takes a long time. . . . Generally, by the time you are REAL, most of your hair has been loved off, and your eyes drop out and you get loose in the joints and very shabby. But these things don't matter at all, because once you are REAL you can't be ugly, except to people who don't understand."

There is a lesson for all health care workers in this old children's story. The residents entrusted to your care may be loose in the joints and shabby in appearance, but they have shaped the communities and the world in which we live. They have families and others who love and value them just as they are: shabby, balding, hard of hearing, slow, confused, even combative. They are worth your investment, even if they don't always appreciate it. They are REAL. ■

- There is a reason for all behavior. What seems like confused behavior may be an acting-out of memories from long ago.
- Acknowledge feelings and memories.

- Disoriented people have the right to express feelings when they can no longer be oriented to reality.
- Living must be resolved in order to prepare for dying.
- Sometimes elderly persons have experienced so many losses during a lifetime that they have no coping abilities left.
- Living in reality is not the only way to live.
- Disoriented elderly have worth. We can give them joy by allowing them to express themselves.
- Within each confused person is a human being who was once a child and later an adult with hopes, joys, sadness, failures, and successes. Each person deserves to be cared for and loved in their final years.

When using validation therapy, allow residents to express their feelings. Reassure them that the feelings are worthwhile. Use a calm, nonthreatening manner. Speak in a loving tone of voice. When the resident describes an emotion, assure him or her that it is okay.

Using validation is an excellent way to communicate with elderly persons. It is also effective for residents with Alzheimer's disease and cognitive impairments. The program is based on the belief that developmental tasks from earlier years must be resolved. If they were not resolved, they will emerge in old age. The elderly person may display many emotions in trying to conclude them. Feil's research has shown that using validation reduces the need for restraints. It helps residents regain feelings of dignity and self-control. Resident response to this therapy can be very encouraging. Seeing positive responses is very rewarding to staff.

Music Therapy

Music therapy is an allied health service similar to occupational therapy and physical therapy. Although it is an enjoyable activity, it is not done strictly for fun and games. Music therapy consists of using music therapeutically to address physical, psychological, cognitive, and social functioning. Music therapy is used successfully with people of all ages and disabilities.

Music therapy dates back to ancient Greece. In that culture, music was part of medical treatment. Think about the effect music has on your own life. Children learn the alphabet by singing the letters. We listen to "oldies" and remember events from our past. You remember the words to songs you have not heard in many years.

Restorative music therapy is used for relieving stress. It can be a planned, formal activity or a spontaneous, informal activity. Singing with residents during bathing and range-of-motion work can be therapeutic and fun for both the resident and the nursing assistant. Studies have shown that participating in music has various mental and physical benefits, including:

- Increased metabolism
- Increased muscle flexibility

- Improved circulation
- Increased lung capacity and improved respirations
- Improved memory, which contributes to reminiscence and satisfaction
- Improvement in mood and emotional states
- Feeling a sense of control over life
- Increased self-awareness
- Anxiety reduction
- Stimulation
- Opportunities to interact socially with others

Sometimes music therapy is part of a planned exercise program. Playing music during exercise makes the activity fun. Music motivates the residents and singing and clapping relieve stress and anxiety. Music teleprompters make it easy for residents to participate even if they do not know the words (Figure 33-25). For relaxation therapy, a portable player and headset may be used.

The activities department may present music activities for other purposes. A professional music therapist may visit the facility regularly to work with residents. Regardless of whether music is used formally as a form of therapy, or informally for recreation, residents respond well to it. Music is a pleasurable activity that maintains or improves residents' physical, mental, social, and emotional functioning. The sensory and intellectual stimulation of music helps maintain residents' quality of life.

Animal-Assisted Therapy

Animal-assisted therapy is also called *pet therapy*. Pets are used in many different ways in the health care environment. Formal programs are developed in which the handler and health care provider consult on specific goals and plan how to accomplish them. With informal pet therapy, an animal is taken to visit residents periodically. Visiting with animals can reduce feelings of loneliness and depres-

FIGURE 33-25 A teleprompter can be used so residents can sing along even if they don't know the words. (Courtesy of Briggs Corporation, Des Moines, IA (800) 247-2343)

sion. Some people become more active and responsive because of visits from pets. The pet may make it easier for the resident to talk. He or she may express thoughts, feelings, and memories. Stroking a dog or cat may reduce a person's blood pressure, and encourages good range of motion of the hands and arms. Animals used in pet therapy must have a health certificate. Some formal groups offer special certifications to pets and handlers based on the experience of the animal/human team and complexity of the working environment. Dogs are commonly used for pet therapy, but other types of animals may be used as well.

REVIEW

A. True/False.

Mark the following true or false by circling T or F.

1. T F Older people have the same emotional needs for good mental health as young people.

2. T F Frustration is an emotion often experienced by the elderly.

3. T F As people age, they become less interested in sexuality.

4. T F Elderly people may not be aware of their need for fluids.

5. T F Infections are not a major concern in the elderly.

6. T F The resident's mouth should be carefully inspected and cleaned each time the dentures are cleaned.

7. T F One of the best approaches when working with persons with dementia is to reason with them and use logic.

8. T F Calories should be increased in the diet of the elderly.

9. T F Elderly persons are fearful of death.

10. T F Daily tub baths or showers are not usually necessary or recommended for elderly residents.

B. Matching.

Choose the correct item from Column II to match each word or phrase in Column I.

Column I

11. _____ dementia
12. _____ validation therapy
13. _____ reminiscing
14. _____ debilitating
15. _____ sundowning

Column II

a. weakening

b. remembering past experiences

c. deficits in thinking, memory, judgment

d. tries to maintain disoriented person's dignity

e. restlessness and increasing confusion of resident with Alzheimer's during evening and night

C. Multiple Choice.

Select the one best answer for each of the following.

16. A characteristic of the nursing assistant that is especially important while caring for older adults is
    a. logical reasoning ability.
    b. kindness.
    c. technical skill.
    d. advanced certifications and training.

17. Characteristics of the elderly include
    a. increased vitality.
    b. decreased night sleep.
    c. increased appetite.
    d. increased mobility and agility.

18. Which of the following nutrients should be increased in the diet of elderly persons?
    a. Fats
    b. Proteins
    c. Calories
    d. Sugar

19. Which statement is true of catastrophic reactions?
    a. They are unavoidable in persons with dementia.
    b. They may be precipitated by too much sensory stimulation.
    c. Providing activity will subdue the catastrophic reaction.
    d. They are always expressions of violence.

20. An appropriate approach to reality orientation is to
    a. ask the resident if he knows your name.
    b. ask the resident what his plans are for the day.
    c. ask the resident if he knows the date.
    d. tell the resident what day it is.

21. Residents in assisted living facilities
    a. need 24-hour nursing care.
    b. require supervision with ADLs.
    c. need skilled rehabilitation.
    d. have mental health needs.

22. Residents in skilled nursing facilities
    a. have complex medical care and rehabilitation needs.
    b. are acutely ill.
    c. require subacute care.
    d. are independent with ADLs.

23. The OBRA regulations
    a. are guidelines that all hospitals follow.
    b. mandate all health care facilities to promote "aging in place."
    c. require facilities to maintain residents at the highest possible level.
    d. do not apply to nursing assistants.

24. Malnutrition
    a. is a risk in certain residents in long-term care facilities.
    b. is a chronic condition in most elderly individuals.
    c. frequently occurs in residents who eat less than all of their meals.
    d. is not a concern for the elderly.

25. When a resident is being tube fed, the head of the bed must be elevated at least:
    a. 10° to 15°.
    b. 25° to 40°.
    c. 30° to 45°.
    d. 50° to 70°.

26. Residents who are at risk of dehydration
    a. drink 6 cups of fluid each day.
    b. are always confused.
    c. have straw-colored urine.
    d. often have difficulty holding a cup.

27. Sepsis is
    a. a serious complication of infection.
    b. a reversible mental illness.
    c. seldom a concern in the elderly.
    d. a complication of malnutrition.

28. Signs and symptoms of delirium are
    a. abdominal pain and nausea.
    b. mental confusion and memory impairment.
    c. catastrophic reaction and reminisence.
    d. headache and sore throat.

29. A resident tells you she is going home to prepare dinner for her children, then proceeds to go toward the front door. Your best response is to walk with her and say
    a. "Don't go outside."
    b. "Your children live in another state."
    c. "Stay inside. What do you like to cook?"
    d. "Your children are spending the night at a friend's house."

30. Validation therapy
    a. helps residents maintain dignity and self-control.
    b. is necessary in physical rehabilitation programs.
    c. orients residents to the season, time, date, and day.
    d. uses music to help residents relax and relieve stress.

D. Nursing Assistant Challenge.

Mr. Delgotti, 83 years old, is one of your assigned patients. Think about the changes that occur with aging and answer these questions.

31. What changes occur in the integumentary system?

32. Because of these changes, what complications could occur during his hospital stay?

33. What actions can you take to avoid these complications?

34. What possible complications can occur in the digestive system?

35. What observations are especially important for all the body systems because of Mr. Delgotti's age?

UNIT 34

The Organization of Home Care: Trends in Health Care

OBJECTIVES

After completing this unit, you will be able to:

- Spell and define terms.
- Briefly describe the history of home care.
- Describe the benefits of working in home care.
- Identify members of the home health team.
- List guidelines for avoiding liability while working as a home health assistant.

- Describe the types of information a home health assistant must be able to document.
- Identify several time management techniques.
- List ways in which the home health assistant can work successfully with client's families.

VOCABULARY

Learn the meaning and the correct spelling of the following words and phrases:

client care records   intermittent care   time/travel records

INTRODUCTION

The health care of persons (clients) in their own homes is an age-old tradition. It was not until the middle of the twentieth century that there was a massive trend to move patient care out of the home and into the community health care facility. The late nineteenth century saw the growth of medical schools and the licensing of physicians. Schools of nursing soon followed. Hospital staffing slots were filled with students enrolled in these programs. Although the permissive laws of the early 1900s gave requirements for nursing licensure, the laws did not restrict nursing practice. There were few legal restrictions on people who provided care in patients' homes. Almost anyone could hire out to provide such care. A few years later, laws were passed to control nurse education. These laws specifically stated the acts that a nurse could and could not perform. Anyone practicing nursing without a license could be held liable.

World War II brought with it:

- A gradual increase in the need for more technical care, as procedures and equipment became more complex.
- Introduction of antibiotics and better techniques of infection control. (Availability of antibiotics was very limited and most were reserved for use in treating military service members.)
- Growth of a new, supplementary force of workers (nursing assistants) to help provide nursing care.
- Construction of many new health care facilities.
- Hospital care of sick people.

Today, the pendulum has swung back once more toward treating acutely ill people in hospitals and providing alternative care (such as home care, day care, or long-term care) for all others (Figure 34-1). Factors that foster this interest in home care include:

- Expensive high technology (Figure 34-2)

FIGURE 34-1 The trend toward home care is growing in response to increased numbers of people requiring continuing care.

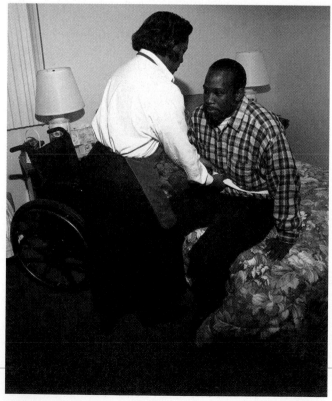

FIGURE 34-2 High technology has increased hospital costs, making home care a practical alternative.

- Introduction of diagnosis-related groups (DRGs), resulting in earlier discharge from hospitals
- Growing population of chronically ill people
- The establishment of hospice care, enabling terminally ill people to choose to stay at home during their last months of life
- The preference of the health care consumer to remain at home if possible

PROVIDERS OF HOME HEALTH CARE

Because of the increasing demand for home care, there are many different types of home care providers:

- Government-sponsored agencies controlled by city or county governments
- Private agencies; some are for-profit and others are nonprofit
- Hospital-sponsored agencies

These providers employ several types of health care workers, including nurses, nursing assistants, therapists, and social workers. Each employer has personnel policies that regulate job descriptions, salaries, and benefits. The employer provides new employees with an orientation to the agency and to their responsibilities.

In addition to working in clients' homes, home care workers may also visit residents in assisted living facilities (ALFs). These facilities do not usually provide nursing services. Residents who become ill or injured may need temporary or short-term nursing care. Rather than moving them from their home in the assisted living facility to a facility that provides a higher level of care, home health care workers visit the resident in the ALF to provide necessary services. Using home care workers in this manner promotes the "aging in place" philosophy of the assisted living facility and enables residents to remain in a familiar environment while they recover.

BENEFITS OF WORKING IN HOME HEALTH CARE

After you have completed your nursing assistant class, you may choose to join a group that provides home health care. There are advantages to working in such agencies:

- Satisfaction of giving complete care to one client at a time
- Satisfaction of caring for the same client over a period of time (Figure 34-3)
- Opportunity to work with greater independence
- Part-time employment, if desired

The person working in home care must have dependable transportation to the homes of the clients. In small towns and rural areas, the worker needs to have a car to get from

FIGURE 34-3 Caring for the same client over a period of time provides great satisfaction.

FIGURE 34-4 The patient and family select a home health agency.

one client to the next. In larger cities, the worker may be able to use public transportation.

SOURCE OF REFERRAL

Most persons using home care are patients being discharged from a hospital or skilled care facility. The health care team at the discharging facility completes a discharge plan and evaluates the person's need for continuing care at home. The physician must then write an order for home health care. The discharge planner at the hospital or long-term care facility provides the patient and family with a list of agencies from which to choose the home care provider (Figure 34-4). (In some areas of the country, only one agency may be available.) The selected agency is given medical information about the patient and then begins to plan care.

PAYMENT FOR HOME HEALTH CARE

Home health care may be paid for by:
- Medicare, for persons over 65 years of age or for those who have been disabled for 2 or more years
- Medicaid (in some states)
- Private insurance companies
- Client's personal funds

Government programs and most insurance companies will only pay for home care that is considered "skilled" and is provided as **intermittent care**. This means that the nursing assistant or other caregiver goes to the home, performs certain procedures or treatments, and then leaves. If a family or client needs a caregiver for several hours a day,

they will probably have to pay for the services with their own money. Because this is very costly, most home care is given on an intermittent basis.

Clients who are members of an HMO must use a home health agency that is affiliated with the HMO. The Medicare program and insurance companies pay for most home health care. To qualify for payment, a home health agency must be approved by the Medicare program. This means that surveyors will regularly inspect the agency to ensure that it meets quality standards. The client's doctor must have approved the need for home health care, and must prepare a plan of care for the home. Medicare pays only for intermittent care and therapy services. It does not cover full-time care.

Medicare defines *intermittent*, or *part-time*, *care* as a maximum of 28 hours per week of skilled nursing and home health aide care combined. Medicare does not pay for home health aide care unless the client is also getting skilled care such as nursing or therapy. In special situations, skilled nursing and home health aide services can be provided for up to a combined total of 8 hours a day, 7 days a week, for several weeks. Likewise, the weekly limit for care may be increased to 35 hours, but these exceptions are for a limited, predictable period of time only. A reduced level of care may be provided after that.

The client must be homebound. A home can be a house or apartment, a relative's home, or an assisted living facility. Facilities that mainly provide skilled nursing or rehabilitation services do not qualify. Absences from home must be infrequent, or of short duration, or to get medical care. A client can be considered homebound if he or she occasionally goes to the barber or beauty shop or for a walk around the block or a short drive.

Age-Appropriate Care ALERT

Clients receiving home care vary widely in age. They are not all elderly. Many are children with serious illness or disabilities. Some will need temporary care, but others will need lifetime care. The needs of some clients are complex, placing great demands on family caregivers. Caregiving can be difficult for family members and loved ones. Having outside caregivers come to the home assists them to maintain the quality of their own lives, and gives them time to take care of their personal affairs. ■

THE HOME HEALTH CARE TEAM

The home health care team consists of the:

- Client (the person in need of care)
  - Clients are of various ages.
  - They need differing levels of nursing and physical care.
  - They may have chronic, progressive ailments.
  - They may be recovering from acute illness, surgery, or childbirth.
  - They need assistance with activities of daily living.
  - They usually require skilled services.
- Family
  - Family members may act as alternate caregivers.
  - They may live in the client's home.
  - They may or may not be supportive of the client.
- Nursing assistant
  - Provides direct client care (Figure 34-5).
  - Provides for the client's safety and comfort.
  - Makes observations and reports them to the nurse.
  - Documents observations and care that was given.
- Supervising nurse
  - Completes periodic client assessments.
  - Plans the care.
  - Teaches and supervises nursing assistants.
  - Coordinates care and members of the home care team.
- Physician
  - Writes orders and acts as a consultant and guide.
- Other specialists, such as:
  - physical therapist (Figure 34-6)
  - occupational therapist
  - speech therapist
  - social worker
  - dietitian

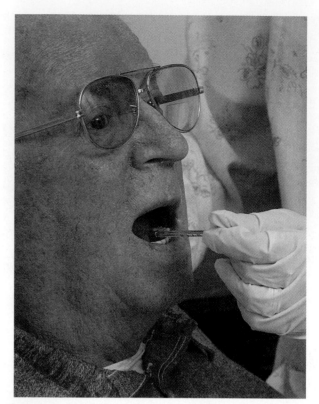

FIGURE 34-5 The home health assistant provides direct client care.

FIGURE 34-6 Many disciplines work together to meet the client's needs. The physical therapist makes home visits several times a week.

THE ASSESSMENT PROCESS

The nurse does an assessment of the client during the first visit. Other health care professionals assigned to the case also complete assessments. After the assessments are finished, the nurse and other team members:

- Identify the client's problems
- Determine approaches to resolve the problems
- Establish goals for the client
- Evaluate the home situation for safety concerns
- Determine the amount of time needed for each visit and the length of time the services may be required

The nurse discusses the plans with the client. The nurse includes the client's wishes as much as possible within the available payment plan. The nurse then develops the assignment for the nursing assistant. You may be assigned to care for several clients or a particular client for a:

- Specified number of hours daily
- Specified period two or three days per week
- Long-term period
- Brief period

The doctor and home health agency personnel review the plan of care as often as necessary, but at least once every 62 days. Professional staff must notify the doctor promptly of any changes in condition that suggest a need to modify the plan of care.

LIABILITY AND THE NURSING ASSISTANT

You need to be aware of the responsibilities involved in home care and how to avoid legal problems associated with caregiving.

RECORDKEEPING

Be sure you know exactly what documentation you are expected to do, what types of records you should keep, and the forms you need to use. All documentation must be accurate, complete, and up-to-date. Medicare and insurance companies frequently audit these records to decide whether to pay for the services.

Two types of records are compiled by the nursing assistant giving home care. They are time/travel records and client care records.

Time/travel records (Figure 34-8) are a record of how you spend your time in the client's home. The information recorded includes:

GUIDELINES *for*
Avoiding Liability

- Be sure you are given a job description upon employment that lists your specific duties and responsibilities. In some areas, home health assistants are only allowed to do certain assigned tasks if they or the employing agency are working with an insurance company or Medicare. Auditors check the tasks assigned and confirm what is actually done in the client's home.
- Carry out procedures carefully and do them as you were taught.
- Always keep safety factors in mind and be on the lookout for possible hazards.
- Be familiar with client's rights.
- Ask for assistance if you are assigned to do a procedure that you have never performed before. Make sure the procedure is within the legal boundaries of nursing assistant practice.
- Do only those tasks that are assigned to you.
- Know how to contact the supervising nurse for questions and issues related to the care of your client. Do not overstep your authority.

- Know how and when to contact emergency services for the client (Figure 34-7).
- Document your care and observations carefully and completely.
- Participate in care conferences with the other team members.

FIGURE 34-7 Home health workers must know how to contact emergency services.

- Time of arrival
- Time of departure
- Length of time required for specific activities
- Travel time if working in more than one home
- Mileage or transportation costs

Keeping a time/travel record requires accuracy and some calculations. Fill in the record as you complete each assignment. Do not wait until the end of the shift and then try to rely on your memory.

To compute mileage (round off to the nearest full mile):

- Record the car odometer reading before starting to your assignment.
- Record the odometer reading when you arrive at the client's home.
- Subtract the starting odometer reading from the arrival reading.
- Record this difference as the mileage.

For example, if the reading on your car odometer before starting was 45,061 and upon arrival at the client's home it is 45,068, the mileage should be recorded as 7 miles (45,068 – 45,061).

Client care records (Figure 34-9) are a record of:

- Care given, such as bathing, positioning, range-of-motion exercises
- Client responses to care
- Housekeeping tasks completed, if assigned to you by the nurse
- Observations:
  - Condition of skin
  - Vital signs
  - Elimination; bowel and urine
  - Food and fluid intake
  - Appetite
  - Incidents such as client falls
  - Any observation that indicates a change in the client's health status
  - Mental status: orientation, alertness, mood, and behavior

You may be expected to keep reports that cover a longer period of time. For example, you may need to keep a weekly or monthly record of daily blood testing results for

RIVERVIEW HOME HEALTH SERVICE
8987 Walkman Ave
Parkhurst, Nebraska
Time and Travel Log

CARE GIVER NAME ___Siadto, Laura CNA___   TITLE ___Home Health Assistant___   EMPT. NO. __62718__   DATE __Aug. 29__

CLIENT NAME/ADDRESS (Last, first)	SERVICE PROVIDED	VISIT CODE	NON BILL CODE	TIME IN	TIME OUT	CLIENT CONTACT TIME	ODOMETER READING	MILES
Volheim, Eleonore	Bedbath, Shampoo	4		8¹⁵	9⁰⁵	50 min	From: 45,061 To: 45,068	7 miles
Jaronello, Sharri		1		9³⁰	9⁴⁵	15 min	From: 45,068 To: 45,083	15 miles
Doyle, Kindra	Enema, bedbath, amb	4		10¹⁰	11³⁰	1 hr. 20 min.	From: 45,083 To: 46,001	18 miles
Hammond, Rachel	Ass't c colostomy cath care, bath, ROM	4		11⁵⁰	1²⁰	1 hr. 30 min.	From: 46,001 To: 46,017	16 miles
Minzey, Aimee		2		1³⁰	1³⁵	—	From: 46,017 To: 46,025	8 miles
Galloway, Rosa		5		1⁵⁰	2⁰⁰	10 min	From: 46,025 To: 46,028	3 miles
							From: To:	

Total Visits __6__   Total Mileage __67__   Parking Fees ___—___

Visit Code
1 IE Initial Eval & Rx   4 HC Home Care
2 FV Follow Up Visit   5 Hospital/Hospice
3 DV Discharge Visit   6 MC Maternal/Child

Supervising Nurse: _Bruce Davenport R.N._

Nonbill Code
1. Refused Care
2. Patient Not Home
3. Non-Bill
4. Expired
5. Delivered Supplies

FIGURE 34-8 Example of a time/travel record

RIVERVIEW HOME HEALTH SERVICE
8987 Walkman Ave
Parkhurst, Nebraska
Client Care Plan / Progress Notes

HOME HEALTH ASSISTANT <u>YOLANDA BROWN, CNA</u>

CLIENT NAME <u>NICHOLAS FRENCH</u>   CLIENT ID # <u>72824C</u>

ADDRESS: <u>529 MAPLE AVE.   PARKHURST, NEBRASKA</u>

	ACTIVITY
0800	Arrived, Determined needs, planned activities Client seemed fatigued "Slept poorly". On nasal O_2 2.5L
0830	Circumoral pallor noted. Vital signs checked. Dyspneic on exertion.
0900	Put laundry into washing machine. Started breakfast. Client ate 1 sl. toast, 8 oz oatbran cereal / milk 6oz orange juice
0930	Prepared equipment for A.M. care – complete bath, shave and denture care.
1000	Asst to commode, soft brown formed stool.
1030	Made comfortable in easy chair. Reading newspaper. Nasal O_2 Cleaned kitchen including refrigerator
1100	Linen changed – dusted and dust mopped bedroom. Vacuumed living room.
1130	Prepared lunch.
1200	Client ate 1/2 chicken sandwich, 8 oz. tea, chocolate pudding, 8 oz. tomato soup.
1230	Client returned to bed for nap
1300	Cleaned lunch dishes and prepared salad, jello for evening meal
1330	Put washed laundry into dryer.
1400	Cleaned bathroom, washed kitchen floor
1400	Put bed linen into washer.
1430	Made out shopping list for A.M.
1500	Client awake. Assisted into living room. Watching T.V. Ordered O_2 tank replacement.
1530	Folded and put clean laundry away. Put washed linens in dryer.
1600	Client seems more rested. Color improved. Resp. easier. Notified supervisor of client's progress.
1630	Left client's home @ 3^{25} P.M.
	Y. Brown CNA

VITAL SIGNS	T	P	R	B/P
	97^4	92	26	116/74
INTAKE	486 mL			
OUTPUT	730 mL			

SUP. SIGNATURE _____

FIGURE 34-9 Examples of client care records

RIVERVIEW HOME HEALTH SERVICE
8987 Walkman Ave
Parkhurst, Nebraska
Client Care Plan / Progress Notes

WT. _146_ TEMP. _98_ BP _114/80_ P _70_ R _14_ MD CONTACT _C. Boylston_

HOMEBOUND DUE TO _Spinal Cord Injury – Paraplegia_ MEN. STATUS _Alert – Coherent_

PROBLEMS	INTERVENTIONS	TIME	PLAN	OUTCOME
① Potential altered	Maintain high-calorie, low-residue, high protein diet		Morning Care	Tol. Well
nutrition: less than	Reduce high calcium and gas-producing foods.	0700	Breakfast	ate entire meal
body requirements	Provide balanced meals and supplements morning and evening	0815	Commode	soft formed stool
		0900	Bath, Cath Care,	
		0945	ROM	
			up in wheelchair	Tolerated well
② Potential for disuse	Exercise to tolerance Avoid fatigue ROM	1030	6oz High Cal drink	
syndrome related to	Turn and reposition q 1 hr.	1045	Returned to Bed	
effects of immobility	Up in wheelchair B.I.D.	1130	Positioned on Rt. Side	
	Encourage self-care activities to tolerance		Positioned on Back	
③ Alteration in bowel	Stool Softener, Glycerine	1230	Lunch	½ tuna sand/tea
elimination: constipation	Suppositories, enemas, PRN.			
	Check for BM q 3 day		up in wheelchair	
		1330	Returned to Bed	
④ Potential for infection	Routine catheter care	1430	Positioned on left side	
related to indwelling	Change per routine schedule		Watching T.V.	
Foley catheter		1500		
⑤ Self-concept disturbance	Encourage verbalization of feelings and fears.			
related to effects of	Encourage independence. Be positive and reassuring.			
limitations				

DAILY SUMMARY

Diet and supplements taken fairly well. Activity tolerated. Muscles soft but some tone. Soft formed stool.

Expressed frustration during transfers from bed to wheelchair. Enjoys reading and watching T.V.

Seems to be gaining some confidence in transfer activities.

Visit Date _____ Pt. Last Name, Employee

Nursing Supervisor Report First Initial _Mitchell, D._ Signature _Ruthy Chek, CNA_

Joint Visit in Home _____ Patient's personal care and comfort measures by home assistant are:

Conference _____ superior _____ ; good _____ ; satisfactory _____ ; need improvement _____ ;

Services provided were appropriate _____ ; inappropriate _____ .

Comments

FIGURE 34-9 *CONTINUED*

a client with diabetes. The physician may change the schedule of insulin based on your long-term report.

TIME MANAGEMENT

As a home health care assistant, you are responsible for planning your assignment and completing the client's care within a certain amount of time. You may have several clients to see during your shift. They will be expecting you at a specific time of the day. There are several actions you can take to make the best use of your time:

- Be sure you have everything you will need for your assignments before you leave home. This might include a thermometer, watch with second hand, stethoscope, blood pressure cuff, forms for documenting, pen.
- Have a work plan in mind before you arrive at the client's home. For example, will you give the client a bath first or help him with his exercises first?
- Organize your supplies before you begin your assignment. Gather together the linens, client clothing, and other items you will need.

- Avoid being distracted by the family. There are many things you may need to discuss with the family, but you probably will not have time for lengthy conversations.
- Call your next client if you find you will be arriving later than expected.
- Avoid getting bogged down in tasks that you are not assigned to perform.

WORKING WITH FAMILIES

Clients may have a spouse or other family members who reside in the home. For other clients, their families may live elsewhere but stop in periodically. In some situations family members may live so far away that they can seldom visit. Family members may call or visit while you are there, seeking information on the client's condition. It is best to let the client speak with them directly if possible. If the client cannot do this, then remember to be objective in your comments. If you do not know the answer to a question, be honest and say so rather than providing false information. Refer all medical questions to the physician or the nurse.

Remember that as a home health assistant, you are a guest of the family and client. You may be assigned to clients who have values and cultural beliefs that are vastly different from yours. It is not your role to try to change this. Report to your supervisor if you feel that there are family practices that are detrimental to the client's well-being and health. Families can be an excellent resource for you. They may be able to give you additional information about the client that will help you to give better care. This can avoid frustration for both you and the client. The family may also be able to tell you how they have cared for the client in the past.

Tact and courtesy are important when communicating with the family. They may wish to be involved in the caregiving, but it is important that you complete the tasks to which you have been assigned. The family has a right to know the progress the patient is making, but there may be some information that the client does not wish you to tell the family. You may need to discuss this issue with your supervisor. Families may feel overwhelmed and discouraged at times, particularly if the client has had a long illness. They need your support, so you must be realistic yet hopeful (Figure 34-10).

If you are spending an entire shift with the client, remember that you are getting paid to spend this time giving care. If all procedures are completed, take your cue from the client or family as to what activities you should complete for the rest of your tour of duty. Some clients may wish to be left alone to read (Figure 34-11) or watch television. Others may seek your companionship for visiting or playing cards. If you are working through the night, ask the client or family if you may read or do quiet activities such as needlework while the client is sleeping. Family

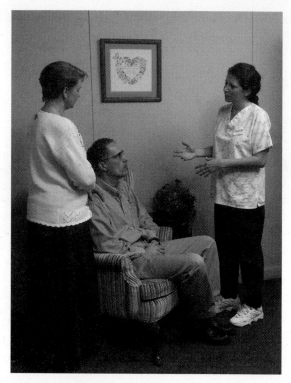

FIGURE 34-10 You must be realistic yet hopeful with families.

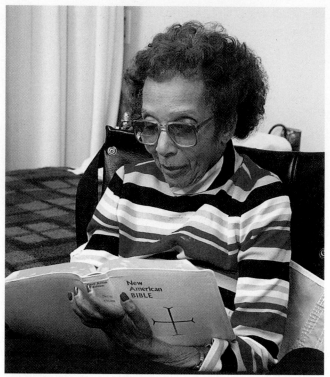

FIGURE 34-11 Some clients may prefer to be left alone to pursue their own interests.

members may ask you to do something that is not part of your assignment. Whether you can meet their request depends on:

- The nature of the request

- The time involved in filling the request
- The policies of the home care agency
- Whether you are assigned to intermittent visits to the client or assigned to work a full shift

REVIEW

A. True/False.

Mark the following true or false by circling T or F.

1. T F World War I stimulated the enrollment of students in hospital-based nursing programs.

2. T F Many new hospitals were built after World War II.

3. T F Only nurses and nursing assistants are employed in home health care.

4. T F The physician acts as care coordinator for the client's home care.

5. T F Home health assistants are expected to provide direct client care.

6. T F Documentation is an important responsibility of the home care assistant.

7. T F The demand for home care has decreased within the last few years.

8. T F The client may receive the services of a physical therapist.

9. T F The home health care assistant may have the opportunity for part-time employment.

10. T F The home health assistant is responsible for completing periodic assessments of the client.

B. Multiple Choice.

Select the one best answer for each of the following.

11. World War II brought about
    a. an increase in the need for more technical care.
    b. widespread use of antibiotics.
    c. a limited supply of health care workers.
    d. construction of hundreds of nursing homes.

12. Home care is increasing because
    a. hospitals are overcrowded.
    b. there are fewer physicians.
    c. people prefer being cared for in their own homes.
    d. families always do some of the nursing care.

13. The person receiving home health care is called the
   a. client.
   b. patient.
   c. resident.
   d. recipient.

14. Members of the home care team include
   a. housekeepers.
   b. the family.
   c. laundry workers.
   d. gardeners.

15. Time management is important because
   a. you can get home earlier.
   b. you may have more than one client to care for during your shift.
   c. the client may have other business to tend to.
   d. the agency will make more money if you work faster.

16. Home care assistants must be able to:
   a. know how to care for family pets.
   b. make accurate observations.
   c. manage the household bills.
   d. drive the client's car.

C. Nursing Assistant Challenge.

You are almost finished with your nursing assistant course and you are thinking about employment. You have been offered jobs in a home health agency and in a hospital and are having trouble making a decision. Your instructor advises you to think about both the advantages and disadvantages of working for each employer. Make a two-column list for each, labeling the columns "advantages" and "disadvantages."

The Nursing Assistant in Home Care

OBJECTIVES

After completing this unit, you will be able to:

- Spell and define terms.
- Describe the characteristics that are especially important to the nursing assistant providing home care.
- List at least 10 methods of protecting your personal safety when working as a home care assistant in the community.

- Describe the duties of the nursing assistant who works in the home setting.
- Describe the duties of the homemaker assistant.
- Carry out home care activities needed to maintain a safe and clean environment.

VOCABULARY

Learn the meaning and the correct spelling of the following words and phrases:

| home health assistant | homemaker aide | homemaker assistant |

THE HOME HEALTH CAREGIVER

In the last unit you learned about the structure of home health care. In this unit you will learn more about the responsibilities of the nursing assistant (home health assistant) working in the client's home.

The nursing assistant is an important part of the health team in the acute hospital and in the long-term care facility. The nursing assistant is part of an equally important team that provides home care.

The nursing assistant may be called:

- **Home health assistant** or home health aide, whose primary role is to provide assistance with nursing care.
- **Homemaker assistant** or **homemaker aide** when the primary role is to do housekeeping chores. The homemaker assistant carries out general household tasks, prepares meals, and runs errands such as food shopping.

The nursing assistant providing health care services may be asked to carry out homemaker assistant duties in some cases.

THE HOME HEALTH ASSISTANT AND THE NURSING PROCESS

You are part of the nursing process. During:

- *Assessment*, your observations and careful reporting can make a valuable contribution to the objective and subjective data from which the analysis of the client's needs is made. Make note of:
  - The client's response to your care
  - The interactions between family members and friends that could lead to stress on the client
  - Support services that may be needed

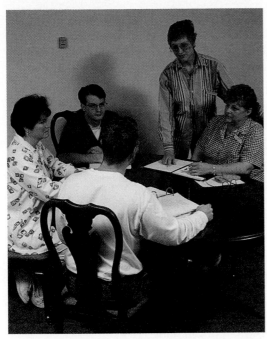

FIGURE 35-1 The home health assistant contributes to the client's care plan.

Clinical Information ALERT

Remember the importance of first impressions. The client and family's first impression of you will set the tone for your future working relationship. Take the time to introduce yourself and explain your responsibilities as a nursing assistant. Many people know what nurses are expected to do, but they are unsure of the nursing assistant's responsibilities on the health care team. Taking the time to introduce yourself and having a quick discussion about your role will help to begin a positive working relationship. ∎

- *Planning,* you contribute as you actively share in care conferences (Figure 35-1).
- *Implementation,* you spend the most time with the client. You are therefore responsible for seeing that the plan is carried out.
  - Report any difficulties in carrying out the plan
  - Develop ways of organizing your work to make the plan more efficient
- *Evaluation,* you once more contribute to the nursing process when you share your observations about the success or lack of success of the care.
  - Be accurate and concise in your reporting

- Be honest in your appraisal of the client's progress and the point at which your services are no longer needed

CHARACTERISTICS OF THE HOME CARE NURSING ASSISTANT AND HOMEMAKER ASSISTANT

The home care nursing assistant and homemaker assistant must have a full measure of the characteristics you have already come to associate with a successful family-based assistant. However, some characteristics should be particularly strong in an assistant who works in clients' homes.

Remember that you will be working directly with the client and her personal possessions, without a supervising nurse constantly with you. This means you must demonstrate:

- Honesty, as you handle the client's possessions and shopping money. Treat the possessions with care and respect. Keep an accurate record of all money spent and receipts received.
- Self-starter ability. You must know and carry out your assigned tasks promptly and efficiently without needing someone to remind you.
- Self-discipline. Do not allow yourself to waste time on activities such as smoking, chatting with friends on the phone, and drinking coffee just because no supervisor is constantly checking on your progress.
- Accuracy and attention to details, so that each task is performed exactly as you were taught.
- Organization, so that you plan your activities to make the best use of your in-home time. Plan your activities around the client's schedule, not your own.
- Maturity, so that judgment and assessments can be made properly.
- Insight that gives you the ability to see the client as a whole person who is an interactive member of a family unit and community.
- Observational skills. Be able to recognize and report abnormal signs and symptoms.
- Adaptability. Although you will need all the physical, emotional, and communication skills you learned and practiced in the clinical setting, you must be creative in adapting them to the home situation. For example, a cut-open plastic bag covered with a towel may be substituted for the bed protectors used in the hospital. Housekeeping chores may be performed as the client rests.
- Acceptance of clients and their home environments. Remember, your clients will be of all ethnic and religious groups and economic levels.
- Ability to perform independently, making decisions within the limits of your responsibilities and the scope of the assignment.

THE NURSING BAG

Most home health care workers carry a nursing bag stocked with the supplies they use routinely in client care. Your bag should be stocked with enough supplies to carry you through the day without having to replenish it. You will probably need it on every visit, and when special treatments or procedures are assigned. Use a tote bag, backpack, or other carrying case that helps you keep your supplies organized and easy to find. The fabric or outside of the bag should be washable or easy to clean. You should clean and restock your bag daily. Bring it in your house at night, or leave in the clinical office. Never leave it in the car. Leaving it in the car invites theft, and heat and cold extremes may damage some of your equipment and supplies. People see the bag and associate it with helping clients. Make it clear to anyone who inquires that the bag does not contain any medications or syringes. When leaving your car for a short period of time, store the bag out of sight and lock the doors.

Nursing Bag Supplies

As you gain experience, you will quickly customize your nursing bag to include items that you find necessary and convenient. Your agency may have a basic supply list. If not, consider your responsibilities and assignments, and pack a basic list of supplies to get started:

- Cell phone
- Phone numbers
- Pens
- Paper or memo book
- Extra forms for documentation
- Waterless (alcohol) hand cleaner
- Small bottle of liquid hand soap (antibacterial or antimicrobial type)
- Street map
- Stethoscope
- Blood pressure cuff
- Thermometer, thermometer sheaths
- Pen light
- Tongue depressors, applicators, plastic bandage strips, adhesive tape, cotton balls, paper tape, 2 × 2 and 4 × 4 dressings if you are responsible for simple dressings

- Alcohol and povidone-iodine swabs
- Safety pins
- Newspapers
- Disposable, plastic aprons
- Paper bag
- Plastic trash bags
- Small plastic bags
- Lubricant jelly or Vaseline
- Bandage scissors
- Rubber bands
- Gloves
- Resuscitation mask
- N95 mask
- Goggles or face shield
- Finger and toenail clippers in sheath
- Orangewood sticks
- Emery boards
- Household disinfectant
- Perineal cleanser ("peri-wash")
- Baby wipes
- Paper towels (carry a few folded dispenser towels, not an entire roll)

Some home health nursing assistants carry personal care items, such as aromatherapy soap, lotion, and shampoo. Grooming and hygiene products of this nature are not required, but they are certainly a bonus for the client's self-esteem.

Surprisingly, some homes do not have running water. Alcohol-based hand cleaner is effective, but the CDC recommends washing hands with soap and water if the hands are visibly soiled. Some workers carry a gallon jug of water in the car for this purpose. Others use premoistened towelettes. In general, towelettes are not as effective for hand cleansing as alcohol gel or handwashing with soap and water. If an alternate method of handwashing must be used, you may want to find a gas station or other facilities and wash your hands with soap and water as soon as possible after leaving the client's home.

When you bring your nursing bag or other supplies into a home, you must place them on a barrier. Many agencies recommend using a piece of newspaper as a barrier. However, some workers avoid newspaper because the newsprint may transfer onto the outside of the nursing bag and the client's bed linen. Some workers use a roll of waxed paper instead, tearing off a sheet each time a barrier is needed. However, waxed paper tends to melt or stick together in a warm car in the summer. Other workers carry disposable underpads ("blue pads") to use as a barrier. These have a plastic backing with a paper surface.

When leaving the home, discard trash, including the barrier pad, into a plastic bag and tie the top closed. Some agencies require workers to bring trash with them, for later disposal at the agency. Discard according to agency policy.

Before using items from your bag:

1. Select a location for placement of your bag that is out of the reach of children. Place your bag on newspaper or another barrier. Prepare a clean area for placement of equipment to use on the client, if necessary. Again, use a barrier if you must place items on a bed or other potentially contaminated area.

2. Wash your hands or use an alcohol hand cleaner.

3. Put on a plastic apron and remove necessary items from your bag. Close the bag.

4. When you are finished, wash and clean reusable equipment. The plastic apron may be left in the client's home or discarded, according to agency policy.

5. Wash your hands and replace equipment in your bag. Store contaminated supplies in a plastic bag for later cleaning and disinfection.
   - If you used bandage scissors, wash them well with soap and water and dry well.

6. Discard contaminated disposable items. It is best if you seal these items in plastic bags and take them to the outside trash cans when you leave for the day. Do not leave contaminated waste in an open waste-basket in the home.
   - Reusable containers in the home, such as plastic wastebaskets, may be used to hold medical waste temporarily, if lined with a plastic bag. Empty the wastebasket daily and replace the bag.
   - If the wastebasket is not lined completely with a plastic bag, it must be washed and thoroughly sanitized each time it is emptied.

PERSONAL SAFETY

Personal safety is always a concern for home care workers. Be alert to conditions and people around you. Inform your employer promptly if you believe unsafe conditions exist. Thousands of nursing personnel make daily home care visits, and incidents of violence are few. However, you must trust your own instincts. If something does not feel right, it probably is not.

Other ways of protecting your own safety are:

- Map out the route in advance so you know where you are going. If you or your agency has online access, print a map with written directions to each new client's residence.

- Inform the patient what time you will be arriving.

- Lock your purse in the trunk of your car at the beginning of your day. Use pockets or a belt-type (fanny) pack for essentials such as driver's license and pens.

- Wear scrubs or clothing that identifies you as a nursing caregiver. Wear your name badge.

- In potentially dangerous areas, ask your agency if you can make joint visits with a coworker or use an escort.

- If neighbors, relatives, or others become a safety problem, make visits when they are away from the home.

- If a patient suggests that a family member escort you, accept the offer, but never get into someone else's car.

- Keep your gas tank full.

- Avoid parking on deserted streets or in dark areas.

- Keep your car windows up and doors locked at all times.

- Attend classes on personal safety and self-defense.

- Consider purchasing a cellular telephone.

HOME HEALTH CARE DUTIES

The duties of the home health care assistant are planned around the family routine. These duties may include:

- Helping with the activities of daily living

- Giving special treatments, such as prescribed exercises

- Providing comfort measures, such as positioning and special mouth care

- Maintaining a safe environment

- Bathing the client

- Changing linen

- Interacting with family members

Homemaker duties may include:

- Light housekeeping

- Shopping for meals (Figure 35-2)

- Preparing meals

You may also have to transport the client to clinic or therapy visits (Figure 35-3). You must have specific permission

FIGURE 35-2 Homemaker duties may include grocery shopping. Prepare a shopping list before going to the store to make sure you get everything.

Difficult SITUATIONS

Sometimes an ice bag is ordered to be applied to a small area, or an area in which a full, large bag causes pain. Try popcorn kernels. Measure a small quantity and place them in a sandwich bag. Tie the bag at the top, then freeze it. The bag can be custom-fitted to small areas, and can be reused when it warms up. Just return it to the freezer. Placing crushed ice in a glove and tying a knot in the end may also work, depending on the area you are treating and the length of the application. Tie the hand opening to the thumb, rather than knotting it closed or using a rubber band. Cover the glove with a washcloth or disposable cover. Gloves that are closed in this manner are less likely to leak than plastic bags. ■

from your agency to perform activities outside of the home. The homemaker duties *do not* include:

- Doing heavy housework such as washing windows, waxing floors, or moving heavy furniture
- Making decisions about food purchases, unless the client is unable to do so

FIGURE 35-3 The home health assistant may have to transport clients to clinics for additional care and therapy.

- Becoming involved in family disputes by offering opinions or taking sides

The skills you learned in the clinical setting can be adapted to the home environment (Figure 35-4). For example:

- Ice bags can be replaced by plastic bags sealed and wrapped in a towel.
- Reusable enema equipment can be substituted for disposable enema equipment.
- Extra pillows can be used to support position changes if the bed position cannot be changed.
- Some equipment may be rented from equipment rental companies (Figure 35-5) or borrowed from church groups or other organizations.
- The entire bed can be raised on blocks, to make caregiving easier if the patient is not ambulatory.
- A cotton blanket or lightweight spread can be used for a bath blanket.
- Plastic covered with a twin-size sheet can be used in place of a drawsheet.
- Making an occupied bed by yourself may be easier if you make a bedroll first. Prepare the linen you will need by laying it out on the table. Then roll it up from side to side, then top to bottom. When the client is on her side, place the roll on the bed and unroll the linen halfway behind the client's back. Turn her on her other side and unroll the rest of the bedroll.
- Apply the principles of standard precautions if contact with blood, body fluids, mucous membranes, or nonintact skin is likely.
- A cardboard box can be cut, taped, and padded for use as a backrest (Figure 35-6A).
- Two lightweight pieces of wood nailed at right angles can be padded and used as a footrest to hold bedding off the toes (Figure 35-6B).
- A bed tray can replace an overbed table for eating and activities.
- A paper bag can be taped to the bed springs to dispose of soiled tissues (Figure 35-6C). The entire bag can then be closed and properly handled for disposal.
- A shoe bag tucked under the mattress and hanging by the bedside (Figure 35-6D) can provide compartments for the patient's personal articles.
- A pillowcase hung on the back of a chair can serve as a laundry bag.
- If you are assigned to do dressing changes on minor skin wounds, use a plastic bag. Place your hand inside the bag and gently remove the dressing. Then turn the bag inside out, with the dressing on the inside. Tie or seal the bag and throw it away. Using this method is simple and prevents contamination. Consider using the plastic bag in this manner any time you handle biohazardous or soiled material.
- Wind two rubber bands tightly around a slippery drinking glass to make it easier for a client to grasp. Place the rubber bands about an inch apart.

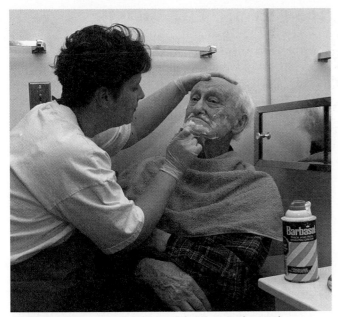

FIGURE 35-4 The skills you have learned may be adapted for care in the home.

FIGURE 35-5 Equipment may be rented or borrowed from other organizations or agencies.

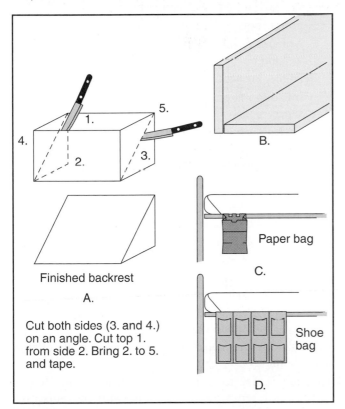

Paper bag

C.

Shoe bag

D.

Finished backrest

A.

Cut both sides (3. and 4.) on an angle. Cut top 1. from side 2. Bring 2. to 5. and tape.

FIGURE 35-6 Make equipment using readily available materials

- Some clients cannot suck forcefully enough to draw liquids up through a straw. Wash and dry your bandage scissors, then cut the straw a few inches shorter. Place the cut end in the bottom of the glass and have the client suck from the smooth end. Removing a few inches is usually enough to enable them to drink the liquid.

- Clients who use walkers and wheelchairs may become frustrated because of their inability to carry items with

them. Attaching an inexpensive cloth tote bag, bicycle basket, or even a plastic grocery sack will work. Position the bag on the front of the walker or on one arm of the wheelchair. If the doorways are narrow, fasten the straps so the bag can be flipped up and held on the client's lap when going through the door. This is a good method for a cordless or cellular phone, or other important items. Although this may seem to be a small step, it is an excellent method of promoting client independence and helping him control the environment.

- A client who uses oxygen continuously is at risk for discomfort and skin breakdown behind the ears from the nasal cannula. To solve this problem, cut a small foam hair curler lengthwise, then wrap the foam around the tubing that rests on the ears. The cheekbones are also a tender area. Wrapping a corn or bunion pad (adhesive side in) around the cannula in the appropriate spot will also relieve pressure.

- If you care for a client who lives with a hard-of-hearing caregiver, suggest that they purchase a baby monitor. Place the receiver in the room near the client's head. Place the speaker in a room (or between two rooms) where the caregiver spends most of her time. Set the unit on "high" so the caregiver can hear it. Another option is to use a wireless or battery-operated doorbell. Give the client the bell button. Plug the bell into whichever outlet is closest to the caregiver.

- To weigh a client who has trouble balancing, ask the client to step onto the scale while holding onto a walker. The client will need to let go for about a second while you get the weight, but having the walker in front of the scale is usually adequate to maintain balance.

- Place a large piece of plastic on the car seat (you can cut a large trash bag, if necessary). The plastic enables the client to slide easily onto or off the seat.

- Use a wire coat hanger to hang a catheter bag on the bed. Slide the hanger between the mattress and box spring, leaving only about an inch of the hook exposed. Hang the loop on the drainage bag on the hook.

- Denture cleaner or dishwasher soap are both effective for removing sediment and stains on the bedpan and urinals. Pour very hot water into the bedpan or urinal and then add one tablet of denture cleaner or 1/4 cup of dishwasher soap. Stir with a tongue blade and let sit for a few minutes. Empty the solution into the toilet and rinse. This eliminates odor and sediment.

- Use a turkey baster (that is reserved for this purpose) and warm water to rinse reusable ostomy pouches and other items.

Difficult SITUATIONS

Dry, sore, burning, itchy eyes are a common problem in the elderly. If they do not clean the eyes regularly, the eyelids fill with matter, which worsens the problem. Washing the eyelids with tearless baby shampoo several times a day and rinsing with warm water clears the condition quickly. A cotton pad is an excellent tool for washing and rinsing the eyes. ■

Difficult SITUATIONS

If the client or a family member informs you of new problems with any of the following when no home care worker is on duty, notify your supervisor: eating, getting in or out of bed, maintaining continence or using the toilet, bathing, or dressing. Clients with new problems related to these activities require further nursing assessment. ■

THE HOME ENVIRONMENT

You are responsible for maintaining a safe and comfortable environment for the client. This means you must:

- Be alert to unsafe situations
- Control the spread of infection
- Care for and maintain the client's furnishings, supplies, and appliances
- Learn the locations of items that may be needed in an emergency (such as a flashlight or fire extinguisher)

SAFETY IN THE HOME

Your first visit to the home gives you an opportunity to check for safety factors. Tell a family member or supervising nurse about safety problems. For example, things to call to the attention of your supervisor include:

- Furniture or other items that obstruct the client's walkway
- Electrical cords that could cause the client to fall
- Stair railings and stair treads that need repair
- Unstable or lightweight chairs
- Highly polished floors that may be slippery
- The need to lock up specific items if the client is disoriented:
  - chemicals such as household cleaning supplies, paints, insecticides, and cleaning fluids
  - medications, both prescription and over-the-counter
  - aerosol cans
  - small appliances like toasters or irons that can be plugged in and used inappropriately
  - power tools
  - weapons or anything that could be used as a weapon
  - fragile, breakable, or valuable items
  - smoking materials that should be used only with supervision
  - electrical outlets that require covering
  - thermostats that may need guards over them
  - stove knobs
- Loose scatter rugs, which might cause a fall as the client ambulates
- Electrical cords that are under rugs, creating a fire hazard
- Lack of smoke detectors and a fire extinguisher
- Overloaded electrical outlets, which might cause a fire when you use equipment such as an electric lift
- Ambulatory aids that need repair or replacement, such as broken straps on braces or worn rubber tips on walkers, canes, and crutches
- Family or client smoking when oxygen is being used in the home

Your job is not to reorganize the client's home but to ensure a safe environment. Discuss with the nurse any other conditions you feel are unsafe. For example, the client may need:

- Handrails installed by the toilet or the bathtub
- A commode to use if the bathroom is not easily accessible
- A raised toilet seat
- A trapeze to assist with bed mobility
- A mechanical lift for transferring out of bed

These items are readily available from durable equipment providers, and most insurance companies and Medicare will pay for equipment that is required for client care. However, the nurse must consult with the physician and an order must be written for the equipment.

Keep a list of emergency numbers close to the telephone. The list should include the:

- Agency
- Supervising nurse
- Physician
- Family member
- Emergency number 911 (in areas where this number is in use)

If the 911 number is not used in your area, you will need numbers for the:

- Ambulance
- Hospital
- Police department
- Fire department

You should find out if the patient:

- uses a medical alert bracelet or necklace.
- has out-of-hospital code papers, advance directives, or a living will.
- has a special storage place in the house for important medical information that would be needed in an emergency. Some people keep these in the refrigerator so they can be easily located.

Assisting with Medications

The physician may prescribe medications for clients receiving home health care. Nursing assistants are not legally responsible for giving medications. However, you may have to supervise the client as she self-administers the medications. The client may need assistance in opening the container. There are many types of containers available that will hold a week's doses in individual sections labeled for the days of the week. These containers simplify the process and it is easy to determine whether the medications have been taken.

ELDER ABUSE

As a home health assistant, you may observe clients who might possibly have been abused. Unit 4 describes the various types of abuse that may be inflicted by staff members, family members, or others. These situations may also occur in the home:

- Some families provide loving, capable care for older, dependent relatives for many years without assistance. They may be emotionally stressed and may have also depleted their financial resources.
- In some cases there has been a long family history of one spouse abusing the other.
- Self-abuse may occur when a disabled person is unable to adequately carry out activities of daily living and is unwilling to accept help.

It is not the responsibility of the nursing assistant to determine if an individual has been abused or what type of abuse has been inflicted. It *is* the nursing assistant's responsibility to report to the nursing supervisor any signs or symptoms that might be the result of abuse. This includes:

- Statements of the client that reflect neglect or abuse
- Unexplained bruises or wounds
- Signs of neglect such as poor hygiene
- A change in personality

Remember, these indications do not necessarily mean that the person is being abused. However, they may signal a need for further investigation by your supervisor.

INFECTION CONTROL

Some of the methods used in daily cleaning help to control the spread of infection. Other requirements are:

- Washing your hands (Figure 35-7) or using an alcohol-based hand cleaner
- Keeping the kitchen and bathroom clean
- Caring for food properly
- Disposing of tissues and other wastes properly
- Cleaning up dirty dishes
- Dusting daily
- Not allowing clutter to accumulate
- Wearing a plastic apron
- Wearing latex gloves for patient care if contact with blood, body fluids, mucous membranes, or nonintact skin is likely
- Wearing utility gloves when cleaning environmental surfaces or doing laundry contaminated with blood, body fluids, secretions, or excretions

Discarding Medical Waste

Your agency will have policies and procedures for discarding disposable, contaminated items, and cleaning permanent items for reuse. Apply the principles of standard precautions and apply personal protective equipment appropriate to the task. Follow your local regulations for disposal of all infectious medical waste. In general:

- Place contaminated supplies in a plastic bag and close tightly.
- Double-bag in a second plastic bag if the outside of the first bag is torn or contaminated.
- Seal the bag by using a twist tie, taping, or tying, or according to agency policy.
- Dispose of double-bagged waste in the household trash. Take it to the outside trash can, if possible, when you leave for the day.
- After discarding trash, wash your hands or use alcohol-based hand cleaner.

FIGURE 35-7 Handwashing is the most important infection control technique in health care. All handwashing rules and guidelines used in facilities also apply to home care.

- Sanitize all contaminated equipment and surfaces appropriately.
- Blood, body fluids, secretions, and excretions may be discarded in the patient's toilet. Pouring should be done slowly and carefully to minimize splashing, spattering, or aerosolizing. Wear eye protection, face mask, and gloves. A gown or plastic apron is also necessary if there is a potential for splashing, spattering, or aerosolizing the fluid.
- Sharp items, such as needles, syringes, fingerstick lancets, and disposable razors, must be placed in a sharps container, which is furnished by the home health care agency and left in the client's home.
  - When the container is 3/4 full, the container should be replaced. This is usually the nurse's responsibility. Inform the nurse when a new container will be needed.
  - When the new container is available, snap the lid of the full container into place, then tape it down. If it is your responsibility to remove it from the home, place the container inside a cardboard box. Seal the box with tape and affix a biohazard emblem, or mark it according to agency policy. Store the box in the trunk of your car. Return it to your agency promptly for disposal. Do not leave it in your car overnight.

HOUSEKEEPING TASKS

In some cases, the homemaker assistant (aide) will perform housekeeping tasks. In other cases, the home health care nursing assistant may be assigned some or all of these duties.

Cleaning the Client's Room

Keeping the client's room clean is a way to prevent infection. It also helps raise the client's morale. Remember that you are not to rearrange the client's things without permission.

- Pick things up so clutter will not accumulate.
- Keep cleaning equipment in one place so you do not waste time gathering it for each job as you move from room to room (Figure 35-8).
- Clean and put equipment away as soon as you have finished with it.
- Dust the room daily.
- Damp-dust noncarpeted floors weekly or vacuum carpeted floors.
- Remove used dishes and glasses when finished and rinse right away.
- Put clean clothes away after laundering. Hang up robes when not in use.
- Line each wastepaper basket with a plastic bag and empty them regularly.

Cleaning the Bathroom

The bathroom can be a source of infection, so you must be careful and thorough in your daily cleaning (Figure 35-9). Use a disinfectant solution (family's choice) to clean the:

- Inside and outside of the toilet
- Shower or tub after each use
- Sink and faucets
- Countertops
- Floor; if carpeted, vacuum daily

Be sure dirty towels are put into the laundry. Replace them with clean towels and washcloths. Use a deodorant to keep the bathroom smelling fresh and clean.

FIGURE 35-8 Keep cleaning equipment together for good organization and efficient time management.

FIGURE 35-9 Clean the bathroom daily.

Cleaning the Kitchen

The kitchen is another area that requires special attention. An unclean kitchen can be the source of infection.

- Clean up after each meal.
- Clean up dirty dishes immediately. Do not allow them to accumulate in the sink.
  - Rinse them and wash by hand in detergent and hot water.
  - Wash glasses first, then silverware, then dishes.
  - Rinse with hot water and allow to dry in drainer.
  - Put away when dry.
- You may wash them in the dishwasher by:
  - Rinsing well.
  - Adding recommended detergent to the dishwasher.
  - Loading washer; but do not run the dishwasher until it is full.
- Wash pots and pans by hand; most are not dishwasher-safe.
- Clean sink, countertops, and stove.
- Dispose of garbage properly. It may be put in an in-sink disposer if one is available. Do not include bones. Wrap those tightly in newspaper and put them in the trash (or compactor if available).
- Sweep the floor after each meal.
- Place leftover foods in small covered containers and refrigerate. Use or discard within a few days.
- Keep the refrigerator clean and keep food covered. Clean spills in the refrigerator immediately (Figure 35-10).

FIGURE 35-10 Wipe spills immediately.

FIGURE 35-11
Wipe the microwave after each use.

- Keep the microwave oven clean (Figure 35-11). Use a damp cloth to wipe up spills immediately and to clean after each use. Make sure you heat food in microwave-safe dishes only. Do not use metal of any kind in a microwave oven. For example, dishes with metallic trim are *not* used.
- Wash the kitchen floor weekly, or more often if necessary.

Ask the client or a responsible family member for instructions on operating appliances before using.

Other Duties

Two other tasks are frequently your responsibility in the home situation. They are food management and laundry.

Food Management. Plan food purchases with the client or a family member. If consultation is not possible, keep these guidelines in mind:

- Plan menus a week in advance. Base them on good nutrition.
- Take into consideration the client's preferences, cultural background, and any religious prohibitions.
- Spend only what the client's budget allows.
- Buy only what you need and what can be used. Large quantities are not a bargain if much of it goes unused or is wasted.
- Look for quality bargains.
- Keep track of all money spent and a list of items purchased; keep receipts.
- Make an accounting of all money handled.

Using the weekly menu, prepare foods in such a way that the client's dietary needs are met. Also:

- Wash fresh fruits and vegetables that are to be used soon and store in the refrigerator; store them unwashed if they are not to be used right away. Remember to wash them before use.
- Keep dairy products and meats refrigerated until use.
- Allow frozen meats to thaw in the refrigerator before use.
- Take into consideration the client's ordered diet, any digestive problems, and preferences.
- Keep dried and canned foods in cabinets.

Laundry. Carefully launder the client's clothes. They represent a sizable investment. This may have to be done daily. Always:

- Read labels before laundering. Some clothes must be dry-cleaned or washed at special temperatures.
- Use the client's choice of detergent and read the label for instructions on amount to use.
- Wear gloves when sorting clothing and loading the washing machine if contact with blood, body fluids, secretions, or excretions is likely.
- Separate light and dark fabrics and wash them separately.
- Wash drip-dry fabrics separately so they can be hung and dried or folded.
- Be sure clothes can be dried in a dryer, and use the proper setting.
- Hang clothes after wiping off the clothesline, if a dryer is not available.
- After laundering, fold, iron, or hang clothes.
- Check for needed repairs and do mending before storing clothes.
- Ask the client or a responsible family member for operating instructions before using washer or dryer.

REVIEW

A. True/False.

Mark the following true or false by circling T or F.

1. T F The home health care nursing assistant may be responsible for both nursing care and household tasks.

2. T F The home health care nursing assistant makes no contribution to the nursing process, because care is given at the client's home and not in the hospital.

3. T F Self-discipline is an important characteristic of the nursing assistant who works in a home.

4. T F When washing dishes, wash the plates first, then the pots and pans, and then the glassware.

5. T F As a home health assistant, your primary role is to do the housework and cooking.

6. T F Your observations are important for monitoring the client's progress.

7. T F Because the client is your responsibility, you need not be concerned with the client's family.

8. T F If the client smokes, it is permissible for the home health assistant to smoke with the client.

9. T F Adaptability is an important characteristic for home health assistants.

10. T F You should clean the bathroom daily.

B. Multiple Choice.

Select the one best answer for each of the following.

11. A special characteristic needed by a home health care nursing assistant working in a home is
   a. honesty.
   b. being a follower.
   c. being a fast worker.
   d. being able to take shortcuts.

12. Which household tasks would the home health care nursing assistant *not* be required to do?
   a. Shop for food
   b. Move heavy furniture
   c. Carry out nursing procedures
   d. Prepare food for the client

13. Home health assistant responsibilities include all but which of these?
   a. Washing windows
   b. Cleaning the bathroom daily
   c. Documenting the care given
   d. Shopping for the client

14. The home health assistant should carry a kit that contains
   a. a change of clothes.
   b. thermometers, stethoscope, blood pressure kit.
   c. gardening gloves.
   d. a policy and procedure manual.

15. Daily tasks may include
   a. sweeping the floor after each meal.
   b. watering the lawn and shrubs.
   c. shampooing the carpets.
   d. washing windows.

C. Nursing Assistant Challenge.

You are working for a home health agency and Mrs. Fernandez is one of your clients. She has had a stroke and needs assistance with all activities of daily living. Your assignment includes: a bath, personal care, dressing, making the bed, making her breakfast, making her lunch so she can have it after you are gone, cleaning the bathroom, and general "picking up" around her apartment. She asks if you will go to the drugstore before you leave to get her prescriptions refilled. Make a work plan that includes all of these tasks, as well as any other routine tasks you need to complete.

- Coma care—weaning off drugs and tubes, **multisensory stimulation** (intense stimulation of sight, sound, touch, smell, pressure, and pain to help the patient awaken and use previously unused portions of the brain), and management of patients in a coma who have respiratory, nutritional, skin and eye care, contracture prevention, and elimination needs

Nursing Assistant Responsibilities

If you work on a subacute care unit, you will participate in special staff development classes to prepare you to meet the needs of patients in your care. A nursing assistant on a subacute unit is expected to:

- Work closely with registered nurses who are specialists in critical care or in a specific area of nursing
- Have extensive knowledge of the types of patients in the unit
- Care for patients receiving complicated treatments
- Have excellent observational skills, because of the complex conditions of the patients
- Be a member of an interdisciplinary team that includes professionals in physical therapy, occupational therapy, speech therapy, respiratory therapy, and social services

It is important that the staff on a subacute care unit be able to provide for patients' emotional well-being. Many of these patients will be able to return to their own homes. For them, this is a time of rejoicing and for making plans for the future. These patients may still have concerns if they will have to rely on community services or family members to meet some of their needs. Other patients will have an uncertain future. For example:

- Will the patient receiving dialysis receive a kidney transplant in time?
- Will the cancer be cured in the patient receiving oncology treatments?
- Will the patient on a ventilator be able to be weaned off the ventilator, or will it be a lifelong need?
- Will the patient receiving rehabilitation recover enough independence to be able to go home?

SPECIAL PROCEDURES PROVIDED IN THE SUBACUTE CARE UNIT

You will be assigned to care for patients who are receiving special treatments because of their health problems. These treatments may require the use of equipment that is unfamiliar to you. As a nursing assistant, you will not be expected to be responsible for these procedures. However, you will be providing the same personal care and procedures that you would with any patients.

Taking Vital Signs in the Subacute Unit

Patients in the subacute unit require close monitoring of their vital signs. When taking vital signs on patients, remember:

- Avoid taking blood pressure on the side affected by a stroke.
- Avoid taking blood pressure in the arm with a dialysis graft or shunt.
- Avoid taking blood pressure in an arm with an IV.
- Avoid taking blood pressure in the arm on the side where a patient recently had a breast removed.
- Avoid taking an oral temperature on patients with tubes in the nose or mouth.
- Report abnormal vital signs to the nurse immediately.

Caring for Patients Connected to Special Equipment

Patients in the subacute unit are frequently connected to electronic monitoring and caregiving devices. Many of these devices are used by patients 24 hours a day and cannot be disconnected while personal care is provided. The nursing assistant must be careful not to accidentally move, bump, or disconnect the equipment. Avoid bending, kinking, or placing traction on tubes entering surgical incisions or body cavities. In most cases, you will not be permitted to adjust or regulate the equipment. If an alarm on a piece of equipment sounds, respond immediately. Notify the nurse without delay.

Rehabilitation

Patients may require intense rehabilitation because they have had:

- A stroke that affected their mobility, their ability to carry out activities of daily living, or their speech
- Orthopedic surgery or an amputation (Figure 36-2)
- An accident that resulted in neurological or orthopedic problems

All caregivers working with these patients must have a knowledge of rehabilitation as well as a knowledge of the underlying condition (stroke, brain injury, etc.). You need to know what the goals are for the patients and what approaches you will be using to help patients reach their goals. Consistency is the key to successful rehabilitation.

Intravenous Therapy

Intravenous (IV) therapy refers to medication or solutions administered directly into a vein. Standard intravenous therapy is given into a peripheral vein (a large vein in the arm). This is called an IV. The IV may consist of a single bag of solution connected to simple tubing with a needle

FIGURE 36-2 Some patients are admitted to learn how to apply and use a prosthesis following an amputation.

Age-Appropriate Care ALERT

Occasionally, a pump error causes fluids to run in very quickly. Elderly and pediatric patients are at high risk for circulatory overload when IV fluids are given rapidly, and should be closely observed during IV therapy. Common signs of circulatory overload are elevated blood pressure, rapid pulse and respirations, coughing, shortness of breath, anxiety, and cyanosis. Inform the nurse immediately if you suspect a problem with a pump. ■

The most common problem of IV therapy is **infiltration**. This occurs when the catheter or needle comes out of the vein and fluid flows into the surrounding tissue. If an IV infiltrates, the drip rate often slows or stops. Monitor the

or small catheter on the end. Sometimes an additional small bag of fluid is attached to tubing that is connected to the main (primary) tubing. This is called a **piggyback**. The small bag contains medication such as an antibiotic that is intermittently dispersed into the vein (Figure 36-3). The IV tubing is usually threaded through an intravenous controller or pump that regulates the flow of solution. These electronic devices fasten to the IV standard and operate by electricity. Most automatically switch to battery mode in the event of a power failure. An alarm will sound for problems such as:

- Air in the line
- Line occlusion
- Problems that interfere with delivery of fluid at the designated rate
- Completion of the infusion
- Low battery

The alarm must always be in the "on" position when fluid is infusing. Sometimes an alarm is touchy and sounds repeatedly for no apparent reason. Although this can be annoying, never turn an alarm off. Some pumps will change to a "keep vein open" rate if the alarm sounds. Some will shut off completely. Respond promptly to the alarm and take corrective action within the limits of your job description, and notify the nurse promptly.

The nurse will immobilize the IV insertion site to prevent the catheter from moving (Figure 36-4). Movement is uncomfortable and increases the risk of catheter dislodgment. The nurse is responsible for the intravenous infusion. However, you must monitor the intravenous site and tubing each time you are in the room.

FIGURE 36-3 The large bag contains intravenous fluid that flows continuously into the vein. The small bag (piggyback) contains medication that is given for a short period of time.

needle insertion site for swelling, cool skin temperature, and a white or pale skin color. The patient may complain of burning or pain. If the patient experiences these problems, or if you are unsure of the infiltration status of the IV, promptly notify the nurse. If infiltration occurs, the nurse will discontinue it and restart it in another area. The nurse may instruct you to apply warm compresses to the area of infiltration.

On the subacute care unit, nursing assistants may be permitted to take limited nursing action if an IV infusion stops dripping. If you are permitted to troubleshoot an IV that has stopped dripping, you should:

- Confirm that fluid is present in the container.
- Check the insertion site for possible infiltration.
- Check the height of the IV solution; it should be at least 30 to 36 inches above the insertion site.
- Check for kinks in the tubing.
- Reposition the arm or patient to see if this affects the flow of solution.
- Straighten the arm with the IV to see if the fluid begins infusing. Monitor the insertion site to see if it begins swelling, which indicates infiltration.

FIGURE 36-4 The nurse will secure the IV insertion site with a transparent dressing or device to prevent movement. Look through the transparent material to check the skin for signs of infiltration. (Photo courtesy of I.V. House, Inc., St. Louis, MO. (800) 530-0400).

If you observe other problems, such as blood backed up in the tubing, inform the nurse promptly. Do not attempt to correct the problem.

Use caution when moving the patient to avoid dislodging the IV line. When caring for the patient, avoid pulling on, kinking, or otherwise obstructing the tubing. Avoid positioning the patient with the tubing under the body. If possible, position the arm with the IV at heart level when the patient is in bed. When the patient is ambulating, instruct him or her to place the arm with the IV across the abdomen. Advise the patient not to comb hair or brush the teeth using the arm with the IV. Notify the nurse immediately if an alarm sounds on an intravenous pump.

Infection Control ALERT

An IV infection can be very serious because, once inside the blood vessel, pathogens can move freely about the body. Organisms on the skin at the insertion site may migrate to the inside or outside of the catheter. To prevent infection, the IV insertion site must be kept dry. If the insertion site gets wet, the risk of infection increases. Although the insertion site is covered with a transparent dressing, it can still get wet. This is problematic for the nursing assistant when the patient is in the tub or shower. If the IV insertion site is in the hand, try cutting the fingers out of an exam glove, leaving about 1/2 inch of each finger. Carefully slip the exam glove over the hand. Although the patient cannot submerge the hand in water, the glove will help keep the insertion site dry. ∎

Central Venous Insertion

IV therapy can also be administered through a **central venous catheter (CVC).** A special catheter is inserted into a vein near the patient's collar bone (Figure 36-5). The catheter tip ends in or near the heart chamber. CV therapy is used to administer medications or to provide total parenteral nutrition.

Peripheral Intravenous Central Catheter Line

A **peripheral intravenous central catheter** or PICC line (Figure 36-6) consists of a catheter that is inserted into a peripheral vein and threaded upward through the vein to the jugular or subclavian vein. It is used to administer medications or to provide total parenteral nutrition.

Infection Control ALERT

Central intravenous catheters have the greatest risk of infection of all IVs. Those that are completely implanted (such as ports) have the lowest risk. Catheters with multiple lumens have a higher risk than single-lumen catheters. The triple-lumen catheter has the greatest infection risk. The insertion site also affects the risk. The sites are listed from highest to lowest risk for infection: femoral, jugular, subclavian, and peripheral (the extremities). Sterile technique is used to care for any insertion site. ■

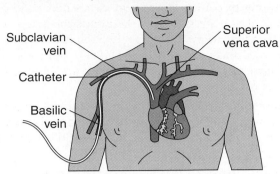

Insertion: Basilic vein (peripheral)
Termination: Superior vena cava

FIGURE 36-6 The PICC is usually inserted into the upper arm. The long catheter is threaded to the superior vena cava of the heart.

Total Parenteral Nutrition

Total parenteral nutrition (TPN) is also called *hyperalimentation*. TPN is given to a patient whose bowel needs complete rest. All required nutrients (carbohydrates, proteins, and fats) are given directly into the vein so the bowel does not have to work to digest food. Patients receiving TPN may need to be weighed daily or every other day. This should be done at the same time of day with the patient wearing the same type of clothing. The patient may be gradually switched over to enteral feedings. With an enteral feeding, liquid nourishment is administered through a tube inserted into the patient's digestive tract (Figure 36-7).

TPN feedings bypass the organs of the digestive system entirely, allowing them to rest and heal. The nurse will

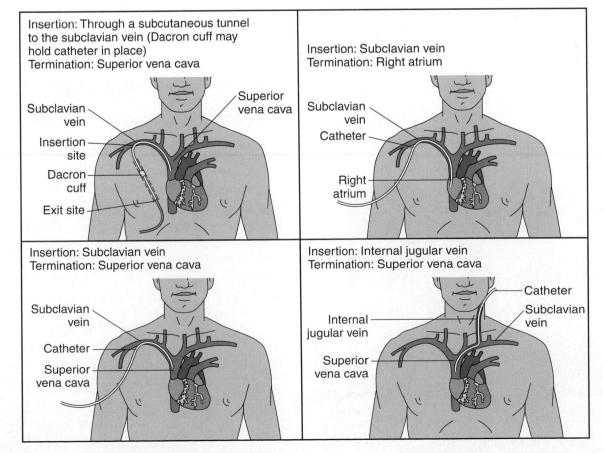

Insertion: Through a subcutaneous tunnel to the subclavian vein (Dacron cuff may hold catheter in place)
Termination: Superior vena cava

Insertion: Subclavian vein
Termination: Right atrium

Insertion: Subclavian vein
Termination: Superior vena cava

Insertion: Internal jugular vein
Termination: Superior vena cava

FIGURE 36-5 Locations for CVC insertion

FIGURE 36-7 Unflavored liquid nutritional supplements are commonly given through a gastrostomy tube that is surgically inserted through the abdominal wall directly into the stomach.

care for the insertion site. Be sure the tubing is not obstructed or kinked. Be very careful to avoid dislodging the tubing when moving or caring for patients. Many health care facilities keep a special clamp, called a **Kelly** (Figure 36-8) at the bedside of patients with central intra-

FIGURE 36-8 The Kelly is used to clamp a broken central line to prevent air from entering the patient's venous system. (Courtesy of Medline Industries, Mundelein, IL (800) MEDLINE).

Safety ALERT

The Kelly should be sealed in a package or covered in plastic. Taping the package on the headboard or over the head of the bed keeps it from being misplaced, and leaves it visible to all if needed in an emergency. ∎

venous lines. Serious complications occur if the tubing breaks or becomes dislodged. The Kelly is used to clamp the tubing close to the patient's body if the line breaks or is accidentally pulled loose. Air in the line can cause fatal complications. The Kelly should be readily available and visible at all times. Avoid storing it in a drawer or removing it from the room.

You may be required to assist the nurse with sterile dressing changes over the intravenous infusion site. When caring for patients with a central venous catheter, notify the nurse immediately if:

- You see blood in the intravenous tubing
- The patient has an elevated temperature or experiences chills
- You observe swelling or redness around the collarbone or near the infusion site
- The patient complains of pain in the neck or chest
- The patient becomes short of breath, develops elevated blood pressure, or edema
- The catheter is broken or cracked
- The alarm sounds on the intravenous infusion pump

PAIN MANAGEMENT PROCEDURES

Pain management may be the major reason why some patients are in a subacute unit. Other patients may be undergoing pain management related to conditions such as recent surgery or cancer. Both drug and nondrug treatments can be successful in helping to prevent and control pain. A 2006 study done at the Cleveland Clinic and Case Western Reserve University showed that listening to music for an hour a day will bring some relief to people suffering from chronic pain. Researchers noted that the kind of music patients listened to had no bearing on the pain relief experienced. Various types of relaxation techniques are also used for pain management.

Patient-Controlled Analgesia

Patient-controlled analgesia (PCA) is used for acute, chronic, or postoperative pain. *Analgesia* means pain relief. A device is inserted into the patient's vein. It is connected to a solution that contains a **narcotic**. A narcotic is a drug such as morphine that is used for pain relief. The dosage is controlled by equipment that has been preset by

---

GUIDELINES *for*

Caring for Patients with Intravenous Lines

- Make sure the solution is flowing. Know the drip rate in the drip chamber. Notify the nurse if the rate changes or the drip chamber is full.
- Avoid pulling or twisting tubing. Make sure the patient does not lie on the tubing.
- Observe the area of needle insertion for signs of swelling, redness, or warmth.
- Note signs of moisture that may indicate the tubing is leaking.
- Make sure all junctions in the tubing are securely connected.
- Always keep the intravenous solution above the needle insertion site.
- Report immediately to the nurse:
  - Signs of dyspnea, cyanosis, chest pain, or back pain
  - If the alarm sounds on an intravenous pump
  - Blood backing up into the intravenous tubing
  - Redness, swelling, or complaints of pain or burning at the needle insertion site
  - Wetness or moisture at the insertion site or where the tubing connects to the intravenous catheter
  - If the solution in the intravenous bag or bottle is empty or low. The container should never run dry.
  - If the intravenous is not dripping, seems to be dripping too fast, or if the drip chamber is completely full
  - If the needle becomes dislodged

  - If the tubing pulls apart from the needle
  - If the solution appears to be leaking
- When caring for patients with any type of IV therapy, NEVER:
  - Change the drip rate
  - Disconnect any tubing
  - Manipulate the needle or tubing. If the tubing or needle accidentally separate, put firm pressure on the needle insertion site with a gloved hand and call for the nurse immediately.
  - Remove, change, or manipulate any dressing over the site
  - Adjust the clamps on the tubing
  - Take a blood pressure in the arm with an intravenous infusion
    Turn off an alarm on an IV pump or other infusion equipment

Infection Control ALERT

Remember that all IV procedures are sterile. If you are assisting a nurse with any of these procedures, you must never contaminate the sterile field or supplies. ∎

the nurse. The patient pushes the PCA button at times of discomfort (Figure 36-9). The pump has preset controls to prevent accidental medication overdose. Report to the nurse if you note any change in the patient's:

- Level of consciousness
- Rate and pattern of respirations
- Pupil size
- Skin color

Other complications of this therapy that you should report to the nurse are:

- Nausea and/or vomiting
- Inability to urinate or difficulty urinating
- Excessive drowsiness
- Confusion
- Itching
- Preset pump alarm sounds

Constipation is a common side effect of narcotic medications. Problems can become serious if not carefully monitored. Encourage patients to eat fiber foods on trays, drink liquids, and be as active as possible in keeping with the plan of care. Carefully monitor and document the patient's bowel activity. Report patient complaints or signs of constipation to the nurse.

Pain Management with an Epidural Catheter

Continuous medication infusion may be used to manage pain after major thoracic, abdominal, and orthopedic surgery. This therapy works by blocking transmission of pain at the spinal cord. Patients receiving continuous epidural analgesia receive stable, consistent doses of pain medication rather than experiencing the peaks and valleys associated with most other control methods. Patients are more

FIGURE 36-9 The patient pushes the button when he needs pain medication. Staff members are not permitted to push the button to dispense medication. As a safeguard, the pump is set to reduce the risk of overdose.

willing to participate in their care plans when they are not having pain, and are usually satisfied with their care.

An **epidural catheter** is implanted beneath the patient's skin. It is inserted into the epidural space near the spinal cord (Figure 36-10). Medication is administered either intermittently or continuously through the catheter into the epidural space. Narcotic pain-relieving medications and local anesthetics are usually given together, but either drug can be given individually. The patient may have leg numbness and weakness for the first 24 hours after the catheter is inserted. Limited mobility in areas not affected by the medication and decreased blood pressure when rising from bed are also common reactions. Instruct the patient to call for assistance when getting out of bed. Elevate the head of the bed 30° or 40°. You may be assigned to monitor the patient's vital signs frequently. The blood pressure and pulse are checked at least every hour for the first 2 hours after the catheter is inserted, then every 2 hours. Respiration is checked every hour for the first day, then every 2 hours.

Report the following to the nurse immediately:

- A catheter becomes dislodged from the insertion site
- Changes in respiration rate and pattern
- Patient complaints of itching
- Vomiting or complaints of nausea
- Dressings covering the catheter become wet from leaking or an external cause
- Respirations decrease to 12 or below
- Oxygen saturation drops below 90%
- The patient's level of consciousness decreases
- Urinary retention; the patient complaints of a need to urinate, but cannot
- Low blood pressure (hypotension)
- Hives
- Rapid pulse (tachycardia)
- Redness, warmth, tenderness, swelling, itching, or drainage at the catheter insertion site
- Patient complaints of inability to move her legs
- Patient complaints of severe low back pain
- Patient complaints of change in sensation or motor function

Implantable Medication Pumps

Implantable medication pumps are sometimes used for long-term medication delivery in both adults and children. The pumps are surgically placed under the abdominal skin. A tiny catheter is threaded under the skin from the pump to the spine (Figure 36-11). Medications are infused directly into the cerebrospinal fluid. This type of therapy has become common for patients with:

- Chronic, severe pain
- Severe **spasticity** (sudden, frequent, involuntary muscle contractions that impair function)
- Treatment for some types of cancer

FIGURE 36-10 The epidural catheter is used for intermittent or constant pain medication.

The medication pump is implanted surgically. The patient will have two surgical sites, one on the abdomen and a smaller one near the spine. A physician or specially trained nurse will use a computer (Figure 36-12) to adjust the medication dose over a period of time until the desired response is achieved.

FIGURE 36-12 A computer sets the dosage and time for medication infusion. The dosage can be varied or constant throughout the day. The computer shows how much medication is left in the pump, and when it needs to be filled. An alarm will sound if the pump volume is low. (Courtesy of Medtronic, Minneapolis, MN. (800) 505-5000).

FIGURE 36-11 The implantable medication pump delivers medication directly into the cerebrospinal fluid. (Courtesy of Medtronic, Minneapolis, MN. (800) 505-5000).

The patient may remain on bedrest for 2 to 20 hours after surgery, depending on physician preference and patient response. An abdominal binder (Unit 29) may be used after surgery. The nurse may instruct you to apply a cool application or ice pack (Unit 27) to the site where the catheter tunnels under the skin. Some physicians permit patients to resume normal activity immediately, if they are able. If you are assisting the patient with transfers, avoid using a transfer belt until the surgical site is fully healed (usually several months after surgery, according to physician order and facility policy). In some facilities, a wide transfer belt is used for these patients, to prevent pressure on the pump or surgical site.

Patients with newly implanted medication pumps may have a complicated medication regimen in which they slowly withdraw from oral medications and depend increasingly on medications administered through the pump. Notify the nurse if the patient:

- Has decreased responsiveness
- Has respirations of 12 or below
- Has a temperature over 100°F orally
- Complains of headache
- Experiences fluid leakage
- Develops a collection of blood or fluid under the skin at the insertion site
- Has redness, warmth, tenderness, swelling, itching, or drainage at the surgical sites
- Complains of a feeling of tightness over the pump site
- Is unable to move the legs
- Has sudden loss of bowel or bladder control

Transcutaneous Electrical Nerve Stimulation

Transcutaneous electrical nerve stimulation (TENS) is a nondrug method of pain relief. Mild, harmless electrical current stimulates nerve fibers to block the transmission of pain to the brain. Electrodes are taped to the patient's skin. The location of the electrodes depends on the areas related to the pain. The electrodes are attached to wires that are in turn attached to a control box (Figure 36-13). The intensity of the stimulation is set on the control box by the nurse.

CARING FOR SUBACUTE PATIENTS WITH RESPIRATORY CONDITIONS

Many patients are admitted to the subacute unit with problems related to the respiratory system. Some conditions are caused by diseases within the lungs. Some patients experience respiratory problems as a result of complications of other conditions. Attention to the patient's oxygenation is a very important responsibility.

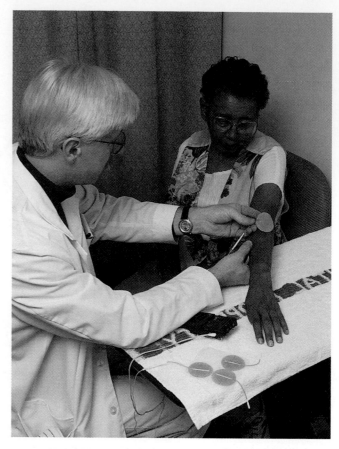

FIGURE 36-13 A TENS unit is used to relieve pain.

The human body eliminates three main waste products. You have learned about problems with urinary and bowel elimination. The third important waste product is carbon dioxide (CO_2). Every cell in the body produces carbon dioxide. It is transported in venous blood. When it reaches the lungs, it is exhaled into the atmosphere. When

Culture ALERT

Many individuals have tongue piercings to make a fashion statement. Many risks accompany this practice. A tongue piercing can be especially problematic if the patient requires an oral airway or endotracheal tube. Notify the nurse promptly if a patient with a tongue piercing has pain, bleeding, increased flow of saliva, swelling, or signs of infection in the mouth. Swelling of the tongue can become severe, closing off the airway. To prevent patient injury, jewelry in tongue piercings will probably have to be removed when an airway is inserted. ■

the body does not eliminate carbon dioxide, chemical reactions cause an acid buildup. Death will result if levels of acid and carbon dioxide become too high. Signs and symptoms that may indicate problems with oxygen use are:

- Unusual skin color, such as dusky, pale, blue, or gray
- Unusual color of the lips, mucous membranes, nail beds, lining or roof of the mouth
- Cool, clammy skin
- Slow, rapid, or irregular breathing
- Shortness of breath or difficulty breathing
- Noisy breathing
- Gasping for breath
- Wet respirations, rattling in the lungs
- Choking on secretions
- Changes in mental status, including decreased responsiveness, drowsiness, sleepiness for no apparent reason, restlessness, increased confusion
- Tachycardia

Patients at Risk of Poor Oxygenation

Certain patients have a known high risk of developing **hypoxemia**. This is a condition in which there is insufficient oxygen in the blood. It can occur in anyone, and is not a disease. Patients who are immobile and those on bedrest have an increased risk of hypoxemia. Other high-risk conditions are:

- Cardiac disease
- Pulmonary disease (Figure 36-14)
- Being a postoperative patient
- Sleep apnea
- Decreased level of consciousness
- Neuromuscular diseases
- Morbid obesity
- Severe kyphoscoliosis (curvature of the spine)

Capillary Refill

Checking capillary refill is a quick, easy, painless test to evaluate how well oxygen gets to the body tissues. **Capillary refill** is an indication of the patient's peripheral circulation and shows how well the tissues are being nourished with oxygen. In a light-skinned person, skin should be pink, indicating an adequate supply of oxygen. The nail beds, mucous membranes in the mouth, and lips are also an indication of how well the patient's body is using oxygen. The color of these areas should also be pink. In a dark-skinned person, you must look at the nail beds, oral mucous membranes, and lips to determine how well the person is using oxygen, because you cannot evaluate the skin. If the skin, nail beds, mucous membranes, or lips are cyanotic, this indicates a problem with oxygen delivery.

FIGURE 36-14 Patients with chronic obstructive lung disease commonly have a barrel chest, and may lean forward to increase lung capacity, making it possible to take in a little more air. (Netter illustration used with permission of Elsevier, Inc. All rights reserved.)

This may be due to lack of oxygen in the blood or poor circulation.

The capillary refill test will help you determine the patient's oxygenation. Delayed capillary refill indicates a problem with oxygen delivery. Perform a capillary refill check on all four extremities, or according to facility policy. Although capillary refill varies with age, skin color should return to normal within 2 to 3 seconds in all patients. The color should be restored to the nail bed in the length of time it takes to say the words *capillary refill*. (Refer to Procedure 87.)

Nail Polish. Several procedures involve using and evaluating the patient's fingernail beds. The color of the fingernails is a good indication of how much oxygen is in the blood. Nail polish will interfere with the ability to evaluate the patient. Follow your facility policy for removing polish. Some facilities remove polish from one finger only. Other facilities remove all nail polish. If a patient has acrylic or sculpted nails, remove the polish with a non-acetone polish remover. Some facilities completely remove the acrylic material from one nail. Know and follow your facility policy.

You can check capillary refill at any time when you are taking vital signs or caring for the patient. If the capillary

PROCEDURE

87

CHECKING CAPILLARY REFILL

1. Carry out initial procedure actions.

2. Insect the nails, noting the color.

3. Press the nail for a few seconds, until the skin underneath blanches, or turns white (Figure 36-15A).

4. Release the nail and evaluate the time it takes for the skin to return to its normal color. With normal oxygenation, this will occur within 2 to 3 seconds (Figure 36-15B).

5. Carry out ending procedure actions.

FIGURE 36-15A Inspect the color of the patient's hand, then pinch the thumb.

FIGURE 36-15B Observe the color again after releasing the thumb.

refill time is greater than 3 seconds, inform the nurse of your findings.

The Pulse Oximeter

Pulse oximetry (Figure 36-16) is another simple, painless test to determine how well oxygen is being carried in the body. The pulse oximeter is an instrument that measures the level of saturation of the patient's hemoglobin with oxygen. Hemoglobin is the part of the blood that carries oxygen to the cells to nourish them. The pulse oximeter measures how full the hemoglobin molecules are with oxygen. The measurement is usually done continuously, but can be intermittent. Having these data readily available enables the nurse to treat the patient quickly. Pulse oximetry will detect critical changes in the patient's oxygen levels before the skin color changes. This makes it a valuable tool that provides details about changes in the patient's condition immediately, as soon as they occur. The patient's outcome is usually better when early treatment is provided. Before applying the pulse oximeter, check the patient's oxygen, if being used. Document the liter flow.

The pulse oximeter is attached to the patient's skin with a sensor. Several different sensors are available. These can be placed on the finger (Figure 36-17A), toe, earlobe, foot,

forehead, or the bridge of the nose (Figure 36-17B). The tip of the finger and the earlobe are most commonly used. In these areas, a clothespin-like sensor is attached to both

Safety ALERT

Always monitor the patient and not the equipment. For example, the pulse oximeter alarm sounds and the oxygen saturation value reads 63%. This suggests that the patient is in distress. However, the patient is visiting with his family, smiling and talking. His color is good, nail beds and mucous membranes are pink, and capillary refill is less than 2 seconds. You are having an equipment problem, not a patient problem. If you cannot identify and correct the problem, ask the nurse or respiratory professional to help. Although your findings indicate an equipment problem, inform the nurse of the problem and your evaluation of the patient and situation. ■

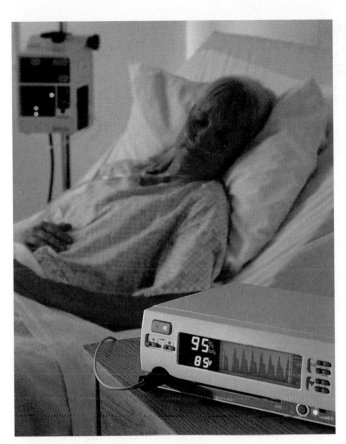

FIGURE 36-16 The pulse oximeter shows the oxygen saturation of the patient's blood as a percentage on the display.

FIGURE 36-17A The finger-clip sensor should be rotated at least every 2 hours.

FIGURE 36-17B The nasal sensor

sides. The finger and toe sensors work best with dark-skinned patients. Poor circulation interferes with use of the pulse oximeter.

The unit has two light-emitting diodes (LEDs). One is red, the other is infrared. The sensor contains a photodetector that measures the light as it passes through the tissue. This measures the amount of oxygen in the patient's arterial blood (Figure 36-18). The pulse oximeter converts this into a percentage, which can be viewed on the digital display. The physician will order what he or she wants the minimum oxygen saturation to be. The nurse will give you this information. A measurement of 95% to 100% is considered normal. Readings below 90% suggest complications. When the reading reaches 85%, there may not be enough oxygen for the tissues. Readings below 70% are life-threatening. The pulse oximeter is not used for patients with known or suspected carbon monoxide poisoning.

The pulse oximeter has an alarm, which is usually preset by the manufacturer to normal limits for adults and children. The nurse will advise you if the alarm settings must be changed. This is done by turning a knob or pressing a button. If you turn the unit off, then back on, the oximeter resets itself to the default values. Before leaving the room, make sure that the alarm is in the "on" position, and is set as ordered. Never turn the alarm off. (Refer to Procedure 88.)

Light-emitting sensor

HgbO$_2$ Hgb HgbO$_2$

Hgb HgbO$_2$ Hgb

Infrared and red light beams

Light-receiving sensor

FIGURE 36-18 The pulse oximeter uses light to measure the amount of oxygen in the arterial blood.

PROCEDURE

88

USING A PULSE OXIMETER

1. Carry out initial procedure actions.

2. Assemble equipment:
   - Pulse oximeter unit
   - Sensor appropriate to the site
   - Adhesive tape, if needed, to secure the sensor

3. Select and apply the sensor. If the sensor has position markings, align them opposite each other to ensure an accurate reading.

4. Fasten the sensor securely (Figure 36-19A), or the reading will not be accurate. Make sure the sensor is not wrapped so tightly with tape that it restricts blood flow.

5. Attach the sensor to the patient cable on the pulse oximeter.

6. Turn the unit on (Figure 36-19B). You will hear a beep with each pulse beat. Adjust the volume as

desired. Some units also use light bars to indicate the strength of the pulse. Note the percentage of oxygen saturation. Inform the nurse and document according to facility policy.

7. Monitor the patient's pulse rate, if the unit provides this reading. Compare with the patient's actual pulse to make sure the unit is picking up each beat. Inform the nurse and document according to facility policy.

8. Monitor the patient's respirations and general appearance. Inform the nurse and document according to facility policy. If the patient's general condition changes at any time, notify the nurse.

9. Carry out ending procedure actions.

FIGURE 36-19A Firmly attach the sensor to the finger.

FIGURE 36-19B Turn the unit on and adjust the volume and other controls.

Monitoring the Patient. You must monitor the patient regularly when a pulse oximeter is being used. Reporting to the nurse is part of your ending procedure actions. In this case, make sure to report the patient's initial pulse oximeter reading and vital signs. This is important information on which the nurse will act. He or she will further assess the patient and provide care for abnormal values. The nurse must know the initial values as a basis for comparison.

If the patient's vital signs or appearance change significantly from baseline values, notify the nurse promptly. Also inform the nurse immediately if the patient's pulse oximetry value is less than the level ordered by the physi-

cian. Monitor the patient's oxygen, if used, each time you are in the room. Make sure it is set at the liter flow ordered by the physician.

Rotate the position of the finger sensor at least every 4 hours. A spring-clip sensor should be moved every 2 hours. Rotating the location of the sensor reduces the risk of skin breakdown and complications related to pressure. If adhesive tape is used to secure the sensor, monitor for signs and symptoms of a reaction to the tape. If a rash, itching, or other signs of tape allergy occur, move the sensor to a different location. Apply a spring-clamp sensor, or attach the sensor with hypoallergenic tape.

Oxygen Therapy

Oxygen is necessary for life. Humans take in oxygen from the air during breathing. Some diseases and conditions prevent the body tissues from getting enough oxygen, so supplemental oxygen is administered. Some patients have normal oxygen levels, but are given oxygen because they are at increased risk of hypoxemia. Oxygen is a prescription item, and a physician's order is necessary to administer it to a patient. The physician will order additional oxygen to be given through an oxygen delivery system. He or she will specify how much oxygen to use and the method of oxygen delivery. Depending on your facility policy, it may also be given at the nurse's discretion, according to protocol or clinical practice guidelines. You should not start, stop, or change the flow rate of oxygen.

The nursing assistant's responsibilities for oxygen administration are determined by facility policy. Most subacute units have a respiratory care practitioner (RCP) on staff to administer oxygen therapy. Nursing personnel monitor patients using oxygen, and notify the RCP as needed. He or she will see the patient one or more times each shift. Although an RCP may be responsible for the patients' oxygen needs, you still must have a working knowledge of oxygen administration. Portable cylinders are used for transporting patients from one area to another, and may be used in emergencies in hallways or other areas without a piped-in oxygen source. You must know where oxygen cylinders are stored, how to assemble them, and how to transport them safely.

Caring for a Patient Who Is Receiving Oxygen Therapy. Elevate the head of the bed when the patient is receiving oxygen. This will make it easier to breathe. A patient using an oxygen mask cannot eat while wearing the mask. The physician may order a nasal cannula at

Safety ALERT

Oxygen is a prescription medication. Using oxygen is safe if you follow facility policies and safety guidelines. Never change the fittings from one type of oxygen bottle to another. Make sure you use the correct adaptor and plug for the unit. If you think that an oxygen tank or liquid oxygen canister is leaking, remove the patient from the room and close the door. Report the problem to the proper person. Never attempt to carry or move an oxygen cylinder or canister if it is leaking. Bed linen can absorb oxygen. Any time oxygen is in use, avoid sparks. Static electricity can start a fire. ■

Safety ALERT

When using cylinder oxygen, identify the contents of the cylinder. Oxygen cylinders are always colored green in the United States. Read the label listing the contents as a double-check. Transport oxygen cylinders carefully. They should be chained to a carrier during transport. Cylinder oxygen should be secured in a base or chained to a carrier or wall. Avoid dropping the tank. Cylinders can explode of the tank is dropped and the cylinder valve is damaged. ■

mealtime. Follow the instructions on the care plan or critical pathway for patient care measures.

Being unable to breathe is very frightening. Patients who are receiving oxygen may need reassurance and emotional support. Check on the patient frequently and spend as much time in the room as possible. Difficulty in breathing also makes it hard to talk. The patient may be unable to hold a normal conversation. Just being with the patient without talking is very reassuring.

You will care for patients using different devices for the administration of oxygen. Carefully check the skin under the device. Make sure it does not become red or irritated from the elastic that holds it in place. Pad the straps with cotton, if necessary. Report problems to the nurse. Because oxygen is drying, patients receiving oxygen will need extra liquids to drink. However, if the patient is short of breath, she may be unable to suck on a straw. Assist the patient by holding the glass, if necessary, and helping her to drink. Patients who use oxygen will also need frequent care of the mouth and nose. Sometimes patients will feel warm and perspire heavily. Extra bathing and linen changes may be necessary. You may need to adjust the temperature in the room and help the patient change into a hospital gown. Cover her with a sheet. The care plan or critical pathway will provide information on patient preferences and needs.

Use of Oxygen in an Emergency. There are several differences between routine oxygen use and use of oxygen in an emergency. In an emergency, high concentrations of oxygen are necessary. Cylinders (Figure 36-20), liquid oxygen, or piped-in oxygen are used. Avoid using an oxygen concentrator, because it cannot supply the high liter flows necessary for emergency care. Some facilities use humidifier bottles when routine oxygen is administered, but this is not necessary. Oxygen may be delivered dry. Do not take the time to search for a humidifier. In an emergency, the patient requires high liter flows of oxygen quickly.

FIGURE 36-20 A portable oxygen tank may be used in an emergency or when the patient is out of the room. No humidification is necessary.

Caring for Patients with Tracheostomies

A **tracheostomy** is a tube that is inserted into a surgical opening in the patient's trachea (windpipe). A tracheostomy is performed when the patient is unable to breathe in air through the nose. The tube allows the patient to breathe, as air goes directly into the trachea and then into the lungs. A person who is on a ventilator for a long time will have a tracheostomy that is connected to the ventilator. The patient may have secretions coming from the chest and through the tube. The nurse will use suction to remove these secretions.

The tube may be made of plastic or metal. Tracheostomy tubes consist of an inner, removable tube called a *cannula* and an outer tube called a *neckplate* that is held in place with neck ties or Velcro. The neckplate rests between the clavicles (breastbones). There is a slot on each side. Tracheostomy ties are inserted here to secure the tube in place (Figure 36-21). Patients with tracheostomies can usually take a bath or shower but must keep the water from entering the opening. Avoid using powders, sprays, or shaving cream around the tube. When you care for a patient with a tracheostomy, observe for:

- Changes in respiratory rate, depth, and quality
- Changes in mental status, such as confusion, restlessness, or irritability, that indicate the patient's brain is not getting adequate oxygen

Report to the nurse immediately if the:

- Tube becomes dislodged from the opening
- Patient is having trouble breathing
- Patient needs suctioning
- Alarm sounds on the respirator

Be sure you know how the patient communicates. The opening in the trachea interferes with the patient's ability to talk. Additional information on caring for patients with tracheostomies and other respiratory conditions is found in Unit 39.

CARING FOR THE PATIENT RECEIVING DIALYSIS TREATMENTS

Dialysis is a process by which the blood is artificially cleansed of liquid wastes when the kidneys are unable to remove the wastes. This procedure is needed when a person has kidney failure. Without dialysis, the person would die as the waste products accumulate in the bloodstream. Dialysis is usually considered a temporary treatment to be used until a suitable organ is found for a kidney transplant. The two types of dialysis are hemodialysis and peritoneal dialysis.

Infection Control ALERT

The nasal hairs and tonsils filter pathogens and other substances from the air, preventing them from reaching the lungs. A patient with a tracheostomy does not have this advantage. The stoma provides a direct, unfiltered passageway to the lungs for irritating foreign substances and pathogens. Practice good infection control techniques when caring for patients with a stoma. ■

FIGURE 36-21 A tracheostomy tube is held in place with ties. Avoid getting lint, dust, powder, or water in the tracheostomy.

Hemodialysis

During **hemodialysis** treatment, the patient's blood is circulated outside of the body into an artificial kidney machine. In the dialysis machine, the blood is cleansed with a liquid substance called *dialysate*. After the waste products have been removed, the blood is returned to the patient's body. Most persons needing hemodialysis are treated in a dialysis center. However, you may care for patients in the subacute unit who go as outpatients to the dialysis center for their treatments. Dialysis is usually done three to four times a week and each treatment takes several hours.

To do dialysis, a connection must be made between the patient's circulatory system and the artificial kidney machine. Minor surgery is done to create either a fistula or a graft. The **fistula** (Figure 36-22A) is created by attaching a vein to an artery, either in an arm or a leg. When a **graft** is used (Figure 36-22B), synthetic material is inserted to form a connection between an artery and a vein. Two needles are inserted for treatment with either a fistula or a graft. The needles are connected to tubes that go to and from the artificial kidney machine (Figure 36-22C).

As a nursing assistant, you are not expected to care for the fistula or the graft. You need to be aware that the patient on dialysis will:

- Have fluid restrictions
- Have dietary restrictions for calories, sodium, protein, potassium, calcium, and phosphorus
- Need all fluid intake and output measured accurately and recorded
- Need to be weighed regularly at the same time of day and with the same type of clothing

- Need to be monitored and have vital signs taken frequently after dialysis. Remember that blood pressure should not be taken in the arm used for dialysis. Patients may be weak when they return from dialysis. Monitor them closely when they ambulate. Watch for dizziness and loss of balance.

Report to the nurse if the patient has:

- Swelling (edema) of the hands, feet, or face
- Changes in vital signs
- Changes in weight
- A change in intake or output measurements
- Shortness of breath
- Complaints of pain at the site of the fistula or graft

Peritoneal Dialysis

Peritoneal dialysis is also a process of cleansing the blood. In peritoneal dialysis, the process takes place within the patient's body in the peritoneal (abdominal) cavity, rather than outside the body in a machine. During dialysis, the dialysate is introduced into the abdominal cavity, allowed to stay in for some time, and then drained

Nearest adjacent vein

Artery

Edges of incision in artery and vein are sutured together to form a common opening.

FIGURE 36-22A The arteriovenous fistula

Ends of natural or synthetic graft sutured into an artery and a vein.

FIGURE 36-22B The arteriovenous vein graft

to vein (8)

from artery (1)

FIGURE 36-22C Hemodialysis is done through the graft or fistula. Most commonly, the patient is fully dressed and sits in a reclining chair during dialysis. Occasionally, it is done at the bedside of an unstable patient.

out (Figure 36-23). As blood flows through the vessels in the peritoneum, waste products are filtered and excess fluids are removed. The nurse instills the dialysate through a catheter that is surgically implanted through the wall of the abdomen into the abdominal cavity. This is done using sterile technique. You may be asked to assist the nurse with sterile dressing changes. The type of dialysis used in the subacute care unit is usually **continuous ambulatory peritoneal dialysis (CAPD)**.

Nursing assistants are not expected to administer peritoneal dialysis. You may be responsible for monitoring the patient's vital signs every 10 to 15 minutes for the first 1 to 2 hours after a treatment and then every 2 to 4 hours. Notify the nurse if there are any changes in vital signs.

Other signs and symptoms to report to the nurse are:

- The dialysate that returns appears bloody or has blood clots in the solution
- The patient complains of abdominal pain
- The dressing becomes wet or soiled
- Fluid leaks around the insertion site

FIGURE 36-23 Waste products and excess fluid are removed as the dialysate flows out of the peritoneal cavity.

*Labels in figure:*
Fresh dialysate solution
Peritoneal catheter
Peritoneal cavity
Adapter
Used dialysate solution

- The tubing or catheter is disconnected
- The solution does not appear to be running, or is running very slowly
- The drainage container is almost full
- The patient is weak or unsteady
- The patient has low blood pressure or complains of dizziness
- The patient is short of breath or complains of difficulty breathing

ONCOLOGY TREATMENTS

Oncology is the care and treatment of persons with cancer. Cancer may be treated with surgery, radiation, chemotherapy, or a combination of any of these. Patients receiving cancer treatment are often cared for in the subacute unit. Care of the oncology patient is described in Unit 47.

WOUND MANAGEMENT

Some patients require wound management for severe pressure ulcers, burns, or surgical wounds. The nurse or physical therapist will perform frequent dressing changes on these areas using sterile technique. You may be required to assist with dressing changes, so a basic knowledge of sterile technique (Unit 51) is necessary. The patient may have special positioning needs related to the injured area of the skin, or may be on a low air loss therapy or another type of specialty bed. You may be required to position the patient hourly, and use special positioning devices and props to promote healing of the injured area. Notify the nurse if any of the following occur:

- The wound appears red, swollen, or has increased drainage
- The dressing becomes saturated with drainage from the wound
- Wound drainage has a foul odor
- The patient complains of increased pain in the wound
- The wound dressing becomes wet, soiled, or falls off

- The wound dressing accidentally becomes contaminated with urine or stool

Care of patients with pressure ulcers and extensive wounds is described in Unit 38.

DOCUMENTATION OF CARE IN THE SUBACUTE UNIT

Reimbursement for care in subacute units is often provided by insurance companies and managed care organizations. In some situations or facilities, reimbursement is based on documentation. The main purpose of documentation is to provide a record of patient care. However, the medical record may also be used to evaluate the level and value of services the facility provides to each patient. The information on the record is used to set payment to the facility.

Payment may be denied if the documentation does not support the care given or what the patient required. The agencies that pay the bills will only pay for care that matches the treatment plan prescribed for the patient. Documentation must reflect the patient's progress toward stated care plan goals and response to treatment provided. You will be responsible for documenting the services you provide. You may also be required to document the patient's response to these services. If you are working with patients on special restorative nursing or therapy programs, you may be required to document additional information. Avoid subjective terms such as good, fair, or poor. Generally, documentation about patient response to services or progress toward care plan goals must be stated in measurable terms, such as:

- "Ambulated 50 feet in hallway with walker."
- "Ate 90% of breakfast meal."
- "Consumed 975 mL of fluid orally this shift."

The facility and its staff depend on payment for services for survival. This is what pays the bills and meets payroll. Therefore, documentation is important for many reasons. Documentation requirements change as reimbursement changes.

Complete, accurate documentation proves that workers have complied with physician orders, complied with the

FIGURE 36-24 Accurate records are important for communication and reimbursement.

law, and met legal standards of care. It shows that the patients received good care. Properly completed records will show that the patients' risks and needs were identified, and that care was given to meet those needs. You will care for several patients each day, and remembering each small detail is difficult. Make notes if necessary, so you do not forget important information (Figure 36-24). Documentation is an important communication tool for all workers who care for the patient. Missing, inaccurate, or absent information may cause problems with communication, reimbursement, facility inspections, or legal actions. Accurate, complete documentation protects both the facility and the individual workers. Your facility will provide instruction on special documentation requirements related to subacute care and reimbursement in the subacute unit.

REVIEW

A. Multiple Choice.

Select the one best answer for each of the following.

1. Subacute care is given to persons who
   a. have been acutely ill.
   b. have had a long, progressive illness.
   c. require only custodial care.
   d. require intensive care.

2. The purpose of subacute care is to
   a. increase the use of long-term care facilities.
   b. discharge patients as quickly as possible.
   c. provide the care a person needs at a lower cost.
   d. provide care to unstable patients.

3. Patients treated in subacute care include persons
   a. who are critically ill.

b. requiring routine long-term care.

c. receiving complex wound care.

d. receiving obstetrical care.

4. A nursing assistant working in subacute care would need to

a. learn how to start intravenous feedings.

b. have excellent observational skills.

c. learn how to administer chemotherapy.

d. instruct patients in pain management techniques.

5. If you accept a position in a subacute care unit, you may need to learn

a. how to administer medication.

b. your responsibilities for patients receiving dialysis.

c. how to prepare special therapeutic diets.

d. to manage unstable patients.

6. The procedure to measure the level of oxygen in arterial blood is called

a. hemodialysis.

b. pulse oximetry.

c. total parenteral nutrition.

d. intravenous therapy.

7. A central venous catheter is inserted into

a. a vein in the patient's foot.

b. an artery in the patient's arm.

c. the jugular or subclavian vein.

d. the epidural space.

8. Total parenteral nutrition (TPN) is used for patients

a. who need to lose weight.

b. who are unconscious.

c. who refuse to eat.

d. whose bowel needs complete rest.

9. The nursing assistant's responsibility for caring for patients with intravenous feedings is to

a. insert the needle into the vein.

b. add medication to the bag of fluid.

c. observe for complications.

d. change the drip rate if it is too fast or too slow.

10. Patient-controlled analgesia is used

a. for acute, chronic, or postoperative pain.

b. for oral medications.

c. to administer medication every 4 hours.

d. for medication delivery on a fixed schedule.

11. An epidural catheter is used for

a. pain management.

b. administering nutrition.

c. emptying the bladder.

d. intravenous feedings.

12. When caring for patients with tracheostomies, you should

a. not allow the patient to bathe or shower.

b. observe for changes in respiratory rate, depth, and quality.

c. maintain the patient on a liquid diet.

d. change the tracheostomy tube daily.

13. Dialysis is a procedure for

a. cleansing the blood of liquid wastes.

b. relieving postoperative pain.

c. administering oxygen.

d. giving total parenteral nutrition.

14. A patient on dialysis will have

a. a regular diet.

b. vital signs taken every hour.

c. weight taken frequently.

d. physical therapy.

15. When caring for patients on dialysis, you should observe for

a. edema of the face, hands, and feet.

b. diarrhea.

c. constipation.

d. thirst.

16. Oncology is the care and treatment of patients with

a. severe wounds.

b. kidney failure.

c. cancer.

d. terminal illness.

17. The nursing assistant should avoid taking blood pressure

a. on a stroke patient's unaffected arm.

b. with an electronic blood pressure unit.

c. on an arm with an intravenous infusion.

d. on the arm with the identification band.

18. Always keep the bag or bottle of intravenous solution

a. below the needle insertion site.

b. exactly 6 feet off the floor.

c. parallel to the needle insertion site.

d. above the needle insertion site.

19. If the intravenous tubing accidentally becomes separated from the needle, the nursing assistant should

a. apply firm pressure to the needle insertion site with a gloved hand.

b. quickly plug the tubing back into the needle or intravenous catheter.

c. wrap the area with a pressure bandage and call the nurse.

d. apply a dressing over the open intravenous catheter and call the nurse.

20. Constipation is a common side effect of
  a. spasticity.
  b. narcotic medications.
  c. peritoneal dialysis.
  d. hypoxemia.

21. Do not use a transfer belt for a patient with a
  a. tracheostomy.
  b. dialysis shunt.
  c. central intravenous catheter.
  d. newly implanted medication pump.

22. Capillary refill is used to evaluate
  a. how much oxygen is in the venous blood.
  b. how well oxygen gets to body tissues.
  c. cyanosis and changes in color.
  d. the strength of the pulse.

23. The normal capillary refill time is
  a. 10 to 12 seconds.
  b. 5 to 7 seconds.
  c. 2 to 3 seconds.
  d. less than 1 second.

24. The normal oxygen saturation is
  a. 95% to 100%.
  b. 85% to 95%.
  c. 80% to 90%
  d. 70% to 80%.

B. Word Choice.

Choose the correct word from the following list to complete each statement in questions 25–38.

CAPD	multisensory stimulation
dialysis	
enteral	narcotic
exacerbation	piggyback
hyperalimentation	pulse oximetry
hypoxemia	spasticity
Kelly	transcutaneous electrical nerve stimulation
	transitional care

25. Subacute care is also called _____.

26. A procedure for removing liquid wastes from the blood is called _____.

27. _____ is used for measuring the oxygen level in arterial blood.

28. A _____ refers to a small bag of fluid containing intravenous medication that is connected with a tube to the primary tubing.

29. Total parenteral nutrition (TPN) is also called _____.

30. A feeding administered through a tube into the patient's stomach is called an _____ feeding.

31. A _____ is a potent drug used for pain relief.

32. The use of electrical current to treat pain is done with a procedure called _____.

33. Using various methods of sight, sound, touch, smell, pressure, and pain to help the patient awaken from a coma is called _____.

34. Worsening of the patient's condition is called _____.

35. A patient with severe _____ has sudden, frequent, involuntary muscle contractions that impair function.

36. A _____ is a curved clamp that is used to occlude central intravenous lines in an emergency.

37. _____ is a condition in which there is insufficient oxygen in the blood.

38. The most common type of dialysis used for subacute patients is _____.

C. Nursing Assistant Challenge.

You have completed your nursing assistant course and have been working the night shift for three months in a skilled care facility. The director of nursing calls you into her office and asks you if you would like to work the day shift in the new subacute care unit of the facility. You tell her you would like to think about it for a day and then give your decision. Consider the types of care that are given in subacute care and then answer these questions.

39. What would your duties be in the new unit?

40. You feel confident of your nursing assistant skills. However, you know you will need to learn some new things to care successfully for subacute care patients. What new information or skills will you need to acquire?

41. How do you plan to obtain this education?

Alternative, Complementary, and Integrative Approaches to Patient Care

OBJECTIVES

After completing this unit, you will be able to:
- Spell and define terms.
- Define alternative medicine.
- Differentiate alternative practices from complementary and integrative practices.

- List five categories of alternative and complementary therapies.
- Define holistic care.
- List at least three ways in which the nursing assistant supports patients' spirituality.

VOCABULARY

Learn the meaning and the correct spelling of the following words and phrases:

acupuncture	chiropractic care	herbs	nutrition therapy
alternative	color therapy	holistic care	osteopathic manipulative
alternative medical	complementary	homeopathy	treatment (OMT)
systems	medicine	hypnotherapy	prayer
Anthroposophically	complementary/alterna-	integrative (integrated)	qigong
Extended Medicine	tive medicine (CAM)	health care	reflexology
(AEM)	cupping	light therapy	Reiki
aromatherapy	dance therapy	massage therapy	relaxation
art therapy	Doctor of Osteopathy	meditation	supplements
Ayurveda	(D.O.)	mind-body therapy	therapeutic touch (TT)
biofeedback	electromagnetic therapy	modalities	traditional Chinese
biological therapy	energy therapy	movement therapy	medicine (TCM)
body-based therapy	guided imagery	moxibustion	visualization
chelation therapy	herbal therapy	Naturopathic medicine	yoga

ALTERNATIVES TO MAINSTREAM HEALTH CARE

When most people in Western society think of medical care, they think of medical, surgical, pharmaceutical, and technological treatment of patients. In the United States, these practices and techniques are the accepted, traditional, mainstream approaches to patient care and healing of illness. Throughout history, people have actively sought

Culture ALERT

Some patients may view an illness as having a supernatural cause. Others may believe that a traditional cure, diet, herb, or therapy is needed for treatment. ■

out other forms of healing the sick. Drawings in caves show early humans practicing healing. Egyptian society (Figure 37-1) was particularly advanced in medical practices. Native American tribes had medicine men. Healing of the sick is mentioned in the Bible. These practices were considered mainstream before twentieth-century advances in technology, research, and medicine. In many ancient cultures, religion and medicine were closely connected. In the Middle Ages, medicine was the concern of either the church or the state. Because of this, many people used folk remedies that included herbs (Figure 37-2). Other religious customs and charms were also used for healing. These methods were more readily available and affordable than medical treatments.

Today, some people prefer natural and spiritual treatments for illness. Others are afraid of the technology, drugs, and surgical procedures of today. Some patients believe that conventional medical treatments are worse than the discomfort of disease. They prefer using other methods of relieving symptoms and eliminating sickness. Because of this, many people use **alternative** health care practices and products to prevent and treat illness. Alternatives are options that are used instead of conventional health care.

FIGURE 37-1 The ancient Egyptians used many natural substances and medical practices that were advanced for their time.

Most alternative strategies use natural products rather than those derived from chemicals. Alternative therapies are used to treat every imaginable symptom and condition, from pain to menopause. Some people use natural products and practices to prevent illness (Figure 37-3). Most towns have at least one health food store that sells alternative products. Many books and magazines are available describing natural alternatives to health care. Some nontraditional practices have proven effective. Others have shown no real benefit, but this is a popular trend. The use of alternative therapy is not a passing fad; it is here to stay.

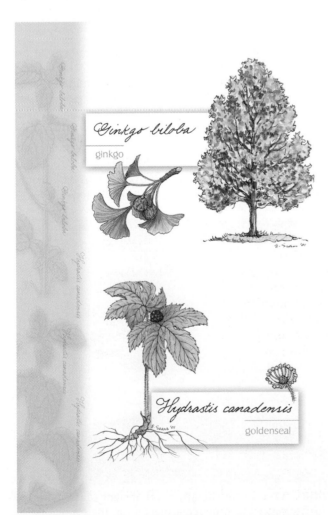

FIGURE 37-2 Herbs are potent natural substances with medicinal properties.

FIGURE 37-3 Many people use natural substances and practices as an alternative to traditional health care, believing that this is more healthful for the body.

Many old remedies, practices, and traditions have been rediscovered and are being used today. Different forms of nontraditional healing are accepted by the public and many medical professionals. These nontraditional methods are called **complementary/alternative medicine (CAM)**. CAM is a group of diverse systems, practices, and products that are not presently considered part of conventional medicine. This is an area of much research and scientific study. Because of this, practices listed as CAM change continually. Safety is always a great concern in health care. Some CAM practices have been proven unsafe or ineffective and are no longer used. Others have proven safe and effective and have moved into mainstream health care. For safety, a CAM program should always be supervised by a physician or other health care practitioner. New practices and techniques are always emerging.

Culture ALERT

Learn the patient's views about health. Accept the patient's practices whenever possible. Inform the nurse of practices that may affect the patient's overall care, and those that pose special health risks, such as taking herbal remedies or eating items not permitted on the diet ordered. ■

Complementary and Alternative Practices

Hundreds of different alternative therapies are used instead of traditional medicine. For example, patients use **herbs** (medicines made from plants), **supplements** (nutritional substances used to make up a deficiency or strengthen the whole), and diet (Figure 37-4) to treat cancer instead of surgery, chemotherapy, and radiation therapy (Unit 47). Nutritional products are usually slow to work and no immediate effect is seen when patients take them. The patient may have to take the preparation for a minimum of three to six months before seeing results.

A degree of caution is necessary when using nutritional preparations. Some are toxic or harmful when taken in large quantities. Some have negative interactions with other medications and foods. Some nutritional products contain combinations of vitamins and nutrients. Taking several combination products increases the risk that the patient will exceed the safe dosage range. An example is vitamin A, which is necessary for good eyesight and night vision. However, when taken excessively, vitamin A can cause blindness. Water-soluble preparations are excreted from the body. Fat-soluble preparations are stored in the tissue for a period of time. Some preparations interfere with drugs and therapies given for other medical conditions. Several have caused serious liver and kidney damage.

FIGURE 37-4 Natural foods are grown and processed without chemicals and pesticides. The heat used in food processing destroys some of the nutrients. Many natural products are processed with low or limited heat.

Complementary medicine is a treatment regimen in which alternative practices are combined with conventional health care. For example, magnets may be used with medications to relieve pain. Various sound and music therapies are used to reduce complications, relieve stress, make patients feel better, and increase their sense of well-being. **Aromatherapy** (using natural scents and smells to promote health and well-being) (Figure 37-5) is used by chemotherapy patients to relieve nausea. Some people use **guided imagery** in combination with cancer

FIGURE 37-5 Aromatherapy is an ancient practice that uses fragrances to produce a reaction in the body. Certain scents are believed to change brain waves, breathing rates, and mood, among other things.

treatment. People who use imagery believe that focusing on and visualizing positive changes causes these changes to occur. **Energy therapies** (Figure 37-6) work with the energy field that allegedly surrounds and penetrates the body. (The existence of this energy has not been confirmed scientifically.) **Relaxation** (techniques and methods of reducing stress) and **meditation** (calming and quieting the mind by focusing attention) are used in combination with heat and medications to relieve pain. Thousands of different treatments and therapies fall under the CAM umbrella. These **modalities** (forms of treatment or uses of therapeutic agents or regimens) can be placed into five broad categories, which are listed in Table 37-1. Most of these practices can be used alone or combined with more conventional treatment. When used alone, they are called *alternative treatments*. When used with other mainstream practices, they are called *complementary therapies*, because they complement the mainstream treatment. Alternative products should never be combined with medical treatment without physician supervision.

Using CAM

Alternative and complementary practices have become very popular in recent years. Many of these therapies are thought to stimulate the body to heal itself. They are also used to strengthen weak body systems, and reduce or eliminate the discomfort of some medical signs and symptoms, such as pain and nausea. Patients with cancer, heart disease, diabetes, and HIV disease commonly use CAM practices. The decision whether to use CAM is an important one that must be made based on accurate information about the benefits and risks of the treatment. The

Etheric or Vital Layer

Emotional Layer

Mental Layer

Intuitive or Spiritual Layer
(also called the astral body)

FIGURE 37-6 The energy field that is said to surround the body

TABLE 37-1 COMMON COMPLEMENTARY AND ALTERNATIVE MEDICINE CATEGORIES

Category	Description	Example
Alternative medical systems	Therapeutic or preventive health care practices that do not follow generally accepted methods and may not have a scientific explanation for their effectiveness. These treatments are usually based on complete systems of medical practice. Many were developed in other countries and have been used for centuries, predating conventional medical practices.	• Traditional Chinese medicine (TCM) • Ayurveda • Homeopathy • Naturopathy
Mind-body therapy	Practices that employ various techniques to enhance the mind's ability to affect bodily function and symptoms (mind-over-matter principle). Many have been accepted by the medical community and are part of integrative health care practices and treatments.	• Meditation • Art therapy • Music therapy • Dance therapy • Patient support groups • Cognitive therapy • Prayer • Guided imagery

TABLE 37-1 *CONTINUED*

Category	Description	Example
Biological therapy	Biologically based practices using natural substances, such as vitamins, herbs, and foods. Other natural products, such as shark cartilage, are also used.	• Herbs • Nutritional products • Dietary supplements
Body-based therapy (may also be called manipulation, or manipulation therapy)	Practices that are based on direct body contact, including manipulation or movement of one or more parts of the body.	• Chiropractic adjustments • Osteopathic manipulation • Massage therapy
Energy therapy	The study of how living organisms interact with electromagnetic energy fields. Although some practitioners believe touch is necessary for healing, others believe they can effect healing by placing the hands within the field. Two types of energy therapy are commonly used. *Biofield* therapies work by laying hands on the body or through its energy field to transfer a healing force. The biofield may also be called an *aura*. The energy field is believed to permeate the body and extends outward for several inches. *Biomagnetic-based* therapy is a form of energy therapy in which the hands are placed in or through the energy field to apply pressure on the body.	• Reiki • Therapeutic touch • Magnet therapy and use of magnetic fields • Pulsed current fields • AC and DC current fields

patient must look beyond advertisers' claims to find reliable, credible information about the method being considered. Authoritative information is difficult to find for some treatments because little research has been done. When evaluating the negatives and positives, ask:

- What are the advantages, disadvantages, risks, side effects, expected results, and length of treatment?
- What is the safety record of the treatment? Are specific safety precautions necessary?
- Is the treatment effective in circumstances similar to mine? Is it harmful in circumstances similar to mine?
- What are the qualifications of the individual providing the treatment (if applicable)?
- Will the CAM therapy interfere with the conventional treatment or medication being used for an acute or chronic medical problem?
- Can I comfortably comply with the directions for using this treatment?

People use alternative therapies and programs for many different purposes. Many do this on their own, without medical supervision. Potential drawbacks of an unsupervised alternative treatment program are:

- Potential for toxicity of herbs and nutritional products
- Self-diagnosis is not always accurate
- Self-treatment does not always work
- The self-treatment regimen may not be appropriate even if the diagnosis is correct

- The regimen may delay necessary medical treatment
- The program may interfere with prescription drugs
- Self-treatment may cure the symptoms, but aggravate other health problems

If you decide to pursue an alternative program, do so under medical supervision. Seek medical help if the condition you are treating does not respond within a week, if the original symptoms worsen, or if new symptoms develop.

INTEGRATIVE (INTEGRATED) HEALTH CARE PRACTICES

Some researchers estimate that at least 50% of the American public uses at least one form of alternative or complementary treatment. Because of this, many hospitals have

Clinical Information ALERT

A four-month study by researchers at Northwestern Memorial Hospital in Chicago showed that art therapy helped alleviate eight of nine symptoms in patients being treated for cancer, including pain, depression, poor appetite, and fatigue. ■

opened specialized units and clinics in which **integrative (integrated) health care** is practiced. Integrative health care involves using both mainstream medical treatments and CAM therapies to treat the patients. Approximately 25% of the hospitals in the United States offer some type of integrative medical services. Most integrative health care programs have two components. The wellness component helps participants stay well and prevent disease. The illness management component helps eliminate uncomfortable symptoms and strengthens the body to overcome the effects of illness. Many patients in the illness track also use approaches from the wellness track to prevent worsening of their conditions. Thus, persons who are well can participate to prevent illness, and those who are ill can participate to aid in their recovery.

Usually, the CAM method is used to enhance mainstream treatment, or to relieve signs and symptoms. Some services combine drug therapy with nutrition, diet, exercise, or other nontraditional therapies. CAM practices that promote relaxation (Figure 37-7) and relieve pain are some of the most commonly used in integrative care. This is based on the belief that when the mind and body are relaxed, pain and unpleasant symptoms decrease, and a healing environment is established within the body. Professionals who practice integrative care are very cautious, and CAM treatments are usually selected only when there is solid evidence of safety. If there is a high risk of harm to the patient, the treatment combination is not used.

Some patients practice integrative care on their own, without the knowledge of their health care provider. This can be dangerous, because some therapies increase the risk of complications when combined with some medical treatments and medications. For example, Mrs. Rosenberg has a strong family history of Alzheimer's disease. She fears she will contract this condition. She has taken herbs regularly for several years, as a preventive measure. Mrs. Rosenberg is hospitalized for a routine surgical procedure. She does not tell the doctor about the herbs, because they are nonprescription, natural products. During surgery, she experiences a large, unexpected blood loss and requires a blood transfusion. Mrs. Rosenberg did not know that the herbs she takes have a blood-thinning effect. Because the physician did not know of the herb use, he did not take measures before surgery to reduce the increased risk of bleeding.

The use of herbs in pregnancy can also be risky. In fact, herbs are very powerful substances that should be treated with caution and respect. They interact with many different prescription and nonprescription medications. Patients should always inform the health care provider if they are using alternative products. If a patient advises you that he or she uses alternatives, always inform the nurse, who will notify the physician.

Holistic Care

Standard medical care focuses on treating single body parts or systems. Most integrative medicine practitioners believe in using **holistic care** (practices that consider the whole person, including mind, body, and spirit). Holistic care (Figure 37-8) is designed to nourish, balance, and vitalize the whole individual. The patient's strengths are used to overcome weaknesses. Nursing care, in its purest form, has always been guided by principles of holistic care. In nursing, we look at the whole person. We know that one weakness can affect the patient's overall health and well-being. By supporting and strengthening all body systems, holistic medical care provides additional tools with which to fight disease.

Practitioners of holistic care also consider the effect that disease has on the patient's family dynamics and relationships. This reaches beyond curing a disease. Holistic care

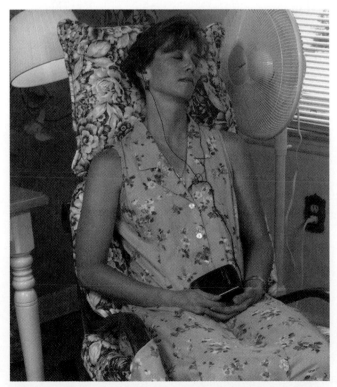

FIGURE 37-7 Some people use music during relaxation and meditation.

Clinical Information ALERT

Nursing schools teaching holistic care have proven that each holistic theory embodies the art and science of nursing, while acknowledging the integrity and wholeness of the individual. They teach to enter each patient's room with healing intent, and recommend stopping outside the door momentarily to clear the mind of one's own concerns, then entering the room with the ability to be fully present and focused on the patient as a whole being. ■

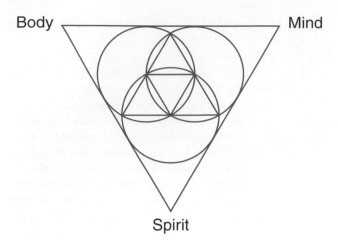

FIGURE 37-8 Holistic care looks at the patient as a person. Practitioners believe that mind, body, and spirit must be balanced for health and wellness.

considers the entire person as a complex being with many problems and needs. The patient is an active member of the health care team, not a passive participant. Besides standard medical care, consideration may be given to:

- Food and nutrition
- Fluid balance
- Elimination of body wastes
- Getting adequate rest and sleep
- Stress-relieving strategies
- Exercise
- Recreation
- Avoidance of unhealthy practices and substances
- Loving relationships and support systems
- Inner strength
- Creative expression
- Spiritual expression and well-being

CAM Practices and Holistic Care

When the patient and physician agree to consider an integrated approach to treatment, the assessment process begins. Integrative health care is based on certain principles:

- Each individual can be empowered to bring greater wellness and healing into his or her own life.
- Complementary therapies can be used to support and strengthen overall health. Some therapies promote healing. Others relieve symptoms, such as pain and nausea.
- The mind affects the healing process.
- Every person is unique and no single set of recommendations will be right for everyone. The integrative program must be individualized to meet the patient's needs and circumstances. More than one supportive therapy may be necessary.

The assessment for a holistic integrative care program will consist of:

- Evaluating the nature of the patient's medical and nursing problems
- Determining if further diagnostic tests are needed (and obtaining tests, if necessary)
- Evaluating the patient's coping resources
- Identifying the patient's goals and expectations
- Evaluating the patient's knowledge about his or her disease
- Evaluating the patient's knowledge about CAM
- Identifying patient teaching needs and developing a patient teaching plan
- Agreeing with the patient on treatments to use and goals of therapy
- Developing an individualized integrative treatment plan
- Making referrals, consultations, and appointments, if necessary

Patient teaching is done so the patient can make informed decisions about his or her care. You may be asked to contribute information to the assessment. You may also reinforce patient teaching when you are caring for the patient. Always follow the plan of care. Teaching is an ongoing process during treatment. The patient's response to treatment will be evaluated frequently, and the treatment plan adjusted as often as necessary to achieve a positive response.

COMMON CAM THERAPIES

Many CAM therapies are being used in health care facilities today. The following lists modalities that are commonly used in integrative practice in hospital units and clinics:

- **Acupuncture** (Figure 37-9) is an ancient practice dating back thousands of years. Acupuncture is used to treat many acute and chronic conditions. Tiny, thin needles are placed in various parts of the body to correct imbalances in energy. It is safe and painless when done by a trained and qualified practitioner.

Clinical Information ALERT

The ancient Chinese believed that every living being has a universal life energy called *chi*. This energy circulates through the body along pathways called *meridians*. The person remains in good health when the energy flows freely. When the flow of energy (chi) is blocked, pain and illness occur. Acupuncture stimulates specific points on the meridians to reprogram and restore normal function. However, acupuncture is only one approach used to treat the patient. It is part of a much larger system of traditional Chinese medicine. ■

FIGURE 37-9
Acupuncture is used to treat many different conditions by correcting energy imbalances throughout the body. The needles are usually left in place from 5 to 20 minutes.

- **Anthroposophically Extended Medicine (AEM)** is a holistic Western system of natural medicine. AEM treats the whole person and not just the disease or symptoms. Practitioners consider the human being as far more than a physical machine. Treatment is designed to harmonize the relationship of body, mind, and spirit. AEM practitioners may use herbal and homeopathic preparations to support and guide the natural healing processes in the body.

- *Aromatherapy* involves using essential oils to stimulate the patient's sense of smell. Smelling the oils stimulates the olfactory nerve, sending messages to the brain. Although this treatment has many uses, it is commonly used to promote relaxation, relieve pain or nausea, and boost the immune system.

- **Art therapy, dance therapy,** and music therapy all focus on use of the senses. Each helps the patient express himself. They provide distraction and stress reduction. Art therapy helps the patient deal with emotional conflict, increase awareness, and express unspoken concerns. Dance therapy uses dance to decrease body tension, reduce pain, improve body image and self-esteem, decrease fear, and express anger. Music therapy has many therapeutic purposes and can be used alone or as part of other programs for relaxation, pain relief, and improved self-esteem.

- **Ayurveda** is a natural system of medicine that originated in India more than 3,000 years ago. Translated, *ayurveda* means "knowledge of life." This system is based on the belief that disease is due to an imbalance in the individual's consciousness. Practitioners encourage certain lifestyle interventions, natural therapies, and regaining a balance between the body, mind, and the environment. It begins with an internal purification process, followed by a special diet, herbal remedies, massage therapy, yoga, and meditation. It is commonly used to treat high blood pressure, reduce stress, and reduce blood cholesterol.

- **Biofeedback** is a method of retraining the mind to control various physical problems and stresses that one would normally not be aware of.

- **Chelation therapy** involves intravenous (IV) injection of an amino acid by a licensed professional. It is commonly used to treat serious circulatory problems and reduced blood flow in the legs because of a buildup on the walls of the blood vessels. The amino acid injection bonds with substances within the blood vessels and removes them into circulation, where they are excreted in the urine. Although chelation therapy is usually considered safe, side effects range from mild to serious. It is usually used in combination with diet and exercise.

- **Chiropractic care** is a common, accepted CAM treatment that many people consider part of the mainstream medical system. Health insurance and Medicare pay for chiropractic visits; they do not pay for treatments for which effectiveness has not been proven. Chiropractic treatment has proven effective in relieving some types of pain, headaches, and menstrual cramps. Chiropractic care is based on the premise that the nervous system must function properly for good health. Because the nerves run through the spinal cord, chiropractic adjustments are done to keep the vertebrae in good alignment. This relieves pressure on nerves, muscles, and joints. Most chiropractors also promote exercise, diet, and good nutrition for overall health.

- Many studies have been done on how color affects the human mind. Some of these have also shown that color affects the body. Color is believed to stimulate many different senses and emotions. Marketing experts and advertisers use color to affect your moods and decisions. The color scheme on the packaging of most products is carefully designed to encourage you to buy. Past due bills are usually pink, which is associated with being very important. Red and orange color themes in restaurants are designed to increase your appetite. Many different alternative health care practices involve the use of **color therapy**. Color therapy is commonly used to affect mood, emotions, relationships, and sense of well-being. Color can be meditated on, gazed at, worn, or beamed in with various lights. Spiritual light and color are used for healing the body and mind. Color is also used for deepening meditation and creating specific effects on the body's energy field.

- **Electromagnetic therapy** is based on the belief that electric and magnetic energy exist within the body. Treatment is given to correct imbalances in the electrical and magnetic fields, which are believed to cause illness and disease. Different forms of electrical energy are used to correct imbalances. Mainstream medicine has adopted many electromagnetic approaches, such as using a defibrillator (Unit 52) to start the heart or a TENS unit (Unit 36) to relieve pain.

- **Herbal therapy** is used throughout the world for its medicinal effect. Many food products we use today are herbs. Herbs are medicines made from plants that provide a different way of treating pain and illness. However, herbs are generally very strong, and some can be very toxic. The use of herbs as medicine should be supervised by a qualified practitioner.
- **Homeopathy** is a practice of medicine that uses a wide range of natural (plant and mineral) substances to stimulate the body's immune system to fight disease. Homeopathic medicines are given to stimulate natural healing abilities of the body.
- **Hypnotherapy** is used to create an altered state of consciousness in which the patient is more open to the power of suggestion. It has many different applications, but in health care it is commonly used to relieve pain, anxiety, depression, addiction, and insomnia.
- **Light therapy** is used to treat mood and sleep disorders, jet lag, and depression. Seasonal affective disorder (Unit 30) is often treated with integrative medicine, and light therapy is an accepted approach. Treatment involves exposing patients to special lights covered with a plastic screen to block ultraviolet rays. The most common treatment involves sitting in front of a light box with the eyes open, but not looking directly into the light. Treatment time is progressively increased up to 90 minutes a day. One treatment involves shining a light behind the patient's knees. Research is being done on using light in the treatment of many conditions, including obesity and premenstrual syndrome.
- **Massage therapy** (Figure 37-10) is provided by licensed massage therapists. Massage stimulates and improves circulation, providing relaxation and pain relief. It is believed to stimulate the immune system to fight disease. Massage increases feelings of well-being and reduces stress and fatigue.
- *Meditation* is a form of body and mind relaxation. It has various applications, ranging from stress relief to

FIGURE 37-10 The massage therapist manipulates various areas of the body to stimulate tissues and promote healing.

pain relief. Meditation is an intensely personal and spiritual experience for most people. To meditate is to turn inward, to concentrate on the inner self. Meditation is a three-step process involving preparation, concentration, and merging with the object of concentration. It is commonly used for personal growth and developing tolerance. Meditation is said to channel awareness into a more positive direction by transforming one's state of mind.

- **Movement therapy** is a form of nonaerobic exercise and breath control that gives patients an awareness of how the body moves. Practitioners learn to alter posture and motion to reduce pain and stress. It is useful in chronic neurological disorders, such as Parkinson's disease, multiple sclerosis, and stroke. It has been used for increasing self-esteem.
- Doctors of **Naturopathic medicine** receive extensive education at one of five schools in North America. Naturopathic care focuses on whole-person wellness, emphasizing prevention and self-care. The doctor looks for the cause of illness, rather than strictly treating symptoms. Naturopathic practitioners cooperate with and refer patients for medical diagnosis and treatment when necessary. They use nontoxic, natural medications that are compounded and individualized to the patient's needs.
- **Nutrition therapy** evaluates the patient's diet to ensure that it contains optimal nutrition for health, wellness, and healing. This may mean eliminating some foods and adding others. Vitamins, minerals, and nutritional supplements may be added for wellness promotion or healing, such as calcium to prevent osteoporosis, or vitamin C to promote pressure-ulcer healing.
- **Prayer** (Figure 37-11) is a CAM technique that is used alone and in combination with other treatments. Some people use it with meditation. Patients have many different religious rituals and activities. Prayer is a connection with a person's higher power. One large study showed that patients who received prayer recovered faster after surgery than patients who were not the recipients of prayer. Many of the study patients were not aware that others were praying for their recovery.
- Practitioners of **qigong** believe that everyone is born with a life force energy, called *qi* or *chi*. This treatment involves physical and mental activities to teach the patient to channel the chi, thereby improving health. It is used to treat a variety of problems, including arthritis, gastric ulcers, insomnia, headaches, allergies, and high blood pressure.
- **Reflexology** (Figure 37-12) is an ancient form of healing used to reduce stress and treat illness. Certain reflex areas in the hands and feet are stimulated. The stimulation affects other parts of the body, reducing stress, stabilizing body functions, and correcting health problems.
- **Reiki** uses touch on various areas of the body to promote health and well-being. The hands are placed in

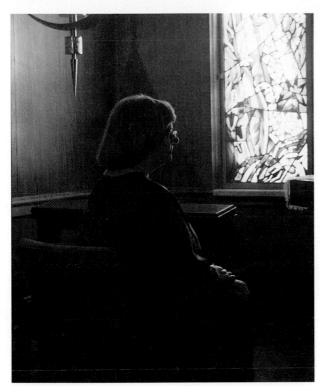

FIGURE 37-11 Prayer is a means of connecting with one's higher power.

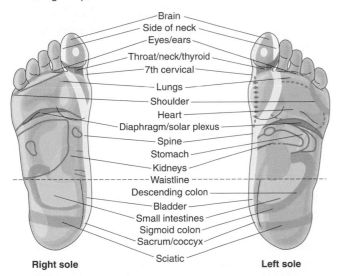

Brain
Side of neck
Eyes/ears
Throat/neck/thyroid
7th cervical
Lungs
Shoulder
Heart
Diaphragm/solar plexus
Spine
Stomach
Kidneys
Waistline
Descending colon
Bladder
Small intestines
Sigmoid colon
Sacrum/coccyx
Sciatic

Right sole   **Left sole**

FIGURE 37-12 Practitioners of reflexology believe that they can heal many areas of the body by manipulating the feet. This is based on the principle that different areas of the foot are connected to different areas of the body, from the internal organs to the ears.

various positions, beginning with the head and working down. The hands are held in place on each area for 3 to 5 minutes. Practitioners believe that sickness drains a person's physical and emotional energy. Reiki is applied to restore energy, enhancing the body's natural healing ability. Reiki practitioners receive special training. It is used to promote spiritual and mental well-being, relieve stress, relieve pain, and promote relaxation.

- **Therapeutic touch (TT)** is a term commonly used to describe touching patients in a caring manner. However, in this context, it is a CAM treatment that involves using the hands to exchange energy and stimulate healing (Figure 37-13A). Therapeutic touch practitioners believe that when energy is unbalanced, disease occurs. TT restores the energy field in the body to create a healing environment. The hands do not touch the patient (Figure 37-13B). The goal is to align the mind, body, and spirit for good health. TT is commonly used in the care of patients with AIDS, chronic pain, anxiety, and high blood pressure.

- **Traditional Chinese medicine (TCM)** is a complete health care system that is thousands of years old. It has changed little over the centuries. The basic idea is that a vital life force surges through the body. Any imbalance in the life force can cause illness. Disease is caused by an imbalance in the opposite and complementary energies that make up the life force, called *yin* and *yang*. The TCM doctor treats disease by restoring the balance between the internal body organs and the

FIGURE 37-13A Therapeutic touch is said to impart healing energy from the practitioner's hands to the patient's body.

FIGURE 37-13B The therapeutic touch practitioner does not touch the patient.

A. Half-spinal twist

B. Cobra

C. Alternate leg stretch

FIGURE 37-14 Many different yoga positions are used, but the focus is on breathing, which is supposed to awaken the consciousness.

external elements of earth, fire, water, wood, and metal. Treatment may involve acupuncture, **moxibustion** (burning herbal leaves on or near the body), **cupping** (use of warmed glass jars to create suction on certain points of the body), massage, herbal remedies, movement, and concentration exercises.

- **Visualization** is one of the practices involved in guided imagery. This technique involves using the imagination to visualize something. Creating images in the mind helps reduce stress, pain, and symptoms associated with many medical conditions. The patient sets health goals and objectives. He or she is guided to visualize and work toward the goals. Two methods are commonly used. Visualization of colors is done to reduce stress. Another method involves visualizing the elimination of health care problems; for example, the patient may imagine a PacMan gobbling up cancer cells in the body.

- **Yoga** (Figure 37-14) means the union between mind and body. Yoga involves a combination of breath control, postures, relaxation, and meditation. It is used to improve lung function and circulation, decrease pain, and reduce anxiety.

Osteopathic Medicine

Some individuals consider osteopathic medicine to be an alternative practice, but over the years, this branch of medicine has been accepted as a form of mainstream medicine. The **Doctor of Osteopathy (D.O.)** has preparation similar to that of a medical doctor (M.D.). A D.O. receives a complete medical education. He or she receives additional training in **osteopathic manipulative treatment (OMT)**, a passive, thrusting motion similar to the chiropractic adjustment. OMT is used to restore normal body movement, in combination with regular medical treatment. For example, a D.O. treats a patient with an

infection of the foot by prescribing antibiotic therapy. Additionally, he provides an OMT treatment to enhance blood and oxygen flow through the body. This is based on the belief that the antibiotic will be more effective in eliminating the infection if the circulation to the foot is not impeded.

Osteopathic Medicine Versus Chiropractic Care. Some people believe that chiropractic and osteopathic treatments are identical, but they are not. Chiropractic care focuses mainly on the spine and involves many very fine maneuvers. The chiropractor focuses on preventing interruptions in nerve flow. The osteopathic physician focuses on how tight muscles and joints affect the function of all body systems. The emphasis is on ensuring proper movement of air (oxygen) and fluid within the body. This is based on the belief that the body works most effectively when:

- All tissues are nourished with oxygen
- Wastes can be removed in body fluids
- The body is in an optimum state of health; healing will occur when it is nourished with oxygen and wastes have been removed

The osteopathic physician uses OMT with regular medical treatment, whereas the chiropractor uses only spinal manipulation. Because of this, the D.O. can treat many conditions that do not respond to chiropractic care.

SPIRITUALITY

Spirituality and religion also have a place in nontraditional health care practices. Many people believe that spirituality and religion are the same thing, but they are not

Religion   Spirituality

FIGURE 37-15A Religion and spirituality have some overlapping aspects.

FIGURE 37-15B Spirituality defines our perceptions of our place in the universe and our responsibilities to others.

(Figure 37-15A). Spirituality is more of an umbrella that defines:

- Our perceptions of our place in the universe (Figure 37-15B).
- A higher power (if any)
- Our responsibilities to others
- Our fears and beliefs about living and dying

The need for spirituality may be fueled by experiences, relationships, opportunities that provide the motivation for deeper healing, and growth throughout life. Illness can be a powerful motivator for eliminating emotional, mental, and physical patterns that limit and restrict spiritual growth. A key to caring for patients' spiritual needs is respecting each patient as an individual, and appreciating that no two people are alike.

When patients use spirituality for healing, they allow the power of the spirit to work more fully in their lives, leading to greater harmony and balance. It is usually a quiet time for introspection and questioning. Healing may require making changes. It involves blending of the physical, mental, emotional, and spiritual aspects of self. When a person experiences deep physical or emotional healing, all parts of the self are changed. Physical problems often involve thoughts and emotions. Patients sometimes have surprises during periods of intense spirituality. They may release a great emotional burden instead of experiencing a physical recovery. The lifting of the emotional burden brings a great sense of inner peace.

Religion

Religion differs from spirituality in that it includes another element for the cause of disease. Religious beliefs vary widely, so making generalizations is difficult. However, members of various religions believe that other factors contribute to the development of disease, such as sin, assault from a demonic power or a lesser god, or the malevolence of others. Another common belief is that disease occurs to help a person learn an important life lesson or overcome a weakness. Most believe that although the higher power allows diseases to occur, that power is in no way responsible for them. Practitioners of some religions believe that the power of prayer, laying-on of hands, or another ritual is necessary to heal the illness. Many believe that the power or intercession of a religious authority (Figure 37-16) is necessary to effect a cure. The patient may practice certain religious rituals, such as fasting and prayer, to promote healing.

Nursing Assistant Actions

The nursing assistant must recognize that all humans are spiritual beings, although we all choose different paths. Be sensitive to the patients' paths and choices. Avoid making judgments about patients' religious, spiritual, ethnic, and cultural practices and choices in health care treatment.

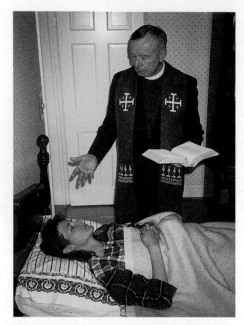

FIGURE 37-16 Practitioners of some religions believe that a religious authority must intercede for them by appealing to the higher power or conducting various practices and rituals. Many believe in the power of prayer and the laying-on of hands.

Although spiritual beliefs are usually considered a private concern, the need for spiritual caring is fundamental when serious health problems occur. The patient may question the meaning and purpose of life, her ability to hope, belief in herself, belief in the caregiver's ability, belief in the physician's ability, and belief in a higher power.

Health care personnel are privileged to have a role in these very personal times of significant stress and turmoil in patients' lives. Pay attention to what the patient is saying. Your role is to listen, to reflect, and to clarify information. Never try to interpret or define spiritual meaning or truth to the patient. Avoid imposing your beliefs on the patient. Avoid pat, uncaring answers to questions. Never give patients false hope. Never use problem-solving techniques to analyze spiritual truths for patients. Admitting that you do not know an answer is all right.

Remember that caring for patients during very private moments is a privilege. Do not be so distracted with your workload or the environment that you fail to show sensitivity when patients express spiritual concerns. Provide privacy and support while they work through challenges to their health and well-being. Inform the nurse or social worker of the patient's concerns. He or she may be able to provide assistance, intervention, or referrals to other sources of help.

REVIEW

A. True/False

Mark the following true or false by circling T or F.

1. T F Alternative practices are unapproved therapies that are used as part of mainstream health care treatment.

2. T F Complementary therapies are used instead of traditional medical treatments.

3. T F Safety is a major concern when considering complementary and alternative methods.

4. T F Some CAM therapies involve manipulation of the body with the hands.

5. T F Herbs are medications made from plants.

6. T F Imagery involves focusing on and visualizing positive changes.

7. T F An osteopathic physician and a chiropractor have similar education and practice.

8. T F The nursing assistant should assist patients in interpreting spiritual issues.

9. T F Complementary therapies have no place in health care.

10. T F Integrative health care involves a combination of mainstream medicine and alternative health care treatments.

11. T F Biofeedback involves training the mind to control physical problems.

12. T F Chiropractic adjustments are done to relieve pressure on nerves.

B. Matching

Choose the correct phrase from Column II to match the words or phrases in Column I.

Column I

13. _____ hypnotherapy

14. _____ homeopathy

15. _____ acupuncture

16. _____ Reiki

17. _____ movement therapy

18. _____ meditation

19. _____ aromatherapy

20. _____ therapeutic touch

21. _____ yoga

22. _____ Ayurveda

23. _____ qigong

24. _____ massage

Column II

a. stimulating sense of smell

b. concentrating on inner self

c. creates awareness of how body moves

d. rubbing body to stimulate circulation, promote relaxation

e. views disease as an imbalance in a person's consciousness

f. activities to teach the patient to channel chi

g. alters the state of consciousness

h. uses natural substances to stimulate immune system

i. begins with hands on head, working down over body

j. restores energy field so healing can occur

k. uses thin needles

l. union between mind and body

C. Multiple Choice

Select the one best answer for each of the following.

25. Holistic care includes
    a. meditation and biofeedback.
    b. using strengths to overcome weaknesses.
    c. freeing nerves from entrapped vertebrae.
    d. focus on the disease process.

26. An integrative care program always begins with
    a. patient teaching.
    b. goal-setting.
    c. assessment.
    d. assisting the patient to cope.

27. Cognitive therapy is a form of
    a. mind-body therapy.
    b. energy therapy.
    c. manipulation.
    d. biological therapy.

28. Chelation therapy is used to
    a. cleanse the mind.
    b. promote rest and relaxation.
    c. relieve stress.
    d. cleanse blood vessels.

29. Yin and yang are concepts used in
    a. Ayurveda.
    b. traditional Chinese medicine.
    c. qigong.
    d. Reiki.

D. Nursing Assistant Challenge

Your patient, Mrs. Matassarin, has been diagnosed with colon cancer. She has chosen an integrative medicine program to treat her illness. She meditates and prays several times each day. The care plan states you are to assist her in preparing to meditate at 3:15 PM each day. You are running a little late. You enter the room at 3:22 PM and find the patient deep in meditation.

30. What nursing assistant action should you take if the patient is meditating? Why?

31. What actions can you use in the future for assisting the patient with the meditation care plan?

32. If you are unsure of what actions to take, how will you find out?

33. Based on your knowledge of integrative health practices, what effect will the meditation have on Mrs. Matassarin?

UNIT 38

Integumentary System

OBJECTIVES

After completing this unit, you will be able to:
- Spell and define terms.
- Review the location and function of the skin.
- Describe some common skin lesions.
- List three diagnostic tests associated with skin conditions.
- Describe nursing assistant actions relating to care of patients with specific skin conditions.
- Identify persons at risk for the formation of pressure ulcers.
- Describe measures to prevent pressure ulcers.
- Describe the stages of pressure ulcer formation and identify appropriate nursing assistant actions.
- List nursing assistant actions in caring for patients with burns.

VOCABULARY

Learn the meaning and the correct spelling of the following words and phrases:

abrasion	decubitus ulcer	lesion	rubra
allergen	dermal ulcer	macule	sebaceous gland
allergies	dermis	malodorous	senile purpura
anaphylactic shock	electrical burn	necrosis	shearing
burns	epidermis	nodule	skin tears
chemical burn	eschar	obese	subcutaneous tissue
contraindicated	excoriation	pallor	sudoriferous gland
contusion	friction	papule	tepid
crust	hematoma	pediculosis	thermal burn
cyanotic	integument	pressure ulcer	vesicle
debride	Kaposi's sarcoma	pustule	wheal

INTEGUMENTARY SYSTEM STRUCTURES

The integumentary system (Figure 38-1) includes:
- Skin
- Hair
- Nails
- Sweat glands
- Nerves
- Oil glands

The outermost layers of the skin make up the epidermis. The dermis lies under the epidermis. The **subcutaneous tissue** that attaches the skin to the muscles lies under the dermis.

The nails are horny cell structures found on the dorsal, distal surfaces of the fingers and toes. They protect the sensitive fingers and toes. The teeth are formed from the tissues of the **integument** (body shell).

Clinical Information ALERT

The skin is the largest organ of the human body. In an average-size adult, the skin weighs approximately 4 kilograms (8.8 pounds). It covers an area of approximately 2 meters (78.4 inches). The average person's skin renews itself every 28 days. Each square inch of human skin consists of approximately 19 million cells, 60 hairs, 90 oil glands, 19 feet of blood vessels, 625 sweat glands, and 19,000 sensory cells. People of different races and skin color have about the same number of cells that produce skin color (melanocytes). A person's skin color depends on how much or how little melanin each melanocyte cell produces. Human skin has about 100,000 bacteria per square centimeter. Ten percent of human dry weight is attributed to bacteria. The normal flora that live on the skin help to protect you from harmful bacteria. ■

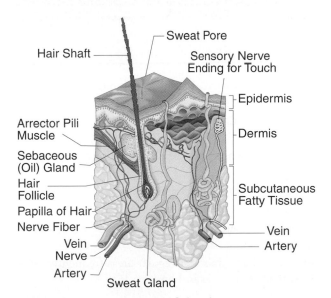

FIGURE 38-1 Cross-section of the skin

Epidermis

The **epidermis** consists of dead outer cells that are constantly shed as new cells move upward from the dermis. There are no blood vessels in the epidermis, so injury to this layer does not cause bleeding. Nerve endings reach into this outer layer. The nerves are sense organs that keep us in contact with changes in the environment. Nerve endings called *receptors* receive information about:

- Heat
- Cold
- Pain
- Pressure
- Temperature regulation—regulates body temperature

Clinical Information ALERT

"Goose bumps" are caused by the contraction of an arrector pili muscle connected to each hair follicle. Although you may not notice it, the contraction also causes the hair to stand on end. ■

Dermis

The **dermis** contains blood vessels, nerve fibers, and two kinds of glands:

- Sweat glands (**sudoriferous glands**)
- Oil glands (**sebaceous glands**)

Clinical Information ALERT

Sweat from the apocrine glands (those located mainly in the underarm and genital areas) is odorless. Body odor is caused by the action of the skin's normal bacteria on the sweat. ■

Sweat Glands

The sweat glands produce perspiration that reaches the skin surface through tubes or ducts that end in openings called pores. Heat from deep in the body is brought to the skin by blood vessels. This heat is transferred to the perspiration. At the skin surface, the perspiration and the heat are lost through the pores to the air. The heat of the body is controlled by changes in the size of the blood vessels in the skin.

- When the central opening of a blood vessel becomes enlarged (dilated), more heat is brought to the body surface.
- When the central opening of a blood vessel becomes smaller (constricted), less heat is brought to the body surface.

Oil Glands and Hair

Oil glands lubricate and keep flexible the hairs found in the skin. Hair covers almost all body surfaces except for the palms of the hands and the soles of the feet.

SKIN FUNCTIONS

The skin has many functions that are critical to the well-being of the body:

- Protection—forms a continuous membranous covering for the body
- Storage—stores fat and vitamins
- Elimination—loses water, salts, and heat through perspiration
- Sensory perception—contains nerve endings that keep us aware of environmental changes

The skin tells us much about the general health of the body.

- A fever may be indicated by hot, dry skin.
- Unusual redness—**rubra**, or flushing of the skin—often follows strenuous activity.
- **Pallor**, which is less color than normal, is a sign associated with many conditions.
- The oxygen content of the blood can be noted quickly by the color of the skin. When the oxygen content is very low, the blood is darker and the skin appears bluish or **cyanotic**.

AGING CHANGES

As a person ages, changes become evident in the skin and its elements. These changes include:

- Glands that are less active
- Decreased circulation
- Dryness, thinning, and scaling
- Thickening of fingernails and toenails
- Loss of fat and elasticity
- Loss of hair color
- Development of skin irregularities such as skin tabs, moles, and warts

SKIN LESIONS

Injury or disease can cause changes in skin structures. These changes are called **lesions**. The lesions may be caused by disease, trauma, wear, or the aging process. When caring for patients with skin lesions, standard pre-

cautions are followed. Some of the most common skin lesions or eruptions are:

- **Macules**—flat, discolored spots, as in measles (Figure 38-2)
- **Nodules**—small, knotlike protrusions; small masses of tissue
- **Papules**—small, solid, raised spots, as in chickenpox
- **Pustules**—raised spots filled with pus, as in acne
- **Vesicles**—raised spots filled with watery fluid, such as a blister (Figure 38-3)
- **Wheals**—large, raised, irregular areas frequently associated with itching, as in hives

FIGURE 38-2 The macules of German measles (Courtesy of the Centers for Disease Control and Prevention (CDC), Atlanta, Georgia)

FIGURE 38-3 The fluid-filled vesicles of poison ivy (Courtesy of the Centers for Disease Control and Prevention (CDC), Atlanta, Georgia)

- **Excoriations**—portions of the skin appear scraped or scratched away
- **Crusts**—areas of dried body secretions, such as scabs

Skin lesions may be a result of systemic responses:

- Communicable disease—diseases that are easily transmitted, directly or indirectly, from person to person. Measles and chickenpox are two such diseases. Each has characteristic skin lesions called *skin eruptions* or *rashes*.
- Immune system problems—Persons whose immune systems are depressed, such as those suffering from HIV infection, may develop a specific type of cancer called **Kaposi's sarcoma** (Figure 38-4). It appears as lesions in the skin and eventually in other organs. The skin lesions begin as macules, papules, or nodules that gradually become bigger and darker. The lesions are reddish-purple to dark blue in color. In addition to

persons with HIV disease, Kaposi's sarcoma (Figure 38-4A and Figure 38-4B) is most common in men over 60 years of age. Recent research suggests that it is caused by a herpes virus, and may be spread by kissing an infected person. Kaposi's lesions can also appear in the mouth and internal organs. Progression of the disease may be slow or rapid.

- **Allergies**—also called *sensitivity reactions*, may have associated skin lesions. The vesicles of poison ivy are well known. The material causing the sensitivity is called an **allergen**. Individuals respond to allergens in different ways.
- **Anaphylactic shock**—a severe, sometimes fatal, sensitivity reaction.

Pediculosis is another term for lice. Three common types of lice are seen on patients in the United States:

- Head lice (*Pediculosis capitis*) (Unit 12) (Figure 38-5A)
  - found on the head, scalp, and behind the ears
- Body lice (*Pediculosis corporis*)
  - found on the body and in clothing of infested people
- Pubic lice (*Pediculosis pubis*) (Figure 38-5B)
  - found in the pubic area; occasionally seen in underarm and eyebrow hair in humans

Another parasite contracted by humans is scabies (Unit 12) (Figure 38-5C). These parasites cause similar signs and symptoms:

- Severe, maddening itching
- Rash
- Sores on body (often caused by scratching)

Pediculosis can be seen with the eye (Figures 38-6A, 38-6B, and 38-6C). Scabies are microscopic (Figure 38-6D) and can only be seen through a microscope. They are spread by direct contact with an infected person. However, they can live for several days without food, so may

FIGURE 38-4A Typical lesions of Kaposi's sarcoma (Courtesy of Daniel J. Barbaro, MD, Fort Worth, Texas)

FIGURE 38-4B Raised lesions of Kaposi's sarcoma (Courtesy of Daniel J. Barbaro, MD, Fort Worth, Texas)

FIGURE 38-5A This image was captured while a head louse was emerging from its egg. After the egg hatches, the shell becomes a more visible dull yellow, still attached to the hair shaft. The nymph looks like an adult head louse, but is about the size of a pinhead, maturing after three molts and becoming an adult about 7 days after hatching. (Courtesy of the Centers for Disease Control and Prevention (CDC), Atlanta, Georgia)

FIGURE 38-5B Pubic lice are generally found in the genital area on pubic hair, but may occasionally be found on other coarse body hair, such as hair on the legs, armpits, mustache, beard, eyebrows, and eyelashes. The tiny brown dots on the skin are blood-filled lice that are firmly attached to the hair shafts with appendages that look like little pinchers on the ends of the legs. (Courtesy of the Centers for Disease Control and Prevention (CDC), Atlanta, Georgia)

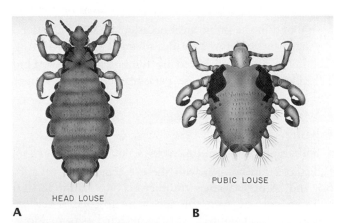

HEAD LOUSE   PUBIC LOUSE

A   **B**

C   **D**

FIGURE 38-6 Parasites that live on the body, and in the clothing or bedding of infested humans. Infestation is common, and is found worldwide. Itching and rash are common with lice infestation. (Courtesy of the Centers for Disease Control and Prevention (CDC), Atlanta, Georgia)

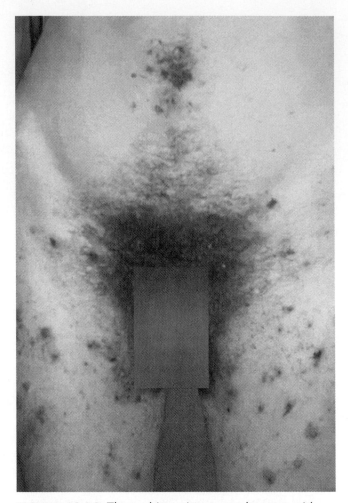

FIGURE 38-5C The scabies mite cannot be seen with the eye. Symptoms of scabies include: (1) pimple-like irritations, burrows, or rash of the skin, especially the webbing between the fingers; the skin folds on the wrist, elbow, or knee; the penis, the breast, or shoulder blades; (2) intense itching, especially at night and over most of the body; (3) sores on the body caused by scratching. These sores can sometimes become infected with bacteria. (Courtesy of the Centers for Disease Control and Prevention (CDC), Atlanta, Georgia).

be contracted by indirect contact through clothing, hair combs, brushes, and accessories, and cracks in furniture. Pediculosis can transmit disease. Another common problem is that all of the parasites are becoming resistant to the chemicals used to treat the pests, making them very difficult to eliminate. Inform the nurse immediately if you suspect that a patient is infected with lice or scabies.

Some lesions commonly occur when the skin is injured:

- **Abrasions** are injuries that result from scraping the skin.
- **Contusions** are mechanical injuries (usually caused by a blow) resulting in hemorrhage beneath the unbroken skin.
- An ecchymosis is a bruise.
- A **hematoma** is a localized mass of blood that is confined to one area.

Clinical Information ALERT

When a bruise occurs, blood becomes trapped under the skin causing a reddish color. The color gradually changes as the body absorbs the spilled blood. ■

- Lacerations are accidental breaks in the skin.
- **Senile purpura** are dark purple bruises on the forearms and backs of hands. These are common in elderly individuals.
- **Skin tears** are shallow injuries in which the epidermis is torn. The shape is often irregular. These injuries are also common in elderly individuals.

Observation of the skin and accurate descriptions of what you see must be carefully charted.

Diagnosing Skin Lesions

Your careful observations and accurate description of any skin lesions provide valuable information about the patient's condition. Several diagnostic tests may be ordered by the physician to help establish the cause of a lesion. These tests include:

- Studying scrapings from the skin lesion under the microscope.
- Culturing the skin lesion if an infection is suspected.
- Performing skin testing if sensitivities are suspected, by introducing small quantities of substances (allergens) known to bring about an allergic (hypersensitivity) reaction in humans. Allergens include pollens, foods, dust, animal dander, and medications.

Care of Skin Lesions

When skin lesions are present, certain general nursing care is indicated. Take the following precautions when caring for these patients.

- Closely observe the patient's skin on admission, but do not remove any dressings. Any changes noted should be reported immediately and described accurately.
- Soap and water and rubbing lotions are often **contraindicated** (not permitted). Check the nursing care plan before bathing the patient or giving a backrub.
- Special products may be used for bathing or soaking the skin, such as *colloidal oatmeal*. This product is used for many different skin conditions to relieve irritation, reduce itching, and moisturize, soften, and protect the skin. When bathing the patient, you may be instructed to use **tepid** (lukewarm) water instead of hot water. Make sure that the patient does not get the treated bath water in the eyes. The product may make the tub slippery. Instruct the patient to use the hand rail when rising from the tub, and provide assistance as needed.

Safety ALERT

Tepid water should be between 80°F and 93°F. The patient may need a therapeutic bath up to three times a day, depending on the severity of the underlying condition. Add the required amount of colloidal oatmeal or other product to the tub *as it is filling*. If the patient complains of feeling sticky after the bath, rinse with a few extra cups of tepid water from the faucet. Pat (do not rub) the skin dry. ■

- Wear gloves when contact with blood, body fluids (including drainage from blisters or skin lesions), or nonintact skin is likely.
- Do not attempt to remove any crusts from skin lesions without special instruction from the nurse.
- Handle the patient gently. Avoid rubbing the skin.
- Special bed linen may be used, such as sterile linen, linen that has been washed in special detergent, or disposable linen. Special bedding will be listed on the care plan.
- A bed cradle (Unit 25) may be placed on the bed to prevent the sheet from contacting the open skin areas.
- Notify the nurse if the:
  - skin lesions are draining
  - nature of the drainage changes
  - amount of drainage increases
  - drainage becomes **malodorous** (having a bad or foul odor)
  - drainage changes in color

Infection Control ALERT

Become familiar with the appearance of scabies and body lice on the skin. These microscopic parasites often appear as numerous, tiny scabs on the skin surface. These areas commonly itch, and the patient may scratch them. If the patient has multiple, tiny, scab-like areas, wear gloves when care requires skin contact. Report the presence of these lesions to the nurse for further assessment. ■

Pressure Ulcers (Dermal Ulcers)

Pressure ulcers, commonly called bedsores or **dermal ulcers**, may occur in patients of any age. You may also hear them called **decubitus ulcers**. This is an older term that continues to be used. It is not as accurate as *pressure ulcers*. *Decubitus* is Latin for lying down. Because ulcers

Clinical Information ALERT

The five most common conditions in which pressure ulcers develop are pneumonia, urinary tract infection, septicemia, aspiration pneumonitis, and congestive heart failure. Patients who are admitted to the hospital for pressure ulcer treatment often have diagnoses of spinal cord injury, paralysis, substance abuse, malnutrition, multiple sclerosis, stroke, and dementia. ▪

can occur when a patient is not in bed, the descriptive terminology was changed to "pressure ulcer" for accuracy. Pressure ulcers are open areas that develop on the skin over a bony prominence as the result of pressure. If there is pressure on the skin for a prolonged period, ulceration can occur, regardless of the patient's position. They are particularly common in patients who are:

- Elderly
- Very thin
- Overweight (**obese**)
- Unable to move
- Incontinent
- Debilitated
- Poorly nourished (eats less than half of meals and snacks)
- Confined to bed or wheelchairs
- Disoriented
- Dehydrated
- In prolonged contact with moisture
- Circulation-impaired
- Has discolored, torn, or swollen skin
- Subjected to shearing

Shearing (Figure 38-7) occurs when the skin moves in one direction while the structures under the skin, such as the bones, remain fixed or move in the opposite direction. This can happen when patients are dragged rather than lifted up in bed, when positions are changed, or when patients slide down in bed or in a wheelchair (Figure 38-8). Blood vessels become twisted and stretched, causing the tissues being served to lose essential oxygen and nutrients, leading to breakdown. In addition, shearing may cause actual tears in fragile skin. These skin tears are painful, a portal of entry for infectious pathogens, and commonly lead to further breakdown. **Friction** (rubbing the skin against another surface, such as bed linen) also contributes to pressure ulcer formation. It usually occurs when the patient is being moved.

Pressure ulcers are caused by prolonged pressure on an area of the body that interferes with circulation. The tissue first becomes reddened. As the cells die (undergo

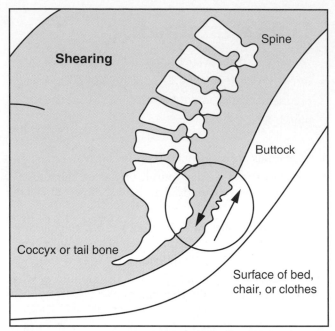

FIGURE 38-7 Shearing occurs when the skin is stretched one direction and the underlying structures move in the opposite direction.

FIGURE 38-8 Shearing occurs when a patient slides down or is improperly pulled up in bed.

necrosis—refer to the photo on page 657) from lack of nourishment, the skin breaks down and an ulcer forms. The resulting pressure ulcers may become large and deep. Pressure ulcers occur most frequently over areas where bones come close to the surface. The most common sites (Figures 38-9A and 38-9B) are the:

- Elbows
- Heels

FIGURE 38-9A Potential areas of pressure when a patient is in bed

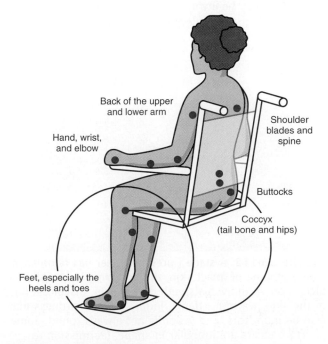

FIGURE 38-9B Potential areas of pressure when a patient is in a chair or wheelchair

- Shoulders
- Sacrum, coccyx
- Hips
- Buttocks
- Ankles
- Ears
- Knees (inner and outer parts)
- Toes

Patients tend to develop pressure ulcers where body parts rub and cause friction. Common sites are:

- Between the folds of the buttocks
- Legs
- Under the breasts
- Abdominal folds
- Ankles
- Knees

The rubbing of tubing and other equipment used in the care of patients over a long period can also cause pressure sores (Figure 38-10).

Clinical Information ALERT

In 2003, government payers were billed for nearly 90% of hospitalizations during which pressure ulcers were noted. The average cost of stays principally for pressure ulcers was $37,800, but charges varied by payer. Medicaid was billed an average of $39,100 per pressure ulcer patient. Pressure ulcers are preventable injuries, and your tax dollars pay for most pressure ulcer care! ■

FIGURE 38-10 Rubbing and pressure from tubes can cause irritation and skin breakdown.

Preventing Pressure Ulcers. Because pressure ulcers are far easier to prevent than to cure, everyone participating in the patient's care has a responsibility to prevent skin breakdown.

When a patient is admitted, the nurse will assess the patient's current status and potential for skin breakdown. This assessment gives a baseline against which all future assessments may be measured. The assessment may be described on the patient's chart in words, pictures, diagrams, or as a score. If a nursing diagnosis of actual or "risk for impaired skin or tissue integrity" is made, every staff member must make extra efforts to prevent skin breakdown, limit any breakdown that has already occurred, and promote the healing process.

Development of Pressure Ulcers

Tissue breakdown occurs in four stages. Nursing intervention at each stage can limit the process and prevent further damage. Remember to continue all preventive measures throughout care.

Clinical Information ALERT

The red area on the patient's skin is believed to be the tip of the iceberg in a stage I pressure ulcer. The damage that cannot be seen below the skin may actually be much larger. Avoid rubbing or massaging red areas that are potentially stage I pressure ulcers. Rubbing will worsen tissue destruction. Inform the nurse of the red area promptly. ■

Stage I. In stage I, the skin develops a redness (Figures 38-11A and 38-11B) or blue-gray discoloration over the pressure area. In dark-skinned people, the area may appear drier, or it may appear dark blue or black. The redness or discoloration does not go away within 30 minutes after pressure has been relieved. The skin is not broken in a stage I area. This stage is usually reversible if the area is detected promptly and pressure is relieved. It has the potential to worsen rapidly.

Legal ALERT

Pressure ulcers are always easier to prevent than to treat. They can worsen rapidly and become seriously infected. Most health care facilities conduct a pressure ulcer risk assessment upon admission, so that patients who are at high risk become known immediately. Once identified, these patients should receive special attention in preventive skin care. Patients who have pressure ulcers are always at high risk of developing additional ulcers. However, patients who are normally healthy, but suddenly become sick and dehydrated, are also at great risk. These patients may be overlooked because of their age or overall good health. They may be fine one day become ill, and quickly develop an unexpected pressure ulcer. Pressure ulcers are a leading cause of lawsuits against health care facilities and providers. Take your responsibility for preventing pressure ulcers very seriously. ■

Stage II. In stage II, the skin is reddened and there are abrasions, blisters, or a shallow crater at the site (Figures 38-12A and 38-12B). The area around the breakdown site may also be reddened. The skin may or may not be broken. The epidermis alone or both the epidermis and the dermis may be involved. If this stage of involvement is neglected, further and deeper damage occurs.

FIGURE 38-11B A stage I pressure ulcer has nonblanchable erythema of intact skin, the heralding lesion of skin ulceration. In individuals with darker skin, discoloration of the skin, warmth, edema, induration, or hardness may also be indicators. The lesion is not always round. Some pressure ulcers are irregular in shape. (Permission to reproduce this copyrighted material has been given by the owner, Hollister, Inc.)

FIGURE 38-11A Cross-section of skin showing damage from stage I pressure ulcer

FIGURE 38-12A Cross-section of skin showing damage from stage II pressure ulcer.

Stage III. In stage III, all the layers of the skin are destroyed and a deep crater forms (Figures 38-13A and 38-13B). The nurse documents the size of the lesion using a commercial scale.

Stage IV. In stage IV, the ulcer extends through the skin and subcutaneous tissues, and may involve bone, muscle, and other structures (Figures 38-14A and 38-14B). At this stage, the patient will experience fluid loss and is at great risk for infection.

FIGURE 38-13A Cross-section of skin showing damage from stage III pressure ulcer

FIGURE 38-13B A stage III pressure ulcer has full-thickness skin loss involving damage to or necrosis of subcutaneous tissue that may extend down to, but not through, underlying fascia. The ulcer presents clinically as a deep crater with or without undermining of adjacent tissue. Although the diameter of this pressure ulcer is not large, the patient has experienced full-thickness skin loss. (Permission to reproduce this copyrighted material has been given by the owner, Hollister, Inc.)

FIGURE 38-12B A stage II pressure ulcer has partial-thickness skin loss involving epidermis, dermis, or both. The ulcer is superficial and presents clinically as an abrasion, blister, or shallow crater. The skin surrounding this ulcer is tender and inflamed and at very high risk for further breakdown. (Permission to reproduce this copyrighted material has been given by the owner, Hollister, Inc.)

Clinical Information ALERT

Pressure ulcers are very painful for the patient. A common health care myth is that stage IV ulcers are not painful because they are below the nerve endings. This is not true. Although the base of the ulcer is stage IV, the nerve endings are exposed around the edges, which are usually the depth of a stage II or III ulcer. The ulcer has passed through stages I, II, and III before becoming a stage IV. In each of these stages, nerve endings were exposed and painful. Depending on the area of the ulcer on the body, even a minor stage I pressure ulcer can be very painful. ■

Actions to Take When Breakdown Occurs.
Nursing assistant actions when skin breakdown occurs include:

- Performing the actions listed in the guidelines to prevent further breakdown
- Following the care plan exactly

FIGURE 38-14A Cross-section of skin showing damage from stage IV pressure ulcer

FIGURE 38-14B A stage IV pressure ulcer has full-thickness skin loss with extensive destruction, tissue necrosis, or damage to muscle, bone, or supporting structures (e.g., tendon, joint capsule). Undermining and sinus tracts also may be associated with stage IV pressure ulcers. (Permission to reproduce this copyrighted material has been given by the owner, Hollister, Inc.)

- Reporting indications of infection, such as fever, odor, drainage, bleeding, and changes in size
- Keeping the area around the breakdown clean and dry
- Assisting with whirlpool baths, if ordered, to keep the area clean

The nurse or physician may perform other procedures to care for areas of skin breakdown. For example:

- The area may be covered with a dry, sterile dressing (DSD). Holding a DSD in place without causing additional injury is not easy. The skin of some patients may be sensitive to regular tape. In this case, silk tape, paper tape, cellophane tape, or other hypoallergenic tape may be used. To prevent injury when removing the tape for a dressing change, a saline solution is applied to loosen the tape.
- Patients may be placed on low air loss mattresses or pressure-reducing mattresses or beds.
- In some facilities, open lesions are packed loosely with gauze soaked in a wound gel. The gel keeps the lesions moist, breaks down dead cells, and promotes healing.

GUIDELINES *for*

Preventing Pressure Ulcers

Nursing assistant actions are vital in identifying potential causes of breakdown and eliminating or minimizing them. The following care should be given:

- Change the patient's position at least every 2 hours. Some patients will require positioning more often. A major shift in position is required. When positioning a patient, be careful to avoid friction, such as sliding the patient over bedclothes or against equipment. Use lifting devices to avoid dragging. The care plan for each patient must be followed carefully. The turning schedule will be posted in the care plan. Figure 38-15 shows an example of the sequence of turns.

- Encourage patients sitting in chairs or wheelchairs to raise themselves every 15 minutes to relieve pressure, or assist patients to do so.

- Encourage proper nutrition and adequate intake of fluids. Breakdown occurs more readily and healing is delayed when the patient is poorly nourished. Proper nutrition may require tube feedings or enriched high-protein and high-vitamin oral supplements. Patients who are able to eat should be encouraged to do so. Adequate fluids are a requirement.

- Immediately remove feces or urine from the skin, because they are very irritating. Wash and dry the area immediately.

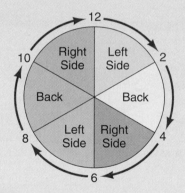

FIGURE 38-15 Example of a turning schedule

- Whenever giving personal care to patients, carefully inspect areas where pressure ulcers commonly form. Report any reddened areas immediately.
- Inspect skin daily and report the condition.
- Keep the skin clean and dry at all times.
- Keep linen dry and free from wrinkles and hard objects such as crumbs and hairpins.
- Bathe patients frequently. Pay particular attention to potential pressure or friction areas. Avoid hot water and friction.
- Keep the skin supple and well-lubricated with lotion. Do not massage directly on the ulcer site and do not use alcohol. Apply moisturizers on dry skin by patting. Do not rub vigorously.

continues

GUIDELINES *continued*

- Do not use lotion on broken skin.
- Separate body areas that are likely to rub together, especially over bony prominences, by using pillows, foam wedges, or folded bath blankets, according to the care plan.
- Use mechanical aids, such as foam padding, sheepskin, or an alternating-pressure mattress, to relieve pressure, friction, and shearing.
- Protect areas at risk, such as heels and elbows.
- Use a turning sheet to move dependent patients in bed. Avoid friction and shearing on the heels when using the draw sheet to position the patient or move him up in bed.
- Elevate the head of the bed no higher than 30°, to prevent a shearing effect on the tissues. If the patient must have the head elevated, such as when a continuous tube feeding is infusing, relieve pressure from the buttocks, hips, and torso regularly. Turn the patient from side to side at least every 2 hours. You will not be able to turn the patient far enough to use the lateral position, but even a slight move and shift to the side is adequate to provide pressure relief. Because the head is up, the patient will not remain positioned for long. Position the patient, then roll one or more pillows behind the back for comfort and support.
- Carry out range-of-motion exercises at least twice daily to encourage circulation.
- Check nasogastric tubes and urinary catheters to be sure they are positioned so as not to be a source of pressure and irritation. Keep the nasal and urinary openings clean and free of drainage. These areas must be checked frequently and carefully.
- Use sheepskin and foam cushions between patients and bottom linen, wheelchair backs, or wheelchair seats where excess pressure may be expected.
- For patients sitting in chairs or wheelchairs, use foam, gel, or air cushions to reduce pressure on buttocks and sacrum. Routinely monitor such patients for skin problems.
- For patients in bed, relieve pressure on heels by supporting feet off the bed. Use a pad between the legs when the patient is on her side.
- Report signs of infection, such as fever, odor, drainage, inflammation, or bleeding, to the nurse.

- The area may be protected and kept moist by using special dressings that have a special covering to keep healing tissue moist and promote healing. A self-adhesive dressing must extend beyond the wound edge. It may be held in place with a frame of hypoallergenic (gentle) tape, if necessary. The dressing is changed every three to five days unless there is leakage or it comes off.
- The wounds may be cleaned by the nurse or physician with saline solution and **debrided** (dead tissue removed) using instruments and proteolytic enzymes (substances that digest skin proteins). Necrotic tissue (Figure 38-16) must be removed before the wound will heal. You may be surprised to see that after the dead tissue is removed, the ulcer looks much larger and deeper than it originally appeared. An ulcer cannot be staged correctly until the necrosis has been removed.
- Antiseptic sprays, antibiotic ointments, and dressings are used to control infection.
- Surgery may be needed to close the ulcerated area in severe cases.

Patients are encouraged to participate to whatever extent is possible in their own care. Attentive nursing care is essential in preventing skin breakdown. Remember that it is far easier to prevent pressure ulcers than to heal them!

FIGURE 38-16 Necrotic tissue is dead, devitalized tissue. It is usually hard, thick, and leathery. It is usually black or brown in color, and is occasionally red. A pressure ulcer cannot be accurately staged until necrosis is removed. Healing will not occur when necrosis is present. (Courtesy of Emory University Hospital, Atlanta, GA)

Blood Circulation to Tissues. Ensuring adequate circulation to tissues is a major factor in preventing skin breakdown. This can be accomplished by:
- Positioning the patient properly
- Using mechanical aids

- Giving backrubs
- Performing active or passive range-of-motion exercises

Positioning. Five basic in-bed positions are used to relieve pressure as the patient's condition permits. Each position must be supported for comfort. The nursing assistant must remember that not all patients are able to assume the full range of positions, because of disabilities such as arthritis, contractures, and breathing limitations. Patients who sit in chairs or wheelchairs for long periods of time must also change position to relieve pressure.

Patients with special problems require extra care when they are positioned in bed. For example:

- Be sure the patient can breathe properly.
- Remember that a fractured hip is never rotated over the unaffected leg.
- If the patient had a stroke, elevate the weak arm to reduce edema.
- Always maintain proper body alignment.
- The patient with a recent stroke is turned on the unaffected side.

The five basic positions patients assume in bed are:

- Supine position
- Semisupine position
- Lateral position
- Semiprone position
- Fowler's position

Note: The prone position is a sixth position, but it is not used by many facilities because some patients do not tolerate it well, and it has the potential to cause respiratory distress. Some facilities permit the use of this position, but a physician's order is required. Remain in the room for 10 to 15 minutes after positioning the patient in the prone position to make sure the patient is able to tolerate it. Know and follow your facility policies for use of the prone position.

Protecting the Feet. Bedfast patients are at very high risk of developing pressure ulcers on the feet and ankles. Patients with hip fractures are at great risk. The skin in the feet and lower legs is thin, and there is little fatty padding. A shallow injury or pressure ulcer can become a deep stage IV ulceration very quickly. The heels and ankles are at greatest risk of ulceration, although occasionally ulcers develop on the toes and the sides of the foot. Foot ulcers are easy to prevent by propping the calves on pillows positioned lengthwise. This suspends the heels over the surface of the bed, relieving all pressure. Follow the patient's care plan and use the pressure prevention measures listed in the guidelines for pressure ulcer prevention. Other measures to prevent pressure ulcers on the feet and ankles are:

- Keep the skin well-lubricated with lotion (but avoid the area between the toes).
- Protect the feet from injury.
- Make sure the patient is wearing properly fit footwear when out of bed. The patient should always wear socks under shoes. He or she should never ambulate barefoot or wearing only socks on the feet.
- Make sure bed linen is not too tight on the feet. Use a bed cradle to keep the bedding away from the skin.
- Make sure footwear is not too tight; if footwear fits tightly, notify the nurse.
- Monitor the skin on the feet and ankles daily and report abnormalities promptly.

Mechanical Aids

Mechanical aids are used to prevent pressure ulcers. Examples are

- Sheepskin pads (or artificial sheepskin).
- Foam pads, pillows, and overlays.
- Protectors for areas such as heels (Figure 38-17A) and elbows (Figure 38-17B) that are subject to friction as the patient moves in bed. Heel protectors prevent friction and shearing, but they do not relieve pressure.
- Bed cradles.
- Alternating-pressure mattresses.
- Flotation mattresses.

FIGURE 38-17A Heel protector (Courtesy of Skil-Care Corporation, Yonkers, NY; (800) 431-2972)

FIGURE 38-17B
Elbow protector
(Courtesy of Skil-Care
Corporation, Yonkers,
NY; (800) 431-2972)

- Air mattresses.
- Pillows.
- Gel-filled mattresses.
- Low air loss beds and other therapeutic beds or mattresses.

Sheepskin Pads (or Artificial Sheepskin). Sheepskin (Figure 38-17C) absorbs moisture and reduces friction and shearing when placed under the patient. It does not relieve pressure. Sheepskin also works well to prevent skin tears and bruises when the patient is up in the wheelchair (Figure 38-17D).

Foam Pads, Pillows, and Overlays. Foam pads and pillows are used to bridge areas to reduce pressure. Foam overlays (Figure 38-17E) are large foam pads that are placed on top of the mattress to provide a pressure-reducing surface. Some of these are cooler than other

pads, which is important because trapped heat contributes to skin breakdown. Many foam overlays and pads lose their fire-retardant properties when washed, and must be replaced if they become soiled. Protect the surface of the overlay with incontinent pads to prevent accidental soiling. Watch patients for signs of disorientation that might be caused by the feeling of weightlessness. Adequate fluid intake to prevent urinary stasis must be provided and conscientious range-of-motion exercises must be carried out.

Bed (Foot) Cradles. Cradles can lift the weight of bedding but must be carefully positioned and may be padded, because injury can occur if the patient strikes them.

Alternating-Pressure Mattress. This type of mattress is used in some facilities. Air pressure is reduced in a different area of the mattress on an alternating basis. The air-pressure alteration reduces pressure against the body so that no skin area is continuously subjected to pressure.

Low Air Loss Therapy Beds and Mattress Overlays. A low air loss bed (Figure 38-17F) provides pressure relief for patients who have pressure ulcers, those who are at risk of pressure ulcers, and some patients with burns. Low air loss therapy beds relieve pressure and keep the patient cooler and drier than other types of beds. Some beds are designed with many special features, such as an instant deflate switch in the event that CPR is necessary. Some are equipped with bed scales. A low air loss mattress overlay (Figure 38-17G) is also available. The overlay is used to replace the mattress on a regular hospital bed. Low air loss beds reduce pressure on the patient's skin, and reduce friction and shearing, which contribute to skin breakdown. These beds use a system of air-filled pillows in which inflation pressure can be adjusted so the characteristics of the support surface are matched to those of the body being supported. The pillows can be inflated and deflated to adjust the level of pressure relief. The design of the bed allows slight air escape upon movement, which reduces pressure.

FIGURE 38-17C A synthetic sheepskin pad prevents friction. It does not relieve pressure. (Courtesy of Skil-Care Corporation, Yonkers, NY; (800) 431-2972)

FIGURE 38-17D Padding the wheelchair with sheepskin protects the skin of patients who are at high risk for conditions such as skin tears. (Courtesy of Skil-Care Corporation, Yonkers, NY; (800) 431-2972)

FIGURE 38-17E A foam mattress overlay has pressure-relieving properties and is comfortable for the patient. (Courtesy of Medline Industries, Inc. (800) MEDLINE)

FIGURE 38-17F The low air loss bed (Courtesy of Hill-Rom, Charleston, SC)

FIGURE 38-17G A low air loss mattress overlay can be used in place of a regular mattress.

FIGURE 38-17H The nylon cover for the low air loss bed is used without sheets in some facilities. Patient and family education regarding the reasons for not using sheets is essential.

FIGURE 38-17I A water or gel-filled mattress reduces the risk of trapped heat and reduces pressure on bony prominences.

Patients using a low air loss bed must be turned and positioned regularly to prevent skin breakdown, which can occur despite the pressure-reducing mattress. Avoid tucking the bottom sheet in tightly, as this increases pressure on the patient's skin. If used, a flat sheet should be loosely applied. Some facilities use these beds with nylon covers only, without sheets. The nylon cover (Figure 38-17H) reduces friction and shearing. Most facilities have several extra covers for each bed, to allow for washing and air-drying. (The nylon cannot withstand the heat of some commercial dryers and must be air-dried.) Special disposable underpads are used with the low air loss bed. Follow the care plan and facility policies.

Flotation Mattress. This is a water bed with controlled temperature (Figure 38-17I). The weight of the patient's body displaces water so that pressure is consistently equalized against the skin. Sheets should not be tucked tightly over a flotation mattress, because this will restrict its function.

> ## OSHA ALERT
>
> The water and gel flotation mattresses are very heavy when filled. Two or more workers are needed to lift, move, and position them correctly on the bed. To prevent injury to your back, never attempt to carry a full mattress by yourself. ■

Special Equipment. Specialized beds or overlays are available for patients who need continuous pressure relief. One type is the Clinitron bed. It is filled with a sandlike material. Warm, dry air circulates through the material to maintain an even temperature and support the body evenly.

Gel-Filled Mattress. The gel in this type of mattress has a consistency similar to body fat. It allows a more equal distribution of body weight because it conforms to the body contours. It is similar in appearance and design to the water-filled flotation mattress. Avoid pins and other sharp objects when using these mattresses. They are punctured easily, and leaks can be difficult to patch.

Pillows. Pillows are used in a technique called *bridging*. In bridging, body parts are supported by pillows so that spaces are left to relieve pressure on specific areas.

Burns

Burns (Figure 38-18) are traumatic injuries to the skin and underlying tissues. They are caused by heat, chemicals, or electricity. A **thermal burn** is caused by heat, fire, or flame. A **chemical burn** is caused by exposure to chemicals that damage the skin and mucous membranes. The most severe burns are those caused by electricity, including lightning. **Electrical burns** are caused by contact with electricity and lightning. They create damage along a pathway in the body that extends from the point of entrance to a point of exit. Location of burns can also be an issue in treatment. For example, burns to the perineum commonly become infected. Burns to the face can cause disfigurement and emotional trauma. Scars and contractures are common complications. Burns are a very painful injury with a very high risk for infection and other serious complications. Extensive treatment is often required.

Whenever large sections of skin are destroyed, the body loses fluids and chemicals called electrolytes, and is vulnerable to infection. Burns commonly cause the loss of large areas of skin.

Classification. The temperature and length of exposure determine the severity of a burn. Prognosis is based on the extent of the burns. Burns are commonly classified as first-, second-, and third-degree. Burns may also be classified according to the depth of tissue involvement:

- *First-degree burns* (partial thickness)
  - Epidermis. When only the epidermis is involved, the skin is pink to red. There may be some temporary swelling and pain. There is usually no permanent damage or scarring.

FIGURE 38-18 Burns are at high risk for infection and many other complications. They are usually very painful and take a long time to heal. Surgery and many other procedures are often necessary to treat the patient. (Courtesy of Emory University Hospital, Atlanta, GA)

- *Second-degree burns* (partial thickness)
  - Dermis. When both epidermis and dermis are involved in the burn, the color may vary from pink or red to white or tan. There is blistering and pain and some scarring.
- *Third-degree burns* (full thickness)
  - When the epidermis, dermis, and subcutaneous tissue are involved, the tissue is bright red to tan and brown. The area is covered with a tough, leathery coat (eschar). There is no pain initially because nerve endings have been destroyed. Later, pain and scarring will result from this injury.
  - When the epidermis, dermis, subcutaneous tissues, muscles, and bones are involved, the tissue appears blackened. Scarring will be extensive.

Management of Burns. Once a burn patient is in the medical facility, the care will involve:

- Assessment of the burn damage
- Analgesia for pain
- Management of fluids and electrolytes
- Prevention of infection
- Clean technique using cap, gown, mask, and gloves
- Complete reverse isolation technique in some cases
- Monitoring the patient for respiratory distress, shock, and anemia
- Cleaning of the burned areas and removal of all debris
- Application of topical antibiotics
- Emotional support

Some hospitals have established burn centers where specially trained personnel care for burn cases. One of two approaches is in common use:

- Open method—the burns are left uncovered. Sterile technique is used to care for the patient.

Clinical Information ALERT

Approximately 2 million people in the United States are treated for burn injuries each year. Of these, approximately 100,000 require hospitalization. Approximately 4,500 people die from burn injuries each year. Burns are the sixth leading cause of death in older adults, with approximately 1,200 deaths a year. Patients' outcome is best when treatment is started immediately. Infection is the leading complication of burns. ■

- Closed method—the burns are covered by special ointments, wrapped in layers of gauze. The body part is checked for circulation distal to the dressing and maintained in proper alignment.

New techniques, such as keeping the patient submerged in a silicone solution, are also being used. Heparin is a chemical produced in the bodies of humans and animals. A synthetic version is used for thinning the blood and preventing blood clots. Researchers have found that it is also an effective treatment for relieving pain and healing burns. It helps heal the body from the inside out, and the patient grows healthy, new skin. Each method of treatment has its advantages and disadvantages. There are four goals of treatment, whatever method is selected:

1. Replacement of lost fluids and electrolytes to combat shock.
2. Relief of pain and anxiety.
3. Prevention of contractures, deformities, and infections. A *contracture* is a shortening of a muscle, which limits motion and causes deformities. Plastic surgery may also be required.
4. Provision of emotional support and motivation.

Nursing Assistant Care. Special care emphasizes:

- Reporting pain so that appropriate analgesics may be prescribed and given
- Maintaining proper alignment
- Gentle positioning, as ordered, to prevent contractures

Note: The burn patient may be on a CircOlectric bed, Stryker frame, or Clinitron bed to permit frequent rotation to relieve pressure.

- Encouraging a high-protein diet
- Carefully measuring intake and output
- Giving emotional support and encouragement
- Carrying out procedures that prevent infection
- Applying the principles of standard precautions and wearing the correct protective apparel if contact with burned skin areas is likely

REVIEW

A. True/False.

Mark the following true or false by circling T or F.

1. T F Obesity is a predisposing cause of pressure ulcer formation.

2. T F The sacrum is a common site for the development of pressure ulcers.

3. T F To avoid pressure ulcers, change the patient's position at least every 2 hours.

4. T F If an area is reddened, massage directly over the area.

5. T F The nails and hair are part of the integumentary system.

6. T F When the epidermis only is damaged by burning, the patient experiences no pain.

7. T F The skin stores carbohydrates and minerals.

8. T F When both the dermis and epidermis are damaged by burns, blisters are apt to form.

9. T F Prevention of infection is an important consideration when caring for a patient with burns.

10. T F The patient with burns needs great emotional support.

11. T F Friction and shearing do not contribute to pressure ulcer development.

12. T F A sheepskin is an excellent pressure-relieving device.

13. T F A stage I pressure ulcer will fade when pressure is relieved for more than 30 minutes.

14. T F Cover the low air loss bed tightly with a sheet to reduce pressure.

15. T F Nodules are small tissue protrusions.

16. T F When assisting with a colloidal oatmeal bath, keep the solution out of the patient's eyes.

B. Matching.

Choose the correct item from Column II to match each word or phrase in Column I.

Column I

17. _____ redness

18. _____ skin

19. _____ thick leathery covering that forms in severe burns

20. _____ bedsore

21. _____ feeling

22. _____ flat, discolored spots, as in measles

23. _____ raised spots filled with watery fluid

24. _____ large, raised areas associated with itching, as in hives

25. _____ areas of dried body secretions such as scabs

26. _____ areas where skin seems to be scraped or scratched away

Column II

a. pressure ulcer

b. rubra

c. tactile sense

d. necrosis

e. integument

f. crusts

g. excoriations

h. vesicles

i. papules

j. macules

k. wheals

C. Multiple Choice.

Select the one best answer for each of the following.

27. Flat, discolored spots such as those seen in measles are called
   a. pustules.
   b. macules.
   c. papules.
   d. vesicles.

28. Raised spots filled with fluid, such as blisters, are called
   a. pustules.
   b. macules.
   c. papules.
   d. vesicles.

29. Anaphylactic shock is
   a. a severe sensitivity reaction.
   b. never fatal.
   c. a communicable disease.
   d. associated with partial-thickness burns.

30. When caring for patients with skin lesions,
   a. rub the skin vigorously.
   b. use soap and water when bathing.
   c. do not attempt to remove any crusts.
   d. use rubbing lotion.

31. To help ensure adequate circulation to prevent skin breakdown, you could
   a. change the patient's position frequently.
   b. position the patient on bony prominences.
   c. rub red areas well.
   d. apply rubbing alcohol to the skin after bathing.

32. Scabies and body lice are commonly spread by
   a. air and droplets.
   b. direct and indirect contact.
   c. fomites and common vehicles.
   d. viruses and bacteria.

33. When assisting a patient with a colloidal oatmeal bath, the nursing assistant should
   a. use tepid water.
   b. give a bedbath.
   c. use very hot water.
   d. scrub the skin well.

34. Safety precautions to follow when assisting a patient with an oatmeal bath include
   a. using sterile water to prevent infection.
   b. scrubbing the lesions well with a sponge.
   c. adding plenty of hot water so the oatmeal will dissolve.
   d. advising the patient to use the hand rail to prevent slipping.

35. In a dark-skinned patient, a stage I pressure ulcer may appear
   a. red or pink.
   b. gray or green.
   c. blue or black.
   d. shiny and oily.

36. Patients using low air loss beds
   a. do not require repositioning, as the bed relieves pressure.
   b. should be turned and positioned at least every 2 hours.
   c. should be turned and positioned twice each shift.
   d. should be turned and positioned every 30 to 45 minutes.

D. Completion.

Complete the statements by filling in the correct word(s).

37. Three nursing assistant actions related to the care of patients with skin lesions are:
   a. _____
   b. _____
   c. _____

38. Three diagnostic tests used to identify skin-related lesions are:
   a. _____
   b. _____
   c. _____

39. Five types of patients at risk for the development of pressure ulcers are:
   a. _____
   b. _____
   c. _____
   d. _____
   e. _____

40. Name five common sites of pressure ulcer formation.

a. _____

b. _____

c. _____

d. _____

e. _____

41. It is especially important to encourage proper nutrition and fluids in patients who have ulcers because _____.

E. Nursing Assistant Challenge.

Agnes Finlay has been transferred to your facility from a long-term care facility. She uses a wheelchair but fell and fractured her arm. You notice a reddened area around the base of her spine. Answer the following by selecting the correct word.

42. People sitting in wheelchairs should raise themselves every _____ minutes.
(60) (15)

43. The head of the patient's bed should not be elevated more than _____ degrees.
(30) (40)

44. While she is in bed, Ms. Finlay's position should be changed at least every _____ hours.
(3) (2)

45. Range-of-motion exercises should be carried out at least _____ a day.
(once) (twice)

UNIT 39

Respiratory System

OBJECTIVES

After completing this unit, you will be able to:
- Spell and define terms.
- Review the location and function of the respiratory organs.
- Describe some common diseases of the respiratory system.
- List five diagnostic tests used to identify respiratory conditions.
- Describe nursing assistant actions related to the care of patients with respiratory conditions.
- Identify patients who are at high risk of poor oxygenation.
- Describe the care of patients with a tracheostomy, laryngectomy, and chest tubes.
- List five safety measures for the use of oxygen therapy.
- Demonstrate the following procedures:
  - Procedure 89 Collecting a Sputum Specimen

VOCABULARY

Learn the meaning and the correct spelling of the following words and phrases:

alveoli	continuous positive	nasal cannula	respiratory care
asthma	airway pressure	nebulizer	practitioner (RCP)
biopsy	(CPAP)	orthopneic position	sputum
bronchi	dyspnea	oxygen	stoma
bronchioles	emphysema	oxygenation	trachea
bronchitis	expectorate	oxygen concentrator	tracheostomy
cannula	high Fowler's position	oxygen mask	tripod position
carbon dioxide	humidifier	pharynx	upper respiratory
chest tubes	incentive spirometer	pleura	infection (URI)
chronic obstructive	laryngectomee	pleural effusion	ventilation
pulmonary disease	laryngectomy	pneumonia	vocal cords
(COPD)	larynx		

INTRODUCTION

Life cannot be maintained without oxygen, and carbon dioxide must be eliminated from the body. Diseases of the respiratory tract that interfere with this vital exchange of oxygen and carbon dioxide bring acute distress. Nursing care is directed toward making breathing easier and preventing transmission of infection.

Clinical Information ALERT

The lungs are the only organs of the body that float in water. Humans breathe 20 times per minute, more than 10 million times per year, and about 700 million times in a lifetime. The lungs contain almost 1,500 miles of airways and more than 300 million alveoli. The average person breathes in 13 pints of air each minute. ■

STRUCTURE AND FUNCTION

The respiratory system (Figure 39-1) is sometimes called the lifeline of the body. It extends from the nose to the tiny air sacs (**alveoli**) that make up the bulk of the lungs.

The organs of the respiratory system include the:

- Nose
- Pharynx (throat)
- Larynx (voice box)
- **Trachea** (windpipe)
- Bronchi
- Lungs

The sinuses, diaphragm, and intercostal muscles between the ribs are called auxiliary structures.

Air is warmed, moistened, and filtered as it passes through the nasal cavities, which are separated by the nasal septum. The air passes through the **pharynx**, a passageway for both air and food, into the larynx and trachea. It then passes into the **bronchi** to join the upper respiratory tract to the lungs. Within the lungs, the bronchi branch into smaller and smaller divisions called **bronchioles**. The

alveoli are tiny air sacs that extend from the bronchioles. The exchange of gases takes place in the alveoli (Figure 39-2).

The alveoli, bronchioles, and the important pulmonary blood vessels form the lungs. The way in which oxygen and carbon dioxide are exchanged between the alveoli and the capillaries is shown in Figure 39-3.

The purpose of this system is to bring **oxygen** (O_2) into the body to meet cellular needs and to expel carbon dioxide (CO_2). **Carbon dioxide** is a gaseous metabolic waste produced by the cells.

Each cell in the body must have a constant supply of oxygen. The oxygen is used to produce the energy for cellular activity:

Nutrients + oxygen yields energy + water + CO$_2$

There is a close connection between the respiratory and circulatory systems. Oxygen is delivered throughout the body by means of the bloodstream. Every cell in the body

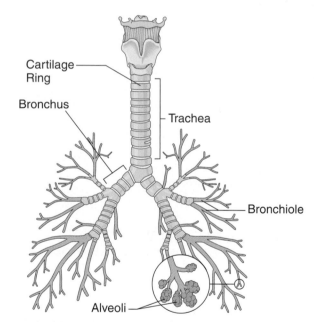

FIGURE 39-2 The lower respiratory tract

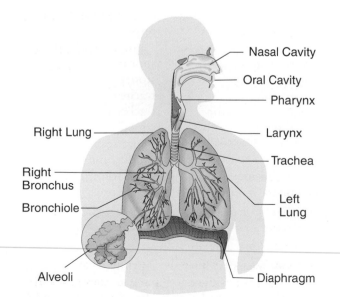

FIGURE 39-1 The respiratory system

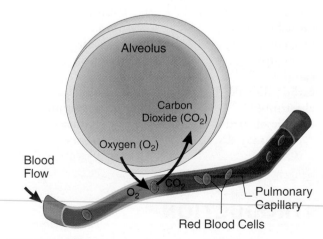

FIGURE 39-3 Oxygen and carbon dioxide are exchanged in the alveoli.

Clinical Information ALERT

The respiratory system is *very powerful*. The air released from an explosive cough moves at speeds up to 60 miles per hour (mph). A sneeze creates a force of air moving nearly 99 mph. It is impossible to sneeze with your eyes open. ∎

produces carbon dioxide. It is transported in venous blood. When it reaches the lungs, it is exhaled into the atmosphere. When the body does not eliminate carbon dioxide, it creates chemical reactions causing an acid buildup. Death will result if levels of acid and carbon dioxide become too high. Signs and symptoms that indicate problems with oxygen use are listed in Table 39-1. Observations to report promptly to the nurse are listed in Table 39-2.

The Act of Respiration

Two lungs are located in the thorax. Each lung is surrounded by a double-walled membrane called the **pleura**. Between the layers of the pleura is a small amount of fluid that reduces friction as the lungs alternately expand and contract, filling with and then expelling air.

The size of the thorax depends on the contraction of the diaphragm and intercostal muscles. As the muscles contract, the thorax enlarges, expanding the lungs. Air carrying oxygen enters the lungs. When the muscles relax, the thorax becomes smaller. Air carrying carbon dioxide leaves the lungs and is breathed out.

- *Inspiration* (or inhalation) is the act of drawing air into the lungs.
- *Expiration* (or exhalation) is the act of expelling air.
- **Ventilation** is the combination of these two actions.
- **Oxygenation** is the movement of oxygen from the lungs and into the blood to be carried to the cells.

Voice Production

The **larynx**, or voice box, is part of the respiratory tract. It is important in voice production. Two membranes called the **vocal cords** stretch across the inside of the larynx. As air moves upward through the larynx, it passes through an opening in the vocal cords. Changes in the shape of the vocal cords and the size of the opening permit controlled amounts of air to reach the mouth, nasal cavities, and sinuses, where specific speech sounds are made when formed by the teeth, lips, and tongue.

PATIENTS AT RISK OF POOR OXYGENATION

Hypoxemia is a condition in which there is insufficient oxygen in the blood. Many of the patients who are at

---

TABLE 39-1 SIGNS AND SYMPTOMS OF DECREASED OXYGENATION

- Respiratory rate below 12 or above 20
- Unusual skin color, such as dusky, pale, blue, or gray
- Unusual color of the lips, mucous membranes, nail beds, lining or roof of mouth
- Cool, clammy skin
- Slow, rapid, or irregular breathing
- Shortness of breath or labored breathing
- Noisy breathing
- Gasping for breath
- Changes in mental status, including decreased responsiveness, drowsiness, sleepiness for no apparent reason, restlessness, increased confusion
- Tachycardia
- Cheyne-Stokes respirations
- Wheezing
- Coughing (dry or moist/productive)
- Retractions

TABLE 39-2 SIGNS AND SYMPTOMS OF INADEQUATE BREATHING TO REPORT TO THE NURSE IMMEDIATELY

- Movement in the chest is absent, minimal, or irregular.
- Breathing movement appears to be in the abdomen, not the lungs.
- Air movement cannot be detected by listening and feeling for breath sounds on your cheek and ear.
- Respiratory rate is too slow or rapid.
- Respirations are irregular, gasping, very deep, or shallow.
- Respirations appear labored.
- Patient is short of breath.
- Patient's skin, lips, tongue, ear lobes, mucous membranes, or nail beds are blue or gray.
- Patient is unable to speak at all, or cannot speak in sentences because of shortness of breath.
- Respirations are noisy.
- Nasal flaring is present during inspiration.
- The muscles below the ribs and/or above the clavicles retract inward during respiration.

Age-Appropriate Care ALERT

Researchers have concluded that a mild decrease of oxygen in the blood, once thought to be of limited harm, contributes to long-term impaired mental function and behavioral disorders, such as attention deficit/hyperactive disorder (ADHD), in children. This is an area of ongoing research and study. ■

high risk for developing hypoxemia are not in the intensive care unit where monitoring is routine. They are on medical and surgical units, in the long-term care facility, or in other patient care areas. Patients who are immobile and those on bedrest have an increased risk of hypoxemia. When hypoxemia develops, immobility makes a positive outcome less likely. Other high-risk conditions are:

- Cardiac disease
- Pulmonary disease
- Being postoperative (for up to a week after surgery)
- Sleep apnea
- Decreased level of consciousness
- Neuromuscular diseases
- Morbid obesity
- Kyphoscoliosis (curvature of the spine)
- Trauma

Checking capillary refill (Unit 36) is a quick means of evaluating how well oxygen is getting to body tissues. A pulse oximeter (Unit 36) may also be used to monitor patients with high-risk conditions.

Respiratory Care

Patients with respiratory disorders have many needs that require highly skilled care. The **respiratory care practitioner (RCP)** is a licensed professional who specializes in the care of patients with disorders of the cardiopulmonary system, respirations, and sleep disorders that affect the patient's breathing. The RCP will be highly involved in the care of the patient and the specialized equipment used for treatment.

UPPER RESPIRATORY INFECTIONS

An **upper respiratory infection (URI)** follows invasion of the upper respiratory organs by microbes. The upper respiratory organs include the nose, sinuses, and throat. A common cold, which is caused by a virus, is an example

of a URI. It is one of the most ordinary illnesses found in people. Symptoms include:

- Elevated temperature (fever)
- Runny nose
- Watery eyes

This usually self-limiting disease is best treated by:

- Use of a drug to reduce fever, such as acetaminophen
- Rest
- Increased fluid intake

Patients with respiratory infections should be taught to:

- Cover the nose and mouth with a tissue when coughing or sneezing.
- Dispose of soiled tissues by placing them in a plastic or paper bag to be burned.
- Turn the face away from others when coughing or sneezing.
- Wash hands after handling soiled tissues.

OSHA ALERT

You have learned that respiratory infections are spread by the airborne and droplet methods of transmission. Secretions containing pathogens make their way to the environment where you pick them up. Good handwashing is the best method of preventing infection, including respiratory infection. ■

You must take special note of and report the following:

- **Dyspnea** (difficult breathing)
- Changes in rate and rhythm of respiration
- Presence and character, color, and amount of respiratory secretions
- Cough
- Changes in skin color, such as pallor or cyanosis

URIs sometimes move down into the chest and develop into bronchitis or even pneumonia.

Pneumonia

Pneumonia is a serious inflammation of the lungs. It can be caused by a variety of infectious organisms. Three common causes of pneumonia are:

- Viruses
- Bacteria
- Protozoa

Pneumocystis carinii is most often seen in patients who have poorly functioning immune systems. Today, most pneumonias, though serious and potentially life-threatening, respond favorably to antibiotic therapy.

CHRONIC OBSTRUCTIVE PULMONARY DISEASE

Chronic obstructive pulmonary disease (COPD) is also called chronic obstructive lung disease (COLD). This term refers to conditions that result in chronic blockage or obstruction of the respiratory system that is not reversible. Several conditions constitute COPD, including:

- Emphysema
- Chronic bronchitis
- Bronchiectasis

It can be very difficult to differentiate asthma from COPD, particularly in older patients.

Asthma

Asthma is a breathing disorder resulting from:

- Constriction of the muscles of the bronchioles
- Swelling of the respiratory membranes
- Production of large amounts of mucus that fill the narrowed passageways

Clinical Information ALERT

Asthma is caused by narrowing and clogging of the bronchi, the small tubes that carry air into and out of the lungs. The bronchi normally narrow during the night, in everyone. This increases resistance to air flow. People who do not have asthma probably will not notice the change. However, in asthmatics the change may be enough to bring on an asthma attack, whether the patient is awake or asleep. ■

A person having an asthma attack has labored breathing and frequent coughing. An attack may result when the person contacts an allergen. Respiratory infections can also cause an asthma attack. Common allergens are:

- Pollen
- Medications
- Dust
- Feathers
- Foods such as peanuts, eggs, or chocolate
- Cigarette and cigar smoke
- Cockroaches
- Dust mites
- Furry pets
- Mold
- Certain chemicals

If a patient has known allergies (hypersensitivity to specific items), they should be marked in the patient's health record. Long-term treatment consists of identifying the allergen and eliminating it. To relieve the attack, the patient is given medication to decrease the swelling and dilate the bronchioles. Low levels of oxygen may also be given.

Age-Appropriate Care ALERT

The incidence of asthma in children is increasing. Children from low-income households, minorities, and children living in inner cities experience higher morbidity and mortality due to asthma. Asthma accounts for at least 14 million lost school days annually. It is the third leading cause of hospitalization among children age 15 and under. Currently, there are no preventive measures or cures for asthma; however, children and adolescents can control their asthma by taking medication and controlling environmental triggers. ■

Chronic Bronchitis

Chronic bronchitis is prolonged inflammation in the bronchi due to infection or irritants. Signs and symptoms include:

- Swollen and red bronchial tissues, resulting in narrowed bronchial passageways
- Persistent cough
- Sputum production
- Respiratory distress

Treatment includes:

- Antibiotics to fight the infection
- Drugs to loosen secretions deep in the respiratory tract
- Techniques to improve ventilation and drainage
- Adequate fluid intake to keep secretions thin so they can be coughed up

Emphysema

Emphysema develops after chronic obstruction of the air flow to the alveoli. The air sacs:

- Become distended
- Lose their elasticity and recoil ability
- Finally become nonfunctional
- Lose the ability to exchange gases

The patient can bring air into the lungs, but it becomes more difficult to expel air from the lungs (Figure 39-4). As a result, there is less and less room for air to reenter.

Risk factors for emphysema are:

- Genetic
- Airways that are very responsive to irritants

FIGURE 39-4 Typical posture for patient with emphysema. The patient leans forward on the arms and purses his lips. (Netter illustration used with permission of Elsevier, Inc. All rights reserved.)

- Exposure to tobacco smoke
- Exposure to dust and chemicals in the workplace
- Exposure to indoor and outdoor air pollution
- Repeated lung infections

Emphysema alone (without chronic bronchitis, which often accompanies it) is a dry disease. There is no sputum production. However, patients with emphysema are at high risk of developing pneumonia. This condition also causes the heart to work harder. The most common sign of respiratory problems in a patient with emphysema is headache. This is caused by increasing carbon dioxide levels in the blood. Other signs and symptoms of emphysema are:

- Fatigue
- Chronic oxygen deprivation
- Difficulty breathing
- Loss of appetite and weight loss

General Care. The care of the emphysema patient includes all the care required of any patient with COPD:

- Assisting with the proper breathing techniques, such as pursed-lip breathing
- Encouraging breathing exercises
- Positioning to improve ventilation
- Assisting with postural drainage (this therapy is not commonly used for emphysema)
- Providing care during low-flow oxygen therapy
- Assisting with and encouraging good nutrition

- Treating infections with antibiotics and drugs to loosen and thin respiratory secretions
- Encouraging fluid intake
- Taking annual flu shots and the pneumonia vaccine at the frequency specified by the health care provider
- Encouraging patients to avoid crowds, especially during the flu season
- Encouraging patients not to smoke

Tips: When caring for patients with COPD, pace activities. Help them to conserve energy as much as possible. Minimize activities in which the patient must raise the arms over the head. Avoid exposing patients to aerosol sprays.

Wear gloves if your hands may contact the patient's respiratory secretions. Wear a gown, goggles or face shield, and a surgical mask if the patient is coughing and spraying respiratory secretions into the air.

Infection Control ALERT

Patients with asthma, bronchitis, COPD, and those with weakened immune systems readily contract fungal infections from pillows. The typical pillow contains many fungi, particularly *Aspergillus*. This pathogen is a common cause of pneumonia. Use disposable pillows, if possible, or make sure the pillow is encased in a plastic pillow cover. ∎

SURGICAL CONDITIONS

Most respiratory problems are not treated with surgery. However, several problems require surgical correction to ensure uninterrupted air flow.

Tracheostomy

A **tracheostomy** (Figure 39-5) is done for some patients who have had head and neck surgery, and some victims of serious trauma. It may also be done for patients who:

- Have required a ventilator to support their breathing for a long time
- Need suctioning to clear airway secretions

A tracheostomy may be temporary or permanent. The external opening on the skin surface is the **stoma.** Eventually, the stoma will heal and remain permanently open. A plastic or metal tube is inserted through the stoma to maintain patency until the stoma has healed open. This tube is the **cannula.** An outer and inner cannula are used. Several types of outer cannulae are available. The most common has an inflatable cuff (Figure 39-6). It seals or reduces the air flow to the nose and throat, so virtually all breathing is done through the tracheostomy. The cuff also

Difficult SITUATIONS

Nonverbal means of communication have long been a source of frustration for patients and hospital personnel. To help solve the communication problem, David Muir, a ventilator-dependent person, developed a positive-closure, one-way speaking valve that has gained widespread acceptance in hospitals and long-term care facilities. The Passy-Muir Tracheostomy and Ventilator Speaking Valve (PMV) opens upon inhalation, enabling the patient to inspire through the tracheostomy tube. The valve closes after inspiration, redirecting the exhaled air around the tube, through the vocal cords, and out the mouth, allowing the patient to speak. A speech language pathologist, RN, and RCP will all be involved in fitting, monitoring, and teaching the patient to use the device. Some patients will only be able to wear the PMV for a few minutes at a time, building up time gradually. When a patient is in an early stage of valve use, monitor blood pressure, pulse, and respirations closely. Inform the nurse at once if the patient shows signs and symptoms of distress, such as a significant change in blood pressure or pulse, increased respiratory rate, dyspnea, diaphoresis, anxiety, uncontrollable coughing, or a pulse oximeter value of less than 90%. ■

helps reduce the risk of aspiration of feedings. Care of the cuff is not a nursing assistant responsibility. The nurse or RCP will inflate and deflate the cuff periodically. The cuff must be inflated before feeding the patient or providing mouth care. A cuffless tube may also be used, but this is less common. Patients with a cuffless tube are able to breathe through the nose, mouth, and tracheostomy. The outer cannula has a flat plate, with a flange on each side that is fastened to twill tape or a Velcro fastener that encircles the patient's neck. The tape helps hold the device securely in place. The inner cannula has an adapter on the distal end that can be attached to the manual resuscitation bag. The parts of the tracheostomy apparatus are shown in Figure 39-7.

Caring for the tracheostomy is the nurse's responsibility. Notify the nurse immediately if the ties are loose or any part of the device comes apart or is removed. The ties can also be too tight. You should be able to slide your finger underneath the tie on either side of the neck. If you cannot, it is too tight, and you should notify the nurse immediately.

Malignancies

Malignant tumors can develop in any part of the respiratory tract. Although the exact causes of malignancy are

FIGURE 39-6 A tracheostomy with the cuff inflated

FIGURE 39-5 The tracheostomy stoma is a surgical opening in the trachea. The cannula keeps the stoma open.

FIGURE 39-7 Parts for the tracheostomy

Infection Control ALERT

The nasal hairs and tonsils filter pathogens and other substances from the air, preventing them from reaching the lungs. Patients with stomas do not have this advantage. The stoma provides a direct, unfiltered passageway to the lungs for irritating foreign substances and pathogens. Practice good infection control techniques when caring for patients with a stoma. ■

Difficult SITUATIONS

If a cannula becomes dislodged, stay with the patient and call for the nurse or RCP immediately. The stoma may close quickly, so this has the potential to become a serious emergency. A second, smaller cannula set is kept at the bedside at all times. The smaller set is used for rapid insertion, to avoid immediate closing of the stoma. A cannula of the original size may not fit. Inform the nurse if the neck ties become moist with secretions or perspiration. ■

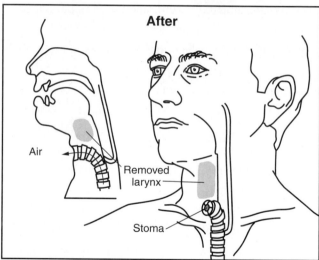

FIGURE 39-8 The anatomy of the face and neck before and after laryngectomy surgery

not fully understood, cigarette smoking and exposure to cancer-producing agents in the environment are known to be contributing factors. Lung cancers are treated by surgery, radiation, or chemotherapy, or a combination of all three therapies.

Cancer of the Larynx

Cancer of the larynx may require removal of the larynx, resulting in loss of the voice. A **laryngectomy** is the surgical removal of the larynx. During this procedure, the airway is separated from the mouth, nose, and esophagus. The patient breathes through an artificial opening in the neck and trachea. A person who has had this surgery may be called a **laryngectomee**. When the larynx is removed, there is no longer a connection between the upper and lower airways (Figure 39-8).

The permanent opening for breathing in the neck and trachea is called a **stoma**. A laryngectomy stoma is a special kind of opening in the neck. Though it may look like a regular tracheostomy, it is very different. If you are caring for a patient with a stoma, you must know whether it is a tracheostomy stoma or a laryngectomy stoma. If the patient has a tracheostomy, the passageway from the mouth and nose through the trachea remains intact.

Patients can still smell odors, blow their noses, and suck on a straw. If a patient has had a laryngectomy, the larynx (voice box) has been removed. The upper airway is no longer connected to the trachea. The patient will not be able to talk, smell, blow his nose, whistle, gargle, or suck on a straw. He retains the ability to swallow, although initially a tube feeding may be used to promote healing and prevent irritation of the esophagus.

Loss of voice is a major trauma for anyone. Just think how frustrated you would feel if you could no longer use your voice to communicate your thoughts, feelings, wants, and needs to others. During the immediate postoperative period, writing is the major form of communication. A "magic slate" is often used. Later, a speech language pathologist will teach the patient to use esophageal speech or electronic speech.

Esophageal Speech. The patient learns to swallow air and then bring it back up through the esophagus into the mouth. Here the air is formed by the teeth and tongue into words, as it would be if it were being exhaled from the lungs. Esophageal speech is difficult to learn, but motivated patients can succeed.

Electronic Speech. Patients who cannot use esophageal speech may be able to use an electronic artificial larynx to create speech. Some patients may use a combination of both techniques.

Patients with laryngectomies need patience and understanding from all health care providers. Communication is possible, but the voice does not sound normal. More time is needed by the patient to formulate the sounds. A difficult psychological adjustment must be made by the patient. The loss of one's voice requires an adjustment similar to that experienced when grieving for the loss of a loved one. Expect periods of depression, anger, and hostility.

Caring for a Patient with a Tracheostomy or Laryngectomy Stoma. When people breathe normally, the structures in the nose and mouth capture microbes and other foreign particles, preventing them from entering the airway. In addition, the body moistens and warms air before it enters the lungs. Inhaling cold, dry air is very uncomfortable, and it irritates the lungs. Because the stoma bypasses the normal breathing structures, the patient's body cannot use its normal protective mechanisms to warm, moisten, and filter the air. Thus, care is designed to replace these body functions. Warm, humidified oxygen may be administered to patients with a stoma.

The stoma now provides a direct passageway into the lungs. Because of this, some patients wear a mask similar to a surgical mask over the opening. The risk of inhaling a foreign particle is greatly increased. Inhaling small objects or water (such as during a shower) can cause serious complications. Check with the nurse or care plan for precautions to take when showering the patient. Avoid getting powder, lint, dust, water, or other objects near or in the stoma.

Likewise, the opening in the neck provides an open pathway for pathogens to enter, causing infection. Use standard precautions and frequent handwashing when caring for a patient with a stoma. Secretions may be expelled from the stoma when the patient coughs. The patient has no control over this. If he or she is expelling secretions, you will also need to wear a gown, mask, and eye protection when caring for the patient.

The stoma in the patient's neck is the primary airway. If the tube becomes blocked, dislodged, disconnected, or otherwise disrupted, the patient's airway will be seriously compromised. Be especially careful when turning and bathing the patient. Monitor the patient's skin color closely. Watch for cyanosis, changes in color of the nail beds or mucous membranes, or respiratory distress. Important, early signs of ineffective airway clearance and poor gas exchange to observe for and report are:

- Restlessness
- Dyspnea
- Anxiety
- Increased heart rate
- Lethargy
- Disorientation

Chest Tubes

Chest tubes (Figure 39-9) are sterile, plastic tubes that are inserted through the skin of the chest, between the ribs and into the space between the pleural membrane that covers the lung and the pleural membrane that lines the chest wall. They are used after surgery to drain any bloody fluid drainage from the chest. These tubes also allow air to escape if there is a leak of air at the suture line after lung surgery.

In subacute care, patients are most likely to have chest tubes for two reasons: one is an air leak after lung surgery that is slow to heal, and the other is to drain fluid that collects around the lungs (often seen in patients who have cancer). This fluid is called a **pleural effusion**.

The chest tube is always attached to a drain of some sort (Figure 39-10). The nurse will manage the system. To help monitor and care for the patient, make sure that nothing pulls on the tube that comes out of the chest. Position the drainage system in an upright position, below the level of the heart at all times. Reposition the patient every 2 hours, or as instructed. Make sure the chest tube is never twisted, kinked, or obstructed. The tubing that connects the chest tube to the drain should be coiled on the bed the same way you would position tubing for a Foley catheter.

If the drain is connected to a vacuum regulator, check with the nurse before you disconnect it to take the patient to the bathroom, for example. Do not hesitate to get the patient up in a chair and to keep him mobile if his condition allows, even though he has a chest tube. The patient with a chest tube should always have oxygen and suction set up at the bedside. A tray of emergency equipment will also be kept in the room. Never remove these items.

Notify the nurse promptly if the:

- Vital signs change
- Pulse oximeter alarm sounds

FIGURE 39-9 The chest tube is securely covered with dressings.

FIGURE 39-10
Make sure the tubing is not obstructed, and that the bottle is lower than the patient's heart.

- Dressing on the chest wall is loose
- Color or amount of drainage from the chest tube changes
- Patient coughs up blood
- Patient becomes short of breath or cyanotic
- Patient develops new swelling on the torso, neck, or face that "crackles" when you touch it
- The tube comes out of the chest wall

DIAGNOSTIC TECHNIQUES

Some techniques used to diagnose problems of the respiratory system include:

- Tissue **biopsy** (microscopic examination of a specimen of tissue removed from the patient)
- Cultures of secretions
- Volume studies that measure the amount of air entering or leaving the lungs during various respiratory movements
- Radiographic techniques such as X-rays, CT scans, and MRIs
- Direct visualization procedures such as bronchoscopy

SPECIAL THERAPIES RELATED TO RESPIRATORY ILLNESS

Nursing assistants aid patient breathing by proper positioning and by helping provide moisture and oxygen. They also are assigned to collect sputum specimens for examinations.

Oxygen Therapy

Oxygen is often ordered by the physician. Remember that when oxygen is in use, special precautions are required to prevent fires and to administer the oxygen safely. Information about general fire control is presented in Unit 14.

Special safety measures must be emphasized in areas where oxygen is being used:

- Be certain that there are no open flames and that no one smokes or has matches.
- Post "no smoking" or "oxygen in use" signs.

Hospitals have a centralized source of oxygen piped to wall units in the patient's room (Figure 39-11). In some facilities, the oxygen is stored in a tank that is brought to the patient's room when therapy is ordered. The amount of oxygen (rate of flow measured in liters) is ordered by the physician. Oxygen is a prescription item, and changing the flow rate is the responsibility of a licensed nurse or RCP.

Caring for a Patient Who Is Receiving Oxygen Therapy. The care plan may instruct you to elevate the head of the bed when the patient is receiving oxygen. This will make it easier to breathe. Patients using oxygen masks cannot eat meals while wearing the mask. The physician may order a nasal cannula at mealtime. Follow the instructions on the care plan or critical pathway for patient care measures.

Being unable to breathe is very frightening. Patients who are receiving oxygen may need reassurance and emotional support. Check on the patient frequently and spend as much time in the room as possible. Difficult breathing makes it hard to talk. The patient may be unable to hold a normal conversation. Just being with the patient without talking is very reassuring. If the patient is having trouble breathing, try to ask questions that can be answered "yes" or "no" so it is easier for the patient to communicate with you.

You will care for patients using different devices for the administration of oxygen. Carefully check the skin under the device to make sure it is not red or irritated from the elastic that holds the oxygen device in place. Report any skin problems to the nurse. Oxygen is drying, so patients

FIGURE 39-11 Oxygen is usually piped in to each unit through a central delivery system.

Communication HIGHLIGHT

Oxygen is a basic need at the lowest level of Maslow's hierarchy of needs. Needs at the lower levels must be fulfilled before needs at the higher levels become important. The patient who is having trouble breathing cannot focus on much else. Keep conversation short and succinct. Give the patient verbal and nonverbal reassurance. Find alternate means of communicating, such as writing, if necessary. ■

FIGURE 39-12 The flow meter shows the amount of oxygen being delivered. The pressure gauge shows the amount of oxygen remaining in the tank.

who are receiving oxygen may need extra liquids to drink. They also need frequent care of the mouth and nose. Sometimes patients feel warm and will perspire heavily. Extra bathing and linen changes may be necessary. You may need to adjust the temperature in the room and help the patient change gowns. Cover him or her with a sheet. The care plan or critical pathway will provide information on patient preferences and needs. When caring for a patient who uses oxygen, you should:

- Wear gloves and apply the principles of standard precautions if contact with the patient's oral or nasal secretions is likely
- Know the oxygen flow rate that was ordered and set for the patient
- Be able to read the flow meter for the rate of oxygen delivery if instructed to check the rate by the nurse
- Notify the nurse immediately if there is a change in the flow rate
- Check that the tubing is not obstructed in any way that would prevent oxygen from reaching the patient
- Check for proper position of the catheter, cannula, or mask and that the elastic band around the head is snug but not constricting
- Check whether straps, cannula, or mask are causing skin irritation
- Provide frequent mouth care
- Use a portable tank to transport the patient to other areas of the hospital. Do not remove the oxygen without permission from the RCP or nurse

If a tank is used as the source of oxygen, be sure that:

- There is sufficient oxygen in the tank. Check the gauge each time you visit the patient (Figure 39-12).
- The oxygen is on.
- An additional tank is available to exchange for the tank in use when it is empty.
- Empty tanks are marked and stored according to facility policy.
- The tank is upright and secure on the carrier or in the stand.

Safety ALERT

In 2001, the FDA sent a warning to all U.S. health care facilities regarding problems created by connecting a gas other than oxygen into the oxygen system. The most significant problems occurred when:

- The person connecting the vessel to the oxygen system did not understand that connection incompatibility is a built-in safeguard.
- The person making the connection did not examine the label to ensure that the product was medical oxygen before connecting it to the oxygen supply system.

Never modify an oxygen system to make the parts fit together. If you cannot connect it readily, seek further help.

The FDA memo also makes recommendations to prevent mixups of medical gases. ■

Humidifiers. In some facilities, a **humidifier** (Figure 39-13) is attached to the oxygen administration equipment if the patient's liter flow exceeds 5 liters. Use of oxygen humidifiers is a controversial subject. Humidification is not necessary with liter flows below 5. Humidifiers are not used at all in some facilities.

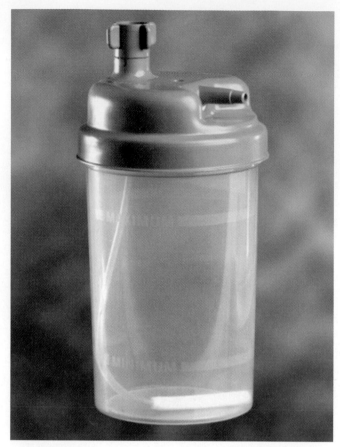

FIGURE 39-13 A humidifier (Courtesy of Hudson RCI, Temecula, CA, USA)

The humidifier is a water bottle that moistens the oxygen for comfort and prevents drying of the mucous membranes in the nose, mouth, and lungs. The bottle screws into a male adapter on the flow meter. Oxygen passes through the water in the humidifier, picking up moisture, before it reaches the patient. The delivery device plugs into a male adapter on the side of the humidifier. The respiratory care practitioner usually cares for the humidifier, but this is a nursing assistant responsibility in some health care settings. If this is the case, you will be responsible for checking or changing the humidifier. Sterile distilled water is always used in the humidifier. Avoid tap water. Inhalation of tap water is associated with an increased incidence of Legionnaire's disease. The water level in the humidifier should always be at or above the "minimum fill" line on the bottle.

When the oxygen delivery system is functioning correctly, the water in the humidifier will bubble. Oxygen will not exit the tubing into the mask or cannula if the tubing is kinked or obstructed. If this occurs, pressure builds up in the unit and discharges through a pressure relief valve. When setting up a humidifier, check this valve by turning the oxygen on and pinching the connecting tubing.

Two types of humidifiers are used. The *prefilled* type of humidifier is commonly used in acute care hospitals. This unit is usually changed once a week, when it is empty, or

according to the manufacturer's directions or facility policies and procedures. Discard the bottle after replacing it with a new one. Your facility may require you to attach a sticker to the bottle listing the date and time it was changed, and your initials.

Refillable humidifiers are washed with soap and water or 2% alkaline gluteraldehyde solution every 24 hours. They are rinsed well, then sterilized. Refill the sterile bottle with sterile distilled water. Never add water to a partially filled humidifier. A sticker may be attached to this bottle showing the date and time it was changed.

Methods of Oxygen Delivery. Oxygen may be delivered to the patient by several different methods. The same basic care is required for each method, with modifications.

- *Nasal cannula:* Delivery of oxygen by **nasal cannula** is the most common method. The oxygen is delivered through a tube that has two small plastic prongs (Figure 39-14). The prongs are placed at the entrance to the patient's nose. A strap around the patient's head holds the cannula in place.
  - Make sure the strap is secure but not too tight.
  - Check for signs of irritation where the prongs touch the patient's nose.
  - Check that mucus has not blocked the prong openings. Clean if necessary.
  - Make sure the cannula is stored when not in use in such a way that it is not contaminated.

- *Mask:* The **oxygen mask** is a cuplike mask held in place by straps around the head The oxygen mask fits over the patient's nose, mouth, and chin. An elastic strap that slips over the back of the head holds the mask in place. A small tube connects the mask to the oxygen source. Masks are available in adult and pediatric sizes. Several different face masks are used, depending on the patient's oxygen needs (Figure 39-15). A special mask fits over a stoma (Figure 39-16). Using an oxygen mask is necessary when high liter flows of oxygen are ordered. Masks may also be used

FIGURE 39-14 Oxygen being administered by nasal cannula

for individuals who breathe through their mouths. A mask is never used with liter flows under 5 because it will cause rebreathing of exhaled carbon dioxide, and has a smothering effect.

– Place the mask over the patient's nose and mouth.
– Adjust the fit by pulling on the ends of the elastic next to the mask so the fit is snug, but not too tight.
– Adjust the metal tab over the bridge of the nose, if needed for comfort.
– Periodically remove the mask. Wash the area under it and dry carefully.
– Some masks have inflatable bags at the bottom (Figure 39-17). The combination of bag and mask increases the amount of oxygen delivered to the patient. The bag should be inflated at all times. Notify the nurse if the bag collapses more than halfway during inspiration. This type of mask provides very high amounts of oxygen and should not be used for more than 24 hours without an evaluation by a health care provider.

FIGURE 39-15 Various types of oxygen masks

FIGURE 39-16 An adult tracheostomy mask

Oxygen Concentrator

An **oxygen concentrator** (Figure 39-18) takes in room air and removes impurities and gases other than oxygen, allowing the oxygen to become concentrated in the unit. The air delivered to the patient from the concentrator is more than 90% oxygen. It is delivered by tubing attached to a nasal cannula. The flow rate is usually 2 liters per minute (L/min).

General Oxygen Concentrator Precautions. Follow these precautions when a concentrator is used to supply oxygen to a patient:

FIGURE 39-17 The nonrebreathing mask is used for severe hypoxemia. The patient's exhaled air escapes through the one-way flaps on the sides, but room air cannot enter because of the one-way design. The bag at the bottom increases the amount of oxygen delivered to the patient. It should not collapse more than halfway when the patient inhales.

FIGURE 39-18 The oxygen concentrator delivers low liter flows. Most concentrators have an attachment for a humidifier, but humidification is not necessary at low liter flows.

- Place the concentrator at least 5 feet away from any heat source and at least 4 inches away from the wall.
- Smoking is not permitted in the same room.
- Be sure the unit is plugged in and grounded.
- Do not use an extension cord with the concentrator.
- Never change the flow meter setting.
- Notify the nurse if the alarm sounds.
- A mask is not used with a concentrator because the exhaled carbon dioxide cannot be expelled with low liter flows of oxygen.
- Wipe the cannula daily with a damp cloth (do not use alcohol- or oil-based products).
- Clean concentrator surfaces using a damp cloth only.
- Remove the filter weekly. Wash in warm soapy water, rinse, squeeze dry, and replace.
- Store the nasal cannula according to facility policy when not in use. Keep it covered and off the floor.
- Some patients may use long oxygen extension tubing so they can move about the room. The tubing presents a trip hazard for both patient and staff. Caution the patient to alert staff entering the room if the tubing is in the walkway. Position the tubing out of the flow of traffic as much as possible.
- Change the cannula every 24 to 48 hours, or according to facility policy, if this is your responsibility. Fold a piece of bandage tape or a label in half over the distal end of the tubing, affixing it to itself. Use a permanent marker to write the date and time the tubing was changed and your initials.
- When changing the cannula, replace the packaging used to store the cannula when not in use.

FIGURE 39-19 The liquid oxygen canister. The portable tank on top is filled from the large tank, then detached.

Safety ALERT

Oxygen concentrators are used only for patients needing low liter flows of oxygen. The concentrator cannot convert room air when high liter flows are necessary. For this reason, an oxygen concentrator should not be used in emergency. If you are sent for an external oxygen source in an emergency, a small tank is best. ■

Liquid Oxygen

Oxygen also comes in a liquid canister (Figure 39-19). Liquid oxygen is made by cooling the oxygen gas. As it cools, it changes to a liquid form. One advantage is that large amounts of liquid oxygen can be stored in small, more convenient containers. These can be filled from the larger unit. However, liquid oxygen cannot be stored for a long period of time because it will evaporate. The canister delivers higher oxygen concentrations than a concentrator, and is portable and convenient. It does not require electricity to operate. The canister is quiet compared with a concentrator, which has an electric motor and makes a humming noise. It is more expensive than using a concentrator.

Safety Precautions for Liquid Oxygen. Liquid oxygen is nontoxic, but will cause severe burns upon direct contact. Avoid opening, touching, or spilling the container. If your skin or clothing contacts the liquid oxygen, flush the area immediately with a large amount of water. When liquid oxygen is used, high concentrations of oxygen build up quickly. Some materials are very flammable when saturated with oxygen. Follow all safety precautions for preventing sparks and fires (Unit 14). Never seal the cap or vent port on the liquid oxygen. Doing so will increase pressure within the system, creating a potentially dangerous situation. If a bottle falls or tips, evacuate yourself and the patient from the room and close the door. Follow facility policies for getting assistance in this type of emergency.

Respiratory Positions

Positioning to permit expansion of the lungs and a straightened airway is helpful to patients with respiratory distress.

High Fowler's Position. In the **high Fowler's position**, the patient is sitting up with the backrest elevated (Figure 39-20).

- Position three pillows behind the patient's head and shoulders. Adjust the knee rest.
- Keep the feet in proper position.
- Check for signs of skin breakdown over the coccyx from shearing forces.

Orthopneic Position. The **orthopneic position** (Figure 39-21) may be used as an alternative to the high Fowler's position. *Orthopnea* means "needing to sit up to breathe comfortably." The patient sits as upright as possible and leans slightly forward, supporting himself with the forearms. This position makes the thorax larger on inspiration, enabling the patient to inhale more air. The **tripod position** (Figure 39-22) is another alternative to improve ventilation.

- The head of the bed is upright, as far as it will go.
- The bedside table is brought across the bed and a pillow or two are placed on top.

FIGURE 39-21 The patient is in the high Fowler's position.

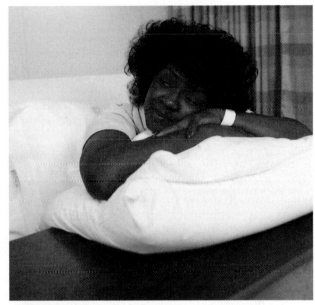

FIGURE 39-22 The tripod position enlarges the chest cavity, making breathing easier.

- The patient leans forward across the table with arms on or beside the pillows.
- Another pillow is placed low behind the patient's back for support.

Another alternative to improve ventilation is to seat the patient on the side of the bed, with the bed in the lowest horizontal position. Make sure the patient's legs are supported on a floor or a stool. The patient can lean across an overbed table, if desired, for additional support.

Incentive Spirometer

The physician may write orders for use of an **incentive spirometer** (Figure 39-23) to help the lungs expand fully. This prevents atelectasis (collapse of the alveoli) and also helps prevent pneumonia.

This procedure may be carried out with the patient in bed, with head and shoulders well supported, if permitted. The procedure usually is taught before surgery.

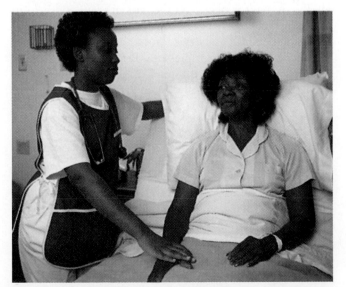

FIGURE 39-20 The patient in the orthopneic position sits straight up, supported on the arms.

FIGURE 39-23 The patient inhales into the incentive spirometer, raising the level of the ball inside the plastic chamber.

- The patient is instructed how to use the incentive spirometer by the RCP or nurse.
- The patient exhales normally and then, with the lips placed tightly around the mouthpiece, inhales through the mouth strongly, enough to raise the balls in the chambers.
- The deep breath should be held as long as possible (or as ordered), thereby keeping the balls suspended.
- The patient then removes the mouthpiece and exhales normally.
- The exercise is repeated as many times as is ordered.

Although this procedure is started by the professional, you too have responsibilities:

- Remind the patient to use the device according to care plan instructions. For example, a postoperative patient may be instructed to use the spirometer 10 times every hour. The RCP will develop this plan of care and set the slide bar to a level on the side of the instrument. The slide bar represents the patient's inhalation goal.
- Observe the patient for correctness of procedure.
- Advise the patient not to take in too many deep breaths in a row, as this will cause dizziness.
- Be sure the patient does not become overly fatigued.
- Encourage the patient to cough and clear the respiratory passages.
- Report to the nurse if the patient seems overly fatigued during the procedure.
- Carefully observe and report any unusual responses, such as pain, dizziness, or throat and airway irritation.
- When the patient has completed the pulmonary exercise, wash the spirometer mouthpiece in warm water, dry it, replace it in the plastic bag, and leave it at the bedside.
- Provide mouth care as needed or desired.

Tips: The incentive spirometer is usually left at the bedside. The patient will be prompted to use it throughout the day. He or she is instructed to take four to five slow, deep breaths using the spirometer, or as ordered. If the patient becomes dizzy or complains of tingling in the fingers, he or she may be breathing too fast. Have the patient relax and breathe normally until the sensation passes. Monitor the patient's breathing before and after the treatment. Report your observations to the nurse.

- Praise patients for their efforts. Many times this encourages greater effort the next time the incentive spirometer is used.

Other Techniques

Aerosol Therapy. Nebulizers deliver moisture or medication deep into the lungs. Drugs that dilate the bronchi are often prescribed. Small-volume nebulizers (Figure 39-24) turn liquid medicine into a mist that can be breathed in by the patient. Typically, drugs are ordered to open up obstructed airways for patients with COPD and asthma. The nebulizer may be powered by oxygen or compressed air. After a nebulizer treatment is given, the patient should be encouraged to cough and assessed by the nurse for improvement after medication delivery.

Continuous Positive Airway Pressure (CPAP)

Some patients stop breathing periodically while they sleep. This condition is called *sleep apnea*. It is commonly caused by a blockage or obstruction in the patient's airway that occurs when the patient falls asleep and the muscles relax. Patients with sleep apnea may stop breathing hundreds of times a night, and they snore loudly when they start to breathe again. This interrupts their sleep, and they are often very tired during the day. Treatment in many cases consists of use of a device that delivers pressure to the airway while the patient sleeps; this pressure holds the airway open.

The device is called **CPAP** (pronounced see-pap) which stands for **continuous positive airway pressure** (Figure 39-25). A mask is placed on the patient's face and held in place with a head strap. Large-diameter corrugated tubing connects the mask to a device (sometimes called a blower) that creates low levels of pressure. Because there is always pressure in the system, the mask must fit tightly against the face. Pressure is usually controlled by an adjustment

FIGURE 39-24 The hand-held, small-volume nebulizer

on the device. The amount of pressure can range from approximately 2 cm H_2O to 20 cm H_2O. This level is ordered by the physician. The device is usually initially set up by an RCP, who works with the patient to determine which type of mask is most effective and most comfortable.

Many patients will put on their own masks at bedtime. Remind them to wash and dry the face thoroughly before putting the mask on so that less skin oil will get on the mask. You should help monitor the patient while he is connected to a CPAP machine. Check to make sure the mask is comfortable. Air leaks around the top can allow air to blow into the patient's eyes, which is very irritating. If this happens, adjust the mask to see if you can reduce the leak. However, if the mask is too tight, the patient may feel pain or there may be redness or skin breakdown on the nose.

If the patient complains of excessive dryness in his nasal passages, the nurse will check with the RCP to see if a humidifier can be added to the CPAP system. The nurse may also get an order for saline spray or nosedrops to reduce the irritation. It is important not to use petrolatum products with respiratory devices. If a patient swallows a lot of air from the mask, belches frequently, and feels pressure in the abdomen, elevate the head of the bed to see if this reduces air swallowing.

Wash the mask each morning, after the patient takes it off. Wash it with soap and water, or according to facility policy. Store the dry mask in a clean plastic bag until use at bedtime.

FIGURE 39-25
The CPAP mask applies pressure to keep the airway open while the patient sleeps, preventing sleep apnea.

COLLECTING A SPUTUM SPECIMEN

You may need to collect a sputum specimen from the patient. **Sputum** is matter that is brought up (**expectorated**) from the lungs. A culture of the specimen identifies the cause of an infection.

You must be sure that the specimen comes from the lungs and is not saliva from the mouth.

If the patient cannot expectorate sputum, suctioning may be needed to obtain the specimen. (The nurse performs this procedure.) It is easier to collect the specimen when the patient wakes up in the morning and after the patient takes two or three deep breaths.

PROCEDURE

89

COLLECTING A SPUTUM SPECIMEN

1. Carry out initial procedure actions.

2. Assemble equipment:
   - Disposable gloves
   - Sterile container and cover for specimen
   - Glass of water
   - Label, including:
     - patient's full name
     - room number
     - patient number
     - date and time of collection
     - physician's name
     - examination to be done
     - other information as requested
   - Tissues

   - Emesis basin
   - Biohazard specimen transport bag
   - Laboratory requisition

3. Wash your hands and put on disposable gloves.

4. Ask the patient to rinse her mouth with water and spit into the emesis basin.

5. Ask the patient to breathe deeply and then cough deeply to bring up sputum. The patient spits the sputum into the container.

   a. While coughing, have the patient cover her mouth with a tissue to prevent the spread of infection.

   b. Collect 1 to 2 tablespoons of sputum unless otherwise ordered.

continues

PROCEDURE 89 CONTINUED

c. Do not contaminate the outside of the container.

d. Avoid touching the inside of the container or lid. Instruct the patient not to touch the inside of the container or lid.

6. Remove your gloves and discard them according to facility policy.

7. Wash your hands.

8. Cover the specimen container tightly and attach a completed label.

9. Place the specimen container in a biohazard transport bag and attach a laboratory requisition.

10. Carry out ending procedure actions.

11. Follow facility policy for transporting specimens to the laboratory.

REVIEW

A. True/False.

Mark the following true or false by circling T or F.

1. T F In asthma, there is increased production of mucus, which blocks the respiratory tract.

2. T F Drugs to reduce fever fight infection.

3. T F An allergen causes a sensitivity reaction.

4. T F URI stands for underrated respiratory injections.

5. T F Use of the incentive spirometer can help prevent pneumonia.

6. T F Always post a sign when oxygen is in use.

7. T F The oxygen flow rate is ordered by the physician.

8. T F Immobility is a risk factor for hypoxemia.

9. T F When oxygen is administered by mask, make sure the straps are very tight.

10. T F In the high Fowler's position, the patient leans forward across the overbed table.

B. Matching.

Choose the correct word from Column II to match each phrase or statement in Column I.

Column I

11. _____ inflammation of the lungs

12. _____ an example of COPD

13. _____ difficult breathing

14. _____ cough up

15. _____ material brought up from lungs

Column II

a. emphysema

b. sputum

c. pneumonia

d. dyspnea

e. spirometer

f. expectorate

C. Multiple Choice.

Select the one best answer for each of the following.

16. Patients with respiratory disease should

    a. cover the nose and mouth when coughing.

    b. turn the face toward others when sneezing.

    c. wash their hands only after toileting.

    d. carry a plastic bag to dispose of soiled tissues.

17. When tank oxygen is in use,

    a. store empty tanks in the patient's room.

    b. attach the tank to the patient's bed.

    c. make sure additional tanks are available.

    d. check the gauge indicating the amount in the tank once each shift.

18. Nursing care for a male patient who is using oxygen includes

    a. keeping the head of the bed elevated 10°.

    b. shaving the patient with an electric razor.

    c. covering the patient with a wool blanket.

    d. providing frequent mouth care.

19. When your patient is receiving oxygen, you should
    a. monitor intake and output.
    b. know the ordered rate.
    c. check the flow rate once each shift.
    d. check the flow rate every 3 hours.

20. When administering oxygen by mask, in addition to routine care and precautions, you should
    a. pull the straps until they are very tight.
    b. provide emotional support and reassurance.
    c. make sure the mask covers only the mouth.
    d. remove the mask for bathing and meals.

D. Nursing Assistant Challenge.

*Mrs. Harvey has had asthma all her life. She is sensitive to many allergens. She is admitted to your facility for emphy-*sema. *She is receiving respiratory assistance with an oxygen concentrator. Complete the following questions related to her care.*

21. The flow rate of the concentrator is usually _____
    (10 L/min) (2 L/min)

22. Smoking in the same room _____ permitted.
    (is) (is not)

23. The flow meter on a concentrator _____ be changed by the nursing assistant.
    (may) (may not)

24. The concentrator should be placed at least _____ from a heat source.
    (2 feet) (5 feet)

25. The concentrator filter should be cleaned _____.
    (daily) (weekly)

Circulatory (Cardiovascular) System

OBJECTIVES

After completing this unit, you will be able to:
- Spell and define terms.
- Review the location and functions of the organs of the circulatory system.
- Describe some common disorders of the circulatory system.

- Describe nursing assistant actions related to care of patients with disorders of the circulatory system.
- List five specific diagnostic tests for disorders of the circulatory system.

VOCABULARY

Learn the meaning and the correct spelling of the following words and phrases:

anemia	congestive heart failure (CHF)	infarction	peripheral
angina pectoris		ischemic	phlebitis
artery	coronary embolism	leukemia	plasma
ascites	coronary occlusion	leukocytes	stent
atheroma	coronary thrombosis	lymph	thrombocytes
atherosclerosis	diuresis	lymphatic vessel	thrombus
atrium	dyscrasia	myocardial infarction (MI)	transient ischemic attack (TIA)
capillary	embolus		varicose vein
cardiac cycle	endocardium	myocardium	vein
cardiac decompensation	erythrocytes	orthopnea	ventricle
compensate	heart block	pacemaker	
	hypertrophy	pericardium	

INTRODUCTION

The circulatory system may be thought of as a transportation system. It takes nourishment and oxygen to the cells and carries away waste products. The closed system is kept in motion by the force of the heartbeat. Diseases that attack any part of this system interfere with overall body function. Long-standing diseases of the cardiovascular system eventually affect the pulmonary system as well.

STRUCTURE AND FUNCTION

The organs of the cardiovascular system include:
1. Heart—a central pumping station
2. Blood vessels
   a. Arteries—tubes that carry blood away from the heart. They
      - have muscular, elastic walls with smooth linings.

  - branch to form arterioles with thinner walls. Arterioles then become capillaries.
  - carry blood with a high concentration of nutrients and oxygen to the body cells.

   b. Veins—tubes that carry blood toward the heart. They
  - have thinner muscular walls.
  - carry blood back to the heart.
  - carry blood with a lower concentration of oxygen, more carbon dioxide, and more waste products.
  - have cuplike valves that help move the blood.

   c. Capillaries—tubes that connect arteries and veins. They
  - have walls only one cell thick.
  - are the site of exchange of nutrients and oxygen from the blood to the cells, and carbon dioxide and waste products from the cells to the blood.

3. Lymphatic vessels—tubes that carry lymph or tissue fluid to the bloodstream. Fluid from the bloodstream passes into the tissue spaces, where it is called *tissue fluid*. Some of the tissue fluid returns to the bloodstream by way of the capillaries. Some of it is first drawn off into the lymphatic vessels, where it is called **lymph**. Eventually the lymph is returned to general circulation and once more becomes part of the blood.

4. Lymph nodes—masses of lymphatic tissue along the pathway of the lymph. They filter the lymph.

5. Spleen—a lymphatic organ. The spleen produces some of the blood cells and helps destroy worn-out blood cells. It acts as a blood reservoir or blood bank.

6. Blood—a connective tissue made up of a liquid (plasma) and cellular elements.

The Blood

Blood is a red body fluid composed of plasma and cellular elements. The body contains 4 to 6 quarts (liters) of blood. Fifty-five percent of the blood is formed of the liquid plasma. **Plasma** is a watery solution containing:

- Antibodies (gamma globulin)—chemicals to fight infection
- Nutrients—such as glucose, amino acids, fats, salts
- Gases—such as oxygen and carbon dioxide
- Waste products—such as urea and creatinine

The blood cells are produced in the bone marrow and lymphatic tissues of the body. The bone marrow, liver, and spleen destroy worn-out blood cells. The blood cells include red blood cells, white blood cells, and thrombocytes.

- Red blood cells (RBC)—**erythrocytes**—carry most of the oxygen and small amounts of carbon dioxide. There are 4.5 to 5 million RBC per cubic millimeter (mm^3).
- White blood cells (WBC)—**leukocytes**—fight infection. There are 7,000 to 8,000 WBC/mm^3.
- **Thrombocytes** (or platelets)—are not whole cells but only parts of cells. They seal small leaks in the walls of blood vessels and initiate blood clotting. There are 200,000 to 400,000 thrombocytes/mm^3.

The Heart

The heart is a hollow muscular organ about the size of a fist (Figure 40-1). It is divided into a right and left side by a muscular wall called the *septum* and into four chambers. There are three layers in the heart wall. The **endocardium** lines the heart chambers. The **myocardium** is the muscle layer. The **pericardium** is a membranous outer covering. The four chambers are:

1. The right **atrium** (RA)—(right upper heart chamber) receives blood from all over the body. This blood has a low oxygen content and a relatively high carbon dioxide level. It is called *deoxygenated blood.*

2. The right **ventricle** (RV)—(right lower heart chamber) receives blood from the right atrium and sends it out to the lungs through the pulmonary artery to pick up oxygen and get rid of the carbon dioxide.

3. The left atrium (LA)—(left upper heart chamber) receives oxygenated blood from the lungs and sends it to the left ventricle.

FIGURE 40-1 The heart

4. The left ventricle (LV)—(left lower heart chamber) receives blood from the left atrium and sends it out through the aorta to the entire body.

Valves separate the chambers. They also guard the exit of the pulmonary artery and aorta to prevent backflow and maintain a constant forward motion. The pulmonary artery carries blood to the lungs. The aorta is the largest blood vessel in the body. The valves are located as follows:

- Tricuspid valve—between right atrium and right ventricle
- Bicuspid (mitral) valve—between left atrium and left ventricle
- Pulmonary semilunar valves—between right ventricle and pulmonary artery
- Aortic semilunar valve—between left ventricle and aorta

Nerve impulses make the heart contract regularly according to body needs. For example, when you run, your body cells need more oxygen. The cells signal the brain that they need more oxygen. The brain sends a signal to the heart through the nerves, telling it to supply more blood. These nerve impulses cause the heart to beat faster. Thus, more oxygenated blood is pumped to the body cells to supply the oxygen required. These impulses cause the heart to beat faster.

The Cardiac Cycle. The heart pumps blood through the body by a series of movements known as the **cardiac cycle**. First, the upper chambers of the heart, called *atria*, relax and fill with blood as the lower chambers contract, forcing blood out of the heart through the aorta and pulmonary arteries. Next, the lower chambers relax, allowing blood to flow into them from the contracting upper chambers. Then the cycle is repeated (Figure 40-2). Each cycle lasts about 0.8 second. This happens about 70 to 80 times per minute.

The pulse you feel at the radial artery corresponds to ventricular contraction. The sounds you hear when listening to the heart and when taking a blood pressure are the sounds made by the closing of the valves during the cardiac cycle.

The rate and rhythm of the cardiac cycle are regulated by the conduction system. The conduction system is made up of special neuromuscular tissue that sends out impulses. The impulses eventually reach the myocardial cells, which respond by contracting.

- The impulses begin at the S-A node in the right atrium and spread across the two atria.
- The atria contract.
- Impulses from the S-A node reach the A-V node in the right atrium.

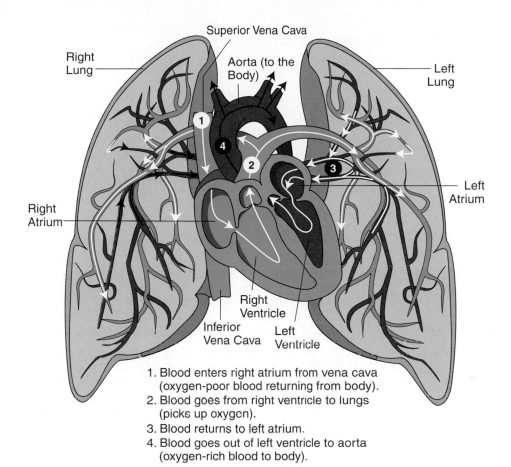

1. Blood enters right atrium from vena cava (oxygen-poor blood returning from body).
2. Blood goes from right ventricle to lungs (picks up oxygen).
3. Blood returns to left atrium.
4. Blood goes out of left ventricle to aorta (oxygen-rich blood to body).

FIGURE 40-2 Blood flows from the heart to the lungs, to the body, and back to the heart to begin the cycle again.

- Messages from the A-V node then spread through the bundle of His in the septum. From there they go through the Purkinje fibers to the walls of the ventricles.
- The ventricles contract, forcing the blood forward.

An electrocardiogram, called an ECG or an EKG, is a test that traces the electrical impulses of the heart. Heart disease may be detected with this test.

Blood Vessels

Many large arteries and veins take their names from the bones they are near or from the part of the body they serve. For example, the femoral artery and vein run close to the femur (thigh bone). The subclavian arteries and veins are found under the clavicle. The axillary arteries and veins are found in the axillary (armpit) area. Figure 40-3 shows the arterial system that distributes blood from the heart. Figure 40-4 shows the venous system that returns blood to the heart.

COMMON CIRCULATORY SYSTEM DISORDERS

Common disorders of this system include:
- Diseases relating to the blood vessels

Clinical Information ALERT

Patients with some types of heart disease will have a fever. This is usually an inflammatory response to heart cell damage after conditions such as a heart attack or acute infection of the heart. Monitor the temperature closely and inform the nurse of abnormalities. ■

- Diseases of the heart
- Blood **dyscrasias** (abnormalities); these diseases can involve the bone, bone marrow, liver, or spleen

Observations the nursing assistant is to report in patients with disorders of the circulatory system are:
- Color change, pallor or cyanosis, redness
- Cool to touch
- Hot to touch
- Changes in pulse rate or rhythm
- Changes in blood pressure
- Edema
- Disorientation

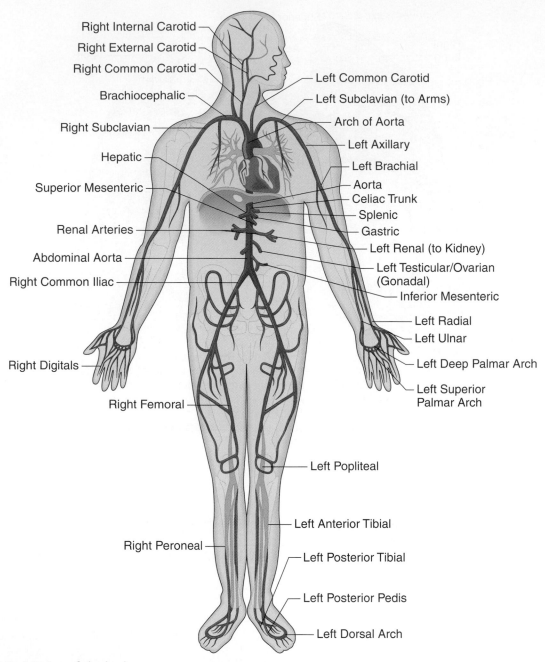

FIGURE 40-3 Arteries of the body

PERIPHERAL VASCULAR DISEASES

The blood vessels that serve the outer parts of the body, particularly those of the hands and feet, are referred to as **peripheral** (toward the outer part) blood vessels. Diseases of these vessels affect the parts of the body through which they pass. The health of these vessels also influences heart function.

Peripheral vascular diseases that affect the arteries diminish the flow of blood to the extremities. Tissues through which the narrowed arteries pass may not get the nourishment they need. Areas affected are the extremities: the arms, legs, and brain. The signs and symptoms associated with decreased peripheral circulation are:

- Burning pain during exercise
- Hair loss over feet and toes
- Thick and rigid toenails
- Dusky red skin or cyanotic, brownish skin
- Dry and scaly or shiny skin
- Chronic edema of the feet and legs
- Cool skin temperature of feet and legs
- Difficulty with ambulation

When the arteries are affected, the blood flow may be seriously interrupted. This condition requires immediate

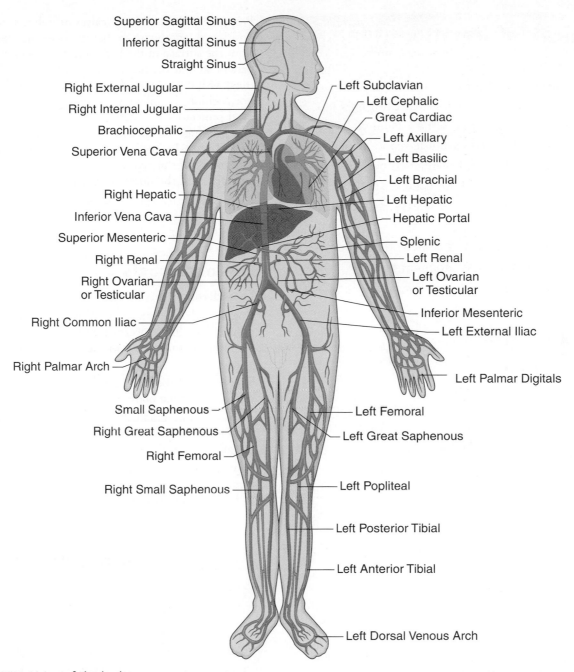

Superior Sagittal Sinus
Inferior Sagittal Sinus
Straight Sinus
Right External Jugular
Right Internal Jugular
Brachiocephalic
Superior Vena Cava
Right Hepatic
Inferior Vena Cava
Superior Mesenteric
Right Renal
Right Ovarian or Testicular
Right Common Iliac
Right Palmar Arch
Small Saphenous
Right Great Saphenous
Right Femoral
Right Small Saphenous

Left Subclavian
Left Cephalic
Great Cardiac
Left Axillary
Left Basilic
Left Brachial
Left Hepatic
Hepatic Portal
Splenic
Left Renal
Left Ovarian or Testicular
Inferior Mesenteric
Left External Iliac
Left Palmar Digitals
Left Femoral
Left Great Saphenous
Left Popliteal
Left Posterior Tibial
Left Anterior Tibial
Left Dorsal Venous Arch

FIGURE 40-4 Veins of the body

medical treatment. Vascular ulcers may occur. These are sores that start because of the poor circulation of the blood in the legs. These ulcers are difficult to treat and may take months to heal.

Treatment is aimed at:

- Increasing local circulation
  - Positioning and specific prescribed exercises can promote arterial flow and venous return.
  - Sometimes an oscillating (rocking) bed is employed to improve the circulatory flow. The oscillating bed rocks up and down in cycles, raising the patient's

feet 6 inches above his head and then lowering them 12 to 15 inches. The steady rhythm provides both passive exercise for the patient and some circulatory stimulation.
  - Nothing that would hamper the patient's circulation is permitted.
- Preventing injuries that may heal poorly.

Protecting the Feet. Patients with impaired circulation are at great risk of ulceration, gangrene (Figure 40-5), and eventual amputation due to pressure or injuries to the feet and ankles. A small injury or ulcer can lead to major

Clinical Information ALERT

Edema develops when the heart cannot pump blood efficiently. In right-sided heart failure, blood backs up into the peripheral veins. Extra fluid has nowhere to go, so it enters the tissues in lower parts of the body, such as the feet and ankles. It may also enter the hands, fingers, and the area over the sacrum. To check for edema, gently press two fingers into the skin and release immediately. If the marks from the fingers remain, the patient has pitting edema. This is a potentially serious problem. Notify the nurse promptly. ■

FIGURE 40-5 The big toe is gangrenous. The toe was eventually amputated, but the foot was saved.

complications. Nursing assistant care for patients with peripheral vascular disease includes:

- Checking the feet and legs daily and reporting abnormalities to the nurse promptly.
- Protecting the feet from injury.
- Making sure the patient is wearing properly fit footwear when out of bed. The patient should always wear socks under shoes. He or she should never ambulate barefoot or wearing only socks on the feet.
- Not cutting toenails; this is a licensed health care provider responsibility. Avoid using sharp objects such as a nail file on the toes.
- Making sure bed linen is not too tight on the feet. Use a bed cradle, if ordered.
- Checking the skin under support hose regularly. Remove the hose periodically, according to the care plan.
- Making sure footwear is not too tight; if footwear fits tightly, notify the nurse.

- Propping bedfast patients' calves on pillows that are positioned lengthwise so that the heels are elevated from the surface of the bed. You may also position the patient so that the heels hang over the end of the mattress, with the soles of the feet against a footboard. Do not position the pillow width-wise under the calves. Heel protectors are excellent for preventing friction and shearing, but they do not prevent pressure on the heels. Other devices are available to keep the heels off the surface of the bed to relieve pressure. Follow the care plan and the nurse's instructions.
- Making sure the feet are supported on footrests when the patient is using a wheelchair; avoid dragging them across the floor.

Atherosclerosis

Atherosclerosis is a common form of vascular disease.

- Roughened areas known as **atheromas**, which are growths developed over deposits of fatty materials, form on the inner walls of the arteries and narrow the vessels.
- The vessels of the heart and brain, and those leading to the legs from the body, are often affected.
- The atheromas gradually grow larger until they eventually block blood flow to the parts and organs served by the affected vessels (Figure 40-6).
- Sometimes clots that have formed over the irregular areas in the vessel walls break off and travel as emboli to block distant vessels.

Clinical Information ALERT

Some patients with cardiac conditions will be alert and oriented. Some will be confused and disoriented. Confusion is caused by decreased oxygen flow to the brain because of poor circulation. Elderly patients are more likely to experience confusion because of advanced arteriosclerotic and atherosclerotic changes to the brain. Report changes in mental status and new-onset or worsening confusion to the nurse promptly. ■

- The narrowing of vessels can lead to serious complications, such as:
  - Formation of blood clots
  - Angina pectoris
  - Myocardial infarction (MI)
  - Strokes (CVA) (also known as brain attacks)
  - Gangrene

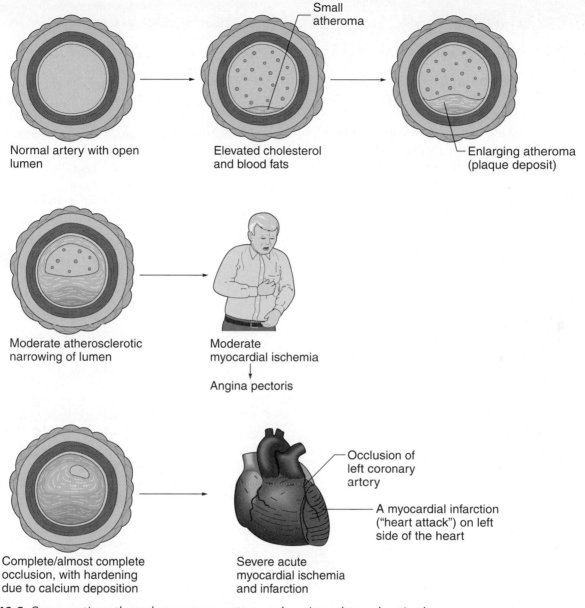

Small atheroma

Normal artery with open lumen

Elevated cholesterol and blood fats

Enlarging atheroma (plaque deposit)

Moderate atherosclerotic narrowing of lumen

Moderate myocardial ischemia

Angina pectoris

Complete/almost complete occlusion, with hardening due to calcium deposition

Severe acute myocardial ischemia and infarction

Occlusion of left coronary artery

A myocardial infarction ("heart attack") on left side of the heart

FIGURE 40-6 Cross-sections through a coronary artery undergoing atherosclerotic changes.

Refer to Figure 40-7 on page 693.

The exact cause of this vascular disease is unknown, but several factors seem to increase the risk that a person will develop it. These factors include:

- Hypertension
- Diabetes mellitus
- Overweight
- Heredity
- Smoking
- Stress
- Lack of exercise
- Diets high in cholesterol and fats

Treatment includes:

- Exercise
- Proper diet
- Reduction of stress
- Control of smoking and obesity

Varicose Veins

The veins can also cause problems. **Varicose veins** form when the valves in the veins in the legs become weakened (Figure 40-8 on page 694). This means:

- The blood does not flow through the veins as it should
- The veins become distended and visible through the skin
- The veins may become inflamed (**phlebitis**)
- A blood clot may form in the vein

Report the following signs:

- Pain or aching in the legs
- Signs of inflammation (warmth and redness)

GUIDELINES *for*
Caring for Patients with Peripheral Vascular Disease

- Elevate the feet when the patient will be sitting in a chair for a long time. When the feet are not elevated, make sure that the patient's feet are flat on the floor. If they are not, support the feet with a footstool. Discourage the patient from crossing the legs when sitting. Discourage the patient from using circular garters or socks with tight elastic tops.
- Discourage smoking—it interferes with circulation.
- Avoid using the knee gatch of the bed.
- Avoid using heating pads or hot water bottles. The patient may not feel temperatures that are too hot.
- Maintain body warmth. Make sure the patient has warm clothes, including socks that fit well. Provide blankets for the bed.
- Prevent injury to the feet:
  - Instruct the patient to wear shoes when out of bed.
  - Check to see that the shoes are in good repair and that they fit well.
  - Avoid pressure to the legs and feet from any source.

- Inspect the feet carefully when you bathe the patient or if the patient complains of any discomfort in the feet. Promptly report any signs of inflammation, injury, or circulatory problems:
  - Broken skin
  - Color change (redness, whiteness, or cyanosis)
  - Heat or coldness
  - Cracking between toes
  - Corns or calluses
  - Swelling
  - Pain
  - Loss of function
  - Drainage
- Bathe the feet regularly.
  - Dry thoroughly and gently between the toes.
  - Use a moisturizing lotion on the feet and legs if the skin is dry.
- Do not cut the toenails of patients who have peripheral vascular disease. In many facilities, nursing assistants are not permitted to clip toenails. Know and follow your facility policies.

Remember that you *never* rub or massage the area of a varicose vein.

Transient Ischemic Attack

Transient ischemic attack (TIA) is a temporary interruption of the blood flow to part of the brain. The patient may experience:

- Weakness or paralysis of any extremity or the face
- Vision problems
- Difficulty with speech
- Difficulty with swallowing

These symptoms come on quickly and may last from just a few minutes to 24 hours. There are no permanent effects. However, a TIA is usually a warning that a stroke will occur at some time. If a patient has any of the symptoms listed, report them to the nurse immediately.

Hypertension

Hypertension is another name for high blood pressure. It may have no known origin, or it may follow illnesses that affect such organs as the:

- Blood vessels

- Kidneys
- Liver

High blood pressure:

- Promotes the development of atherosclerosis, which further narrows the vessels. This increases the blood pressure even more.
- Increases the stress on the heart.
- Increases the damage to the blood vessel walls, so they are more apt to rupture.
- Further limits blood flow to the organs of the body.

Treatment may consist of:

- Drugs that lower the blood pressure
- Diet low in sodium
- Diet that promotes weight loss
- Regular exercise program
- Quitting smoking
- Moderation in lifestyle
- Biofeedback techniques to lower the blood pressure

Report immediately any of the signs and symptoms of hypertension:

- Flushed face
- Dizziness

AFFECTED SITE

COMPLICATION

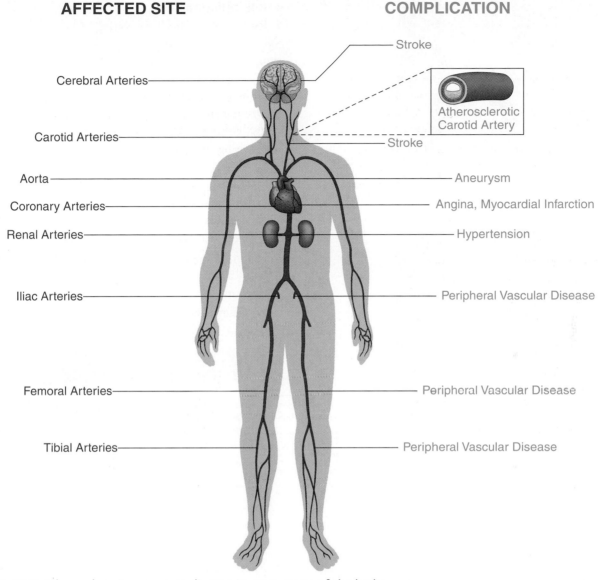

FIGURE 40-7 Atherosclerosis can cause disease in many parts of the body.

- Nosebleeds
- Headaches
- Changes in speech patterns
- Blurred vision

HEART CONDITIONS

Heart disease may sometimes be due to an infection, but most heart disease develops because of changes in the blood vessels. As the openings of the blood vessels become smaller, the heart must work harder and harder to do its job of pumping blood to the body.

Tips: Always take patient complaints of chest pain seriously. If a patient complains of chest pain, assist her to stop all activity and assume a comfortable position. Notify the nurse promptly.

Clinical Information ALERT

Poor circulation is common in patients with disorders of the cardiovascular system. The poor circulation causes reduced blood flow to body organs and systems. Pain is a common sign of reduced blood flow, which in this case is called *ischemia*. Chest pain is caused by ischemia of the heart muscle. Pain in the legs is also common. This is caused by lack of oxygen in the leg muscles. Observe cardiovascular patients for pain. If noted, inform the nurse promptly. ■

FIGURE 40-8 Veins contain valves to prevent the backward flow of blood. A. External view of the vein shows wider area of valve. B. Internal view with the valve open as blood flows through. C. Internal view with the valve closed. D. Vein with weakened valve that causes a varicose vein.

Angina Pectoris

Angina pectoris is known as cardiac "pain of effort." You will recall that the blood vessels nourishing the heart are the coronary arteries. These vessels often are the site of atherosclerotic changes. In an angina attack, the vessels are unable to carry enough blood to meet the heart's demand for oxygen. This may develop:

- Gradually over a period of time, as atheromas develop
- Suddenly, as the vessels constrict

Factors that precipitate (bring on) an attack include:

- Exertion
- Heavy eating
- Emotional stress

The signs and symptoms of angina pectoris that you should immediately report include:

- Pain when exercising or under stress. Stress causes a need for an immediate increase in coronary circulation. The pain is described as dull, with increasing intensity. It is usually centered under the breast bone (sternum), spreading to the left arm and up into the neck.

- Pale or flushed face.
- Patient who is freely perspiring.

Signs and symptoms may differ with individuals, but the symptoms are usually the same each time a person experiences an attack.

Treatment of angina pectoris consists of:

- Diagnosing hidden causes. A treadmill stress test is one method of doing this.
- Teaching the patient to avoid stress and sudden exertion.
- Drugs that relax the coronary arteries.
- Coronary artery bypass surgery.
- Angioplasty, a surgical procedure to open the vessels.

You may assist the patient who has angina pectoris by:

- Helping the patient to avoid unnecessary emotional or physical stress
- Encouraging the patient not to smoke
- Reporting any signs or symptoms of an attack to the nurse at once

Clinical Information ALERT

Patients with cardiac conditions may have skin color or temperature changes. Make sure you have good light when checking the skin. You will see cyanosis on the lips and mucous membranes of the mouth, as well as on the earlobes, skin, and nail beds. Caucasian patients with pallor may appear as if they have no blood. In African American, Asian, and Hispanic patients, pallor may show as a gray color. If the patient has a circulation problem, check the arms and legs. Make sure the skin color and temperature are equal on both sides of the body. Thick toenails and little to no hair growth on the legs indicates a circulatory problem. Varicosities may also be present. ■

Myocardial Infarction (Coronary Heart Attack)

The term **myocardial infarction (MI)**, or heart attack, refers to a period in which the heart suddenly cannot function properly. There are different kinds of heart attacks. They differ in severity and prognosis (expected outcome). Remember that the heart is muscle tissue and may become tired just as any muscle may tire. The cells of the heart require nourishment and oxygen like all other cells.

An acute myocardial infarction occurs when the coronary arteries, which nourish the heart, are blocked. Part of the heart muscle supplied by these vessels becomes **ischemic** (loses its blood supply). Unless circulation is restored quickly, the cells die (**infarction**). If too much tissue dies, the person cannot survive. Coronary heart attack is also called:

- **Coronary occlusion**—blockage of coronary arteries
- **Coronary thrombosis**—when a **thrombus** (stationary blood clot) forms at the site, blocking the blood flow
- **Coronary embolism**—when a moving clot or insoluble particle (**embolus**), which originated elsewhere and has moved, becomes lodged in the artery

Signs and Symptoms. The signs and symptoms of a heart attack include:

- Pain—may resemble severe indigestion. It is often described as "crushing" chest pain that radiates to the jaw and left arm (Figure 40-9).
- Nausea/vomiting.
- Irregular pulse and respiration.
- Perspiration (diaphoresis).
- Feelings of anxiety and weakness.
- Indications of shock, which include drop in blood pressure and pallor.
- Shortness of breath.
- Syncope (fainting).
- Restlessness.
- Cyanosis or gray skin color.

The signs and symptoms of a heart attack vary with the individual. The pain may be in the chest in some patients, and radiate to the jaw or either arm. If a patient has chest pain combined with any other signs or symptoms, he should be evaluated by a health care professional. Have the patient stop any activity immediately and assume a

FIGURE 40-9 The patient having a heart attack usually experiences crushing chest pain that is described as "the worst pain I've had in my life," or "It feels like an elephant is standing on my chest."

comfortable position. Stay with the patient and call for assistance.

Immediate treatment has saved many people. The treatment is directed toward:

- Relieving the pain
- Reducing heart activity
- Altering the clotting ability of the blood
- Administering drugs to dissolve the clot

Nursing Care. During the acute stage, heart attack patients require professional care. Many hospitals provide intensive and/or cardiac care units for these patients. Nursing care supports the therapy ordered. Special attention must be given to:

- Noting signs of a recurrence and reporting immediately to the nurse
- Watching for bleeding and reporting immediately
- Assisting with activities of daily living
- Monitoring vital signs
- Patient teaching to eliminate risk factors

Congestive Heart Failure (CHF)

The heart, like any other muscle, will enlarge and tire if it has to work against increasing pressure. When blood vessels narrowed by atherosclerosis increase the resistance to blood flow, and when there is severe damage to major organs like the liver and spleen, it is more difficult to maintain the circulation. The heart is not pumping well enough to meet the body's demands for oxygen. The heart muscle may also have been damaged and weakened by myocardial infarction. Other common causes are heredity, longstanding high blood pressure, alcohol abuse, and viral infection. The heart must pump harder to maintain the internal flow of blood.

At first, the heart enlarges (**hypertrophy**) and makes up (**compensates**) for the additional workload. Eventually, however, it reaches a point when it can no longer compensate. Heart failure follows.

This form of heart disease is known as **congestive heart failure (CHF)** or **cardiac decompensation**. The condition got its name because of *failure* of the *heart* to pump efficiently, which results in *congestion* of the lungs. The heart tries to compensate for the problem, but this worsens the condition.

Signs and Symptoms. The signs and symptoms are the result of the heart being unable to pump the blood with sufficient force.

- Hemoptysis (spitting up blood).
- Cough.
- Dyspnea (difficulty breathing).
- **Orthopnea** (difficulty in breathing unless sitting upright).
- **Ascites** (fluid collecting in the abdomen).
- Neck vein swelling.

- Fatiguing easily.
- Hypoxia (hypoxemia; inadequate oxygen levels).
- Confusion.
- Edema (swelling), which develops in dependent tissues and slows blood flow, congesting the vessels and allowing more fluid to enter the body spaces and tissues. It is most common in the abdomen, ankles, and fingers.
- Waking up at night with breathlessness.
- Being unable to lie flat at night.
- Fluid accumulation in the lungs.
- Cyanosis, which occurs because fluid in the lungs makes gas exchange less efficient.
- Irregular and rapid pulse.
- High blood pressure.
- Palpitations (galloping heartbeat).
- Kidney malfunction in later stages.
- Liver malfunction.

Treatment. Treatment involves:

- Drugs to help the heart beat more strongly and regularly and to increase the output of fluids (**diuresis**) by the kidneys.
- Minimally invasive procedures may be done to open the arteries. These involve inserting a long tube into an artery in the groin. The tube is threaded through the system to the heart. A balloon on the tube is inflated to open blocked arteries (Figure 40-10A). The balloon-tipped catheter is removed and replaced with a **stent** (Figure 40-10B), a device that keeps the arteries open. This procedure pushes the fatty deposits back against the artery walls, making more room for blood to flow through and preventing heart attack.
- Low-sodium diet.
- Restriction of fluids, if ordered.
- Weighing the patient daily to monitor level of fluid retention.
- Monitoring the apical pulse and observing for pulse deficit (Figure 40-11).
- Positioning the patient in orthopneic position or high Fowler's supported by pillows, or supported in a chair. The position must be changed frequently, but changes in position should be made slowly. Padded footboards help keep the weight of the bedding off the toes.
- Applying elasticized stockings or *TED hose* (Unit 29). TED hose are elastic anti-embolism stockings. TED hose and Ace bandages help channel blood to the deeper vessels. They must be checked often and reapplied every 6 to 8 hours. Check the extremities carefully for adequate circulation. The skin should be normal color and warm.
- Assisting with activities of daily living as needed.
- Attending to general hygiene. Complete bathing is tiring, but partial baths can stimulate circulation and provide comfort. Special attention must be given to the

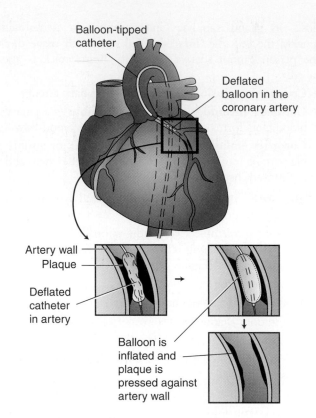

FIGURE 40-10A The balloon presses the plaque against the wall of the artery, making the vessel larger.

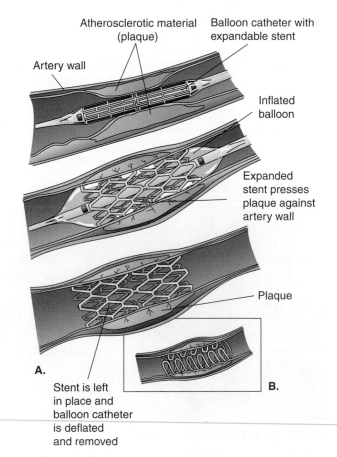

FIGURE 40-10B The stent is left in place to keep the artery open, and the balloon is removed.

FIGURE 40-11 Ineffective heart contractions may cause a pulse deficit.

A.

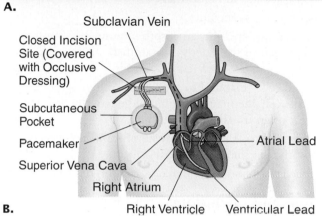

Subclavian Vein

Closed Incision
Site (Covered
with Occlusive
Dressing)

Subcutaneous
Pocket

Pacemaker

Superior Vena Cava

Right Atrium

Atrial Lead

B.

Right Ventricle   Ventricular Lead

FIGURE 40-12 The electronic pacemaker sends electrical impulses to the heart muscle, causing it to contract. A. A typical pacemaker. B. The pacemaker is inserted under the skin with the electrode placed inside the heart, resting on the heart muscle. (Photo courtesy of Medtronic, Inc.)

skin because the combination of position, edema, and poor circulation contributes to tissue breakdown. Allow the patient to be as independent with bathing as possible, unless you are instructed otherwise. Bathing is not normally a strenuous activity, but the patient with CHF may tire easily. Check the patient frequently while he or she is bathing. Be prepared to take over and complete the bath if the patient becomes short of breath or too tired.

- Assisting with oxygen therapy. Oxygen therapy may be provided either by face mask or nasal cannula. Because cardiac patients often breathe through the mouth, the mouth tends to be very dry. Special mouth care may be needed.
- Providing for elimination. A bedside commode is convenient. The use of a commode is less tiring for the patient than using a bedpan for elimination.
- Encouraging adequate nutrition. Small, easily digested meals should be provided. You may need to assist in feeding the patient to prevent fatigue.
- Monitoring and recording fluid intake. Patients with acute heart failure may be given drugs that increase the output of urine and alter the heart rate. Measuring the intake and output and taking daily weights are ways of determining if fluid is being retained. The patient may be on fluid restriction (Unit 26) in the acute phase of the illness.
- Regularly checking vital signs. Sometimes the force of heart contraction, which propels the blood forward into the blood vessels, does not have enough strength to make the vessels expand.
- Keeping the feet elevated when the patient is up in a chair or wheelchair.
- Encouraging regular rest periods throughout the day.
- Assisting with exercise, as specified on the care plan.

Heart Block

Heart block is a condition that develops due to interference in the electrical current through the heart. (The flow

of electrical current through the heart muscle makes the normal cardiac cycle possible.)

An electronic device called a **pacemaker** (Figure 40-12) is implanted under the chest muscles or in the abdomen. An electrode carries electrical current from the pacemaker directly into the heart muscle to replace the lost control. The electrical current signals the heart to contract. Some pacemakers send messages only if normal messages carried by the conduction system are delayed. This type of pacemaker is called a *demand pacemaker*. Other pacemakers send regular signals to keep the heart contracting at a preset rate.

When caring for a patient who has a pacemaker:

- Count and record the pulse rate
- Report any irregularities or changes below the present rate
- Report any discoloration over the implant site
- Report hiccupping, because this may indicate problems
- Keep the patient away from microwave ovens and cellular phones, because they may disrupt the function of the pacemaker

Patients usually function very well with pacemakers as long as they are adequately monitored.

BLOOD ABNORMALITIES

Blood abnormalities are often called *blood dyscrasias*.

Anemia

Anemia is a condition that results from a decrease in the quantity or quality of red blood cells. There are several causes, such as:

- Poor diet
- Low production of new red blood cells
- Blood loss, as in hemorrhage

Types of anemia include:

- Pernicious—inability to absorb vitamin B_{12} (most often seen in the elderly). Vitamin B_{12} is required by the body to produce red blood cells.
- Sickle cell—inability to form normal hemoglobin. Sickle cell anemia is transmitted genetically. It is seen most often in African Americans.
- Deficiency—inadequate intake of iron, inability to absorb iron, or excessive loss of iron.
- Dietary—inadequate intake of iron or vitamins in diet.

Signs and Symptoms. The person with anemia may:

- Have little energy
- Be pale or jaundiced
- Have dyspnea
- Experience digestive problems
- Have a rapid pulse
- Complain of light-headedness
- Feel cold
- Experience dizziness
- Have an increased respiratory rate

Treatment. Treatment is aimed at:

- Improving the quantity and quality of the blood by giving iron supplements
- Eliminating the basic cause of the disease
- Giving blood transfusions as needed
- Providing nutrients and nutritious meals

Leukemia

Leukemia is sometimes called cancer of the blood. The causes of the many forms of leukemia are not known. This disease may strike young or old. The number of white blood cells increases, but the white blood cells may be of poor quality. The number of erythrocytes and platelets decreases. Patients with leukemia are highly susceptible to infection. During the course of the disease, even minor trauma causes bleeding.

Treatment. Treatment is aimed at:

- Easing symptoms and keeping the patient comfortable.
- Maintaining normal blood levels. Transfusions may be needed to combat the anemia that accompanies the condition.
- Combating infection by using antibiotics.
- Slowing the production of abnormal white cells through chemotherapy and/or radiation therapy.

Infection Control ALERT

Patients with leukemia are at high risk of infection because the immature white blood cells do not protect the body effectively. Conscientiously apply the principles of standard precautions in all patient care. Notify the nurse promptly of signs or symptoms of infection. ∎

Special Care

Patients who have cancer or anemia require special care. You must:

- Check vital signs
- Encourage rest
- Handle the patient very gently
- Encourage good nutrition and fluid intake
- Give special mouth care, because the mouth and tongue become sensitive
- Be sure to report any signs of bleeding, such as bruises or discolorations, because further blood loss makes the condition worse
- Keep the patient warm
- Protect the patient from falls that may result from dizziness or weakness
- Change the patient's position often, at least every 2 hours
- Provide emotional support

DIAGNOSTIC TESTS

Some techniques used to diagnose problems of the cardiovascular system include:

- Blood chemistry tests, such as electrolyte panels
- Complete blood cell count (CBC)
- Electrocardiogram (ECG or EKG)
- Cardiac catheterization and angiogram—introduction of catheter and dyes into the vascular system under fluoroscopy
- Ultrasound—sound waves are bounced against tissues to reflect variations in tissue density

REVIEW

A. True/False.

Mark the following true or false by circling T or F.

1. T F Smoking is not harmful to the person with atherosclerosis.

2. T F The treadmill test is done to detect hidden cardiac stress.

3. T F When warmth is needed by someone with peripheral vascular disease, a heating pad should not be used.

4. T F Another name for a heart attack is coronary infarction.

5. T F In leukemia, there is an increase in white cells.

6. T F The heart muscle shrinks as it undergoes hypertrophy.

7. T F An embolus is a moving blood clot.

8. T F Anemia is an example of a blood dyscrasia.

9. T F Hypertension is best treated with a high-sodium diet.

10. T F The person with CHF should be monitored for pulse deficit.

B. Matching.

Choose the correct word from Column II to match each phrase in Column I.

Column I

11. _____ inflammation of a vein

12. _____ death of the heart muscle

13. _____ another term for stroke

14. _____ high blood pressure

15. _____ blocking of the blood supply to the heart

Column II

a. hypertension

b. edema

c. myocardial infarction

d. plasma

e. phlebitis

f. CVA

g. hypotension

h. coronary occlusion

C. Multiple Choice.

Select the one best answer for each of the following.

16. Which of the following is not a predisposing cause of atherosclerosis?
    a. Emboli
    b. Diabetes mellitus
    c. Heredity
    d. Stress

17. You suspect the patient needs immediate attention for a possible heart attack because the person
    a. has chest pain.
    b. complains of not feeling well.
    c. has ankle edema.
    d. has pink nailbeds.

18. Nursing care of the patient with anemia might include
    a. bloodletting.
    b. good nutrition.
    c. pacemaker.
    d. chemotherapy.

19. The patient with anemia has a
    a. high energy level.
    b. pink, rosy skin.
    c. low energy level.
    d. slower than normal respiratory rate.

20. An attack of angina pectoris could be brought about by
    a. bathing in the evening.
    b. resting in bed.
    c. emotional stress.
    d. walking in the hallway.

D. Completion.

Complete the statements in the spaces provided.

21. Five specific tests used to diagnose cardiac, vascular, or blood abnormalities are:
    a. _____
    b. _____
    c. _____
    d. _____
    e. _____

22. Six predisposing factors for atherosclerosis are:

    a. _____

    b. _____

    c. _____

    d. _____

    e. _____

    f. _____

E. Nursing Assistant Challenge.

Mrs. O'Brien is only 38 years old, but has been diagnosed with hypertension. Recently she experienced dizziness and weakness and had difficulty speaking for a short period. The doctor suspects she had a TIA. Complete the statements in questions 23–30 by choosing the correct word from the following list.

blurred vision	low
brain	permanent
discouraged	potassium
encouraged	sodium
exercise	stroke
high	temporary
hypertension	

23. Hypertension means this patient has _____ blood pressure.

24. The TIA means there was a _____ interruption of the blood flow to the _____.

25. The diet for this patient should be low in _____ .

26. Smoking should be _____.

27. The TIA indicates that a _____ will probably occur in the future.

28. Treatment for hypertension includes regular

    _____.

29. _____ is a sign that should be reported immediately.

30. Nosebleeds are a danger sign for people with

    _____.

UNIT 41

Musculoskeletal System

OBJECTIVES

After completing this unit, you will be able to:

- Spell and define terms.
- Describe the location and functions of the musculoskeletal system.
- Describe some common conditions of the musculoskeletal system.
- Describe nursing assistant actions related to the care of patients with conditions and diseases of the musculoskeletal system.

- List seven specific diagnostic tests for musculoskeletal conditions.
- Demonstrate the following procedures:
  - Procedure 90 Procedure for Continuous Passive Motion
  - Procedure 91 Performing Range-of-Motion Exercises (Passive)

VOCABULARY

Learn the meaning and the correct spelling of the following words and phrases:

abduction
abduction pillow
adduction
amputation
arthritis
atrophy
avulsion fracture
bursae
bursitis
cardiac muscle
cartilage
cervical traction
closed (simple) fracture
comminuted fracture
compartment syndrome
complete fracture
compound (open) fracture
compression fracture
continuous passive motion (CPM)

countertraction
degenerative joint disease (DJD)
depressed fracture
discectomy
dorsiflexion
ecchymosis
eversion
exacerbation
extension
fibromyalgia
flexion
fracture
fusion
gout
greenstick fracture
impacted fracture
incomplete fracture
insertion
inversion
involuntary muscle

laminectomy
ligament
oblique fracture
open (compound) fracture
open reduction/internal fixation
origin
osteoarthritic joint disease (OJD)
osteoporosis
passive range of motion (PROM)
pathologic fracture
pelvic belt traction
phantom pain
plantar flexion
pronation
radial deviation
range-of-motion (ROM) exercises

remission
rheumatoid arthritis (RA)
rotation
simple (closed) fracture
spica cast
spiral fracture
stimulus
supination
tendon
total hip arthroplasty (THA)
transverse fracture
ulnar deviation
vascular
vertebrae
visceral muscle
voluntary muscle

THE MUSCULOSKELETAL SYSTEM

The bony frame of the body is called the *skeleton*. Tissue that is made up of contractile fibers (fibers that contract and relax) or cells that produce movement are called *muscles*. Together, the skeleton and muscles are termed the musculoskeletal system.

The musculoskeletal system includes:

- Skeletal muscles
- Bones
- Joints
- Tendons
- Ligaments

The system functions to:

- Give shape and form to the body
- Protect and support organs and body parts
- Permit movement

Clinical Information ALERT

Babies are born with 300 bones, but by adulthood we have only 206 in our bodies. The face has 14 bones; the human hand has 27. Humans and giraffes have the same number of neck bones, but the giraffe's bones are much longer. The seventh cervical vertebra is the most prominent in the spine. A child's kneecaps do not fully develop until 2 to 6 years of age. The least fractured bone is the scapula. The most fractured bone is the clavicle. The most mobile joints are in the shoulders. The least mobile joints are the sutures in the skull. The longest bone is the femur, which makes up about 25% of your height. The span of your outstretched arms is approximately equal to your height. However, you shrink slightly during the day because of the compression of intervertebral disks. The smallest bone is the stapes in the ear, which is approximately $\frac{1}{10}$ of an inch long. The hip joint is the strongest joint in the body. Most people have 12 pairs of ribs. One person in 20 has an extra rib. The only bone in the body that is not connected to another bone is the hyoid, a V-shaped bone located at the base of the tongue between the mandible and the voice box. The purpose of this bone is to support the tongue and its muscles. ∎

- Produce some blood cells
- Store calcium and phosphorus

When muscles, bones, or joints have been injured, a long period of rest and inactivity may be required for the part to heal. During this period, it is important that all other moving parts get sufficient exercise. Bones that are not stressed lose calcium and become less functional.

Structure and Function

Bones. It will be helpful for you to learn the names and general location of the bones of the body. To learn the names, study the skeleton in Figure 41-1A and the skull in Figure 41-1B. Note that the same number and kinds of bones are found on one side of the midline as on the other.

The bones:

- Number 206
- May share the same name. For example, there are:
  - 24 ribs helping to form the chest
  - 56 phalanges, the finger bones
  - 2 femurs, the thigh bones

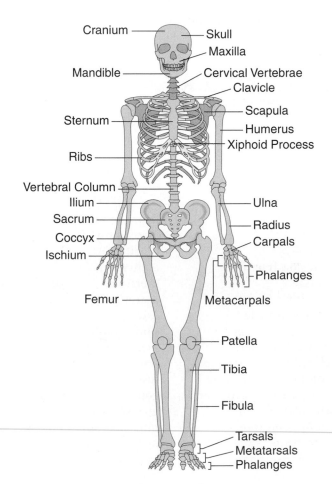

FIGURE 41-1A The human skeleton anterior

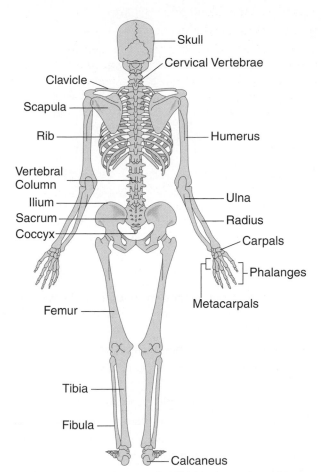

FIGURE 41-1A *CONTINUED* The human skeleton posterior

- 31 bones (**vertebrae**) in the spinal column. Small discs or pads of **cartilage** with soft, gel-like centers between the vertebrae help to cushion these bones. The anterior (front) of the vertebrae support the head and body. The posterior (rear) portions form a tunnel that surrounds the delicate spinal cord and nerves.
- Are of different shapes and sizes, such as
  - long, like the femur, humerus, ulna, and radius
  - short, like the phalanges, carpals, and tarsals
  - flat, like the scapula and cranial bones
  - irregular, like the vertebrae and mandible
- Meet one another to form joints

Joints. Joints are points where bones come together and there is the possibility of movement. Without movable joints, walking, bending, lifting, and sitting would not be possible. Joints are capable of different movements depending the type of joint (Figure 41-2). **Ligaments** are strong bands of fibrous tissues that hold the bones together and support the joints. **Bursae** are small sacs of synovial fluid that are located around joints and help reduce friction.

Special terms are used to describe the different movements in a diarthrotic joint.

- **Flexion**: Decreasing the angle between two bones (Figure 41-3A). For example, bending the elbow.

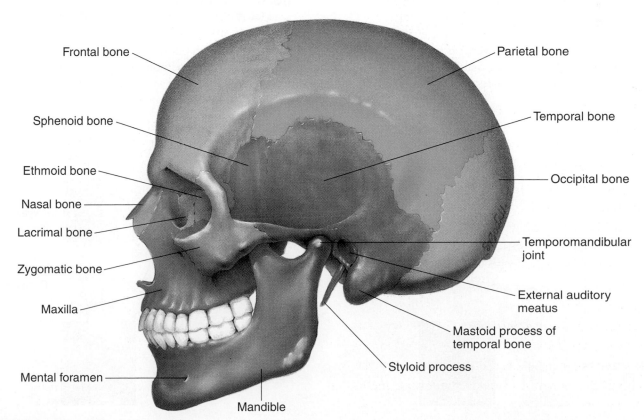

FIGURE 41-1B Bones of the skull

FIGURE 41-2 Types of joints: A. Ball joint. B and C. Hinge joints

- **Extension**: Increasing the angle between two bones (Figure 41-3B). For example, straightening the elbow.
- **Rotation**: Circular motion in a ball-and-socket joint (Figure 41-3C). For example, the shoulder and hip joints, which can move in all directions.
- **Abduction**: Moving away from the midline (Figure 41-3D).
- **Adduction**: Moving toward the midline (Figure 41-3E).

Muscles. There are about 650 muscles in the body (Figures 41-4A and 41-4B on page 706). The muscles work in groups. There are three kinds of muscles:

1. **Cardiac muscle** forms the wall of the heart.
2. **Voluntary muscles** are skeletal muscles that are attached to bones. When we wish to pick up something, for instance, we can make our muscles contract and perform the necessary movements.

3. **Involuntary** or **visceral muscles** form the walls of organs. These muscles operate without our conscious control.

Muscles receive their names in three ways:

1. Their location. For example, rectus femoris near the femur
2. Their shape. For example, trapezius—trapezoidal shape
3. Their action. For example, flexors—bring about flexion

You can easily locate the major muscle groups responsible for an activity if you remember that:

- Muscles can only shorten (contract) and lengthen (relax). Contraction occurs when nerves bring the message (**stimulus**) to the muscle cells. Muscles relax when there is no stimulus.
- Muscles have two points of attachment to the bone. As they stretch from one point (**origin**) to the other (**insertion**), they cross over one or more joints.

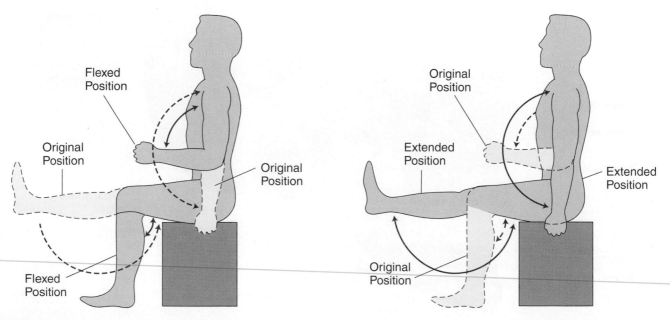

FIGURE 41-3A Flexion—bending a joint

FIGURE 41-3B Extension—straightening a joint

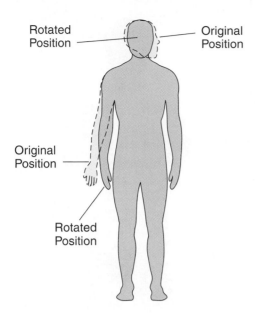

FIGURE 41-3C Rotation—moving a joint in a circular motion

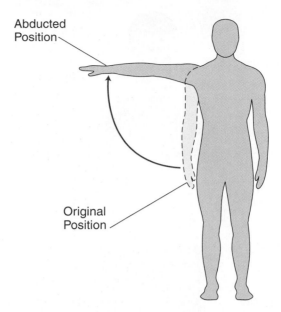

FIGURE 41-3D Abduction—moving an extremity away from the body

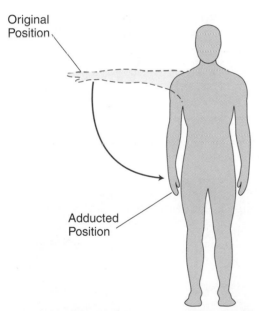

FIGURE 41-3E Adduction—moving an extremity back toward the body

- Muscles are not inserted directly into bones. Rather, they are connected to the bone by strong, fibrous bands of connective tissue called **tendons**. Ligaments support bones at joints.
- As muscles contract, they shorten, pulling their points of origin and insertion closer together. For example, bending the forearm at the elbow takes place when the biceps muscle contracts. The biceps muscle is on the anterior arm and extends from the shoulder to below the elbow. At the same time, the triceps muscle relaxes. This muscle is attached to the posterior shoulder and to the arm below the elbow. To straighten the arm at the elbow, the triceps contracts and the biceps relaxes.

Clinical Information ALERT

There about 650 skeletal muscles in the body, which provide approximately 23% of a female's and 40% of a male's body weight. There are more than 230 movable and semimovable joints in the body. There are 30 muscles in the face. It takes 17 muscles to smile and 43 muscles to frown. The smallest muscle is the stapedius. The largest muscle is the gluteus maximus, and the strongest is the masseter. The jaw muscles provide about 200 pounds of force to bring the back teeth together when chewing food. If all the body muscles pulled in one direction simultaneously, 25 tons of force would be created. The longest muscle in the body is the sartorius, which enables you to sit cross-legged. The smallest motor unit (3 muscle cells) is an external eye muscle. The external eye muscle is the most active muscle in the body. Scientists estimate that this muscle may move more than 100,000 times a day. Contraction of skeletal muscles provides the greatest source of body heat. ■

- The more muscles are used, the more powerful they become. The less muscles are used, the weaker they become.

FIGURE 41-4A Major muscles of the body, anterior view

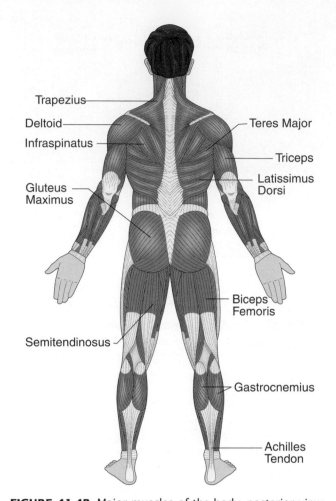

FIGURE 41-4B Major muscles of the body, posterior view

COMMON CONDITIONS

Many conditions can affect the bones, muscles, tendons, ligaments, and joints. Often, when one of these structures is diseased or injured, the surrounding tissues are also involved.

Bursitis

Bursae are small sacs of fluid found around joints. They help to reduce friction when muscles move. At times, the bursae can become inflamed and the tissues around a joint may become painful. This condition is known as **bursitis**. Treatment of bursitis includes:

- Applications of heat to promote healing
- Immobilization so that the joint cannot move, to relieve pain around the joint
- Removal of excess fluid from the joint by aspiration with a needle
- Administration of steroids

Arthritis

The term **arthritis** (Figure 41-5) means inflammation of the joints. It may develop following an acute injury, or it

FIGURE 41-5 These deformities, caused by rheumatoid arthritis, make hand movement difficult.

may be chronic and progressive. The most common forms of chronic arthritis are:

1. **Rheumatoid arthritis (RA)** affects the joint tissues and the joint lining, and can affect any other body system. It is a serious form of arthritis that can occur

in persons of any age. The cause is not specifically known. It is believed to be an autoimmune response. It usually follows an intermittent course. RA has **exacerbations**, or times in which the condition seems to worsen, and **remissions**, or times in which the disease appears stable. The involved joints may feel hot to touch. The condition causes reduced joint function and deformities. These can be severe and disabling.

2. **Osteoarthritic joint disease (OJD)** or **degenerative joint disease (DJD)** affects the cartilage covering the ends of the bones that form a joint. Cartilage breaks down and the ends of the bones rub together, causing pain and deformity. The joints most often affected are the weight-bearing joints. Several factors seem to contribute to the disease process, including:

   – aging
   – trauma
   – obesity

   The most common symptom of osteoarthritis is pain. This is usually described as a deep, aching pain that occurs after exercise, weight bearing, or exertion. It is often relieved by rest. Changes in the weather may also cause pain. Other symptoms include limited ability to move and stiffness, particularly upon arising in the morning. This also may occur after strenuous exercise or physical overactivity. In some individuals, an audible grating sound can be heard in the joints during movement. Osteoarthritis may cause redness and swelling in the joints. Conditions such as obesity and stress aggravate the symptoms.

3. **Gout** (gouty arthritis) is a metabolic disease that can be severely disabling. It is caused by increased uric acid in the bloodstream, which deposits in the joints and forms crystals that cause pain. It can occur in any joint, but is most common in the feet and legs. The great toe is often the first joint affected. Gout also follows a course of remission and exacerbation. It can lead to complete disability, hypertension, and chronic renal disease. The cause is unknown, but it is thought to be caused by a genetic defect in the ability to metabolize uric acid. The affected joints may be red or cyanotic in appearance. The patient may have a low-grade fever during this time. After the initial,

painful period, symptoms subside. The condition goes into remission and the patient will be pain-free for a period of time. The next attack is usually more painful and severe than the first. Eventually, chronic disease sets in. It is marked by pain, tenderness, and swelling in the joints. Other body systems may be affected in this stage. Dietary restrictions are used to reduce the uric acid level in the blood. The dietitian will plan a diet that restricts the amount of red meat and foods rich in purines.

Arthritis can cause mild discomfort to severe deformities and disability. Patients with arthritis are at high risk of contractures (Figure 41-6). If permitted by your facility, place patients with this condition in the prone position periodically. This reduces the risk of contractures of the hips and knees. Avoid placing pillows under the knees or elevating the knee area of the bed. Using a small, flat pillow under the head and neck is best. A large pillow pushes the neck into a position of flexion. You may be assigned to perform range-of-motion exercises on patients with arthritis. Be very gentle. Avoid moving joints past the point of resistance.

Treatment of arthritis includes:

- Relief of pain
- Balance of rest and exercise
- Joint immobilization where there is pain
- Weight control to relieve pressure on the joints
- Medication to relieve pain and reduce the inflammation
- Physical therapy when inflammation subsides, to maintain joint mobility
- Replacement of badly damaged joints by surgery
- Use of splints, braces, and adaptive equipment to enable the patient to get the most range of motion from injured joints
- Exercise of arthritic joints in warm water (with or without whirlpool action) to maintain function and relieve pain
- Prevention of deformities and contractures

FIGURE 41-6 This patient has many problems with her legs, including arthritic deformities and contractures.

Osteoporosis

Osteoporosis is a metabolic disorder of the bones. It is most common in elderly females, but can occur in males. Bone mass is lost, causing bones to become porous and spongy (Figure 41-7). Because of this, affected bones are at very high risk for fracture. Fractures can occur spontaneously, such as when the patient is walking. They can also occur when the patient is moved or turned in bed or during transfers.

The cause of osteoporosis is unknown. It is thought to result from years of inadequate calcium intake. Other potential causes are declining adrenal function, faulty protein metabolism, estrogen deficiency, and lack of exercise or activity.

Signs and Symptoms. The first sign of osteoporosis is usually a fracture. Commonly, the patient moves or lifts something and hears a "pop" or snapping sound in a bone. This frequently occurs in the lower back or hip. The patient who is walking may suddenly fall. In this case, the fall is the *result* of the fracture; in most falls, the opposite is true. After the initial incident, the area is very painful, particularly upon movement. Sometimes the onset of osteoporosis begins with a curvature of the spine and loss of height. The back progressively weakens, straining the neck, hips, and low back. Spontaneous fractures may occur during movement or as a result of a minor injury.

Treatment. The goals of treatment are to prevent further fractures and control pain. Gentle range-of-motion and other exercises may be ordered. Splints, braces, and other devices may be ordered to support weakened bones. Female patients may be given estrogen replacement and other drugs to replace calcium and bone mass. For bone to withstand mechanical stresses, old bone mass is constantly being broken down and new bone formed. This is called *bone remodeling*. Disruption of bone remodeling can lead to osteoporosis and other disorders. *Bisphosphonates* are a class of medications that inhibit the breakdown of bones. These drugs are a newer method of preventing and treating osteoporosis. Patients taking drugs in this category have specific requirements for eating, drinking, and maintaining an upright position. The nurse and the care plan will provide information about special monitoring.

You must handle the patient very gently. If you are assigned to perform range-of-motion exercises, do so slowly and carefully. Avoid stretching the joint past the point of resistance. Use a mechanical lift for transfers whenever possible. This is less traumatic than pulling on the patient. Make sure you have extra help for all procedures in which you will be moving or positioning the patient. Follow the care plan exactly in the care of the patient.

Fibromyalgia

Fibromyalgia is a common chronic pain syndrome for which there is no known cause or cure. It affects more women than men. The area between the shoulder blades and the bottom of the neck is often painful. The pain is described as either a general soreness or a gnawing ache, and stiffness is usually worst in the morning. Although this is a common problem, it is very controversial. Some physicians believe that there is no physical cause, and that psychiatric problems or sleep disorders are responsible for the patient's symptoms. The condition can be very painful and interfere with the patient's quality of life and daily activities. To be diagnosed with this condition, the patient must meet certain criteria, such as:

- Having pain on both sides of the body
- Having pain both above and below the waist
- Having pain upon palpation in at least 11 of 18 specified body sites (Figure 41-8)

Signs and Symptoms. Signs and symptoms of fibromyalgia are:

- Pain and stiffness
- Feeling abnormally tired
- Waking up tired
- Pain upon touch in certain areas of the body

Treatment. Treatment involves pain medications and exercise. Muscle-relaxant medications and antidepressants are sometimes used. Some patients use alternative and complementary therapies to relieve pain and stiffness. The most common complementary therapies used to treat this condition are:

- Massage
- Biofeedback
- Acupuncture
- Hypnosis

FIGURE 41-7 Bone loss from osteoporosis causes painful, disabling fractures in both sexes. About 40% of women and 13% of men will suffer a bone fracture due to osteoporosis in their lifetime. (Courtesy of Sharmila Majumdar, PhD, Professor, University of California, San Francisco)

FIGURE 41-8 The patient must have pain at 11 of 18 specific areas of the body for a diagnosis of fibromyalgia.

- Relaxation, meditation, and other forms of stress management

Because the cause of fibromyalgia is not known, there is no prevention or cure for this condition. Fibromyalgia complicates treatment for many other medical problems because of the underlying pain and difficulty in assuming some positions necessary for examination and treatment.

Tips: Most patients with fibromyalgia are middle-aged women. They are often very deconditioned because pain and fatigue have caused them to limit movement and stop exercising. The pain and fatigue of fibromyalgia often improve with mild exercise, and the physician will usually order some type of exercise program. Encourage the patient to adhere to the program, but not to push to the point of exhaustion. Patients should start exercising slowly, and should not try to keep the same exercise pace as they did before the fibromyalgia developed. A restful night's sleep will improve comfort and mood. Be attentive to the patient's needs for uninterrupted sleep. Plan your care to allow the patient to sleep for prolonged periods without interruption.

Fractures

A **fracture** is any break in the continuity of a bone. Falls are the most common cause of fractures. Fractures (Figure 41-9) are classified by the type of break in the bone and whether or not the skin is broken:

- A **complete fracture** involves a break across the entire cross-section of the bone. It is often displaced, or improperly aligned, and must be reduced and straightened.
- An **incomplete fracture** involves only part of the cross-section of bone.

- A **closed** or **simple fracture** (Figure 41-9A) occurs when the skin is intact and not broken.
- An **open** or **compound fracture** (Figure 41-9B) occurs when the skin over the fracture is broken. The bone may or may not protrude.
- A **pathologic fracture** is a fracture in a diseased bone. It occurs as a result of osteoporosis, a tumor, or cancer.

The pattern of a fracture describes the manner in which the bone is broken:

- A **greenstick fracture** (Figure 41-9C) occurs when only one side of the bone is broken and the other side is bent. This fracture is common in children, whose bone growth is incomplete. The bones tend to bend like young trees; hence the name "greenstick" fracture.
- A **transverse fracture** (Figure 41-9D) breaks completely across the bone.
- An **oblique fracture** (Figure 41-9E) runs at an angle across the bone.
- A **spiral fracture** (Figure 41-9F) twists around the bone.
- A **comminuted fracture** (Figure 41-9G) involves shattering and splintering of the bone into more than three fragments.
- A **depressed fracture** (Figure 41-9H) is seen only in fractures of the skull and face. This type of fracture depresses the bone and drives fragments inward.
- A **compression fracture** (Figure 41-9I) is seen only in the vertebrae of the spine. This type of fracture collapses the bone inward.
- An **avulsion fracture** (Figure 41-9J) occurs when a bone fragment is pulled off at the point of ligament or tendon attachment.
- An **impacted fracture** (Figure 41-9K) occurs when a fragment from one bone is wedged into another bone.

Signs and Symptoms. Signs and symptoms of fractures will vary with the type of fracture and location. Fractures are painful conditions. Movement is limited, or the patient may be unable to move the injured area. The skin surrounding the fracture may appear deformed. Edema is common. **Ecchymosis**, or bruising, may occur. Some parts of the body, such as the area over the femur, are very **vascular**. Areas that are vascular contain many blood vessels. They bleed readily under the skin. An ecchymosis the size of an adult's fist over the femur indicates loss of approximately one pint of blood.

Treatment. A new fracture is usually treated in the hospital emergency department. Admission for surgical correction of the fracture may be necessary. The immediate goals of care are to:

- Control pain
- Prevent complications of immobility
- Prevent or reduce edema
- Keep the fracture in good alignment
- Keep the fractured extremity immobile

(A) Closed (simple, complete)

(B) Open (compound)

(C) Greenstick (incomplete)

(D) Transverse

(E) Oblique

(F) Spiral

(G) Comminuted

(H) Depressed

(I) Compression

Fracture

(J) Avulsion

(K) Impacted

FIGURE 41-9 Types and patterns of fractures

Fractures of any kind are treated by keeping the part that is injured immobilized in proper position until healing takes place. Injured bones take from several weeks to several months to heal. Immobilization is achieved through the use of:

- Pins (Figure 41-10)
- Screws
- Splints
- Bone plates
- Casting
- Traction

Special beds and attachments are used to make nursing care easier. The patient may be placed on a Stryker frame or a CircOlectric bed.

Be sure you know how to operate each bed and attachment before attempting care. In many facilities, a nurse must be present when the bed is turned. Know and follow the policy of your facility.

FIGURE 41-10 Certain fractures are repaired using plates, pins, or screws.

You will assist patients who have fractures with range-of-motion exercises several times each day. Check with the nurse or care plan for specific instructions. In most cases, you will not exercise the fractured extremity. You may be assigned to exercise the patient's joints above and below the cast to keep them mobile. For fractured arms and legs, you may be permitted to exercise fingers and toes. Exercising the rest of the patient's body is important. The exercise prevents complications related to immobility and inactivity.

You may also assist the patient with coughing and deep breathing exercises to prevent pneumonia. When working with patients with fractures, encourage adequate fluid intake. The increased fluid liquefies secretions that accumulate in the lungs. Coughing and deep breathing exercises are the same as those used in postoperative care. A *trapeze* (Figure 41-11) may be attached to the bed to assist the patient with movement. The nurse will teach you how to move and reposition the patient without interfering with the traction. The casted extremity is elevated on pillows if traction is not used.

Treatment for patients with fractures begins soon after admission. The type of treatment is determined by the location and type of fracture, and method of fracture reduction. Patients with fractures will be evaluated by physical and occupational therapists. Therapists will design rehabilitation programs to meet the patients' needs and help them to regain as much mobility as possible.

Care of Patients with Casts. Two types of cast materials are commonly used:

1. Plaster of Paris, which can take up to 48 hours to dry completely
2. Fiberglass, which dries very rapidly

FIGURE 41-11 The overhead trapeze helps the patient to move in bed. The trapeze is not used by patients with some back injuries and back surgeries, because independent positioning can worsen the condition or cause further injuries.

Cast material is wet when it is applied. During the drying period, the cast gives off heat. Special care for the newly casted patient includes:

- Supporting the cast and body in good alignment with pillows covered by cloth pillowcases, and keeping the cast uncovered.
- Elevating the casted extremity on a pillow as instructed. When positioning a patient with a leg cast, elevate the foot higher than the hip. The fingers should be higher than the elbow. Avoid placing the cast on a flat surface. Avoid placing anything plastic under a wet cast. Check the skin distal to the cast frequently for signs of poor circulation.
- Turning the patient frequently to permit air circulation to all parts of the cast. Maintain support. Use the palm of your hand, not your fingers, to support the wet cast.
- Not positioning the cast against the footboard or side rail. Leaving the cast open to air until it dries is best. If the patient is cold, cover the cast loosely with a sheet. Avoid tucking the sheet under the mattress. A bed cradle may be used, if necessary. The greatest area of heat loss is the head. Covering the upper body and back and top of the head with a blanket may help keep the patient warm.

Clinical Information ALERT

To warm a patient quickly, fashion a hat using 6-inch stockinette. This is the sock-like material that is used to protect a leg before a cast is applied. Cut a length of stockinette, then fasten it closed with a rubber band. Warm the hat in the blanket warmer or microwave, if available. Applying a warm hat helps to warm and comfort a cool patient quickly, and he or she will appreciate your concern. ■

- Closely observing the uncasted areas of the extremities, such as the fingers and toes, for signs of decreased circulation. Report coldness, cyanosis, swelling, increased pain, numbness, or tingling immediately.
- Closely observing skin areas around the cast edges for signs of irritation (Figure 41-12). Rough edges should be covered with adhesive strips to prevent skin irritation.

Recall the following key of reportables when checking the patient:

- C = color
- M = motion
- E = edema
- T = temperature

FIGURE 41-12 Check the skin around the edges of the cast regularly for signs of irritation. Check the circulation in the toes.

FIGURE 41-13 The spica cast is a full body cast that is commonly used to treat hip fracture and after hip surgery in children.

Safety ALERT

A fiberglass cast dries immediately. A plaster arm or leg cast will take 24 to 48 hours to dry completely. A plaster body or spica cast will take 48 to 72 hours to dry. Proper positioning of the cast is essential during the drying period to prevent depressions that can cause pressure and edema. Never use a table or hard object to support the cast during the drying period. Avoid rubber or plastic pillows, which increase heat under the cast. When the cast is dry, it will look white and shiny. It will not appear soft or damp. ■

Special Care After the Cast Is Dry. After the cast has dried completely:

- Turn the patient to the noncasted side. This is particularly important in moving a patient with a body cast (**spica cast**) (Figure 41-13), because turning to the casted side may crack the cast.
- Always support the cast when turning or moving a patient.
- Encourage use of a trapeze to assist the patient in helping herself.
- Tape edges of casts to prevent pressure and abrasive areas, if edges were not covered when the cast was applied.
- Use plastic to protect cast edges that are near the genitals and buttocks, to help prevent soiling during toileting.

After the cast dries, you may observe changes that indicate infection or ulceration under the cast:

- Odor from the cast
- Drainage through the cast

The care plan may instruct you to keep the casted extremity elevated to prevent edema. A sling (Figure 41-14) may

be used to elevate an arm cast when the patient is out of bed. A wheelchair with an elevated leg rest is used for patients with leg casts. Cover the cast with plastic during bathing. Keep small objects from getting inside the cast. The patient may complain of an itching sensation under the cast. Discourage him or her from placing objects down the cast to scratch. This could cause a skin injury and infection. Report complaints of itching to the nurse.

Care of Patients in Traction. Traction is designed to pull two body areas slightly apart to:

- Relieve pressure.
- Help tightly contracted (spasmodic) muscles relax.
- Keep them in proper position as healing takes place.

Traction is of two types:

FIGURE 41-14 A sling may be ordered to elevate the hand and wrist.

- Skin traction, where traction is applied to the skin or outside of the body (Figure 41-15)
- Skeletal traction, where traction is applied through the skin to the bone

Traction is applied by attaching weights to a part of the body above or below the area to be treated. The patient's body weight serves as **countertraction** by pulling in the direction opposite to the traction. Belts, head halters, or tapes may be applied to the patient's skin to hold the traction. Traction may be applied continuously or intermittently.

Skeletal traction (Figure 41-16) uses tongs or pins placed into bones with weights applied to the tongs or pins. Skeletal traction is always continuous once applied. The weights for skeletal traction must not be lifted or removed until the traction is to be discontinued.

When patients are in traction:

- Review the correct placement of straps and weights with the therapist or nurse. Get instructions for mov-

ing the patient up in bed and turning to the sides, as ordered.

- Do not disturb the weights or permit them to swing, drop, or rest on any surface. Avoid moving, dropping, or releasing the weights. They should not touch the bed, swing back and forth freely, or rest upon any object or surface. The water bag or weight hangs motionless at the end of the bed.
- Keep the patient in good alignment in the center of the bed. Make sure that the body is acting properly as countertraction by keeping the head of the bed low. The feet should not rest against the end of the bed.
- Check under straps and belts for areas of pressure or irritation.
- Make sure straps and belts are smooth, straight, and properly secured.
- Keep bed covers off ropes and pulleys.

Not all patients remain in traction continually. If **pelvic belt traction** (Figure 41-17), or **cervical traction** with a head halter (Figure 41-18), is to be discontinued, take the following steps:

FIGURE 41-16 Skeletal traction immobilizes a body part by attaching weights directly to the patient's bones with pins, screws, wires, or tongs.

Water Weight Bag

FIGURE 41-15 Buck's traction is a type of skin traction that may be used for a hip fracture. It may be used to stabilize the bone before surgery, or until the fracture heals in patients who are not candidates for surgery.

FIGURE 41-17 Pelvic belt traction. A bag filled with water is often used as a weight. This treatment is not commonly used. Other methods of treating low back pain have proven more effective.

FIGURE 41-18 Cervical traction. This method is infrequently used, but is effective in relieving pain and spasticity in some patients.

- Slowly raise the weights to the bed. Avoid abrupt or jerking movements, as this may cause the patient pain. If two sets of weights are being used, raise them at the same time and rate.

- Remove the weight holder and weights from the connection with the halter or belt and place them on the floor. Remove the head halter or pelvic belt.

- To reapply traction, reverse the procedure.

- Remember never to jerk or drop the weights quickly or lower them unevenly. Always apply weights smoothly to avoid causing the patient pain.

Bedmaking. Bedmaking for orthopedic patients varies according to the type of traction.

- Two half sheets are often used in place of a large sheet for the bottom.

- Bottom linens may be changed from top to bottom rather than side to side.

- The top linen is arranged according to the patient's special needs. Half sheets and folded bath blankets can be worked around the traction to keep the patient covered and comfortable.

Fractured Hip

Hip fractures are the most common type of fracture in the elderly. It is not unusual for a patient to be admitted to the hospital for treatment of another problem, then fall and break a hip. The most common cause of hip fractures is falls, but fractures may also occur because of osteoporosis. In this case, the patient may hear a popping sound in the bone, then fall. An X-ray will reveal a fracture. The term "hip fracture" really is not accurate. This term refers to a fracture anywhere in the upper third or head of the femur.

Signs and Symptoms of Hip Fracture. A patient with a fractured hip is usually found on the floor. He or she will be unable to get up or move the injured leg. The leg on the affected side may be shortened and in a position of external rotation. In this position, the toes point outward. The shortening and rotation occur because the strong muscles in the upper leg contract. This causes the bone ends to override each other.

The patient will complain of severe pain in the hip. The pain of a hip fracture is usually localized in the hip. Some patients complain of pain in the knee. This may be confusing or misleading. Edema and ecchymosis may be present in the hip, thigh, groin, or lower pelvic area.

Emergency Care. Avoid moving the patient until you are instructed to do so by a nurse. You will use a sheet, backboard, or other device to move the patient. Avoid excessive movement, which can worsen the injury. Moving a patient with a hip fracture requires four or five individuals. The patient is logrolled onto the lifting device. The device is lifted to the bed or stretcher. You may be assigned to monitor the patient's vital signs and check for signs of shock. Some patients are treated with Buck's traction.

Open Reduction/Internal Fixation. The most common treatment for a fractured hip is a surgical procedure called **open reduction/internal fixation**. This means the surgeon makes an incision, manipulates the fractured bone into alignment, and then inserts a device such as a nail, pin, or rod to hold the ends of the fractured bone in place. If you are assigned to a patient who has had this surgery, you must:

- Know how to position the patient in bed. It is important to avoid adduction and internal and external rotation of the affected hip.

- Know the correct procedure if the patient is allowed to ambulate. The patient is usually not allowed to bear weight on the affected side for a few weeks after surgery.

Difficult SITUATIONS

A patient who has had hip surgery will probably have physician orders for anti-embolism hosiery and an incentive spirometer. A pressure-relieving mattress may be ordered. Following hip surgery, the patient will be at high risk for pressure ulcer development, particularly on the heels. Take active measures to prevent pressure. Follow the care plan. Check the skin regularly for redness, irritation, and breakdown. ■

Total Hip Arthroplasty

Total hip arthroplasty (THA), or insertion of a hip prosthesis (artificial body part), is a common procedure. This surgery is done because the patient:

- Has fractured a hip and the bone cannot be set by traditional methods

- Has degenerative arthritis that has caused the hip joint to deteriorate

The patient's hip joint is surgically removed and a metal or synthetic ball and socket are inserted (Figure 41-19).

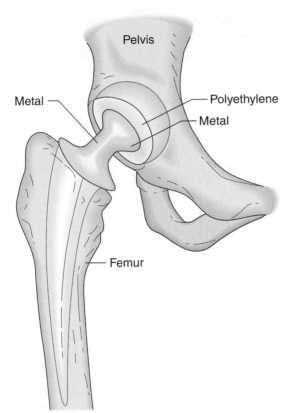

FIGURE 41-19 A hip prosthesis replaces the ball of the femur and the socket when the patient has a total hip arthroplasty.

There are specific body positions that the patient must avoid to prevent damage to the new joint.

Caring for the Patient with Hip Surgery.

After hip surgery, the following general procedures are commonly ordered:

- A trapeze is attached to the bed to assist with movement. The patient is instructed not to press down on the foot of the affected leg when using the trapeze.
- Anti-embolism stockings are applied.
- A fracture bedpan is used initially for elimination. When the patient is able to use the toilet, an elevated toilet seat is used.
- The head of the bed is not elevated more than 45° without a specific order.
- Avoid acute flexion of the hip and legs. The physician will give directions for positioning and the degree of flexion permitted.
- Patients who have had hip replacement surgery will usually have a special pillow, called an **abduction pillow**, to keep the legs apart (Figure 41-20). This is particularly important when the patient is turned on the side. The patient will be instructed to avoid crossing the legs, which can cause a dislocation. Keep the pillow in place when the patient is turned to the side. Support the lower leg on pillows, if necessary.

FIGURE 41-20 An abduction pillow is commonly used after hip surgery to keep the legs from crossing over at the ankles or adducting.

- Maintain the affected leg in good alignment without internal or external rotation.
- Avoid rolling the affected leg toward the other leg when turning the patient. Make sure the abduction pillow is in place during turning to prevent the legs from crossing.
- Support the affected leg when moving the patient to the side of the bed.
- Instruct the patient to:
  - avoid sleeping on the stomach or operative side.
  - avoid crossing the legs, as this may cause hip dislocation.
  - avoid sitting on low chairs or couches. Position the patient only in chairs with arms where the knees remain lower than the hips.
  - avoid leaning forward while sitting, and avoid picking up items from the floor or bending to put on shoes and socks.
  - avoid flexing the hips more than 80° or rotating the foot and leg inward.
  - avoid raising the knee higher than the hip on the operative side.
  - keep the legs at least 3 to 6 inches apart when sitting, or use the abduction pillow.
  - avoid stretching the affected hip back.
  - avoid kneeling on one knee.
  - avoid turning the foot outward on the affected side.
  - avoid twisting the body away from the affected hip.
  - avoid standing with the toes pointed outward; keep the toes of the affected leg pointed forward when standing, sitting, or walking.
  - avoid swinging the affected leg outward away from the body.
  - avoid assuming a straddling position.

The physician will specify how long the patient must avoid weight bearing after surgery. The physical therapist will work with the patient to restore mobility. Some patients are able to ambulate soon after surgery. A walker, crutches, or cane are commonly used for a period of time after surgery. Some physicians do not permit full weight bearing for as long as four to six weeks. Initially, you will assist with procedures to prevent the complications of immobility. These include range-of-motion exercises of the unaffected extremities, turning and repositioning, and coughing and deep breathing exercises. Patients with hip surgery are at very high risk of developing heel pressure ulcers. Follow the care plan and get specific instructions from the nurse for positions and techniques to use for turning and repositioning the patient. Relieve pressure from the heels and check the patient's skin carefully each day for signs of red or open areas.

Total Joint Replacement

Sometimes joints are completely replaced because of arthritis or severe damage to the joint. The goal of joint replacement surgery is to relieve pain, which is often so severe that the patient avoids using the joint as much as possible. This weakens the muscles and worsens the problem. Hip and knee replacements are the most common, but joint replacement surgery can be done on the ankle, foot, shoulder, elbow, and fingers. Postoperative care will vary with the surgical procedure. General care for joint replacement surgery includes:

- Preventing infection
- Preventing blood clots
- Administering anticoagulant medication to thin the blood
- Applying anti-embolism hosiery (Unit 29)
- Doing exercises to increase blood flow in the leg muscles, if not contraindicated
- Using sequential compression therapy (Unit 29)

Continuous Passive Motion. Continuous passive motion (CPM) therapy (Figure 41-22) may be ordered following joint replacement and other orthopedic procedures. Moving a joint is painful for most patients postoperatively. If the patient fails to move the joint, stiffness and limited range of motion will occur. Months of physical therapy will be necessary for the patient to fully recover. CPM therapy prevents stiffness by delivering a form of passive range-of-motion exercise so the joint is moved without the patient's muscles being used. CPM therapy is effortless for the patient. A machine moves the affected joint through a prescribed range of motion for an extended period of time. CPM therapy:

GUIDELINES *for*

Caring for Patients with THA

The patient should **not:**

- Flex the hip more than 90° (Figure 41-21A).
- Cross the affected leg over the midline of the body, whether in bed or sitting in a chair (Figure 41-21B).
- Internally rotate the hip on the affected side (Figure 41-21C).

Never do passive range-of-motion exercises on a joint that has had surgery, unless you are specifically instructed to do so—and then only if you have been given instructions as to which actions can safely be performed.

The patient will have limited weight bearing on the affected leg for several days or weeks after surgery.

FIGURE 41-21B The patient with a new hip prosthesis should never cross the affected leg over the midline of the body.

FIGURE 41-21A The patient with a new hip prosthesis should never flex the affected hip more than 90°.

FIGURE 41-21C The patient with a new hip prosthesis should never internally rotate the hip on the affected side.

Difficult SITUATIONS

A patient who has had hip replacement surgery may usually have the head of the bed elevated up to 45° for comfort. Never elevate the head more than this without specific permission from the nurse. Some physicians permit greater elevation. Try to limit elevation of the head to 30 minutes at a time, if possible. In any event, do not let the patient remain in a position of hip flexion for more than 90 minutes, because longer periods increase the risk of prosthesis dislocation. Positioning the patient in the supine position, with the affected leg in extension, for 1 hour three times a day will help prevent contractures of the hip joint. ∎

FIGURE 41-22 The continuous passive motion (CPM) machine performs passive range-of-motion exercises on the affected joint without straining the patient's muscles. (Courtesy of OrthoRehab, Inc.)

- Enhances circulation, which lowers the risk of blood clots
- Reduces edema
- Promotes collagen formation within the joint, which enhances healing
- Reduces scarring
- Decreases stiffness
- Improves range of motion (which decreases postoperatively without movement)
- Reduces the risk of complications in the joint, such as contractures and adhesions
- Helps reduce pain

Many orthopedic surgeons prescribe CPM therapy following knee replacement and other surgical procedures. CPM devices are available for the knee, ankle, toes, jaw, shoulder, elbow, wrist, and hand. Indications for using CPM therapy are:

- Crush injuries of the hand without fractures or dislocations
- Burn injuries
- Stable fractures
- Joint and tendon repair
- Surgical release of contractures
- Knee or hip replacement
- Reconstructive surgery on bone, cartilage, tendons, and ligaments
- Prolonged joint immobilization

The physician prescribes how the CPM unit should be used. He or she orders the settings on the CPM unit that control the speed, duration of use, range of motion, pause settings, hours of use per day, and rate of increase of motion. The directions for use will vary slightly depending on the body area being treated, the type of CPM machine used, and physicians' orders. In some facilities, this procedure is done only by licensed nurses. In others, the nursing assistant can set up the unit, but the nurse must check the settings for accuracy. This is a key step. Improper settings can damage reconstructive work in the joint. Follow your facility policies and procedures.

Contraindications for CPM therapy include:

- Untreated infections
- Unstable fractures
- Known or suspected blood clots (deep vein thrombosis)
- Hemorrhage

If the patient develops any of the following signs or symptoms upon using the device, stop the unit and inform the nurse promptly:

- Fever
- Increasing redness or irritation
- Increasing warmth
- Edema
- Bleeding
- Increased or persistent pain

Do not proceed with treatment until the nurse informs you that the physician has approved continued use of the device.

Check the patient periodically when using the CPM machine. Each time the settings are changed, stay with the patient for several cycles to be sure she tolerates the change. Check the skin every 2 hours for signs of redness, irritation, or breakdown. Report problems and abnormalities to the nurse.

Safety ALERT

Make sure the side rail is up on the side where the CPM unit is placed. Position the edge of the tibia sling slightly above the support bar. ∎

PROCEDURE

90

ASSISTING WITH CONTINUOUS PASSIVE MOTION

 Note: Be sure this is a nursing assistant procedure at your facility.

 Note: These instructions are generic and are not device-specific. The person setting up the device should be trained in use of the specific device, and have an operating manual for that device.

1. Carry out initial procedure actions. Apply the principles of standard precautions during this procedure if contact with wound drainage or nonintact skin is likely.

2. Gather equipment:
   - CPM unit
   - Soft goods kit, if available OR
   - Sheepskin foot pad
   - Tibia/femur sling
   - Hip pad
   - Velcro fasteners

3. Check the unit for safety and stability. Make sure that the attachments are tight, the frame is stable, and the electric controls work. Have the nurse adjust the settings according to the doctor's orders, or follow facility policy for setting the speed and degree of flexion. (In some facilities, assistants are permitted to adjust the settings. If this is the case, have the nurse check the settings before proceeding.) Stop the machine in full extension.

4. Raise the side rail on the side of the bed where you will be placing the unit.

5. Position the CPM unit on the bed and secure the attachment, depending on the type of device being used.

6. Fasten the foot pad to the foot plate with a Velcro fastener.

7. Attach the tibia/femur sling (wide section toward the footrest). Fasten the Velcro closures under the sling.

8. Apply the hip pad to the hinge area of the adjustment bar. Position the femur sling straps over the hinges, then fasten underneath with Velcro.

9. Fit the CPM machine to the patient's leg length by lengthening or shortening the frame.

10. Align the knee joint with the knee hinge, then position the knee approximately 1 inch below the knee joint line (Figure 41-23A).

11. Center the leg on the unit. Avoid pressure on the side and middle of the knee joint.

12. Adjust the foot pad so the patient's foot is comfortable and well supported (Figure 41-23B). The leg should be lifted at the thigh with no pressure on the foot. Secure the Velcro straps across the thigh and top of foot (Figure 41-23C).

13. When the leg is in the proper position, give the patient the control (Figure 41-23D). Instruct the patient to start the unit. Instruct the patient to turn the unit off and use the call signal if the exercise causes extreme pain, or the unit malfunctions.

FIGURE 41-23A Position the leg straight, with the toes upright. Line the knee up with the marking at the hinge.

FIGURE 41-23B Make sure the foot is comfortable and well supported. Add padding if needed for patient comfort.

continues

PROCEDURE 90 CONTINUED

FIGURE 41-23C Secure the straps across the leg and foot. Make sure the strap is not too tight.

14. Stay with the patient for at least two full cycles to make sure she tolerates the procedure.

15. Return to check on the patient frequently when the unit is in use. Some devices have compliance monitors that allow you to check usage of the device. After the patient is experienced in the use of the CPM machine, he or she may be instructed to keep a record of the times the unit is used, or you may be required to document this information.

16. Carry out ending procedure actions.

FIGURE 41-23D Show the patient how to turn the unit on, then give her the switch. Stay in the room until the machine goes through at least two cycles if the unit is being used for the first time. (Courtesy of OrthoRehab, Inc.)

Compartment Syndrome

Compartment syndrome is a very painful condition that occurs when pressure within the muscles builds up, preventing blood and oxygen from reaching muscles and nerves. This is a serious complication that may develop following an injury or surgical procedure. It may also occur following athletic injuries, burns, snake bites, IV infiltration, frostbite, and musculoskeletal conditions in which there is no fracture. Patients of all ages can be affected.

Compartment syndrome is usually seen after a traumatic injury, such as a long bone fracture. It may develop if an injury or surgical site swells after a cast has been applied. A tough membrane, called *fascia*, surrounds the muscles in the arms and legs. Fascia does not expand readily. Compartment syndrome develops gradually over several hours. Bleeding or swelling occurs in the muscle tissue, under the fascia. In some cases, pressure from a cast or compression device also increases the pressure from the outside. If the swelling is not relieved, pressure on the muscles and nerves builds. Eventually, the pressure inside the fascia compartment will exceed the blood pressure, causing the capillaries to collapse. Blood flow to the muscles and nerves stops. If it is not restored promptly, tissue death begins.

Signs and Symptoms. The most common symptom of acute compartment syndrome is severe pain, especially when the muscle is moved. The pain may seem out of proportion to the injury. The patient may also complain of

- Severe pain when the muscle is gently stretched
- Tenderness when the area is touched gently
- Pain during deep breathing
- Tingling
- Burning
- Numbness
- Feeling tight or full in the affected muscle
- Abnormal sensations in the affected area
- Weakness or inability to use the muscle

You may observe:

- The color of the extremity may appear pale, cyanotic, or red
- The skin of an extremity with no cast may feel warm to touch
- The fingers or toes of a casted extremity may feel cool to touch
- Edema (swelling)

Difficult SITUATIONS

The most common location of compartment syndrome in adults is in a fractured tibia. The most common location of compartment syndrome in children is the humerus. ■

Loss of the pulse in the extremity is a late sign. Rapid identification and treatment of this condition is necessary.

Nursing Assistant Responsibilities. Follow the care plan and monitor patients with musculoskeletal injuries and casts frequently. Monitor for changes in the extremity. Check the color and temperature of the extremity distal to a cast. Notify the nurse if the color is abnormal. Ask the patient if he is able to move the fingers or toes. Notify the nurse promptly of any unusual findings. If the patient complains of severe pain, or if the pain is not relieved after the patient receives pain medication, notify the nurse promptly. This condition is frightening for the patient. Provide emotional support.

Compartment syndrome is a surgical emergency. The nurse will assess the patient and notify the physician of the findings. If compartment syndrome is suspected, the patient will be taken to surgery quickly to relieve the pressure. Follow facility policies and the nurse's instructions for preparing the patient for surgery.

Ruptured or Slipped Disc

It is possible for a disc to bulge (slip) out of place or for the soft center to rupture. In either case, pressure is placed on the spinal nerves (Figure 41-24). Depending on which disc is injured, the patient may experience, in different parts of the body:

- Pain
- Numbness
- Tingling
- Weakness of one or more muscles

Treatment. Treatment attempts to relieve pressure on the nerve roots. Early treatment is very conservative and includes rest, medication, ice, compresses, physical therapy, and exercise. Some people use complementary and alternative therapies, most commonly:

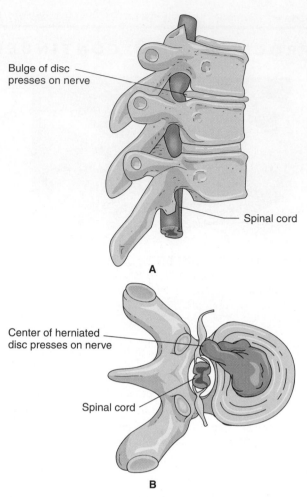

FIGURE 41-24 A. Uneven pressure causes the disc to bulge, putting pressure on the nerve root (slipped disc). B. A herniated (ruptured) disc applies pressure on the nerve root as the gel-like center oozes backward.

- Acupuncture
- Chiropractic
- Massage
- Yoga
- Biofeedback

If conservative attempts to relieve pressure fail, other methods will be used to relieve pressure on the spinal cord. These are:

1. Traction. This is an older treatment that is seldom used.
2. The physician may order a firm mattress or bedboards.
3. Surgery to remove the protruding portion of the disc (**laminectomy**). The surgery sometimes includes a fixation (**fusion**) of the vertebral bones.
4. A surgical procedure called **discectomy**. This is a minimally invasive procedure with rapid recovery. In this procedure, a tiny wand is inserted through the back into the disc. Tissue is removed through the wand, and the channel is thermally sealed. The wand is then removed. This may be done as an outpatient surgery in some facilities.

GUIDELINES *for*

Caring for Patients After Spinal Surgeries

- Monitor vital signs as ordered.
- Assist with coughing, deep breathing, and incentive spirometer treatments, as ordered.
- Monitor the dressing for bleeding and clear fluid leakage. If noted, inform the nurse promptly.
- Use the fracture bedpan for elimination.
- Inform the nurse if the patient is unable to void or voids less than 240 mL in 8 hours.

Caring for Patients with Cervical Surgery

- Do not remove the cervical collar.
- Encourage the patient to keep the head straight in midline position; avoid turning to sides.
- Support the patient's head, neck, and upper shoulders when repositioning or moving from lying to sitting to standing position, and when getting into and out of a chair.
- Observe for and report complications on one side of the body:
  - abnormal drooping of the eyelid
  - constricted pupil
  - eye that appears to be sinking into the orbit
  - lack of perspiration on one side of the face

Caring for Patients with Lumbar Surgery

- Turn every 2 hours or more often; logroll the patient when turning (Unit 15).
- Keep the spine in good alignment at all times.
- Advise the patient to call for help with moving; he or she should avoid turning self.
- Instruct the patient to avoid twisting the back.
- During the first postoperative week, the patient should sit in a straight-backed chair.
- Teach the patient to avoid prolonged sitting and avoid slumping.
- Remind the patient to use good body mechanics and bend from the knees and hips, not the waist.

Lower Extremity Amputation

You may care for patients who have had one or both legs surgically removed (amputated). A leg may have to undergo **amputation** because of circulatory problems, a malignancy, or an accident in which the leg was severely damaged.

It is common for people to experience **phantom pain** after the removal of a limb. Patients with phantom pain may feel pain or tingling where the limb used to be. These feelings may persist for months. The pain is real, although it is difficult to explain.

When you are positioning a patient who has had an amputation of the lower extremities, remember:

- Avoid abduction and flexion of the patient's hip— because the weight of the lower leg is not there, the hip on the affected side will quickly become contracted if flexion is allowed.
- If the patient has a below-the-knee amputation (BKA), avoid flexion of the knee, so that a contracture does not form.
- Avoid placing pillows under the amputated extremity. Position the leg flat on the bed.
- Avoid elevating the head of the bed for prolonged periods.
- Keep the legs in a position of adduction. A trochanter roll is helpful. Avoid positioning the patient with pillows between the legs.
- Assist the patient to lie in the prone position twice a day, if permitted.
- Encourage and assist the patient to move in bed frequently.

After the surgery, the patient will either have the stump wrapped with elastic bandage or will wear a stump shrinker. It is important that these be on at all times except during the bath. It is the nurse's responsibility to apply either of these items. If you notice that the bandage or shrinker is loose or needs to be reapplied, notify the nurse. The purpose of these items is to make sure that the stump heals in the appropriate shape.

If you bathe a patient with an amputation:

- Gently wash the stump with soap and warm water, rinse well, and pat dry.
- Observe the stump for:
  - redness
  - swelling
  - drainage from the incision
  - open areas in the incision or anywhere else on the stump
- Do not apply lotion to the stump. Lotion softens the skin, making safe prosthesis use difficult.
- Make sure the skin is protected before applying the prosthesis. Never apply a prosthesis over unprotected skin.

After an amputation, some patients are fitted with an artificial leg (prosthesis). They have to learn how to walk and sit when the prosthesis is worn. A prosthesis is custom-made for the person who will be wearing it. A special health care professional measures the patient and makes the prosthesis. The physical therapist teaches the patient how to apply the prosthesis and how to use it. If you are responsible for helping a patient put on a prosthesis, be sure you know how to attach and secure it, because each device is different.

Safety ALERT

Make sure that the stump shrinker, sock, or wrap is smooth, with no wrinkles or exposed skin. Inform the nurse promptly if the patient complains of throbbing under the stump shrinker. Throbbing is an indication of impaired circulation, a potentially serious complication. ■

Difficult SITUATIONS

When the stump is healed and the patient prepares to use the prosthesis, the physician may order special care. This involves not shaving the stump, as shaving increases the risk of rash and irritation. Bathing of the stump may be ordered for bedtime, because warm water may increase swelling and make application of the prosthesis difficult. The physician may also order alcohol rubs to the stump several times a day to toughen the skin. Avoid powders and lotions, which soften the skin. Monitor the stump for irritation and report to the nurse, if present. The stump sock may require frequent changing to avoid wetness. The socks must be handwashed. Muscle-strengthening exercises will be ordered to prepare the patient to lift the weight of the prosthesis. ■

Various types of materials are used to make prostheses. They need to be cleaned regularly, and the method of cleaning depends on what materials were used to make the prosthesis.

Wipe the inside of the prosthesis daily with a damp, soapy cloth to remove sweat and body oils. Rinse with a second damp cloth. Dry the inside of the socket well. Avoid placing a damp prosthesis on a patient. Never attempt to adjust the prosthesis. Consult the nurse if you believe an adjustment is necessary.

RANGE OF MOTION

Patients who have been ill or confined to bed are not as active, so joints may not move through the normal range of motion daily. Weakness and muscle wasting from lack of use is called **atrophy**. Over time, muscles become rigid. The joints do not move as freely as they once did. Joint movement may be painful because the muscles have shortened from lack of use. When the joint moves, the muscle stretches. This causes discomfort or pain, and the patient may move even less because of it.

Contractures and deformities develop when the patient is immobile. *Contractures* are disfigurements caused by muscle shortening. They are serious, painful complications of inactivity. Contractures make caring for the patient more difficult. There is a direct relationship between contractures and pressure ulcers. Patients with contractures of the knees, feet, and ankles cannot walk. A footboard should be used with all bedfast patients to prevent contracture development. If permitted, placing patients in the prone position for 15 to 30 minutes daily helps to stretch the muscles, which prevents contractures. Avoiding the sitting position for prolonged periods also helps prevent flexion contractures.

Patients' joints must be moved regularly to prevent complications. If patients cannot move independently, you will be responsible for exercising their joints. All patients should be exercised regularly to prevent deformities. This includes patients with no potential for rehabilitation. Like pressure ulcers, contractures are much easier to prevent than to reverse. However, they can be reversed, particularly in the early stages. Reversing contractures requires a diligent effort by staff. Reversing a contracture also takes a long time—much longer than it took for the contracture to develop.

Other complications of inadequate exercise are:

- Mineral loss from bones.
- Slowing of general body circulation.

Active **range-of-motion (ROM) exercises** are done by the patient during activities of daily living. **Passive range-of-motion (PROM)** exercises are performed for patients when independent movement is impossible. Passive range-of-motion exercises maintain movement and prevent deformities. They do *not* strengthen the muscles. You will perform PROM for patients with conditions such as:

- Paralysis
- Contractures
- Orthopedic conditions
- Neurologic disorders
- Severe cognitive impairment

Passive range-of-motion exercises are also ordered when active movement:

- Increases spasticity
- Causes pain
- Creates excessive stress on the heart
- Makes patients unable to move joints safely

The patient must be comfortable and relaxed during the exercises. Each joint is taken through the normal range of movement.

The nurse will instruct you as to the type or limitation of range-of-motion exercises to be done. These exercises are usually done during or after the bath and before the bed is made. They may be carried out at other times as well.

Precautions and Special Situations

Patients with certain conditions require special care and handling. Avoid exercising extremities with fractures or dislocations. When assisting patients with healed hip or other joint replacements, avoid internal rotation. Also avoid adduction beyond the midline. Some patients have bones that break easily. Patients with osteoporosis can sustain fractures with little or no trauma. You have learned that patients with this condition may develop spontaneous fractures. Check with the nurse and the care plan when your patient has a special situation or osteoporosis.

If the patient has a wound or pressure ulcer, check to see if exercise will harm the healing tissue. If a patient is combative or resists exercise, avoid forcing him. Gently explain and demonstrate the procedure. Try to coax the patient into participating. Sometimes singing an old song will distract the patient. Encourage the patient to sing along with you. If distracted, she may allow you to perform the exercises. The patient may even have fun! Performing range-of-motion exercises in the bathtub or whirlpool may also be an option, if permitted. Notify the nurse if the patient continues to refuse.

Some patients have muscle spasms and rigidity. When exercising patients with these conditions, move the joint slowly and smoothly. Stop at the point of pain or resistance. Apply gentle, steady pressure until the muscle relaxes (Figure 41-25). Avoid rapid, jerking movements. Do not stretch the joint too far. These activities cause pain and worsen the condition. Suspect muscle spasms if resistance progressively increases during exercise. Rigidity presents as resistance to movement in any direction. Slow, continuous, sustained movements help prevent spasticity and rigidity. If rigidity and muscle spasms develop, hold steady, gentle pressure on the muscle. Avoid forcing the muscle past the point of resistance. This should enable you to complete the exercise. Report the problems to the nurse. The nurse or therapist will provide specific instructions.

FIGURE 41-25 Apply steady, gentle pressure to reduce spasticity.

GUIDELINES *for*

Assisting Patients with Range-of-Motion Exercises

- Check the care plan or ask the nurse for specific guidelines and limitations.
- Explain the procedure to the patient.
- Before beginning, make sure the patient is comfortable.
- Position the patient in good body alignment, in the supine position, before beginning.
- Elevate the bed to a comfortable working height.
- Use good posture and apply the principles of good body mechanics.
- Encourage the patient to assist, if able, but keep your hands in position to provide support.
- Make sure you have enough space for full movement of the extremities.
- Expose only the part of the body you are exercising.

- Support each joint by placing one hand above and one hand below the joint.
- Move each joint slowly and consistently. Stop briefly at the end of each motion.
- Work systematically from the top of the body to the bottom.
- Never push the patient past the point of joint resistance. Move each joint only as far as it will comfortably go.
- In many facilities, the neck is not exercised without a physician's order. Know and follow your facility policy.
- Perform each joint motion five times, or according to facility policy.
- Stop the exercise and report to the nurse if the patient complains of pain. Watch the patient's body language and facial expression for signs of pain.

continues

GUIDELINES *continued*

- Be alert for changes in the patient's condition during the activity. If you feel that the activity is harming the patient, stop. Notify the nurse. Changes that suggest a potential problem are pain, shortness of breath, sweating, and change in color.

- Help the patient relax during exercise.

- Use the session as quality time to communicate with the patient.

- For patients who are stiff or combative, consider doing the exercise in the bathtub or whirlpool. Check with the nurse.

PROCEDURE

PERFORMING RANGE-OF-MOTION EXERCISES (PASSIVE)

Legal ALERT

Passive range of motion that involves the neck is usually carried out by a physical therapist or a nurse. Patients who can exercise this area themselves are encouraged to do so. Check your facility policy regarding ROM neck exercises. ∎

FIGURE 41-26 Shoulder abduction and adduction. Support the arm at the elbow and wrist, then bring the entire arm out at a right angle from the body.

Note: This procedure may be carried out as an independent procedure or as part of the bath. Repeat each action five times.

1. Carry out initial procedure actions.

2. Assemble equipment:
   - Bath blanket

3. Position the patient on his back close to you.

4. Adjust the bath blanket to keep the patient covered as much as possible.

5. Supporting the elbow and wrist, exercise the shoulder joint nearest you as follows:
   a. Bring the entire arm out at a right angle to the body (horizontal abduction) (Figure 41-26).
   b. Return the arm to a position parallel to the body (horizontal adduction).

6. a. With the arm parallel to the body, roll the entire arm toward the body (internal rotation of shoulder).

   b. Maintaining the parallel position, roll the entire arm away from the body (external rotation of shoulder).

7. With the shoulder in abduction, flex the elbow and raise the entire arm over the head (shoulder flexion) (Figure 41-27).

8. With the arm parallel to the body (palm up— supination), flex and extend the elbow (Figures 41-28A and 41-28B).

9. Flex and extend the wrist (Figure 41-29). Flex and extend each finger joint (Figure 41-30).

10. Move each finger, in turn, away from the middle finger (abduction) (Figure 41-31A) and toward the middle finger (adduction) (Figure 41-31B).

11. Abduct the thumb by moving it toward the extended fingers (Figure 41-32).

continues

PROCEDURE **91** CONTINUED

FIGURE 41-27 Shoulder flexion. With the shoulder in abduction, flex the elbow and raise the entire arm over the head.

FIGURE 41-28A Elbow extension and flexion. Support the upper arm and wrist, then straighten the elbow.

FIGURE 41-28B Flex the lower arm toward the upper arm.

FIGURE 41-29 Wrist extension and flexion. Supporting the arm above the wrist and hand, straighten the wrist.

FIGURE 41-30 Finger extension. Slip your fingers over the patient's flexed fingers, then straighten the fingers.

FIGURE 41-31A Abduction of the fingers

12. Touch the thumb to the base of the little finger, then to each fingertip (opposition) (Figure 41-33).

13. Turn the hand palm down (**pronation**), then palm up (supination).

14. Grasp the patient's wrist with one hand and the patient's hand with the other. Bring the wrist toward the body (**inversion**) and then away from the body (**eversion**) (Figure 41-34).

continues

PROCEDURE 91 CONTINUED

FIGURE 41-31B Adduction of the fingers

FIGURE 41-32 Abduction and adduction of the thumb and fingers. Supporting the hand, draw the thumb toward and away from the extended fingers.

FIGURE 41-33 Thumb opposition. Supporting the hand, touch each finger with the thumb.

FIGURE 41-34 Wrist inversion (supination) and eversion (pronation). Grasp the patient's wrist with one hand. Grasp the patient's hand with your other hand. Bring the wrist toward the body, then away from the body.

15. Point the hand in supination toward the thumb side (**radial deviation**), then toward the little-finger side (**ulnar deviation**).

16. Cover the patient's upper extremities and body. Expose only the leg being exercised. Face the foot of the bed.

17. Supporting the knee and ankle, move the entire leg away from the body center (abduction) (Figure 41-35) and toward the body (adduction).

18. Turn to face the bed. Supporting the knee in bent position (flexion), raise the knee toward the pelvis (hip flexion) (Figure 41-36A). Straighten the knee (extension) (Figure 41-36B), as you lower the leg to the bed.

19. a. Supporting the leg at the knee and ankle, roll the leg in a circular fashion away from the body (lateral hip rotation).

FIGURE 41-35 Abduction of the hip. Supporting the patient's knee and ankle, move the entire leg away from the center of the body.

continues

PROCEDURE 91 CONTINUED

FIGURE 41-36A Hip and knee flexion. Supporting the leg, return toward the center of the body.

FIGURE 41-36B Knee extension. Supporting the knee and ankle, straighten the leg.

FIGURE 41-37A Ankle flexion. Grasp the patient's heel with one hand, using your upper arm to support the foot. Dorsiflex the ankle by bringing the toes and foot toward the knee.

FIGURE 41-37B Plantar flex the ankle by drawing the foot in a downward position.

    b. Continuing to support the leg, roll the leg in the same fashion toward the body (medial hip rotation).

20. Grasp the patient's toes and support the ankle. Bring toes toward the knee (**dorsiflexion**) (Figure 41-37A). Then point the toes toward the foot of the bed (**plantar flexion**) (Figure 41-37B).

> 📝 **Note:** The patient may be more comfortable if the knee is slightly flexed during this motion.

21. Gently turn the patient's foot inward (inversion) (Figure 41-38) and outward (eversion).

FIGURE 41-38 Foot inversion. Grasp the patient's foot and gently turn it inward.

continues

PROCEDURE 91 CONTINUED

FIGURE 41-39A Toe abduction. Move each toe away from the second toe one at a time.

FIGURE 41-39B Toe adduction. Move each toe toward the second toe one at a time.

22. Place your fingers over the patient's toes. Bend the toes (flexion) and straighten them (extension).

23. Move each toe away from the second toe (abduction) (Figure 41-39A) and then toward the second toe (adduction) (Figure 41-39B).

24. Cover the leg with the bath blanket. Raise the side rail and move to the opposite side of the bed.

25. Move the patient close to you and repeat steps 5 through 23.

DIAGNOSTIC TECHNIQUES

Some techniques used to diagnose problems of the musculoskeletal system include:

- Radiographic techniques such as X-ray.
- Electromyography (EMG) test to measure the effectiveness of muscle/nerve interaction.
- Measurements of alkaline and acid phosphatases.
- Bone marrow examination, when a sample of the bone marrow is removed and evaluated.

- CAT scan to check for bone, muscle, and joint conditions.
- Radioisotope scanning, a technique that often can detect early bone and joint changes.
- Arthroscopy for direct visualization of a joint.
- Magnetic resonance imaging (MRI) to show conditions of tissues around bones. This helps to diagnose tumors, a ruptured disc between two vertebrae, and other conditions.

REVIEW

A. True/False.

Mark the following true or false by circling T or F.

1. T F Osteoporosis is a type of arthritis in which joint deformities are common.

2. T F If ROM is not carried out faithfully, the patient's future mobility may be threatened.

3. T F When carrying out ROM, always support the parts being exercised at the joint.

4. T F The nursing assistant will carry out special corrective exercises.

5. T F Aging is a contributory factor in osteoarthritis.

6. T F When the patient has a painful arthritic joint, it should be exercised vigorously.

7. T F An overbed bar (trapeze) will assist orthopedic patients to move more easily and enable them to help themselves.

8. T F A fracture is any break in a bone.

9. T F Before operating beds or attachments used with orthopedic patients, the nursing assistant must be sure of her competency to operate this equipment.

10. T F It only takes a few moments for a plaster cast to dry completely.

11. T F Patients recovering from fractured hips are generally not allowed to bear weight on the affected side for several weeks.

12. T F If a patient has an open reduction/internal fixation for a fractured hip, it means a cast will have been applied.

13. T F Phantom pain after an amputation is imaginary and of no concern to caregivers.

14. T F The nursing assistant is responsible for teaching patients with prostheses how to use them.

15. T F It is important to prevent contractures after an amputation.

B. Matching.

Choose the correct word from Column II to match each phrase in Column I.

Column I

16. _____ correct position

17. _____ small fluid-filled sacs found around joints

18. _____ name given to a cast covering hips and one or both legs

19. _____ fracture where bone breaks through skin

20. _____ inflammation of joints

Column II

a. arthritis

b. spica

c. closed

d. bursae

e. simple

f. alignment

g. open

C. Multiple Choice.

Select the one best answer for each of the following.

21. When assigned to perform ROM, you should
   a. exercise every joint.
   b. exercise joints to the point of pain.
   c. check with the nurse for any limitations before starting.
   d. perform each exercise four times.

22. A greenstick fracture
   a. occurs mainly in children.
   b. fragments the bone.
   c. occurs mainly in the elderly.
   d. twists around the bone.

23. While a leg cast is drying,
   a. cover it tightly so moisture will not be lost.
   b. maintaining general alignment is not important.
   c. carefully observe the extremities for circulation.
   d. use only fingertips to handle the cast.

24. When caring for the patient in traction,
   a. maintain proper alignment.
   b. lift the weights rapidly.
   c. allow weights to rest on the floor.
   d. position the patient's feet against the footboard.

25. Your patient has a ruptured disc. You should note and report
   a. crossing of the legs.
   b. ambulation in the room.
   c. numbness and tingling.
   d. complaints of feeling tired.

26. The most common symptom of osteoarthritis is
   a. swollen joints.
   b. pain.
   c. redness.
   d. limited mobility.

27. Gout is caused by
   a. renal disease.
   b. hypertension.
   c. arthritic changes in aging.
   d. elevated uric acid levels in the blood.

28. When positioning a patient with hip replacement surgery, you should
   a. elevate the head of the bed at least 60°.
   b. cross the legs at the ankles.
   c. avoid elevating the head more than 45°.
   d. position the hips and knees in complete flexion.

29. Compartment syndrome is a
   a. serious surgical emergency.
   b. normal side effect of a fracture.
   c. chronic condition related to arthritis.
   d. side effect of medications.

30. Position the patient with a leg amputation
   a. with both legs in abduction.
   b. with pillows between the legs.
   c. with the head elevated at least 90°.
   d. with the legs in adduction.

D. Nursing Assistant Challenge.

You are assigned to care for Mrs. Nellie Goldstein, 62 years old, who had a total hip arthroplasty two days ago. She will be starting rehabilitation today and will continue her therapy as an outpatient after she is discharged in three more days. Mrs. Goldstein is a very active person and is eager to be "up and going."

31. What restrictions do you need to be aware of when taking care of Mrs. Goldstein?

UNIT 42

Endocrine System

OBJECTIVES

After completing this unit, you will be able to:
- Spell and define terms.
- Review the location and functions of the endocrine system.
- List five specific diagnostic tests associated with conditions of the endocrine system.
- Describe some common diseases of the endocrine system.

- Recognize the signs and symptoms of hypoglycemia and hyperglycemia.
- Describe nursing assistant actions related to the care of patients with disorders of the endocrine system.
- Perform blood tests for glucose levels if facility policy permits.
- Perform the following procedure:
  - Procedure 92 Obtaining a Fingerstick Blood Sugar

VOCABULARY

Learn the meaning and the correct spelling of the following words and phrases:

acetone
Addison's disease
adrenal glands
assimilate
Cushing's syndrome
diabetes mellitus
endocrine glands
estrogen
fingerstick blood sugar
  (FSBS)
glucagon
glucose
glycated hemoglobin
  (A1C)

glycogen
glycosuria
gonads
hormones
hypercalcemia
hyperglycemia
hypersecretion
hyperthyroidism
hypertrophy
hypoglycemia
hyposecretion
hypothyroidism
insulin

insulin-dependent
  diabetes mellitus
  (IDDM)
iodine
islets of Langerhans
lancet
non–insulin-dependent
  diabetes mellitus
  (NIDDM)
ovaries
ovum
parathormone
parathyroid gland
pineal body

pituitary gland
polydipsia
polyphagia
polyuria
progesterone
scrotum
simple goiter
sperm
testes
testosterone
tetany
thyrocalcitonin
thyroid gland
thyroxine

STRUCTURE AND FUNCTION

The **endocrine glands** (Figure 42-1):

- Secrete **hormones**, chemicals that regulate the body's activities
- Control body activities and growth
- Are found as distinct glands or clusters of cells
- Are subject to disease that can result in **hyposecretion** (underproduction) or **hypersecretion** (overproduction) of hormones

Pituitary Gland

Because it controls most of the other glands, the **pituitary gland** is called the master gland. The pituitary gland has two portions called *lobes*. Each of the lobes secretes more than one hormone.

1. The anterior lobe secretes:
   - STH (somatotropic hormone)—a growth hormone that stimulates the growth of long bones
   - TSH (thyroid-stimulating hormone)—stimulates the thyroid gland

Clinical Information ALERT

Hormones from the endocrine system travel through the bloodstream to various body sites. The human body produces more than 30 hormones regulating such things as hunger, body temperature, stress reactions, and growth. The purpose of some hormones is to stimulate other glands to secrete their own hormones. Regardless of external factors, hormones are responsible for regulating organ function and normalizing the body, keeping it in a balanced, normal state. Of the glands in the endocrine system, the adrenal glands produce the greatest number of hormones. The parathyroids are the smallest endocrine glands (there are 4 of these), and the largest pure endocrine gland is the thyroid. The thymus is the largest at birth. ■

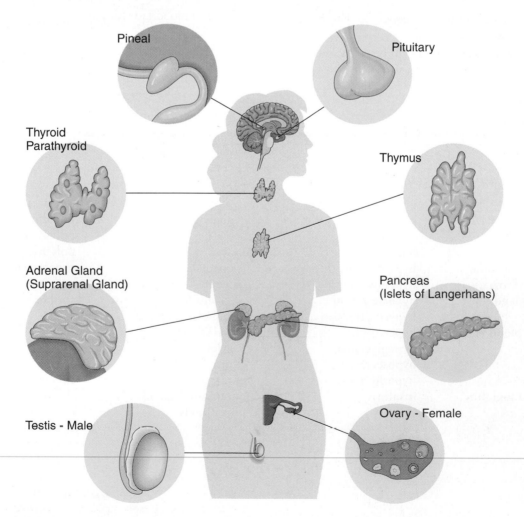

FIGURE 42-1 Endocrine system

– FSH (follicle-stimulating hormone)—promotes growth of the ovarian follicle in which the egg develops during the menstrual cycle

– ACTH (adrenocorticotropic hormone)—stimulates production by the adrenal gland

– LH (luteinizing hormone)—in females, helps stimulate ovulation during the menstrual cycle

– ICSH (interstitial cell-stimulating hormone)—stimulates the male testes

– Lactogenic hormone (LTH)—stimulates milk production in pregnant women

2. The posterior lobe secretes:

– ADH (antidiuretic hormone)—acts on kidneys to prevent excess water loss

– Pitocin (oxytocin)—stimulates uterine contractions during childbirth

Pineal Body

The **pineal body** is a small gland that is also located in the skull beneath the brain. Very little is known about this gland. It is thought to be related to sexual growth, because it tends to get smaller at maturity. It produces:

● Glomerulotropin, which influences the adrenal gland

● Serotonin, which acts in the brain

● Melatonin, which keeps sexual maturity from occurring too early and may affect the sleep/wake cycle

Adrenal Glands

There are two **adrenal glands**. One gland is located on top of each kidney. Each gland has two distinct portions that secrete separate hormones.

1. The adrenal medulla (inside) produces norepinephrine (noradrenalin) and epinephrine (adrenalin), which stimulate the body to produce energy quickly during an emergency.

Clinical Information ALERT

The adrenal glands are responsible for the "flight or fight" reaction when we perceive a threat. In this reaction, adrenalin flows throughout the body, causing changes that your body needs to react quickly for possible defense. The senses sharpen, so you feel more alert. The pupils dilate, enabling you to see more clearly. Hairs stand on end; heart rate and respirations increase. Blood supply to the muscles increases and blood flow to nonessential organs is reduced. ■

2. The adrenal cortex (outside) produces:

– Glucocorticoids—elevate blood sugar levels and control the response of the body to stress and inflammation. They also depress inflammation.

– Mineral corticoids—manage sodium and potassium levels.

– Gonadocorticoids—influence both male and female sex hormones.

Gonads

The term **gonads** refers to the male and female sex glands. The female gonads (two **ovaries**):

● Are located within the pelvic cavity on either side of the uterus.

● Produce two hormones, **estrogen** and **progesterone**. These hormones are responsible for the development of female characteristics such as:

– breast development

– pubic and axillary hair

– onset and regulation of menstruation

– pregnancy

The male gonads (two **testes**):

● Are located on the outside of the body in a pouch called the **scrotum**.

● Produce the hormone **testosterone**. This hormone is responsible for secondary male characteristics such as:

– muscular development

– deepening voice

– hair growth

The male and female gonads also produce special cells—in the female, the **ovum**, and in the male, the **sperm**. These cells unite during fertilization to form the embryo that becomes a new human being.

Thyroid Gland

The **thyroid gland** has two lobes and is found in the neck, anterior to the larynx. Hormones secreted by this gland are thyroxine and thyrocalcitonin. **Thyroxine** regulates metabolism. **Iodine** is an important component of this hormone. **Thyrocalcitonin** regulates calcium and phosphorus levels.

Parathyroid Glands

The tiny **parathyroid glands** are embedded in the posterior thyroid gland. The hormone they manufacture is called parathormone. **Parathormone** helps control the body's use of two minerals, calcium and phosphorus. Insufficient amounts of calcium result in severe muscle spasms or **tetany**. Untreated tetany can lead to death.

Islets of Langerhans

The **islets of Langerhans** are small groups of cells found within the pancreas. These cells produce two hormones: insulin and glucagon. **Insulin** lowers blood sugar. **Glucagon** elevates blood sugar.

COMMON CONDITIONS OF THE THYROID GLAND

The thyroid gland may secrete too much or not enough hormones. Either situation is treatable. If not treated, severe illness or death will occur.

Hyperthyroidism

Hyperthyroidism, or overactivity of the thyroid gland, results in production of too much thyroxine (hypersecretion). The person shows:

- Irritability and restlessness
- Nervousness
- Rapid pulse
- Increased appetite
- Weight loss
- Sensitivity

Nursing Assistant Actions. When caring for these patients, the nursing assistant must be understanding and have patience. The room should be kept quiet and cool. The patient's increased nutritional needs should be met with foods that the patient likes.

Treatment. Treatment of hyperthyroidism is designed to reduce the level of thyroxine through:

- Surgical thyroidectomy
- Radiation to reduce the number of functional cells

Thyroidectomy. It may be necessary to treat hyperthyroidism with surgery. You may be assigned to assist in the postoperative care. Following surgery:

- The patient is placed in a semi-Fowler's position, with neck and shoulders well supported. Remember at all times to support the back of the neck. Hyperextension of the neck may damage the operative site.
- Assist with oxygen, if ordered, using all oxygen precautions.
- Give routine postoperative care.
- Check for and report the following:
  - Any signs of bleeding (this may drain toward the back of the neck). The pillows behind the patient should be checked, as well as the dressings.
  - Signs of respiratory distress.
  - Inability of the patient to speak. Initial hoarseness is common, but any increase should be reported.
  - Greatly elevated temperature and pulse, pronounced apprehension, or irritability.
  - Numbness, tingling, or muscular spasm (tetany) of the extremities.

Hypothyroidism

Hypothyroidism results in an undersecretion of thyroxine. Recall that iodine is an essential component of thyroxine. A lack of iodine in the diet can result in low thyroxine production.

- The condition is called **simple goiter.**
- The thyroid gland enlarges (**hypertrophies**).
- Secretions produced have low thyroxine content.

Hypothyroidism can usually be successfully managed with thyroxine replacement.

COMMON CONDITIONS OF THE PARATHYROID GLANDS

Parathormone, secreted by the parathyroids, regulates the levels of electrolytes, calcium, and phosphates. Hypersecretion of this hormone results in:

- Excessively high levels of blood calcium (**hypercalcemia**)
- Developmental of renal calculi (kidney stones)
- Loss of bone calcium

Hypersecretion is usually caused by tumors. Tumors can be treated by surgical removal.

Hyposecretion can lead to:

- Abnormal muscle-nerve interaction
- Severe muscle spasm (tetany)

This can be an emergency situation, requiring management of the muscle spasms and administration of calcium. In the chronic state, calcium replacements and increased dietary calcium are prescribed.

COMMON CONDITIONS OF THE ADRENAL GLANDS

Adrenal gland secretions regulate:

- Development and maintenance of sexual characteristics
- Carbohydrate, fat, and protein metabolism
- Fluid balance
- Electrolyte levels of sodium and potassium

Hypersecretion results in **Cushing's syndrome**, which is characterized by:

- Weakness due to loss of body protein
- Increased blood sugar levels (hyperglycemia)
- Edema
- Hypertension
- Loss of potassium and retention of sodium
- Masculinization of a female

Therapy is primarily surgical and supportive.

Hyposecretion results in **Addison's disease**, which is characterized by:

- Loss of sodium and retention of potassium
- Abnormally low blood sugar (hypoglycemia)
- Dehydration
- Low stress tolerance

Addison's disease is treated by hormone replacement therapy and techniques to combat dehydration.

DIABETES MELLITUS

In the United States, 20.8 million people (7% of the population) had diabetes by 2005. Of these, 14.6 million had been diagnosed, but 6.2 million were not diagnosed yet. About 176,500 people aged 20 or younger have type 1 diabetes. This is about one in every 400 to 600 children and adolescents in this country. Diabetes occurs in people of all ages and races, but is most common in African Americans, Native Americans, Latinos, Asian Americans, Alaska Natives, and Pacific Islanders. The incidence of diabetes increases with age.

Diabetes mellitus is a chronic disease that results from a deficiency of insulin or a resistance to the effects of insulin. The problems with insulin cause the body to be unable to properly process food into energy. The glucose from the food breakdown remains in the blood, resulting in elevated blood sugar. Persistent, elevated glucose levels affect the blood vessels and nerves, making the person with diabetes more likely to develop heart attack, stroke, blindness, renal disease, and other serious complications and conditions.

Clinical Information ALERT

Almost 1 in 20 people worldwide are diabetic. Approximately 2,000 cases are diagnosed every day. Before developing type 2 diabetes, most people develop a condition called *prediabetes*. In this condition, the blood glucose is higher than normal, but not high enough to be called diabetes. Damage to the body associated with diabetes may be caused in this stage. People with prediabetes may be able to delay or prevent type 2 diabetes through diet and exercise. ∎

The reason why diabetes develops is not fully understood. Factors that seem to play a role in the incidence of diabetes are:

- Heredity
- Obesity
- Age
- Diet
- Lack of exercise

All diabetics should wear or carry a Medic Alert identification so that proper and immediate care can be provided in an emergency. It is also recommended that diabetics carry food that provides a quick source of carbohydrates.

Disease Mechanism

In diabetes, the normal metabolism of fats, carbohydrates, and proteins is unbalanced. Normally, when carbohydrates are absorbed into the bloodstream, the blood sugar (glucose) level rises. The pancreas responds to an increase of **glucose** by secreting more insulin. Insulin is the hormone primarily responsible for:

- Lowering the blood sugar level by allowing glucose to cross the cell membrane.
- Increasing the oxidation of glucose by the tissues.
- Stimulating the conversion of glucose to glycogen by the liver. **Glycogen** is a storage form of energy.
- Decreasing glucose production from amino acids.
- Stimulating glucose formation into fat for storage.

In diabetes, there is insufficient insulin for these metabolic functions.

- Glucose cannot be properly utilized for energy.
- Fats and proteins are incompletely broken down. This leads to an accumulation of ketone bodies and nitrogenous waste products.
- The excess glucose is eliminated, along with water and salts, through the kidneys. This causes dehydration and electrolyte imbalance.
- The characteristic symptoms of excessive thirst, hunger, and increased urination are directly related to the loss of fluids, electrolytes, and sugar.

Types of Diabetes Mellitus

Diabetes mellitus is typed and named according to the need for insulin. Examples are insulin-dependent diabetes mellitus (IDDM) and non–insulin-dependent diabetes (NIDDM). IDDM appears more commonly in the young and NIDDM is more common in older people.

Insulin-dependent diabetes mellitus (IDDM) (type 1) accounts for approximately 5% to 10% of diabetes. This type tends to run in families. It is most common in children and young adults. Initial symptoms may mimic the flu in young children. People with type 1 diabetes must take daily insulin injections to stay alive. Typical signs and symptoms are:

- **Polyuria** (excessive urination)
- **Polydipsia** (thirst)
- **Polyphagia** (hunger)
- **Glycosuria** (sugar in the urine)

Non–insulin-dependent diabetes mellitus (NIDDM) (type 2) is a metabolic disorder that occurs when the body does not make enough insulin, or does not properly use insulin. This is the most common form of diabetes. It accounts for 90% to 95% of all diabetes. It is said to be nearing epidemic proportions due to the high incidence of obesity and sedentary lifestyles. Type 2 diabetes was once seen only in adults. Over the past decade, the incidence has risen dramatically in young people. By 1999, type 2 diabetes was accounting for 8% to 45% of new childhood diabetes cases. Today, many physicians are diagnosing more new cases of type 2 diabetes in children than type 1. Although there are no firm statistics, experts say that approximately 39,000 U.S. adolescents may have type 2 diabetes and more than 2.5 million may have prediabetes.

People may not be aware they have the condition until symptoms become severe or complications develop. The risk for type 2 diabetes increases with age. More than 20% of the United States population aged 65 and older has diabetes. Common signs and symptoms of type 2 diabetes are:

- Easy fatigue
- Skin infections
- Slow healing
- Itching
- Pruritus vulvae (itching of the vulva)
- Burning on urination
- Vision changes
- Obesity

Often only one or two symptoms are apparent in the elderly person. The older person may:

- Complain of constant fatigue
- Have a skin lesion that takes an unusually long time to heal
- Experience vision changes that may be mistakenly attributed to aging

Care of the diabetic is directed toward maintaining a normal blood glucose level so that complications may be prevented. To regulate blood glucose, the diabetic person must:

- Eat a healthful, well-balanced diet as prescribed by the physician
- Exercise regularly in a manner appropriate for the person's age and ability
- Check the blood sugar regularly
- Use insulin or oral antidiabetic agents correctly if ordered by the physician

For some persons, this may require lifestyle changes. Nurses and dietitians are responsible for teaching patients who are newly diagnosed with diabetes how to care for themselves. People with diabetes who are knowledgeable about the disease and who are willing to manage their lives accordingly can live happily and productively (Figure 42-2).

Diet

Diet is an important part of diabetic treatment. Physicians do not fully agree as to how strictly a diet must be followed by all patients.

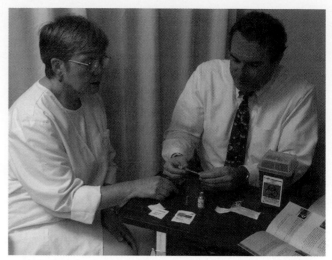

FIGURE 42-2 Patients are taught to manage their diabetes by the nurse.

- Weight reduction is favored.
- Weight reduction alone may be sufficient to bring the condition under control in NIDDM.

Meal Planning. The dietitian is a key member of the health care team for patients with diabetes. The dietitian helps the patient plan meals in keeping with the patient's goals, lifestyle, laboratory values, caloric and nutritional needs, and food preferences. Many diabetics use the USDA food guide pyramid for daily meal planning. The pyramid that was introduced in 2005 is designed to be individualized to meet each person's needs. Because of this, it is an excellent tool for diabetics. The American Diabetes Association (ADA) supports the USDA's effort to balance food intake with physical activity. Such a balance is essential in promoting health, including the prevention of diabetes and its complications. The Diabetes Prevention Program (DPP) proved that type 2 diabetes can be prevented or delayed by keeping weight in control and by increasing physical activity. Those wishing to use the interactive food pyramid technology can visit http://www.mypyramid.gov/.

The goals of the diet include maintaining near-normal blood sugar, optimal fat levels, and adequate calories based on individual needs. Meal plans are flexible. The diet should be well balanced, with sufficient fiber.

The diabetic exchange system of foods was formulated by a committee with representatives from the American Diabetic Association and the diabetic branch of the U.S. Public Health Service. The exchanges are available through the registered dietitian or diabetes educator. Although the exchange list system has been used for years, it is regularly updated to reflect new trends. The lists provide maximum flexibility in planning a healthy diet. The dietitian teaches the patient the importance of reading food labels, and how to interpret them. Common household measures are used to determine portion size.

Exercise

Exercise (Figure 42-3) is an important part of the overall treatment. The amount and type of exercise the patient routinely engages in are balanced by the food intake and insulin or hypoglycemic drug requirements.

Hypoglycemic Drugs

Diabetes mellitus is treated by one of two main drug groups. One is administered subcutaneously or intravenously. The other is given orally.

At present, there are several types of insulin. They vary in:

- Speed of action
- Duration
- Potency or strength

Insulin is:

- Administered by the nurse. The nurse rotates the administration sites.
- Given by injection.
- Increasingly given through use of an insulin pump. The insulin pump delivers a prescribed amount of insulin on a regular basis into the patient's body.
- Used to treat IDDM and some patients with NIDDM.

Persons living at home are taught to administer their own insulin.

Note: When insulin is self-administered, it is important to report any missed injections or signs of infection around the administration site.

Oral hypoglycemic drugs are:

- Administered by the nurse
- Given by mouth
- Used to treat NIDDM

Inhaled insulin was approved by the FDA in 2006 for the treatment of type 1 and type 2 diabetes. Type 1 diabetics can use the product in combination with longer-acting injected insulin. Type 2 diabetics can use it as an alternative to rapid-acting insulin or oral diabetes drugs, or in combination with oral drugs or injected insulin. Smokers (including those who have quit smoking in the past 6 months) should not use the product. Also, it is not recommended for persons with COPD. Other inhaled insulins are currently in development, as are other alternatives, including mouth sprays and insulin patches.

Islet cell transplantation is occasionally used as a treatment for type 1 diabetes. It is still considered an experimental therapy, so it is not widely available. Currently, 17 U.S. centers are participating in islet cell research programs. The ADA recommends that transplantation be performed only in these centers, which are best equipped to handle the complex needs of transplant patients.

Some people use CAM therapy to treat diabetes. Products such as chromium, magnesium, brewer's yeast, and vanadium are the most commonly used alternatives. Several herbs are also used, but little is known about their long-term safety or efficacy in treatment of diabetes. Currently, there are no formal recommendations for use of alternatives.

Complications

Because persistently high glucose levels cause damage to the nerves and blood vessels, the following complications can occur:

- Renal disease
- Circulatory impairments that often result in gangrene (Figure 42-4) and amputation
- Poor healing
- Hypertension
- Cardiovascular problems
- Diabetic coma
- Vision problems and blindness

FIGURE 42-3 Exercise and sufficient water intake are important factors in maintaining good health.

Difficult SITUATIONS

Persons with diabetes are at very high risk for skin breakdown and pressure ulcers. Ulcers on the feet can be very serious in patients with diabetes, eventually leading to amputation. Pay close attention to risk factors. Relieve pressure from the feet and check the feet each day for abnormalities. ■

Hypoglycemia (Low Blood Sugar)

Hypoglycemia occurs when the blood glucose level is below normal. It:

- May occur rapidly
- Is referred to as *insulin reaction* or *insulin shock* when due to an overdose of insulin

FIGURE 42-4 Gangrene of the feet and toes will require amputation. In most cases, the leg is amputated below the knee. (Courtesy of Centers for Disease Control and Prevention)

Hypoglycemia can be brought on by:
- Skipping meals
- Unusual activity
- Stress
- Vomiting
- Diarrhea
- Omission of planned snack or meals
- Interaction of drugs
- Too much insulin or antidiabetic medication

Signs and Symptoms. The signs and symptoms of hypoglycemia include:
- Complaints of hunger, weakness, dizziness, shakiness
- Skin cold, moist, clammy, pale
- Rapid, shallow respirations
- Nervousness and excitement
- Rapid pulse
- Unconsciousness
- No sugar in the urine
- Low blood sugar test results

If the patient is awake and alert, treatment includes intake of orange juice, milk, or another easily absorbed carbohydrate such as hard candy. If the patient is unconscious, the physician or nurse may give glucagon, which causes a rapid elevation of blood sugar.

Hyperglycemia (High Blood Sugar)

Hyperglycemia (diabetic coma):
- Occurs when there is insufficient insulin for metabolic needs

- Usually develops slowly, sometimes over a 24-hour period
- May be seen as confusion, drowsiness, or a slow slippage into coma in a patient who is confined to bed

Hyperglycemia may be brought on by:
- Stress
- Illness such as infection
- Dehydration
- Injury
- Forgotten medication
- Intake of too much food

Signs and Symptoms. The signs and symptoms of diabetic coma include:
- Early headache, drowsiness, or confusion
- Sweet, fruity odor to the breath
- Deep breathing, labored respirations
- Full, bounding pulse
- Low blood pressure
- Nausea or vomiting
- Flushed, dry, hot skin
- Weakness
- Unconsciousness
- Sugar in the urine
- High blood sugar test results

Treatment includes administration of insulin, fluids, and electrolytes.

Other Complications

Persons with diabetes should have regular health monitoring so that complications may be detected early and treated promptly. Health monitoring should include:
- Eye examinations by an ophthalmologist for early detection of diabetic retinopathy, which can lead to impaired vision and eventually blindness
- Urinalysis and other urological examinations to evaluate the condition of the kidneys
- Cardiac evaluation; monitoring of heart action and blood pressure
- Circulatory evaluation
- Care and treatment of any wounds
- Blood sugar monitoring
- Regular tooth cleaning and evaluation by a dental professional

Difficult SITUATIONS

People with diabetes need to pay special attention to care of the teeth. A 2005 study showed that periodontal disease was a strong predictor of mortality from heart disease and kidney disease. ■

Nursing Assistant Responsibilities

- Know the signs of insulin shock and diabetic coma.
- Be alert for the signs of diabetic coma or insulin shock and report them immediately to the nurse.
- Know the storage location of orange juice or other easily **assimilated** (absorbed) sources of carbohydrates.
- Keep easily assimilated carbohydrates, such as orange juice, crackers, hard candy, or Karo syrup, available if caring for a diabetic patient at home.
- Make sure you serve the patient proper trays of food.
- Do not give extra nourishments without permission.
- Document food consumption on the patient's chart, and report uneaten meals to the nurse (Figure 42-5).
- Give special attention to care of the diabetic patient's feet.
  - Wash daily, carefully drying between toes.
  - Inspect feet closely for any breaks or signs of irritation.
  - Report any abnormalities to the nurse.
  - Do not allow moisture to collect between toes.
  - The toenails of a diabetic should be cut only by a nurse or a podiatrist, a specialist who is licensed to provide foot care.
  - Shoes and stockings should be clean, be free of holes, and fit well. Anything that might injure the feet or interfere with the circulation must be avoided.
  - Do not allow the patient to go barefoot.

Difficult SITUATIONS

Attention to personal hygiene, oral care, and cleanliness is particularly important in individuals with diabetes. Diabetics must bathe regularly to prevent localized skin infections. However, they should avoid prolonged soaking in a tub, which can soften the tissues and lead to breakdown. If you observe unusual areas, such as yellowish pimples or boils on a diabetic patient's skin, or red areas in skin folds (such as under the breasts, underarms, or groin), inform the nurse. Assist the patient with toothbrushing and flossing. The teeth have five surfaces, and toothbrushing only reaches three. Flossing effectively cleans the areas that are not accessible with the brush. Good foot care and drying well between the toes are essential. Report signs and symptoms of infection, even if they seem minor. ■

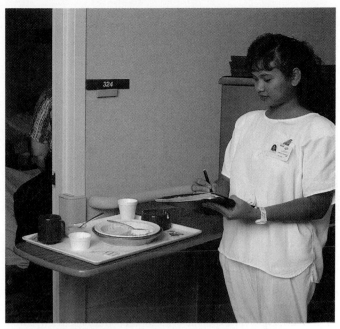

FIGURE 42-5 The amount and type of food consumed by diabetic patients is closely observed and recorded.

DIAGNOSTIC TECHNIQUES

Techniques used to diagnose problems of the endocrine system include:

- Blood analysis for hormone levels
- Urine analysis for hormone levels
- Radioisotope scanning for thyroid disease
- Radioactive iodine uptake for thyroid function
- Basal metabolic rate (BMR) to measure the speed of oxygen uptake

BLOOD GLUCOSE MONITORING

Glycated Hemoglobin

Glycated hemoglobin is a term used to describe a series of stable minor hemoglobin components formed from hemoglobin and glucose. It is commonly called "A1C." The A1C test is a measurement of glucose levels in the blood over a prolonged period of time. It differs from the fingerstick blood sugar because it provides a snapshot of the patient's diabetic control over the past two to three months. The percentage of A1C in whole blood is approximately:

- 50% from the most recent 30 days
- 25% from the previous 30 to 60 days
- 25% from the previous 60 to 90 days

The A1C test is not a screening test. It is used only for testing ongoing glucose control in persons who have been diagnosed with diabetes. If testing is done regularly, it helps predict and control the risk for development of many serious, chronic complications. The ADA recommends A1C testing twice a year for patients who are meeting treatment goals, and four times a year for patients who are not meeting treatment goals, or those who need more intensive monitoring. Home testing kits are now available. Single-use, disposable kits are also being used in physicians' offices, and as a point-of-care bedside test in the hospital and long-term care facility.

Having the A1C profile information enables the physician to evaluate the patient's control; order additional diagnostic tests, if necessary; regulate medications; and establish a monitoring routine. Patient teaching is a very important part of care for patients with diabetes. Knowing the degree of diabetic control enables the nurse and certified diabetes educator to plan and provide specific patient teaching targeted toward normalizing the blood sugar and maintaining good control. The information helps the dietitian to assist the patient with diet management, food preparation, and methods of meeting the patient's individual dietary wants and needs.

Bedside glucose testing has become very common in the management of patients with diabetes. Many individuals perform this testing at home several times each day. The antidiabetic medication may be adjusted according to the patient's blood sugar. A blood sample is taken from a capillary. The test meter will display the blood sugar value in one minute or less. This is a convenient, accurate method of monitoring the blood sugar. Nursing assistants perform this procedure in some facilities. Know and follow your facility policy.

The physician will order specific times for blood sugar testing. The specimen may be collected at a fixed time, such as before meals. The nurse may administer insulin to the patient based on the blood sugar value. Collect the capillary sample exactly as ordered. Specimens that are not collected at the proper time can cause misinterpretation of the results. Always report the value to the nurse, and document according to facility policy.

If the nurse suspects that a patient is having complications related to diabetes, he or she may ask you to obtain a stat blood sugar. This test must be performed immediately. Report the results immediately.

Safety ALERT

In 2005, the FDA issued a warning that in some cases, mistaken blood glucose readings have resulted in diabetics' blood sugar becoming dangerously high. This occurred because the meters were accidentally switched to report the blood sugar level in the foreign standard of units, millimoles per liter, instead of milligrams per deciliter, which is the value of measure used in the United States. The switch can occur:

- When the time and date on the meter are set
- If the meter is dropped
- During battery replacement

Make sure the meter you are using is set for the correct value. ■

Infection Control ALERT

In 2005, the CDC reported three incidents of hepatitis B infection that developed as a result of a shared glucose meter in a long-term care facility. Other diseases may also be spread in this manner, such as hepatitis C and human immunodeficiency virus, the virus that causes AIDS. These viruses are stable on environmental surfaces at room temperature, and infected patients often have no symptoms. Because of this, viruses may easily be passed to workers and other patients if improper techniques are used. This emphasizes the need for education, use of standard precautions, and careful monitoring of diabetes care procedures in all health care settings.

Some hospitals issue a new, individual glucose meter to each patient, who takes the meter home upon discharge. All facilities have policies and procedures for disinfecting meters to be reused after each use. Take your responsibility for cleaning the equipment very seriously. ■

Fingerstick Blood Sugar

Fingerstick blood sugar (FSBS) testing is done by collecting a sample of capillary blood with a **lancet**, or tiny needle. The blood is transferred to a reagent strip or other test strip. For most reagent strips, you must place a hanging drop of blood onto the reagent pad. Avoid smearing the strip against the finger. The Multistix (Figure 42-6) and Chemstrip BG can be read visually, by comparing the color on the reagent strip with the key on the bottle.

Many new meters do not use a reagent strip. After making the fingerstick, a drop of blood is transferred to the test strip, which is inserted into the meter before beginning. The tiny tube draws blood to the inside on contact. This feature works well with patients from whom it is difficult to obtain a hanging drop of blood. An audible beep informs you when the tube has collected enough blood.

FIGURE 42-6 Multistix are used for many different blood tests.

Many different blood glucose meters are available. All are accurate and simple to use. Each meter has its own reagent or test strip. For accuracy, make sure the strip is compatible with the meter you are using (Figure 42-7). Also, check the expiration date on the bottle or package. Do not use strips that are beyond the expiration date. Follow the directions for the meter and reagent strips you are using. All are slightly different.

Many different lancets are also available for performing blood glucose checks. Retractable lancets, which are spring-loaded, have the lowest incidence of injury. The needle withdraws after the finger has been punctured, reducing the chance of needlestick injuries. Discard lancets into a puncture-resistant sharps container. Many health care workers have been injured by lancets that were inadvertently dropped in the bed or on the floor.

The normal blood sugar values vary with the health care facility. The normal fasting range in most facilities is somewhere between 65 and 120, with the normal value commonly being 70 to 110. Values below 70 usually suggest hypoglycemia. Fasting values above 110 suggest hyperglycemia. Learn the normal values for your facility. Values that are well above or below the normal range suggest potentially serious diabetic problems. Notify the nurse immediately of blood sugar values outside of the normal range or other signs and symptoms of blood sugar problems, such as:

- Inadequate food intake
- Eating food not permitted on diet
- Refusal of meals, supplements, or snacks
- Nausea, vomiting, or diarrhea
- Inadequate fluid intake
- Excessive activity
- Complaints of dizziness, shakiness, racing heart

Infection Control ALERT

When doing a fingerstick test, ask the patient to wash the hands under warm, running water. This reduces the risk of infection and increases blood flow to the hand. After piercing the skin with the lancet, squeeze lightly. Avoid prolonged pressure, as this may cause incorrect results by introducing tissue fluids. The fingerstick should be deep enough so that hard pressure is not required. If gentle pressure is not effective to start blood flow, repeat the puncture. ∎

Some blood glucose meters do not have a wide range. Typically, hand-held blood glucose meters will read a blood sugar value as low as 40. A few measure blood sugars as low as 20. For values below the lowest meter reading, the screen will display the word "low." On the high end, most meters do not read values above 400 or 500. If the FSBS exceeds the meter capacity, the display will read "high." If the screen displays the word *low* or *high*, there is potential for serious complications. The patient's condition may deteriorate quickly. Inform the nurse immediately.

Difficult SITUATIONS

Ketone bodies are created when body fat is burned for fuel instead of sugar. The ketone bodies cause a chemical imbalance, resulting in accumulation of acids and upset of the patient's buffer system. If a patient's blood sugar is over 250 mg/dL, the nurse may instruct you to check the patient's urine for ketones. If the patient is very ill, the nurse may request a ketone test even if the blood sugar is not high. ∎

FIGURE 42-7 The reagent strips must be compatible with the glucose meter.

PROCEDURE

OBTAINING A FINGERSTICK BLOOD SUGAR

Legal ALERT

Be sure this is a nursing assistant procedure in your facility. ■

FIGURE 42-8A
Pierce the side of the finger with the lancet.

📝 **Note:** This procedure is generic and applies the principles used for most blood glucose meters. Follow the directions for the meter and strip you are using. The operating directions are slightly different for each.

1. Carry out initial procedure actions.

2. Assemble equipment:
   - Disposable exam gloves
   - Alcohol sponge
   - Lancet
   - Blood glucose meter
   - Reagent strip or test strip for the blood glucose meter being used
   - Sharps container
   - Plastic bandage strip
   - Plastic bag for used supplies

FIGURE 42-8B
Insert the strip in the meter.

3. Wipe the patient's finger with the alcohol sponge. Allow the alcohol to dry.

4. Pierce the sides of the middle or ring finger using the lancet (Figure 42-8A).

5. Discard the lancet in the sharps container.

6. Squeeze the sides of the finger gently to obtain a drop of blood.

7. Hold the puncture site directly over the reagent strip, and place a hanging drop of blood onto the reagent pad. If using capillary tube (straw-like) strips, peel the package back to open it. Hold the package firmly with your thumb and forefinger over the test end (patient end) of the strip. Insert the strip into the meter (Figure 42-8B). Remove and discard the package. Hold the strip next to the puncture site to draw blood into the straw (Figure 42-8C).

FIGURE 42-8C
This strip is like a straw that will draw blood into the base.

8. Insert the strip into the meter, if this was not done previously.

continues

PROCEDURE 92 CONTINUED

FIGURE 42-8D
Read the meter after the designated period of time.

9. Wipe the patient's finger with the alcohol sponge and allow to dry. Apply pressure until bleeding stops. Apply a bandage strip, if necessary.

10. Wait the designated period of time for the meter you are using. An audible beep will indicate when the blood sugar value is displayed on the screen (Figure 42-8D).

11. Carry out ending procedure actions.

Acetone Monitoring

You may be expected to test the patient's urine for acetone. **Acetone** is a substance that accumulates in the body when the blood glucose is out of balance. A simple urine test detects the presence of acetone. Some blood glucose meters also check for ketones in the blood. However, urine monitoring is still done when the ketone level must be measured.

REVIEW

A. True/False.

Mark the following true or false by circling T or F.

1. T F The person with polyphagia has a high urine output.

2. T F In type 2 diabetes, the body does not make enough insulin, or does not properly use insulin.

3. T F Glucose is another name for blood sugar.

4. T F The person with hyperthyroidism is slow-moving and lethargic.

5. T F Hyperthyroidism causes people to lose weight.

6. T F You should keep the room of a patient with hyperthyroidism quite warm.

7. T F Obesity may play a role in the incidence of diabetes mellitus.

8. T F If the patient with IDDM appears drowsy and confused, you should suspect the possibility of hyperglycemia.

9. T F Foot care is especially important for the diabetic patient.

10. T F Disposable gloves should be worn when testing urine for ketones.

B. Matching.

Choose the correct item from Column II to match each word or phrase in Column I.

Column I

11. _____ chemical messenger

12. _____ diabetic coma

13. _____ excess thirst

14. _____ sugar in urine

15. _____ produces hormones

16. _____ excess hunger

17. _____ blood sugar

18. _____ overweight

19. _____ master gland

20. _____ located above kidneys

Column II

a. polydipsia

b. polyphagia

c. glycosuria

d. endocrine gland

e. hormone

f. obesity

g. hyperglycemia

h. glucose

i. adrenal glands

j. pituitary gland

C. Multiple Choice.

Select the one best answer for each of the following.

21. Your patient has had a thyroidectomy. You should
    a. keep the patient flat in bed.
    b. watch for and report signs of respiratory distress.
    c. carry out ROM exercises immediately.
    d. position the patient in a left Sims' position.

22. Lack of iodine in the diet can result in
    a. hypothyroidism.
    b. hyperthyroidism.
    c. diabetes mellitus.
    d. ketosis.

23. The pituitary gland is responsible for secreting hormones that
    a. stimulate ovulation during the menstrual cycle.
    b. manage sodium and potassium levels.
    c. control calcium and phosphorus.
    d. regulate blood sugar.

24. Your patient is an insulin-dependent diabetic. You know this
    a. is a stable form of the disease.
    b. affects only older persons.
    c. requires oral hypoglycemic drugs.
    d. is a less stable form of the disease.

25. Insulin is an important hormone because it
    a. lowers blood sugar.
    b. raises blood sugar.
    c. stimulates the conversion of glycogen to glucose.
    d. breaks fat down to form glucose.

D. Nursing Assistant Challenge.

You are assigned to two patients who both have diabetes. Sally Sakowski is 29 years old and has had diabetes for 10 years. She is considered to be IDDM. Ruth Young is 72 years old and has just been diagnosed with NIDDM. Although these patients both have diabetes, there may be many differences in their signs, symptoms, and problems. Consider these questions:

26. What differences would you see in the signs and symptoms experienced by these two women?

27. What differences would you expect in their treatment?

28. Knowing the difference in their ages, how would you expect the disease to affect the lifestyle of each woman?

29. Hypoglycemia and hyperglycemia may be a complication for either patient. List the differences in the signs and symptoms of both complications.

UNIT 43

Nervous System

OBJECTIVES

After completing this unit, you will be able to:

- Spell and define terms.
- State the location and functions of the organs of the nervous system.
- List five diagnostic tests used to determine conditions of the nervous system.
- Describe 15 common conditions of the nervous system.
- Describe nursing assistant actions related to the care of patients with conditions of the nervous system.

- Explain the proper care, handling, and insertion of an artificial eye.
- Explain the proper care, handling, and insertion of a hearing aid.
- Demonstrate the following procedures:
  - Procedure 93 Caring for the Eye Socket and Artificial Eye
  - Procedure 94 Applying Warm or Cool Eye Compresses

VOCABULARY

Learn the meaning and the correct spelling of the following words and phrases:

absence seizure
akinesia
amyotrophic lateral sclerosis (ALS)
aphasia
aura
autonomic dysreflexia
axon
brain attack
brain stem
cataract
cerebellum
cerebrospinal fluid (CSF)
cerebrovascular accident (CVA)
cerebrum
chorea
cochlea
cognitive impairment

conjunctiva
convulsion
cornea
dendrite
diplegia
emotional lability
epilepsy
eustachian tube
expressive aphasia
flaccid paralysis
generalized tonic-clonic seizure
Glasgow Coma Scale
glaucoma
global aphasia
grand mal seizure
hemianopsia
hemiparesis
hemiplegia
Huntington's disease (HD)

intention tremor
intracranial pressure
iris
lacrimal gland
Lhermitte's sign
macular degeneration
meninges
meningitis
monoplegia
multiple sclerosis (MS)
nerve
neuron
neurotransmitter
nystagmus
ossicle
otitis media
otosclerosis
paralysis
paraplegia
Parkinson's disease

petit mal seizure
position sense
post polio syndrome (PPS)
pupil
quadriplegia
receptive aphasia
retinal degeneration
semicircular canal
spastic paralysis
spatial-perceptual deficit
status epilepticus
stroke
synapse
tetraplegia
tremor
tympanic membrane
unilateral neglect
vertigo

STRUCTURE AND FUNCTION

The nervous system controls and coordinates all body activities, including the production of hormones. Special parts of the nervous system are concerned with maintaining normal day-to-day functions. Other parts act during emergency situations. Still others control voluntary activities. Neurological conditions require highly specialized nursing care. You will assist with the less technical aspects of that care.

Clinical Information ALERT

There are 31 pairs of spinal nerves and 12 pairs of cranial nerves. One nerve can send up to 1,000 impulses per second. A nerve impulse travels at approximately 224 miles per hour. One square inch of skin on the back of your hand has 12,000 nerve endings. There are 45 miles of nerves in the skin of a human being. If all the nerves in the body were laid out end to end, they would measure 167 miles. There are 30 times more pain receptors than cold sensors. The body is more sensitive to pain late in the afternoon. ■

Neurons

Cells of the nervous system are called **neurons** (Figure 43-1A). They are specialized to conduct electriclike impulses. The neuron has extensions called **axons** and **dendrites**. Impulses enter the neuron only through the dendrites and leave only through the axon.

Although neurons do not actually touch each other, the axon of one neuron lies close to the dendrites of many

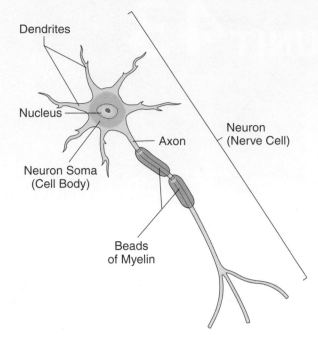

FIGURE 43-1A The neuron

other neurons. In this way, impulses may follow many different routes. The space between the axon of one cell and the dendrites of others is called a **synapse**. Axons and dendrites in the periphery are covered with *myelin*, which acts as insulation.

Neurotransmitters

Neurotransmitters are chemicals that enable messages (nerve impulses) to pass from one cell to another (Figure 43-1B). If the chemicals are not produced in the right amounts, the message pathway becomes confused or blocked.

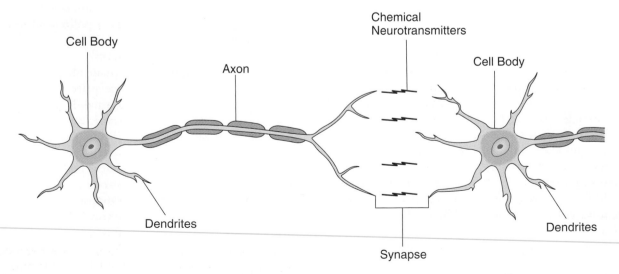

FIGURE 43-1B Chemicals called neurotransmitters help pass the message across the synapse from one neuron to another.

Lateral ventricles (2)
Skull
Frontal lobe
Temporal lobe
Pituitary gland
Midbrain
Pons
Medulla oblongata
Spinal cord

Parietal lobe
Convolutions (gyri)
Sulci
Dura mater
Arachnoid — Meninges
Pia mater
Third ventricle
Cerebral
Fourth ventricle
Cerebellum
Cerebrum

FIGURE 43-2 The central nervous system is composed of the brain and the spinal cord.

Nerves

Some axons and dendrites are long. Others are short. Axons and dendrites of many neurons are found in bundles. The bundles are held together by connective tissue. These bundles resemble telephone cables and are called **nerves**. The cell bodies of the axons and dendrites in these nerves may be found far from the ends of the nerves in clusters called *ganglia*.

Sensory nerves are made up of dendrites. They carry sensations to the brain and spinal cord from the various body parts. Feeling is lost when these nerve impulses are interrupted. Motor nerves carry impulses from the brain and spinal cord to muscles that cause body activity. Paralysis or loss of function occurs when these nerves are damaged.

For easier study, the nervous system can be divided into two parts: the central nervous system (CNS) and the peripheral nervous system (PNS). The CNS is composed of the brain and spinal cord (Figure 43-2). The PNS is composed of the 12 pairs of cranial nerves and 31 pairs of spinal nerves that reach throughout the body (Figure 43-3). Remember, though, that the nervous system is one interwoven system, a complex of millions of neurons.

The Central Nervous System

The brain and spinal cord are:

• Surrounded by bone

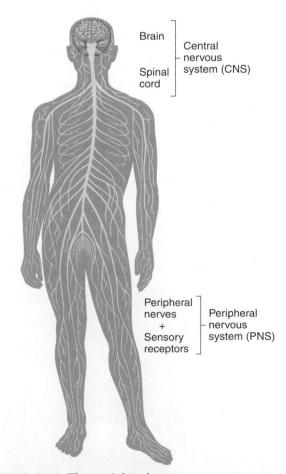

Brain
Spinal cord
Central nervous system (CNS)

Peripheral nerves + Sensory receptors
Peripheral nervous system (PNS)

FIGURE 43-3 The peripheral nervous system connects the central nervous system to the various structures of the body. Messages are relayed from these structures back to the brain through the spinal cord.

- Protected by membranes called *meninges*
- Cushioned by cerebrospinal fluid

The brain and spinal cord are a continuous structure found within the skull and spinal canal. The spinal cord is about 17 inches long. It ends just above the small of the back. Nerves extend from the brain and the spinal cord.

The Brain

The brain (encephalon) is a large, soft mass of nerve tissue contained within the cranium. It is composed of gray matter and white matter. Gray matter consists principally of nerve-cell bodies. White matter consists of nerve cells that form connections between various parts of the brain.

The brain can be further subdivided into the:

- **Cerebrum**—The largest portion of the brain. The outer portion is formed in folds known as convolutions and separated into lobes. The lobes take their names from the skull bones that surround them (Figure 43-4).
  - The outer portion, the cerebral cortex, is composed of cell bodies and appears gray.
  - The inner portion is composed of axons and dendrites and so appears white.
  - All mental activities—thought, direction of voluntary movements, interpretation of sensations, and experience of emotions—are carried out by cerebral cells (Figure 43-5). Certain activities are centered in each lobe.

Clinical Information ALERT

The brain is 85% water. The adult brain has 14 billion nerve cells, yet weighs less than 3 pounds. It uses 25% of the body's total oxygen supply. It also consumes more energy than any other organ, approximately one-fifth of the total food taken in. The cerebral hemispheres make up 83% of the brain's weight. It is supported by cerebrospinal fluid, or it would flatten out. It is the least sensitive organ in the body. The most sensitive parts of the brain are the meninges. It operates on the same amount of electricity as a 10-watt light bulb. The brain triples in size during the first few years of childhood. The center of the brain is the warmest part of the body. The brain has a separate area controlling the thumb. The motor neuron from the spinal cord to the big toe is the largest cell in the body. The myelinated fiber tracts make up the whitest part of brain. The collections of neuronal cell bodies make up the grayest part of the brain. ■

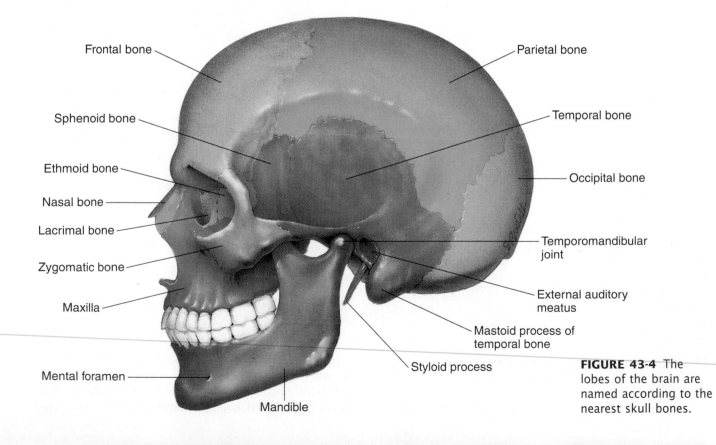

FIGURE 43-4 The lobes of the brain are named according to the nearest skull bones.

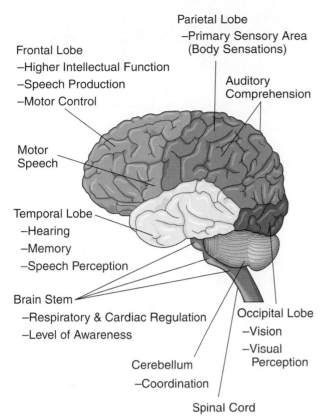

Frontal Lobe
–Higher Intellectual Function
–Speech Production
–Motor Control

Parietal Lobe
–Primary Sensory Area
(Body Sensations)

Auditory
Comprehension

Motor
Speech

Temporal Lobe
–Hearing
–Memory
–Speech Perception

Brain Stem
–Respiratory & Cardiac Regulation
–Level of Awareness

Occipital Lobe
–Vision
–Visual
Perception

Cerebellum
–Coordination

Spinal Cord

FIGURE 43-5 Each lobe of the brain is responsible for a different function.

- In general, the right side of the cerebrum interprets for and controls the left side of the body and vice versa.
- **Cerebellum**—Found beneath the occipital lobe of the cerebrum. It too has an outer layer of gray cell bodies. This portion of the brain coordinates muscular activities and balance.
- **Brain stem**—The midbrain, pons, and medulla are in the brain stem. They are composed mainly of axons and dendrites. These fibers serve as connecting pathways between the control centers in the cerebrum and cerebellum and the spinal cord. Control centers are found within the brain stem for involuntary movements of such vital organs as the:
  - Heart
  - Blood vessels
  - Lungs
  - Stomach
  - Intestines

The Spinal Cord

The spinal cord (Figure 43-6) extends from the medulla to the second lumbar vertebra in the spinal canal, which is above the small of the back, a distance of about 17 inches. Nerves entering and leaving the spinal cord carry impulses to and from the control centers. Certain reflex activities performed without conscious thought are controlled within the cord. Pulling your hand away from something hot is an example of this type of reflex activity (Figure 43-7).

The Meninges

Three membranes, called **meninges**, surround both the brain and the spinal cord. They are the dura mater, the arachnoid mater, and the pia mater.

The dura mater is the tough outer covering. The arachnoid mater is the middle, loosely structured layer. It is filled with cerebrospinal fluid. The pia mater is the innermost, delicate layer. It is very vascular (contains many blood vessels) and clings to the brain, spinal cord, and nerve roots.

Cerebrospinal Fluid

Ventricles are cavities within the cerebrum that are lined with highly vascular tissue. These tissues produce **cerebrospinal fluid (CSF)**, which flows around the brain and the spinal cord. The cerebrospinal fluid bathes the central nervous system as tissue fluid and cushions it against shock and possible injury.

Special Relationships: The Autonomic Nervous System

The phrase *autonomic nervous system (ANS)* refers to special pathways in cranial and spinal nerves (Figure 43-8). The control center is in the brain stem. The pathways begin in the CNS and reach out to the glands, smooth muscle walls of organs, and heart.

The autonomic nervous system consists of two parts: sympathetic fibers and parasympathetic fibers. Sympathetic fibers stimulate activities that prepare the body to deal with emergency situations. This is the mechanism of "fight or flight." Parasympathetic fibers control the usual functions of moderate heartbeat, digestion, elimination, respiration, and glandular activity.

Sensory Receptors

The ends of the dendrites carrying sensations to the central nervous system are found throughout the body.

- Some begin in joints and bring information about body positions to the brain.
- Others in the skin carry sensations of pain, heat, pressure, and cold.
- Those in the nose carry the sense of smell.
- The dendrites in the tongue carry the sense of taste.

Sensory dendrites also receive stimulation through two very special end organs, the eye and the ear. All of these structures are called sensory receptors because they carry

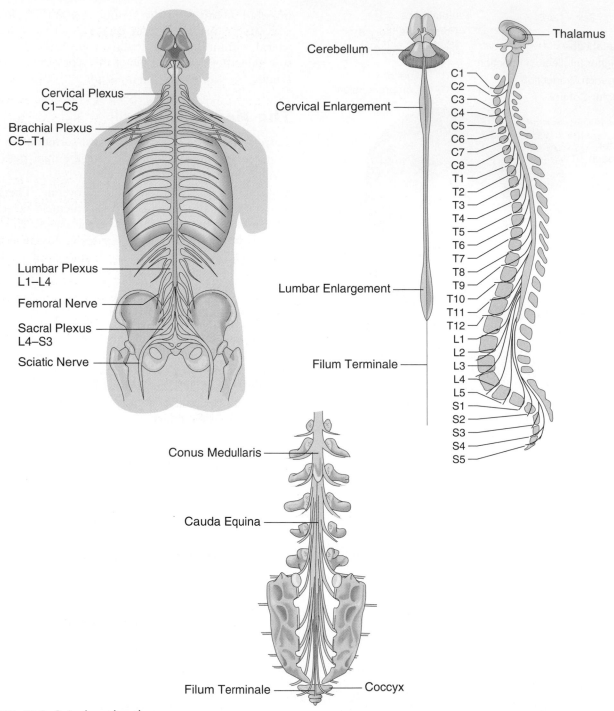

FIGURE 43-6 Spinal cord and nerves

information about the outside world to the brain. The brain interprets and processes the information.

The Eye

The eye (Figures 43-9A and 43-9B) is a hollow ball filled with two liquids called the *aqueous humor* and the *vitreous humor*. The wall of the eye is made up of three layers:

- The sclera: A tough, white outer coat that is protective. The **cornea** is the transparent portion in the front. Light rays pass through the cornea into the eye.

- The choroid: The nutritive layer found beneath the sclera. The choroid nourishes the eye tissues through its large number of blood vessels.

- The retina: The innermost layer is made up of neurons that are sensitive to light. The neurons join together and their axons leave the eye as the optic nerve. The two nerves cross beneath the brain and carry their impulses to the occipital lobe of the cerebrum to let us know what we are seeing.

Seeing. We see as light enters the eye through the cornea. The amount of light entering the eye is controlled

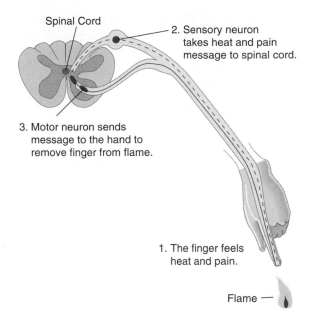

2. Sensory neuron takes heat and pain message to spinal cord.

Spinal Cord

3. Motor neuron sends message to the hand to remove finger from flame.

1. The finger feels heat and pain.

Flame —

FIGURE 43-7 Reflex arc

Special senses (controls pupil size)

Respiratory system (controls respiratory rate)

Cardiovascular system (controls heart rate and blood flow)

Digestive system (controls functions of stomach and small intestine)

Digestive system (controls flow of pancreatic juices)

Endocrine system (adrenal glands stimulate the sympathetic nervous system)

Digestive system (controls functions of large intestine)

FIGURE 43-8 Autonomic nervous system

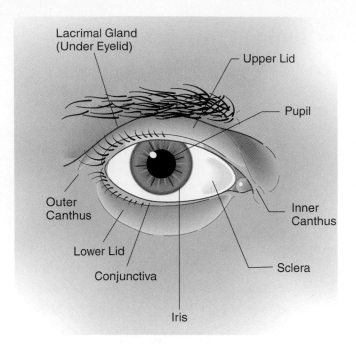

FIGURE 43-9A External view of the eye

by the iris. The **iris** is the colored portion of the eye. It is found behind the cornea. Fluid between the cornea and iris helps to bend the light rays and bring them to focus on the retina. The opening in the iris is called the **pupil**. The pupil appears black because there is no light behind it. Directly behind the iris is the lens. Small muscles pull on either side of the lens to change its shape. The changing shape of the lens makes it possible for us to adjust the range of our vision from far to near or from near to far.

The eye is:

- Held within the bony socket by muscles that can change its position.
- Covered by a mucous membrane, the **conjunctiva**. The conjunctiva lines the eyelids and covers the eye.

- Protected by the eyelids and eyelashes. Tears are manufactured by the **lacrimal glands** found beneath the lateral side of the upper lid. Tears protect the eye as they wash across the eye, keeping it moist, and then drain into the nasal cavity.

The Ear

Just as the eye is sensitive to light, the ear is sensitive to sound (Figure 43-10). The ear functions in hearing and equilibrium (balance). The ear has three parts: the outer ear, the middle ear, and the inner ear. The outer ear consists of the visible external structure known as the *pinna* and a canal, which directs sound waves toward the middle ear. At the end of the canal is the eardrum, or **tympanic membrane**. Sound waves cause the eardrum to vibrate.

The middle ear is made up of three tiny bones called **ossicles**. The ossicles form a chain across the middle ear from the tympanic membrane to an opening in the inner ear. These bones are known as the:

- Incus or anvil
- Malleus or hammer
- Stapes or stirrup

Small tubes, called the **eustachian tubes**, lead from the nasopharynx into the middle ear to equalize pressure on either side of the eardrum. Sound waves pushing against the tympanic membrane cause the ossicles to vibrate and push against the opening of the inner ear. This motion starts fluid moving in the inner ear.

The inner ear is a very complex structure. It has two main parts: the cochlea and three semicircular canals. The **cochlea** looks somewhat like a coiled snail shell. Within the cochlea are the tiny dendrites of the hearing or auditory nerve. Fluid covers the dendrites. When the fluid is set in motion by the vibration of the middle ear bones, it stimulates the dendrites with sound sensations. The auditory nerves, one from each ear, carry the sensations to the

FIGURE 43-9B Internal view of the eye

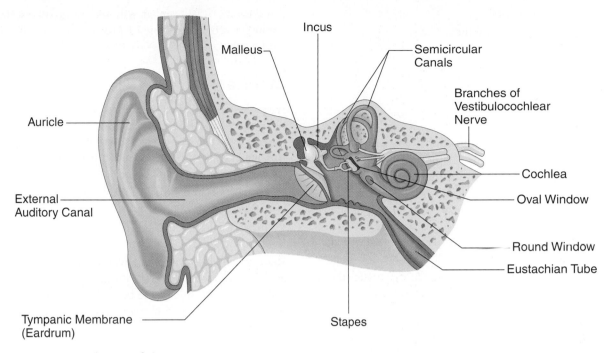

Incus
Malleus
Semicircular Canals
Branches of Vestibulocochlear Nerve
Auricle
Cochlea
External Auditory Canal
Oval Window
Round Window
Eustachian Tube
Tympanic Membrane (Eardrum)
Stapes

FIGURE 43-10 Internal view of the ear

temporal lobe of the cerebrum to let us know what we are hearing.

The three **semicircular canals** also contain liquid and nerve endings. When these nerve endings are stimulated, impulses about the position of the head are sent to the brain. This helps us keep our balance.

COMMON CONDITIONS

The nervous system usually remains healthy. However, injury or disease to the brain, spinal cord, or nerves requires appropriate treatment.

Increased Intracranial Pressure

The structures within the skull normally exert a certain amount of pressure, called the **intracranial pressure**. The pressure is due to:

- Nervous tissue
- Cerebrospinal fluid
- Blood flowing through cerebral vessels

Any change in the size or amount of these components changes the pressure. Increased intracranial pressure can result from:

- Head injury. Bleeding from damaged blood vessels and edema puts pressure on the delicate nervous tissue.
- Inflammation or infection plus edema.
- Intracranial bleeding due to ruptured blood vessels. This is called a cerebrovascular accident (CVA).
- Toxins.
- High temperature.

- Blockage of the normal flow of cerebrospinal fluid.
- Tumors.

Signs and Symptoms. Indications of increased intracranial pressure include:

- Alteration in pupil size and response to light. In the normal eye, the pupil becomes smaller when a flashlight is directed at each eye. The equality of the pupils and their ability to react to light is an important observation when a head injury occurs.
- Headache.
- Vomiting.
- Loss of consciousness and sensation.
- **Paralysis**—loss of voluntary motor control.
- **Convulsions** (seizures)—uncontrolled muscular contractions that are often violent.

How long all or part of the symptoms remain depends on the extent and cause of damage to the brain cells. Remember also that paralysis is not always accompanied by sensory loss.

Specific Nursing Care. Patients who are acutely ill with head injuries or increased intracranial pressure require skilled nursing care. The nurse is responsible for monitoring the patient's:

- Level of consciousness
- Degree of orientation to time and place
- Reaction to pain and stimuli
- Vital signs

If you note any change in the patient's response or behavior as you are assisting in care, bring it to the nurse's attention immediately. Changes that might be very significant include:

- Incontinence (new onset)
- Uncontrolled body movements
- Disorientation
- Deepening or lessening in the level of consciousness
- Dizziness
- Vomiting
- Alterations in speech
- Change in ability to follow directions

Once improved, the patient may be moved from a critical unit to an intermediate unit. From there, the patient may go to a long-term care facility for a possibly long period of convalescence. The patient may require extensive rehabilitation to regain functional skills. The nursing measures first established in the critical care unit must be maintained throughout this extended period.

Loss of sensation and decreased mobility make these patients more prone to pressure ulcers, infection, and contractures. You must continue to:

- Give special skin care.
- Carry out range-of-motion exercises.
- Check skin over pressure points frequently.
- Change the patient's position regularly.
- Report early signs of infection.
- Monitor elimination. Loss of muscle tone and inactivity may lead to constipation and impaction.
- Check drainage tubes such as indwelling catheters. They must receive careful attention.
- Provide reality orientation as needed.
- Be alert to any signs of mood change and plan extra time to provide essential support. Patients recovering from these illnesses often experience anxiety and depression.
- Keep a careful check on vital signs of any patient with a head injury. A special record (neurological monitoring record) may be kept for recording all observations.

The **Glasgow Coma Scale** is used to monitor neurologic problems after trauma, stroke, and other illnesses and injuries. The examiner determines the best response the patient can make to stimuli. The score is determined by adding the total of all three categories. Higher point values are assigned to responses that indicate increased awareness and arousal. A score of less than 8 indicates a neurological crisis. A score of 9–13 indicates moderate dysfunction, and a score of 13–15 indicates moderate to minor dysfunction.

Transient Ischemic Attack

A *transient ischemic attack (TIA)* is a temporary period of diminished blood flow to the brain. The attack comes on rapidly and may last from 2 to 15 minutes or for as long as 24 hours. Symptoms are similar to those of a stroke but are temporary and reversible. Transient ischemic attacks may occur once or several times in a lifetime. Persons experiencing TIAs are at risk for eventually suffering a stroke. A scoring system to predict the risk of having a stroke appears in Table 43-1.

Stroke

A **stroke** is also called a **cerebrovascular accident (CVA)** or **brain attack**. It affects the vascular system and the nervous system. The complete or partial loss of blood flow to the brain tissue is frequently a complication of atherosclerosis or brain hemorrhage. Causes of CVA include:

- Vascular occlusion due to a thrombus, atherosclerotic plaques, or emboli that obstruct the flow of blood
- Intracranial bleeding as blood vessels rupture, releasing blood into the brain tissue

Remember, most nerve pathways cross. Therefore, damage on one side of the brain results in signs and symptoms on the opposite side of the body. Symptoms vary depending on the extent of interference with the circulation and

TABLE 43-1 PREDICTING STROKES

Factor	Score
Age over 60	1
Elevated blood pressure	1
Symptoms	
weakness on one side of body	
speech difficulty	2
weakness on one side of body (only)	1
neither	0
Duration of Symptoms	
more than 60 minutes	2
10 to 59 minutes	1
less than 10 minutes	0

Total Score

Risk of stroke within 7 days of a TIA:

Score	Risk
1–3	0.0%
4	1.1%
5	12.1%
6	31.4%

SOURCE: Rothwell, P. M., Giles, M. F., Flossmann, E. et al. (2005). A simple score (ABCD) to identify individuals at high early risk of stroke after transient ischaemic attack. *Lancet, 366,* 29–36.

Clinical Information ALERT

The average stroke takes 10 hours to evolve and involves 54 milliliters (about 3 cubic inches) of brain tissue. Oxygen deprivation causes the brain to age about 3.6 years each hour; 1.9 million nerve cells in the brain die each minute after a stroke. Getting rapid treatment is essential to preventing further damage to the brain. A popular saying is "Time is brain," suggesting that outcomes decline when treatment is delayed. Stroke is the leading cause of long-term disability in the United States, affecting more than 2.5 million people, and killing nearly 200,000 a year. When the patient with a suspected stroke arrives at the hospital, doctors will determine what type of stroke he or she is having (Figure 43-11). About 80% of strokes are *ischemic* strokes, in which a blood clot travels along an artery in the brain until it gets stuck and blocks the flow of blood. About 15% of all strokes are bleeding (*hemorrhagic*) strokes, which occur when a blood vessel in the brain ruptures. Ischemic strokes can be treated with newer, clot-busting drugs if the patient arrives at the hospital quickly. Hemorrhagic stroke is more deadly and difficult to treat. ▪

on the area and amount of tissue damaged. Patients with damage to the right side of the brain will exhibit:

- **Spatial-perceptual deficits.** This means it is difficult to distinguish right from left and up from down. The world may appear "tilted" to the person with right-brain damage. The patient will have problems propelling a wheelchair, setting down items, and carrying out the activities of daily living.
- Change in personality. The individual with right brain damage becomes very quick and impulsive.

If the left side of the brain is damaged, you will note:

- **Aphasia**—an inability to express or understand speech.
- Change in personality. The individual becomes very cautious, anxious, and slow to complete tasks.

Other symptoms may be present with either right- or left-brain damage. These include:

- **Hemiparesis** (weakness) or **hemiplegia** (paralysis) on one side of the body, on the opposite side from the area of the brain in which the stroke occurred. You will notice a difference when comparing the sides of the

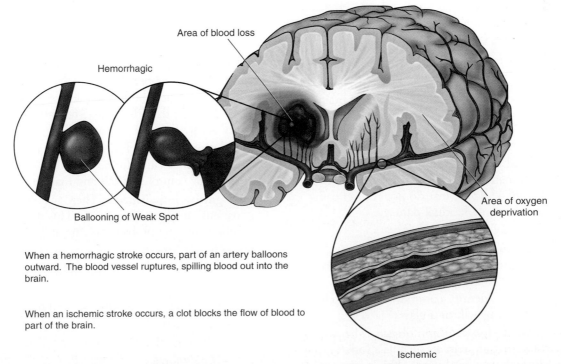

Area of blood loss

Hemorrhagic

Ballooning of Weak Spot

Area of oxygen deprivation

When a hemorrhagic stroke occurs, part of an artery balloons outward. The blood vessel ruptures, spilling blood out into the brain.

When an ischemic stroke occurs, a clot blocks the flow of blood to part of the brain.

Ischemic

FIGURE 43-11 Although there are no definite rules, thrombotic strokes usually occur more commonly in older adults, and hemorrhagic strokes are more common in younger persons. "Clotbuster" drugs may be given to treat a thrombotic stroke if the condition is identified and treated rapidly, usually within 3 hours of the onset of symptoms. No comparable drugs are available to treat hemorrhagic stroke, and the prognosis is not as good.

A. Normal

B. Stroke on left side of brain (right side of picture)

A. Normal

B. Stroke on left side of brain (right side of picture)

FIGURE 43-12 Compare the right and left sides of the patient's body. Weakness or paralysis occurs on the face, arm, and leg on the opposite side of the area of the brain in which the stroke occurred.

body, from head to foot (Figure 43-12). With early, aggressive treatment, some patients make a partial recovery (Figure 43-13). Most do not recover completely, and have some residual damage.

- Sensory-perceptual deficits
  - Loss of **position sense**. The person cannot tell, for example, where an affected foot is or what position it is in without looking at it.
  - The inability to identify common objects such as a comb, a fork, a pencil, or a glass.
  - The inability to use common objects. The patient may know what an item is, such as a fork, but be unable to pick it up and use it. This is not a result of paralysis but is due to brain damage.
- **Unilateral neglect.** The patient ignores the paralyzed side of the body. For example, the affected arm may

hang over the side of the wheelchair without the patient realizing where the arm is.

- **Hemianopsia.** This is impaired vision. Both eyes have only half vision. For example, if the patient has left hemiplegia, the left half of both eyes is blind (Figure 43-14). Remember this if a patient who has had a stroke eats the food on one side of the tray and leaves the food on the other side. The patient probably cannot see it. Turn the tray around.
- **Emotional lability.** Patients who have had a stroke may start to cry or laugh for no apparent reason. They have very little control over this and may be embarrassed.
- **Cognitive impairments.** There may be changes in the patient's intellectual function. This may affect memory, judgment, and problem-solving abilities.

Nursing Care. The goals of poststroke care include:

1. Maintaining the skills and abilities that the patient has left.
2. Preventing complications caused by immobility:
   - Contractures
   - Pressure ulcers
   - Pneumonia
   - Blood clots
3. Helping the patient regain functional abilities:
   - Activities of daily living (Figure 43-15)

FIGURE 43-13 This woman had a stroke on the left side of the brain, affecting the right side of her body. She is able to walk with a cane and is making a good recovery.

FIGURE 43-14 Hemianopsia is a common problem after a stroke. The patient is blind in one-half of the visual field. Unrecognized, this is a serious problem at mealtime, because the patient cannot see half the food, so does not eat it, resulting in significant weight loss. The problem is easily solved by turning the plate around. The patient may not remember to do it, even if instructed, because of brain damage from the stroke.

- Bowel and bladder control
- Mobility
- Communication skills

FIGURE 43-15 The patient who has had a stroke may need to relearn activities of daily living. Depending on the area of brain damage, she may need to learn to do her ADLs in a different way than she did previously.

Clinical Information ALERT

We care for patients during their most vulnerable moments and try to be empathetic. Patients view caregivers as compassionate, talented, professional healers who accept patients' loss of independence with grace and dignity. Unfortunately, patients often do not accept their losses well. Each time we touch them, they want us to make it all right and ease their pain, which is often emotional. Understanding how tangible independence is, along with the dynamics, grief, and pain associated with a loss of this magnitude, will enhance your insight into patients' needs. It will give you insight into why some patients take risks. Their physical, mental, emotional, and psychosocial challenges are often enormous. ■

During Recovery. Recovery from a stroke is often a very frustrating experience for the patient. Caregivers must be patient. In your approach to the patient, remember two things:

1. The patient has more than enough frustration for both of you, so be careful not to let yours show. The last thing the patient needs is your silent reinforcement of his helplessness.

2. The degree and speed of recovery are directly related, in most cases, to the patience and encouragement of the caregivers with whom the patient has close contact.

Other interventions during recovery include:

- Physical therapy to increase independent mobility: bed movement, getting to the side of the bed, standing by the side of the bed, transferring out of bed and into a chair, and ambulation.
- Occupational therapy to regain the ability to perform the activities of daily living, such as bathing, grooming, dressing, and eating, with little or no assistance.
- Speech therapy to regain or to learn different methods of communication. The speech therapist also works with swallowing problems caused by the stroke.
- Nursing care to:
  - implement bowel and bladder training programs, or give catheter care if necessary
  - implement pressure ulcer prevention programs
  - reinforce the therapy programs
- Care to prevent contractures by:
  - positioning the patient appropriately and changing positions at least every 2 hours
  - performing passive range-of-motion exercises as directed
  - applying splints or braces as ordered

Communication HIGHLIGHT

Try to develop rapport with the patient on your first contact. At times, this is difficult because a stroke often causes mood changes. If the patient is newly dependent, he may also have mood or behavior problems. Be consistent and avoid becoming discouraged. Try to remember that the illness is causing the problem. Find the most effective means of communicating the information you need to convey. Ask yes or no questions whenever possible. Avoid treating the patient like a child and do not correct his speech. If you must repeat yourself, do so quietly and calmly. Use gestures, if necessary. ■

All staff can help with rehabilitation efforts by:

- Encouraging the patient to communicate
- Maintaining a positive and supportive attitude at all times
- Providing only the assistance that the patient needs
- Following approaches consistently as outlined in the patient's care plan

Convalescence is often long. The nursing care is demanding, requiring much patience and understanding.

Aphasia

Stroke victims often suffer from aphasia or language impairment. They have difficulty forming thoughts or expressing them in coherent ways. This is extremely frustrating and frightening for the patient and family.

- **Receptive aphasia** means that the person cannot comprehend communication.
- **Expressive aphasia** means that the person cannot properly form thoughts or express them coherently.
- **Global aphasia** means that the person has lost all language abilities.

Review Unit 7 for guidelines for communicating with patients with aphasia.

Parkinson's Disease

Parkinson's disease is believed to be caused by not having enough neurotransmitters (dopamine) in the brain stem and cerebellum. The symptoms are progressive over many years. Some people will show minor changes. Others will have much more obvious symptoms (Figure 43-16).

Signs and Symptoms. Signs and symptoms of Parkinson's disease include:

- **Tremors** (uncontrolled trembling). Tremors of the hands commonly affect the fingers and thumb in such a way that an affected person will appear to be rolling a small object (such as a pill) between them. These tremors occur frequently. They usually begin in the fingers, then involve the entire hand and arm, and finally affect an entire side of the body. Starting on one side, the tremors eventually involve both sides of the body. Tremors are more evident when the person is inactive. A typical posture of a patient suffering from Parkinson's disease is shown in Figure 43-17.
- Muscular rigidity (loss of flexibility). The muscular rigidity is more evident when the patient is inactive. It seems to be lessened when the person sleeps or engages in activities such as walking or other exercises that require large-muscle involvement. The rigidity makes the person with Parkinson's disease more prone to falls and injury.
- **Akinesia** (difficulty and slowness in carrying out voluntary muscular activities). Persons with advanced Parkinson's typically have:
  - a shuffling manner of walking
  - difficulty starting the process of walking
  - difficulty stopping smoothly once walking has started
  - affected speech, causing words to be slurred and poorly spoken (enunciated)
  - facial muscles that lose expressiveness and emotional response

FIGURE 43-17 The typical posture of a patient with Parkinson's disease. In addition to the standing posture, note the patient's hands.

FIGURE 43-16 Progression of Parkinson's disease. A. The patient leans slightly forward and develops flexion of affected arm. B. The patient stoops forward slightly and walks with a shuffling gait. C. As the disease progresses, the patient needs support to prevent falling. The patient tends to shuffle faster and faster, leaning farther forward until he falls on his face. D. The disease progresses to the point of needing assistance for ambulation. E. The patient has profound weakness and severe tremors. Ambulation becomes impossible.

- Loss of autonomic nervous control. Because of loss of autonomic nervous control, persons with Parkinson's may:
  - drool
  - become incontinent
  - become constipated
  - retain urine
- Mood swings and gradual behavioral changes. A patient may appear happy and positive one moment, and then be depressed the next. The depression tends to be progressive. Personality and behavioral changes may occur that cause psychotic breakdowns and dementia in later stages.

Treatment. The treatment consists of:

- Surgery for patients who qualify
- Drug therapy
- Therapy to limit the muscular rigidity and to meet basic physical and emotional needs

Nursing Care. Nursing care of the person with Parkinson's disease includes:

- Maintaining a calm environment. Symptoms are more intense when the patient is under stress.
- Assisting and supervising the activities of daily living. For example, directing food into the mouth and then keeping it there to be chewed and swallowed is very difficult for many persons with Parkinson's disease.
- Providing emotional support and encouragement.
- Carrying out a program of general and specific exercises.
- Providing protection for patients with dementia.

Difficult SITUATIONS

Patients with Parkinson's disease may have inconsistent needs for physical support and assistance. If the patient is tired, he may need more support than when he is rested. When the patient is stressed, the tremors may worsen, increasing the need for hands-on assistance. ■

Huntington's Disease

Huntington's disease (HD) is also called Huntington's chorea. This is a hereditary disease. In recent years, a genetic test has become available. The test shows if individuals with a family history of the disorder have the Huntington's gene. If the gene is present, development of the disease is inevitable. Some people with a family history are not tested, because they do not want to know if they will develop the condition. They have seen family members with the disease and fear the diagnosis.

Signs and Symptoms. Clinical signs of the disease usually begin when individuals are in their 40s or 50s. In some individuals, symptoms of the disease first appear in childhood or young adulthood. The disease is progressive and there is no cure. Disability and death occur within 15 to 20 years. Abnormal movements, called **chorea**, are the primary sign of HD. The movements are subtle early in the course of the illness. The individual will appear anxious or restless. He appears to move frequently. Most people are aware of this movement. The patient may try to disguise the activity with voluntary movements, such as scratching the head or crossing the legs. As the disease progresses, rapid, jerking choreiform movements develop. These movements involve the entire body. The patient will eventually lose voluntary control of all movement.

She also loses control of the bowel and bladder. The involuntary movement increases with stress and attempts to control the choreiform motions.

Nursing Care. There is no known treatment or cure for HD. Patients with Huntington's disease are commonly admitted to the long-term care facility because they cannot function safely at home. They may be hospitalized for complications, such as aspiration and pneumonia, which are common with this condition. Urinary tract infection and pressure ulcers are also problematic. As the disease progresses, the patient's response to pain and heat and cold sensitivity may be delayed. The nursing assistant should anticipate these sensation abnormalities and monitor food and bath water temperature closely. Nursing care is designed to:

- Maintain a consistent routine, avoiding change as much as possible
- Keep the patient as independent as possible for as long as possible
- Maintain the person's current abilities
- Prevent weight loss by replacing calories used by the spastic movement
- Promote safe swallowing and prevent choking
- Prevent falls and other injuries
- Maintain the patient's ability to communicate

Poor muscular control makes communication difficult. The speech therapist will assess the patient and establish a communication program. The patient will be taught to use either hand signals, cards, or a communication board. Give the patient feedback when he speaks. Repeating what the patient says is a good way to show that the communication was successful.

Ambulation and Mobility. As the disease progresses, the patient will develop a strange gait in which she sways back and forth and extends the hips in an attempt to balance. If the patient is ambulatory, she is at very high risk of falls. If the person can walk, allow her to do so, but provide support and assistance, if necessary. Sitting in a chair may be difficult for some patients. The involuntary movements may cause the patient to fall out of the chair and onto the floor. Approaches to assist with mobility are:

- Supervise ambulation for safety
- Ambulate with a gait belt

A recliner with adaptations and padding may be necessary to enable the person to be out of bed. A seat belt may also be necessary when the patient is in the chair. When the patient is in bed, the side rails should be well padded to prevent injury caused by banging arms and legs into the rails because of spasticity.

Cognitive Changes. Individuals with HD develop mental changes. Early in the condition, the individual becomes nervous, suspicious of others, and irritable. Mood swings are common, as is depression. As the condition progresses, the individual develops dementia. He becomes totally dependent on others.

Loss of control, power, and autonomy are major issues in HD. The patient loses impulse control with disease progression and may become angry at caregivers' efforts to protect him. Some patients view cigarette smoking as a bridge between independence and dependence. They insist on smoking because it is "the last remaining pleasure" they have. Unfortunately, with their impaired safety judgment, they may exhibit unsafe smoking behavior. They lose sensitivity to heat and cold, and may burn themselves when lighting a cigarette, or when smoking down to the filter. Give patients as much control over daily routines as possible, and empower them by offering choices. Other approaches are to:

- Treat the patient with dignity and respect.
- Monitor smoking behavior carefully.
- Inform the nurse if you find smoking materials in a HD patient's room.
- Despite cognitive changes, the patients usually know what is going on around them. Avoid treating them like children or making insensitive remarks.

Nutrition. The rapid movements burn many calories. The patient is at very high risk for weight loss. Extra nutrition and hydration will be ordered. The patient may have difficulty with the texture of some foods. Saliva may run from the mouth, and the tongue may be difficult to control. The patient will develop difficulty swallowing and is at very high risk for choking. She may need to be spoon-fed. Increased movements of the tongue may tend to push the food out of the mouth, making chewing and swallowing difficult. Assist the patient at mealtime by:

- Keeping mealtime as stress-free as possible.
- Applying a clothing protector; avoid calling this garment a bib.
- Allowing extra time for the patient to eat. You may have to reheat the food.
- Serving a mechanical soft or pureed diet or foods that are easy to swallow.
- Feeding slowly.
- Encouraging use of adaptive utensils listed on the care plan to help maintain independence.
- Seating the patient completely upright at meals to prevent choking.
- Following the care plan:
  - the care plan may instruct you to remind the patient to tuck the chin when swallowing.
  - remind the patient to keep the chin down near the chest during swallowing, to prevent choking.
  - remind the patient to cough after each mouthful. This clears the throat of any remaining food.
- Avoiding conversation at mealtime. Limit conversation to cues and instructions for eating.
- Checking the mouth for retained food after each meal.

- Providing oral hygiene after meals. This is important because of the risk of aspiration of food particles and saliva.

Multiple Sclerosis

Multiple sclerosis (MS) generally occurs in young adults. It is the result of the loss of insulation (myelin) around central nervous system nerve fibers. This interferes with the ability of the nerve fibers to function.

The cause of MS is unknown. Many individuals live the usual life span even though they have this chronic condition. The symptoms are variable and may not be the same for all individuals. Symptoms may include:

- Loss of sensation with regard to temperature, pain, and touch
- Feelings of numbness and tingling
- **Vertigo** (a spinning or dizzy sensation)
- **Lhermitte's sign** (a tingling, shock-like sensation that passes down the arms or spine when the neck is flexed)

Problems with vision occur in almost half of the people who have MS. The problem may be temporary or permanent. Vision symptoms may include:

- Blurriness, color blindness, or difficulty seeing objects in bright light
- Double vision
- **Nystagmus** (jerky eye movements)

Mobility is usually affected:

- Pain in the legs that disappears with rest.
- **Paraplegia** (paralysis of both legs) and **quadriplegia** (paralysis of all four extremities) in advanced cases. Another term for paralysis of the arms and legs is **tetraplegia**. When a person is paralyzed, voluntary movement, strength, and sensation are limited or absent. This condition involves much more than ability to move a body part.
- Spasticity of muscles.
- **Intention tremor** (shaking of the hands that gets worse as the individual tries to touch or pick up an object).

In severe MS, speech is affected because of the weakness of the muscles in the chest, face, and lips. The speech may be slow, with poor articulation. The mind usually remains alert. Incontinence of bowel and bladder are common in advanced cases.

One of the most disabling features of MS is fatigue. The fatigue is very real and is not psychological.

MS may follow one of four courses:

- *Benign course:* mild attacks with long periods of no symptoms.
- *Exacerbating-remitting:* Severe attacks (exacerbations) followed by periods of partial or complete recovery (remissions). Often the periods of exacerbation get longer and more severe with shorter periods of remission.

- *Slowly progressive:* slow, steady deterioration.
- *Rapidly progressive:* deterioration is rapid and progressive and may be life-threatening.

Nursing Care. Nursing care of the patient with multiple sclerosis includes:

1. Implement a pressure ulcer prevention program.
2. Implement contracture prevention programs through consistent changes of position and passive range-of-motion exercises. Apply splints correctly, if ordered.
3. Pay careful attention to catheter care if the patient has an indwelling catheter, to prevent bladder infections.
4. Encourage independence. Follow instructions from the nurse or the therapists for specific techniques to use.
5. Help the patient maintain a balanced schedule of rest and activity.
6. Provide emotional support and encouragement.

Treatment. There is no known way to stop the progression of the disease. Treatment consists of maintaining functional ability as long as possible through general health practices and physical therapy.

Difficult SITUATIONS

A warm bath or shower is often very relaxing to a patient with multiple sclerosis. However, you must make sure that the water is not too hot, which temporarily intensifies some symptoms of MS. Keeping bath water at about 100°F to 105°F is best. Take your responsibility for assisting with range-of-motion exercises seriously. ROM is especially important in patients with MS to maintain joint mobility and muscle tone, reduce spasticity, improve coordination, and boost self-esteem. ■

Post Polio Syndrome (PPS)

Polio is a very serious neurological disease that has been with us since at least 1350 B.C. This disease is caused by a virus that attacks the motor neurons in the spinal cord. Muscles affected by these neurons no longer function properly, resulting in weakness and paralysis. Some patients had respiratory paralysis, and needed a special ventilator to breathe. Others had speech and swallowing problems. Most had paralysis and weakness in the arms and legs. Many people died as a result of polio. Most of those who survived learned to overcome their disabilities and lead productive lives.

There were large annual outbreaks of polio in the United States every summer. The largest was in 1952. In 1955,

an injectable vaccine became available to prevent polio. Because of the severity of the condition, most children received the vaccination. In 1962, an oral polio vaccine was introduced. Both vaccines continue to be used today. Because of the effectiveness of the vaccines, infectious polio has been eliminated in the United States.

Post polio syndrome (PPS) is a neurologic condition marked by increased weakness and abnormal muscle fatigue in persons who had polio many years earlier. Estimates are that 30 to 70% of all polio survivors will develop this condition. There are several theories about the cause of PPS. The most common involves the motor neurons. Most polio survivors have about half as many motor neurons as others who were not affected by polio. It is believed that motor neurons that were not destroyed by the initial polio infection compensated by sprouting new connections. Some of the new neurons adapted to innervate areas that are five to seven times larger than normal. These neurons may be slowly dying, perhaps because of years of overuse. As the neurons die, they lose their muscle connections, and muscles stop responding.

Signs and Symptoms. Signs and symptoms of PPS range from annoying to debilitating. Onset may be gradual or sudden, following trauma, infection, surgery, a fall, or a stressful event. The new injury puts stress on the remaining motor neurons, causing further reduction in function, pain, and fatigue. Signs and symptoms include:

- Fatigue that may be debilitating.
- New joint and muscle pain.
- New weakness in muscles affected by polio; unaffected muscles are also affected. The new weakness may be more prominent on one side of the body.
- New dyspnea and other respiratory problems.
- Severe cold intolerance, even with mild cold exposure. This causes the muscle weakness to worsen, the arms or legs to become pale or cyanotic, and the extremities to feel cold to the touch.
- Muscle spasms and cramps that are sometimes severe and painful.
- Difficulty swallowing.
- Difficulty falling asleep and waking frequently during the night.

Some PPS patients become anxious when they are hospitalized. Emotional expressions of discouragement and displays of anger are fairly common. The patient may be fearful. Health care practices and attitudes were very different during the era of the polio epidemic. Many PPS patients were children during the original infection. They were in the hospital for a long time, and may have been forcibly separated from their parents. This was traumatic and caused them to feel isolated. Sadly, some were physically, emotionally, and sexually abused by hospital personnel. When a person with PPS is in the hospital, old feelings and fears sometimes return. The patient may experience feelings of fear and powerlessness that she cannot or will not talk about. Provide reassurance and emotional support, and report the patient's behavior to the nurse.

Most PPS patients experience pain daily. Muscle spasms often worsen the pain. Use nursing comfort measures, such as positioning and a backrub, to relieve pain. Inform the nurse of the patient's complaints of pain. Reducing strain and adjusting activities to conserve energy also help relieve pain. You may be asked to provide a heat treatment, which also relieves pain.

Many polio survivors have disturbed sleep because of muscle spasms, pain, or anxiety. Some experience sleep apnea, but are not aware of it. Body positioning is important during sleep to support weakened areas and deformities. Certain positions may be painful for the patient and extra pillows may be needed for support. Observe the patient's sleep at night and manage problems as they arise. Report your observations to the nurse.

Fatigue occurs daily, and can be debilitating. It may worsen as the day progresses. Some require more sleep than others who are not affected by PPS. Encourage the patient to rest and nap periodically throughout the day. Help the patient pace her activities and use measures to conserve energy. Therapy may be ordered to teach the patient to conserve energy.

About one-fifth of all PPS patients have swallowing problems. This increases the risk of choking. Position the patient as upright as possible while he is eating, and for 30 to 60 minutes after meals. Monitor the patient while eating and teach him to avoid talking while eating. Encourage him to alternate food and fluid, and to avoid swallowing when the head is tipped back. Assist with oral care after meals to remove retained food particles.

Patients with PPS have serious problems with cold because the nerves that control blood vessel size were destroyed by the virus. The legs and feet are commonly affected. One theory is that people with PPS function as if it were 20° colder than the actual temperature. Their legs and feet turn bright red following a hot bath. When the patient stands up, she may become dizzy or faint as blood pools in the legs, causing the blood pressure to drop. If the patient complains of cold, assist her with socks or extra blankets. You may be instructed to soak the feet in warm water, or assist with a warm bath. Caution the patient to call for help before getting out of the tub.

Surgical Procedures. Post polio patients who are admitted for surgery have many special needs. They are much more sensitive to anesthesia than persons who have not had polio. They require less medication and half the anesthesia, yet take twice as long as other patients to recover from the anesthesia. Because of this, the patient with PPS must be monitored closely for other problems. Patients may:

- Shiver violently after surgery. Provide warm blankets.
- Have side effects from common drugs. Monitor closely for abnormalities, and report to the nurse promptly.

- Have problems from blood loss, even a small amount. Monitor the operative site and vital signs carefully and report to the nurse.
- Have respiratory problems because of muscle weakness and lung problems. Encouraging the patient to cough and deep breathe after surgery is very important.
- Be unable to reposition themselves in bed. Assist the patient as needed.
- Have positioning problems because of deformities or discomfort. Do your best to make the patient comfortable. Use pillows and props for comfort and support.
- Vomit. This may cause fainting if the patient is upright. Monitor for choking. Report nausea or vomiting to the nurse.
- Choke on secretions. Position the patient on his side until he is fully awake. Monitor closely.
- Have problems with transfers and ambulation after surgery. Instruct the patient to call when she is ready to get out of bed. Have the patient dangle before rising. Use a transfer belt for safey.

Difficult SITUATIONS

Patients with post polio syndrome are fiercely independent, sometimes to their detriment. They may not complain because most were taught that part of their recovery includes being "normal." Asking for help may be very difficult for these patients. ■

Nursing Assistant Care. Patients with post polio syndrome are usually in the hospital for treatment of another condition. The problems caused by PPS are seldom severe enough to require hospitalization. However, they complicate the care of other conditions and procedures. Remember that these patients have lived with their condition for years and have found ways to adapt to it. Overall, they are experts in their own care. Respect their expertise. Coping with the new problems from PPS is often much more difficult than recovery from the original illness. Be prepared to help with activities of daily living, bed mobility, transfers, and ambulation. Patients with post polio syndrome may have many special needs.

Most PPS patients have their homes arranged so they can function independently. Temporarily staying in a different environment, such as a hospital, can be very troublesome for the patient. She may need help with tasks that she could do independently at home. Most PPS patients fear becoming dependent on others. The patient may have great difficulty asking for help. Anticipate her needs and ask if assistance is needed. Do not be surprised if the patient refuses your offer of help. Respect the refusal, but advise the patient that accepting assistance is different from being dependent. In fact, assistance may help the patient to remain independent. Even if the patient refuses your help, stand by to see if he can perform the task or procedure safely. Adapt the environment, whenever possible, for optimal independent function. You may do this by moving furniture, or bringing a bedside commode, for example. Most polio survivors are in tune to what their bodies are telling them. If the patient says she cannot do something, pay attention.

Amyotrophic Lateral Sclerosis (ALS)

Amyotrophic lateral sclerosis (ALS) is a progressive neuromuscular disease that causes muscle weakness and paralysis. It is a disease of the motor nerves that control voluntary movement. The cause is unknown. There seems to be a familial link in about 10% of the cases. ALS occurs in all races and both genders, although it is more common in men. The most common age of onset is 55, but it can occur in persons of any age. It is a progressive condition for which there is no cure. ALS is almost always fatal. In the United States, ALS is also called Lou Gehrig's disease, after a famous baseball player. Other names may be used in other countries. About half of the patients diagnosed with ALS die within 18 months, although some may live for many years. One drug has been successful in slowing progression of the disease, but there is no known cure. Some medications are used to relieve the symptoms.

Signs and Symptoms. ALS takes months to diagnose because the signs and symptoms are similar to those of other neurologic conditions. Common signs and symptoms of ALS are:

- Stumbling, tripping, and falling
- Loss of strength and muscle control in hands, arms, and legs
- Difficulty speaking
- Difficulty swallowing
- Drooling
- Breathing becoming progressively more difficult
- Muscle cramping, shaking, and twitching, progressing to spasticity
- Muscle weakness and atrophy
- Abnormal reflexes

ALS is not a painful disease, but the effects of ALS often cause pain. These are:

- Muscle cramps
- Contractures
- Constipation
- Burning eyes
- Swelling feet
- Muscle aches
- Pressure ulcers

ALS does not affect the entire body. The patient's mental acuity is intact. Depression is common. The heart, bowel and bladder control, and sexual function are not affected. The muscles controlling eye and eyelid movement are the last muscles affected. Sometimes they are not affected at all.

Progression of ALS. Progression of ALS varies with the patient. Worsening occurs over several months to several years. A common pattern is:

- Difficulty walking, causing the patient to use a cane, then a walker, then a wheelchair
- As the legs weaken, the hands and arms also become weaker
- The patient loses the ability to write and feed herself
- The patient experiences difficulty speaking, chewing, swallowing, and talking
- Eventually a feeding tube becomes necessary
- The patient needs an alternate communication system
- Chest and diaphragm muscles weaken, causing lung problems
- The patient needs a ventilator to stay alive

Nursing Assistant Care. Most ALS patients are cared for at home, with brief hospitalizations to manage complications. Because of this, ALS often involves the whole family. Patients are taught to manage their own illness. Allow the patient to be in control of daily routines, and respect his intelligence. Adaptive equipment is used to maintain independence for as long as possible.

Many ALS patients are not bedridden, despite being completely paralyzed. Special wheelchairs and portable ventilators are often used so patients can get out of bed. Follow the patient's care plan for mobility. If the patient does not get out of bed, reposition and turn her at least every 2 hours, or more often, as instructed.

Nursing care is designed to prevent complications of immobility. The most common problems are constipation, contractures, and pressure ulcers. You will also take measures to prevent choking and infection. Care of the patient is largely determined by the stage of the patient's disease at hospital admission. Follow the care plan and the nurse's instructions. Care of the typical ALS patient involves:

- Attention to positioning. An upright position (such as high Fowler's) may be ordered to ease respirations.
- Range-of-motion and light exercises to prevent deformities and maintain the strength of muscles that are not yet affected.
- Assisting the patient to use the incentive spirometer (Unit 39).
- Having the patient rest before meals to conserve muscle strength and reduce the risk of choking.
- Providing small, frequent feedings.
- Taking swallowing precautions when feeding the patient. The speech therapist may have taught the

patient positions and techniques to use to prevent choking. Commonly, the patient is as upright as possible, with the neck flexed slightly forward.

- Not washing solid foods down with liquids. This increases the risk of choking and aspiration in ALS patients.
- Checking the mouth after meals to make sure that no food particles remain. They can cause choking later. Provide mouth care promptly after each meal.
- Scheduling rest and activities to preserve the patient's strength and energy.
- Using good infection control measures, handwashing, and standard precautions to reduce the risk of infection.

Difficult SITUATIONS

ALS is a particularly cruel disease that causes fairly rapid degeneration of the nervous system, making the patient dependent. The mind remains intact and alert, so the patient is aware of each small change and its implications. Strive to develop a good rapport with the patient and provide generous emotional support and compassion. ■

Seizure Disorder (Epilepsy)

Seizure disorder (convulsions, **epilepsy**) involves recurrent, transient attacks of disturbed brain function. It is characterized by various forms of convulsions called *seizures*. Not all seizures are alike. A seizure occurs when one or more of the following is present:

- An altered state of consciousness, which may be momentary or prolonged
- Convulsive uncontrolled movements
- Disturbances of feeling or behavior

Seizures may develop:

- Congenitally, associated with a difficult birth
- Following a head injury
- As a result of increased intracranial pressure
- As a result of lesions of the brain such as tumors
- As a result of cerebrovascular accidents
- As a result of high fever or infection, especially in infants and children
- From taking certain medications or street drugs

Some persons experience an aura just before the seizure occurs. An **aura** involves one of the senses. The person may smell an unusual odor or hear a sound. The aura is usually consistent and remains the same each time it is experienced. For some people the aura serves as a warning so the person can get to a safe place. Other people may not remember the aura.

Some people have service dogs that warn them of an impending seizure so they can take safety precautions before the seizure begins. A dog's sense of smell is much more sensitive than a human's. It is believed that the dog smells a chemical reaction that signals the onset of a seizure. All states have access laws regarding service animals, but these vary widely. Your facility will have policies regarding the use of service animals while patients are hospitalized.

There are many different types and categories of seizure activity. The most common are classified as follows:

- Partial seizures
  - There may or may not be loss of consciousness.
  - Seizures generally begin in one part of the body and involve only one side of the body.
- Generalized seizures (Figure 43-18)
  - These include **grand mal seizures**. A newer name is **generalized tonic-clonic seizures**. There is bilateral generalized motor movement and muscular rigidity. Consciousness is lost and special awareness may or may not precede convulsive movements. The sensory awareness or aura may be in the form of lights, sounds, or aromas and is part of the seizure. When this seizure begins, the patient cries out, then falls to the floor. The muscles stiffen (tonic phase), then the extremities begin to jerk and twitch (clonic phase). The patient may lose bladder control. Consciousness returns slowly. After the seizure, the patient may feel tired, or be confused and disoriented. This state may last from a few minutes to several hours or days. The patient may fall asleep, or gradually become less confused until full consciousness returns.
  - **Petit mal seizures** are characterized by momentary loss of muscle tone. A more recent name is **absence seizures**. The seizure begins without warning, and consists of a period of unconsciousness, in which the patient blinks rapidly, stares blankly, breathes rapidly, or makes chewing movements. The seizure lasts 2 to 10 seconds, then ends abruptly. The patient usually resumes normal activity immediately. Because these seizures are mild, they may go unnoticed. Children with absence seizures may have learning problems if the seizures are not identified and treated.
- **Status epilepticus** is a seizure that lasts for a long time or repeats without recovery. It is a serious medical emergency. Death may result if the patient is not treated immediately. Status epilepticus can be convulsive (tonic-clonic) or nonconvulsive (absence). A person in nonconvulsive status epilepticus may become confused or appear dazed. The highest incidence of status epilepticus occurs during the first year of life and after age 60. In elderly adults, most cases are related to cerebrovascular accidents.

Nursing Care During Seizures. The main nursing focus during a seizure is to:

- Prevent injury by:

FIGURE 43-18 Generalized tonic-clonic seizures involve the entire body. Side rails should be padded for patients with seizure disorder. Side rails in this picture are down for clarity only.

– staying with the person
– assisting the person to lie down, if there is time
– making no attempt to restrain the person's movements or to put anything in her mouth
– moving away any object the person might hit, to protect the person from injuring herself
● Maintain an airway by:
– loosening clothing, particularly around the neck
– turning the person's head or body to one side so that saliva or vomitus drains out
– opening the airway, if necessary, by using the head-tilt, chin-lift method (Unit 52), or lifting the person's shoulders and allowing the head to tilt back

If you find a person who is having a seizure:
● Do not leave the person.
● Do not move the person.
● Do not put anything in the person's mouth.
● Maintain an airway.
● Ring or call for assistance.
● Protect the person from self-inflicted injury.

Difficult SITUATIONS

Patients with epilepsy commonly take a drug called phenytoin to prevent seizures. This drug causes hyperplasia of the gums, a condition in which the normal cells increase, causing excess bulk and thickness. This condition can be relieved to some degree by consistent, conscientious attention to oral hygiene and mouth care. Do not overlook this important activity of daily living in patients with epilepsy or seizure disorder. ■

● Watch the person carefully.
● Apply standard precautions when caring for a patient with seizure activity. There is a high probability of contact with blood, body fluids, secretions, and excretions during the care of this patient.

Observation of the patient should be made during and following the seizure. Breathing should be carefully monitored. Ring for assistance, if possible, but do not leave the patient alone. As much as possible, protect the patient from injuring herself during the seizure.

Nursing Care After a Seizure. When the seizure stops, tell the patient where she is and what happened. Assist her to bed. The patient will be very tired. Allow her to sleep. She may be confused and require periodic reorientation. Leave the patient in a position of comfort and safety with the call signal and needed personal items within reach. Other care includes:

- Providing incontinent care, if necessary
- Checking the vital signs as instructed; you may take vital signs frequently until the patient is stable
- Monitoring the patient closely for return of seizure activity
- Assisting the nurse to administer oxygen or suctioning, if needed

Report to the nurse:

- Any change in the patient before the seizure, such as an aura, confusion, or change in behavior
- A description of the way the seizure looked, including the body parts involved
- Loss of bowel or bladder control, eyes rolling upward, rapid blinking, biting tongue
- The time the seizure started and stopped, if known
- Condition of the patient after the seizure
- Vital signs

Spinal Cord Injuries

Injuries to the spinal cord result in loss of function and sensation below the level of the injury. These patients are particularly prone to contractures and pressure ulcers.

Paralysis is seen in many medical conditions, but is most commonly associated with spinal cord injury. Paralysis may involve a single muscle, but usually involves an entire region of the body. In spinal cord injury, paralysis occurs as a result of damage or trauma to the spinal cord. This causes loss or impaired function resulting in reduced mobility or feeling (sensation) below the level of the injury to the cord. The word *lesion* is a general term used to describe an alteration or change in tissue, which may be due to many causes. The most common of these are wounds and injuries. The damage to the spinal cord is also called a lesion. Terms used to describe paralysis are:

- **diplegia**—paralysis affecting the same region on both sides of the body (such as both arms)
- *hemiplegia*—paralysis on one entire side of the body (such as the arm and leg)
- **monoplegia**—paralysis affecting one limb only
- *paraplegia*—paralysis of the trunk (usually below the waist) and both legs
- *tetraplegia* (*quadriplegia*)—paralysis of the trunk (usually below the neck), both arms, and both legs

Flaccid paralysis involves loss of muscle tone and absence of tendon reflexes. Some patients have **spastic paralysis**. These patients have no voluntary movement. The extremities move in an involuntary pattern, similar to muscle spasms. The patient is aware of the movements, but cannot stop them. The type of paralysis is determined by the level of injury. Patients with upper motor injuries are more likely to exhibit spastic paralysis.

Signs and Symptoms. Signs and symptoms of paralysis vary with the level of the injury. The patient will be paralyzed below the level where the spinal cord was damaged. For example, an injury to the upper vertebrae in the neck will cause respiratory depression. The patient will be unable to move the arms and legs. He or she will lose bowel and bladder control. An injury near the waist will also cause loss of bowel and bladder control. The patient will be unable to move the legs.

Treatment. Treatment depends on the level of injury. Overall, treatment is directed at:

- Keeping the lungs clear
- Preventing complications of immobility
- Preventing deformities
- Restoring the patient to the highest degree of independence possible

Responsibilities of the Nursing Assistant. Patients with spinal cord injury need long-term nursing care, which includes:

- Listening. Many persons with spinal cord injury are taught to give directions to caregivers who are doing for the person what the individual cannot do for himself.
- A consistently calm and patient approach, because the loss of sensory and motor functions often makes self-care difficult.
- Acceptance of the patient's expressions of anger, fear, and depression, as well as clumsy attempts at self-care.

Clinical Information ALERT

In the United States, the term *quadriplegia* was used for many years to describe paralysis. It is derived from a combination of Greek and Latin words. In Europe, the term used to describe this condition has always been *tetraplegia*. In 1991, the American Spinal Cord Injury Classification system was revised and the terminology thoroughly researched. Since then, the American Spinal Cord Association has recommended that the term *tetraplegia* be used so that there are not two different words in English referring to the same thing. ∎

Remember that the patient's ability to think is not necessarily impaired. Frustration is even greater because these patients can no longer will their actions.

- Careful skin care, because:
  - incontinence not only causes the patient embarrassment and discomfort but also makes the skin prone to breakdown
  - the lack of nervous stimulation decreases circulation to the skin
  - pain and pressure cannot be felt
- Attention to elimination needs. For example, suppositories may be given daily. A catheter may be inserted into the bladder, so catheter and drainage care will be needed. Special pads within plastic incontinence pants may also be used.
- Avoidance of contractures and deformities, which occur rapidly after the onset of paralysis. When moving and positioning patients with paralysis, move the extremities slowly and gently. Rapid, rough movements will cause spasticity. If a patient's extremities move into a position of flexion, position them in extension. If the extremities move into a position of extension, position them in flexion. Positioning devices may be necessary to maintain position. Attention to proper positioning is very important. This is a major key to preventing contractures and deformities in these high-risk patients.
- Provision of ROM exercises. These will be needed for the rest of the patient's life.
- Proper attention and care to prevent:
  - respiratory infections
  - urinary tract infections
  - pressure ulcers

Autonomic Dysreflexia. Autonomic dysreflexia (Figure 43-19) is a potentially life-threatening complication of spinal cord injury. It usually occurs in patients with injuries above the mid-thoracic area. It indicates uncontrolled sympathetic nervous system activity. Problems that seem minor can trigger this condition. As a rule, injuries that would normally cause pain below the level of spinal injury can set this life-threatening chain of events in motion. For example:

- Overfull bladder (this is the most common cause)
- Urinary retention
- Urinary tract infection
- Blocked catheter
- Overfilled urinary drainage bag
- Constipation or fecal impaction
- Hemorrhoids
- Infection or irritation in the abdomen, such as appendicitis or acute abdominal conditions
- Pressure ulcers

FIGURE 43-19 In autonomic dysreflexia, lower motor neurons sense a painful stimulus and send a signal to the brain. However, the signal cannot penetrate the area of spinal cord injury. This causes the signal to be interrupted so it cannot reach the brain. This triggers hypertension, pounding headache, gooseflesh (goosebumps) below the injury, and generalized pallor, visual changes, and anxiety. The body tries to notify the brain of the hypertension, but again the message cannot penetrate the spinal cord injury. This triggers the vagus nerve to slow the heart rate, and the patient develops bradycardia as a result of the body's attempt to normalize internal conditions.

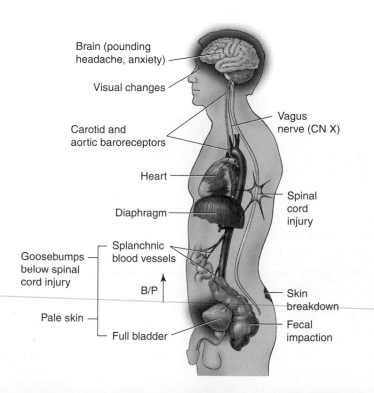

Brain (pounding headache, anxiety)
Visual changes
Carotid and aortic baroreceptors
Vagus nerve (CN X)
Heart
Spinal cord injury
Diaphragm
Splanchnic blood vessels
Goosebumps below spinal cord injury
B/P
Pale skin
Full bladder
Skin breakdown
Fecal impaction

- Prolonged pressure by an object in the chair, shoe, wrinkled clothing, and the like
- Minor injury, such as a cut, bruise, or abrasion
- Ingrown toenails
- Burns, including sunburn
- Pressure on skin from tight or constrictive clothing
- Menstrual cramps
- Labor and delivery
- Overstimulation during sexual activity
- Fractured bones

Signs and symptoms of autonomic dysreflexia are:

- Extremely high blood pressure, over 200/100
- Severe headache
- Red, flushed face
- Red blotches on the skin above the level of spinal injury
- Sweating above the level of spinal injury
- Stuffy nose
- Nausea
- Bradycardia (pulse below 60)
- Goosebumps below the level of injury
- Cold, clammy skin below the level of injury

If you observe any of these signs and symptoms, notify the nurse immediately. Treatment for this condition involves identifying the offending stimulus and removing it. If you believe something has triggered the condition, inform the nurse. Remove tight and constricting clothing and shoes. Check the catheter and drainage bag. Follow the nurses' instructions.

Meningitis

Meningitis is an inflammation of the meninges. It is usually caused by viruses or bacteria.

The signs and symptoms of meningitis are:

- Headache
- Nausea
- Stiffness of the neck
- Seizures
- Chills
- Elevated temperature

If the cause is bacterial, meningitis is treated with antibiotics. If it is communicable, droplet precautions are used.

Cataracts

Cataracts (Figure 43-20) are the leading cause of vision loss in adults over the age of 55. Because of this, cataract surgery is one of the most common surgeries in the United States today.

Cataracts cause the normally clear lens of the eye to become cloudy. The cloudy (opaque) lens will not allow light rays to pass through. Therefore, the person is no longer able to see.

FIGURE 43-20 When the patient develops a cataract, the lens is cloudy instead of transparent. (Photo courtesy of Linda Jaakobovitch, Cincinnati Eye Institute)

Treatment. Removal or replacement of the lens permits light rays to enter the eye. Sight is then restored. The lens is needed to adjust vision to different distances. The latest innovations in cataract surgery increase comfort and convenience for the patient. Until recently, most surgery for cataracts involved removing the center (nucleus) of the lens through a large incision. Currently, most surgeons remove cataracts with a small incision and ultrasound.

The surgery is performed either as an outpatient procedure or in a day surgery center. The patient is admitted to the center in the morning and remains for one to two hours after the surgery, or until vital signs are stable. Eye drops are used to numb the eye. In this surgery, the cataract is removed. A plastic, silicone, or hydrogel lens is usually implanted (Figures 43-21A and 43-21B), and the incision is naturally sealed. Stitches are not used. Some surgeons apply a patch to the eye, but most do not.

Nursing Care. Nursing care of the cataract patient includes:

- Routine postoperative care.
- Relief of pain. Discomfort is usually mild. If pain worsens, the patient complains of sharp pain, or vision decreases, promptly notify the nurse.
- Being sure all needed items, such as signal cords, are within easy reach.
- Taking extra precautions if the patient is confused or restless.
- Checking vital signs until stable.
- Keeping the surgical site undisturbed. After surgery, the patient may feel as if something (such as an eyelash) is in the eye. The patient may complain of itching. Slight fluid discharge may be present, and the eye may be sensitive to light and touch. Instruct the patient not to rub, scratch, or squeeze the eye.
- Helping the patient to adapt to temporarily blurred vision. This is normal due to the bright lights used in surgery and drops used to dilate the eyes. The problem should resolve on its own promptly.

Lens Implant Surgery for Cataracts

A. Cataract

Cataract-clouded lens

Posterior capsule

Plastic lens implant

Posterior capsule

B. Following surgery

FIGURE 43-21A The lens is removed and the plastic intraocular lens is permanently placed in the eye.

FIGURE 43-21B The lens implant is left in place. The patient cannot feel it after the eye heals. The lens implant is similar to a contact lens and smaller than a dime. (Photo courtesy of Linda Jaakobovitch, Cincinnati Eye Institute)

- Assisting the patient with initial ambulation, if needed. Many patients are able to walk without help immediately after surgery.

After the patient is stable, he is usually discharged home. Orders regarding postoperative activity usually include:

- Protecting the eye from injury for the first 4 weeks.
- Avoid straining activities such as bending over, lifting objects that weigh more than 20 pounds, or strenuous coughing. Bending increases pressure in the eye. The patient can usually walk, climb stairs, and do light housework. The surgeon or nurse will instruct the patient on the level of activity.

- Using medicated eye drops for several weeks to promote healing and control pressure. These may sting a little, but the medication is necessary to promote a successful outcome.
- Wearing an eye shield at night, if instructed by the doctor.
- Informing the physician if there is an increase in pain or loss of vision.

Glaucoma

Glaucoma is a condition of increased pressure within the eye. The most common type of glaucoma is *open angle glaucoma*, a slowly progressive, chronic condition. There are no early signs and symptoms. As the problem progresses, the patient begins to experience vision loss. The problem causes gradual loss of peripheral vision. The patient:

- Develops eye pain
- Has difficulty adjusting to darkness
- May be unable to detect color
- Sees halos around lights

Untreated, it progresses to loss of central vision and blindness. The problem is usually detected during a routine eye examination. Untreated, the condition compresses the lens into the vitreous humor. This places pressure on the neurons in the retina, leading to blindness. Open angle glaucoma commonly occurs in both eyes at the same time.

An acute glaucoma, called *closed angle glaucoma*, is less common. This type usually occurs in one eye. When the pressure within the eye increases, the iris will bulge out. The patient usually has severe pain and vision loss in the eye. Other signs and symptoms are:

- Nausea and vomiting
- Headache
- Feeling very tired
- Blurred vision
- Rainbow-like halos around lights

This is an emergency situation that must be promptly treated.

Care of the Patient with Glaucoma. Glaucoma is treated with medications and special eye drops that reduce pressure. Surgery may be done to drain fluid and relieve pressure. The patient must have regular eye examinations to measure the pressure within the eye. Care of the patient with glaucoma includes:

- Monitoring accurate intake and output if the patient is on intravenous medication to reduce eye pressure
- Checking vital signs every 2 to 4 hours
- Reporting complaints of eye pain promptly to the nurse
- Arranging needed items so the patient can see them; avoid moving things unless the patient gives permission
- Avoiding strain and exertion that will increase intraocular pressure

- Keeping the patient from stooping or lifting
- Avoiding tight and constrictive clothing, which also increases pressure
- Keeping the patient safe, if vision is limited

Retinal Degeneration

Breakdown of the retina, known as **retinal degeneration** or **macular degeneration**, occurs over a period of months or years. The incidence increases with age. Central vision is progressively lost as the macula (area of acute central vision) is damaged. Subretinal hemorrhages lead to scarring of this important area.

Early treatment with laser therapy can seal the tiny capillaries to prevent further damage to the macula.

Vision Impairment

Cataracts, glaucoma, retinal degeneration, eye infections, and other eye conditions, such as ocular tumors, can cause blindness. Persons who are legally blind may still have partial vision. The degree of visual limitation must be considered when giving care. It is also important to consider the patient's attitude to the limitations. Adjustment to blindness is both a physical and an emotional process.

Allow the person who is blind or nearly blind the opportunity to do as much as possible in personal care and other activities. Many blind people are capable and independent. In fact, most blind people do well with minimal help and support once they are fully oriented to their surroundings.

Review Unit 7 for guidelines for working with persons who have visual impairments.

Artificial Eye

Situations such as severe injury to the eye or untreatable cancer may require surgical removal of an eye. An eye prosthesis (artificial eye) is usually inserted after the surgery. The care plan should provide information if the patient has an artificial eye.

Some patients remove the artificial eye at night. Others prefer not to remove the eye at all. You may be responsible for removing the eye. If the eye is to remain out of the socket, store it in a marked cup in contact lens disinfectant solution or sterile saline (Figure 43-22) (Procedure 93). The socket is usually cleansed and irrigated when the eye is removed. Irrigation of the socket may be a licensed nursing procedure in your facility. Know and follow your facility policy. Apply the principles of standard precautions when caring for the artificial eye and mucous membranes in the eye socket.

FIGURE 43-22 Many different products and solutions are used to clean, disinfect, and remove protein deposits from the artificial eye. Most of these were developed to be used in the care of contact lenses. They are safe and useful for eye prostheses. The patient must bring the eye in to be polished once or twice a year.

PROCEDURE

93

CARING FOR THE EYE SOCKET AND ARTIFICIAL EYE

1. Carry out initial procedure actions.

2. Assemble equipment:
   - Eye cup or clean denture cup
   - Prescribed solution, if ordered
   - Small plastic bag
   - 4 to 6 cotton balls
   - 2 4 × 4 gauze pads
   - Emesis basin with lukewarm water
   - Disposable gloves
   - Towel

3. Place the patient in supine position, if tolerated. Place a towel across the patient's chest.

4. Put on disposable gloves.

5. Moisten cotton balls in lukewarm water in the emesis basin.
   a. Ask the patient to close his eyes.
   b. Wipe the upper lid of the affected eye from the inner corner of the eye to the outer edge. Repeat with a clean cotton ball until the area is clean and free of mucus.

continues

PROCEDURE 93 CONTINUED

6. Dispose of the used cotton balls in a plastic bag.

7. Place a 4 × 4 gauze pad in the bottom of the eye cup or denture cup.

8. Remove the artificial eye:

   a. Gently pull down the lower eyelid with your thumb (Figure 43-23A). Open the upper lid with your index finger.

   b. Grasp the artificial eye as it comes out of the eye socket and place it on the gauze in the cup.

   c. Some patients use a small suction cup to remove the eye. Gently hold the eye open with the fingers of one hand. Depress the suction cup between your thumb and index finger (Figure 43-23B). Place the suction cup in the center of the artificial eye. Release the pressure. Gently pull the eye from the socket (Figure 43-23C).

9. Use clean cotton balls moistened with water or solution as ordered and clean the empty eye socket. Dry gently with clean, dry cotton balls. Use a new cotton ball for each wipe. Pat the patient's face dry, as needed. If the external eyelid has mucus, secretions, or other crusty matter on the skin surface, you may wash it gently with warm water and baby shampoo.

10. Carry the cup with the artificial eye to the sink. Fill the sink one-third full with lukewarm water.

11. Wash the eye under lukewarm running water, or use the prescribed solution. Use gauze if necessary to loosen and remove any accumulation from the eye. Wipe gently to avoid scratching the eye.

12. Rinse the eye and place it on a dry 4 × 4 gauze pad, or store the eye in sterile water or the prescribed solution, according to the care plan. (Do not dry an artificial eye.)

13. Discard the water or solution in the eye cup and rinse the cup.

14. Remove your gloves. Wash your hands. Carry the artificial eye to the patient's bedside.

15. Explain to the patient what you are going to do.

16. Insert the artificial eye into the eye socket:

   a. Carry out initial procedure actions.

   b. Put on disposable gloves.

   c. Clean and rinse the artificial eye with the prescribed solution, if you have not already done so. The eye should be moist for insertion. Do not attempt to insert it dry.

FIGURE 43-23B Squeeze the cup, place it against the eye, then release the suction.

FIGURE 43-23A To loosen the eye, pull the lower lid down, then push back up slightly.

FIGURE 43-23C Pull the eye down gently from the socket. Never try to pull it straight out.

continues

PROCEDURE 93 CONTINUED

d. Position the notched edge of the eye toward the patient's nose (Figure 43-23D).

e. Gently open the upper eyelid. Bring the prosthesis up past the lower lid and under the upper lid. Set it flush once it is past the lower lid and touching the upper tissues (Figure 43-23E).

f. Place your index finger on the prosthesis and slip it up under the upper lid (Figure 43-23F).

g. Release the upper lid.

h. Draw the edge of the lower lid forward, covering the lower edge of the eye. Press down lightly.

17. Carry out ending procedure actions.

Note: Some professionals advise their patients to remove the eye only occasionally unless special problems, such as having a cold, having excessive secretions, a dusty environment, or other environmental conditions are present. Removing the eye increases the potential for introducing pathogens into the eye socket. Many patients reinsert the prosthesis immediately after cleaning because the socket contracts slightly when the eye is removed. After several hours, the prosthesis may be more difficult to reinsert. Some patients complain of discomfort when the eye is reinserted. Although it should be rinsed well after cleaning, the problem may be from lack of natural lubrication, not the products used. It may take up to several days for the body to make sufficient natural lubricants for the eye to feel comfortable. Until then, the patient may use an artificial tears preparation or lens wetting solution to lubricate the eye for comfort. If you have questions about the prosthesis, the patient or a family caregiver should be able to provide information.

FIGURE 43-23E Gently move the artificial eye up past the lower lid.

FIGURE 43-23F Using your index finger, push the eye the rest of the way up and under the upper lid.

Large Portion

Point

Iris

Right Eye   Left Eye

FIGURE 43-23D The notched part of the eye is positioned next to the patient's nose.

Warm and Cool Eye Compresses

Many elderly patients have dry, itchy eyes. This may be caused by allergies, irritants, squinting, rubbing, or blinking the eyes. The eyes may appear red, with swollen eyelids. If patients rub or scratch their eyes, they may become infected. Patients with dry, itchy eyes may complain of:

- Burning
- Scratchy feeling
- Itching
- Light sensitivity
- Difficulty moving eyes
- Excess mucus production

- Severe pain
- Blurred vision
- Seeing halos

Observe the patient for:

- Drainage from the eyes
- Redness of eyelid rims
- Scaly, flaky skin around the eyes

- Edema of the eyelids

Report your observations to the nurse. You may be instructed to apply warm or cool soaks to the eyelids. Apply the principles of standard precautions when performing this procedure. If an infection is suspected, use separate gloves and equipment for each eye. This will prevent the infection from spreading.

PROCEDURE

94

APPLYING WARM OR COOL EYE COMPRESSES

1. Carry out initial procedure actions.

2. Assemble equipment:
   - Disposable exam gloves
   - Towel
   - Small bottle of sterile saline
   - Small sterile basin
   - Sterile gauze pads
   - Ice, if cool compresses are ordered
   - Plastic bag for used items

3. Position the patient for comfort. For warm compresses, assist the patient to a Fowler's or high Fowler's position, if possible. (This position helps reduce edema.) Cover the neck and shoulders with a bath towel.

4. Heat the bottle of sterile saline under hot running water, or place it in a second bowl of hot water. The solution should become comfortably warm, not hot. Check the temperature with a thermometer. It should be approximately 105°F.

    Note: Never use the microwave to heat water for heat treatments.

   If cool compresses are ordered, cool the bottle of saline by packing it in ice.

5. Pour the warm or cool solution into the small, sterile basin.

6. Wash your hands, or use alcohol-based cleaner.

7. Apply disposable gloves.

8. Place the gauze pads into the bowl.

9. Remove a gauze pad from the bowl, squeezing out the excess solution.

10. Instruct the patient to close her eyes.

11. Apply one compress to the affected eye (Figure 43-24).

12. Remove a second gauze pad from the bowl, squeezing out the excess solution.

13. Apply the second compress on top of the first.

14. Repeat with the other eye, as directed.

15. If the patient complains that the compress is too hot or cold, remove it immediately.

16. Change the compresses every few minutes for the prescribed length of time. The treatment should not last longer than 15 to 20 minutes. Check the skin under the compress each time you change it.

17. You may be directed to cover the compress with an ice pack or warm pack. Make a small ice pack

FIGURE 43-24 Instruct the patient to close her eyes. Apply one compress to the affected eye. Follow with a second compress.

continues

PROCEDURE 94 CONTINUED

by placing ice chips in a sandwich bag or disposable glove. Squeeze the air out of the bag and tie the end. Keep the pack size small. Cover the compress with the pack, as directed. Remove it immediately if the patient complains of pain.

18. After 15 to 20 minutes, or as directed, remove the compresses. Discard them in the plastic bag.

19. Use clean gauze pads to dry the eye. Pat gently from the inner corner to the outer corner. Use each gauze pad once, then discard in the bag.

20. Carry out ending procedure actions.

Otitis Media

Otitis media is an infection of the middle ear. Infections of the nose and throat can move along the eustachian tube to the middle ear, causing inflammation. Fluid and pus form within the middle ear. This may result in fusion (locking) of the middle ear bones. Increased pressure may cause the eardrum to rupture. Both conditions decrease the ability to transmit sound waves. This condition, which is rare in adults, is common in children.

Antibiotics are usually given. A surgical opening (myringotomy) is sometimes made in the eardrum to drain the pus. Small tubes may be inserted for drainage.

Otosclerosis

Otosclerosis is a progressive form of deafness of unknown cause. The process involves the growth of new, abnormal bone in the bony labyrinth. This growth prevents the stapes from vibrating properly.

Hearing is improved by the use of a hearing aid. Surgery (stapedectomy) removes the excess bone and replaces it with a prosthesis.

Hearing Impairment

Some of your patients will be hard of hearing or completely deaf. A hearing aid (Figures 43-25A and 43-25B) will sometimes improve the patient's level of hearing and comprehension. Lip reading or sign language may be needed to communicate. Review Unit 7 for guidelines on working with persons who have hearing impairments.

FIGURE 43-25A Parts of a behind-the-ear hearing aid. The ear mold is placed in the ear canal. The rest of the hearing aid is worn outside and over the top of the ear.

FIGURE 43-25B This hearing aid is worn inside the outer ear canal.

Caring for Hearing Aids

A hearing aid is a delicate and expensive prosthesis. It requires safe handling and regular care.

GUIDELINES *for*

Caring for a Hearing Aid

- Store hearing aids at room temperature when they are not being worn. Temperature extremes can damage hearing aids. They should not be worn for more than a few minutes in very cold weather.

continues

GUIDELINES *continued*

- Keep hearing aids dry. If an aid is worn accidentally in the shower, ask the nurse how to dry it. Avoid exposing them to hair dryers. The heat will damage the aid and the noise is very annoying to the patient.

- Store extra batteries in a cool, dry place. Remove the batteries from the hearing aid at night or open the battery compartment. This allows trapped moisture to evaporate.

- Keep hearing aids safe. They break easily if dropped on a hard surface.

- Remove the hearing aid if hair spray is being used, as the spray may cause damage.

- Turn the hearing aid off when it is not in use. Turn the aid off before removing it.

- Wipe in-the-ear aids daily with a dry tissue.

- Check regularly to make sure the opening of the aid or ear mold is free of wax. In-the-ear types come with a cleaning tool. This should be used only by someone who has been instructed how to use it. Never use a toothpick, paper clip, or other sharp object to clean the hearing aid.

- Insert the hearing aid properly. Sometimes the shape of the ear changes with aging and the hearing aid may have to be refitted. If the patient complains of pain or the aid is difficult to insert, this may be the problem. Advise the nurse if this occurs.

- When communicating with the patient, follow the same guidelines that you use when communicating with a patient who has hearing impairment.

- Check bed linen carefully before placing it in the soiled linen hamper. A hearing aid is small, expensive, and easily lost. It will not survive a trip through the washer and dryer!

- Always shave the male patient with an electric razor *before* the hearing aid is put in the ear, or remove the hearing aid before using the electric razor. The hearing aid will amplify the noise from the razor, making it quite loud and annoying.

GUIDELINES *for*

Troubleshooting Hearing Aids

If the aid is not producing sound, before inserting it in the patient's ear:

- Check to make sure the "+" (positive) side of the battery is next to the "+" inside the hearing aid battery case or compartment.

- Try a new battery—the old one may be dead. Hold the hearing aid in the palm of your hand. Turn the volume all the way up. Cup the aid between your hands. You should hear a loud whistle. A weak or absent sound indicates that the battery is low.

- Before changing the battery, check the position of the old battery so you can put the new one in the same way. When inserting a new battery, place it in the unit gently. If you meet resistance, do not force it. Consult the nurse.

- Check the ear mold to see if it is plugged with wax.

- Make sure the hearing aid is set on "M" (microphone), not "T" (telephone switch).

- If the hearing aid works intermittently or makes a scratchy sound, check for dirt under and around the battery. Also check the volume control and connections. If the hearing aid has a connecting wire, make sure it is plugged in tightly and is not cracked or bent.

If the hearing aid is making squealing sounds:

- If the hearing aid is in the patient's ear and makes a loud, whistling sound, check the position. The aid should be securely in the ear. Make sure that hair, ear wax, or clothing are not interfering with the position. Check the tubing (if any) for cracks. Whistling usually indicates an air leak.

- Determine if the ear mold fits properly. It should be completely in the ear. If it does not fit well, report it to the nurse.

- Check the volume on the aid. If it is too high, turn it down until the squealing stops.

- Check the plastic tubing on a behind-the-ear aid. If it is cracked or split, it must be replaced.

DIAGNOSTIC TECHNIQUES

Numerous tests and techniques help physicians diagnose problems of the nervous system. Diagnostic tests include:

- Magnetic resonance imaging (MRI)
- Computerized axial tomography (CAT) scan
- Electroencephalogram (EEG) to measure electrical activity of the brain
- Myelogram, which introduces dye or contrast material into the spinal canal so an X-ray can be done
- Tonometry to measure intraocular pressure
- Audiometry to evaluate hearing
- Spinal puncture to collect cerebrospinal fluid

Spinal Puncture

Spinal or lumbar punctures are done to withdraw cerebrospinal fluid (CSF) for examination or to introduce medication or anesthetic into the spinal column. The physician inserts a long, sterile needle between the lumbar vertebrae into the fluid-filled space between the arachnoid mater and pia mater. The pressure of the CSF is measured. A sample is withdrawn and placed in a sterile test tube. This test may be performed in the patient's room with nurses or nursing assistants helping with the procedure. The patient is placed in a position that will make it easier for the needle to enter the spinal column. It is important that the patient not move during the procedure. The patient may be placed in a lateral position:

- The patient is placed on the side facing away from the physician
- The knees are drawn up to the abdomen, with the head bent down on the chest
- The arms are comfortably flexed (Figure 43-26)

The patient may also be placed in a sitting position (Figure 43-27)

- The patient is seated on the edge of the bed facing away from the physician
- The shoulders are hunched forward
- The patient may lean on an overbed table for support
- It is important for someone to steady the table to prevent the patient from falling

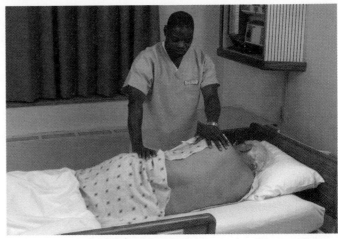

FIGURE 43-26 The patient may be positioned on his her side with the upper body and legs flexed for a cerebrospinal puncture.

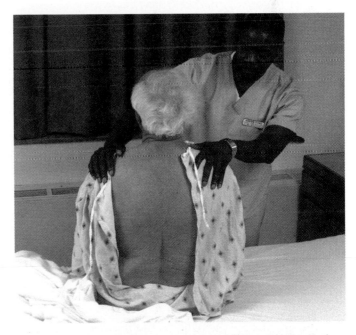

FIGURE 43-27 An alternate position for cerebrospinal puncture. The patient may be more comfortable leaning on a pillow on an overbed table. However, you must make sure that the table does not slip.

REVIEW

A. True/False.

Mark the following true or false by circling T or F.

1. T F The patient with right-brain damage will not be able to speak.

2. T F If a patient has aphasia, it is not necessary to speak to him because he cannot understand anyway.

3. T F The patient suffering from a CVA will need assistance in carrying out ROM exercises.

4. T F Hemiplegia is a paralysis on one side of the body.

5. T F The patient with Parkinson's disease characteristically has a "pill-rolling" tremor in the hands.

6. T F   Status epilepticus is a serious condition.

7. T F   The Parkinson's disease patient often has mood swings.

8. T F   The person with tetraplegia is paralyzed on one side of the body.

9. T F   Fluid may be withdrawn from the spinal canal for examination.

B. Multiple Choice.

Select the one best answer for each of the following.

10. The brain and spinal cord make up the
  a. central nervous system.
  b. peripheral nervous system.
  c. sensory organs.
  d. cerebrospinal fluid space.

11. Neurotransmitters are
  a. neurons.
  b. special nerves.
  c. chemicals that help pass messages.
  d. brain cells.

12. The brain stem controls
  a. voluntary movement.
  b. thinking.
  c. vital functions of the body.
  d. emotions.

13. A condition that causes the lens of the eye to become cloudy and impair vision is called
  a. glaucoma.
  b. macular degeneration.
  c. diabetic retinopathy.
  d. cataract.

14. Hearing aids should be kept
  a. wrapped in tissue.
  b. dry.
  c. disassembled.
  d. in the refrigerator when not in use.

15. Persons with Parkinson's disease generally have
  a. pain.
  b. rigidity.
  c. spasticity.
  d. hearing impairment.

16. A person who has had a stroke on the left side of the brain will
  a. have left hemiplegia.
  b. become quick and impulsive.
  c. have aphasia.
  d. have no personality changes.

17. The person who has had a stroke on the right side of the brain will
  a. have left hemiplegia.
  b. have aphasia.
  c. become slow, anxious, and cautious.
  d. have hearing loss in the right ear.

18. Patients with stroke
  a. need proper positioning to prevent contractures.
  b. must be repositioned every 4 hours.
  c. will be unable to speak during the acute phase.
  d. will always be NPO during the acute phase.

19. Multiple sclerosis occurs because
  a. the myelin sheath of the neuron is damaged.
  b. of a hemorrhage in the brain.
  c. of a lack of a certain neurotransmitter.
  d. of muscle damage.

20. Patients with multiple sclerosis may experience
  a. hemiplegia.
  b. no obvious signs or symptoms.
  c. loss of sensation to temperature, pain, and touch.
  d. inability to swallow.

21. Increased intracranial pressure can develop from
  a. Parkinson's disease.
  b. head injuries.
  c. ruptured disc.
  d. post polio syndrome.

22. If you are assisting in the care of a patient with a head injury, you should note and report
  a. blood pressure of 112/74.
  b. pulse rate of 96.
  c. changes in levels of consciousness.
  d. skin warm and dry.

23. You come into a room and find a patient having a seizure. You should
  a. leave and find help.
  b. restrain the patient's movements.
  c. raise the foot of the bed.
  d. remove any object the patient might hit.

24. The patient with post polio syndrome experiences
  a. nausea and vomiting.
  b. visual disturbances and facial droop.
  c. cold intolerance and weakness.
  d. hemiplegia.

25. After surgery, patients with post polio syndrome
  a. often take longer to recover from the anesthesia than other patients.
  b. usually experience bowel and bladder incontinence.

c. do not feel pain as acutely as other patients.

d. commonly experience tachycardia for 24 hours.

26. Patients with ALS commonly experience

a. hemiplegia.

b. muscle weakness and atrophy.

c. difficulty hearing.

d. mental confusion.

27. When caring for a patient with ALS, the nursing assistant should

a. encourage the patient to feed himself so he does not lose this ability.

b. allow the patient to set the routines, because his mental clarity is unaffected.

c. keep the patient in bed and as still as possible.

d. limit fluids to prevent choking and aspiration.

28. Autonomic dysreflexia can be caused by

a. hunger.

b. thirst.

c. overfull bladder.

d. drowsiness.

29. Autonomic dysreflexia is

a. a life-threatening condition.

b. a minor complication of surgery.

c. very painful.

d. common in patients with multiple sclerosis.

30. Glaucoma is

a. a clouding of the lens of the eye.

b. caused by chemical exposure.

c. related to retinal degeneration.

d. a condition caused by very high pressure in the eye.

31. When caring for a patient with glaucoma, the nursing assistant should

a. apply patches to the patient's eyes at bedtime.

b. perform tasks that would strain or exert the patient.

c. apply eye drops to the affected eye.

d. apply cool eye compresses every 2 hours.

C. Matching.

Choose the correct item from Column II to match each word or phrase in Column I.

Column I

32. _____ uncontrolled trembling

33. _____ CVA

34. _____ difficulty and slowness in carrying out voluntary muscular activities

35. _____ language impairment

36. _____ convulsion

37. _____ aura

38. _____ nystagmus

Column II

a. akinesia

b. aphasia

c. tremors

d. seizure

e. sclera

f. stroke

g. involuntary movement of the eye seen in multiple sclerosis

h. sensation experienced by some persons just before having a seizure

D. Nursing Assistant Challenge.

You are assigned to care for Mr. Johnson, who has had a stroke. You learn from his care plan that he has right hemiplegia and aphasia. Consider these questions:

39. From this information, you know that which part of Mr. Johnson's brain was affected by the stroke?

40. What does right hemiplegia mean?

41. What will you expect from Mr. Johnson's attempts to communicate verbally?

42. What complications is he at risk for? What can you do to prevent these complications?

43. What observations would indicate cognitive impairment?

UNIT 44

Gastrointestinal System

OBJECTIVES

After completing this unit, you will be able to:

- Spell and define terms.
- Review the location and functions of the organs of the gastrointestinal system.
- List specific diagnostic tests associated with disorders of the gastrointestinal system.
- Describe some common disorders of the gastrointestinal system.
- Describe nursing assistant actions related to the care of patients with disorders of the gastrointestinal system.

- Identify different types of enemas and state their purpose.
- Demonstrate the following procedures:
  - Procedure 95 Collecting a Stool Specimen
  - Procedure 96 Giving a Soap-Solution Enema
  - Procedure 97 Giving a Commercially Prepared Enema
  - Procedure 98 Inserting a Rectal Suppository

VOCABULARY

Learn the meaning and the correct spelling of the following words and phrases:

abdominal distention	diarrhea	hernia	proctoscopy
bile	duodenal resection	herniorrhaphy	pyloric sphincter
bolus	duodenal ulcer	hydrochloric acid (HCl)	sigmoidoscopy
cholecystectomy	enema	ileostomy	stool
cholecystitis	fecal impaction	incarcerated (strangu-	suppository
cholelithiasis	fecal material	lated) hernia	ulcer
chyme	flatus	nasogastric tube (NG	ulcerative colitis
colon	gastrectomy	tube)	urgency
colostomy	gastric resection	occult blood	
constipation	gastric ulcer	pepsin	
defecation	gastroscopy	peristalsis	

INTRODUCTION

The digestive tract extends from the mouth to the anus. It receives the help of the teeth, tongue, salivary glands, liver, gallbladder, and pancreas in breaking food into simpler substances. These substances are used by the body cells to carry on their work of supplying nutrition and eliminating wastes.

STRUCTURE AND FUNCTION

The gastrointestinal system is also called the GI or digestive tract. It extends from the mouth to the anus and is lined with mucous membrane (Figure 44-1). The organs along the length of this system change food into simple forms that can pass through the walls of the small intestine and into the circulatory system. The circulatory system

In the digestive system:

● Proteins are changed to amino acids
● Carbohydrates are changed to simple sugars like glucose
● Fats are changed to fatty acids and glycerol

These changes are brought about by mechanical action and chemicals called *enzymes*. The nondigestible portions of what we eat are moved along the intestines and are finally excreted from the body as feces. Several organs contribute to the digestive process and many disease conditions affect them.

Mouth

In the mouth (Figure 44-2), food is chewed so it can be swallowed easily. The digestive process begins with the help of the:

FIGURE 44-1 Digestive system

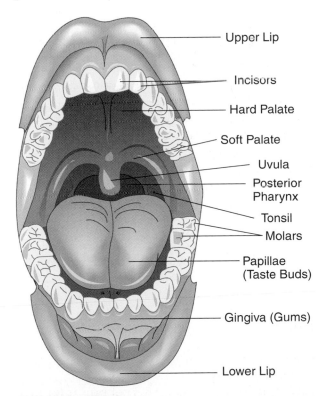

FIGURE 44-2 Mouth

then carries the nutrients to the body cells. The gastrointestinal system includes the:

● Mouth, teeth, tongue, salivary glands
● Pharynx
● Esophagus (gullet)
● Stomach
● Small intestine
● Liver, gallbladder, pancreas
● Large intestine

- Tongue—a skeletal muscle that is covered by tastebuds. The tongue pushes the food between the teeth to be broken up. It assists in mastication (chewing). It propels the food backward toward the pharynx to assist in swallowing. It also aids in speech formation.
- *Papillae*—tiny bumps on the tongue that are commonly called tastebuds. Humans can detect five known tastes, but this is an area in which further study is needed. The areas that have been identified are:
  - sweet
  - salt
  - bitter
  - sour
  - *umami* (first established as a taste in 2000. It was formerly considered a "flavor enhancer." Umami is a Japanese word for a savory, meaty, or protein taste. Examples of umami tastes are steak and sauteed mushrooms.)
- Salt and some other substances amplify the response of the tastebuds, probably by acting as an electrical conductor. Tastebuds are lost with age, beginning with sweet and salt. This helps explain why some elderly persons put a great deal of sugar and salt on their food. To a younger person with intact tastebuds, the amount used seems excessive.
- Salivary glands—secrete saliva containing a digestive enzyme called salivary amylase.
  - Salivary amylase begins carbohydrate digestion
  - $1^1/_2$ quarts of saliva are secreted daily
  - Saliva moistens food to help in swallowing
- Teeth—mechanically break up food into smaller particles, forming a **bolus** of food. The bolus is then swallowed. There are two natural sets of teeth. The first set (deciduous or temporary) numbers 20. The second set (permanent) numbers 32 and gradually replaces the deciduous set.
- Pharynx—allows the passage of both food and air. It leads to the esophagus.
- Esophagus—a tube 10 to 12 inches long that carries the food to the stomach. Strong muscular contractions called *peristaltic* waves move the food along the tract. These waves begin in the esophagus and continue throughout the intestinal tract.

The Stomach

The stomach
- Is a hollow, muscular, J-shaped organ
- Is found in the peritoneal cavity
- Is two-thirds to the left of the midline
- Is just below the diaphragm
- Has circular muscles at either end that hold food while it is thoroughly mixed with digestive enzymes
- Begins the chemical process of digestion

Clinical Information ALERT

The digestive system is open at both ends and is about 25 to 30 feet long. The narrowest part of the digestive system is the esophagus and the widest part is the stomach. The stomach can stretch to 50 times its empty size and can hold about a gallon (4 liters). Hydrochloric acid in the stomach is the most acidic substance in the body. The stomach must produce a new layer of mucus every 2 weeks; otherwise it would digest itself. ■

- Holds food between 3 to 4 hours

The stomach has three parts:
1. Fundus—the area above the entrance of the esophagus.
2. Body—holds food.
3. Pylorus—the long, narrowly tapered distal end that connects with the small intestines. The muscle guarding this exit point is called the **pyloric sphincter**. Sometimes in babies this muscle is so tight (pyloric stenosis) that milk cannot get through and the muscle must be cut surgically.

The stomach cells produce gastric juice, which contains:
- Proteolytic enzyme (**pepsin**) to begin protein breakdown
- Hydrochloric acid (HCl)
- Intrinsic factor, needed for the absorption of vitamin B_{12}

The Intestines

When food leaves the stomach, it is in a semiliquid form called **chyme**. Chyme enters the small intestine, where any undigested nutrients are broken down by intestinal and pancreatic enzymes and bile from the liver.

Clinical Information ALERT

The liver is the largest gland in the body. The pancreas is the source of the most diverse mixture of digestive enzymes. The jejunum has the richest blood supply in the digestive system. The cells in the digestive system with the shortest life span are those found on the epithelium of the duodenum. These cells live for approximately 3 days. The small intestine is about 23 feet long, making it the largest internal organ in the body. ■

Materials continue to be moved through the intestines by waves of **peristalsis**. Food digestion is completed in the small intestine. Most of the nutrients and food the body needs are absorbed into the bloodstream through the walls of the small intestine.

The small intestine is about 23 feet long. It coils within the peritoneum. There are three main portions:

1. The duodenum—about 12 inches long. Has an opening in the back to receive the bile and pancreatic secretions.

2. The jejunum—about 8 feet long.

3. The ileum—the last 12 to 13 feet. Terminates in the ileocecal valve and is connected to the large intestine. The ileocecal valve prevents food from traveling backward into the small intestine.

The large intestine (colon) is $4^1/_2$ feet long. It is divided into several sections:

- Cecum
- Ascending colon
- Transverse colon
- Descending colon
- Sigmoid colon
- Rectum
- Anus

No digestive enzymes are secreted in the colon. The colon is the place where:

- Some vitamins are absorbed into the circulatory system.
- More complex carbohydrates are acted upon by bacteria.
- Much of the remaining water is absorbed through the walls of the large intestine, changing wastes to a more solid form. In this way, the large intestine helps to maintain the water balance of the body.

Peristalsis continues to move waste through the large intestine until it reaches the rectum. When a certain amount has been collected in the rectum, it is eliminated as feces through the anus. This process is called **defecation**.

The Appendix

The appendix is located in the lower right quadrant, attached to the cecum. Its function is not known. When it becomes inflamed, the condition is called *appendicitis*.

Liver and Gallbladder

The liver is a large gland with four lobes. It is located just beneath the right diaphragm. It carries on numerous metabolic functions. For example, the liver helps control the amount of protein and sugar in the blood by changing and storing excess amounts. It produces blood proteins such as prothrombin and fibrinogen, which are important factors in the blood clotting process. The liver also produces bile, which is carried directly to the small intestine for use in digestion or to the gallbladder for storage. Bile prepares (emulsifies) fats for digestion.

The gallbladder is a small hollow sac that is attached to the underside of the liver. It holds about two ounces of bile that it receives from the liver. It releases bile into the small intestine to help digest a fatty meal. The presence of bile in the digestive tract gives solid wastes their usual brown color.

The Pancreas

The pancreas is a glandular organ that produces both exocrine secretions (digestive enzymes) and endocrine secretions (insulin and glucagon). It extends from behind the stomach into the curve of the duodenum. It manufactures pancreatic juice. The pancreatic juice is sent into the duodenum to aid in the digestion of foods. The pancreas also produces insulin and glucagon. Both insulin and glucagon are sent directly into the bloodstream.

COMMON CONDITIONS

The tublike mucous membrane structure of the alimentary canal lends itself to the possibility of malignancies, ulcerations, obstructions, and herniations.

Malignancy

Malignancies (cancers) of the gastrointestinal tract are very common. The symptoms they cause depend on their location. Among the symptoms are:

- Obstruction. Blocking of the passageway is sometimes the first major indication of a long-growing tumor.
- Indigestion.
- Vomiting.
- Constipation.
- Changes in the shape of the **stool** (bowel movement).
- **Flatus** (gas).
- Blood in the stool.

Treatment. Malignancies of the intestinal tract are usually treated surgically by removing the affected part. For example:

- Esophagectomy—removal of the esophagus
- Subtotal gastrectomy—removal of part of the stomach
- Colectomy (bowel resection)—removal of a part of the **colon** (large intestine).
- **Colostomy**—creation of an artificial opening in the abdominal wall and bringing a section of the colon to it for the elimination of feces
- **Ileostomy**—creation of an artificial opening in the abdominal wall and bringing a section of ileum through it for the elimination of waste

Ulcerations

An **ulcer** (sore or tissue breakdown) can occur anywhere along the digestive tract. Common places are the:

- Colon—**ulcerative colitis**. In colitis, malnutrition and dehydration are brought about by loss of fluids in frequent, watery, foul-smelling stools with mucus and pus.
- Stomach—**gastric ulcer**.
- Duodenum—**duodenal ulcer**.

Treatment. Treatment of ulcerative colitis includes:

- Medication to slow peristalsis (the wave-like contractions of the intestines) and reduce patient anxiety.
- Modification of diet to include high protein, high calories, and low residue. The low-residue diet is one in which the foods are almost completely digested. There is little waste with this type of diet.
- Medication (steroids) to reduce inflammation.
- Antibiotics to control infection by the microorganism *H. pylori*.

Patients with gastric or duodenal ulcers have periodic burning pain about 2 hours after eating. Most patients improve when they are placed on a diet in which foods that cause distress are not served. Medications are given to neutralize the **hydrochloric acid (HCl)**, to coat the stomach, and to decrease anxiety. It is sometimes necessary to remove part of the stomach (**gastrectomy** or **gastric resection**) or duodenum (**duodenal resection**). Following such surgery, the patient is:

- NPO. Special mouth care is therefore needed.
- Placed on gastrointestinal drainage. A **nasogastric tube (NG tube)** (Figures 44-3A and 44-3B) is inserted through the patient's nose and into the stomach. The tube is attached to a drainage bottle. Additional tubes are inserted into the intestinal tract. Be careful not to disturb the tubes. Check frequently to ensure that the drainage is not blocked. If drainage becomes blocked, report it to the nurse at once. The type and amount of drainage are noted and recorded.

Hernias

A **hernia** results when a structure such as the intestine pushes through a weakened area in a normally restraining wall. The danger of such abnormal protrusions is that some of the protruding tissue can become trapped in the weakened area. Circulation then becomes limited so that the tissue is in danger of dying. This is called an **incarcerated (strangulated) hernia**.

Frequent sites of herniation are:

- Groin area (inguinal hernia)
- Near the umbilicus (umbilical hernia)
- Through a poorly healed incision (incisional hernia)
- Through the diaphragm (hiatal hernia)

Hernias are usually repaired surgically with a **herniorrhaphy**.

FIGURE 44-3A Materials for feeding tube insertion

FIGURE 44-3B The nurse is taping the nasogastric tube securely. Be cautious when turning or moving the patient, to avoid dislodging or pulling on the tube.

Gallbladder Conditions

Two common conditions affecting the gallbladder are:

- **Cholecystitis**—an inflammation of the gallbladder.
- **Cholelithiasis**—the formation of stones in the gallbladder. The stones may obstruct the flow of **bile** (fluid that aids digestion), giving rise to signs and symptoms such as:
  - Indigestion
  - Pain
  - Jaundice (yellow discoloration of the skin and whites of the eyes)

Treatment. Cholecystitis and cholelithiasis may be treated by:

- Low-fat diet.
- Surgery to remove the gallbladder and stones. This surgical procedure is called a **cholecystectomy**.
- Laser therapy to break up the stones.

Drains are often placed in the operative areas. Initially, large amounts of yellowish-green drainage may be expected.

In addition to routine postoperative care:

- Position the patient in a semi-Fowler's position

- Do not disturb drains
- If you notice fresh blood on the dressing, increased jaundice, or dark urine, report it immediately to the nurse

COMMON PROBLEMS RELATED TO THE LOWER BOWEL

The frequency of bowel elimination varies with the individual. Some people have more than one bowel movement (BM) a day, but others have a BM every two or three days. **Fecal material** (solid body waste, bowel movement, BM) is normally brown, but the color can be affected by certain foods, medications, and diseases. The bowel movement is normally soft and formed. If it passes through the colon too quickly, it is loose and watery. Multiple watery stools is called **diarrhea**. If stool passes through the colon too slowly, the fecal material becomes hard, dry, or sticky and pasty in consistency. This is referred to as **constipation**.

Certain foods, medications, infections, and diseases can cause constipation and diarrhea. As foods move through the gastrointestinal tract by peristalsis, gas is formed. When the gas is expelled from the body, it is called "passing flatus" or flatulence. If the gas is not passed, it accumulates in the intestine. The abdomen will enlarge and appear bloated. This is called **abdominal distention**, and is an important observation to report to the nurse. Abdominal distention may also be caused by constipation and urinary retention.

Changes in Function of the Gastrointestinal System Associated with Aging and Disease

Change in bowel function may be caused by aging, disease, surgery, diet, and medications. Lack of privacy may also affect the patient's ability to have a bowel movement. As a person ages, movement in the colon is decreased. Food absorption is slowed and fewer digestive juices are produced. Constipation is a common problem. Other factors that affect bowel function are:

- Bedrest
- Inactivity
- Inadequate exercise
- Inability to chew foods properly
- Loose or missing teeth
- Inadequate fluid intake
- Stress
- Change in environment
- Change in diet
- A diet that does not contain enough fiber, fruits, or vegetables

Observations to Make when Assisting Patients with Bowel Elimination

You must observe the amount/quantity, color, odor, character, and consistency of the patient's bowel movement before discarding it. Notify the nurse if the fecal material has an unusual color or odor, if there is an unusual amount, or if there is blood, mucus, parasites, or food particles (except corn and raisins) in the stool. If you think a stool is abnormal, save it for the nurse to assess.

Constipation and Fecal Impaction

Report problems with constipation to the nurse. The patient is probably constipated if he has not had a bowel movement in more than three days, strains, or passes hard, marble-like stools. **Fecal impaction** (Figure 44-4) is the most serious form of constipation. It is caused by retention of stool in the rectum, where water is absorbed. Over time, the stool becomes hard and dry. The patient may be unable to pass it. The dried waste irritates the bowel. Mucus dissolves the hard, outer part of the mass. The rectum becomes so full that fluid escapes around the impaction and is eliminated from the rectum as diarrhea. The patient may complain of:

- Abdominal or rectal pain
- Nausea
- Loss of appetite
- Feeling the need to have a bowel movement, but being unable

Other signs and symptoms of impaction are:

- Passing excessive flatus
- Bloating and abdominal distention
- Frequent urination
- Inability to empty the bladder
- Leaking around the catheter
- Mental confusion
- Fever
- Liquid stool or mucus seeping from the rectum

Fecal impaction is a very serious condition that is usually treated by manual removal of the mass by the nurse or advanced care provider. Laxatives and enemas are also used to treat fecal impaction. The best thing to do is observe the patient's bowel elimination carefully and prevent fecal impaction from developing. Document bowel elimination according to facility policy. Alert the nurse if a patient has not had a BM for 3 days.

Diarrhea

Diarrhea occurs when peristalsis in the intestines is very rapid. The need to defecate is usually very urgent if the patient has diarrhea. Some patients may become incontinent because of the force with which the fecal material

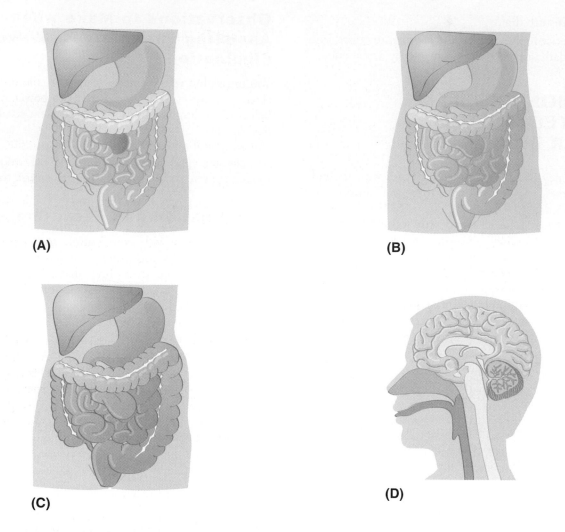

FIGURE 44-4 Progression of a fecal impaction, a life threatening condition: A. A fecal impaction blocks the rectum. The rectum and sigmoid colon become enlarged. B. The colon continues to enlarge. C. Fecal material fills the colon. Digested and undigested food back up into the small intestines and stomach. The patient has signs and symptoms of acute illness, including lethargy, distention, constipation, and dull, cramping pain. D. The entire system is full, and the patient vomits fecal material. The feces are commonly aspirated into the lungs.

Infection Control ALERT

C. difficile is usually transmitted on workers' hands after they touch feces or contaminated surfaces. The pathogen and spores can survive under fingernails, in skin folds, and on jewelry. *C. difficile* is then spread to patients by direct contact. Workers' hands may also contaminate bathrooms, faucets, clean linen, side rails, call buttons, and toilets. Remember not to use alcohol-based hand cleaner if the patient is suspected of having infectious diarrhea that is spread by spores. ∎

Diarrhea can cause dehydration and other serious medical problems if undetected or untreated. Most health care facilities have a definition of diarrhea, such as three or more loose stools within a defined period of time. One loose stool is not diarrhea. Remember to be objective in reporting your observations. When reporting loose stools to the the nurse, report the color, odor, consistency, character, amount, and frequency of stools. Also report any patient complaints of pain or other discomfort.

Bowel Incontinence

Bowel incontinence is involuntary passage of fecal material from the anus. It has many causes, including trauma, neurological diseases, inability to reach the toilet on time, and mental confusion. It is not as common as urinary incontinence. Fecal material is very irritating to the skin, so the patient must be cleansed well after each episode of incontinence. Skin exposed to fecal material will break

moves through the intestines. The patient may also complain of abdominal pain and cramping.

Clinical Information ALERT

Moisture from urinary and fecal incontinence increases the risk of friction and shearing on the skin. Continued exposure to moisture weakens the skin and reduces its protective function. This sets the stage for more irritation and continued weakening of the skin. Enzymes pass through the digestive system in feces. These enzymes break down food during digestion. They also break down the skin during prolonged exposure to stool, such as in diarrhea, an ostomy, or incontinence. Studies have shown that fecal incontinence is a contributing factor to more than half of all pressure ulcers in the torso and buttock area. ■

Communication HIGHLIGHT

Remember that bowel activity is a normal body function. Do not show disgust in your facial expressions or body language when assisting patients with elimination. Documenting bowel activity is a very important responsibility. Unrelieved constipation is a serious, uncomfortable condition. The nurse depends on the accuracy of your documentation in the elimination record. The nurse will use this record to contact the physician, and administer medications and other treatments related to bowel elimination. ■

down quickly. Bowel incontinence may lower the patient's self-esteem. Be professional, compassionate, and understanding when assisting patients with bowel elimination and incontinence.

Patients with bowel incontinence may be placed on a bowel retraining or incontinence management program. If this is ineffective, a fecal incontinence collector may be used.

Role of the Nursing Assistant in Assisting Patients with Bowel Elimination

Assisting with bowel elimination is a very important responsibility. Always apply the principles of standard pre-cautions when assisting with elimination. Avoid contaminating environmental surfaces with your gloves. Wear a gown, eye protection, and face mask if splashing is likely. If an adult must wear a protective garment to contain incontinence, avoid calling the garment a "diaper," which is a demeaning term for an adult. Use another term, such as brief, adult brief, or clothing protector, or call the garment by the product name, such as Depends.

Stool Specimens

A specimen of stool is a sample of fecal material (solid body waste or bowel movement) collected in a special container. The specimen is then sent to the laboratory for examination. In the laboratory, stool may be examined for:

GUIDELINES *for*

Assisting Patients with Bowel Elimination

- Apply the principles of standard precautions when assisting with bowel elimination. Avoid environmental contamination from your gloves.
- Encourage patients to consume an adequate amount of fluid. Maintaining fluid intake is as important for bowel elimination as it is for urinary elimination.
- Encourage patients to eat a well-balanced diet.
- Allow adequate time for patients to eat meals.
- Encourage patients to chew food well. Cut it into small pieces if necessary. Report chewing problems to the nurse for further assessment.

- If you observe that a patient has not eaten fiber foods, fruits, or vegetables, offer a substitute. The dietitian may visit the patient to discuss likes and dislikes and ensure that the patient will eat the foods served.
- Encourage exercise and activity, as allowed and tolerated.
- Assist patients with toileting at regular intervals and provide privacy.
- Position patients in a sitting position, if allowed, for bowel elimination.

continues

GUIDELINES *continued*

- Use a bath blanket to cover a patient who is using the bedpan or commode, for privacy and warmth.
- Leave the call signal and toilet tissue within reach and respond to the call signal immediately.
- Allow adequate time for defecation.
- Provide perineal care as needed, or according to facility policy. Feces are very irritating to the skin and prolonged contact promotes skin breakdown and infection.
- Assist patients with cleaning the anal area (this may be called the rectal area by some health care providers).
- Assist patients with handwashing and other personal hygiene after bowel elimination.

- Monitor bowel elimination and report irregularities.
- Record bowel movements on the flow sheet or other designated location. If a patient is independent with bowel elimination, ask each day if she has had a bowel movement.
- Report to the nurse: frequent stools, absence of stools, pain, cramping, excessive flatulence, abnormal color or consistency of stool, extremely small amounts of stool, hard, dry stool, or enlargement of the abdomen.
- Specific abnormalities in stools to report are presence of blood, pus, mucus, black or other unusual color, undigested food (except corn and raisins), or presence of parasites.

Clinical Information ALERT

Sometimes the doctor will order stool specimens X3 for Ova and Parasites (O&P). These specimens should be 24 hours apart, unless otherwise ordered. A 12-hour minimum may be acceptable, depending on the circumstances. Always check with the nurse:

- Before discarding a specimen
- If the patient just had a lower GI series (barium enema)
- After the administration of a prep for lower colon X-rays
- After the nurse has given a laxative or suppository

Normal saline enema specimens are acceptable, but must be labeled "saline enema specimen." If in doubt about the preparation for the specimen, check with the nurse. ■

- Pathogenic microorganisms (germs)
- Parasites
- **Occult blood** (hidden blood or blood that cannot be seen with the eye)
- Chemical analysis

Unit 51 sets out the advanced procedure of testing for occult blood using Hemoccult and developer.

SPECIAL DIAGNOSTIC TESTS

Some techniques used to diagnose problems of the gastrointestinal system include:

- Gastrointestinal (GI) series—a liquid called barium is either swallowed (upper GI series) or given as an enema (lower GI series). X-rays are then taken.
- Direct visualization procedures:
  - **Proctoscopy**—visualization of the rectum
  - **Sigmoidoscopy**—visualization of the sigmoid colon
  - **Gastroscopy**—visualization of the stomach

In preparation for the tests, the entire GI tract must be emptied before the X-rays.

- No food is permitted for 8 hours or longer
- Enemas are given before the series until only the clear liquid returns
- Laxatives are given the night before the test

Cholecystogram (Gallbladder Series)

A gallbladder (GB) series is an X-ray examination similar to the GI series except that the dye tablets are swallowed. Orders for preparing patients for this test vary. Cleansing enemas may be ordered. A special diet may also be required beforehand.

Ultrasonography

Ultrasound is very high frequency sound that cannot be heard. When concentrated in a beam and directed at body organs and tissues, the ultrasound moves at different speeds through the tissues, because of the varying tissue

PROCEDURE

95

COLLECTING A STOOL SPECIMEN

1. Carry out initial procedure actions.

2. Assemble equipment:
   - Disposable gloves
   - Bedpan and cover or collection container
   - Specimen container and cover
   - Biohazard specimen transport bag
   - Label, including:
     - patient's full name
     - room number
     - date and time of collection
     - physician's name
     - examination to be performed
     - other information required
   - Toilet tissue
   - Tongue depressors
   - Basin

3. Wash your hands and put on disposable gloves.

4. Uncover the container that was used to collect the bowel movement (bedpan or commode receptacle). (If a toilet insert is used, the specimen will be collected from the insert.) If the patient is incontinent of feces, use tongue depressors to obtain a specimen from bed linens, adult brief, or protective padding. A specimen may also be obtained from a fecal incontinence collection bag when the bag is changed.

5. Following defecation, the patient washes his hands. Fill a basin with water at 105°F. Assist the patient if needed. If the patient is incontinent, carefully clean and dry the area around the anus. Change bed linens as needed.

6. Take the container with the bowel movement to the bathroom. Use tongue blades to remove a specimen and place it in a specimen container (Figure 44-5). Do not contaminate the outside of the specimen container or the cover. If possible, take a sample (about 1 teaspoon) from each part of the specimen.

7. Empty the collection container into the toilet. Clean or dispose of the collection container according to facility policy. If the patient was incontinent, dispose of the soiled brief or padding as biohazardous waste. Place soiled linen in the proper hamper.

8. Remove and dispose of your gloves according to facility policy.

9. Wash your hands.

10. Cover the container and attach the completed label. Make sure the cover is on the container tightly. Place the container in a biohazard transport bag.

11. Take or send the specimen to the laboratory promptly. (Stool specimens are never refrigerated.)

12. Carry out ending procedure actions.

FIGURE 44-5 Use tongue blades to transfer the specimen from the collection device to the specimen cup.

density. This permits a picture to be made of the tissues being examined. *Ultrasonography* is the use of sound to produce an image of an organ or tissue.

ENEMAS

A cleansing **enema** is the technique of introducing fluid into the rectum to remove feces and flatus (gas) from the colon and rectum. (Refer to Procedures 96 and 97.) Enemas are given:

- To aid illumination during X-rays
- Before surgery
- Before testing
- During bowel retraining programs
- To relieve constipation and impaction
- To instill drugs

The fluids often used for enemas are:

- Soap solution (SSE)
- Salt solution (saline)
- Tap water (TWE)
- Phosphosoda

These solutions create a feeling of urgency in the patient's bowel. **Urgency** is the term used to describe the need to empty the bowel. Solutions are expelled a short time after they are given. When enemas are given in preparation for diagnostic X-rays or to instill drugs, the fluid is retained as long as possible.

Culture ALERT

Patients from some cultures may be resistant to using a bedpan or urinal, or may refuse to use it at all. A bedside commode may be much more acceptable, particularly when a treatment such as an enema or suppositories is necessary. Some of these individuals may try to avoid having BMs while hospitalized, and will return home feeling very constipated. Monitor elimination carefully and report no BM in 3 days to the nurse. Members of these cultures (Central American, Chinese American, Cuban, Filipino, Gypsy, Haitian, Iranian, Mexican American, Puerto Rican, and Samoan) are often very modest. They may avoid discussing issues related to elimination, sex, or sexuality. ■

General Considerations

Some general considerations to keep in mind are:

- Apply the principles of standard precautions. Avoid environmental contamination from your gloves.

- Administer an enema only upon the direction of a licensed nurse.
- If the patient is to get up following the enema and use the bathroom, make sure the bathroom is available and not in use before giving the enema.
- When possible, the enema should be given before the patient's bath or before breakfast.
- Do not give an enema within an hour following a meal.
- Consult the care plan or the nurse for the amount and type of solution to use, and any special instructions.

Tips: Avoid giving an enema within an hour after meals, because the increased peristalsis makes it difficult for the patient to retain the solution. Avoid administering an enema to a patient in a sitting position, such as on the toilet. The solution will not flow high into the colon when administered to a patient who is seated. It will cause the rectum to enlarge, causing rapid expulsion of the fluid.

Position

The best position for the patient to receive an enema is in the left Sims' position. Fluid flows into the bowel more easily when the patient is in this position. The left Sims' position and several alternative positions are shown in Figure 44-6.

At times, the enema may have to be administered with the patient on the bedpan in the supine position. The supine position can be used if the patient is unable to hold the fluid or to assume Sims' position.

- The patient's knees are flexed and separated.
- An orthopedic (fracture) bedpan is more comfortable than a regular bedpan. It may have to be padded when the patient is very thin.

Disposable Enema Units

Disposable enema units are available to give:

- Soap-solution enema
- Commercially prepared enema
- Phosphosoda enema
- Oil-retention enema

Administration of disposable enemas is simple. Time is saved in preparing and cleaning the equipment. The techniques for using reusable equipment for oil-retention or soap-solution enemas are the same.

Giving an Enema with a Commercially Prepared Chemical Enema Solution

Commercially prepared enemas are convenient to administer and more comfortable for the patient. The enema may be either an oil-retention enema or a phosphosoda

Sims' (left-lateral) Position   Knee-Chest Position

Position for Self-Administration   Child's Position

FIGURE 44-6   Alternative positions for enema administration

PROCEDURE

96

GIVING A SOAP-SOLUTION ENEMA

 Note: Be sure this is a nursing assistant procedure in your facility.

1. Carry out initial procedure actions.

2. Assemble equipment:

- Disposable gloves
- Disposable enema equipment, consisting of a plastic container, tubing with rectal tube, clamp, and lubricant (equipment is commercially available as a kit)
- Bedpan and cover
- Bed protector
- Toilet tissue
- Bath blanket
- Castile soap packet
- Towel, soap, basin

3. In the utility room:

a. Connect the tubing to the solution container (Figure 44-7A).

FIGURE 44-7A
Attach the tubing to the container.

b. Adjust the clamp on the tubing and snap it shut (Figure 44-7B).

c. Fill the container with warm water (105°F) to the 1,000-mL line (500 mL for children) (Figures 44-7C and 44-7D).

continues

PROCEDURE 96 CONTINUED

FIGURE 44-7B Slip the clamp over the tubing.

FIGURE 44-7C Fill the container with warm water.

FIGURE 44-7D Use a bath thermometer to make sure the temperature is about 105°F.

d. Open the packet of liquid soap and put the soap in the water (Figure 44-7E).

e. Using the tip of the tubing, mix the solution (mix gently so that no suds form) or rotate the bag to mix. Do not shake.

f. Run a small amount of solution through the tube to eliminate air and warm the tube (Figure 44-7F). Clamp the tubing (Figure 44-7G).

4. Place a chair at the foot of the bed and cover it with a bed protector. Place the bedpan on it.

5. Elevate the bed to a comfortable working height. Be sure the opposite side rail is up and secure for safety.

6. Cover the patient with a bath blanket and fanfold linen to the foot of the bed.

7. Wash your hands and put on gloves.

8. Place a bed protector under the patient's buttocks.

9. Help the patient turn on the left side and flex the knees.

FIGURE 44-7E Add soap from the packet.

FIGURE 44-7F Run a small amount of water through the tubing to expel air.

FIGURE 44-7G Clamp the tubing.

continues

PROCEDURE 96 CONTINUED

10. Place the container of solution on the chair so the tubing will reach the patient.

11. Adjust the bath blanket to expose the anal area.

12. Expose the anus by raising the upper buttock.

13. Lubricate the tip of the tube. The patient should breathe deeply and bear down as the tube is inserted, to relax the anal sphincter. Insert the tube 2 to 4 inches into the anus.

14. Never force the tube. If the tube cannot be inserted easily, get help. There may be a tumor or a mass of feces blocking the bowel. The mass of feces is known as an *impaction*.

15. Open the clamp and raise the container 12 inches above the level of the anus so that the fluid flows in slowly (Figure 44-7H).

    ● Ask the patient to take deep breaths to relax the abdomen.

    ● If the patient complains of cramping, clamp the tube and wait until the cramping stops. Then open the tubing to continue the fluid flow.

16. Clamp the tubing before the container is completely empty.

17. Tell the patient to hold his breath while the upper buttock is raised and the tube is gently withdrawn.

18. Wrap the tubing in a paper towel. Put it in the disposable container.

19. Place the patient on a bedpan or assist him to the bathroom.

20. Using a paper towel, so your glove does not contaminate the control or crank, raise the head of the bed to a comfortable height if the patient is on the bedpan. Raise the side rail for safety if needed.

21. Place toilet tissue and the signal cord within reach of the patient. If the patient is in the bathroom, stay nearby. Caution the patient not to flush the toilet.

22. Discard disposable materials as biohazardous waste, according to facility policy.

FIGURE 44-7H Raise the container above the anus so the flow of fluid is unobstructed.

23. Remove your gloves and discard according to facility policy. Wash your hands.

24. Return to the bedside. Put on fresh gloves.

25. Remove the bedpan. Place it on a bed protector on the chair and cover it.

26. Cleanse the patient's anal area.

27. Remove the bed protector and discard according to facility policy.

28. Remove gloves and wash your hands.

29. Give the patient soap, water, and towel to wash and dry his hands.

30. Replace the top bedding and remove the bath blanket.

31. Put on gloves. Take the bedpan to the bathroom. Dispose of contents according to facility policy or, using a paper towel, flush the toilet.

32. Remove gloves and dispose of according to facility policy.

33. Wash your hands.

34. Air the room and leave the room in order.

35. Unscreen the unit.

36. Clean and replace all other equipment used according to facility policy.

37. Carry out ending procedure actions.

enema and is followed by a cleansing (soap-solution) enema.

- The solution is already measured and ready to use.
- A small amount of fluid will remain in the container after administration.
- The solution in a phosphosoda enema draws fluid from the body to stimulate peristalsis.
- The oil-retention enema solution softens the feces, making them easier to expel.

- The amount of solution administered is about 4 ounces.
- The tip of the container is prelubricated.
- The enema solution is in an easy-to-handle plastic container.
- The solution is sometimes used at room temperature.
- You may be asked to warm the solution by placing the container in warm water before administration. Check with the nurse regarding your facility's policy.

PROCEDURE

GIVING A COMMERCIALLY PREPARED ENEMA

 Note: Be sure this is a nursing assistant procedure in your facility.

 Note: Use this procedure when giving an oil-retention or a phosphosoda enema.

1. Carry out initial procedure actions.

2. Assemble equipment:
   - Disposable gloves
   - Disposable prepackaged enema
   - Bedpan and cover
   - Bed protector
   - Pan of warm water (if enema solution is to be warmed)

3. Open the package and remove the plastic container of enema solution. Place the solution container in warm water (if it is to be warmed).

4. Lower the head of the bed to a horizontal position and elevate the bed to a comfortable working height. Raise the side rail on the opposite side of the bed for safety.

5. Put on gloves.

6. Place a bedpan and cover on the chair close at hand.

7. Assist the patient to turn to the left side and flex the right leg.

8. Place a bed protector under the patient.

9. Expose only the patient's buttocks by drawing the bedding upward in one hand.

FIGURE 44-8 Remove the cover from the prelubricated tip of the container.

10. Remove the cover from the enema tip (Figure 44-8). Gently squeeze to make sure the tip is undamaged (patent).

11. Separate the buttocks, exposing the anus, and ask the patient to breathe deeply and bear down slightly.

12. Insert the lubricated enema tip 2 inches into the rectum.

13. Gently squeeze and roll the container until the desired quantity of solution is administered (Figure 44-9). A small amount of solution will remain in the container. Avoid releasing pressure on the container, or the solution will return.

14. Remove the tip from the patient and place the container in the box. Encourage the patient to hold the solution as long as possible.

continues

PROCEDURE 97 CONTINUED

FIGURE 44-9 Squeeze the bottle from the bottom. A small amount of fluid will remain in the container.

15. Remove gloves and dispose of properly. Wash your hands.

16. Discard the used enema as biohazard waste.

17. Provide privacy. This enema should be retained for 20 minutes. Give the patient the call signal and leave.

18. When the patient feels the urge to defecate, lower the bed and assist the patient to the bathroom or commode, or position the patient on the bedpan.

19. Raise the head of the bed to a comfortable height if the patient is using a bedpan.

20. Place toilet tissue and the signal cord within reach of the patient. Raise the side rail for safety if the bed is left in high position. If the patient is in the bathroom, stay nearby. Caution the patient not to flush the toilet.

21. Return to the patient when signaled. Wash your hands. Lower the nearest side rail, if it is up. Put on gloves.

22. Remove the bedpan and place it on the bed protector covering the chair. Observe the contents of the bedpan. Cover the bedpan.

23. Clean the anal area of the patient, if required.

24. If the patient has used a commode or toilet:

a. Clean the anal area, if required.

b. Observe the contents of the commode or toilet.

c. Flush the toilet using a paper towel, or cover the commode.

d. Remove gloves and discard according to facility policy. Assist the patient into bed.

25. Put on gloves. Take the bedpan or commode container and equipment to the bathroom. Dispose of contents according to facility policy.

26. Remove and dispose of gloves properly. Wash your hands.

27. Give the patient soap, water, and a towel to wash her hands. Return equipment. Leave the side rails down unless needed for safety and leave the bed in low position.

28. Carry out ending procedure actions.

Rectal Suppositories

Rectal **suppositories** are used to stimulate bowel evacuation or to administer medication. Medicinal suppositories must be inserted by the nurse. You may be asked to insert the type of suppository that softens stool and promotes elimination. (See Procedure 98.) Check your facility policy to be sure this is a nursing assistant function. The suppository must be placed beyond the rectal sphincter (circular muscle that controls the anal opening) and against the bowel wall so it can melt and lubricate the rectum.

Rectal Tube and Flatus Bag

The rectal tube is used to reduce flatus (gas) in the bowel. Placing a rectal tube into the rectum provides a passageway for the gas to escape. Flatus distends the intestines, causing pain and stress on incisions.

You can assist the patient as follows:

- Encourage activity.
- Promote regularity.
- Accept the expulsion of gas as a natural body function. Do not contribute to the patient's embarrassment.
- Use flatus-reducing procedures when ordered.
- Insert a rectal tube with flatus bag if ordered. (Remember that your facility policies must state that nursing assistants can perform this procedure.)

The disposable tube is used once in a 24-hour period for no more than 20 minutes.

- Relief may occur as soon as the tube is inserted.
- Check the amount of abdominal distention (stretching).
- Question the patient about the amount of relief.

PROCEDURE

98

INSERTING A RECTAL SUPPOSITORY

 Note: Be sure this is a nursing assistant procedure in your facility.

1. Carry out initial procedure actions.

2. Assemble equipment:
   - Disposable gloves
   - Suppository as ordered
   - Toilet tissue
   - Bedpan and cover, if needed
   - Lubricant
   - Bed protector

3. Wash your hands and put on gloves.

4. Help the patient turn on the left side and flex the right leg. Place a bed protector under the patient's hips.

5. Adjust bed linen to expose the buttocks only.

6. Unwrap the suppository.

7. With your left hand, separate the patient's buttocks, exposing the anus.

8. Apply a small amount of lubricant to the anus and to the suppository and insert the suppository. The suppository must be inserted deeply enough to enter the rectum beyond the sphincter (approximately 2 inches) (Figure 44-10).

9. Encourage the patient to take deep breaths and relax (until the need to defecate is felt in 5 to 20 minutes).

10. Remove gloves and dispose of properly. Wash your hands.

11. Adjust the bedding and help the patient to assume a comfortable position.

12. Place the signal cord near the patient's hand, but check every 5 minutes.

13. Wash your hands and put on gloves.

14. Assist the patient to the bathroom or commode, or position the patient on a bedpan.

15. Provide privacy. Once the patient is finished, assist with hygiene if necessary.

FIGURE 44-10 Lubricate the anus and insert the suppository beyond the sphincter muscle.

16. Observe results and note any unusual characteristics of the stool. If stool is unusual, save it and report to the nurse.

17. Dispose of stool and clean equipment according to facility policy. Store equipment as required.

18. Remove and dispose of gloves according to facility policy. Wash your hands.

19. Carry out ending procedure actions.

REVIEW

A. True/False.

Mark the following true or false by circling T or F.

1. T F A herniorrhaphy is the surgery performed when there is bowel malignancy.

2. T F The drainage from a new cholecystectomy incision is normally yellowish-green.

3. T F The patient is placed on the left side, if possible, for enema administration.

4. T F When a prepackaged enema is administered, approximately 4 ounces are given.

5. T F Be sure the bathroom is free before giving an enema.

6. T F A flatus tube is used to reduce abdominal distention from gas.

7. T F An enema may be given only upon direction from the nurse.

8. T F When giving a soap-solution enema, approximately 2,000 mL are used.

9. T F Gastric ulcers are located in the esophagus.

B. Matching.

Choose the correct word from Column II to match each word or phrase in Column I.

Column I

10. _____ gas

11. _____ yellow discoloration of skin

12. _____ large bowel

13. _____ feces

14. _____ gallstones

Column II

a. stool

b. flatus

c. cholelithiasis

d. cyanosis

e. cholecystectomy

f. colon

g. jaundice

C. Multiple Choice.

Select the one best answer for each of the following.

15. A sign of possible gastrointestinal malignancy is
    a. good appetite.
    b. change in stool color.
    c. weight gain.
    d. nausea.

16. Your patient has just returned from surgery for gallstones. She will be most comfortable in the
    a. dorsal recumbent position.
    b. lithotomy position.
    c. semi-Fowler's position.
    d. left Sims' position.

17. Enemas are given
    a. after the patient showers.
    b. at bedtime.
    c. before diagnostic testing.
    d. after surgery.

18. The oil-retention enema is usually
    a. preceded by a soap-solution enema.
    b. retained for 1 hour.
    c. followed by a soap-solution enema.
    d. given in the semi-Fowler's position.

19. Urgency is a term that means
    a. inability to have a BM.
    b. need to eliminate.
    c. pain from flatus.
    d. need to vomit.

D. Completion.

Complete the statements in the spaces provided.

20. The enema given to soften feces is known as _____.

21. The purpose of a soap-solution enema is to _____.

E. Nursing Assistant Challenge.

Mr. Rayburn has been admitted with a provisional diagnosis of gastric ulcers. He had been complaining of a burning sensation in his stomach halfway between meals. He is scheduled for an upper GI series at 8:00 AM tomorrow morning. Answer the following questions regarding Mr. Rayburn and his care.

22. What acid is naturally found in Mr. Rayburn's stomach?

23. Before the GI series, will it be all right to serve Mr. Rayburn breakfast in the morning?

24. What procedure will you be asked to carry out before the test?

25. Will Mr. Rayburn swallow the barium, or will he be given a barium enema?

26. Will X-rays be taken?

UNIT 45

Urinary System

OBJECTIVES

After completing this unit, you will be able to:

- Spell and define terms.
- Review the location and function of the urinary system.
- List five diagnostic tests associated with conditions of the urinary system.
- Describe some common diseases of the urinary system.
- Describe nursing assistant actions related to the care of patients with urinary system diseases and conditions.
- Demonstrate the following procedures:
  - Procedure 99 Collecting a Routine Urine Specimen
  - Procedure 100 Collecting a Clean-Catch Urine Specimen

- Procedure 101 Collecting a 24-Hour Urine Specimen
- Procedure 102 Routine Drainage Check
- Procedure 103 Giving Indwelling Catheter Care
- Procedure 104 Emptying a Urinary Drainage Unit
- Procedure 105 Disconnecting the Catheter
- Procedure 106 Applying a Condom for Urinary Drainage
- Procedure 107 Connecting a Catheter to a Leg Bag
- Procedure 108 Emptying a Leg Bag

VOCABULARY

Learn the meaning and the correct spelling of the following words and phrases:

Bowman's capsule	glomerulus	nephritis	suprapubic catheter
catheter	hematuria	nephron	ureter
condom catheter	hydronephrosis	pelvis	urethra
cortex	indwelling catheter	pyelogram	urinalysis
cystitis	intravenous pyelogram	renal calculi	urinary bladder
cystoscopy	(IVP)	renal colic	urinary incontinence
dialysis	kidney	retention	urinary meatus
dysuria	lithotripsy	retrograde pyelogram	void
Foley catheter	medulla	suppression	

INTRODUCTION

The urinary system consists of the kidneys, ureters, bladder, and urethra. The functions that this system performs are vital. It:

- Excretes liquid wastes

- Manages blood chemistry
- Manages fluid balance

Because the chemistry of the blood and urine reflect the chemistry of the cells, many tests are performed on urine specimens. It is important that urine samples be obtained and preserved properly.

Clinical Information A

An average human drinks about 16,000 gallons of water in a lifetime. The human body is about 66% water. Death will result if you lose 12% of your body fluids. An average person urinates 6 times per day. The yellow color of urine is caused by pigment derived from bile. The left kidney is slightly higher than the right. About 440 gallons of blood flow through the kidneys each day. If all the renal tubules were laid end to end, they would measure about 66 yards. The kidneys have about a million structures that filter out liquids and wastes in the blood. ∎

STRUCTURE AND FUNCTION

The urinary system is shown in Figure 45-1. As the name implies, the organs of this system produce urine—liquid waste—that is excreted from the body. The urinary system also helps to control the vital water and salt balance of the body. Inability to secrete urine by the kidneys is known as **suppression**. Inability to excrete urine that has been produced by the kidneys is called **retention**. The organs of this system include:

- **Kidneys:** Organs that produce the urine.
- **Ureters:** Tubes that carry the urine from the kidneys to the urinary bladder. These tubes are 10 to 12 inches long and about ¼-inch wide.
- **Urinary bladder:** Holds the urine until expelled. The urge to urinate (micturate or void) occurs when 150 to 300 mL of urine are in the bladder, although the bladder can hold more urine than this.
- **Urethra:** The tube that carries the urine to the outside. The female urethra is about 1½ inches long. The male urethra is about 6 to 8 inches long. The opening to the outside is called the external **urinary meatus**. The meatus is guarded by a round sphincter muscle that relaxes to release the urine.

The Kidneys

The two bean-shaped kidneys are located behind the peritoneum. They are held in place by capsules of fat. Each kidney weighs about 5 ounces. The outer portion of the kidney is called the **cortex**. This area produces the urine.

FIGURE 45-1 Structures of the urinary system

The middle area is known as the **medulla**. It is a series of tubes that drain the urine from the cortex. The **pelvis** of the kidney receives the urine and directs it to the ureter.

Urine Production. The renal arteries carry blood to each kidney. Their many branches pass through the medulla to the cortex. In the cortex, urine is produced in filtering units called **nephrons** (Figure 45-2). It is estimated that each kidney contains 1 million nephrons.

Blood arriving at the kidneys carries waste products such as acids and salts. These waste products must be eliminated from the body. Urine is a liquid waste solution containing water and dissolved substances. In the kidneys:

- Waste products, helpful products, and large quantities of water are passed (filtered) through the capillary walls of the **glomerulus** (capillary bed) into **Bowman's capsule**, forming a liquid called *filtrate*.
- The filtrate moves slowly along the convoluted tubules where some water and helpful substances like sugar are reabsorbed into the blood.

- The liquid remaining in the convoluted tubules is urine, which contains wastes.
- The urine passes into the collecting tubules of the medulla, then out of the kidney to the ureter and into the urinary bladder.
- Normal urine is acidic and pale to deep yellow in color.
- Dilute urine has more water and fewer dissolved substances, so it is colorless to pale yellow.
- Concentrated urine has less water and more dissolved substances, so it is darker in color and has a stronger odor.
- The amount of urine produced depends on the amount of intake and various physical conditions. Inadequate water intake leading to dehydration results in a small amount of concentrated urine.

The substances in the urine provide good information about the chemistry of the body and how well it is functioning. Tests are frequently performed on the urine (**urinalysis**).

COMMON CONDITIONS

Common conditions affecting the urinary system include inflammations due to ascending or descending infections and obstructions to the normal flow of fluids through the tube structure.

Cystitis

Cystitis, or inflammation of the urinary bladder, is fairly common. It is particularly common in women because the female urethra is so short. Signs and symptoms of cystitis include:

- Frequent urination
- **Hematuria** (blood in the urine)
- **Dysuria** (painful urination and/or burning upon urination)
- Bladder spasm

Treatment. Treatment is aimed at relieving the symptoms and eliminating the cause. Treatment includes:

- Sitz baths
- Rest
- Bacteriostatic agents
- Increased fluid intake
- Antibiotics

Nephritis

Nephritis means inflammation of the kidney. Nephritis:

- May follow an attack of infectious disease or may result from general arteriosclerosis. In either case, kidney cells are destroyed. This results in decreased urine production.

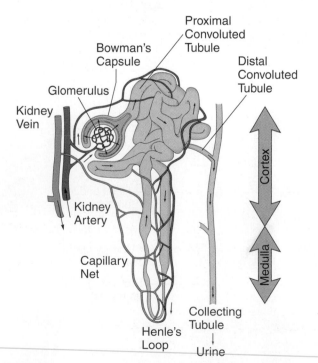

FIGURE 45-2 Nephron and related structures. Arrows indicate the flow of blood through the nephron. The urine produced by the nephron flows through the collecting tubule.

- May follow a disease course that is acute (rapid) or chronic (slow).
- Causes hypertension and edema.

Signs and symptoms of nephritis are:

- Edema
- Hematuria
- Proteinuria (protein in urine)
- Hypertension
- Oliguria (occasionally) (decreased urination)

Treatment. Treatment includes:

- Absolute bedrest
- Low-sodium diet
- Restricted fluid intake, at times
- Frequent checks on vital signs
- Accurate intake and output (I/O) measurement
- Steroid medication in some cases

If both kidneys are involved, the patient will require regular dialysis until the diseased kidney can be replaced with a healthy kidney (kidney transplant). **Dialysis** is the process of removing the waste products from the blood with a hemodialysis machine, commonly called an artificial kidney.

Many patients on dialysis receive treatment in a hospital dialysis unit or in special outpatient dialysis centers. Portable equipment is brought to the patient's bedside, if necessary. Other patients receive dialysis at home, using portable dialysis machines. The patient's overall physical condition is an important factor in determining if home dialysis is an option.

Renal Calculi

Renal calculi are kidney stones. They can cause obstructions when they become lodged in the urinary passageways.

There may be no sign of the development of renal calculi until some obstruction develops. Then:

- The pain is sudden and intense. It is called **renal colic**.
- Calculi may be passed in the urine.
- As stones pass along the tract, tissue damage may occur, resulting in hematuria (blood in the urine).

Treatment. The goal of treatment is to relieve the blockage and eliminate the stones.

- Encouraging fluids increases urine output. This helps to move the stones along the tract.
- All urine must be strained through gauze or filter paper, which is inspected for stones before it is discarded (Figure 45-3). Stones that are found can be analyzed. With information from the stones, the diet can sometimes be changed to make the formation of stones less likely.
- When it is impossible for the patient to pass the stones, surgery may be necessary. This type of surgery can be done by passing a cystoscope through the ure-

thra or through a surgical incision. With the cystoscope, the physician is able to see inside the bladder and locate the stones. The stones may then be crushed so they can be flushed out in the urine.

- At other times, the stones can be reached and removed only through a surgical incision. When a surgical incision is made, the patient usually returns from surgery with two drainage tubes in place. One tube is inserted in the urinary bladder. The other tube is inserted in the ureter or kidney.
  - The nurse will see that proper drainage is established.
  - In addition to routine postoperative care, you must check frequently to be sure the drainage is not blocked by kinks in the tubes or by the patient's body lying on the tubes.
  - The amount and type of drainage from each area should be carefully noted.
- **Lithotripsy** is a technique that uses carefully directed sound waves to crush the stones without the need for any surgical incision. The patient receiving this form of treatment is usually in the hospital less than 24 hours.

Clinical Information ALERT

Kidney stones may develop anywhere in the urinary tract from mineral salts collecting around bacteria, blood clots, or other particles. They are a complication of immobility, but there are other causes, such as excess calcium in the diet, inadequate intake of fluids, dehydration, and heredity. Although tiny, the stones are very painful for the patient. The size ranges from microscopic to several centimeters. Renal calculi may be various colors, each of which has diagnostic value. If the patient has an indwelling catheter, strain all urine each time the drainage bag is emptied. ■

Hydronephrosis

Hydronephrosis results from accumulation of fluid within the kidney. The increasing amount of urine causes pressure on the kidney cells. As a result, kidney cells are destroyed. The fluid accumulates in the kidney because something is blocking its flow. The flow may be blocked by:

- Renal calculi
- Kinking or twisting of the ureters
- Tumors, especially benign prostatic hypertrophy
- Distended bladder

Symptoms may be acute and similar to those of renal calculi, or they may occur so gradually that they go unnoticed until much damage has been done.

FIGURE 45-3 When the physician writes an order to strain urine, each voiding is poured through filter paper to retrieve kidney stones.

Treatment. The condition is treated by draining the urine above the blockage to relieve pressure and then correcting the cause.

RESPONSIBILITIES OF THE NURSING ASSISTANT

Be sure you understand the orders for each individual patient before you assist in nursing care. Orders regarding positioning, drainage, and activity for urological (urinary) patients vary.

There are some important measures that will apply to most urinary patients in your care:

- Accurately measure intake and output (Figure 45-4).
- Promptly report signs and symptoms of:
  - Bleeding
  - Chilling
  - Elevated temperature
  - Reduced output
  - Increased edema
  - Pain
- Properly care for urinary drainage.
- Know the proper steps to take for encouraging fluid intake (forcing fluids) and for limiting fluids.
- When assisting with urination, collecting a urine sample, or recording I/O, note and report the following:
  - Amount of urine
  - Color of urine

FIGURE 45-4 Accurately measure and record intake and output.

- Odor of urine
- Presence and type of sediment

URINARY INCONTINENCE

Urinary incontinence (loss of control of urination) may be due to one or a combination of factors. It is not unusual to find more than one factor present at the same time.

- Any interruption of cerebral control can lead to incontinence, including stroke, brain damage that destroys the control centers or pathways, confusion and decreased awareness due to general cerebral degeneration, or aphasia leading to the patient's inability to communicate the need for help.
- Incontinence may occur simply because the patient is unable to reach the proper facilities in time. The condition may be related to fecal impaction. Fecal impaction acts as a mechanical obstruction, causing the urine to be retained. The incontinence in this case is actually overflow. Perhaps the most common reason for incontinence is infection. Inflammation irritates sensory nerve endings in the bladder. Mucosal and bladder contractions are increased, causing the incontinence.

Age-Appropriate Care ALERT

Incontinence is up to 5 times more common in persons over age 50 than in younger adults. However, incontinence is not a normal aging change. It is always associated with another medical or psychological problem. Approximately one-third of all hospitalized adults are incontinent of stool. About half of all long-term care facility residents are incontinent of urine. ∎

- Incontinence may be temporary, lasting only a few days. For example, after a period of illness, continence may improve as the patient becomes more able to respond to the environment. Attention to the underlying causes and the temporary use of incontinence pads may be all that is needed. Every effort should be made to help the patient become continent as soon as possible, with little reference to the temporary incontinence. You can give a great deal of emotional support and reassurance to the patient.

- Incontinence of an established nature continues even though the patient is ambulatory. This is a more difficult, but still not impossible, form of incontinence to treat. Drugs are sometimes used to achieve bladder control. Retraining may also be needed.

DIAGNOSTIC TESTS

Techniques used to diagnose problems of the urinary tract include:

- Magnetic resonance imaging (MRI).
- CAT scan.
- Urinalysis—one common method of learning about the condition of the kidneys is to examine and test the urine.
- **Cystoscopy**—a test usually performed during surgery. It enables the physician to look inside the bladder. An instrument called a cystoscope is inserted through the urethra. Following this examination, frequency of urination is to be expected, but heavy bleeding or a complaint of sharp, intense pain should be reported at once.
- **Pyelogram**—an X-ray examination of the urinary tract, similar to the GB and GI series. The dye may be given intravenously (**intravenous pyelogram** or **IVP**) or inserted during cystoscopy (**retrograde pyelogram**) through the urethra. Preparation of the patient usually includes cleansing enemas. Satisfactory results of the X-ray examination depend largely on proper patient preparation.
- Blood chemistry tests
  - Blood urea nitrogen (BUN)
  - Creatinine

continues

GUIDELINES *for*

Caring for the Patient with Incontinence

Nursing assistant responsibilities include:

- Assisting patients who need help to toilet regularly.
- Answering call lights promptly.
- Always being courteous and patient when assisting patients with toileting.
- Maintaining a positive attitude when changing soiled garments and bed linen and never being critical.
- Performing good perineal care and being sure skin is clean and dry.
- Checking the skin for signs of irritation whenever toileting or bathing a patient or performing perineal care.
- Giving special attention to patients who are confused or forgetful, because they may be unable to clearly state their need for assistance.
- Changing wet linen immediately. This limits discomfort and embarrassment of the patient. Prolonged exposure of the skin to urine is a major cause of skin breakdown. In addition, pathogens grow rapidly on the warmth and moisture and can quickly move upward through the urinary tract, causing life-threatening infection.
- Helping the patient become continent. Little reference should be made to the temporary incontinence. Nursing assistants can do much to give emotional support and reassurance to patients who are incontinent.

PROCEDURE

COLLECTING A ROUTINE URINE SPECIMEN

1. Carry out initial procedure actions.
2. Assemble equipment:
   - Disposable gloves
   - Bedpan/urinal with cover
   - Bed protector
   - Toilet tissue

PROCEDURE 99 CONTINUED

- Small plastic bag
- Specimen container and cover
- Label, including:
  - patient's full name
  - room number
  - facility identification
  - date and time of collection
  - physician's name
  - examination to be done
  - other information requested or required
- Graduate pitcher
- Laboratory requisition slip, properly filled out
- Biohazard specimen transport bag

3. Completely fill out the label of the specimen container.

4. Wash your hands and put on disposable gloves.

5. If the patient cannot ambulate, offer the bedpan or urinal.

6. Instruct the patient not to discard toilet tissue in the pan with the urine. Provide a small plastic bag in which to place the soiled tissue.

7. After the patient has voided, cover the pan and place it on the bed protector on the chair. Offer wash water to the patient.

8. If the patient can ambulate to the bathroom, place a specimen collector in the toilet.

9. Assist the patient to the bathroom. Ask the patient to void into the specimen collector. Remind the patient to discard soiled toilet tissue in the plastic bag provided. Tissue must not be placed in the collector.

10. Provide privacy.

11. Put on gloves. Remove the specimen collector from the toilet. If the patient is on I&O, note the amount of urine (Figure 45-5). If the patient used a bedpan, pour the urine into a graduate to measure it. Note the amount. Remove gloves and discard according to facility policy. Wash your hands.

12. Remove the cap from the specimen container, and place it (inside up) on a shelf or other flat surface in the bathroom or utility room. Do not touch the inside of the cap or container.

FIGURE 45-5 Remove the collection device. Note the total amount if the patient is on I&O.

13. Put on gloves. Carefully pour about 120 mL of urine into the specimen container from the collector (Figure 45-6).

14. Remove and discard gloves according to facility policy.

15. Wash your hands.

16. Place the cap on the specimen container. Do not contaminate the outside of the container. Attach

FIGURE 45-6 Carefully pour the specimen into the container.

continues

PROCEDURE 99 CONTINUED

the completed label to the container (Figure 45-7). Place the specimen container in a biohazard specimen transport bag and attach a laboratory requisition slip (Figure 45-8).

17. Carry out ending procedure actions.

18. Follow facility policy for transporting the specimen to the laboratory.

FIGURE 45-8 The properly labeled container is placed in a transport bag with the laboratory requisition attached.

FIGURE 45-7 After placing the cap on the container, apply the label.

PROCEDURE

100

COLLECTING A CLEAN-CATCH URINE SPECIMEN

1. Carry out initial procedure actions.

2. Assemble equipment:
- Disposable gloves
- Small plastic bag
- Sterile specimen container and cover
- Label for container, with:
  - patient's full name
  - room number
  - facility identification
  - date and time of collection
  - physician's name
  - type of specimen test to be performed
  - any other information requested
- Gauze squares or cotton
- Antiseptic solution
- Laboratory requisition slip, properly filled out
- Biohazard specimen transport bag

3. Wash your hands and put on disposable gloves.

4. Wash the patient's genital area properly or instruct the patient to do so. If the area is soiled due to incontinence, perform perineal care.

a. *For female patients:*

i. Using the gauze or cotton and the antiseptic solution, cleanse the outer folds of the vulva (folds are also called *labia* or *lips*) from front to back. Use a separate cotton/gauze square for each side. Discard the gauze/cotton in the plastic bag.

ii. Cleanse the inner folds of the vulva with two pieces of gauze and antiseptic solution, again from front to back. Discard used gauze/cotton in the plastic bag.

iii. Cleanse the middle, innermost area (meatus or urinary opening) in the same manner. Discard the gauze/cotton in the plastic bag.

continues

PROCEDURE 100 CONTINUED

    iv. Keep the labia separated so that the folds do not fall back and cover the meatus.

  b. *For male patients:*

    i. Using the gauze/cotton and the antiseptic solution, cleanse the tip of the penis. Begin at the meatus, working outward and using a circular motion. Wash the remainder of the penis using downward strokes.

    ii. Discard the gauze/cotton in the plastic bag.

5. Open the container. Place the cap on the counter with the clean inside facing up. Do not touch the inside of the cup or lid with your hands.

6. Instruct the patient to void, allowing the first part of the urine to escape. Then:

  a. Catch the urine stream that follows in the sterile specimen container.

  b. Allow the last portion of the urine stream to escape.

Note: If the patient is on I&O, or if the amount of urine passed must be measured, catch the first and last part of the urine in a bedpan, urinal, or specimen collection container.

7. Place the sterile cap on the urine container immediately to prevent contamination of the urine specimen.

8. Allow the patient to wash hands.

9. With the cap securely tightened, wash the outside of the specimen container. Dry the container.

10. Remove and dispose of gloves according to facility policy.

11. Wash your hands.

12. Attach a completed label to the container and place the specimen in the transport bag.

13. Carry out ending procedure actions.

14. Follow facility policy for transporting the specimen to the laboratory.

Urine Specimens

Routine Urine Specimen. Urinalysis is the most common laboratory test. The specimen is usually taken when the patient first **voids** (urinates) in the morning. The properties of fresh urine begin to change after 15 minutes. Therefore, it is important that you immediately take the sample to the laboratory or refrigerate it until delivery can be made.

Catheterized Urine Specimen. When a urine specimen is needed that is free of contamination from organisms found in areas near the urinary meatus (opening), the specimen may be collected by inserting a sterile tube (**catheter**). The nurse will perform this procedure.

Twenty-Four-Hour Specimen. If a 24-hour urine specimen is ordered, all urine excreted by the patient in a 24-hour period is collected and saved. A 24-hour urine specimen requires that the patient start the 24-hour time period with an empty bladder. For this reason, the first specimen is discarded.

- All urine is saved in a large, carefully labeled container that is supplied by the laboratory and may contain a preservative.

- The container is usually surrounded by ice. If the patient has an indwelling catheter, place the catheter bag in a container surrounded by ice. Empty the bag into the container supplied by the laboratory.

- The patient is asked to void. This first urine is discarded so that the bladder is empty at the time the test begins.

- All other urine is saved, including that voided as the test time finishes.

- No toilet tissue should be allowed to enter the container.

- If you or the patient forget to save a specimen during the test period, report it immediately to the nurse. The test must be discontinued and started again for another 24 hours.

Remember to put on disposable gloves and remove and dispose of them properly each time you collect a specimen.

Urine Testing

The HemaCombistix is used to test for the presence of protein, blood, and glucose, and for pH (acidity) of urine.

RENAL DIALYSIS

As a result of disease or trauma, the kidneys may not be able to carry out their life-sustaining function of filtering impurities from the blood. In this case, mechanical dialysis is substituted to remove wastes from the blood.

PROCEDURE

COLLECTING A 24-HOUR URINE SPECIMEN

1. Carry out initial procedure actions.

2. Assemble equipment:
- Disposable gloves
- 24-hour specimen container (supplied by health care facility)
- Label
- Bedpan, urinal, or commode, or specimen collector for toilet
- Plastic bag
- Sign for patient's bed
- Biohazard bag

3. Label the container with:
- Patient's name
- Room number
- Test ordered
- Type of specimen
- Time started
- Time ended
- Date
- Physician's name

4. Emphasize to the patient the necessity of saving all urine passed.

5. Place the specimen collection container in the bathroom in a pan of ice (Figures 45-9A and 45-9B). The ice will keep the specimen cool for 24 hours.

6. Put on disposable gloves.

7. Allow the patient to void.
- **a.** Assist with the bedpan or urinal as needed.
- **b.** Measure the amount of urine passed if the patient is on I&O.
- **c.** Discard the urine specimen.
- **d.** Note the date and time of voiding. This time will mark the start of the 24-hour collection.

8. Place a sign on the patient's bed to alert other health care team members that a 24-hour urine specimen is being collected. (The sign may read: *Save all urine—24-hour specimen.*)

9. From this time on, for a period of 24 hours, all urine voided is added to the specimen container (Figure 45-9C). The container is kept on ice when not in use. Check facility policy regarding handling of the specimen container.

10. Instruct the patient not to discard toilet tissue into the specimen collection container. Provide small plastic bags for this purpose.

11. At the end of the 24-hour period:
- **a.** Put on disposable gloves.
- **b.** Ask the patient to void one last time.
- **c.** Add this urine to the specimen container.

FIGURE 45-9A Close the container with the plastic fastener. Place the 24-hour specimen container in the patient's bathroom in a pan of ice.

FIGURE 45-9B Some facilities use plastic containers for collecting a 24-hour specimen.

FIGURE 45-9C Open the mouth of the container wide to avoid spilling the specimen.

continues

PROCEDURE **101** CONTINUED

12. Remove the sign from the patient's bed. Check the container label for accuracy and completeness. Attach the appropriate requisition slip.

13. Remove and dispose of gloves according to facility policy.

14. Place the specimen in a protective biohazard bag for transport.

15. Carry out ending procedure actions.

16. Clean and replace all equipment used, according to facility policy.

17. Follow facility policy for transporting the specimen to the laboratory.

OSHA ALERT

Most facilities do not permit personnel to wear gloves or other PPE in the hallway. This is because the OSHA Bloodborne Pathogen Standard states PPE must be removed prior to leaving the work area. In this situation, the patient's room is the work area. Some facilities allow staff to use the one glove technique (Unit 13) to carry wet or soiled linen and other items into the hallway in close proximity to a patient's room. Know and follow your facility policies. ■

Patients requiring this treatment usually have tubing permanently placed in the arm to make it easier to connect to the dialysis machine. The graft attaches to an artery and a vein to provide ready access to the circulatory system. When not in use, the tubing from the artery and the tubing from the vein are joined.

 Note: The nursing assistant should never use the arm with a dialysis access site to measure blood pressure.

When dialysis is performed, the two sections of tubing are separated and attached to the dialysis machine. Blood passes from the artery to the machine, where impurities are filtered out. The blood is then returned to the patient's vein by way of the graft. The process takes 6 to 8 hours. It is usually performed 2 to 3 times per week. Patients with chronic renal failure may be maintained in this manner for some time, often for more than one year.

Sometimes a compatible kidney can be obtained from a donor and transplanted into the person with renal failure. If the kidney is not rejected, it will take on the life-sustaining role of the original kidneys.

URINARY DRAINAGE

Many patients with urinary problems will have a catheter for urinary drainage.

- Urine is drained from the bladder through a tube called a *catheter*.
- French catheters or straight catheters (Figure 45-10A) are hollow tubes. They are usually made of soft rubber or plastic. These catheters are used to drain the bladder. They do not remain in the bladder.
- **Foley catheters** (Figure 45-10B) have a balloon surrounding the neck. The balloon is inflated after the catheter is introduced into the bladder. This is known as an **indwelling** or retention **catheter**. Sometimes the patient will complain of feeling the urge to urinate after the catheter is inserted. This is due to the pressure of the balloon on the internal sphincter of the urethra. The pressure feels the same as the sensation of urine pressing on the sphincter. If the patient with a catheter complains of feeling the urge to void, notify the nurse.

FIGURE 45-10A A straight catheter is inserted to collect a specimen, then removed.

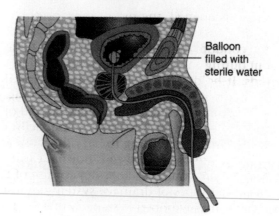

Balloon filled with sterile water

FIGURE 45-10B An indwelling (Foley) catheter is left in place to empty the bladder. The balloon is inflated with sterile water to hold the catheter in place.

- A **suprapubic catheter** (Figure 45-11) is inserted surgically through the abdominal wall directly into the bladder.
- A **condom catheter** is an external catheter used on males. It is applied over the penis and attached to drainage tubing.

The insertion of a catheter is a sterile procedure. It is performed by the nurse or advanced care provider. Closed urinary drainage systems protect the patient from infection.

Infection Control ALERT

As many as 28,000 patients die each year in the United States because of catheter-related infections. Careful handling and attention to technique when caring for and emptying the catheter will reduce the risk of infection. Catheters should be used only as a treatment of last resort because of the risk of complications. Possible complications are urinary tract or kidney infections, blood infections (septicemia), urethral injury, skin breakdown, bladder stones, and blood in the urine (hematuria). After many years of catheter use, bladder cancer may also develop. ■

FIGURE 45-11 The suprapubic catheter is surgically inserted through the abdominal wall. The urethra is not functional.

You have definite responsibilities when patients are using urinary drainage:

- Apply the principles of standard precautions.
- Keep the urinary meatus clean.
- Wash the area around the meatus daily with a solution approved by your facility.
- Check regularly for signs of irritation or urinary discomfort and report them to the nurse.
- Secure the tubing so that there is no strain on the catheter or tubing. A catheter strap should be applied to the leg to secure the tubing.
- Maintain the drainage bag below the level of the bladder.
- When the patient is in bed, the closed drainage bag is attached to the frame of the bed, never the side rail.
- When the patient is in a chair or wheelchair, the closed drainage bag is attached to the frame of the chair.
- Many facilities use cloth catheter bags for privacy. The cloth bag is connected to the bed or chair frame, and the urinary drainage bag is placed in it.
- When the patient is ambulating, the tubing and drainage bag are carried below the level of the bladder.
- Secure the catheter with a strap or tape. Some facilities secure the catheter to the leg in women and the abdomen, using tape, in men. When securing the catheter to the leg, it is positioned on the top side. Avoid placing the catheter under the leg, which may pinch and obstruct the flow of urine. Know and follow your facility policy.
- Attach the tubing to the bed with a rubber band and plastic clip.
- Use care when lifting, moving, and transferring patients with catheters to avoid accidentally dislodging the catheter by pulling on the tubing.
- Do not open a closed system.
- Make sure the tubing is not kinked or obstructed.
- Ensure that the collection bag does not touch the floor.
- Measure the amount of drainage in the collection bag at the end of each shift, note the character of the urine, and report and record the information. (See Procedure 104.)
- In certain medical conditions, the physician will order an hourly output measurement. In this situation, a catheter drainage bag with a *urimeter* (Figure 45-12) will be used. The urine drains into the small chamber. You will empty this chamber every hour and inform the nurse of the output measurement.
- Check the entire drainage setup each time care is given and at the beginning and end of your shift (see Procedure 102).
- Monitor the level of urine in the drainage bag. Most people excrete about 50 to 80 mL of urine each hour. If the level of urine in the bag does not change, if the

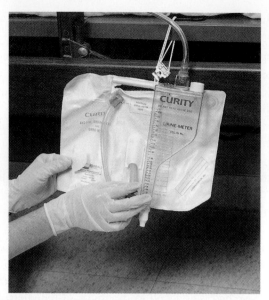

FIGURE 45-12 The drainage bag with a urimeter is used when the physician orders hourly output measurements.

catheter is leaking, if no urine is present in the bag, or if the urine has an abnormal color, odor, or appearance, inform the nurse.

Difficult SITUATIONS

Unless the patient is on a fluid restriction, encourage the catheterized patient to drink fluids each time you are in the room. Make sure that ice in the water pitcher is refilled regularly. If the patient does not like to drink water, offer fluids of choice, as permitted. Increasing fluid consumption to 2,500 mL a day is best when the patient has an indwelling catheter. The increased fluid prevents sediment formation and flushes the catheter. Check the level of urine in the drainage bag each time you are in the room. Empty the bag if it is full. ∎

- Notify the nurse if redness, irritation, drainage, crusting, or open areas are present at the catheter insertion site.
- Notify the nurse if the patient complains of pain, burning, tenderness, or has other signs or symptoms of urinary tract infection.

PROCEDURE

102
ROUTINE DRAINAGE CHECK

OBRA

1. Carry out initial procedure actions.

2. Wash your hands. Put on gloves.

3. Raise the bedding to observe the tubing.

4. Check the condition of the catheter and the meatus.

5. Keep the drainage tubing coiled on the bed so there is a direct drop to the collection bag (Figure 45-13).

6. The collection bag must be lower than the patient's hips.

7. Keep the end of the drainage tube above the urine level in the bag. Check to be sure that neither the tubing nor the drainage bag is touching the floor.

8. Be sure the drainage bag is attached to the bed frame (not the side rail).

9. Note the color, character, and flow of urine.

10. Measure urine using proper technique.

FIGURE 45-13 A Velcro strap is used to fasten the catheter to the leg. Coil the tubing on the bed. These measures prevent the catheter from moving and accidentally being pulled out during movement or transfers.

11. Remove gloves and discard according to facility policy.

12. Carry out ending procedure actions.

Catheter Care

Once the Foley catheter is inserted, the urinary meatus must be kept clean and free of secretions. The area around the meatus is washed daily with a solution approved by your facility or with soap and water. In some facilities, this procedure may be performed on each shift. This care is called indwelling catheter care.

Indwelling catheter care may be performed during routine morning care, as part of perineal care, or as a separate procedure (see Procedure 103). Report signs of irritation or complaints of discomfort, and changes in the character or quantity of drainage.

Ambulating with a Catheter

When patients are ambulatory or using a geri-chair or wheelchair, you must be careful about placement of the urinary drainage bag. Remember that the drainage bag must always be lower than the bladder so the urine cannot flow back into the bladder. The bag may be secured to the patient's leg or clothing when the patient ambulates.

When the patient is seated in a wheelchair, the tubing should run below and under the wheelchair so the drainage bag can be secured to the wheelchair back. The drainage bag or tubing must never touch the floor.

PROCEDURE

GIVING INDWELLING CATHETER CARE

1. Carry out initial procedure actions.

2. Assemble equipment:
   - Disposable gloves
   - Bed protector
   - Bath blanket
   - Plastic bag for disposables
   - Daily catheter care kit (if available)
   - Washcloth, towel, basin, and soap if kit is unavailable
   - Antiseptic solution
   - Sterile applicators
   - Tape or Velcro strap

3. Raise the bed to a comfortable working height. Be sure the opposite side rail is up and secure. Position the patient on his or her back, with legs separated and knees bent, if permitted.

4. Cover the patient with a bath blanket and fan-fold bedding to the foot of the bed.

5. Ask the patient to raise the hips. Place a bed protector underneath the patient.

6. Position a bath blanket so that only the genitals will be exposed.

7. Arrange a catheter care kit on the overbed table. Open the kit. Position the open bag at the foot of the bed.

8. Wash your hands. Put on gloves and draw the drape or bath blanket back.

9. *For the male patient:*
   - Gently grasp the penis and draw the foreskin back, if not circumcised (Figure 45-14).
   - Using a new applicator dipped in antiseptic solution for each stroke, cleanse the glans from the meatus toward the shaft for approximately 4 inches.
   - After each stroke, dispose of the used applicator in a plastic bag.
   - **Alternate action:** Clean around the catheter first and then around the meatus and glans. Wash with soap and water, using a circular motion. Dry in the same manner. Make sure to return the foreskin (if not circumcised) to its proper position.

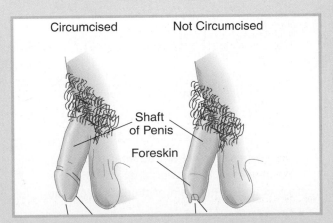

FIGURE 45-14 Comparison of circumcised and uncircumcised penis

continues

PROCEDURE 103 CONTINUED

For the female patient:

- Separate the labia.
- Using a new applicator dipped in antiseptic for each stroke, cleanse from front to back. Begin at the center, then cleanse each side.
- After each stroke, dispose of the used applicator in a plastic bag.
- Clean the catheter down about 4 inches.
- Dry carefully.

10. Remove gloves and discard in plastic bag. Wash your hands.

11. Check the catheter to be sure it is secured properly to the leg (see Figure 45-13). Readjust the Velcro strap for slack, if needed. If a Velcro strap is not available, use tape (Figure 45-15).

12. Check to be sure the tubing is coiled on the bed and that it hangs straight down into the drainage container. Empty the bag and measure the contents, if necessary. Do not raise the bag above the level of the patient's hips. Check to be

FIGURE 45-15 The catheter tubing may be taped to the thigh. The nurse may instruct you to tape the catheter to the abdomen in male patients.

sure that neither the tubing nor the drainage bag is touching the floor.

13. Replace bedding and remove the bath blanket.

14. Fold the bath blanket and store, or put it in the linen hamper.

15. Lower the bed. Adjust side rails for safety.

16. Carry out ending procedure actions.

PROCEDURE

 OBRA

104

EMPTYING A URINARY DRAINAGE UNIT

1. Carry out initial procedure actions.

2. Assemble equipment:
   - Disposable gloves
   - Graduated container
   - Sterile cap or sterile 4 × 4 pad (needed if container has no bottom drain tube)
   - Antiseptic wipes

3. Wash your hands and put on gloves.

4. Place a paper towel on the floor under the drainage bag. Place a graduate on the paper towel under the drain of the collection bag.

5. Remove the drain from the holder (Figure 45-16) and open the drain. Allow the urine to drain into the graduate, using aseptic technique. Do not

allow the tip of the tubing to touch the sides of the graduate (Figure 45-17).

6. Close the drain and replace it in the holder. If accidental contamination occurs, wipe the drain tip with an antiseptic wipe before returning it to the holder. Dispose of used antiseptic wipes in a plastic bag.

7. Check the position of the drainage tube.

8. Pick up the paper towel, touching the top surface only, and discard it.

9. Take the graduate to the bathroom and empty it.

10. Wash and dry the graduate and store it according to facility policy.

continues

PROCEDURE 104 CONTINUED

FIGURE 45-16 Place a paper towel on the floor.

FIGURE 45-17 Center the graduate under the drainage spout. If the spout accidentally contacts your fingers or the edge of the graduate, wipe it with an alcohol sponge before returning it to the drainage bag.

11. Record the amount of urine and note its character.

12. Remove gloves and discard according to facility policy.

13. Carry out ending procedure actions.

There are times when you may have to disconnect the catheter. Follow your facility policies for performing this procedure. In some facilities, a licensed nurse must give permission to disconnect a closed drainage system.

Infection Risk

You must follow the procedure for disconnecting the catheter carefully. The patient who has an indwelling catheter is at risk for infection. There are several sites where infection can enter the drainage system (Figure 45-18):

- Urinary meatus, where the catheter is inserted
- Connection between the catheter and the drainage tube
- Connection between the drainage bag and the drainage tubing
- Opening used to empty the drainage bag

Disconnecting the Catheter

It is preferable never to disconnect the drainage setup, but at times it is necessary. If sterile caps and plugs are avail-able, they should be used. If not, the disconnected ends must be protected with sterile gauze sponges.

External Drainage Systems (Male)

External urinary drainage systems are preferred for male patients who require long periods of urinary drainage. In external drainage, a catheter is not inserted in the urethra. Thus, there is less danger of infection. A condom (sheath) catheter is connected, or some other type of external drainage appliance is applied to the penis (see Procedure 106).

Other complications, ranging from minor irritation to circulatory impairment, can occur. The external catheter is applied over the penis. It is usually attached with an adhesive strip. The strip should always be wrapped in a spiral. If it completely encircles the penis, severe injury can result. Some external catheters have a self-adhesive film on the inside, making the adhesive strip on the outside unnecessary. About one inch of the catheter should extend beyond the tip of the penis and attach to the drainage tubing. Always apply the principles of standard precautions when caring for an external catheter.

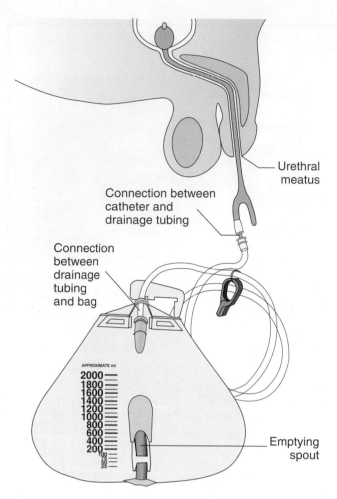

FIGURE 45-18 Handle the closed drainage system carefully to avoid accidental contamination of these areas.

The condom is attached to drainage tubing and a collection bag. The condom is removed every 24 hours and the penis is washed and dried. Different types of drainage systems are available. Urine may be collected in a bag that hangs from the bed or wheelchair or in a bag attached to the patient's leg.

Difficult SITUATIONS

Inspect the condom catheter periodically to make sure it is not twisted or obstructed. If the catheter becomes twisted, the urine will collect inside the catheter, causing irritation. As the urine accumulates, the catheter will expand until it eventually comes off. ■

Leg Bag Drainage

Some patients find it easier to ambulate when urine drainage is collected in a leg bag instead of the larger urinary drainage bag. The leg bag is held to the patient's leg by Velcro straps, around either the thigh or the lower leg (Figure 45-22 on page 816). Points to keep in mind when patients use a leg bag are:

- The leg bag is smaller and must be emptied more often
- The bag must be placed so there is a straight drop down from the catheter

PROCEDURE

105

DISCONNECTING THE CATHETER

1. Carry out initial procedure actions.

2. Assemble equipment:
   - Disposable gloves
   - Antiseptic wipes
   - Gauze sponges
   - Sterile caps/plugs
   - Clamps

3. Wash your hands and put on gloves.

4. Clamp the catheter.

5. Disconnect the catheter and drainage tubing. Do not put the ends down or allow them to touch anything. If accidental contamination occurs,

wipe the ends with antiseptic wipes before inserting the plug or placing the cap. Dispose of used antiseptic wipes in a plastic bag.

6. Insert a sterile plug in the end of the catheter. Place a sterile cap over the exposed end of the drainage tube (Figure 45-19).

7. Secure the drainage tube to the bed frame so that the tube will not touch the floor.

8. Remove and dispose of gloves according to facility policy. Wash your hands.

9. Carry out ending procedure actions.

continues

PROCEDURE 105 CONTINUED

Note: Reverse the procedure to reconnect the catheter. If you find an unprotected, disconnected tube in the bed or on the floor, *do not reconnect it. Report it at once.*

FIGURE 45-19 A. Sterile catheter plug and protective cap. B. Plug and protective cap in place.

PROCEDURE
106

APPLYING A CONDOM FOR URINARY DRAINAGE

1. Carry out initial procedure actions.

2. Assemble equipment:
   - Disposable gloves
   - Basin of warm water
   - Washcloth
   - Towel
   - Condom with drainage tip
   - Bed protector
   - Bath blanket
   - Towel

3. Arrange equipment on the overbed table.

4. Raise the bed to a comfortable working height. Be sure the opposite side rail is up and secure for safety.

5. Lower the side rail on the side where you will be working.

6. Cover the patient with a bath blanket and fan-fold bedding to the foot of the bed.

7. Wash your hands and put on gloves.

8. Place a bed protector under the patient's hips.

9. Adjust the bath blanket to expose the genitals only.

10. Carefully wash and dry the penis. Observe for signs of irritation. Check to see if the condom has a "ready stick" surface.

11. Apply the condom and drainage tip to the penis by placing the condom at the top of the penis and rolling toward the base of the penis. Leave space between the drainage tip and the glans of the penis to prevent irritation (Figure 45-20). If the patient is not circumcised, be sure that the foreskin is in normal position.

12. Spiral-wrap the tape provided with the condom to secure it to the penis (Figure 45-21).

13. The condom is now ready to be connected to drainage tubing leading to a collection bag.

14. Remove gloves and discard according to facility policy.

15. Wash your hands.

continues

PROCEDURE 106 CONTINUED

FIGURE 45-20 Leave room between the glans penis and the drainage tip on the condom to prevent irritation and allow sufficient space for drainage. Roll the condom down to the base of the penis.

16. Adjust bedding and remove the bath blanket. Fold the bath blanket and store it in the room, or place it in the laundry hamper.

17. Lower the bed. Adjust the side rails for safety.

18. Carry out ending procedure actions.

19. To change the catheter, remove the adhesive strip and roll the condom back over the tip of

FIGURE 45-21 Correctly applied and secured condom catheter ready to be attached to the drainage tubing

the penis. Discard it in a plastic bag, or according to facility policy.

a. Observe the skin on the penis for redness, irritation, swelling, and open areas. If noted, report your observations to the nurse before applying a new condom catheter.

b. After the catheter has been removed, it is not reapplied. A new catheter is used each time.

c. Provide perineal care before applying another external catheter.

FIGURE 45-22
The leg bag is held in place by adjustable straps. The bag is smaller than a bed collection bag and must be emptied more often.

- Tension on the catheter tubing must be minimal
- Care must be taken not to introduce germs when connecting and disconnecting the bag and catheter

Infection Control ALERT

Avoid putting the patient to bed while he is wearing a leg bag. The urine may flow back into the bladder from the bag when the patient is in bed. Disconnect the leg bag and connect the catheter to the regular drainage bag when the patient is in bed. ■

PROCEDURE

107

CONNECTING A CATHETER TO A LEG BAG

 Note: Always check with the nurse before using a leg bag.

1. Carry out initial procedure actions.

2. Assemble equipment:
   - Disposable gloves
   - Antiseptic wipes
   - Leg bag and tubing
   - Emesis basin
   - Bed protector
   - Sterile cap/plug
   - Clamp

3. Wash your hands and put on gloves.

4. Place a bed protector under the connection between the catheter and the drainage tube.

5. Clamp the catheter.

6. Disconnect the catheter and drainage tubing. Do not put them down or allow them to touch anything.

7. Insert a sterile plug in the end of the catheter. Place a sterile cap over the exposed end of the drainage tube.

 Note: If accidental contamination occurs, wipe the area with antiseptic wipes before inserting a sterile plug or replacing a sterile cap over the exposed end of the drainage tubing. Dispose of used antiseptic wipes in a plastic bag.

8. Secure the drainage tube to the bed frame. The drainage tube must not touch the floor.

9. Remove the catheter plug.

10. Insert the end of the leg bag tubing into the catheter (Figure 45-23).

11. Release the catheter clamp.

12. Secure the leg bag with Velcro straps to the patient's leg so there is no tension on the tubing. Be sure there is a straight drop down from the catheter to the bag for urine flow. Check for leakage.

13. Remove the bed protector and discard it.

14. Remove gloves and discard according to facility policy. Wash your hands.

15. Assist the patient to get out of bed. The single-use leg bag should be discarded in a biohazardous waste container.

16. Carry out ending procedure actions.

 Note: To reconnect the regular drainage bag, reverse this procedure.

FIGURE 45-23 Carefully connect the catheter to the leg bag. Avoid touching anything against the end of the catheter. The drainage tubing on the bed bag is covered with a sterile cap that is left in place until it is reconnected to the catheter.

Abdominal Drainage

People with some medical conditions use a catheter all the time. Patients with permanent suprapubic or indwelling urethral catheters may wear a device called an abdominal urine bag ("belly bag," Figure 45-24) at home. If a patient is admitted to the hospital with this system in place, it may be left in place unless the physician orders a change in the drainage system. Verify this information by checking the care plan or with the nurse. The belly bag is contraindicated with a condom catheter because the combination of devices increases the risk for irritation and infection. The bag and belt are disposable and are intended for a single use only. The bag is removed and a new bag applied every 3 to 4 weeks during home use. The used bag is discarded. Creams and lotions containing petroleum products should be avoided in the area of the catheter and bag, as they have the potential to damage either device.

PROCEDURE

EMPTYING A LEG BAG

1. Carry out initial procedure actions.

2. Assemble equipment:
   - Disposable gloves
   - Antiseptic wipes
   - Emesis basin
   - Graduate pitcher
   - Paper towels

3. Position the patient safely.

4. Wash your hands and put on gloves.

5. Release the Velcro straps holding the leg bag so the bag can be moved away from the patient's leg.

6. Place a paper towel on the floor under the drainage outlet of the leg bag.

7. Place a graduate on the paper towel under the drainage outlet.

8. Remove the cap, being careful not to touch the tip. Drain the collected urine into the graduate.

Do not put the cap down and do not touch the inside of the cap. If accidental contamination occurs, wipe the area with antiseptic wipes before replacing the cap. Dispose of used antiseptic wipes in a plastic bag.

9. Wipe the drainage outlet with an antiseptic wipe and replace the cap.

10. Refasten the straps to secure the drainage bag to the leg.

11. Make sure the patient is comfortable and safe.

12. Discard the paper towel.

13. Measure the urine and note the amount, if required.

14. Discard the urine. Clean the graduate and store it.

15. Remove gloves and discard according to facility policy.

16. Carry out ending procedure actions.

FIGURE 45-24 The disposable abdominal drainage bag is removed and a new bag applied after 3 to 4 weeks of home use. Users of this bag say it is superior to other types of drainage systems. (Courtesy of Medline Industries, Inc. (800) MEDLINE)

The abdominal drainage bag may be worn 24 hours a day. It has a soft backing, so it does not irritate the skin. It is worn at the waist, under the clothing, and has many advantages over traditional drainage systems. A belt holds the bag in place. An antireflux valve behind the catheter port prevents backflow of urine from the bag into the bladder. The bag is emptied through a drainage tube that is in the approximate position of the urethra. It is twisted open and closed. Most patients sleep with the bag in place. Patients who use this type of bag find it superior to bed and leg drainage bags and may refuse to use anything else while hospitalized. Consult the nurse before using any substitute bag that you are not familiar with. Become familiar with the use instructions for the bags stocked by your facility or provided by the patient.

REVIEW

A. True/False.

Mark the following true or false by circling T or F.

1. T F Insertion of a sterile catheter into the urinary bladder is a routine nursing assistant task.

2. T F Gloves should be worn when emptying a urine collection bag.

3. T F It is preferable never to disconnect a urinary drainage setup.

4. T F The pain associated with kidney stones is referred to as renal colic.

5. T F If you find an unprotected, disconnected catheter or tubing on the floor, you should reconnect it immediately.

6. T F The hemodialysis machine takes the place of nonfunctioning kidneys.

7. T F Ample fluid intake encourages increased output, which is important in treating kidney stones.

8. T F A catheter with an inflatable balloon is called a French catheter.

9. T F Foley catheters are indwelling catheters.

10. T F Cystitis is a fairly common problem for women.

B. Matching.

Choose the correct term from Column II to match each word or phrase in Column I.

Column I

11. _____ indwelling catheter
12. _____ inability to expel formed urine
13. _____ urinate
14. _____ inflammation of the bladder
15. _____ blood in the urine

Column II

a. void
b. hematuria
c. cystitis
d. retention
e. dysuria
f. Foley catheter
g. suppression

C. Multiple Choice.

Select the one best answer for each of the following.

16. Your patient has a diagnosis of nephritis. Your care will include
    a. keeping the patient very active.
    b. serving a high-sodium diet.
    c. measuring I&O accurately.
    d. eliminating vital sign measurements so the patient can rest more.

17. Your patient has renal calculi. One of your responsibilities will be
    a. saving all urine.
    b. straining urine.
    c. limiting fluids.
    d. inserting a catheter.

18. A common cause of hydronephrosis is
    a. renal calculi.
    b. pain in the bladder.
    c. bladder infection.
    d. drinking too much fluid.

19. Important signs and symptoms to report when there is a diagnosis involving the urinary system include
    a. hunger.
    b. thirst.
    c. temperature elevation.
    d. voiding every 3 to 4 hours.

20. Indwelling catheter care is
    a. a licensed nurse responsibility.
    b. performed during AM care.
    c. safely omitted as long as the patient is in bed.
    d. performed twice a week.

D. Completion.

Complete the following statements.

21. The nursing assistant who finds a disconnected catheter in the bed should _____ .

22. A routine check of a patient who uses urinary drainage should include _____ .

E. Nursing Assistant Challenge.

Mr. Starkman is 68 years of age. An external urinary condom is to be applied. Answer the following regarding his care while the condom is being applied.

23. You should wear gloves to apply the condom.

_____

(yes) (no)

24. The condom should be applied by _____ of the penis.

(pulling it up toward the tip)
(rolling it down toward the base)

25. When applying the condom, you should _____ space between the drainage tip and the glans of the penis.

(leave) (not leave)

Reproductive System

OBJECTIVES

After completing this unit, you will be able to:

- Spell and define terms.
- Review the location and functions of the organs of the male and female reproductive systems.
- Describe some common disorders and conditions of the male reproductive system.
- Describe some common disorders and conditions of the female reproductive system.
- List six diagnostic tests associated with conditions of the male and female reproductive systems.
- Describe nursing assistant actions related to the care of patients with conditions and diseases of the reproductive system.
- State the nursing precautions required for patients who have sexually transmitted diseases.
- Demonstrate the following procedures:
  - Procedure 109 Giving a Nonsterile Vaginal Douche

VOCABULARY

Learn the meaning and the correct spelling of the following words and phrases:

amenorrhea	endometrium	metrorrhagia	salpingectomy
benign prostatic hypertrophy	epididymis	oophorectomy	seminal vesicles
biopsy	fallopian tubes	orchiectomy	sexually transmitted disease (STD)
brachytherapy	genitalia	ovary	simple mastectomy
chancre	gonorrhea	oviduct	sperm
chlamydia	hemorrhoid	ovulation	sterility
climacteric	herpes simplex II	ovum	syphilis
clitoris	hysterectomy	panhysterectomy	testes
colporrhaphy	labia majora	Pap smear	trichomonas vaginitis
Cowper's glands	labia minora	pelvic inflammatory disease (PID)	uterus
cystocele	leukorrhea	penis	vagina
dilatation and curettage (D & C)	lumpectomy	prostatectomy	vas deferens
douche	mammogram	prostate gland	venereal warts
dysmenorrhea	mastectomy	puberty	vulva
ejaculatory duct	menopause	radical mastectomy	vulvovaginitis
	menorrhagia	rectocele	
	menstruation		

STRUCTURE AND FUNCTION

Both the male and female reproductive organs have dual functions. They:

1. Produce reproductive cells. The male produces **sperm**. The female produces the **ovum**.
2. Produce hormones that are responsible for sex characteristics.
   a. Males produce testosterone.
   b. Females produce estrogen and progesterone.

In the reproductive process, the:

- Male and female engage in sexual intercourse.
- Male ejaculates (propels) the sperm and the seminal fluid in which they swim into the female vagina.
- Sperm and egg meet in the female fallopian tube. One sperm penetrates the egg and conception takes place.
- Baby (fetus) develops in the uterus until birth.
- Female breasts (mammary glands) produce milk to nourish the newborn.

The Male Reproductive Organs: Structure and Function

The male organs (Figure 46-1) include the:

- **Testes:** Two glandular organs located in the scrotum. The testes produce sperm and the hormone testosterone.

- **Epididymis:** A 20-foot-long coiled tube located on the top and back of each testis. The epididymis stores the sperm and allows them to mature.
- **Vas deferens:** A tube that leads from the epididymis. It carries the sperm upward into the pelvic cavity to the seminal vesicles during ejaculation. The vas deferens is accompanied by nerves and blood vessels. Together, they form the spermatic cord.
- **Seminal vesicles:** Located behind the bladder. They receive and store the sperm from the vas deferens. They contribute nutrients to the seminal fluid. The

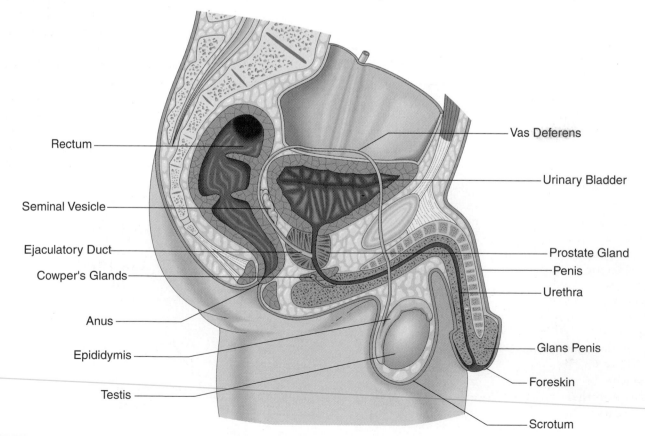

FIGURE 46-1 Cross-section of the male reproductive system

small ejaculatory duct leads from the seminal vesicles to the urethra just below the prostate gland.

- **Ejaculatory duct**: Carries the fluid produced in the seminal vesicles. Fluids are added as the sperm are propelled forward. The sperm and fluid form the seminal fluid or ejaculate. The fluid contains nutrients and other substances needed by the sperm.

- **Prostate gland**: Found just below the urinary bladder surrounding the urethra. It secretes a fluid that increases the ability of the sperm to move in the seminal fluid. Enlargement of the prostate gland may impede or prevent urine from passing through the urethra. This is a fairly common occurrence in older men.

- **Cowper's glands**: Two small glands located beside the urethra. They produce mucus for lubrication.

- **Penis**: Composed of special tissue that can become filled with blood, making the organ enlarge and become stiffened so that it may enter the vagina to deposit seminal fluid. Loose-fitting skin (the prepuce or foreskin) covers the penis.

The male urethra passes through the penis and serves two purposes. It carries:

- Reproductive fluid during intercourse
- Urine during voiding

The two activities cannot occur at the same time because they are under the control of different parts of the nervous system.

The Female Reproductive Organs: Structure and Function

The external female structures (**genitalia**) (Figure 46-2) include the:

- **Vulva**: Made up of two liplike structures, the **labia majora** and **labia minora**. When the labia are separated, other external structures may be seen.

- **Clitoris**: A very sensitive structure found just behind the juncture of the labia minora. It functions during sexual stimulation to begin the rhythmic series of contractions associated with female climax (orgasm).

- **Urinary meatus**: The opening of the urethra to the outside.

- **Vaginal meatus**: The opening to the vagina or birth canal.

The Internal Female Structures

The internal female reproductive organs (Figures 46-3 and 46-4) include the following structures.

- **Ovaries**: Two small glands, found on either side of the uterus, at the ends of the oviducts (fallopian tubes) in the pelvis. They produce two hormones, estrogen and progesterone, and the egg (ovum). The eggs are contained in many little sacs called follicles. About once each month, a follicle matures and releases an ovum. The ovum makes its way into one of the 4-inch-long oviducts. This process is called **ovulation**. The cells of the follicles that are left produce progesterone. The progesterone causes changes within the uterus, readying it for the possibility of receiving a fertilized ovum.

- **Fallopian tubes (oviducts)**: Two tubes, approximately 4 inches long, that serve as a pathway between the ovary and uterus. The sperm and egg meet in the tubes. Fertilization takes place here.

- **Uterus**: A hollow, pear-shaped organ. Its walls are made up of involuntary muscles. It is lined with special tissue called **endometrium**. The uterus has three main parts: the fundus, body, and cervix. The body and the fundus can stretch enough to hold a fetus, the amniotic sac, and the afterbirth (placenta). The cervix extends into the vagina. During labor, the cervix opens up to allow the baby to be delivered.

- **Vagina**: Found between the urinary bladder and the rectum. Its muscular walls are capable of much stretching. It is lined with mucous membrane. Two glands known as Bartholin's glands are found on either side of the external vaginal opening. They provide lubrication.

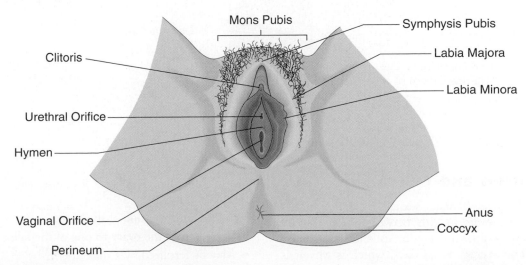

FIGURE 46-2 External female reproductive organs

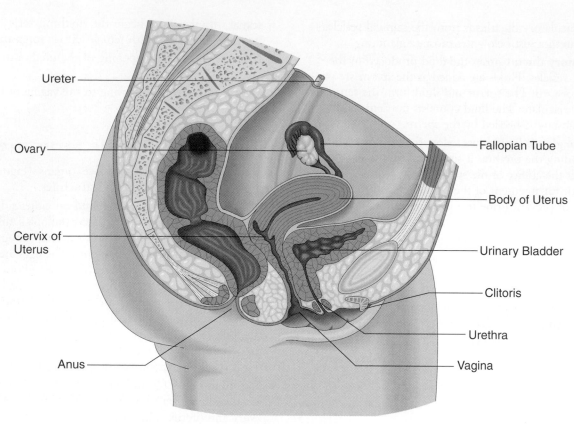

FIGURE 46-3 Cross-section of internal female reproductive system

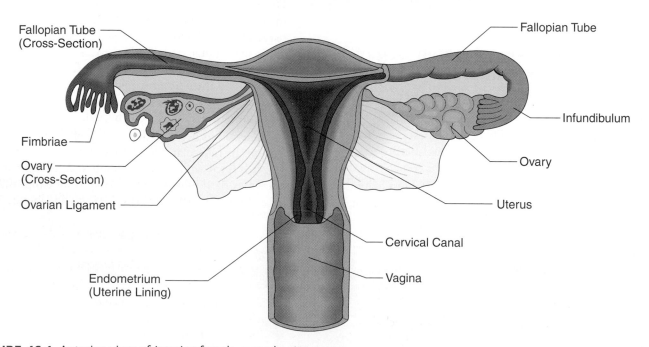

FIGURE 46-4 Anterior view of interior female reproductive organs

Menstruation and Ovulation

The menstrual cycle (female sexual cycle) begins at **puberty**. Puberty occurs in girls between the ages of 9 and 17. The cycle varies in length, usually between 25 and 30 days. The average is 28 days, which is why it is considered a monthly cycle.

During the menstrual cycle, a mature egg, or ovum (plural, ova):

- Is released from one of the ovaries
- Travels from the ovary to one of the fallopian tubes
- May be fertilized by a male sperm

At the same time that the ovum is being matured and expelled from the ovary (ovulation), the lining of the uterus (endometrium) is being built up and made ready to receive the fertilized ovum. If fertilization does not occur, the endometrium is no longer needed, so it is carried out of the body as the menstrual flow. This process is known as **menstruation**.

Unlike the sperm cells, all the special cells that will become the ova exist when a woman is born. When the last ova are released, the menstrual cycle ceases and **menopause** begins.

Menopause

As women age, the menstrual cycle becomes irregular and gradually ceases altogether. This is called the menopause, or **climacteric**, or change of life.

Menopause usually occurs around the age of 55 and involves a natural series of changes that stops the menstrual cycle. These changes are not abrupt, but usually take place over a period of years. Because eggs are no longer being matured and released, pregnancy cannot occur.

Some women may undergo menopause earlier in life after surgical removal of the ovaries.

CONDITIONS OF THE MALE REPRODUCTIVE ORGANS

The male organs are subject to the same kinds of disease processes that affect other body parts. Examples of these conditions are tumors and infections. A very common problem experienced by many men involves the prostate gland.

Prostate Conditions

Benign prostatic (of the prostate gland) **hypertrophy** *hyperplasia* (Figure 46-5) is an enlargement of the prostate gland without tumor development. It:

- Causes narrowing of the urethra, which passes through the center of the prostate gland
- Can cause sufficient enlargement to cause urinary retention.
- Is noncancerous.

Signs and symptoms of prostate conditions include difficulty in starting the stream of urine or in emptying the bladder completely.

Prostate cancer is the second leading cause of cancer deaths in males. A blood test, the prostate specific antigen (PSA), is used to screen for abnormalities. Because of the widespread use of the blood test, many prostate cancers are caught early, and the outcome is usually favorable. Prostate cancer usually grows very slowly. In the early stages, there may be no symptoms. As the condition progresses, signs and symptoms develop. The most common are:

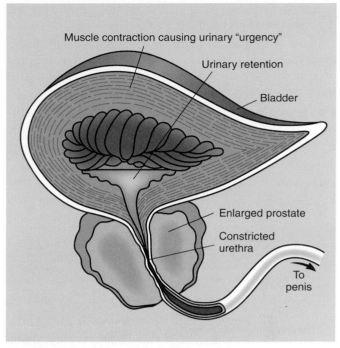

FIGURE 46-5 Cell growth causes the prostate to enlarge, constricting the urethra. The bladder may not empty completely, causing discomfort and increasing the risk of infection.

- Difficulty with urination
- Decreased force of the urine stream
- Frequency of urination
- Urgency (an intense need to urinate)
- Urinary retention
- Repeated urinary tract infections
- Blood in the urine or semen

Treatment. Various surgical approaches are used to remove all or part of the prostate gland (**prostatectomy**) to relieve urinary retention.

- Transurethral prostatectomy (TURP)—only enough of the gland is removed, working from inside the urethra, to permit urine to pass.
- Perineal prostatectomy—the entire gland is removed through surgical incisions in the perineum.
- Suprapubic prostatectomy—an incision is made just above the pubis and part of the gland is removed.

Radiation therapy consists of 5 to 7 weeks of treatments in which radiation is directed to the prostate gland. **Brachytherapy** is another form of radiation therapy in which tiny radioactive seeds or pellets are implanted directly inside the prostate gland. This treatment is very successful and preferred over traditional radiation therapy because it has fewer side effects.

Hormone therapy is used to treat some prostate cancers. This treatment suppresses the male sex hormone (testosterone) that stimulates the cancer to grow.

Patients are likely to be disturbed by the necessity of prostate surgery. Men often fear that they will not be able to have sexual intercourse after a prostatectomy. They feel that their manhood is threatened.

Urinary incontinence is also a common problem and a great concern. In most cases, the rate of leakage decreases over time. Nevertheless, incontinence has a substantial impact on quality of life.

Postsurgical Care. In addition to routine postoperative care, the prostatectomy patient:

● Will have a Foley catheter in place following the surgery
● May have a suprapubic drain through the suprapubic incision
● May have a perineal drain in the perineal incision

Difficult SITUATIONS

After prostate surgery, the patient may have a three-way catheter with continuous irrigation. Inform the nurse if the bottle is low. Monitor the tubing for the presence of blood clots. Monitor the patient for signs of excess bleeding, cold or clammy skin, pallor, restlessness, falling blood pressure, or rapid pulse. If noted, report promptly. ■

The nursing assistant should:

● Wear personal protective equipment and apply the principles of standard precautions if contact with blood, body fluids, mucous membranes, or nonintact skin is likely.
● Be careful that the tubes do not become twisted, stressed, or dislodged when positioning the patient.
● Carefully note the amount and color of drainage from all areas.
● Report at once any sudden increase in bright redness or the appearance of clots that seem to block the tube.
● Report to the nurse if dressings become wet with urinary drainage.
● Be patient and understanding of the patient's emotional stress.
● Refer questions about possible sexual limitation and urinary incontinence to the nurse so that the patient can get information and support.

At times, it will be necessary to irrigate (wash out) the drainage tubes. This is a sterile procedure that will be carried out by the nurse or physician.

Cancer of the Testes

Cancer of the testes is fairly common. Treatment may require removal of the testicles (**orchiectomy**). This procedure is performed when there is testicular malignancy. When an early diagnosis is made, treatment can be started early. Orchiectomy can then be avoided.

CONDITIONS OF THE FEMALE REPRODUCTIVE ORGANS

Like the male organs, female reproductive organs are subject to disease processes, including tumors and infections.

Rectocele and Cystocele

Rectoceles and cystoceles are hernias. They usually occur at the same time.

● **Rectoceles** (Figure 46-6) are a weakening of the wall shared between the vagina and the rectum. These hernias frequently cause constipation and **hemorrhoids** (varicose veins of the rectum).
● **Cystoceles** (Figure 46-7) are a weakening of the muscles between the bladder and the vagina. Cystoceles cause urinary incontinence.

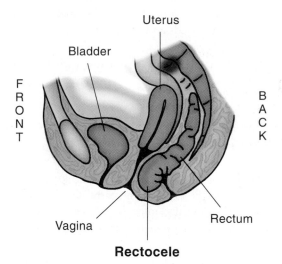

Rectocele

FIGURE 46-6 A rectocele causes the rectum to bulge into the vagina.

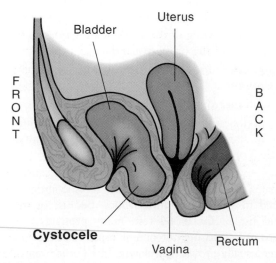

FIGURE 46-7 A cystocele causes the bladder to bulge into the vagina.

Treatment and Nursing Care. A surgical procedure called **colporrhaphy** tightens the vaginal walls.

In addition to routine postsurgical care, you may assist in:

- Applying ice packs
- Giving sitz baths
- Giving vaginal douches (irrigations) (see Procedure 109)
- Checking carefully for signs of excessive bleeding or foul discharge

Vulvovaginitis

Vulvovaginitis is most often caused by a fungal infection of *Candida albicans*.

- There is a thick, white, cheesy vaginal discharge
- Inflammation and itching are intense
- Douches are not given for this condition
- Special drugs and creams are prescribed to fight the infection

Tumors of Uterus and Ovaries

Benign and malignant tumors of the uterus and ovaries are frequent. Malignancies of the cervix are very common. The cure rate is very high if treated in time.

The most common indications of tumors of the uterus and ovaries are changes in the menstrual flow, such as:

- **Menorrhagia** (excessive flow)
- **Amenorrhea** (lack of menstrual flow)
- **Dysmenorrhea** (difficult or painful menstrual flow)
- **Metrorrhagia** (bleeding at completely irregular intervals)

Ovarian cancer is very dangerous because there are no symptoms until it is well advanced and has spread beyond the ovaries. Even then, the symptoms are often mild, such as bloating, and may be attributed to other problems. It usually cannot be detected by a pelvic examination. This cancer accounts for more deaths than any other cancer of the female reproductive system. The disease has a strong familial link, and is most common in women over age 50. Women who have never had children and those who have taken fertility drugs are also at high risk. Women who take birth control pills have a lower risk.

Signs and Symptoms of Ovarian Cancer. Signs and symptoms of ovarian cancer may include:

- Abdominal discomfort and pain
- Bloating
- Nausea
- Diarrhea
- Frequent urination
- Sudden weight gain or loss
- Abnormal vaginal bleeding

Treatment. Several different types of procedures may be performed to treat tumors of the female reproductive tract, including chemotherapy, radiation, and surgery. Some surgical procedures are:

- Total **hysterectomy**—removal of the entire uterus, including the cervix.
- **Oophorectomy**—removal of an ovary. In younger women, at least a portion of the ovary is left to continue hormone production whenever possible.
- **Salpingectomy**—removal of a fallopian tube.
- **Panhysterectomy**—removal of the uterus and both ovaries and tubes. The surgical approach may be abdominal or vaginal. If a panhysterectomy is performed, the patient experiences surgically induced menopause. The more uncomfortable symptoms of menopause are usually relieved with hormone supplements.

If cancer is present, nonsurgical forms of treatment may be used, including radiation therapy and chemotherapy.

Postoperative Care. In addition to the usual postoperative care, the care following a hysterectomy will include:

- Caring for catheter drainage
- Possibly caring for a nasogastric tube, which may be in place to relieve abdominal distention and nausea
- Giving special attention to maintaining good circulation, because slowing of the blood supply to the pelvis may result in clot formation
- Introducing fluids and foods gradually after the initial nausea subsides
- Carefully observing the patient for low back pain
- Monitoring urine output and bleeding
- Checking both the abdominal incisional area and the vagina for presence and type of drainage
- Providing emotional support

Tumors of the Breast

Tumors, both benign and malignant, are commonly found in the breasts. Breast cancer is the second most common cancer in women. However, men can also develop breast cancer. Signs and symptoms of breast tumors include:

- Painless lump or mass
- Nipple discharge
- Retraction of nipple
- Scaly skin around nipple
- Dimpling of the skin
- Enlarged lymph nodes

Treatment. **Mastectomy** means removal of the breast. All or part of the breast tissue may be removed in a mastectomy.

- A **simple mastectomy** removes the breast tissue only.
- A **radical mastectomy** includes the breast tissue, underlying muscles, and the glands in the axillary area. This procedure is not performed as often as it was previously.

- A **lumpectomy** removes the abnormal tissue and only a small amount of the breast tissue.

Nonsurgical forms of treatment include:

- Radiation therapy
- Chemotherapy
- Hormonal chemotherapy, which blocks estrogen from entering the breast cancer cells

Any form of mastectomy requires a great deal of psychological adjustment for the patient. There is the fear of disfigurement and the fear of loss of femininity. Many excellent breast forms are now available to restore the outward physical appearance of the mastectomy patient. Breast implants are another way of restoring the physical form of the breast. There are also support groups to aid in the psychological adjustment.

Postoperative Care. In addition to routine postoperative care, you will:

- Wear personal protective equipment and apply the principles of standard precautions if contact with blood, body fluids, mucous membranes, or nonintact skin is likely.
- Avoid taking the blood pressure on the side where the surgery was done.
- Realize that because a large amount of blood can be lost during a mastectomy, transfusions are likely to be ordered. Monitor a blood transfusion as you would monitor an intravenous infusion.
- Check pressure dressings frequently for signs of excess bleeding.
- Check the bed linen, because blood may drain to the back of the dressing.
- Report immediately numbness or swelling in the arm of the operative side.
- Be ready to offer support; walking may be difficult for the patient, who may feel unbalanced.
- Offer your fullest emotional support.
- Assist the patient in rehabilitative exercises.
- Refer questions about disfigurement and loss of femininity to the nurse, who will see that the patient is provided with accurate information and support.

SEXUALLY TRANSMITTED DISEASE (STD)

Sexually transmitted diseases (STDs) affect both men and women. Although most sexually transmitted diseases can be treated and cured, patients do not develop immunity to repeated infections. It is possible to transmit the organisms causing STDs from:

- Mucous membrane to mucous membrane (Figure 46-8A), such as from genitals to mouth or genitals
- Mucous membrane to skin, such as genitals to hands (Figure 46-8B)

FIGURE 46-8A This person contracted an STD through genital to oral contact. (Courtesy of Centers for Disease Control and Prevention)

FIGURE 46-8B Although less common, lesions on the hands can develop as a result of contact with the genitalia of an infected person. (Courtesy of Centers for Disease Control and Prevention)

- Skin to mucous membrane, such as hands to genitals

Using standard precautions correctly will protect the nursing assistant from contracting these diseases when caring for patients.

Any disease that is transmitted mainly in this way is an STD. There are many sexually transmitted diseases. Some are seen more commonly than others. It is important to realize that patients may:

- Not always be aware that they have been infected
- Be too embarrassed to tell you about the problem
- Not realize the serious damage these infectious diseases can do to the body

The most common sexually transmitted diseases are gonorrhea, herpes simplex II, and syphilis. Other sexually transmitted diseases are caused by chlamydia, human papillomavirus, HIV, and the trichomonas parasite.

Trichomonas Vaginitis

Trichomonas vaginitis is caused by a parasite, *Trichomonas vaginalis*. This condition:

- Is sexually transmitted
- May affect the male reproductive tract with no signs and symptoms
- In females, causes a large amount of white, foul-smelling vaginal discharge called **leukorrhea** (Figure 46-9)
- Can be controlled with medication
- Requires that both sex partners receive treatment

Gonorrhea

Gonorrhea is a serious STD caused by the bacterium *Neisseria gonorrheae*. The disease causes an acute inflammation. In the male:

- Greenish-yellow discharge appears from the penis within two to five days after contact
- There is burning on urination
- The disease can spread throughout the reproductive tract, causing **sterility** (inability to reproduce)

In the female:

- 80% may have no signs or symptoms for quite a while. Thus, it is possible to spread the disease before the woman is aware of being infected.

FIGURE 46-9 *Trichomonas vaginalis* is the most common pathogenic protozoan of humans in industrialized countries. It resides in the female lower genital tract and the male urethra and prostate. This magnified view is from a case of *trichomonas vaginitis* with copious purulent (pus-like) discharge from the cervix of the uterus. (Courtesy of Centers for Disease Control and Prevention)

- **Pelvic inflammatory disease** (PID) can lead to formation of abscesses and sterility.

It is important for all sex partners to be treated with antibiotics (Figure 46-10). When a pregnant woman has gonorrhea, her baby's eyes may be permanently damaged if they are contaminated by the disease during birth. As a preventive measure, all babies' eyes are routinely treated with silver nitrate drops or antibiotics shortly after birth.

Syphilis

Syphilis is caused by the microorganism *Treponema pallidum*. Both sexes show the same effects of the disease. If untreated, this disease passes through three stages.

1. First stage—a sore (**chancre**) (Figure 46-11A) develops within 90 days of exposure. The chancre heals without treatment. Because it is not painful, it may go entirely unnoticed.

2. Second stage—may be accompanied by a rash, sore throat, or other mild symptoms suggestive of a viral infection (Figure 46-11B). Again, the signs and symptoms disappear without treatment. The disease is infectious during the first and second stages and may be transmitted to a sexual partner. By this time, the microorganisms have gained entrance into vital organs such as the heart, liver, brain, and spinal cord.

3. Third stage—permanent damage is done to vital organs, though the damage may not appear for many years. Patients in this stage are usually cognitively impaired, but there is no way to differentiate cognitive impairment caused by syphilis from impairment due to other causes. Aside from this, the patient usually has no other signs or symptoms, and

FIGURE 46-10 This patient was not treated for gonorrhea, and the infection spread throughout the body, causing conjunctivitis (pink eye) of the right eye. The most common symptoms of untreated gonorrhea are rash and joint pains and conjunctivitis, but other symptoms may also occur. (Courtesy of Centers for Disease Control and Prevention)

FIGURE 46-11A Although this lesion is open, it is painless and will disappear on its own in about 3 to 6 weeks. The lesion develops at the spot where the infective bacteria enter the body. If the person is not treated, the syphilis infection will remain in the body, where it continues to cause serious damage. (Courtesy of Centers for Disease Control and Prevention)

FIGURE 46-11B This person has a rash on the hands as a result of untreated syphilis infection. The second stage starts when one or more areas of the skin break into a rash that appears as rough, red or reddish-brown spots. These usually occur on the palms of the hands and the bottoms of the feet. Without treatment, the rash will clear up by itself. (Courtesy of Centers for Disease Control and Prevention)

FIGURE 46-11C The signs and symptoms of third-stage syphilis include loss of coordination, dementia, paralysis, numbness, and gradual blindness. Occasionally, the patient develops a painless, nodular, ulcerative lesion, such as the one pictured. The lesion can occur anywhere on the body. The patient is not contagious in this stage, but the damage is serious enough to cause death. (Courtesy of Centers for Disease Control and Prevention)

Infection Control ALERT

There are several closely related strains of herpes viruses. Oral herpes and genital herpes are caused by different strains. However, they can be cross-infected with each other. Touching a cold sore, then touching the genital area will transmit the herpes virus to the genitalia, and vice versa. Because of this, persons with the herpes virus must use very careful handwashing, and avoid hand contact with the lesions as much as possible. The virus will occasionally spread when no signs and symptoms are present. The virus usually lies dormant in nerves near the infection site until lesions erupt on the skin during an outbreak. The outbreak may be preceded by tingling, itching, and pain. ∎

the diagnosis of tertiary syphylis is usually made after a routine blood test shows an abnormality. Occasionally, the person will develop painless lesions (*gumma*) on various parts of the body (Figure 46-11C). The patient is not infectious in this stage.

An additional danger of syphilis during pregnancy is that the microorganism can attack the fetus, causing it to die or be seriously deformed.

Herpes

Herpes simplex II (genital herpes) is an infectious disease caused by the herpes simplex virus. It is transmitted primarily through direct sexual contact. The person who has herpes:

- May develop painful, red, blister-like sores on the reproductive organs (Figure 46-12A)

FIGURE 46-12A One out of every four women and one out of every five men in the United States have genital herpes. The lesions appear as one or more painful blisters on or around the genitals or rectum. The blisters eventually break, leaving tender ulcers that may take 2 to 4 weeks to heal the first time they appear. Oral herpes can be spread to the genital area just as genital herpes can be spread to the mouth. (Courtesy of Centers for Disease Control and Prevention)

- Has sores that are associated with a burning sensation
- Usually has sores that heal in about 2 weeks
- Must remember that the fluid in the blisters is infectious
- May transmit (shed) organisms even when an outbreak is not present

One in five American adults has genital herpes and may not know it. People with the herpes infection may have only one episode or may have repeated attacks. In many cases, repeated attacks are milder. Individuals who have weakened immune systems often develop chronic cases of herpes (Figure 46-12B). In addition to the local discomfort:

- There seems to be a greater incidence of cancer of the cervix and miscarriages among female sufferers than among women who do not have this condition.
- Newborn children can be infected when the mother gives birth. This is why the baby of a mother with an active case of herpes simplex II is usually delivered by cesarean section.

Because herpes is caused by a virus, there is no cure. Oral medications are available to stop the replication of the virus, which makes an outbreak subside more quickly.

FIGURE 46-12B Chronic herpes in an AIDS patient. (Courtesy of Daniel J. Barbaro, MD, Fort Worth, Texas)

Topical creams are available to relieve discomfort and reduce the danger of spreading the infection.

Venereal Warts

Venereal warts are caused by a virus.

- Lesions develop on the genitals, on both skin and mucous membranes (Figure 46-13).
- The warts are cauliflower-shaped, raised, and darkened
- They may be removed by ointments or surgery but often recur
- They may cause discomfort during intercourse and may cause bleeding when dislodged
- Warts predispose the patient to development of cancerous changes
- Venereal warts are one of the most rapidly growing forms of STD

FIGURE 46-13 *Condylomata acuminata* may be called venereal or genital warts. This STD is caused by the human papilloma virus (HPV). It appears as bumps or warts on the genitalia or within the perineal region. This male patient has venereal warts in the anal region. (Courtesy of Centers for Disease Control and Prevention)

Chlamydia Infection

Chlamydia are small infectious organisms that can invade mucous membranes of the body. These organisms can be:

- Introduced into the eyes, infecting the conjunctiva. This causes inflammation (conjunctivitis) and a more serious condition called trachoma. Trachoma can lead to blindness.
- Sexually transmitted; this commonly causes infections of the reproductive tract.
- The cause of serious pelvic inflammatory disease (PID), with scarring and even systemic infections. The scarring can result in sterility.
- Responsible for signs and symptoms similar to those of gonorrhea, except that the discharge is usually yellow to whitish in color.
- Treated with antibiotics.

Patients with pelvic infections are usually checked for gonorrhea. If they are found negative for gonorrhea, they are frequently diagnosed as having nongonorrheal urethritis (NGU) or nonspecified urethritis (NSU), because many different organisms may cause the infection. However, chlamydia organisms are the most common cause.

Human Immunodeficiency Virus (HIV) Disease

HIV is a viral disease (Figure 46-14). It is transmitted primarily through direct contact with the bodily secretions of an infected person. Therefore, it can be transmitted through direct sexual contact when infected blood, semen, or vaginal secretions come in contact with an uninfected person's broken skin or mucous membranes. HIV disease destroys the immune system. There is no

FIGURE 46-14 This picture of the HIV virus is magnified many times. The small spheres on the surface of the cells are called virions. (Courtesy of Centers for Disease Control and Prevention)

cure for this condition, although drugs can slow the damage to the body. If the disease progresses, the immune system is severely weakened. This stage of HIV disease is called AIDS (acquired immune deficiency syndrome). A discussion of AIDS is found in Unit 12.

DIAGNOSTIC TESTS

Techniques used to diagnose problems of the reproductive system include:

- Cultures for microorganisms.
- Urinalysis for hormone levels.
- **Pap smear**—test using cells from the cervix to detect possible cancer of the cervix. The test:
  - is painless.
  - can be performed in the physician's office during the routine pelvic examination.
  - should be done regularly.
- **Dilatation and curettage** (**D & C**)—a surgical procedure used to help diagnose conditions of the uterus, including tumors. In a D & C, the opening of the cervix is stretched open (dilated) and the uterus is scraped with a surgical instrument known as a curette.
- **Biopsy** (examining a sample of living tissue) is used to make a diagnosis. The biopsy sample is obtained through a needle. The procedure may be performed in the physician's office or in the hospital.
- Blood tests for cancer of the prostate.
- MRI and CT scans to help define the presence and extent of tumors.
- Ultrasound, a painless diagnostic tool that uses sound waves to diagnose ovarian cancer and other tumors.
- Cystoscopy—used to evaluate prostate conditions.
- Self-examination.
  Breast self-examination should be performed:
  - by all adult females.
  - each month on the last day of the menstrual flow.
  - on one selected day of the month, after menopause.
  - faithfully in a routine manner.
  Testicular self-examination should be performed:
  - by all adult males.
  - at least once each month.
  - during a warm shower so the scrotum will be relaxed.
  - with soapy fingers.
  - by palpating each testis between the fingers and thumb.
- Mammography—X-rays of the breasts. A **mammogram**:
  - can identify the presence of tumors up to 2 years before the tumor can be felt during self-examination.

- should be performed when the woman is between the ages of 35 and 40 years, to provide a baseline evaluation.
- thereafter, should be performed every 1 to 2 years until age 50.
- should be performed yearly after age 50.

VAGINAL DOUCHE

A vaginal **douche** is an irrigation of the vagina with fluid or medication. It is done by physician's order.

A vaginal douche requires standard precautions. When a douche is given to administer medications, it is given by the nurse. Other douches may be given by the nursing assistant if it is the policy of the facility. Be sure to check. Vaginal douches are given to:

- Remove odor or foul discharge
- Stop bleeding
- Relieve inflammation and pain
- Neutralize vaginal secretions
- Disinfect the vagina
- Cleanse the vagina before surgery or examination
- Administer antiseptic drugs

PROCEDURE

109

GIVING A NONSTERILE VAGINAL DOUCHE

1. Carry out initial procedure actions.
2. Assemble equipment:
   - Disposable gloves
   - Disposable douche container or kit
   - Bed protector
   - Toilet tissue
   - Bath blanket
   - Cotton balls
   - Disinfectant
   - Cup
   - Irrigating standard
   - Bedpan and cover
   - Plastic bag
3. Pour a small amount of the specified disinfecting solution over the cotton balls in the cup.
4. Measure water into the douche container. The temperature should be about 105°F. Add powder or solution as ordered.
5. Hang the douche bag on the standard. Close the clamp on the tubing. Leave the protector on the sterile tip.
6. Place a bed protector on the chair and assemble equipment where you can reach it. Screen the unit.
7. Elevate the bed to a comfortable working height and put up the side rails for safety.
8. Wash your hands and put on gloves. Lower the side rail on the working side.

9. Assist the patient into the dorsal recumbent position.
10. Place a bed protector beneath the patient's buttocks.
11. Remove the perineal pad (if used) from front to back and discard it in a plastic bag.
12. Drape the patient with a bath blanket (Figure 46-15). Fanfold top bedding to the foot of the bed.
13. Place a bedpan under the patient and ask her to void. Follow facility policies for emptying the bedpan, if necessary.

FIGURE 46-15 Drape the patient.

continues

PROCEDURE **109** CONTINUED

14. Cleanse the patient's perineum.
    - Use one cotton ball with disinfectant for each stroke.
    - Cleanse from the vulva toward the anus.
    - Cleanse the labia majora first.
    - Expose the labia minora with your thumb and forefinger and cleanse.
    - Give special attention to folds.
    - Discard used cotton balls in a plastic bag.

15. Replace the bedpan, if necessary. Position the patient in the dorsal recumbent position and readjust the bath blanket, if necessary. Elevate the head slightly for comfort, if desired.

16. Open the clamp to expel air. Remove the protector from the sterile tip of the disposable douche.

17. Allow a small amount of solution to flow over the inner thigh and then over the vulva. Do not touch the vulva with the nozzle.

18. Allow solution to continue to flow and insert the nozzle slowly and gently into the vagina, with an upward and backward movement, for about 3 inches.

19. Rotate the nozzle from side to side as solution flows.

20. When all solution has been given, remove the nozzle slowly and clamp the tubing.

21. Have the patient sit up on the bedpan to allow all the solution to return.

22. Remove the douche bag from the standard and place it on the bed protector.

23. Dry the perineum with tissue. Discard used tissue in the bedpan.

24. Cover the bedpan and place it on the bed protector on the chair.

25. Have the patient turn on her side. Dry her buttocks with tissue.

26. Place a clean pad over the vulva from front to back. Do not touch the inside of the pad.

27. Remove the bed protector and bath blanket. Replace with top bedding.

28. Observe the contents of the bedpan. Note the character and amount of discharge, if any. Discard the contents of the bedpan according to facility policy. Care for equipment according to facility policy. Remove gloves and dispose of them according to facility policy. Wash your hands.

29. Carry out ending procedure actions.

REVIEW

A. True/False.

Mark the following true or false by circling T or F.

1. T F D & C is a surgical procedure that can help establish a diagnosis related to the female reproductive system.

2. T F Following a panhysterectomy, you should check the patient for increased bleeding.

3. T F Salpingectomy means removal of the ovaries.

4. T F Foul-smelling leukorrhea is associated with the condition called trichomonas vaginitis.

5. T F The female with gonorrhea may not know she has been infected with the disease.

6. T F Untreated gonorrhea passes through three stages.

7. T F Syphilis is caused by a bacterium.

8. T F AIDS may be sexually transmitted.

9. T F The discharge in gonorrhea is white and very irritating.

B. Matching.

Choose the correct term from Column II to match each phrase in Column I.

Column I

10. _____ inability to reproduce

11. _____ inflammation of the vagina

12. _____ painful menstruation

13. _____ removal of a breast

14. _____ whitish discharge

Column II

a. dysmenorrhea

b. mastectomy

c. circumcision

d. leukorrhea

e. sterility

f. vaginitis

C. Multiple Choice.

Select the one best answer for each of the following.

15. You are to give a nonsterile douche. You will remember to

a. place the patient in a high Fowler's position.

b. use a solution with a temperature of about 115°F.

c. insert the nozzle about 3 inches into the vagina.

d. allow the nozzle to touch the vulva.

16. Breast self-examination should be performed

a. daily.

b. weekly.

c. monthly.

d. yearly.

17. Your patient has just returned from a suprapubic prostatectomy. You know that

a. there will be no incision.

b. there will be a Foley catheter drain.

c. the patient must be assisted to void every 2 hours.

d. the patient will be NPO for 2 to 3 days.

18. Testicular self-examination should be

a. done daily.

b. performed while lifting the commode.

c. performed with soapy fingers.

d. performed only by males over age 50.

D. Completion.

Complete the following statements.

19. The type of precautions to be used when caring for patients with STD is _____.

20. Women over the age of 50 should have a mammogram _____.

21. Breast self-examination should be performed _____.

E. Nursing Assistant Challenge.

Mrs. Forstein is 39 and has been admitted for a large pelvic mass. Her doctor suspects that she has a large tumor in her left ovary. She has experienced menorrhagia, dysmenorrhea, and pelvic pain. She is scheduled for an oophorectomy after tests are complete.

Briefly answer the following questions:

22. How else might you have described her menorrhagia and dysmenorrhea?

23. Does the doctor plan to remove the entire uterus, including the cervix?

24. What type of pain would be very significant following surgery?

25. What two areas would you check for drainage?

26. Why is it so important to maintain good circulation postoperatively?

Expanded Role of the Nursing Assistant

UNIT 47

Caring for the Patient with Cancer

OBJECTIVES

After completing this unit, you will be able to:

- Spell and define terms.
- List methods of reducing the risk of cancer.
- Explain the importance of good nutrition in cancer prevention and treatment.
- List seven signs and symptoms of cancer.
- Describe three types of cancer treatment.
- Describe nursing assistant responsibilities when caring for patients with cancer.

VOCABULARY

Learn the meaning and the correct spelling of the following words and phrases:

alopecia	carcinogen	immunotherapy	palliative care
anorexia	chemotherapy	malignant	radiation isolation sign
benign	dosimeter	metastasis	radiation therapy
cancer			

INTRODUCTION

Cancer is a disease in which the normal mechanisms of cell growth are disturbed. Cells grow abnormally, invade surrounding tissues, and use oxygen and nutrition intended for normal cells. Cancers that stay in one location and do not spread are **benign**. Benign cancers usually grow slowly. Some types of cancer cells spread to other parts of the body through the blood and lymphatic systems. This is called **metastasis**. When metastasis occurs, a tumor will eventually grow in another area. Cancers that spread to other parts of the body are **malignant**. Many patients die from metastasis instead of the original tumor. Some malignant cancers spread very rapidly. A **carcinogen** is a substance that causes cancer. Tobacco is one common carcinogen. The incidence of cancer and death rates vary with geographic location, sex, race, and age.

Risk Factors

Many factors increase the risk of developing cancer. Some cancers tend to be genetic. This means they run in families. Breast cancer, ovarian cancer, stomach cancer, and pancreatic cancer are examples of cancers that seem to have a hereditary component. Other common risk factors for cancer are:

- Age—this is the most common risk, with most cancers occurring in persons over the age of 55
- Lifestyle and habits:
  - smoking (Figure 47-1) and using smokeless or chewing tobacco
  - alcohol consumption
  - diet
- Family history, genetics
- Environmental pollution

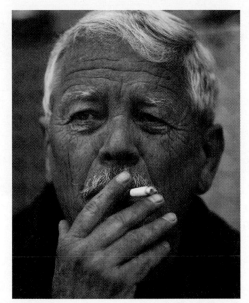

FIGURE 47-1 Lifestyle and habits such as cigarette smoking increase the risk of cancer. Smoking and sun exposure also increase facial wrinkles and give the appearance of premature aging.

- Harmful substances in the environment
  - asbestos
  - benzene
- Chemicals
- Radiation
- Prolonged sun exposure
- Infections and some viruses

Nutrition and Cancer

There is a direct relationship between intake of certain foods and the development of certain types of cancers. Table 47-1 lists various types of cancers and their relationship to certain food items. Obesity is associated with cancer of the gallbladder, uterus, colon, and breast. The American Cancer Society recommends following the food guide pyramid. These dietary guidelines will help prevent cancer:

- No more than 30% of total calories from fat
- Total cholesterol from diet should not exceed 300 mg a day
- At least 55% of total calories should come from complex carbohydrates, such as fruit, vegetables, cereals, and grains
- Salt from all food sources should not exceed 1 teaspoon a day

CANCER PREVENTION AND DETECTION

The American Cancer Society recommends certain lifestyle changes and preventive measures. These include:

TABLE 47-1 CANCER AND FOOD

Type of Cancer	Relationship to Food
Breast	High-fat diet
Prostate	High-fat diet
Colon	High-fat diet, low intake of fruits and vegetables, low fiber, low intake of complex carbohydrates
Esophagus	Low intake of fruits and vegetables, low fiber, low intake of complex carbohydrates, salt-cured foods; also drinking alcoholic beverages
Bladder	Low intake of fruits and vegetables, low fiber, low intake of complex carbohydrates
Stomach	Low intake of fruits and vegetables, low fiber, low intake of complex carbohydrates, high intake of salt-cured food
Larynx	Low intake of fruits and vegetables, low fiber, low intake of complex carbohydrates
Lung	Low intake of fruits and vegetables, low fiber, low intake of complex carbohydrates

- Not smoking
- Limiting the intake of alcoholic beverages
- Following the food guide pyramid and eating a healthy diet
- Regular exercise (Figure 47-2)
- Maintaining a healthy weight
- Avoiding sun exposure, particularly between 10:00 AM and 3:00 PM
- Getting genetic testing and counseling if at risk for familial cancers

Some patients take various drugs to reduce the risk of cancer. Natural substances, such as vitamin E and selenium, are being researched for their cancer prevention properties.

Signs and Symptoms of Cancer

Each type of cancer has its own signs and symptoms. General signs and symptoms that may indicate cancer spell the word CAUTION:

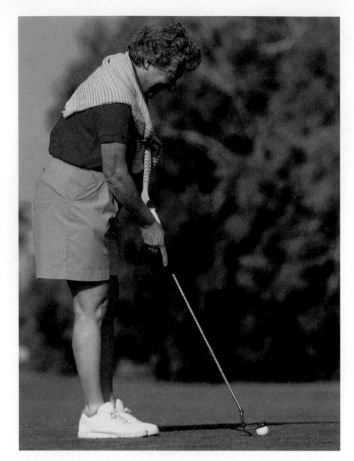

FIGURE 47-2 Regular exercise reduces the risk of cancer and many other diseases.

C = Change in bowel or bladder habits

A = A sore that does not heal (Figure 47-3)

U = Unusual bleeding or discharge

T = Thickening or lump in the breast, testicles, or any part of the body

I = Indigestion or difficulty swallowing

O = Obvious change in a wart, mole, or skin condition (Figure 47-4)

N = Nagging cough or hoarseness

FIGURE 47-3 A sore that does not heal should be examined by the doctor.

FIGURE 47-4 Change in a wart or mole warrants further investigation.

People with one or more of these warning signs should see a doctor right away.

Screening

Regular screening (Figure 47-5) for cancer is a key to survival, because the outcome is better if the disease is detected early. Many different professional organizations have guidelines for cancer screening. These vary slightly from one group to the next. Screening is based on a person's age, gender, risk factors, family history, ethnicity, and history of exposure to carcinogens in the environment. Some personal screening tests are recommended monthly, such as breast self-examination for women and testicular self-examination for men. Other routine screening tests are done by physicians.

TREATMENT

Many different treatments are used for cancer. In addition, some people use alternative and complementary therapies. The type of treatment is determined by:

- The type of cancer
- Location of the cancer

FIGURE 47-5
Regular health screening and early cancer detection are key to survival.

- Whether the cancer is malignant
- The stage (how advanced the cancer is)
- General condition of the patient

Surgery

A biopsy is a minor surgery that is sometimes done to diagnose a cancer. A biopsy involves removing a small piece of tissue from a suspicious area. The tissue is sent for laboratory examination. If the biopsy is positive for cancerous cells, a surgical procedure is done with the goal of completely removing the cancer. This may involve removing all or part of an organ, such as a lung, breast, or the uterus. Lymph nodes in the area may also be removed. The surgeon removes as much cancerous tissue as possible. If it is not possible to remove the entire cancerous area, a portion is left and is usually treated with other methods.

Reconstructive surgery may be done for cosmetic repair of an area. Sometimes this is done early, or even with the initial surgery. Other times reconstruction is done long after the original surgery. An example of reconstructive surgery is breast reconstruction. Preventive surgery may involve a radical procedure that is done when there is a strong genetic link to cancer. For example, the breasts or ovaries may be removed because of a high risk of developing cancer. Preventive surgery is also done to remove areas, such as rectal polyps, that may develop into cancer later.

Chemotherapy

Chemotherapy uses medications or drugs to destroy the cancer. Unfortunately, healthy cells may also be destroyed. The goals of chemotherapy vary, depending on the type of cancer, stage, and situation. Goals might be to:

- Completely eliminate the cancer
- Control and slow the growth of cancer to prolong the patient's life
- Reduce the size of the cancer to eliminate pain and improve quality of life

Chemotherapy is given by many different routes. Some patients are able to take oral medications. Others must receive the drugs in the muscles, veins, or other organs and body cavities. If the drugs are given intravenously, a central intravenous catheter (Figure 47-6) is often inserted to avoid repeated needlesticks and reduce the risk of vein irritation and collapse. Chemotherapy drugs are very potent and can irritate the skin, eyes, and mucous membranes of caregivers. Because of this, special measures are used to handle the drugs. Never eat, drink, or chew gum in an area where chemotherapy is being prepared. If you accidentally contact a chemotherapy drug with your hands or mucous membranes, flush well with water and seek medical attention. These drugs and the containers they are dispensed in require special handling and disposal.

FIGURE 47-6 The central intravenous catheter is commonly inserted to deliver intravenous chemotherapy. (Photo provided by Bard Access Systems. Hickman® is a registered trademark of Bard Access Systems.)

Side Effects of Chemotherapy. Chemotherapy targets rapidly regenerating cells, such as cancer cells. The drugs cannot differentiate cancer cells from normal cells, so other cells that regenerate rapidly may also be affected. Other cells in the body that are commonly affected are:

- Blood cells, such as red blood cells, white blood cells, and platelets
- Hair and nail cells
- Gastrointestinal cells

Side effects of cancer drugs can range from mild to life-threatening. Patients receiving these drugs need special monitoring. Sometimes the dose and scheduling must be changed to reduce side effects. Common side effects are:

- **Alopecia** (hair loss). This commonly starts within 2 weeks after chemotherapy begins. It may take up to 5 or 6 months to regrow the hair.
- Nausea and vomiting, depending on the drugs used. Sometimes nausea occurs immediately, but it may be delayed until several days after the drug is given.
- **Anorexia**, or loss of appetite. This sometimes occurs because the drugs cause changes in the tastebuds. In other patients, loss of appetite is due to nausea.
- Anemia, a deficiency of the red blood cells. This is caused by changes in the body due to the chemotherapy drugs. Sometimes special medications are given to reverse the anemia.
- Fatigue. Patients often become very tired. Anemia and reduced number of red blood cells are the most likely cause.
- Low white blood cell count, which increases the risk of infection. This usually starts within a week of the beginning of therapy, and it may last a long time. Precautions are taken to prevent exposure to infection.
- A reduction in the number of platelets in the blood, which increases the risk of bleeding. Precautions must be taken to prevent injury.

- Destruction of the mucous membranes of the mouth. This causes burning, pain, redness, and breakdown inside the mouth.

Many other side effects are caused by chemotherapy drugs. The nurse will advise you what to watch for in each patient. Having chemotherapy treatments can be physically and emotionally taxing. The patient will need a great deal of emotional support.

Disposal of Body Fluids and Wastes. Patients receiving chemotherapy may excrete the drugs in their waste and body fluids. The care plan will list special instructions for wearing PPE, if any, during patient care procedures. Discard gloves and other protective apparel, if worn, in a leakproof container. Follow facility policies for discarding PPE in a biohazardous waste or other contaminated area. Because the drugs are excreted in body waste, linens that have contacted blood, body fluids, or excretions require special handling. Wear gloves when handling linen, and always apply the principles of standard precautions. Soiled items should be put in specially marked bags before you send them to the laundry.

Special Care of the Chemotherapy Patient. Observe chemotherapy patients for side effects of the drugs and report any possible problems to the nurse promptly. Provide nursing comfort measures, such as good mouth care and daily bathing. Routinely take precautions to prevent injuries and infection. For example, you may be instructed to remind the patient to cough and deep breathe to keep the lungs clear. You may be asked to take vital signs every 4 hours. Rectal temperatures should not be taken in some patients. Check with the nurse before taking a rectal temperature. Report a fever over 101°F or chilling to the nurse immediately. Other signs of infection to report are:

- Swelling, redness, or irritation inside the mouth
- Rectal pain or tenderness
- Change in bowel or bladder habits
- Pain or burning on urination
- Redness, swelling, open area, or pain on the skin
- Cough or shortness of breath
- Decreased level of consciousness
- Decreased urine output
- Warm, flushed, dry skin
- Hypotension (below 100/60, or as instructed)

Because of the risk of bleeding, patients may have to take special precautions, such as blowing the nose gently and using an electric razor. A very soft toothbrush will probably be necessary. Special mouthwash products may be ordered. The care plan and the nurse will provide special directions.

Promoting good nutrition and hydration is very important. You may be asked to serve the patient six small meals a day. High-protein drinks may also be ordered. Encourage fluids, and record intake and output, including emesis. Alternate periods of rest with periods of activity, to reduce fatigue. Plan your care to allow frequent rest periods. Inform the nurse if the patient:

- Has nausea or vomiting
- Is not eating or drinking
- Complains of changes in the tastebuds, affecting the ability or desire to eat
- Constipation or diarrhea
- Has white patches or unusual areas inside the mouth (Figure 47-7)
- Complains of signs of a vaginal infection
- Develops bruising or bleeding (Figure 47-8)

Because the chemotherapy drugs are so toxic, you must observe the patient closely when he or she is receiving them. Inform the nurse promptly if there is:

FIGURE 47-7
Monitor for and report white patches in the mouth to the nurse. (Courtesy of Daniel J. Barbaro, MD, Fort Worth, Texas)

FIGURE 47-8
Report bruises to the nurse promptly.

- Any sign of IV infiltration, such as redness, swelling, or pain at the needle insertion site
- Change in mental status
- Change in vital signs

Assisting the Patient with Body Image. Cancer surgery and chemotherapy may change body appearance. This is often very upsetting to the patient. Hair loss may be especially traumatic, particularly in females. Be calm and reassuring. The hair will grow back, although the color or texture may be different. Assist the patient to wear a turban, scarf, or wig, if desired.

Radiation Therapy

Radiation therapy involves the use of high-energy, ionizing beams at the site of the cancer (Figure 47-9). The objective is to destroy the cancerous tissue without damaging healthy tissue. Several different types of radiation therapy may be used. Common side effects of radiation that should be reported to the nurse are:

- Fatigue
- Nausea, vomiting
- Loss of appetite
- Diarrhea
- Skin redness, irritation, peeling
- Change in ability to taste
- Irritation of mucous membranes
- Cough
- Shortness of breath

Special Care of the Radiation Therapy Patient. The patient may have markings on the skin at the site where radiation is delivered. Do not wash these off. The radiation may be very irritating to the patient's skin. Check the skin daily for problems and report them to the nurse, if found. Special skin care may be listed on the care plan. You may be instructed to:

- Wash the patient with lukewarm water and mild soap, using a soft washcloth; in some situations no soap is used
- Avoid rubbing or creating friction on the skin
- Avoid shaving areas near the treatment field
- Avoid tape on the patient's skin near the treatment field
- Avoid lotions and cosmetics near the treatment field
- Avoid tight-fitting garments; dress the patient in loose, comfortable clothing
- Avoid heat and cold treatments to the irradiated area

Brachytherapy

Brachytherapy is another form of radiation therapy in which tiny radioactive seeds or pellets are implanted directly inside the body. This treatment is very successful and preferred over traditional radiation therapy for some patients because it has fewer side effects. Brachytherapy is used to treat patients with breast, prostate, lung, cervical, and endometrial cancers, and some cancers of the head and neck. It is used for cancers that are localized. The small radioactive seeds are implanted directly into the tumor. The dosage varies with the area being treated and the type of cancer. Treatment may last from several hours to several days. The brachytherapy seeds used to treat prostate cancer may be left in place permanently. Brachytherapy may be used in combination with traditional radiation therapy.

Care of the Patient Receiving Brachytherapy. If a source of radiation is implanted inside the patient's body, you will be instructed in special precautions to follow to reduce your risk of radiation exposure. The patient will be in a private room. Usually, the hospital has designated rooms that are used only for radiation therapy patients. The patient may be on bedrest to prevent dislodgment of the radioactive device(s). To prevent radiation exposure, visitors will be restricted with regard to how close they may get to the patient and how long they may stay in the room. Pregnant women and children under the age of 18 are not permitted to enter the room. A patient who has permanently implanted seeds will be instructed to stay away from pregnant women and children for a designated period of time, such as 6 months.

If you will be caring for radiation therapy patients, you will be assigned a personal monitoring badge, called a **dosimeter**. This is a small instrument that measures the radiation dose to which each individual is exposed when working with the patient. Always wear the badge between your waist and collar when you enter the room. Never borrow someone else's badge. Use only the badge that was issued to you. Do not take the badge home. When off duty, store it according to facility policy, away from sources of radiation.

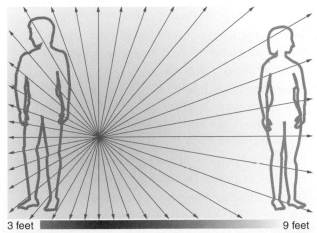

3 feet   9 feet

FIGURE 47-9 Radiation therapy is used to treat certain cancers.

Difficult SITUATIONS

A lead-lined container and long-handled forceps will be stored in a corner of the room of a patient with a radiation implant. Radiation safety personnel will mark a "safe line" on the floor with masking tape approximately 6 feet from the bed. The line is a warning to visitors to minimize their radiation exposure; they should remain behind the line when visiting the patient. The radiation safety department may also place a portable lead shield in the back of the room to use when providing care. If the patient has an implant in the neck or mouth, an emergency tracheotomy tray will be placed in the room. Do not store it in a drawer or cupboard. The tray should be visible at all times. ■

Immunotherapy

Immunotherapy is another cancer treatment that is done to alter the patient's immune response and eliminate the cancer. Various biologic agents are given to change the normal immune response. The vital signs are regularly and closely monitored when these agents are given. Side effects of therapy usually cease within a week after treatment. Care of the patient receiving immunotherapy involves:

- Monitoring vital signs every 4 hours, or more often if instructed
- Monitoring capillary refill as instructed
- Advising the patient to remain in bed if the systolic blood pressure is below 100, or according to the nurse's instructions
- Weighing the patient daily and informing the nurse of weight gain

Notify the nurse promptly if the patient:

- Has fever or chills

GUIDELINES *for*

Working with Radiation Therapy and Brachytherapy Patients

- If you think you may be pregnant, do not enter the room. Inform the nurse.
- Plan and organize your time before entering the patient's room. Provide necessary care, but try to minimize time spent with the patient.
- You may be required to apply gloves and shoe covers when entering the patient's room. Remove them before leaving.
- Wear a mask if the patient has a tracheostomy or signs of a respiratory infection.
- Work behind mobile shields whenever possible.
- Work no closer to the patient than necessary. Stay at least 3 feet away from the patient unless direct care is being given.
- Think about what you are doing. Conscientiously apply the principles of standard precautions for all patient care.
- A separate sink may be designated for handwashing. If so, use only this sink.
- Follow all special instructions on the patient's care plan. Consult the nurse if you are unsure of something or have questions.
- The care plan, critical pathway, or **radiation isolation sign** will list where to find special safety pre-

cautions, including the maximum length of time to remain in the room. The radiation isolation sign is not an infection control sign. After the radioactive material has been given to the patient, he or she will be restricted under "Radiation Precautions." A sign bearing a radiation symbol (Figure 47-10) will be posted on the door to the room. This sign has a black or magenta tri-blade on a white or yellow background, with the words "Caution: Radioactive Material." No one should enter the room without consulting medical, nursing, or radiation safety staff. Become familiar with the precautions for each patient, and follow them carefully.

- Monitor the length of time visitors stay in the room. Inform the nurse if they stay beyond the specified time.
- Chairs and other furniture in the room will be located a certain distance away from the patient. Do not move the furniture. Instruct visitors not to move chairs closer to the patient.
- Explain the purpose of the mobile safety shield and ask visitors to remain behind it.
- Do not allow pregnant women or children under the age of 18 into the radiation isolation room to visit.

continues

GUIDELINES *continued*

FIGURE 47-10 The radiation precautions sign has a black or magenta tri-blade on a white or yellow background, with the words "Caution: Radioactive Material." No one should enter the room without first consulting medical, nursing, or radiation safety staff.

- Follow facility policies for cleaning the room, serving, and removing meal trays. In many facilities, personnel from the dietary and housekeeping departments are not permitted to enter the room.
- Do not remove items from the room without permission from radiation safety personnel.
- If a radiation source becomes dislodged from the patient, avoid touching it. Ask visitors to leave the room. Try to move the source to a corner by using a tool such as a yardstick. Inform the nurse or radiation safety personnel.
- Find out if special precautions are necessary for handling soiled linens, tissues, or dressings.
- Strain all urine of patients with brachytherapy seeds near the bladder. Some seeds may be lost through urination. Follow facility policies for straining urine in a catheter bag. In some facilities, careful visual inspection of the catheter bag is sufficient. If a seed is found, do not attempt to remove it. Inform the nurse or radiation safety personnel.
- Place a small radioactive-labeled container in the patient's bathroom. Do not remove it. The container will be used to dispose of dislodged seeds, if any.
- Follow the nurse's instructions if you are directed to obtain a urine specimen after brachytherapy seeds have been implanted.

- Patients receiving certain types of therapy will require special urine collection. Bottles and special collection shields will be provided. Teach the patient to be responsible for urine collection, if possible. The urine collection bottles will be removed by radiation safety personnel.
- Notify radiation safety personnel if there is a large spill of urine.
- Contaminated items must be incinerated if possible. A separate container will be used to discard these items, such as tissues, gauze sponges, shoe covers, and gloves.
- Use a separate, designated laundry bag for items that have been contaminated with body fluids, such as vomitus, incontinence, wound drainage, or profuse perspiration.

When the patient is discharged:

- Discard disposable utensils, such as bedpans, urinals, and basins, with the radioactive waste.
- You will use the same permanent-equipment items for the patient from admission until discharge. Wash them well with soap and running water. Radiation safety personnel must check the items before they are returned to floor stock.
- Wear utility gloves when washing potentially contaminated equipment. When you have finished, wash the gloves with soap and water, then dry them *before* removing them. (This is the only exception to the rule that you should never wash your gloved hands. It is a radiation precaution, not an infection control problem.)
- The room will require special cleaning. Follow the radiation safety department's instructions. The room must not be used again until after it has been cleared by the radiation safety department.

- Has rapid pulse (over 100, or according to nurse's instructions) or rapid respirations (over 24, or according to nurse's instructions)
- Becomes cyanotic
- Is short of breath
- Is restless or apprehensive
- Has diarrhea, nausea, or vomiting
- Complains of itching

PAIN

Pain is the most common symptom in patients with cancer. The pain may be caused by the cancer, or be a result of the treatment. The pain may cause difficulty sleeping, loss of appetite, depression, and anxiety. Pain over an extended period of time reduces the patient's quality of life. The World Health Organization (WHO) analgesic ladder (Figure 47-11) is used as a model for pain management.

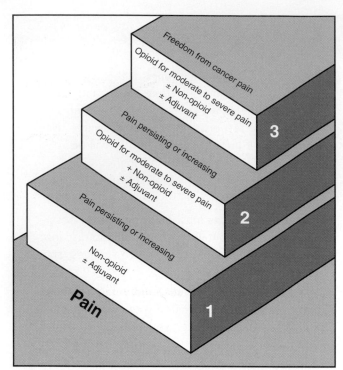

FIGURE 47-11 The WHO three-step analgesic ladder is used as a model in pain management. (Courtesy of World Health Organization, Geneva, Switzerland. Used with permission.)

Cancer patients should be evaluated for pain regularly. A pain scale (Unit 10) is usually used. Narcotic pain-relieving medications may be necessary to control the pain. These are not withheld out of fear of addiction. The incidence of addiction in cancer patients is very low. Pain should be treated before it becomes severe and out of control. Notify the nurse promptly if a patient complains of pain, or the patient tells you that pain medication was ineffective.

MENTAL AND EMOTIONAL NEEDS

Patients with cancer have a life-altering disease. They commonly fear dying. They may be anxious or depressed, and they often go through the grieving process (Unit 32). Nursing assistant measures to assist with mental and emotional needs include:

- Spending as much time as possible with the patient if he wants to talk
- Allowing the patient to talk about feelings and fears

- Being proficient at providing physical care and assistance with ADLs.
- Anticipating patients' needs before they ask
- Respecting the patient's beliefs and wishes
- Providing emotional support
- Respecting the patient's privacy if she wants to be alone
- Making the patient feel respected and valued as a person

Avoid giving the patient false hope. If you think a patient is losing control, inform the nurse. Just being with the patient and allowing him to talk is very helpful.

Communication HIGHLIGHT

A cancer diagnosis evokes strong feelings and emotions in patients and their families. These may be difficult to understand and cope with. Patients or families may lash out in anger at you or their loved ones. They are not angry with you. They are angry with their circumstances. Avoid responding with anger. Keep your temper even, and do not take comments personally. Saying, "I see you are upset," or validating their feelings is the best way to respond. Providing compassionate care, listening, and giving sincere, solid emotional support will help patients and family members cope with this difficult time. ■

PALLIATIVE CARE

Some patients with cancer elect to have **palliative care**. This care is designed to treat the symptoms of discomfort, but not the disease. The patient will have an advance directive and do not resuscitate (DNR) order. The patient is kept comfortable until death occurs. A hospice (Unit 32) may be involved in the patient's care. One goal of this care is to maintain the patient's quality of life for as long as possible.

Your care is designed to keep the patient clean and comfortable. Use nursing measures, such as positioning and backrubs, to enhance the patient's comfort. Spend time with the patient and allow her to talk, if she wants. Respect the patient's wishes. Provide emotional support. Inform the nurse if the patient is short of breath, anxious, or complains of pain.

REVIEW

A. True/False.

Mark the following true or false by circling T or F.

1. T F Benign tumors spread rapidly to other parts of the body.

2. T F A carcinogen is a cancer-producing substance.

3. T F Most cancers occur in persons over the age of 65.

4. T F In a healthy diet, no more than 30% of daily calories comes from fat.

5. T F Lifestyle modification may reduce the risk of cancer.

B. Matching.

Choose the correct word from Column II to match the phrase or statement in Column I.

Column I

6. _____ cancer that spreads

7. _____ tissue sample

8. _____ medications or drugs

9. _____ changes immune response

10. _____ comfort care

Column II

a. chemotherapy

b. malignant

c. palliative

d. biopsy

e. immunotherapy

C. Multiple Choice.

Select the one best answer for each of the following.

11. The most common risk factor for cancer is
    a. cigarette smoking.
    b. heredity.
    c. poor nutrition.
    d. age.

12. Complex carbohydrates should make up _____ % of the daily caloric intake.
    a. 20
    b. 30
    c. 55
    d. 85

13. Lifestyle changes that will reduce the risk of cancer include
    a. drinking herbal tea daily.
    b. getting a complete physical exam every 5 years.
    c. a regular exercise program.
    d. consuming at least 800 mL of water daily.

14. Females should perform a breast self-examination
    a. weekly.
    b. monthly.
    c. every 6 months.
    d. yearly.

15. Males should perform testicular self-examination
    a. monthly.
    b. every 3 months.
    c. every 6 months.
    d. annually.

16. The use of medications to destroy cancer cells is
    a. brachytherapy.
    b. radiation therapy.
    c. chemotherapy.
    d. complementary therapy.

17. A deficiency of red blood cells that is a common side effect of cancer therapy is
    a. alopecia.
    b. anemia.
    c. anorexia.
    d. metastasis.

18. Radiation therapy is a cancer treatment that uses
    a. high-energy ionizing beams.
    b. chemicals.
    c. medication.
    d. change in the immune response.

19. A patient returns from a radiation treatment with markings on the skin. You should
    a. wash the markings off with soap and water.
    b. scrub the area vigorously.
    c. apply lotion to the area.
    d. leave the markings alone.

20. The most common symptom of patients with cancer is
    a. nausea.
    b. vomiting.
    c. pain.
    d. alopecia.

D. Nursing Assistant Challenge.

Mr. Weiss is a 37-year-old patient who was recently diagnosed with breast cancer. He had a breast surgically removed and is undergoing chemotherapy. You take his vital signs early in the shift, but he refuses to speak to you. A few hours later, you bring his meal tray to the room and set it on the overbed table. Mr. Weiss sweeps the tray off the table with his arm, and food and dishes fly everywhere. He yells at you, shouting "You know I am not hungry. Now get out of here and leave me alone."

21. Why do you think Mr. Weiss is acting this way?

22. Is he mad at you?

23. What action should you take immediately?

24. What will you report to the nurse?

25. Should you leave Mr. Weiss alone for the rest of the shift?

UNIT 48

850 SECTION 12 Expanded Role of the Nursing Assistant

• Rehabilitation is usually given to improve the ... condition and safety awareness. Restorative ... may be provided to prevent the ... phy between worsening. Thus, the ... from worsening. Thus, the ... tion experts are ... designed ...

OBJECTIVES

After completing this unit, you will be able to:

- Spell and define terms.
- Compare and contrast rehabilitation and restorative nursing care.
- Identify five members of the interdisciplinary team.
- Describe the role of the nursing assistant in rehabilitation and restorative care.
- Describe the principles of rehabilitation.

- List the elements of successful rehabilitation/restorative care.
- List six complications resulting from inactivity.
- Identify four perceptual deficits.
- Describe four approaches used for restorative programs.
- List the guidelines for implementing restorative programs.

VOCABULARY

Learn the meaning and the correct spelling of the following words and phrases:

activities of daily living (ADLs)	geriatric	perceptual deficit	restoration
	handicap	physiatrist	restorative
adaptive device	mobility skills	rehabilitation	self-care deficit
disability			

INTRODUCTION TO REHABILITATION AND RESTORATIVE CARE

The term **rehabilitation** refers to a process in which the patient is assisted to reach an optimal level of ability. That means we are concerned with helping patients be the best they can be: physically, mentally, and emotionally. Rehabilitation and restorative care are similar processes, but there are some differences:

- Rehabilitation is usually more aggressive and intensive than restorative care (Figure 48-1). Therapies are planned for a period of several weeks. Restorative care is a slower process; it may be planned for weeks or months or go on indefinitely.

- Rehabilitation requires the skills of many disciplines, including nursing and various therapies. **Restorative** care is basically a nursing responsibility, carried out with consultation from therapists and other health professionals.
- Rehabilitation services are given from 1 to 4 hours a day, depending on the setting and patient's needs. They are typically provided 5 days a week. Therapy is not available on weekends in some facilities. Restorative care may be given 24 hours a day, 7 days a week, or as often as the service is needed. The difference is that restorative nursing addresses services the patient may need at any time of the day or night. Restorative approaches are integrated into the regular nursing care and are used each time the patient needs the service. This care is not a separate service.

patient's
ive nursing
patient's condition
is a difference in philoso-
ation and restorative. Rehabilita-
required by payers to develop programs
to cause rapid, significant improvement in the
patient. Those who practice restorative care maintain patients at their highest level, even if the patients have no potential for improvement. The patient benefits because restorative maintenance programs prevent declines (worsening of the patient's condition).

- Rehabilitation services may be provided in a general acute care hospital, a rehabilitation center, a skilled care facility, a subacute care unit, or the patient's home. Most restorative care is given in a skilled care facility or in the patient's home.

- OBRA regulations require that restorative services be provided to patients in skilled care facilities. Nursing assistants in these facilities must have the knowledge and skills to participate in this process.

The goals of both rehabilitation and restorative care are to:

- Increase the patient's physical abilities. This may include **mobility skills** (Figure 48-2) and the ability to carry out **activities of daily living (ADLs)**. Activities of daily living are the tasks that we learn as children and do throughout life. These tasks include: bathing,

FIGURE 48-2 Rehabilitation and restorative nursing both work on increasing mobility and independence.

oral care, hair and nail care, dressing and undressing, eating, toileting, and mobility.

- Prevent complications such as pressure ulcers and contractures.

- Maintain the patient's current abilities.

- Help the patient adapt to limitations imposed by a disability.

- Increase the patient's quality of life.

The information in this unit applies to both rehabilitation and restorative care. These services complement each other. When you follow the restorative program established by the therapist to complement the rehabilitation program, this reinforces what the therapists are teaching, and the patient masters the skill more quickly. This process is called **restoration**.

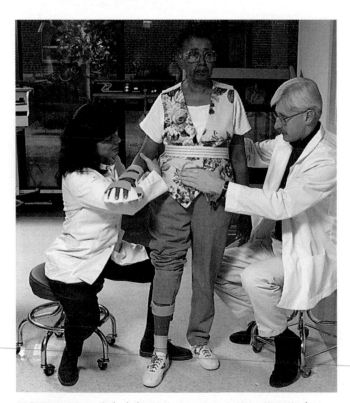

FIGURE 48-1 Rehabilitation is more aggressive and intensive than restorative care.

REASONS FOR REHABILITATION/ RESTORATIVE CARE

A person may need rehabilitation because of a **disability**. A disability exists when the person has an impairment that affects the ability to perform an activity that a person of that age would normally be able to do. Adults, for example, are able to dress and undress independently. If a person is unable to do this because of a disease or injury, a disability exists. A disability may be temporary or permanent.

A **handicap** exists if the disability limits or prevents the person from fulfilling a role that is normal for that person. This might include such functions as holding a job, managing a household, and raising a family.

If a disability is permanent, such as tetraplegia (paralysis from the neck down) from a spinal cord injury, it is unrealistic to expect that rehabilitation will enable the patient to walk again. In these situations, the interdisciplinary team will teach the patient to:

- Adapt to the present circumstances.
- Use adaptive devices to increase independence.
- Learn new ways of doing routine tasks, such as dressing or bathing.
- Become as independent as possible in light of the disability. Patients with severely limiting conditions, such as tetraplegia, are taught to assume responsibility for personal well-being, including verbally directing caregivers to accomplish the results the patient wants.

Impairments or disabilities result from trauma or disease. Disorders of the musculoskeletal system, such as amputation (Figure 48-3) of an extremity or arthritis, may require rehabilitation. Stroke, spinal cord injury, and brain injuries are examples of nervous system disorders that will benefit from rehabilitation. A patient who has been in bed for a long time because of a serious illness, such as heart disease, may require rehabilitation for reconditioning or to restore the individual to a previous level of ability.

THE INTERDISCIPLINARY HEALTH CARE TEAM

Physicians who specialize in rehabilitation are called **physiatrists**. Nurses and nursing assistants who work in rehabilitation receive additional specialized education. Many other disciplines may be involved in the rehabilitation process. For instance, a person who has had a stroke may receive:

- Physical therapy to learn how to walk again
- Occupational therapy to relearn the activities of daily living
- Speech therapy to learn new communication or swallowing methods
- Nursing services for bowel and bladder management, prevention of pressure ulcers, and other complications
- Dietitian services to help the patient learn to manage new dietary restrictions for a low-sodium diet (to reduce blood pressure), and to plan and prepare meals
- Psychological support to adapt to the sudden changes brought about by the stroke
- Social services to plan for the impending discharge

Each discipline has specific responsibilities, but all disciplines work together with the patient and family to resolve problems and to plan care.

There are many subspecialties in rehabilitation. Health care professionals may choose to work in **geriatric** (care of the elderly) or pediatric rehabilitation. Others may specialize in the care of patients with strokes, spinal cord injuries, brain injuries, amputations, or arthritis.

THE ROLE OF THE NURSING ASSISTANT IN REHABILITATION AND RESTORATIVE CARE

The nursing assistant who works in rehabilitation will assist the nurses with

- Procedures to prevent complications: passive range-of-motion exercises and positioning
- Mobility skills: transfers and ambulation
- Bathing and personal care procedures
- Bowel and bladder management programs
- Maintaining the patient's nutritional status
- Programs to increase the patient's independence

FIGURE 48-3 Patients who have had an amputation often benefit from intensive rehabilitation.

PRINCIPLES OF REHABILITATION

Four principles form the foundation of successful rehabilitation or restorative care.

- *Treatment begins as soon as possible.*

  This means that plans for maintaining or increasing abilities begin as soon as the patient's condition is stable. For example, if a patient has had a stroke, passive exercises and positioning techniques are initiated in the critical care unit to prevent contractures, pressure ulcers, and other complications that would prohibit or delay rehabilitation.

- *Stress the patient's ability, not disability.*

  Care providers must think in terms of what the patient can do, not what the patient cannot do. The patient's strengths are used to help in adapting to any limitations. A *strength* refers to anything the patient is able to do. Perhaps a patient whose dominant hand is paralyzed cannot use that hand to feed himself—but instead of having nursing staff feed him, he can be taught to use the other, stronger hand. Use the restorative philosophy when communicating with patients. Avoid statements such as, "You *can't* use your right hand." Instead, say, "You *can* use your left hand." Allow the patient to struggle a little, but avoid letting him progress to the point of frustration before you step in to assist.

- *Activity strengthens and inactivity weakens.*

  Complications result from physical and mental inactivity. These can cause further disability or even be life-threatening. A rehabilitation or restorative plan of care always includes approaches and goals for both physical and mental activity.

- *Treat the whole person.*

  When we are giving care to patients, we are not concerned only with their physical well-being. We also must attend to their emotional and mental health needs (Figure 48-4). An angry or depressed patient will not be able to concentrate on the work involved in rehabilitation. We must also work with the patients' families. They directly influence the emotional and mental health of the patients.

The elements of successful rehabilitation/restorative care require that members of the team:

- Have a positive attitude about patients and their capabilities
- Have confidence in their own abilities as caregivers
- Be willing to learn from other care providers, patients, and their families
- Use problem-solving skills in place of unproductive coping methods
- Use all available tools and resources to give effective care

FIGURE 48-4 The patient's mental and emotional state are as important as her physical condition.

- Work with other staff as team members
- Realize that ideal working situations seldom exist, but strive to bring ideal and real closer together
- Continually learn and acquire new skills by participating in educational programs
- Accept the need for change to improve the quality of care for all patients.

Keys to success in rehabilitation and restorative nursing programs are:

- Use of the care plan. All staff are familiar with the patient's problems, goals, and approaches to use.
- Consistency of care. All staff use the same approaches (as listed on the care plan) when caring for the patient.
- Continuity of care. There is a smooth progression and flow between caregivers and between shifts.
- Good communication among all caregivers, the patient, and interested family members.

COMPLICATIONS FROM INACTIVITY

People with disabilities may be unable to move about at will. The inactivity or immobility can result in numerous complications affecting body systems:

1. Musculoskeletal system.
   - Muscles become weak and atrophy (decrease in size and strength).
   - Contractures can form, making any movement impossible. A contracture (Figure 48-5) occurs when a joint is in a permanent state of flexion.
   - Disuse osteoporosis develops. This means that calcium drains from the bones, causing them to become brittle. Fractures can occur even without trauma.

Clinical Information ALERT

Elderly and chronically ill patients usually lose independence by degrees. Loss of independence as a result of trauma can be devastating for the patient. Imagine being normal one minute, then having an auto accident that leaves you completely paralyzed. This type of injury immediately changes the lives of the patient and her entire family. Therapists work with patients who are struggling to regain their self-help skills. Most will tell you the job is sometimes difficult and frustrating for both patient and caregiver. Some patients will regain all or part of their independence, but most have to adjust activities and routines to disability. Because their bodies now work differently, they must learn to do things differently. This is also difficult and frustrating. Being completely unable to perform ADL is even more frustrating. Despite the best medical and rehabilitative care, an unfortunate few will be completely dependent on others for the rest of their lives. ■

FIGURE 48-5 Contractures are a painful complication of immobility. This patient has foot drop, a serious contracture of the feet.

2. Integumentary system.
   – Pressure ulcers develop over bony prominences.
3. Cardiovascular system.
   – The heart takes longer to return to a normal pace after activity.
   – Blood does not circulate as efficiently. This can lead to thrombus (a stationary blood clot) or embolus (a blood clot that moves through the circulatory system).

   – Edema may be caused by lack of movement.
   – The heart must work harder to pump blood through the body.
   – Changes in the blood vessels may cause dizziness and fainting when the patient is placed in the upright position.
4. Respiratory system.
   – The lungs do not expand as fully as they did when the person was active. Secretions collect in the lungs and cause pneumonia.
   – Respiratory tract infections are more common.
5. Gastrointestinal system.
   – Appetite decreases, causing weight loss.
   – The risk of pressure ulcers increases with weight loss and lack of nutrition.
   – Peristalsis slows down, causing indigestion and constipation.
   – Indigestion and heartburn may result if the patient is not positioned properly during and after meals.
   – The patient is at risk of choking and aspiration unless positioned upright during and after meals.
6. Urinary system.
   – The bladder does not empty completely. This increases the risk of bladder infection.
   – Incontinence can result from inability to get to the bathroom.
   – Urinary stones may develop from calcium in the bloodstream resulting from osteoporosis.
7. Nervous system.
   – Weakness and limited mobility.
   – Insomnia may result from sleeping too much during the day, then being unable to sleep at night.
8. Psychosocial reaction.
   – Depression can occur from physical and mental inactivity and feelings of helplessness.
   – Inactivity and lack of sensory stimulation can cause disorientation.
   – Irritability, boredom, and lethargy may result from the patient's frustration.

Activities of Daily Living

One purpose of restorative care is to increase the patient's physical abilities. This includes mobility skills and the ability to carry out activities of daily living.

These tasks or skills are taught to us as children. Healthy adults do these tasks automatically. If the patient cannot complete any or all of the ADLs, a **self-care deficit** exists. Adults may have self-care deficits because of:

- Diseases such as multiple sclerosis, post polio syndrome, arthritis, Parkinson's disease, or Alzheimer's disease

- Injuries causing damage to the extremities, brain, or spinal cord
- Vision impairment
- Emotional illness

Deficits are caused by problems that limit the patient's ability to do self-care. Examples of these problems are:

- Decreased strength
- Lack of endurance
- Limited range of motion
- Depression
- Disorientation
- Perceptual deficits

There are many types of **perceptual deficits**. These usually occur because of damage to the brain from disease or injury. Here are some examples of perceptual deficits:

- An inability to organize a task. ADLs cannot be completed unless the individual is able to prepare for the task, get the necessary items together, and then do it.
- An inability to sequence a task. When putting on clothing, for example, a slip must go on before the dress and socks before shoes.
- Lack of judgment. This deficit may be noted if a patient puts on a wool coat in hot weather (when appropriate clothing is available).
- An inability to identify common objects, such as eating utensils and grooming items (*agnosia*). The patient may try to use a fork to comb her hair, for example.
- An inability to use common items (*apraxia*). The patient may be able to identify the item but be unable to use it (even though there is no physical reason such as paralysis).
- An inability to initiate a task.

Patients with self-care deficits are evaluated by therapists and nurses. The results of evaluation will determine whether a patient's functional (physical) abilities can be increased. In other words, can the interdisciplinary team help this person to relearn an activity of daily living? This is discussed with the patient and the family.

RESTORATIVE PROGRAMS

If the patient has the potential to relearn an ADL and is motivated to try, a restorative program is planned. These

Difficult SITUATIONS

Disabilities can take many forms. Some forms, such as speech, hearing, or language problems, interfere with communication. Other problems, such as physical impairments, may make you uncomfortable. You may be unsure of how to avoid offending the patient. Individuals who are newly disabled are more sensitive to their problems than people who have lived with a disability for a long time. People with disabilities are like you are. They have the same wants and needs. Their problems are no different from yours. However, having a disability makes living with these same problems much more difficult and creates additional problems. People with disabilities can do many of the same things you can. However, they may need to adapt the environment to do them. Changing things to meet a patient's needs is called providing *reasonable accommodation*. People with disabilities may perform a task differently than you do. However, the outcome of a task is the same. Their bodies just work differently! As a rule, persons who have disabilities do not want to be treated differently from anyone else. Many are self-sufficient. All are valuable and equal members of society. Emphasize the uniqueness, value, and worth of each patient. Avoid comparing people. Treat people with disabilities the way you like to be treated. ■

Clinical Information ALERT

We normally think of the grieving process in relation to death and dying. However, the process applies to any major loss. Patients and families experience the grieving process because of disability and loss of independence. The stage of grieving often affects rehabilitation and safety. Some patients are in denial and use poor safety judgment, taking risks because of anger or indifference. They may take risks during the bargaining stage to test their higher power. During the depression stage, they may say they are giving up because rehabilitation is much too difficult. Some health care workers label the patients as being "difficult" or "trying" when in fact they are grieving. Avoid stereotyping and labeling patients. Recognize the stages of the grieving process and use the skills you learned in Unit 32 to support the patient. ■

programs are sometimes called retraining programs or ADL programs.

When the patient is unable to do any of the ADLs independently, it is generally best to concentrate on just one at a time. The first step is to find out what the patient wants to work on first. The interdisciplinary team then works with the patient and family to plan the process. They will:

- Establish goals. Each ADL consists of several steps, as shown in Table 48-1. The patient will not be able to do all steps right away. Some patients may never be able to do all of the steps. Goals, therefore, are very small. For example, if the patient is in a restorative program for eating, the first goal may be to hold a glass and drink from it. All goals are functional. Instead of saying the patient will walk 30 feet, the goal will state: "Patient will walk to the dining room for breakfast."
- Plan approaches. The approaches include the techniques and procedures carried out by the interdisciplinary team. The approaches are planned to help the patient relearn the ADL.

Approaches Used in Restorative Programs

The approach to use will be listed on the care plan. It is important that the same approach be used consistently.

- *Setup.* Patients with self-care deficits are not able to set up or prepare for activities of daily living. You may need to provide the setup (Figure 48-6). Example for bathing: collect all needed items, prepare the bathtub or shower, help the patient into the tub or shower.
- *Verbal cues.* The care provider uses short, simple phrases to prompt the patient. Example: give the patient a prepared washcloth and then say, "Please wash your face" (Figure 48-7). If a complete task, such as washing the entire face, is overwhelming, break it down into a series of smaller tasks, such as washing the forehead, then the left cheek, and so forth.
- *Hand-over-hand techniques.* Example for eating program: Place a glass in the patient's hand. Place your hand over the patient's hand. Guide the glass to the patient's mouth (Figure 48-8).
- *Demonstration.* Act out what you want the patient to do. Example: Before giving the patient a toothbrush, make the motions of brushing your teeth with the toothbrush (Figure 48-9).

Adaptive Devices

Adaptive devices are sometimes used to simplify an ADL. **Adaptive devices** are ordinary items that have been modified for use by patients with various types of problems.

A person with a disability may be unable to perform certain ADLs. Sometimes adding a device that changes the way the task is done will enable the patient to perform it

TABLE 48-1 FUNCTIONAL STEPS OF ACTIVITIES OF DAILY LIVING

Bathing	• Gets to tub/sink/shower
	• Regulates water flow and temperature
	• Washes/rinses upper body
	• Washes/rinses lower body
	• Dries body
Dressing/Undressing	• Obtains/selects clothing
	• Puts on/takes off slipover top
	• Puts on/takes off cardigan-style top
	• Manages buttons, snaps, ties, zippers
	• Puts on/takes off skirt/pants
	• Buckles belt
	• Puts on socks/shoes
Eating	• Gets to table
	• Uses spoon, fork, knife appropriately
	• Opens/pours
	• Brings food to mouth
	• Chews, swallows
	• Uses napkin
Toileting	• Gets to commode/toilet
	• Manipulates clothing
	• Sits on toilet
	• Eliminates in toilet
	• Cleans self
	• Flushes toilet
	• Gets clothing back in place
	• Washes hands
Mobility	• Gets self to side of bed
	• Maintains upright position
	• Comes to standing position
	• Places self in position to sit in chair
	• Locks wheelchair brakes
	• Turns body to sit
	• Lowers self into chair
	• Propels wheelchair
	• Repositions self in chair
	• Raises self from chair
	• Places self in position to sit on edge of bed
	• Walks alone/with assistance
	• Uses assistive device

FIGURE 48-6 This patient is able to feed herself if the nursing assistant sets up the tray.

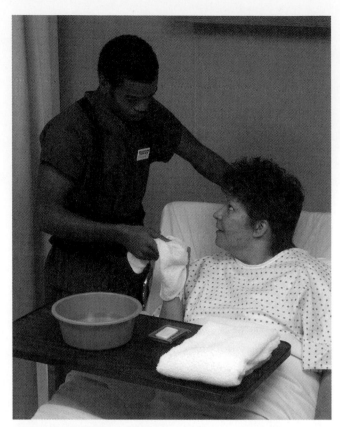

FIGURE 48-7 The nursing assistant uses verbal cues to assist the patient with ADLs.

FIGURE 48-8 Hand-over-hand technique is another approach that helps patients relearn essential skills.

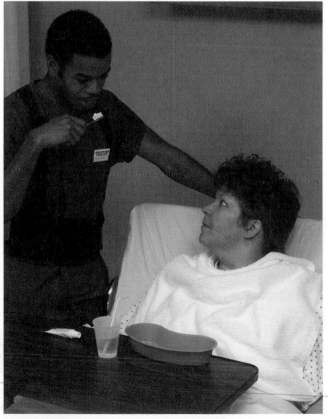

FIGURE 48-9 Demonstrating the activity is a good way to help the patient understand the directions.

independently. Adaptive devices are usually prescribed by the occupational therapist or restorative nurse based on an evaluation of the patient's individual needs. The patient is taught how to use the device for everyday tasks (Figure 48-10). Your role as a nursing assistant is to make sure the device is clean, available, and used by the patient. You may need to work on the skill with the patient when she is learning to use the device. The care plan will provide instructions on the types of devices the patient uses.

Adaptive Devices for Eating. The most common adaptive devices are used to enable patients to feed themselves. Many individual devices are available to meet patients' needs. The most common devices are adaptive silverware (Figures 48-11A and 48-11B), plates (Figure 48-11C), plate guards, and cups (Figure 48-11D). Other items, such as a straw holder (Figure 48-11E), may also be necessary.

Adaptive Devices for Dressing. Dressing aids are also commonly used (Figures 48-12). These devices make it easier for patients to dress themselves. Using these adaptive devices may appear awkward to you, but for patients, being able to dress themselves is important for self-esteem.

Adaptive Devices for Grooming and Hygiene. Being able to bathe and groom oneself are important skills. Everyone has a personal hygienic routine. Grooming and hygiene are very private activities. Using adaptive

FIGURE 48-11 A. Many types of adaptive utensils are available to meet individual needs and enable patients to feed themselves. B. The wrist cuff enables the patient to hold silverware and eat independently. C. Adaptive plates and bowls have raised edges so patients can scoop food easily. D. An adaptive cup. E. The straw holder centers the straw and holds it in place. (Courtesy of Maddak, Inc.)

FIGURE 48-10 The patient learned how to use this device by working with the occupational therapist. Now she uses it independently to put her shoes on each day.

devices (Figure 48-13) permits the patient to perform these skills and increases self-esteem and comfort.

The Restorative Environment

All patients benefit from living in an environment that attempts to improve the quality of life. The interdisciplinary team can help promote this environment:

- Give the patient a sense of control and opportunities to make decisions.
- Remember that mental and physical activity are essential to the patient's well-being.
- Encourage and assist patients to be well dressed and well groomed.
- Use touch freely in appropriate ways with patients.
- Provide cues for orientation throughout the building.
- Respect patients' identity, individuality, and privacy at all times.
- Respect and understand the patient's sexuality and need for intimacy.
- Give patients opportunities to help others.

A. LONG-HANDLED SHOEHORN

B. SHOE GRABBER AND SHOE HORN

C. STOCKING AID

D. TROUSER AID

E. DRESSING STICK

F. BUTTON LOOP

G. ZIPPER AID

FIGURE 48-12 Various adaptive devices enable patients to dress independently.

A. TOOTHBRUSH HOLDER TO APPLY TOOTHPASTE WITH ONLY ONE HAND

B. LONG-HANDLED SPONGE

C. LONG-HANDLED BRUSH AND COMB

D. COMBINATION NAIL CLIPPER AND FILE FOR ONE-HANDED USE

E. AEROSOL CAN ADAPTER WITH TRIGGER TO PUSH BUTTON

F. GROOMING AIDS WITH BUILT-UP HANDLES FOR EASIER GRIPPING

FIGURE 48-13 These devices enable the patient to be independent with grooming and personal hygiene.

- Encourage and assist patients to remain a part of the community.
- Create an environment that is safe, serene, and colorful.

Not all patients are candidates for restorative programs. For those who are not, the goals are to prevent complications and maintain remaining abilities as long as possible. Some patients reach the point where even maintenance is difficult. We are then basically concerned with preventing complications and maintaining the highest quality of life possible.

GUIDELINES *for*

Implementing Restorative Programs

- Know why the patient has the self-care deficit.
- Do the task at the normal time of day the task should be done. For example, most men shave in the morning. Do the task in the morning, not afternoon, or according to patient preference.
- Make the task part of the regular routine so it is purposeful. Avoid making it look like "busy work."
- Use the restorative care plan approaches each time the task must be done. Some tasks must be done multiple times each day.
- Keep your directions simple but not childish.
- Avoid distractions. Do the ADL in a private area.
- Be consistent. Read the care plan and follow the specific directions each time you work with the patient. The patient benefits from this consistency. When all staff use the same care plan approaches, the patient masters the task much faster.
- Use adaptive devices consistently and correctly.
- Do not show impatience. Be encouraging and give praise.
- Treat the patient with dignity at all times.
- Realize that the patient's progress may be uneven and inconsistent. Compliment the patient for making progress even if the gains are small.
- It is better for the patient to complete even part of a task than it is for you to do it. Allow the patient to do what she can, then finish the task without complaint. Avoid making the patient feel like a failure because she could not finish the task.

REVIEW

A. True/False.

Mark the following true or false by circling T or F.

1. T F Rehabilitation services are provided only in special hospitals.

2. T F OBRA regulations require that restorative services be provided to patients in skilled care facilities.

3. T F Rehabilitation and restorative services both strive to prevent complications.

4. T F Persons with disabilities will never recover their lost skills.

5. T F All persons with disabilities are considered to be handicapped.

B. Multiple Choice.

Select the one best answer for each of the following.

6. A patient with a permanent disability is
   a. taught to adapt to the present circumstances.
   b. not a good candidate for rehabilitation.
   c. given much sympathy.
   d. encouraged to be helpless.

7. Disabilities may result from
   a. too much exercise.
   b. getting inadequate sleep.
   c. spinal cord injury.
   d. not drinking enough water.

8. A patient who is unable to communicate verbally will be treated by a
   a. physical therapist.
   b. occupational therapist.
   c. nursing assistant.
   d. speech language pathologist.

9. Physical inactivity is *most likely* to cause
   a. pressure ulcers.
   b. dehydration.
   c. pain.
   d. infection.

10. Agnosia is a perceptual deficit in which the patient cannot
    a. organize a task.
    b. identify common items.
    c. sequence a task.
    d. initiate a task.

11. Adaptive devices are
    a. inappropriate for patients receiving rehabilitation.
    b. used by nursing assistants to feed patients.
    c. ordinary items modified for use by patients with self-care deficits.
    d. used only by occupational therapists.

12. Placing your hand over the patient's hand to guide the patient's actions is an approach called
    a. giving verbal cues.
    b. demonstration.
    c. hand-over-hand technique.
    d. setting up.

C. Completion.

Complete the statements by choosing the correct word from the following list.

activities of daily living	handicap
atrophy	mobility skills
contracture	physiatrist
disability	rehabilitation
disuse osteoporosis	self-care deficit
embolus	verbal cues
geriatric	

13. The process used to help a patient reach an optimal level of ability is _____.

14. Ambulation and transfers are examples of _____.

15. Dressing and undressing are examples of _____.

16. An impairment that affects the ability to perform an activity that a person of that age would normally be able to do is called a/an _____.

17. When the impairment limits or prevents the person from fulfilling a role that is normal for that person, a/an _____ exists.

18. A person who chooses to work with rehabilitation of the elderly is specializing in _____ rehabilitation.

19. A physician who specializes in rehabilitation is called a/an _____.

20. A/An _____ occurs when a joint is in a permanent state of flexion.

21. _____ occurs when a muscle shrinks and loses strength.

22. Physical inactivity can cause calcium to drain from the bones, resulting in _____.

23. A/An _____ is a blood clot that moves through the circulatory system.

24. A/An _____ exists when an adult cannot complete one or more activities of daily living.

25. Using short, simple phrases to prompt the patient to complete an activity of daily living is called _____.

D. Nursing Assistant Challenge.

You are working as a nursing assistant in the rehabilitation unit of a subacute care section of a skilled nursing facility. Think about what you have learned in this unit and answer the following questions:

26. What types of patients will you see?

27. What kinds of disabilities will the patients have?

28. What may be the cause of the self-care deficits experienced by your patients?

29. What kinds of problems can limit a patient's ability to do self-care?

30. What are the differences between rehabilitation and restorative care?

31. What are the responsibilities of the nursing assistant when giving restorative care?

UNIT 49

Obstetrical Patients and Neonates

OBJECTIVES

After completing this unit, you will be able to:

- Spell and define terms.
- Assist in prenatal care of the normal pregnant woman.
- List reportable observations of patients in the prenatal period.
- Define *doula* and identify the role and responsibilities of the doula as a member of the childbirth team.
- Assist in care of the normal postpartum patient.
- Properly change a perineal pad.
- Recognize reportable observations of patients in the postpartum period.

- Recognize reportable signs and symptoms of urine retention in the postpartum patient.
- Assist in care of the normal newborn.
- Demonstrate three methods of safely holding a baby.
- List measures to prevent inadvertent switching, misidentification, and abduction of infants.
- Assist in carrying out the discharge procedures for mother and infant.
- Demonstrate the following procedures:
  - Procedure 110 Changing a Diaper
  - Procedure 111 Bathing an Infant

VOCABULARY

Learn the meaning and the correct spelling of the following words and phrases:

amniocentesis	endoscope	involution	prenatal
amniotic fluid	engagement	isolette	quickening
amniotic sac	episiotomy	labor	rooming-in
Apgar score	expulsion stage	lactation	status
cesarean	fetal monitor	lochia	trimester
circumcision	fetoscopy	neonate	ultrasound
colostrum	fetus	obstetrical	umbilical cord
dilation stage	foreskin	placenta	vaginal examination
doula	fundus	placental stage	
efface	gestational age	postpartum	

INTRODUCTION

When a baby is ready to be born, it is normally upside down in the mother's uterus with its head toward the birth canal (Figure 49-1). Before the baby is born, it is known as a **fetus**. It is surrounded by a membranous bag

called an **amniotic sac**. The fetus floats in a liquid called **amniotic fluid**.

The fetus gets nourishment from the mother through the **umbilical cord**. The umbilical cord is attached to the fetus and the **placenta** (afterbirth). The placenta is attached to the wall of the mother's uterus.

After the baby is born and separated from the umbilical cord, the placenta, amniotic sac, and remaining cord are expelled as the afterbirth. After a period of time, the mother's uterus, or womb, which was greatly stretched to accommodate the pregnancy, will return to its normal size and shape.

There are three phases of pregnancy:

- **Prenatal** (before birth)
- Labor and delivery
- **Postpartum** (after birth)

The specially trained nursing assistant helps provide care and support throughout each phase.

PRENATAL CARE

The care of the mother begins in the prenatal period, when she first learns she is pregnant. You may meet her as you work in a doctor's office or in an **obstetrical** (pregnancy) clinic.

A normal pregnancy lasts about 280 days and is divided into **trimesters** (3 months). Each trimester is noted by specific signs and symptoms:

First trimester (1 through 12 weeks)

- Absence of menstrual period
- Nausea and vomiting (usually in the morning)
- Swelling and tenderness of breasts
- Frequent urination
- Constipation
- Positive pregnancy test within 7 to 10 days after conception
- Softening of uterus and cervix, and bluish color of vagina noted by examiner
- Increased vaginal secretions

Second trimester (13 through 27 weeks)

- Weight gain
- Abdominal enlargement

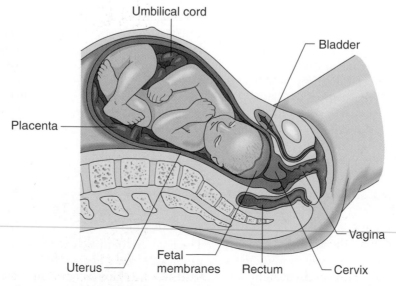

FIGURE 49-1 The usual position of the fetus at birth. This is known as the vertex position.

Clinical Information ALERT

A fetus acquires fingerprints at the age of 3 months. Fingerprints serve a purpose other than identification: they provide traction for the fingers to grasp things. ■

- Stretch marks may be noted on abdominal skin
- Breast enlargement—colostrum may be noted at about 20 weeks
- Hemorrhoids may be noted
- Uterus and fetus enlargement noted by examiner—mother will feel **quickening** (movements of fetus) about the 20th week

Clinical Information ALERT

The head is the widest part of the developing fetus's body. One in every 2,000 babies is born with a tooth. Babies are born with 300 bones. By adulthood, there are only 206 bones in the body. Humans have 46 chromosomes. Peas have 14 and crayfish have 200. ■

Third trimester (28th through 40th week)
- Mother feels occasional painless uterine contractions (the contractions are strengthening the uterus for labor)
- Uterus and fetus increase in size; this may cause indigestion, insomnia, and shortness of breath
- Mother may have backaches related to posture changes due to weight of fetus
- Edema of ankles may be present
- Varicose veins may appear

Care of the mother throughout pregnancy is important to ensure the birth of a healthy baby. The first trimester is an especially critical time. During the first 3 months, the fetus is very susceptible to the negative effects of tobacco, alcohol, caffeine, and other drugs, as well as to viruses and bacteria. Exposure to any of these may cause physical and/or mental harm to the developing fetus.

The pregnant woman is usually advised to visit the physician, nurse practitioner, or midwife at least once a month during the first trimester. During the first visit, the examiner will complete a very thorough history and physical examination, which will include:

- Routine information: age, occupation (to determine exposure to any hazards), education, race (some genetic diseases such as sickle cell anemia are found only in certain races), religion (this may affect mother's health care practices)
- History of menstruation, contraception, pregnancies
- Medical and family history
- Nutritional status
- Examination of fetus

Visits become more frequent as the pregnancy progresses (Figure 49-2). Routine procedures during the visits include:

- Weighing the mother
- Taking the blood pressure and pulse
- Urine testing
- Counseling and teaching the mother about diet, lifestyle, and signs and symptoms that she should report to the physician
- Palpating the abdomen to check fetal size
- Listening for fetal heart tones

You should call anything unusual to the attention of the nurse. Examples of items to report are:

- Complaints of persistent headache
- Elevated blood pressure
- Vaginal bleeding
- Complaints of dizziness
- Swelling of the hands and feet

PREPARATION FOR BIRTH

Both parents are encouraged to participate fully in the birth of their baby. Special training for the birth begins in the prenatal period. It prepares the parents to participate in the birthing process. Many parents elect to use natural childbirth. This technique of birthing:

FIGURE 49-2 This diagram shows approximate uterine height throughout the pregnancy.

- Allows the mother to be awake and fully participate in the birth.
- Encourages the father or an alternative support person to act as coach for the mother.
- Necessitates little, if any, pain-controlling medication. One of the most popular of these methods is called the Lamaze method.

Training Classes

In birth training classes:

- The father or some other person learns to act as a coach for the mother
- The mother learns ways of cooperating with her body during labor and delivery, using special breathing and relaxation techniques
- The couple sees films of the birth process
- Vaginal and cesarean deliveries are discussed
- There are opportunities to ask questions of a trained professional

PRENATAL TESTING

Congenital abnormalities (those present at birth) can sometimes be identified through prenatal testing. Testing methods include:

- **Ultrasound**—a technique of using sound waves to identify **gestational age** (time of development) and defects in the structure of fetal organs (Figure 49-3).
- **Amniocentesis**—a procedure in which a sterile needle is inserted into the fetal sac and cells are withdrawn for examination. Some genetic defects may be identified in this way.
- **Fetoscopy**—a direct visualization of the fetus in the uterus through a small visualization instrument (**endoscope**). Blood abnormalities may also be identified from samples of the fetal blood that is withdrawn.

LABOR AND DELIVERY

At the end of 40 weeks (within 2 weeks more or less), the signs of impending **labor** will be noted:

- **Engagement** or lightening (the fetus moves downward—sometimes referred to as "dropping")
- Mucous plug is expelled from cervix; the mucous plug is usually referred to as the "bloody show"
- Dilation of cervix begins
- Amniotic membranes may rupture just before actual labor begins, or may rupture during labor
- Uterine contractions begin
  - Irregular at first
  - Stronger, more regular, and closer together as labor progresses

The mother is taught during her pregnancy when she should go to the hospital.

The Doula

You may encounter patients who come to the hospital in labor accompanied by both the spouse and a **doula**. The

FIGURE 49-3 The ultrasound test is done to check fetal development and detect potential defects in development of fetal organs. (Courtesy of Jackson Community College, Jackson, MI)

word *doula* is derived from Greek, and means "woman's servant." Doulas have been available throughout history, but in the past decade there has been increasing awareness of their role and responsibilities in the birth process. They are represented by a large, active professional association and locator service. A doula may work for a physician or midwife. Some are self-employed. A few work for hospitals. They do not provide hands-on care or assist with clinical procedures. They are responsible for supporting and comforting the mother and enhancing communication between the mother and medical professionals. There are two types of doulas providing services to families during the childbirth process, although many doulas are qualified to do both jobs:

- A *birth doula* is trained and experienced to provide support and nurture the mother before, during, and just after childbirth. The doula also supports the patient's spouse or significant other during childbirth. The doula will remain with the patient throughout labor and birth. Many use CAM techniques, such as massage and relaxation, to comfort the mother.

- A *postpartum doula* nurtures the parents in their new roles. When working with a postpartum family, the role of the doula changes daily, as the needs of the family change. The doula does whatever the mother needs to help her care for and enjoy the new addition to the family. He or she makes sure the new mother takes in sufficient food and fluids. The doula also provides information about caring for the baby, breastfeeding, and related subjects. She makes sure the mother is comfortable. As the parents succeed and become confident in caring for the infant, the role of the doula decreases.

View doulas as members of the childbirth team. The doula is not a caregiver. He or she provides a valuable service to the mother and father during an exciting, but sometimes difficult and stressful, time.

Dilation

The **dilation** (opening) **stage** begins with the first regular uterine contractions. It ends when the cervix is fully dilated or opened. This may take 18 to 24 hours in a first pregnancy. The labor in each successive pregnancy is often shorter. An exception is when five or more years pass between the first and second pregnancies. In this case, the second labor may be as long as the first, but it is seldom longer.

As the labor progresses, the cervix also thins (**effaces**) so that the fetus may move downward into the birth canal and out of the mother's body. The degree of dilation at any given time is measured by the nurse or physician. The nurse or physician places a gloved finger in the patient's vagina and measures (approximately) the size of the cervical opening and amount of effacement. This procedure is called **vaginal examination**.

Relief of Discomfort

Drugs may be given to the mother in the labor and delivery phase to reduce pain. When anesthesia is used, the patient will not feel an episiotomy or its repair, but she will still be able to move her legs. The type of pain relief given to the mother during labor and delivery determines the postpartum care she will receive.

Fetal Monitors

In most hospitals, a **fetal monitor** (instrument to check the well-being of the baby during labor) (Figure 49-4) is attached either to the mother's abdomen or to the baby's head.

Culture ALERT

Women who are members of the Latter Day Saints Church may wear a special one-piece undergarment. This garment has very special religious significance. It should not be cut for emergency childbirth, if at all possible. Many Mormons believe this garment must touch their bodies at all times. Ask the mother how she wants the garment handled, and respect her wishes. ■

Expulsion

Expulsion stage is the period extending from the point of full cervical dilation until the baby is delivered. This may be 1 to 2 hours or more.

The baby moves down the birth canal. The mother is encouraged to help the process by "bearing down" with

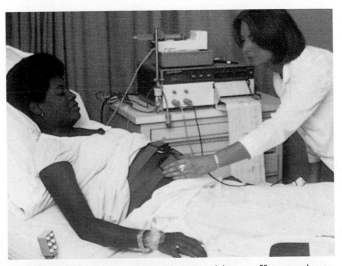

FIGURE 49-4 The fetal monitor enables staff to evaluate the infant's condition during labor. (Courtesy of Memorial Medical Center of Long Beach, CA)

her abdominal muscles with each contraction. Figure 49-5 and shows the baby being assisted in delivery and rotated as the shoulders are presented.

During delivery, it may be necessary to enlarge the vaginal opening. This is done by making a cut in the perineum. The cut is called an **episiotomy** (Figure 49-6) The episiotomy is sutured (sewn up) after delivery.

Forceps may be used at this stage to assist in delivery of the head. Once delivered, the baby is held head down to clear the respiratory tract. The baby is then usually placed on the mother's abdomen while the cord is clamped and cut.

Placental Stage

The **placental stage** lasts from delivery of the baby through the delivery of the placenta (Figure 49-7). This is a short period. The placenta is usually delivered within an hour of delivery of the baby.

In this stage, the placenta separates from the wall of the uterus. Uterine contractions push it downward and out through the birth canal. After delivery of the placenta:

FIGURE 49-7 The placenta is delivered.

- If an episiotomy was needed, it is repaired.
- The mother's uterus is checked for firmness. Drugs may be given to help it contract to control bleeding.
- Both mother and child are identified with name tags (Figure 49-8) before being separated.
- The baby is footprinted (Figure 49-9) along with the mother's thumbprint.
- The baby's eyes are treated to prevent infection (Figure 49-10).

FIGURE 49-5 The baby's head emerges.

FIGURE 49-6 An episiotomy may be done to prevent tearing of the perineum.

FIGURE 49-8 The mother and infant are given identifying bands. In some hospitals, fathers are also given an identification band. This is a security feature to reduce the risk of an infant abduction.

FIGURE 49-9 The infant's footprints are taken soon after delivery.

FIGURE 49-10 Silver nitrate is placed in the eyes to reduce the risk of infection that the infant may have contracted during the birthing process.

In most hospitals today, the labor, delivery, and postpartum (period after delivery) care are all carried out in the same room. Keeping the newborn in the same room with the mother is called **rooming-in.** The baby can be taken to the nursery if the mother has complications or is unable to rest with the baby in the room. The usual length of stay for the new mother and baby is about 2 days, unless there are complications. After the mother has recovered from anesthesia and any medications that were given during labor, she is encouraged to do as much self-

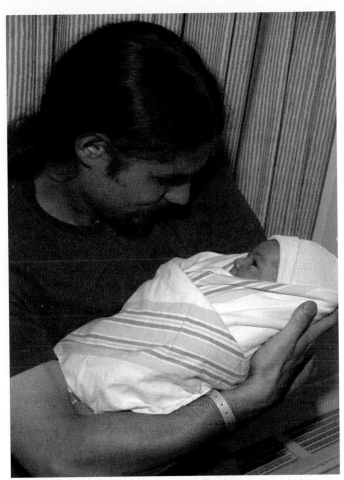

FIGURE 49-11 The father is getting to know the infant. Note the father's identification band.

care as possible. She is allowed to get out of bed soon after delivery if there are no complications.

The father or another supportive person who has attended the prenatal classes with the pregnant woman is encouraged to participate in the labor, delivery, and care of the newborn. The baby's siblings, grandparents, and other family members are allowed to visit during the postpartum period and to hold and love the baby (Figure 49-11). Many hospitals serve the new parents a special, private meal the evening before discharge.

In the last several years there has been a trend toward:

- Making the delivery a family affair
- Having the delivery take place at home or in a home-like environment
- Continuing to provide for the safety of both mother and infant

CESAREAN BIRTH

Cesarean section is another way of delivering a baby. The baby is delivered through an incision in the abdomen rather than through the birth canal. Between 20 and 30% of all births in the United States occur in this way.

A spinal or epidural anesthetic is administered before the surgery. This type of procedure introduces drugs into the cerebrospinal fluid and blocks sensation from the upper abdomen down to the toes. Until the anesthetic wears off, the patient will not be able either to feel or move her legs.

After the delivery, the mother sometimes is given a general anesthetic that allows her to sleep during the rest of the procedure.

Cesarean deliveries may be performed when there is:

- Fetal distress
- A preterm infant
- Breech (non-headfirst) presentation
- Prolonged rupture of the membranes
- Prolapsed cord
- Genital herpes
- Premature separation of the placenta
- Placenta previa
- Failure of labor to progress
- A mother who has already had a cesarean section

The incision in the abdominal wall may be:

- Vertical, along the midplane
- Transverse, across the lowest and narrowest part of the abdomen (bikini cut)

The mother's coach or partner is encouraged to be in the operative area to offer emotional support while the cesarean is being done. The same basic activities are carried out in the operating room as are followed after a vaginal delivery.

After the surgery is complete, the baby is usually admitted to the nursery (Figure 49-12). The mother is moved to the recovery room for immediate postanesthesia care. If the infant is in distress, she will be taken to the neonatal intensive care unit (Figure 49-13).

FIGURE 49-12 Babies are transported in their own bassinets from the delivery room to the nursery. (Courtesy of Memorial Medical Center of Long Beach, CA)

FIGURE 49-13 This infant has been moved to the neonatal intensive care unit. The eyes are covered to protect them. (Courtesy of Memorial Medical Center of Long Beach, CA)

POSTPARTUM CARE

You may be assigned to assist in caring for the mother during the postpartum period.

With other team members, you will assist the mother from the stretcher into bed. A protective pad (bed protector or incontinent pad; may be called a "blue pad" or Chux) may be placed under the patient's buttocks.

Always wear gloves and follow standard precautions when caring for the postpartum patient. There is a high probability of contact with blood, mucous membranes, urine, and breast milk. All of these body fluids are considered potentially infectious.

Safety ALERT

You may be assigned to monitor patients' vital signs immediately after delivery, and every 2 to 4 hours after that. Position the mother in the same position each time. After childbirth, it is not unusual for the blood pressure to drop when the mother changes position from lying to sitting or sitting to standing. For safety, monitor the mother for dizziness during position changes. ■

Anesthesia

If an anesthetic was used, follow the procedures for postoperative care of surgical patients (Unit 29).

- Keep the patient flat on her back.
- Make sure the patient has a fresh gown and clean bed linen.

- Check blood pressure, pulse, and respirations as ordered until the patient is stable.
- Continue to monitor vital signs every 4 hours for 24 hours.
- If the patient complains of being cold, an extra blanket may provide comfort. If the patient does not become comfortable, inform the nurse.
- Record the first voiding. Inform the nurse if the patient has not voided by the end of your shift.

Drainage

Carefully check the condition of the perineum and the perineal pad for the amount and color of drainage.

- When removing the pad, always lift it away from the body from front to back.
- Red vaginal discharge, called **lochia**, is expected. *Lochia rubra* is the name given to the discharge that occurs during the first 3 days after delivery. The amount of discharge and any clotting should be reported.

Clinical Information ALERT

If the patient has been in bed for a long time, lochia pools in the vagina. When the patient stands, she may have very heavy flow. This is normal. Exercising vigorously will also increase the flow. If the flow is heavy, inform the nurse. ■

Initially, the lochia is bright red and moderate in amount (Figure 49-14). Over the next week, the lochia will lessen and become pink to pink-brown in color. A discharge that is yellowish-white or brown may continue for 1 to 3 weeks after delivery and then stop. Note and report:

- Signs of tenderness
- Signs of inflammation
- Presence of an episiotomy
- Presence of large blood clots
- Foul-smelling lochia
- Saturation of a pad in 15 to 30 minutes (Figure 49-15)

FIGURE 49-14 Moderate lochia is normal during the first few days.

FIGURE 49-15 Heavy lochia must be promptly reported to the nurse.

Clinical Information ALERT

Notify the nurse if the patient complains of severe pain on the perineum. This may be a symptom of complications. The patient may also be restless, lean to the side when sitting, or be unable to find a comfortable position. If a complication has developed, the signs and symptoms may seem out of proportion to the injury to the perineum. ■

The Uterus

The size and firmness of the uterus should be checked and reported. A soft and enlarging uterus indicates excessive bleeding.

Massaging. The top of the uterus, the **fundus**, is massaged in a circular fashion while the opposite hand is held against the pubic bone (Figure 49-16). Massaging the fundus stimulates the uterine muscles to contract, firming the uterus.

Measuring Height of Uterus. The level of the fundus is measured by placing the fingers lengthwise across the abdomen between the fundus and the navel. On the first postpartal day, the level of the fundus is usually at the umbilicus or one to two fingers'-width below.

FIGURE 49-16 Both hands are used to massage the fundus.

Cramping. As the uterus begins to return to its normal size (**involution**), the patient may experience strong uterine contractions or cramps. Cramping may also be associated with breast feeding. This is normal, but be sure to report any complaints of pain to the nurse, who can administer medication for relief.

Voiding

The new mother should be encouraged to void within the first 6 to 8 hours after the delivery. Check carefully for signs of urine retention. These include:

- A uterus that is unusually high or pushed to one side
- Swelling just above the pubis
- Complaints of urgency (the need to void), but with voidings of 200 mL or less

Be sure to report:

- Signs of possible urine retention immediately, so the patient's recovery will not be impeded
- Any inability to void within the first 8 hours postpartum
- Voidings of less than 100 mL

This is important because a full bladder can cause postpartum hemorrhage.

TOILETING AND PERINEAL CARE

The mother may be:

- Provided with a squeezable bottle filled with warm tap water.
- Instructed to rinse the genitals and perineum after voiding or defecating.
- Instructed to gently pat, not wipe, the perineal area containing the stitches with tissue or special medicated pads—once only, from front to back. The tissue is discarded in the toilet.
- Taught to wash her hands before applying a fresh perineal pad.
- Taught not to touch the inside of the perineal pad.

Infection Control ALERT

Peri pads are normally packaged in sterile containers. Teach the mother to handle the pad only on the ends. She should avoid touching the center part of the pad, so that the part that contacts the perineum remains sterile. ■

If the perineum is very uncomfortable:

- Specially medicated pads may be used for cleansing. The procedure is always the same—front to back and discard.

- Anesthetic sprays may be ordered.
- Ice packs may be used to reduce edema and relieve discomfort.

Infection Control ALERT

Infection occurs in about 6% of all postpartum patients. When assisting patients with toileting, have the patient stand up before flushing the toilet. This prevents spraying with contaminated water. Inform the nurse promptly if a patient has an elevated temperature, chills, foul-smelling lochia, or other signs and symptoms of infection. ■

Patients should be cautioned to apply anesthetics and ointments after cleansing. The nurse will give the mother a can of topical anesthetic spray and instruct her how to use it to reduce discomfort from the episiotomy.

Sitting may be uncomfortable when an episiotomy has been performed. Instruct the mother to squeeze her buttocks together and hold them in this position until she is seated upright. This reduces tension on the suture line.

BREAST CARE

The mother's first milk is called **colostrum**. The colostrum:

- Is watery.
- Carries protective antibodies to the child.
- Usually begins to flow about 12 hours after delivery. **Lactation**, the flow of milk, does not begin until the second or third postpartum day.

Keeping the breasts clean is especially important when the mother is planning to breast-feed her baby.

- The mother's hands and nipples should be washed just prior to feeding the baby.
- During the shower, the mother should wash the breasts, using a circular motion from the nipples outward.
- Creams are sometimes used between feedings to help the nipples remain supple.
- Breast pads absorb milk leakage. They should be changed frequently.
- The breasts should be supported by a well-fitted brassiere.

Even if the mother chooses not to breast-feed, the breasts should be washed daily with soap and water. The breasts should also be supported continuously by a well-fitted brassiere. Medication to suppress milk production is sometimes ordered.

When delivery is uncomplicated, mothers and healthy newborns do not stay in the hospital very long. They are usually able to go home within 2 days.

GUIDELINES *for*
Assisting with Breast-Feeding

A recent trend holds that "the breast is best," and many mothers elect to breast-feed their newborns. Assist the mother by:

- Instructing her to wash the nipples and areolae with clear water on a cotton ball before nursing. She should begin at the nipple, working outward in a circular motion.

- Helping to position the baby. The football hold (Figure 49-17A) or cradle hold (Figure 49-17B) is usually easiest.

- Gently stroking the infant's cheek near the mouth to get the baby to open the mouth and turn toward the breast.

- Instructing the mother to place the nipple and areola into the baby's mouth. The infant should begin to suck and swallow.

- Checking the position of the breast. Advise the mother to press and hold the breast back, if necessary, so it does not obstruct the baby's nose.

- Allowing the baby to nurse for 5 to 7 minutes, if he or she has not stopped by then.
  - If the infant has not stopped nursing, avoid pulling it from the breast. Break the infant's suction by placing a finger into the side of the mouth and moving the breast. Instruct the mother to burp the infant.

- Switching to the other breast after the infant has burped. Help the mother reposition the infant and get the baby started nursing on the opposite breast.

- The infant should stop nursing when he or she is full. Have the mother burp the baby again.

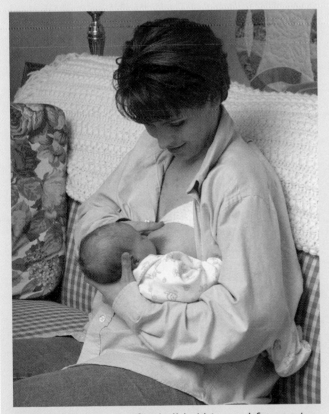

FIGURE 49-17A The football hold is used for nursing and other activities when the baby must be supported well, such as when washing the hair.

FIGURE 49-17B The cradle hold is also a comfortable position for nursing.

NEONATAL CARE

After the newborn is admitted to the nursery, some procedures not carried out in the delivery room are completed.

The physician or nurse will examine the baby and make an evaluation of the baby's condition, or **status**.

Apgar Scoring

The **Apgar score** is an evaluation of the **neonate**. It is made at 1 minute, 5 minutes, and 10 minutes after birth. The areas evaluated are:

- Heart rate
- Respiratory effort
- Muscle tone
- Reflex, irritability
- Color

A number value is applied to each assessment and recorded on a special form. For example, the neonate who has a heart rate of less than 100, has slow respirations, offers slight resistance to limb extension, has a weak cry, and is pale and cyanotic would be rated as follows:

Heart rate	1
Respiratory effort	1
Muscle tone	1
Reflex, irritability	1
Color	0
Total	4

Totals indicate the infant's condition. A score of 7 to 10 indicates that the infant is in good condition. A score of 4 to 6 indicates a fair condition. A score of 0 to 4 indicates a poor condition.

Care of the Newborn Infant

In the nursery, the baby's vital signs are determined. Measurements of length and weight are also taken. The infant's axillary temperature is monitored and recorded every 30 to 60 minutes until stable, then every 4 hours or according to the nurse's instructions.

When the newborn's status becomes stable:

- If the eyes were not treated with silver nitrate drops or antibiotics in the delivery room, or the footprints were not taken, these procedures are done at this time.

- The baby is cleaned. Sometimes an admission bath using an antiseptic soap or oil is administered, but procedures for bathing newborns vary from hospital to hospital. In some hospitals, the bath is omitted and the cheesy material known as *vernix caseosa* is allowed to remain on the skin. The area around the umbilical cord is carefully cleaned with a solution prescribed by the facility (Figure 49-18).

- The baby must be kept warm because a newborn's temperature has not yet stabilized. The baby is dressed according to facility policy. A stockinette cap is placed on the head because much body heat can be lost through this surface.

- The baby is placed in a crib or **isolette** (Figure 49-19).

- Feeding is not usually started for 4 to 6 hours after birth. During these hours, the baby is monitored and observed carefully for successful, independent life. After 4 to 6 hours, the baby is either taken to breast-feed or started on feedings of glucose and water. Babies whose mothers are unable to feed them will be fed in the nursery.

- Male babies may be circumcised before discharge. In **circumcision**, the excess tissue (**foreskin**) is cut from the tip of the penis (Figure 49-20). This procedure is usually performed based on the parents' personal choices, as well as cultural, ethnic, and religious traditions. For members of some faiths, circumcision is a religious ceremony performed at another location within the first few weeks of life.

- Babies who are jaundiced may have their eyes protected and be placed under a special light (bili light) to help clear the levels of bilirubin in the skin.

Handling the Infant

Take care when lifting, carrying, and positioning an infant. Remember to:

- Lift the baby by grasping the legs securely with one hand while slipping the other hand under the baby's

FIGURE 49-18 The cord is carefully cleaned to cause it to dry and to prevent infection.

FIGURE 49-19 Some babies are cared for in the controlled environment of the isolette. (Courtesy of Memorial Medical Center of Long Beach, CA)

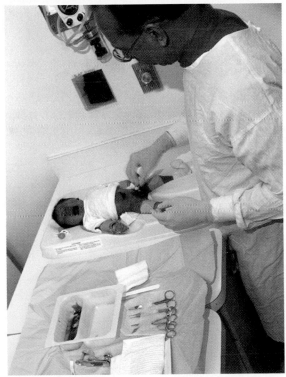

FIGURE 49-20 The infant is circumcised shortly after birth at the parents' request.

FIGURE 49-21A Always support the infant's bottom and neck.

FIGURE 49-21B Shoulder hold

back to support the head and neck (Figures 49-21A and 49-21B). You may also use the cradle hold or football hold.

- Hold the baby securely.
- Support the head, neck, and back at all times.
- Back through doorways when carrying a baby.
- Never turn your back on an infant when the infant is on an unprotected surface.

PKU Test

The baby's blood is tested to detect the presence of phenylketonuria (PKU). PKU is a congenital, hereditary abnormality. It may lead to mental retardation if undetected and not treated early. In PKU, normal protein digestion is not possible. The disorder cannot be cured, but it can be controlled by a special diet.

Eye Care

The first eye treatment is performed by the nurse. Silver nitrate ($AgNO_3$) in a 1% solution is commonly used, but other medications such as antibiotics may be ordered.

Elimination

The passage of urine and stool in a newborn infant are important observations. A normal newborn will urinate

FIGURE 49-22A The first stools are meconium stools.

FIGURE 49-22B A yellow stool from a breast-fed infant

6 to 10 times a day. Elimination activity is recorded and the color of stool documented. Stools should change from dark, meconium stools (Figure 49-22A) to brown-yellow, pasty transitional stools, then finally to yellow stools that are slightly loose (Figure 49-22B).

Postcircumcision Care

The circumcision should be checked each time the diaper is changed and should be a routine part of that care. Observe the incision site for bleeding and report anything

PROCEDURE

CHANGING A DIAPER

1. Carry out initial procedure actions.

2. Assemble equipment:
   - Clean diaper
   - Gloves
   - Plastic bag or container for trash
   - Damp washcloths, wipes, or cotton balls for cleansing
   - Mild soap, if used
   - Supplies for cord care and/or circumcision care, according to facility policy

3. Remove the soiled diaper and observe for color, consistency, and quantity of elimination.

4. Roll the soiled diaper so the clean outer side faces out. Put it in the trash or place it out of reach of the infant.

5. Cleanse the diaper area with wipes or a damp washcloth. Clean from the front toward the back

in a female infant, and from the tip of the penis toward the scrotum for a male infant. Cleanse all folds of the groin and anus. Discard the wipes or washcloth.

6. Lift the buttocks with one hand and slide the new, open diaper underneath.

7. Pull the diaper between the legs. Fold the top edge of the diaper down so it is positioned under the umbilical cord. Fasten the tape snugly on each side.

8. Perform cord care with alcohol or antiseptic according to facility policy.

9. Change other clothing, blanket, or crib linen if soiled or wet.

10. Discard the soiled diaper and your gloves, if not done previously.

11. Carry out ending procedure actions.

unusual. The crib identification should note the new circumcision. A note should also be included on the nursery record as to the condition of the circumcision and first voiding after circumcision.

Bathing the Infant

The infant may be bathed after the temperature has stabilized. Bathing is done daily, and as needed. The nurse will teach the parents how to bathe the infant as part of the discharge instructions.

SECURITY

All infants must be identified to prevent inadvertent switching, misidentification, and abduction. The nurse will

Difficult SITUATIONS

Babies are normally dressed in a long-sleeved T-shirt and a diaper. They are covered with a receiving blanket, and often have a stockinette cap covering the head. Despite these measures, some newborns have trouble maintaining temperature. This is especially problematic with premature infants. To keep a newborn warm, add a second long-sleeved T-shirt over the diaper. Place the baby's legs in the armholes and pull up the shirt to create leggings. ■

PROCEDURE

BATHING AN INFANT

Note: Before beginning the procedure, check with the nurse to make sure the infant's temperature is stable enough for bathing. Keep the infant warm throughout the procedure.

1. Carry out initial procedure actions.

2. Assemble equipment:
   - Clean diaper
   - Gloves (if this is the infant's first bath, wear gloves for the entire procedure; change them before contact with mucous membranes or nonintact skin, according to the principles of standard precautions)
   - Washbasin with warm water (98°F to 100°F)
   - Plastic bag or container for trash
   - Washcloths (2–3)
   - Towel
   - Cotton balls
   - Liquid infant cleanser/shampoo
   - Supplies for cord care and/or circumcision care, according to facility policy
   - Blankets
   - Sheet

3. Place the infant in a bassinet with sides. Arrange the supplies within reach.

4. Check the infant's skin for dryness, peeling, or signs of infection. If present, notify the nurse and obtain instructions for care.

5. Check the site of the umbilical cord for redness, drainage, drying, and bleeding. If present, notify the nurse and obtain instructions for care.

6. Remove the infant's clothing. Cover the infant with a blanket for warmth.

7. Moisten a cotton ball with plain water. Cleanse the eye from inner to outer canthus, in one wipe. Repeat with a new cotton ball for the other eye.

8. Wash the external ears with plain water and a cotton ball or twisted end of the washcloth.

9. Make a mitt with the washcloth. Wash the face and neck with plain water, with attention to areas behind the ears and creases in the neck.

10. Pat the face and neck dry with a towel.

11. Pull the blanket down to expose the upper body.

12. Cleanse the upper body with soap and a washcloth. Rinse soap from the hands quickly, then rinse the remainder of the upper body. Pat dry with a towel.

13. Cleanse the area around the umbilicus. Rinse the area. Keep the cord dry. Pat dry. Follow the nurse's instructions for cord care.

continues

PROCEDURE 111 CONTINUED

14. Cover the upper body with the blanket. Pull blanket up to expose the lower body.

15. Wash the legs and outer buttocks with soap and water. Rinse well and pat dry.

16. Obtain a fresh washcloth.

17. Cleanse the genitalia with plain water.
    - *Female infant:*
      - Spread labia gently. Wash from front to back toward the anus. Turn the washcloth so a separate part is used for each wipe.
      - Wash the remaining portions of the labia and the folds in the groin.
      - Rinse and pat dry.
    - *Uncircumcised male infant:*
      - Avoid retracting the foreskin.
      - Wash from the urethra outward, then down toward the scrotum.
      - Wash the remaining portions of the scrotum and the folds in the groin.
      - Rinse and pat dry.
    - *Circumcised male infant:*
      - Care for the circumcision according to the nurse's instructions.
      - Check for bleeding.
      - Gently cleanse the area with warm water and cotton balls.
      - Apply petroleum jelly gauze dressing, or according to facility policy.

18. Cleanse the anal area with soap. Rinse and pat dry.

19. Diaper the infant.

20. Wrap the infant in the blanket.

21. Pick up the infant, using the football hold. Hold the head over the basin.

22. Wet the scalp well with a washcloth and water.

23. Lather and gently wash the scalp with baby shampoo or gentle cleanser.

24. Rinse the scalp by pouring water from a small cup over the scalp and into the washbasin, or rinse well using a washcloth.

25. Pat dry.

26. Comb the infant's hair. Cover the head, according to facility policy.

27. Dress the infant.

28. Replace the damp blanket and sheets.

29. Carry out ending procedure actions.

Difficult SITUATIONS

When bathing a newborn for the first time after delivery, you may have trouble rinsing blood from the hair. Apply a solution of 1 tablespoon of baby oil to 2 tablespoons of water to wet hair. Slowly comb the hair with a soft baby comb. Blood is easily removed and the infant will have clean and shiny hair. ■

Safety ALERT

Your facility will issue photo identification to all personnel working in the maternity department. Many staff do not like others to see their pictures, so they turn the card around so only the back side shows. This is an unsafe practice that most likely violates hospital policy. Wear your identification badge on your upper body, with the picture on the front side. The hospital will inform mothers that they must request to see the worker's identification badge if someone tries to remove the infant from the room for any reason. ■

apply identification bands to the infant's wrist and ankle while in the delivery room. The mother is given a matching wrist band. In some facilities, the father is also given a wrist band. The identification bands must be checked each time the infant is brought to the mother for feeding or rooming-in. Crib cards and other documents are also used for infant identification. Each facility has policies for checking identification. In some, the identification is also checked at the beginning and end of each shift.

Infant Abduction

Unfortunately, a number of infant abductions occur each year. Nursing personnel will be expected to wear an identification badge. Reinforce your identity and position to the mothers each time you provide care. The mother will be instructed not to hand the infant over to someone she does not know. Hospitals have various security measures in place to prevent abduction. Some apply magnetic-sensor ankle bands in the delivery room, similar to an anti-shoplifting device. An alarm will sound if the infant is removed from the unit. A few are using global tracking systems (GPS). The mother's written permission may be required for other friends or relatives to hold or feed the infant. If the infant must be transported to another area of the hospital, nursing staff must remain with the child, then return the child to the original location.

Each hospital has a policy and procedure to follow in the event of an infant abduction. You must become familiar with the procedures to follow in case this occurs. Taking a proactive position is best, however. Be aware of safety and security measures, and practice them daily.

DISCHARGE

To carry out the discharge procedure from a facility:

- Match the baby's identification with the mother's.
- Dress the child in his or her own clothing (Figure 49-23). This may be done in the nursery or in the mother's room.
- Wrap the baby in a blanket, using the technique of "papoosing," as shown in Figures 49-24A through 49-24D.
- Check to be sure that the mother has received and understands any special discharge instructions. If not, inform the nurse.

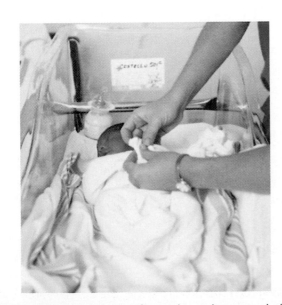

FIGURE 49-23 Dress the infant in his or her own clothing.

- Check to be sure equipment or needed formula is ready when the parents and newborn are ready to go home (Figure 49-25).
- Transport the mother, carrying her baby, by wheelchair to the discharge area. Make sure the infant is strapped into a properly secured car seat. Stay with them until they leave.
- Record the discharge information on the charts of both mother and child. Include the condition of each and the time of release.

FIGURE 49-24A Position the receiving blanket under the infant so the corners are at the head and feet. Bring the bottom corner up over the infant.

FIGURE 49-24B Fold one side corner over the infant.

FIGURE 49-24C Bring the corner from the other side over the infant.

FIGURE 49-24D Tuck the final corner under the infant, who is now ready for discharge.

FIGURE 49-25 Parents prepare to leave the hospital with the newborn.

Home Care

The discharged mother faces many new challenges. It will take approximately 6 weeks for her reproductive organs to recover. Home care of the mother includes:

- Providing adequate nutrition
- Allowing for sufficient rest
- Attending to proper elimination
- Providing emotional support during any transitory depression
- Providing breast care, if she is nursing the baby

REVIEW

A. True/False.

Mark the following true or false by circling T or F.

1. T F You are responsible for noting and reporting the first postpartal voiding.

2. T F Care of the mother begins in the prenatal period.

3. T F The nurse or physician monitors the progress of labor by performing a vaginal examination.

4. T F Immediate postpartum lochia should be yellowish-white.

5. T F Massaging the cervix stimulates the uterine muscles to contract.

6. T F A congenital abnormality is one that is present at birth.

7. T F Ultrasound is a technique used to examine the baby before birth.

8. T F In the first pregnancy, the period of labor and delivery called expulsion lasts 18 to 24 hours.

9. T F As labor progresses, the uterine cervix becomes more and more tightened.

10. T F The shoulder hold is a safe way to hold and support an infant.

11. T F The first feeding for the newborn is usually given 12 hours after birth.

12. T F The mother's hands and nipples should be washed before she nurses the baby.

B. Matching.

Choose the correct term from Column II to match each phrase in Column I.

Column I

13. _____ surgery to remove the foreskin

14. _____ maintains an even temperature for the fetus

15. _____ mother's first postpartum breast secretions

16. _____ attachment between baby and placenta

17. _____ vaginal discharge following delivery

Column II

a. lochia

b. umbilical cord

c. fundus

d. lactation

e. colostrum

f. circumcision

g. vernix caseosa

h. isolette

i. placenta

C. Nursing Assistant Challenge.

You are working in a prenatal clinic for a nurse practitioner. One of the patients is Mrs. McDonnel, who is coming in today for her first appointment. She tells you she has missed two menstrual periods. Answer the following questions.

18. What signs and symptoms do you expect to see today and for the next month or so?

19. Because this is the patient's first visit, what equipment and supplies do you need to have ready for the nurse practitioner?

20. What signs and symptoms will you observe during the second trimester?

21. What signs and symptoms will you observe during the third trimester?

22. Which procedures would be completed at each visit?

23. What statements by the patient would you report immediately?

Pediatric Patients

OBJECTIVES

After completing this unit, you will be able to:

- Spell and define terms.
- Describe how to foster growth and development of hospitalized pediatric patients.
- Describe how to maintain a safe environment for the pediatric patient.
- Discuss the problem of childhood obesity and identify special problems and complications that occur as a result of this condition.
- Discuss the role of parents and siblings of the hospitalized pediatric patient.
- Demonstrate the following procedures:
  - Procedure 112 Admitting a Pediatric Patient

- Procedure 113 Weighing the Pediatric Patient
- Procedure 114 Changing Crib Linens
- Procedure 115 Changing Crib Linens (Infant in Crib)
- Procedure 116 Measuring Temperature
- Procedure 117 Determining Heart Rate (Pulse)
- Procedure 118 Counting Respiratory Rate
- Procedure 119 Measuring Blood Pressure
- Procedure 120 Bottle-Feeding an Infant
- Procedure 121 Burping an Infant
- Procedure 122 Collecting a Urine Specimen from an Infant

VOCABULARY

Learn the meaning and the correct spelling of the following words and phrases:

adolescence	developmental mile-	foster parent	regress
adoptive parent	stones	initiative	stepparent
autonomy	developmental tasks	legal custody	
biological parent	family	legal guardian	

INTRODUCTION

Children, like adults, get sick and need hospitalization for diagnosis and treatment of their illnesses. But children are different. They are not just small adults. Children differ in age, size, and developmental level. When you work with children, you will also be working with their parents or those responsible for their upbringing. When a child is sick and hospitalized, the illness affects the entire family.

The family is an important part of the child's life regardless of the child's age.

In today's society, the words *parents* and *family* can have different meanings. A child may live with one or both parents. The words *biological*, *adoptive*, *foster*, and *step* refer to the various types of parents that may be part of a child's family. The terms are defined as follows:

- **Biological parent**—birth (genetic) parent

- **Adoptive parent**—person who has legally assumed responsibility for parenting
- **Foster parent**—person who carries out parenting duties under the authority of a legal agency
- **Stepparent**—person who assumes the parenting role by marrying a birth or adoptive parent

Families may also include combinations of parents. For example, a child may live with a biological father and an adoptive mother or stepmother. Or a child may live with a single parent, who could be either biological, adoptive, or foster. Other family arrangements may include the child living with a relative while the parent maintains legal custody of the child. **Legal custody** refers to the person who has the right to give consent for hospitalization and for the procedures that may be needed while the child is hospitalized. This person is known as the **legal guardian**. The child may live with someone other than the legal guardian.

The word **family** refers to the household unit in which the child lives. Members of the family may include the parents, siblings (biological, adoptive, or step), and/or other relatives or persons in the household.

As a member of the health care team, it is important for you to identify the child's caretakers as well as the person who has legal custody. Depending on the child's age, some hospitals require at least one family member to remain at the hospital during the child's stay. This person may be required to stay in the room at all times, and cannot leave the child alone.

This unit provides guidelines for care of the hospitalized child. The nursing assistant must recognize that hospitalization may interrupt the child's normal growth and development. This is a traumatic time for the child. Suggestions are given to show how the nursing assistant can assist and encourage the child's development during hospitalization.

Safety is an important part of providing care. This unit presents guidelines for creating a safe environment for each pediatric age group. Because families are important, suggestions are also made on creating a family-centered approach to pediatric health care.

PEDIATRIC UNITS

Pediatric units are typically set up in one of two ways:

1. By specific age groups of children
2. By types of patient, such as surgical, orthopedic, cardiac, and so on

Regardless of the ages of the children, working in pediatrics offers many rewards and challenges.

When a child is admitted to the hospital, you may be involved in the admission procedure. A nurse will obtain a medical and social history from the parents. Information obtained will include the child's nickname, the ages and names of siblings, the child's likes and dislikes, and normal times and routines for meals, naps, and bedtimes. Any information that will make the child's hospital stay easier is marked in the history. Once the history is complete, you can continue with the admission procedure (Figure 50-1).

This unit gives guidelines for caring for children by age groups. The groups are:

- Infancy (0–1 year)
- Toddler (1–3 years)
- Preschooler (3–6 years)
- School-age (6–12 years)
- Adolescent (12–18 years)

DEVELOPMENTAL TASKS

For each age group, it is expected that the child will have reached a certain developmental level. Each level is characterized by physical and psychological tasks that the average child in the group can perform. Review the developmental tasks for the pediatric age group in Unit 9. If you understand the **developmental tasks** for each age group, it will be easier to find ways to encourage the child's development during hospitalization. The approaches suggested here should be personalized for each patient. Some children may appear younger than their stated age due to medical and/or emotional problems. It is also normal for children to **regress** (go backward) when hospitalized.

CARING FOR INFANTS (BIRTH–1 YEAR)

During the first year of life, the normal infant will:
- Double her birth length
- Triple her birth weight
- Show progress in gaining mastery over gross motor behavior, beginning with the head and moving down the trunk toward the feet

FIGURE 50-1 Make the child feel comfortable during the admission process.

PROCEDURE

ADMITTING A PEDIATRIC PATIENT

1. Carry out initial procedure actions.

2. Introduce yourself and escort child and parents to the child's room and familiarize them with unit.

3. Explain what you will do.

4. Wash your hands.

5. Place an identification band on the child.

6. Dress the child in his own pajamas or hospital clothing.

7. Obtain the child's height and weight. Record according to hospital policy.

8. Measure the child's vital signs.

9. Obtain a urine specimen.

10. Wash your hands.

11. Assist the physician or nurse with examination of the child as necessary.

12. Explain rooming-in and visiting policies to the parents. Comfort the child if parents leave.

13. Carry out ending procedure actions.

The normal infant begins by gaining head control. The infant then progresses to rolling over, sitting up, crawling, and walking. These motor skills generally occur within specific weeks or months of the infant's life. Achievement of these skills is referred to as reaching the infant's **developmental milestones**.

Learning to trust is the primary psychosocial developmental task for the infant. All infants depend on others for survival; others must meet all their basic needs. How the infant's needs are met lays the foundation for the infant's developing personality.

Normally, the mother is the caregiver and prime source for developing trust. However, when the infant is hospitalized, the hospital caregivers may assume the role of substitute mother. A caregiver can continue to develop the infant's trust by responding to her cry and her needs. Trust is fostered by feeding, holding, touching, and talking to the infant (Figure 50-2), in addition to keeping her warm and dry.

It is important for the infant to have consistent mothering. Therefore, it is ideal to have the mother room-in with her infant. If this is not possible, an alternative approach is to use the same caregivers for an infant. This means that every time a nurse or nursing assistant works, he will care for the same infants. Besides being consistent for the infant, it also allows the caregiver to become familiar with the infant as a unique person. Consistency is especially important when an infant is between 6 and 7 months of age. At this age, the infant normally begins to display a fear of strangers.

Communicating with Infants

Working with infants can be challenging because the infant cannot tell the caregiver in words what he wants or

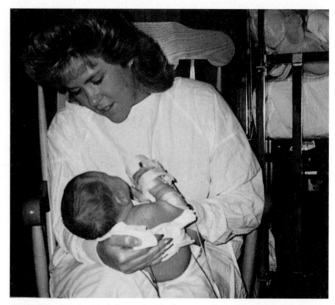

FIGURE 50-2 Holding the infant and making good eye contact promotes trust, security, and affection.

needs. The infant communicates with his cry and body movements. The cry can vary depending on needs. Just as a mother learns to interpret the sound of her infant's cry,

Communication HIGHLIGHT

An infant's senses of touch and hearing are important. Babies are naturally curious. Talk to babies when you are giving care. Although the infant will not understand, a tone of calm reassurance in your voice makes the baby feel safe. ■

the caregiver will also learn to interpret the meanings of the cry by caring for the infant.

Infants respond to voices, faces, and touch. You should talk to the infant (Figure 50-3) whenever you are giving personal care such as bathing, feeding, or holding.

The Waking Hours

When the infant is awake, she needs to explore the environment. Age-appropriate toys are provided so that the infant can continue development while in the hospital. Appropriate toys include colorful mobiles, rattles, and mirrors.

Importance of Families

Siblings of the infant should be allowed to visit while the infant is hospitalized. Toddlers and preschoolers engage in "magical thinking." In other words, they believe that if they wish the infant to be sick, it happens, or if they wish the baby to be gone she won't be back. Therefore, it is important for both toddlers and preschoolers to see their infant sibling. If the mother is rooming-in with the infant, it is also important for toddlers and preschoolers to see and talk to their mother.

Routine Procedures

When carrying out routine care of the infant, be sure that you hold the infant properly (Figure 50-4). (Refer to Unit 49.)

Before feeding the infant, organize his care so that he can be allowed to digest his food and sleep after he has eaten. You should not move him unnecessarily, as it may cause him to vomit what he has just eaten. In organizing the care, you would weigh, bathe, diaper, and dress him. Then change the crib linens, weigh him, and feed him.

The routine procedures covered here may apply to all pediatric patients. They include taking vital signs, measuring weight, and changing crib linens.

Weighing the Infant

Routine care includes weighing the infant. This procedure should also be done before feeding.

Tips: Put clean paper on the scale before using it, to prevent chilling. Balance the scale with the paper in place. Keep your hand on the infant to prevent accidents. Work quickly to prevent heat loss in the infant. Disinfect the scale each time it is used, to prevent cross-contamination.

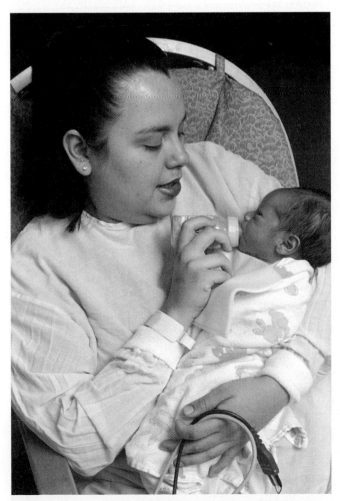

FIGURE 50-3 Talk to the infant each time you provide care.

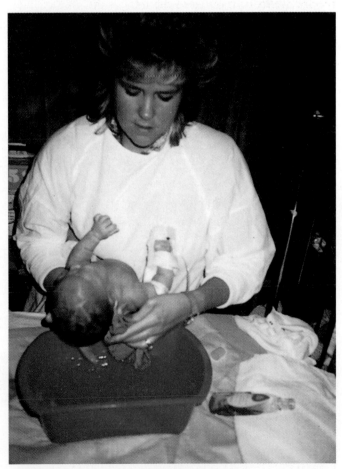

FIGURE 50-4 Hold the infant properly when giving care. The nursing assistant is supporting the head during the bath.

PROCEDURE

WEIGHING THE PEDIATRIC PATIENT

Infant

1. Wash your hands.

2. Place a small sheet or receiving blanket on the scale and balance the scale with the blanket on it.

3. Check the infant's previous weight.

4. Check the infant's identification band.

5. Remove the infant's diaper and shirt.

6. Place the infant on the scale, keeping a hand over the infant to prevent falling (Figure 50-5).

7. Move the bar to the correct weight until the scale balances.

8. Return the infant to the crib. Diaper and dress the infant.

9. Record the infant's weight according to hospital policy.

10. Remove the linen from the scale and place it in a laundry receptacle.

11. Return the scale to its proper storage place.

12. Wash your hands.

Toddler to Adolescent

1. Use an upright scale if the child is able to stand. Bring the scale to the bedside, if possible, and balance it.

2. Wash your hands.

3. Check the child's identification band.

4. Check the child's previous weight.

5. Weigh the child in as few clothes as possible. Remove any diaper and shoes or slippers.

FIGURE 50-5 Maintain light hand contact with the infant while adjusting the weights with the other hand.

6. Have the child stand on the scale. Move the bar to the correct weight until the scale balances.

7. Record the weight according to hospital policy.

8. Return the child to bed.

9. Return the scale to its proper storage place.

10. Wash your hands.

Alternate Action: If the toddler is unable to stand on his own, pick him up and step on the scale. Obtain the combined weight. Put the toddler back in bed, weigh yourself, and subtract your weight from the combined weight. The toddler's weight is the difference in weights.

PROCEDURE

CHANGING CRIB LINENS

1. Wash your hands.

2. Gather supplies:

- Disposable gloves
- Sheet

continues

PROCEDURE 114 CONTINUED

- Blanket
- Shirt
- Diaper
- Pad

Do steps 1 and 2 before bathing the infant.

3. When bathing the infant, apply the principles of standard precautions as you would with an adult.

4. After bathing the infant, diaper and dress her.

5. Place the infant in a stroller, playpen, or other safe place.

6. Strip the linen from the crib. Wear gloves if linen is soiled. Dispose of soiled or used linen according to facility policy.

7. Remove gloves and discard according to facility policy.

8. Wash your hands.

9. Place clean linen on the bed and open the sheet, hem side down.

10. Make one side of the crib; miter the corners top and bottom, and tuck in the side (Figure 50-6A).

11. Pull down the crib top (Figure 50-6B). Pull up the crib side (Figure 50-6C).

12. Repeat step 10 on the opposite side of the crib.

13. Place a diaper pad on top of the sheet, according to hospital policy.

14. Place a clean blanket at the bottom of the bed.

15. Arrange bumper pads around the sides of the crib.

16. Wash your hands.

17. Return the infant to the crib, cover her with the blanket (if appropriate), and pull up the crib side.

FIGURE 50-6A Make one side of the crib. Miter corners at the top and bottom and tuck under mattress.

FIGURE 50-6B Pull the crib top down.

FIGURE 50-6C Pull the side up and check for security.

PROCEDURE 115

CHANGING CRIB LINENS (INFANT IN CRIB)

1. Wash your hands.

2. Gather linens
   - Sheet
   - Blanket
   - Shirt
   - Diaper
   - Bathing equipment
   - Disposable gloves

   Do steps 1 and 2 before bathing the infant.

3. After bathing the infant, diaper and dress him.

4. Pick up the infant and hold him in one arm.

continues

PROCEDURE 115 CONTINUED

5. With your free hand, strip the old linen off the crib. Wear gloves if linen is soiled.

6. Place the clean linen on the mattress and open the sheet, placing the hem side down. Place the infant on the sheet.

7. Place one hand on the infant and keep it on him at all times.

8. Make one side of the crib. Miter the corners, top and bottom, and tuck in the side.

9. Remove your hand from the infant and pull up the crib side.

10. Go around to the other side of the crib.

11. Take down the crib side, place one hand on the infant, and repeat step 8.

12. Place a diaper pad under the infant and cover him with the blanket, if appropriate.

13. Arrange bumper pads around the crib, if appropriate.

14. Pull up the crib side.

15. Wash your hands.

Determining Vital Signs

The infant's vital signs must be measured as outlined in the care plan. It is normal for an infant's heart to beat faster than an adult's. The normal ranges of heart rates and respiratory rates for each age group are listed in Table 50-1. An increase in the infant's heart and respiratory rates can be caused by stress (crying, fever, or infection). Therefore, the pulse and respiratory rates should be taken when the infant is quiet, either awake or sleeping.

Feeding

Feeding is important to the infant because it satisfies her hunger and sucking needs. Sucking provides the infant with a pleasant sensation, whether she receives food with her sucking or not. The amount of time an infant needs to suckle will vary with each infant. Always provide the infant with the opportunity to suck. This is even more important if the infant cannot eat.

When feeding an infant:

- Hold the infant unless there is a medical reason not to. Holding the infant during a feeding allows close, physical contact with the person feeding her.

- If an infant cannot be held, you should still hold the bottle for her while she eats.

- Never leave an infant in a crib with a bottle propped in his mouth. This is dangerous because the infant could get too much formula at one time, vomit, and choke.

During feeding and following feeding, the infant should be burped. (This section on feeding continues on pages 890–891.)

Note: If an infant cannot be fed, she should still be held and allowed to suck on a pacifier unless a medical reason prevents removal of the infant from the crib.

TABLE 50-1 NORMAL VITAL SIGNS

| Age | Heart Rate | Respirations | Blood Pressure | |
			Systolic	Diastolic
Infants	120–160	30–60	74–100	50–70
Toddlers	90–140	24–40	80–112	50–80
Preschoolers	80–110	22–34	82–110	50–78
School-age	75–100	18–30	84–119	54–80
Adolescents	60–90	12–24	94–119	62–88

Note: Pulse and respiration are taken for a full minute. The apical pulse is used with infants and young children.

PROCEDURE

116

MEASURING TEMPERATURE

Temperatures on children 5 years of age and under are usually taken rectally or by the tympanic method unless there is a medical reason not to. Axillary temperature can be taken in place of rectal temperature.

Rectal Temperature

All other vital signs should be measured before the temperature if a rectal temperature is to be measured.

1. Wash your hands and put on gloves.

2. Check the patient's identification band.

3. Explain to the parents and child what you are going to do.

4. Inspect the thermometer for breaks.

5. Shake down the thermometer.

6. Cover the thermometer with a disposable sheath.

7. Lubricate the thermometer sheath, if it is not prelubricated.

8. Lay the child on his back on bed (Figure 50-7A) or on her stomach across your lap (Figure 50-7B).

9. Insert the thermometer 1/2 inch into the child's rectum and hold. Hold the child securely and gently so the child does not move about.

10. Leave the thermometer in place for the required amount of time (3 to 5 minutes). Follow your facility's policy.

FIGURE 50-7B
Infant in prone position

11. Remove the thermometer. Discard the sheath according to facility policy.

12. Remove gloves and wash your hands.

13. Record.

14. Report any deviations from normal according to hospital policy.

FIGURE 50-7A
Infant in supine position

Safety ALERT

Check with the nurse before taking a rectal temperature on a newborn infant. In some facilities, the first rectal temperature must be taken by the nurse, to ensure that the rectum is patent. After that, axillary or tympanic temperature may be the method of choice. Know and follow your facility policy. When taking a rectal temperature, grasp the child's ankles gently, but firmly, with one hand. Cover the penis of a male infant with a diaper. Insert the lubricated thermometer while holding the ankles. Continue to hold the ankles with one hand and the thermometer with the other throughout the procedure. ∎

continues

PROCEDURE 116 CONTINUED

Oral Temperature

1. Explain to the parents and child what you will be doing.

2. Check the patient's identification band.

3. Wash your hands.

4. Inspect the thermometer for breaks.

5. Shake down the thermometer.

6. Cover the thermometer with a disposable sheath.

7. Apply gloves.

8. Instruct the child to hold the thermometer under his tongue. If the child cannot hold the thermometer in his mouth, then obtain either a rectal, tympanic, or axillary temperature.

9. Leave the thermometer under the child's tongue for the required amount of time (usually 5 to 8 minutes).

10. Remove the thermometer. Discard the sheath according to facility policy.

11. Read the thermometer.

12. Remove gloves and discard according to facility policy.

13. Wash your hands.

14. Record the temperature.

15. Report any deviations from normal according to hospital policy.

Axillary Temperature

1. Explain to the parents and child what you are going to do.

2. Check the patient's identification band.

3. Wash your hands.

4. Inspect the thermometer for breaks.

5. Shake down the thermometer.

6. Cover the thermometer with a disposable sheath.

7. Place the thermometer in the child's armpit.

8. Hold the child's arm close to her chest for the required amount of time (10 minutes).

9. Remove the thermometer. Discard the sheath according to facility policy.

10. Read the thermometer.

11. Wash your hands and record the temperature value.

12. Report any deviations from normal according to hospital policy.

> **Note:** If an electronic thermometer is used, follow the manufacturer's directions supplied with the equipment.

Tympanic Temperature

1. Explain to the parents and child what you are going to do.

2. Check the patient's identification band.

3. Wash your hands.

4. Check the lens on the thermometer to make sure it is clean and intact.

5. Set the appropriate mode on the thermometer.

6. Place a clean probe cover on the probe.

7. Position the patient so you will have access to the ear you will be using.

8. If the patient is under age 1, pull the ear straight back, then down. In children over age 1, pull the ear up and back. While gently tugging the ear, fit the probe snugly into the canal, aiming at the tympanic membrane. Point the probe tip at the midpoint between the eyebrow and sideburn on the opposite side of the face. The probe tip should penetrate at least one-third of the ear canal and form a complete seal.

> **Note:** Tympanic thermometers measure temperature by aiming an infrared light beam on the tympanic membrane. Light does not go around corners. If the ear canal is not fully straightened when the thermometer is inserted, the value will not be accurate. Because of this, step 8 is very important to the accuracy of this procedure.

9. Press the activation button. Leave the thermometer in place until the display blinks or signals that the temperature is final.

10. Remove the thermometer. Discard the probe cover.

11. Wash your hands and record the temperature.

12. Report any deviations from normal according to hospital policy.

Difficult **SITUATIONS**

When taking vital signs on an infant or small child, take the rectal temperature *last*. Taking the rectal temperature first may cause the infant to cry, which will accelerate the pulse and respirations. ■

PROCEDURE

DETERMINING HEART RATE (PULSE)

With infants and children, the easiest way to find the heart rate is to place the stethoscope over the heart (Figure 50-8). This is called the apical pulse. It should be done when the child is quiet or at rest because stress and crying can result in a reading that is higher than normal.

1. Wash your hands.

2. Check the patient's identification band.

3. Explain the procedure to the patient and/or his parents. Clean stethoscope earpieces and diaphragm with an antiseptic wipe and dry them. (Allow a child to play with the stethoscope first.)

4. Rub the diaphragm of the stethoscope to warm it so that it will not be cold when placed on the infant's chest.

5. Place the stethoscope over the infant's heart and count the number of beats you hear in a minute.

6. Clean the stethoscope earpieces and diaphragm with an antiseptic wipe and dry them.

7. Wash your hands and record the results.

FIGURE 50-8 Measuring the apical pulse

8. Report rates higher or lower than the normal for the appropriate age group, according to hospital policy.

Note: The radial pulse can be used for children 6 years and over. The procedure used is the same as for adults. Refer to Procedure 37 in Unit 19.

PROCEDURE

COUNTING RESPIRATORY RATE

Infants and toddlers use their abdominal muscles for breathing. To count the respiratory rate for this age group, look at the abdomen and chest and count the respirations for a full minute.

To obtain the respiratory rate for preschoolers and older children, follow Procedure 39 in Unit 19, as for adults, but count the respirations for a full minute.

PROCEDURE

MEASURING BLOOD PRESSURE

A blood pressure measurement may not always be required for all pediatric patients. If blood pressure is to be recorded, you must have the correct size cuff for the child. The cuff should cover two-thirds of the upper arm.

1. Select the correct cuff size for the patient.

2. Assemble all equipment. Clean stethoscope earpieces and diaphragm with an antiseptic wipe and dry them.

3. Wash your hands.

4. Check the patient's identification band.

5. Explain the procedure to the child, using language such as, "This will feel like a tight hug on your arm."

6. Wrap the cuff securely around the upper arm.

7. Feel for the brachial pulse.

8. Place the stethoscope earpieces in your ears and place the diaphragm near the pulse point.

9. Pump up the cuff until you no longer hear the pulse. Release the valve and listen for systolic and diastolic sounds.

10. Wash your hands and record the results according to hospital policy.

Infection Control ALERT

The formula and bottle should be sterile for bottle-feeding a newborn infant. Wash your hands well before feeding the infant. Avoid touching the nipple or the inside of the cap with your hands. Keep the nipple covered with the cap until you are ready to begin feeding. Check the expiration date on the bottle to make sure the formula has not expired. ▪

Safety ALERT

Shake the bottle slightly to ensure that the formula is mixed well. Invert the bottle and drop a few drops of formula on your wrist to check for temperature of formula and patency of the nipple. Formula should drip freely, but not come out in a stream. If the formula runs out in a stream, change the nipple before proceeding. Elevate the child's head and shoulders slightly during feeding to prevent aspiration of formula and allow air to rise to the top of the stomach, where it is expelled more readily. Keep the nipple filled with formula at all times, to prevent ingestion of air. A steady stream of bubbles should rise in the bottle during feeding. If the infant pushes the nipple out with her tongue, reinsert it. This is a normal reflex and does not mean the child is full or does not want to eat. ▪

Burping

The frequency with which you burp the infant will depend on the infant's age and medical condition. Burping is important because bottle-fed infants swallow a lot of air while sucking. The infant can be burped as frequently as after every half-ounce of formula. Older infants can be burped after 1 to 2 ounces during feeding and at the conclusion of feeding. Refer to your hospital policy for the frequency of burping. There are two methods of burping an infant.

Breast-Feeding

If the rooming-in or visiting mother is breast-feeding, she should be directed to an area where she can be assured of privacy as well as comfort. As a nursing assistant, you may be responsible for weighing the infant before and after feeding, according to your hospital policy. (See Procedure 113.) When returning the infant to his crib after feeding, place him on his back or side. A rolled blanket can be used to keep him on his side.

PROCEDURE

120

BOTTLE-FEEDING AN INFANT

1. Wash your hands.

2. Gather the infant's formula and diaper pad, washcloth, or bib.

3. Check the infant's identification band.

4. Pick up the infant and hold her to feed her, unless there is a medical reason not to.

5. Sit in a chair or rocker.

6. Hold the infant in the crook of your arm, with the infant's head slightly raised (Figure 50-9).

7. Place a diaper, washcloth, or bib under the infant's chin, covering the chest.

8. Tip the bottle so the nipple is filled with formula.

9. Stroke the side of the infant's cheek closest to you. The infant will automatically turn toward the side stroked and open her mouth. Place the nipple in the infant's mouth.

10. If the nipple is in the mouth but the infant is not sucking, gently lift up under the infant's chin to close her mouth on the nipple.

11. Hold the bottle so the nipple stays filled with formula while the infant feeds.

12. Feed the infant the ordered amount of formula and burp according to the infant's age and hospital policy. (See Procedure 121.)

13. If the infant starts to vomit while feeding, remove the bottle and turn the infant to the

FIGURE 50-9 Hold the infant with the head elevated during bottle-feeding. Keep the nipple filled with fluid while the infant sucks, to prevent excess air in the stomach, which is painful.

side, with her head lowered, to prevent aspiration. Seek help as needed.

14. After feeding, return the child to the crib and place her on her back or side.

15. Pull up the crib side.

16. Wash your hands.

17. Record the amount of formula the infant took, according to hospital policy.

PROCEDURE

121

BURPING AN INFANT

Burping (Method A)

1. Place a diaper or cloth over your shoulder.

2. Lift the infant up to your shoulder, holding the infant close to your chest (Figure 50-10).

3. Holding the infant in place with one hand, use the other hand to gently rub or pat the infant's back until the infant burps.

Burping (Method B)

1. Place a diaper, cloth, or bib under the infant's chin.

2. Place the child in a sitting or upright position. Put one hand on the infant's chest, supporting the infant's weight (Figure 50-11). With the other hand, gently rub or pat the infant's back until the infant burps.

continues

PROCEDURE 121 CONTINUED

FIGURE 50-10 Burping the infant during and after feeding helps eliminate swallowed air. Gently rub or pat the infant's back.

FIGURE 50-11 An alternative method of burping is to sit the infant on your lap with a cloth or bib under the chin.

Age-Appropriate Care ALERT

The pediatric urine collection device is fastened to the perineum with a self-adhesive surface. It should not be used for children with diaper rash, inflamed or broken skin, or those who are allergic to adhesive tape. If any of these conditions exists, check with the nurse before proceeding. If a clean specimen is needed, another option may be to place several sterile cotton balls directly over the external urinary meatus, then replace the diaper. After the child has voided, collect and use the urine squeezed from the cotton balls into a specimen cup (with your gloved hands). If using the pediatric collection bag or cotton balls is not possible, try applying a disposable diaper inside out. After the child voids, remove the diaper carefully. Pour the urine from the plastic outer surface (which is facing inside) into a specimen collection cup or test tube. ■

Collecting a Urine Specimen

Urine specimens are needed for various diagnostic tests. The presence of a urinary tract infection is very important, and in infants and small children, it may indicate an abnormality that was not identified previously. When collecting a specimen from an older child, use the same procedures as are used for adults (Unit 45). To collect a urine specimen from infants and toddlers who are not potty-trained, a self-adhesive pediatric urine collection bag is used (Figure 50-12). After the child voids, the contents of the bag are emptied into a specimen collection cup. In some facilities, the specimen is withdrawn into a syringe, then transferred into a urine specimen cup. Some facilities cap the syringe and send it to the lab as is. Follow your facility policy for specimen handling. Because an infant or toddler cannot urinate on demand, it is a good idea to give the child fluids that he or she likes every 15 to 30 minutes until the specimen is collected.

To keep the bag in place, make sure the skin is clean, dry, and free of lotions, oils, and powder. Remove the backing from the collection bag and position the opening over the penis in the male and the labia in the female. Press gently to secure the adhesive. Replace the diaper. Remove the collection bag after the child voids. After the specimen has been collected, carefully pour the contents of the bag into a specimen collection cup. Sometimes the bag becomes

FIGURE 50-12 The pediatric urine collection device has an adhesive backing. The hole in the bag is placed over the external urinary meatus.

dislodged, especially if the infant is active. If you cannot collect a specimen on the first attempt, try again. If you are unsuccessful after two tries, inform the nurse. Ask for the nurse's permission before using other techniques.

Restraints

It is generally not necessary to obtain a physician's order to restrain an infant or a child. Restraints can be used for the child's safety. Restraints are used to protect the child from injury to herself or to others, or to protect the child from injury by equipment used in care. Any child who is restrained in any way should be freed from the restraints every 2 hours and allowed to exercise the extremities under supervision. Restraints should never be tied to a crib side or bed rail, only to the bed or crib frame.

A *jacket restraint* is a sleeveless cloth garment. It is fitted to the child's chest and crosses in the back, out of the child's reach. It has long straps that can be tied under the mattress or through a chair. When tied this way, the child can

PROCEDURE

COLLECTING A URINE SPECIMEN FROM AN INFANT

1. Wash your hands.

2. Assemble supplies:
   - Disposable gloves (at least 2 pair)
   - Soap and water, or cleanser used by facility
   - Cotton balls or washcloth to cleanse perineum
   - Towel
   - Clean diaper
   - Bed protector
   - Plastic bag
   - Pediatric urine collection bag
   - Syringe to withdraw specimen from collection bag, if this is facility policy
   - Urine specimen cup with label(s)
   - Transport bag

3. Remove the infant's diaper.

4. Wash the perineum with soap and water. Make sure to remove powder or ointment.

5. Rinse the perineum and dry well.

6. Discard the used diaper, cotton balls, and other used supplies in the plastic bag.

7. Apply the urine collection bag by removing the paper backing to expose the adhesive and positioning the center of the hole in the bag over the external urinary meatus in a female, or over the penis in a male.

8. Gently press the bag in place to seal the adhesive.

9. Reapply the diaper, leaving the bag unfolded. In some facilities, the bag is pulled through to the outside of the diaper, or a hole is cut in the diaper so the bag can be pulled through to the outside.

10. Remove gloves and discard in the plastic bag.

11. Wash your hands.

12. Prepare the specimen labels and attach them to the specimen cup and transport bag, or according to facility policy. Set aside.

13. Remove the collection device immediately after the child voids.

14. Place the collection device on a bed protector or other clean area. Put the bag down and

continues

PROCEDURE 122 CONTINUED

position the hole in the center carefully to avoid spilling the contents.

15. Cleanse the infant's perineum and apply a clean diaper.

16. Leave the infant in a position of comfort and safety.

17. Open the specimen collection cup. Place the lid on the table, with the clean inner side facing up. Avoid touching the inside of the lid or specimen container.

18. Carefully pour the specimen into the collection container, or withdraw it with a syringe (with no needle attached) and gently push the plunger to move the specimen to the cup.

19. Apply the lid to the specimen cup. Place the cup in the transport bag.

20. Carry out ending procedure actions.

---

move the extremities, sit up, lie down in bed, or turn side-to-side without falling.

An *extremity restraint* may be used on the child's arms, hands, legs, or feet. Commercial restraints are available in sheepskin, Velcro, or disposable materials. This restraint is placed on the child's extremity according to hospital policy and procedure and manufacturer's directions. The ties are tied to the frame of the crib. For very small infants, the ties may be pinned to the mattress.

Summary of Nursing Assistant Tasks and Responsibilities When Caring for Infants

- Maintain a safe environment
- Provide information to the health team through monitoring of vital signs (temperature, pulse, respiration), weight, intake, and output
- Provide routine care such as bathing, feeding, and changing
- Collect and test specimens
- Assist with treatments, examinations, and procedures
- Provide warmth, security, and affection

Safety ALERT

Avoid use of restraints whenever possible. Consider alternatives, such as distraction, before applying restraints. If restraints are necessary, the nurse should make the decision regarding the type of restraint to use. Remove and reapply the restraint every 2 hours. Elevate the head of the bed every 30 minutes. Offer comfort measures, including food, fluids, and toileting as appropriate. Provide distraction and touch. ■

CHILDHOOD OBESITY

Some children may be admitted for complications of obesity. More than 10% of preschool children (ages 2 to 5) are considered overweight. An Institute of Medicine (IOM) report issued in 2005 states that there are approximately 9 million children nationwide over the age of 6 who are considered obese (Figure 50-13). This is signifi-

---

GUIDELINES *for*

Ensuring a Safe Environment for Infants

- Always keep crib side rails up.
- Always keep one hand on the infant when the crib side rail is down.
- Use crib bumpers or rolled blankets to prevent injury.
- Never tie balloons or toys to cribs.
- Never use toys with small removable parts or pointed objects.
- Never prop bottles.
- Never tape pacifiers in an infant's mouth.

FIGURE 50-13 This 11-year-old has battled with his weight since he was 5. He is a well-adjusted middle child and a good student who enjoys his membership on the soccer team.

cant because the number has tripled in the past 20 years. An increase in obesity causes an increase in health care costs. Health care professionals are seeing diseases in children that were previously limited to the adult population, such as:

- Type 2 diabetes
- Sleep apnea
- Hypertension
- Skin disorders
- Weight-related orthopedic problems
- Gallstones
- Depression
- Risk factors for atherosclerosis and other cardiac problems

Sleep apnea is a special concern. Researchers have known for years that interrupted sleep inhibits a child's ability to learn. Performance in school, on verbal skills tests, and on IQ tests is not as good as that of children with no sleep problem. It is also suspected that sleep disorders reduce cognitive function. This is important because the damage is being done while the child is growing.

Several studies suggest that obese children almost always become obese adults. About half of those studied who were overweight at age 6 became overweight adults. About 80% of overweight adolescents become overweight adults. Because of the severity of the problem, childhood obesity is being studied to identify causes and potential solutions to the problem.

Identifying and correcting family eating patterns is often necessary. Educating children and parents about healthy nutrition, exercise, and positive lifestyle choices are some of the methods used to correct overweight. When used in combination with behavior modification, this approach has met with some success in solving the obesity problem. Bariatric surgery (Unit 31) is a very limited option considered only when other methods have failed.

Overweight and obese children are often teased and tormented by their peers. Many suffer from low self-esteem. Treat them with compassion and sensitivity when you care for them.

CARING FOR TODDLERS (1–3 YEARS)

The years between 1 and 3 can be a difficult time for a child to be hospitalized. This is the age when a child is trying to be independent and in control. Between $1\frac{1}{2}$ and 3 years of age, the child:

- Increases motor coordination
- Becomes more verbal
- Becomes more curious about the world

At the same time, her parents are trying to toilet-train her. They also are beginning to set limits on her behavior. The developmental task for the toddler is **autonomy** (independent action).

When caring for the toddler, allow her as much independence and choice as possible (within hospital policy guidelines). Avoid situations that could create a struggle between the caregiver and the child. Expect delays when the toddler is feeding herself or bathing. Be sure to allow the toddler time to do these activities.

The Hospital Environment

When a toddler is hospitalized, it is important to provide an environment that allows as much independence and control as possible while ensuring safety. An example of this is the choice of bed (crib) for the toddler. If a crib is to be used, it should have a top and sides to prevent the child from climbing out and possibly falling (Figure 50-14). If the child has been sleeping in a bed at home, then it is more appropriate to provide a child-sized hospital bed with side rails, if available. Hospital policies vary, so check your hospital policy with reference to toddlers.

If the child is toilet-trained, it is important to know the words the child uses for urination and bowel movements. It is also important to know if the child uses a potty chair or the toilet at home. You should try to provide the same arrangement for toileting in the hospital. It is not uncommon for a hospitalized child to regress. You should not be surprised if a toddler who is toilet-trained starts to have "accidents" while in the hospital. Do not scold the child if this happens. The incident should be treated in a matter-of-fact manner. In addition, a hospitalized toddler may ask for a bottle or pacifier. Even though the toddler may

FIGURE 50-14 The crib must provide a safe environment, yet be large enough to allow freedom of movement.

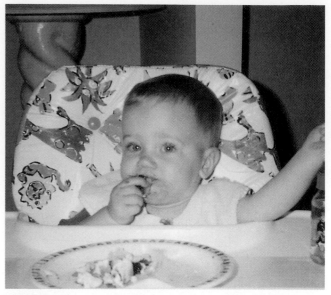

FIGURE 50-15 The nursing assistant must help the toddler when necessary, but allow the toddler as much independence as possible. Most toddlers do well with finger foods, although they often make a mess.

have been weaned from them, treat the request as normal. Do not try to reason with the child.

The Toddler's Need for Autonomy

The toddler is learning to be independent. He may want to feed, dress, and wash himself while in the hospital. It will be your responsibility to help the toddler with these activities (Figure 50-15). Allow him his independence. At the same time, you must keep him safe. For example, when bathing the toddler in the bathtub, you must never leave him alone, even for a minute. Before you put the toddler in the tub, check the temperature of the bath water.

Emotional Reaction to Illness

Another important area in the care of toddlers concerns their feelings of responsibility for their own illnesses. You must stress that the illness is not the toddler's or anyone else's fault.

To overcome anxiety about routine procedures, allow the toddler to handle equipment whenever possible. A few extra minutes spent familiarizing the toddler with the equipment to be used may make the difference between a frightened child and an interested one (Figure 50-16). The toddler will have a difficult time if separated from the mother. One way to prevent this is to permit the mother to room-in. If this cannot happen, either because a parent cannot stay or because hospital policy does not permit it, then parents should be encouraged to visit frequently. If a parent is not going to stay:

FIGURE 50-16 Explain what you are doing in a language the child understands. You may ask a child who can read to tell you what the numbers are. This child is very interested in learning about weight.

- Reassure the child that she will not be alone
- Tell her the names of the people who will care for her
- Encourage each person caring for the toddler to introduce himself when entering the room
- Whenever possible, place the toddler who does not have a parent staying with her in a room near the nurses' station
- Encourage parents who cannot visit to call, or you can call the parents so the child can talk to them

Routine Activities

Routines are important to toddlers. Ask the parents to describe the child's normal day. Try to follow the child's

Age-Appropriate Care ALERT

Treatments are not done in the child's room, which should be viewed as a "safe place." If the unit has a playroom, this is also considered "safe." When painful treatments are necessary, most hospitals use a special treatment room in the unit or take the child to another area of the hospital for the procedure. ■

usual schedule as much as possible for eating, naps, toileting, and other activities. Ask the parents about the child's nickname, likes, dislikes, names of siblings and pets, and anything else the parents feel the nursing assistant should know about the child.

Toddlers love to play but, because they have short attention spans, they cannot play with one toy for a long time. Plan a variety of activities to keep the toddler amused. For example:

- Finger painting
- Moving toy cars or trucks (Figure 50-17)
- Coloring
- Handling blocks
- Push-pull toys
- Reading of stories

Educational toys that teach how to dress, button, and zip can also be fun for the toddler. Stethoscopes, masks, and gloves make good hospital toys because they can allow the toddler to work out his fears. Do not leave the child alone with these items, because of the risk of accident or injury. Toddlers will not play together, but they will play near or next to each other.

FIGURE 50-17 Toddlers and preschool children often enjoy playing with cars, trucks, and toys with wheels.

Temper tantrums are common with toddlers. If they occur, ignore the tantrum as long as the child cannot hurt herself or others. If a toddler is misbehaving, set limits in a firm, consistent manner.

When working with the toddler, remember that he is trying to be independent. Allow the toddler as much choice as possible. For example, at snack time ask if he wants an apple or a cracker. If no choice can be given, be firm and say what will occur. For example, "It's time to take your nap now." It is best to be truthful and to give simple explanations to toddlers. If the child is having a blood test, tell him just before it happens. It does not do any good to prepare toddlers in advance because they do not have any concept of time. Such advance warning only increases their anxiety.

The toddler has great natural curiosity and loves to explore. It is important to maintain a safe environment in the hospital.

Summary of Nursing Assistant Tasks and Responsibilities When Caring for Toddlers

- Maintain a safe environment
- Apply standard precautions if contact with blood, body fluids, mucous membranes, or nonintact skin is likely

GUIDELINES *for*

Ensuring a Safe Environment for Toddlers

- All poisonous liquids should be kept in a locked container or cabinet.
- All open electrical sockets should have protective covers. Never leave toddlers unattended or unsupervised.
- Never leave toddlers alone in the bathtub or bathroom.
- Keep thermometers out of toddlers' reach.
- Keep crib sides and side rails up when the toddler is in bed.
- Never allow toddlers to play with balloons unless supervised.
- Avoid toys with sharp edges, long strings, or small removable parts.
- Keep doors to stair, kitchen, treatment, and storage areas closed and locked whenever possible.
- Keep doors to linen chutes locked.

- Provide information to the health team through monitoring of vital signs (temperature, pulse, and respiration), weight, intake, and output
- Supervise and assist with routine care such as bathing, feeding, and dressing
- Collect and test specimens
- Assist with treatments, examinations, and procedures
- Provide and assist with opportunities for play
- Provide warmth, security, and affection (Figure 50-18)
- Promote independence by providing opportunities for choices

CARING FOR PRESCHOOL CHILDREN (3–6 YEARS)

Developmental Tasks

Between the ages of 3 and 6 years, the child's language, fine motor skills, and gross motor skills continue to increase with activity. The preschooler continues to develop independence, but the primary developmental task for the age group is **initiative** (doing things themselves). Children in this age group need to be able to initiate physical and intellectual activities to feel more competent.

FIGURE 50-18 Showing affection and allowing the child to become familiar with your equipment will help relieve anxiety.

The preschooler learns her sex role in life by imitating the behavior of the same-sex parent.

The preschooler needs his independence, but he still needs to feel safe and secure. The caregiver must provide the correct balance of independence and control for the preschooler. This is normally the job of the parents, but when the preschooler is hospitalized, you will be considered the caregiver.

Emotional Reactions to Illness

Preschoolers normally have many fears. One fear is that their body parts will be injured or changed. For example, a preschooler may fear that if an adhesive bandage is taken off, some of her will "leak out." Preschoolers cannot tell the difference between a "good hurt" and a "bad hurt"; that is, pain from a procedure versus pain from a spanking. Therefore, it is important to use simple, honest explanations when telling the preschooler what to expect.

Fear of the dark, of night time, and of being alone are other normal fears for a preschooler. You can help reduce this fear by leaving a nightlight on. Another child in the room can also ease his fears. Be sure to leave the call bell within reach. Sitting with him until he falls asleep will also help. Like the toddler, the preschooler can also benefit from having his mother room-in, because he still fears separation.

"Magical thinking" and fantasy are still present in this age group. Therefore, it is important to stress to the preschooler that it is not her fault that she is sick, and that she is not sick because she was bad. The preschooler needs to know that she will return home. She will not be forgotten and left in the hospital. Siblings should be allowed and encouraged to visit (Figure 50-19). In addition to eas-

FIGURE 50-19 Having siblings visit the hospitalized child is important.

ing separation from the family, this can also be a way of assuring the child that no one is taking her place at home.

Explaining Procedures

When telling a preschooler what to expect, simple, honest explanations work best. Choose your words carefully because the preschooler takes things literally (exactly as said).

- If surgery is being planned, show and tell the child what parts of his body will be involved in the procedure (Figure 50-20).
- Preschoolers have a limited concept of time, so when you explain when something will occur, use time references that are familiar to the child (such as mealtime, nap time, or the time of a favorite TV show). For example, if the child is scheduled for an X-ray in the late morning, tell her that she will have it after breakfast or before lunch.
- Always explain to the preschooler what you are going to do. Do not assume that he will remember what you told him before.
- The preschooler needs to maintain some control. Therefore, allow him to make as many decisions as possible. Give him the opportunity to make a choice. Allow the preschooler to do as much of her own care as she can, to make her feel independent.

Age-Appropriate Care ALERT

Preschoolers and young school-age children enjoy stories. Make up or tell childhood stories to entertain them, or to teach them about the procedures you will be doing and reduce fear. Using hand or finger puppets is another enjoyable, effective approach to care. ■

Activities

Imagination and fantasy are part of the preschooler's world. Imaginary playmates are normal for the preschooler. These playmates may find their way to the hospital with the child. The playmates can vary in age and sex. They often have different or unusual-sounding names. If the child talks about his imaginary friend, treat it matter-of-factly and listen. However, be realistic. Do not say that you see or hear this playmate. Just say that you know this playmate exists only in the child's imagination.

Play is important for the hospitalized preschooler. Play may give you clues about what the preschooler is thinking. The preschooler is more coordinated and can enjoy

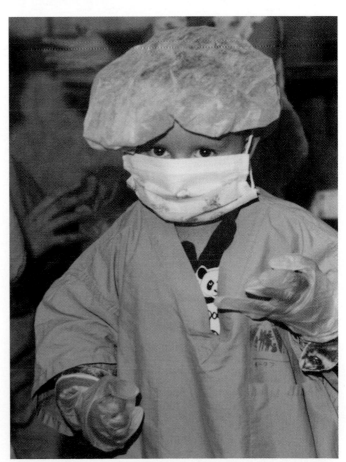

FIGURE 50-20 Surgery can be very frightening for children of all ages. Explaining what will happen and allowing them to play with supplies helps calm their fears.

activities such as puzzles, coloring, and drawing. The pre-schooler enjoys imitating roles and playing with other children (Figure 50-21). Playing house and doctor is especially fun for this age group. Hand puppets are also a good way to talk to preschoolers, because they relate easily to the character of the puppet.

You can help the preschooler deal with her hospital stay by maintaining consistency in her schedule and in the limits put on her behavior. Positive reinforcers such as hugs or stickers should be used as rewards for appropriate behavior.

Summary of Nursing Assistant Tasks and Responsibilities When Caring for Preschoolers

- Maintain a safe environment
- Apply standard precautions if contact with blood, body fluids, mucous membranes, or nonintact skin is likely

G U I D E L I N E S *for*

Ensuring a Safe Environment for Preschoolers

- Keep toys from cluttering walkways, to prevent falls.
- Keep side rails on the bed up at night.
- Keep beds in low position.
- Keep doors to kitchen and storage areas closed.
- Keep a nightlight on.
- Never leave the child unattended in the tub.
- Never allow children to run with popsicles or lollipops in their mouths.

FIGURE 50-21 Playing "hospital" or "doctor" with children is a good way of teaching them, as well as allaying their fears.

- Provide information to the health team through monitoring of vital signs (temperature, pulse, and respiration), weight, intake, and output
- Supervise and assist with routine care such as bathing, feeding, and dressing
- Collect and test specimens
- Assist with treatments, examinations, and procedures
- Provide and assist with opportunities for play
- Provide warmth, security, and affection

CARING FOR SCHOOL-AGE CHILDREN (6–12 YEARS)

In general, the school-age years are a time of exceptionally good health. School-age children are more active, stronger, and steadier than younger children. They have either had most of the childhood illnesses or have been immunized against them. The most common problems of these times involve the gastrointestinal system (for example, stomach aches) and the respiratory system (for example, colds and coughs).

Developmental Tasks

In this period, the child is striving to achieve a sense of accomplishment through an increasing number of tasks and completion of projects. He also continues to increase control over his environment and his independence. It is important to remember these tasks when caring for the school-age child.

The school-age child's reaction to hospitalization will be significantly different from that of the younger child. The school-age child is better able to handle the stress of illness and hospitalization. In fact, hospitalization presents the school-age child with an opportunity to:

- Explore a new environment
- Meet new friends (Figure 50-22)
- Learn more about her body

FIGURE 50-22 School-age children usually enjoy meeting and playing with new friends.

Psychosocial Adjustment

Separation from parents will not be as difficult for the school-age child. However, those just entering this period may regress to a preschool level. These children will need their parents' presence.

The school-age child has left the security of home and entered the school system. In school, the child has begun to develop relationships with other children. In the hospital, she may respond more to the separation from her peers than from her parents. It is important to give these children opportunities to communicate with their schoolmates. For example, they can be helped to write letters and make phone calls. When possible, friends can visit.

The older school-age child may welcome the opportunity to be away from his parents. In this situation, the child can test newly developed skills and increase independence. Children of this age group also need privacy—but if the parents are there, they may not get it. Some parents may need to have their child's opposition to their staying explained in this context, because they may think the child is angry with them.

Roommate selection is especially important for this age group. A roommate of approximately the same age will act as a diversion. With a roommate of the same age, the child will be able to continue work on the developmental task of learning to get along with others. Because the school-age child is seeking more independence, she may be reluctant to ask for help even when she needs it. Her feelings may show themselves in different ways, such as:

- Irritability.
- Hostility toward her siblings.
- Other behavior problems. It is important that you, as a caregiver, observe and note these behaviors and bring them to the attention of the nurse.

Resistance to bedtime may also become a problem during these years. In the hospital, it is important to be aware of the parents' rules and follow them. Learning rules is another developmental task of the school-age years.

Adjustment to Illness

Fears or stresses associated with an illness and subsequent hospitalization contribute to the school-age child's feelings of loss of control. By involving the child in her own care, you will help her to be a more cooperative patient (Figure 50-23). Procedures that we routinely do without explanation or without providing options, such as using the bedpan, are particularly upsetting to the school-age child. This child is trying hard to act grown up but is not being given the chance. It is also important for this child's self-esteem that you do not scold him when he does lose control. It is best to just overlook the episode.

The school-age child is able to reason. She also understands the impact of her illness and the potential for disability and death. These children take an active interest in health and enjoy acquiring knowledge. You can help them

FIGURE 50-23 Explaining procedures boosts self-esteem, gives the child a sense of independence, and lets him feel that he is a participating team member.

gain information and deal with their fears by explaining all procedures in simple terms. This is also an appropriate age for playing with hospital equipment such as a stethoscope (Figure 50-24).

Pain is passively accepted by the school-age child. He is able to tell you where his pain is located and what it feels like. This child will hold rigidly still, bite his lip, or clench his fists when in pain, in an effort to keep in control and to act brave. This child does well with distraction during painful procedures. During procedures, you should stay with him whenever possible to talk him through them. This child also tries to postpone all major procedures. For example, when it is time to go to a test, he will need to go to the bathroom. The caregiver needs to put limits on the number of postponements the child is allowed.

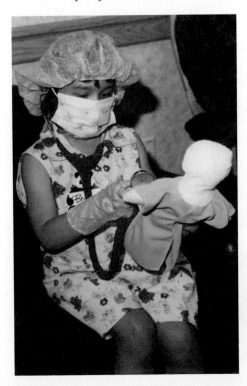

FIGURE 50-24 Showing the child how to use the equipment and enabling her to play with it is a good learning experience.

Age-Appropriate Care ALERT

Children aged 6 to 12 enjoy games. Make up games to teach them how you will perform a procedure, or challenge them to do a task, to reduce fear. Allow them to win, when possible, and praise them for trying and/or doing their best. Take the time to play age-appropriate board games, when possible. ■

GUIDELINES *for*

Ensuring a Safe Environment for School-Age Children

- Never leave poisonous materials within reach.
- Keep side rails up when children are in bed.
- Monitor toys to ensure that they are not dangerous.

Activities

Increased physical and social activities are characteristic of this period. Hospitalization does not usually provide school-age children with adequate diversions. School-age children may also miss the activities of school, although they usually deny this.

You should allow these children time during the day for their own work. This includes schoolwork and visits with friends and other patients. Competitiveness is also characteristic of this period. It adds to the school-age child's need to stay up-to-date with schoolwork (Figure 50-25). Having the play therapist at the hospital provide appropriate activities will help to reduce the stress the child feels.

Caregivers should encourage the child to take part in her own care as part of her work. Helping to make her bed or clean her room will make her feel useful. She should be held responsible only for tasks that are within her capabilities.

Physically, this child has entered a period of slow, steady growth. Although growth has slowed, it is still important to maintain a balanced diet. School-age children tend to be less picky about what they eat and they are more willing to try new foods.

Summary of Nursing Assistant Tasks and Responsibilities When Caring for School-Age Children

- Maintain a safe environment
- Apply standard precautions if contact with blood, body fluids, mucous membranes, or nonintact skin is likely
- Provide information to the health care team through monitoring of vital signs (temperature, pulse, and respiration), weight, intake, and output
- Supervise and assist with routine care
- Collect and test specimens
- Assist with treatments, examinations, and procedures
- Provide explanations using proper names of body parts, drawings, and books (Figure 50-26)
- Encourage socialization with other children in the same age group
- Provide time for schoolwork and tutors

CARING FOR THE ADOLESCENT (12–18 YEARS)

Adolescence is the transitional period from childhood into adulthood. Like school-age children, adolescents are relatively healthy. The major health problems of this period are usually related to the drastic physical changes that occur during this time, to accidents, to sports injuries, or to chronic and/or permanent disabilities.

Psychosocial Development

Dealing with adolescents is especially difficult for health care providers because:

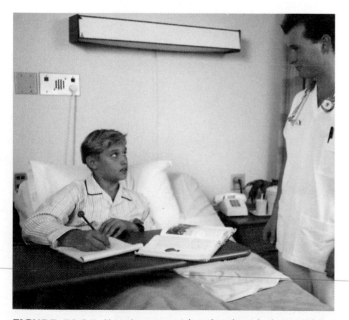

FIGURE 50-25 Keeping up with schoolwork during the hospitalization is important.

FIGURE 50-26 Sometimes children write or draw pictures depicting new information they have learned, or as a means of describing their fears. Injections are a common cause of anxiety for many children.

FIGURE 50-27 Adolescents may have a difficult time relating to those in authority.

- The adolescent is developing an identity and becoming increasingly independent.
- Being hospitalized forces the adolescent into a situation where she is dependent on others to meet her needs. Because of this, it is important to allow the adolescent to make as many of her own decisions as possible. When this is not possible, keep the adolescent involved in the decision-making process.
- Adolescents have a difficult time with authority figures (Figure 50-27). As the caregiver, you will represent authority to this child. You should not get into struggles with the adolescent. Limit restrictions whenever appropriate.
- Adolescents are usually uncooperative. The best approach is to let the adolescent know, in a nonthreatening way, what the rules of the unit are (Figure 50-28). It is best to do this at the time of admission. Speak to adolescents as you would to adults. Be as flexible as possible. For example, instead of struggling through the morning trying to get the adolescent up and washed, give him a list of things that have to be accomplished by a certain time. Then allow him the freedom to do things his way and in his order. At the time you decided on, check back with the adolescent to see that the tasks have been completed.

The most important people to adolescents are their friends. A hospital stay makes it more difficult for the adolescent to see friends. It is essential that you:

- Allow the adolescent time for visits
- Permit phone calls (Figure 50-29).
- Introduce them to other patients their age

Recognize that adolescents may not want to visit with others if illness has changed their appearance in any way. Body image is important at this age. You can promote a

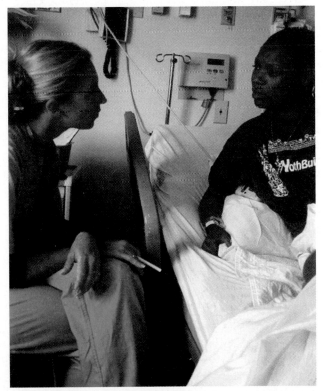

FIGURE 50-28 Taking the time to talk to the adolescent on her level is an excellent way of learning her fears and explaining unit rules. This two-way exchange is better received than lecturing or dictating to the child.

positive image by encouraging the adolescent to continue a normal grooming routine in the hospital. Also encourage the adolescent to wear clothes or her own pajamas. This will make her look and feel better about herself. Use the opportunity to teach good hygiene practices if the hospitalized adolescent does not already practice them. Ask a nurse to help if you note that this is a problem for a patient.

FIGURE 50-29 Staying in contact with friends is very important.

Keep in mind that the adolescent is very aware of the changes taking place in his body, whether they can be seen or not. It is important to provide the adolescent with privacy. Keep him covered as much as possible during procedures and examinations.

Nutrition and Activity

Adolescents go through a growth spurt. Girls are usually 2 years ahead of boys. Adequate nutrition and rest continue to be important. In the hospital, the importance of proper eating habits should be stressed to the adolescent. You should:

- Permit the adolescent to continue to make decisions about what and when she will eat, unless it is medically unsafe.
- Recognize that adolescent girls are often on diets. Emotional problems related to weight are common.
- Be aware that adolescents frequently skip breakfast.

The adolescent often stays up late and likes to sleep late in the morning. Sleep requirements are decreased, but a good night's sleep is essential. It is important to explain the routines of the unit and yet provide flexibility for the adolescent. For example, if the television must be turned off at a certain time, the adolescent should be encouraged to find another quiet activity (such as listening to music with headphones) if he does not want to go to sleep. Many hospitals have lounges exclusively for the use of this age group, for their own activities and for socializing. Check with the nurse to find out if there is a specific area for adolescents.

Summary of Nursing Assistant Tasks and Responsibilities When Caring for Adolescents

- Maintain a safe environment
- Apply standard precautions if contact with blood, body fluids, mucous membranes, or nonintact skin is likely
- Orient the adolescent to unit and hospital rules
- Provide information to the health team through monitoring of vital signs (temperature, pulse, and respiration), weight, intake, and output
- Provide simple explanations to the adolescent
- Assist with body hygiene to help maintain positive self-image
- Collect and test specimens
- Assist with treatment, examinations, and procedures
- Promote independence; allow adolescents as much control as possible over schedule of treatments, procedures, and so on
- Encourage socialization with other adolescents

GUIDELINES *for*

Ensuring a Safe Environment for Adolescents

- Carefully check all electrical equipment that the adolescent brings to the hospital—radios, hair dryers, and so on—to ensure that it is appropriate and safe to use. Review hospital guidelines regarding use of electrical equipment with the patient.
- Review smoking policies with all adolescents.
- Reinforce to adolescents that alcohol and other drugs are illegal and are not permitted.
- Provide assistance with showers and bathing if the patient is incapacitated or weakened in any way. The adolescent may not ask for assistance.
- Reinforce the use of shoes or slippers to prevent injuries to the feet.
- Remind adolescents to keep staff informed of their whereabouts.
- Keep beds in low position to prevent falls.

REVIEW

A. True/False.

Mark the following true or false by circling T or F.

1. T F It is normal for a child to regress when hospitalized.

2. T F The nursing assistant can foster an infant's sense of trust by keeping him warm and dry.

3. T F The nursing assistant may assume the role of substitute mother.

4. T F Between the ages of 6 and 7 months, the infant loses her fear of strangers.

5. T F Following a feeding, the infant should be encouraged to play.

6. T F Routine weighing of the infant should be carried out right after the 10:00 AM feeding.

7. T F Pulse and respirations should be measured when the child is quiet or asleep.

8. T F The school-age child has an average heart rate of 90 to 140 beats per minute.

9. T F The respiratory rate of the toddler averages 30 to 60 respirations per minute.

10. T F The systolic blood pressure of the child increases with age.

11. T F Preschoolers normally have many fears.

12. T F The preschooler learns his or her sex role in life by imitating the behavior of the opposite-sex parent.

13. T F The most common physical complaints of a school-age child are stomach aches and colds.

14. T F The school-age child would be most comfortable sharing a room with a teenager.

15. T F It is best to overlook the loss of self-control exhibited by the school-age child.

16. T F The best way to measure a pulse rate in an infant or child is the apical method.

17. T F The temperature of a child under 5 years of age should be measured using the rectal method.

18. T F Sucking should be encouraged only when the infant is hungry.

19. T F It is proper to prop a bottle so the infant can eat in his crib if you are very busy.

20. T F After a feeding, the infant should be placed carefully on her back.

21. T F To entertain an infant, tie a bright red balloon to the crib.

22. T F The toddler should be placed in a crib with a top and sides as a safety measure.

23. T F It is permissible to allow a toddler to play unsupervised in a bathtub for a short time before bathing him, as long as the water is warm.

24. T F Adolescents have a difficult time dealing with authority figures.

25. T F Adolescents are particularly sensitive about changes in their body images.

B. Matching.

Choose the correct word from Column II to match each phrase in Column I.

Column I

26. _____ physical and psychological achievements

27. _____ achievement of skills characteristic of a specific age group

28. _____ a person married to a biological parent

29. _____ to move backward developmentally

30. _____ person who has the right to consent to procedures and hospitalization of a minor

31. _____ birth parent

32. _____ self-determination

Column II

a. autonomy   **e.** biological parent

b. regress   **f.** developmental milestone

c. legal guardian   **g.** stepparent

d. developmental tasks

C. Nursing Assistant Challenge.

You are assigned to take vital signs. The nurse manager just asked the maintenance department to check a problem with the tympanic thermometer, so it is not available. An electronic thermometer is available on the unit, as are oral and rectal glass thermometers. Select the appropriate thermometer and route or method for taking temperatures on these patients:

33. Joey, a 3-week-old infant who was admitted for surgery.

34. Brittany, a 15-month-old child who was admitted with an upper respiratory infection.

35. David, a 4-year-old child who was admitted with diarrhea.

36. Maria, a 6-year-old with cystic fibrosis, who is having difficulty breathing.

37. Lisa, an 8-year-old admitted with leukemia.

38. Robert, a 13-year-old who had his appendix removed earlier today.

UNIT 51

Special Advanced Procedures

OBJECTIVES

After completing this unit, you will be able to:

- Spell and define terms.
- State the reasons for removing an indwelling catheter as soon as possible.
- List the guidelines for caring for an ostomy.
- List at least six procedures in which sterile technique is used.
- State nursing assistant responsibilities for the care of patients with advanced airways.
- Demonstrate the following procedures:
  - Procedure 123 Testing for Occult Blood Using Hemoccult and Developer
  - Procedure 124 Collecting a Urine Specimen Through a Drainage Port
  - Procedure 125 Removing an Indwelling Catheter
  - Procedure 126 Giving Routine Stoma Care (Colostomy)
  - Procedure 127 Routine Care of an Ileostomy (with Patient in Bed)
  - Procedure 128 Setting Up a Sterile Field Using a Sterile Drape
  - Procedure 129 Adding an Item to a Sterile Field
  - Procedure 130 Adding Liquids to a Sterile Field
  - Procedure 131 Applying and Removing Sterile Gloves
  - Procedure 132 Using Transfer Forceps

VOCABULARY

Learn the meaning and the correct spelling of the following words and phrases:

appliance	endotracheal tube (ET tube)	oropharyngeal airway	ventilator
bag-valve-mask		ostomy	Yankauer catheter
colostomy	ileostomy	port	
endotracheal intubation	nasopharyngeal airway	stoma	

INTRODUCTION

The responsibilities of nursing assistants vary throughout the nation. The scope and type of assignments that are given to nursing assistants are influenced by:

- Basic preparation
- Experience
- Specific advanced training in procedural skills
- Facility policy
- State laws that specify the range of practice of nursing assistants

Important principles to keep in mind are that:

- Some procedures that are considered routine for some workers would not be appropriate or permitted in other situations. Even basic procedures such as bed bathing might be restricted to nurses if the situation or patient conditions warrant such precautions.

- Under no circumstances can it be assumed that because the following procedures are included in this textbook, they should be assigned to all nursing assistants.
- Each facility has established policies and supervisory practices that are consistent with legal regulations and that ensure competency on the part of the caregiver and safety for the patient.
- These procedures are to be carried out only after adequate practice, with supervision, and only in accord with specific facility policy. Additional information supporting these advanced procedures may be found in the units indicated.

URINE AND STOOL TESTS

Special tests performed on urine and stool samples may be part of your responsibility. Additional information appears in Units 44 and 45.

Collecting a Specimen from a Closed Urinary Drainage System

At some time, it may be necessary to collect a fresh specimen of urine when the patient is on a closed urinary drainage system. Keep in mind that the:

- Urine sample must be fresh
- Urine in the bag has accumulated over a period of time

PROCEDURE

123

TESTING FOR OCCULT BLOOD USING HEMOCCULT AND DEVELOPER

1. Wash your hands and assemble equipment:
   - Disposable gloves
   - Bedpan with fresh specimen
   - Hemoccult slide packet
   - Hemoccult developer
   - Tongue blade
   - Paper towel

2. Place the paper towel on a flat surface and open the flap of the Hemoccult packet, exposing the guaiac paper.

3. Put on gloves.

4. Using a tongue blade, take a small sample of feces and smear it on the paper area marked A (Figure 51-1A).

5. Repeat the procedure, taking the fecal sample from a different part of the specimen and making a smear in area B.

6. Close the tab and turn the packet over.

7. Open the back tab.

8. Apply two drops of Hemoccult developer directly over each smear (Figure 51-1B). Time the reaction.

continues

PROCEDURE 123 CONTINUED

FIGURE 51-1A A small stool specimen is placed on a special area of the card for an occult blood test.

9. Read the results 30 to 60 seconds later.

FIGURE 51-1B Apply drops of Hemoccult developer on the exposed guaiac paper.

10. The presence of blood is indicated by a blue discoloration around the perimeter of the smear.

11. Dispose of the specimen.

12. Clean the bedpan according to facility policy and dispose of the paper towel, packet, and tongue blade.

13. Remove and dispose of gloves according to facility policy. Wash your hands.

• The specimen may not be taken from the bag
• The specimen must be taken from the catheter

The procedure to be followed is determined by the type of Foley catheter that is in place. If the catheter has a **port**

(opening) for fluid withdrawal, follow Procedure 124. The procedure must be carried out using proper techniques, to avoid introducing infectious organisms into the system.

PROCEDURE

124

COLLECTING A URINE SPECIMEN THROUGH A DRAINAGE PORT

1. Carry out initial procedure actions.

2. Assemble equipment:
   • Disposable gloves
   • Tube clamp
   • Laboratory requisition
   • Completed label
   • Emesis basin
   • 10-mL syringe
   • Specimen cup and lid

   • 21-gauge or 22-gauge needle
   • Sharps container
   • Alcohol wipe
   • Bed protector
   • Biohazard specimen transport bag

3. Go to the bedside half an hour before the sample is to be collected.

4. Clamp the drainage tube.

continues

PROCEDURE 124 CONTINUED

5. Wash your hands. Return to the bedside after 30 minutes.

6. Put on gloves.

7. Place a bed protector on the bed and place an emesis basin on the bed protector under the catheter drainage port.

8. Wipe the drainage port with an alcohol wipe (Figure 51-2).

9. Carefully remove the cap on the syringe. Do not contaminate the tip.

10. Attach the needle carefully. Do not contaminate the needle tip.

11. Open the package with the specimen container. Remove the lid and lay it, inside up, on the bed-

side stand. Do not touch the inside of the cup or the lid with your hands.

12. Insert the needle into the port and withdraw the specimen (Figure 51-3).

13. Carefully withdraw the needle.

14. Wipe the port with the alcohol wipe.

15. Transfer the urine sample to the specimen container (Figure 51-4).

16. Handling the lid by the top only, cover the container.

17. Do not recap the needle. Do not detach the needle from the syringe. Discard the needle and syringe into the sharps container at the bedside.

18. Remove gloves and dispose of according to facility policy. Wash your hands.

Infection Control ALERT

Unless you are instructed otherwise, select a sterile specimen collection cup for this procedure. Avoid touching the inside of the cup and the lid with your hands. When you open the cup, place the lid with the clean, inner side up on the table. Make sure the clamp is removed from the drainage tube before you leave the room after collecting the specimen, or urine will back up into the patient's bladder, causing discomfort and increasing the potential for infection and other complications. ∎

FIGURE 51-3 Draw the specimen into the needle.

FIGURE 51-2 Wipe the port with an antiseptic wipe or alcohol sponge.

FIGURE 51-4 Transfer the specimen to the container.

continues

PROCEDURE 124 CONTINUED

FIGURE 51-5
Place the specimen in the biohazard transport bag, seal the bag, and attach the laboratory requisition.

19. Remove the catheter clamp.

20. Complete the information on the label and put the label on the container. Compare the label to the requisition to be sure that the information is complete and accurate.

21. Place the specimen container in a biohazard transport bag, seal the bag, and attach the completed laboratory requisition (Figure 51-5).

22. Carry out ending procedure actions.

23. Follow instructions for care and transport of the specimen.

REMOVING AN INDWELLING CATHETER

An indwelling catheter is removed as soon as possible to reduce the risk of infection. A catheter must also be removed if it is obstructed, or for a routine change ordered by the physician. If a new catheter is not reinserted by the nurse, you must monitor the patient's voiding after catheter removal. Follow your facility policy for reporting to the nurse. If the patient has not voided within 4 to 6 hours, or if she complains of abdominal pain, notify the nurse.

PROCEDURE

REMOVING AN INDWELLING CATHETER

1. Carry out initial procedure actions.

2. Assemble equipment:
   - Disposable exam gloves, 2 pair
   - 10-mL syringe
   - Underpad
   - Plastic bag for used supplies
   - Washcloth
   - Towel
   - Washbasin
   - Soap

3. Position the underpad under the patient's buttocks.

4. Remove the tape or Velcro strap that secures the catheter to the leg.

5. Manipulate the tubing so that any urine in the tubing flows into the drainage bag.

6. Open the syringe. Attach the syringe to the inflation port.

7. Allow the inflation balloon to deflate into the syringe on its own. Follow facility policy for pulling on the plunger to withdraw fluid. If this method is used, pull very gently to avoid collapsing the inflation tube. (When the inflation tubing is collapsed, deflation of the balloon cannot occur.) The amount of fluid in the balloon may be marked on the catheter. Make sure you remove this amount. Depending on the catheter used, the port may flatten when the fluid is withdrawn. Empty the fluid from the syringe, reinsert the needle, and attempt to remove fluid again. When you are satisfied that the balloon is empty, proceed to the next step.

continues

PROCEDURE 125 CONTINUED

8. Grasp the catheter close to the perineum. Gently pull the catheter. If you feel resistance, stop. The balloon may not be completely deflated. Repeat steps 6 and 7.

9. If no resistance is met, withdraw the catheter. Observe the tip for the presence of sediment, blood, or mucus. If present, inform the nurse, who may request a culture.

10. Disconnect the catheter from the drainage tubing. Discard the catheter in the plastic bag, or according to facility policy.

   Note: Some facilities culture the tip of the catheter after it is removed. If this will be done, you will need a sterile specimen cup and sterile scissors. After removing the catheter, hold the end over the open specimen cup, and clip it 3 inches from the tip. Cover the cup and discard the remainder of the catheter.

11. Remove gloves and discard in the plastic bag.

12. Wash your hands.

13. Apply clean gloves.

14. Perform perineal care according to facility policy.

15. Empty the catheter bag and measure output. Discard the empty bag in the plastic bag, or according to facility policy.

16. After the catheter is removed, instruct the patient to drink fluids, if permitted. Offer to take the patient to the bathroom, or offer the bedpan or urinal in 2 to 4 hours. Inform the nurse if the patient cannot void, or has complaints of urgency, pain, or burning.

17. Carry out ending procedure actions.

OSTOMIES

The surgical removal of a section of diseased bowel requires the creation of an artificial opening (**ostomy**) in the abdominal wall for elimination of solid waste and flatus.

Care of the Patient with a Colostomy

When the colon is brought through the abdominal wall, the opening is called a **colostomy**. The mouth of the opening is called a **stoma** (Figure 51-6). The ostomy may be temporary or permanent. The location of the ostomy (Figure 51-7) determines if the feces are formed, soft and mushy, semiliquid, or liquid.

The patient with a colostomy does not have normal sphincter control. This means the patient cannot voluntarily control emptying of the bowel in the same manner as emptying through the anus. If the colostomy is located in the bowel where stool is formed, regularity of elimination may be established. As elimination is controlled, the stoma may be covered with a simple dressing between evacuations. Liquid to mushy fecal drainage from a stoma is collected in a disposable drainage pouch, called an **appliance**, that is attached over the stoma. (Refer to Procedure 126.) Proper stoma care is required to maintain healthy tissue, because the area around the opening comes into contact with liquid or semiliquid stool. At the stoma, there may be problems of:

- Leakage
- Odor control
- Irritation of the surrounding area

You can assist the patient who has a colostomy by:

- Keeping the area clean and dry
- Performing routine stoma care, including removing drainage and/or replacing the appliance if your facility allows you to assist or give this care after you have had special training

Remember:

- Initial irrigations will be performed by the nurse
- If the colostomy is to be permanent, patients are taught to carry out the irrigation procedure for themselves

FIGURE 51-6 Typical colostomy stoma

Fluid to Semifluid Feces

Ascending Colostomy

Mushy Feces

Transverse Colostomy

Semimushy to Solid Feces

Descending Colostomy

Solid (Formed) Feces

Sigmoid Colostomy

FIGURE 51-7 The location of the ostomy determines the character of the feces.

Difficult SITUATIONS

The two-piece system has an outer ring that snaps onto the pouch. The size of the ring in the pouch is very important. An improper fit can injure the stoma. It must seal the appliance around the stoma, but not fit so tightly that it squeezes the stoma. An improperly applied belt may also injure the stoma. Read the directions and make sure you understand how to use the type of device you have. ■

Difficult SITUATIONS

Having an ostomy alters the way a patient eliminates waste. This alteration of body image can be very traumatic for the patient. Covering the pouch with an attractive cover (check with the enterostomal therapy nurse) may help the patient's self-esteem. The ostomy may also have a profound effect on the patient's sex life. Be supportive and empathetic. Occasionally, a patient may become aroused or feel sexual pleasure when the ostomy is touched. Remain calm and professional and do not overreact. Avoid sending the patient mixed sexual messages, even in a joking manner. If the patient persists, inform him or her that sexual advances are not appropriate. The patient will most likely be very embarrassed about becoming involuntarily sexually aroused. ■

GUIDELINES *for*
Caring for an Ostomy

- Apply the principles of standard precautions. Avoid environmental contamination with your gloves.

- Remove and apply the ostomy appliance gently to prevent irritation to the skin. It may help to apply gentle traction to the skin next to the appliance when you are removing the adhesive.

- Empty the reusable bag and wash it thoroughly with soap and water after each bowel movement. Secure the clamp at the bottom of the bag to prevent leaking. Discard a disposable bag in the biohazardous waste and replace it with a new bag.

- Observe the stoma and surrounding skin for redness, irritation, and skin breakdown; report to the nurse, if present.

- After the appliance has been removed, gently wipe the area surrounding the stoma with toilet tissue. Discard the tissue in the toilet or a plastic bag. If a plastic bag is used, discard it in the biohazardous waste.

- Wash the skin around the stoma with mild soap when the appliance is removed. Rinse well and gently pat dry.

- Apply skin barriers, lubricants, or medicated creams to the area surrounding the stoma as stated on the care plan. Apply only a thin layer. Avoid caking any products on the skin.

- You may be required to cut an opening into the appliance before applying it to the skin. Cut the area about 1/8 inch larger than the size of the stoma.

- When reapplying a new appliance, seal the entire area surrounding the stoma, to prevent leaking.

- Observe the color, character, amount, and frequency of stools, and report abnormalities to the nurse.

PROCEDURE

126

GIVING ROUTINE STOMA CARE (COLOSTOMY)

1. Carry out initial procedure actions.

2. Assemble equipment:
   - Disposable gloves
   - Washcloth and towel
   - Basin of warm water
   - Bed protectors
   - Bath blanket
   - Disposable colostomy bag and belt
   - Bedpan
   - Skin lotion as directed
   - Prescribed solvent and dropper
   - Cleansing agent
   - Adhesive wafer
   - 4 × 4 gauze square
   - Toilet tissue
   - Plastic bag

3. Place a bath blanket over the patient. Fanfold the top bedding to the foot of the bed.

4. Wash your hands and put on disposable gloves.

5. Place a bed protector under the patient's hips.

6. Place a bedpan and cover on a bed protector on the chair.

7. Remove the soiled disposable stoma bag (appliance) and place it in the bedpan or plastic bag—note the amount and type of drainage.

8. Remove the belt that holds the stoma bag and save it, if clean.

9. Gently clean the area around the stoma with toilet tissue to remove feces and drainage (Figure 51-8). Dispose of used tissue in the bedpan or plastic bag.

continues

PROCEDURE 126 CONTINUED

10. Wash the area around the stoma with soap and water. Rinse thoroughly and dry.

11. If ordered, apply barrier cream lightly around the stoma. Too much lotion may interfere with proper sealing of the fresh ostomy bag.

12. Position a clean belt around the patient. Inspect the skin under the belt for irritation or breakdown.

13. It may be necessary to remove the adhesive wafer. To select the proper size of wafer, you can use a commercial guide to size the stoma (Figure 51-9).

14. Replace the adhesive wafer (Figure 51-10). Place a clean ostomy bag over the stoma and secure the belt.

15. Remove the bed protector. Check to be sure the bottom bedding is not wet. Change it if necessary.

16. Remove gloves and discard according to facility policy. Wash your hands.

17. Replace the bath blanket with the top bedding, and make the patient comfortable.

18. Using a paper towel to protect your hands, gather and cover the soiled materials and bedpan or plastic bag. Take them to the utility room. Dispose of materials according to facility policy.

19. Empty, wash, and dry the bedpan. Store it according to facility policy.

20. Carry out ending procedure actions.

FIGURE 51-8 The area around the stoma is cleansed gently, then dried before a new appliance is applied.

FIGURE 51-9 Check the stoma size to make sure the correct size barrier is used.

FIGURE 51-10 Apply a new barrier adhesive wafer around the stoma.

Difficult SITUATIONS

Most ostomy appliances are odor-free. If odor control is a problem, consult the nurse. Commercial products are available to eliminate odors in the bag. Leave a small amount of air in the bag when changing it, to allow stool to fall to the bottom. ■

Care of the Patient with an Ileostomy

An **ileostomy** is a permanent artificial opening in the ileum (Figure 51-11) that drains through a stoma on the surface of the abdomen. The drainage from the ileum is in liquid form and contains digestive enzymes that are irritating to the skin. (Refer to Procedure 127.)

Considerations for caring for a patient with an ileostomy include:

- The licensed nurse cares for the patient with a new ileostomy.
- Routine care may be given by nursing assistants.
- The drainage from an ileostomy is very irritating to the skin, so care of the skin surrounding the stoma is crucial.
- The fit of the ileostomy ring is important so that leakage does not occur. This is true for both the disposable and reusable types of appliances (Figure 51-12).

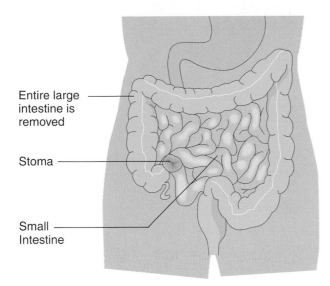

FIGURE 51-11 An ileostomy brings a section of the ileum through the abdominal wall.

Entire large intestine is removed

Stoma

Small Intestine

A. Adhesive ring seals around stoma to prevent leakage
B. Opening placed over stoma
C. Collection bag
D. Drainage end of bag
E. Secures drainage end of bag to prevent leakage

FIGURE 51-12 Stoma protector and collection bag (Courtesy of Hollister, Inc, Libertyville, Illinois)

PROCEDURE

ROUTINE CARE OF AN ILEOSTOMY (WITH PATIENT IN BED)

1. Carry out initial procedure actions.

2. Assemble equipment:
   - Disposable gloves
   - Basin of warm water
   - Bed protector
   - Bath blanket
   - Bedpan and cover
   - Fresh appliance and belt
   - Clamp for appliance
   - Prescribed solvent and dropper
   - Cotton balls
   - Deodorant (if permitted)
   - Cleansing agent
   - Karaya ring
   - 4 × 4 gauze squares
   - Toilet tissue
   - Paper towels
   - Plastic bag

3. Raise the opposite side rail for safety. Elevate the head of the bed and assist the patient to turn on the side toward you.

4. Replace bedding with a bath blanket.

5. Wash your hands. Put on disposable gloves.

6. Place a bed protector under the patient.

7. Place a bedpan on the bed protector against the patient.

8. Place the end of the ileostomy bag in the bedpan or plastic bag. Open the clamp and allow the bag to drain (note the clamp in Figure 51-12). Note the amount and character of drainage.

continues

PROCEDURE 127 CONTINUED

9. Wipe the end of the drainage sheath with toilet paper and move it out of drainage. Place used tissue in the bedpan. Cover the bedpan.

10. Disconnect the belt from the appliance and remove the belt from the patient. Place it on paper towels.

11. With a dropper, apply a small amount of solvent around the ring of the appliance. This will loosen it so it can be removed. Wait a few seconds. Do not force the appliance free.

12. Cover the stoma with gauze.
    - Carefully inspect the skin area around the stoma.
    - If the area is irritated or the skin is broken, cover the patient with a bath blanket, raise the side rail, and lower the bed.
    - Remove gloves and dispose of properly.
    - Wash your hands.
    - Report to the nurse for instructions.
    - Put on fresh gloves before continuing the procedure.

13. Remove the gauze from the stoma and place it on paper towels.

14. If an appliance is used with a Karaya ring, moisten the ring, allow it to become sticky, and apply it to the stoma. If the appliance uses a paper-covered adhesive strip around the stoma opening, remove the paper and apply the strip around the stoma.

15. Clamp the appliance bag and apply it to the ring.

16. Remove gloves and dispose of properly. Wash your hands.

17. Adjust a clean belt in position around the patient and connect it to the appliance.

18. Remove the bath blanket and assist the patient to wash hands.

19. Wash your hands. Put on gloves.

20. Clean the patient's bathroom. Wash the belt and appliance, if reusable, and allow them to dry.

21. Carry out ending procedure actions.

STERILE TECHNIQUE

In many facilities, only licensed nursing personnel perform procedures using sterile technique. However, there are times when a nursing assistant may be asked to assist with a sterile procedure. Common nursing procedures in which sterile technique is used are:

- All invasive procedures
- Procedures in which the skin is broken, such as injections and insertion of intravenous needles or catheters
- Procedures in which body cavities are entered, such as catheterization and tracheal suctioning
- Changing surgical dressings
- Changing dressings on central intravenous catheters (Unit 36)
- Procedures involving patients with severe destruction of the skin, such as burns and trauma

Only sterile supplies contact the patient's body during sterile procedures. Sterile gloves are worn. Masks are worn during some sterile procedures. Follow Procedure 2 for applying a mask. In some procedures, the patient also wears a mask. In others, a mask is not necessary. Check with the nurse if you are not sure whether to wear a mask.

Environmental Conditions

Before using a sterile item, or creating a sterile field, check the environment. The surface on which you open the sterile package must be clean, dry, flat, and stable. The area must be free from airborne contamination. Patients can accidentally contaminate sterile supplies and trays. Explain the procedure to the patient before beginning. Instruct him or her to avoid touching sterile supplies, crossing over the sterile field, or talking, coughing, or sneezing over sterile articles. Remind the patient during the procedure, as necessary.

Setting Up a Sterile Field

A *sterile field* is a sterile surface that you create to use as a work area for sterile procedures. A 1-inch border around the outside edge of the field is considered not sterile. Avoid placing sterile items in this border area. Only the top surface of the work area is considered sterile. A sterile drape often hangs over the edges of the table. The area below the table top is not sterile. Sterile supplies can touch only the sterile field. Avoid touching the field or items on it with your hands.

GUIDELINES *for*
Sterile Procedures

- Always wash your hands before beginning a sterile procedure.
- Check the expiration date on the package. Avoid using items that are beyond the expiration date.
- If the sterility of an item is in doubt, consider it unsterile and avoid using it.
- If a sterile package is cracked, cut, or torn, it is contaminated and should not be used.
- If a sterile item or package becomes wet, it is contaminated.
- If a sterile item contacts an unsterile item, the sterile item is contaminated.
- Follow your facility policy. You may be asked to sanitize and dry the table or other surface that sterile supplies will be placed on before establishing a sterile field.
- The outside of a sterile wrapper is not sterile. It may be handled with your hands. Avoid touching the inside of the wrapper or items inside the package with your hands.

- The inside of a sterile package can be used as a sterile field.
- Never turn your back on a sterile field.
- Avoid reaching across or touching a sterile field. If you must add an item to the sterile field, drop it onto the field from the sterile package.
- Avoid touching unsterile articles when wearing sterile gloves. Avoid touching the outside of sterile packages when wearing sterile gloves. Make sure you can see your hands at all times. Keep them above your waist. Avoid touching your clothing or body. If the gloves become torn or contaminated, change them immediately.
- If sterile gloves touch an unsterile item, such as the outside of a package, they are contaminated. Change them before proceeding.
- Keep sterile items above waist level.
- Avoid talking, coughing, or sneezing over a sterile field.

PROCEDURE 128

SETTING UP A STERILE FIELD USING A STERILE DRAPE

1. Wash your hands.
2. Open the sterile package containing the sterile drape.
3. With the thumb and index finger of your dominant hand, grasp the folded top edge of the drape.
4. Lift the drape out of the package. Extend your arm, holding the drape away from your body. Allow it to unfold. Make sure it does not touch any other surface, your body, or clothing as it unfolds.
5. Pick up the top corner on the other side of the drape after it is unfolded. Avoid touching the drape to your body, clothing, or other surfaces.
6. Beginning with the side opposite your body, slowly lay the drape across the table (Figure 51-13).
7. Open the other packages and add necessary items to the sterile field.

FIGURE 51-13 Beginning on the opposite side of the table, slowly position the drape.

PROCEDURE

129

ADDING AN ITEM TO A STERILE FIELD

1. Wash your hands.

2. Open the sterile package.

3. With one hand, grasp the package from the bottom. Using your free hand, pull the sides of the package away from the sterile field (Figure 51-14A). If you are using a peel-away package, peel the sides apart and drop the inner package onto the sterile field (Figure 51-14B).

4. Drop the sterile item onto the sterile field. Avoid touching the sterile field with the package wrapper.

5. Discard the wrapper.

FIGURE 51-14A Pull the sides of the outer wrap back so they do not touch the sterile field. Drop the inner sterile package onto the sterile field.

FIGURE 51-14B Peel the sides of the outer package back, then drop the sterile inner package onto the sterile field.

PROCEDURE

130

ADDING LIQUIDS TO A STERILE FIELD

1. Wash your hands.

2. Inspect the container. The seal should be intact, and the container should not be broken or cracked.

3. Open the container of liquid.

4. Place the cap upright on the table, with the outside of the cap resting on the table surface and the clean inner side facing up.

continues

PROCEDURE 130 CONTINUED

5. Pour a small amount of the solution into the sink or wastebasket to rinse the lip. When adding the solution to the sterile field, pour from the same side of the container. This is done to remove any microbes that might be on the lip.

6. Hold the bottle at an angle, 6 to 8 inches above the sterile bowl or other sterile container. Avoid reaching across the sterile field with your arm or hand.

7. From the clean side of the container, slowly pour the liquid to prevent splashing (Figure 51-15). If the liquid is spilled or splashed, the field is contaminated because moisture soaks through to the nonsterile surface beneath.

8. Replace the cap on the bottle.

9. Write the date and time the container was opened on the bottle. Write on the label, or use a separate piece of tape. Avoid writing directly

FIGURE 51-15 Pour the liquid slowly into the cup to prevent splashing.

on the plastic bottle. The ink from a pen or marker may bleed through the plastic, contaminating the solution.

If a small surface is needed, the inside of a sterile package can be used as a sterile field. If a larger surface is needed, a sterile drape is used as the foundation for the sterile field.

Sterile Gloves. Using sterile gloves is essential when using aseptic (sterile) technique. Wearing sterile gloves permits you to touch sterile items without contaminating them.

PROCEDURE

APPLYING AND REMOVING STERILE GLOVES

1. Wash your hands.

2. Check the glove package for sterility.

3. Open the outer package by peeling the upper edges back with your thumbs.

4. Remove the inner package containing the gloves and place it on the inside of the outer package.

5. Open the inner package, handling it only by the corners on the outside (Figure 51-16).

6. Pick up the cuff of the right-hand glove using your left hand (Figure 51-17). Avoid touching the area below the cuff.

7. Insert your right hand into the glove. Spread your fingers slightly, sliding them into the glove

FIGURE 51-16 Carefully fold the edges of the package back without touching the inside of the package or the gloves.

continues

PROCEDURE 131 CONTINUED

FIGURE 51-17 With your fingertips, carefully lift the edges of the cuff, then slide the opposite hand into the glove.

FIGURE 51-18 Protect the right-hand glove by sliding the fingers under the cuff of the left glove. Slide your left hand into the glove. Once both hands are gloved, adjust both gloves for comfort and fit.

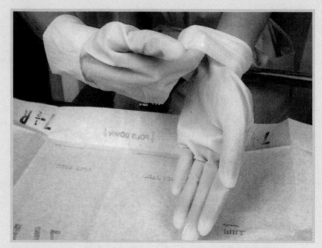

FIGURE 51-19 Carefully adjust the cuffs. Avoid touching your wrists.

fingers. If the glove is not on correctly, do not attempt to straighten it at this time.

8. Insert the gloved fingers of your right hand under the cuff of the left glove (Figure 51-18).

9. Slide your fingers into the left glove, adjusting the fingers of the gloves for comfort and fit. Because both gloves are sterile, they may touch each other. Avoid touching the cuffs of the gloves.

10. Insert your right hand under the cuff of the left glove and push the cuff up over your wrist (Figure 51-19). Avoid touching your wrist or the outside of the cuff with your glove.

11. Insert your left hand under the cuff of the right glove and push the cuff up over your wrist. Avoid touching your wrist or the outside of the cuff with your glove.

12. You may now touch sterile items with your sterile gloves. Avoid touching unsterile items.

To remove the gloves:

13. Grasp the outside of the glove on your nondominant hand at the cuff. Pull the glove off so that the inside of the glove faces outward. Avoid touching the skin of your wrist with the fingers of the glove.

14. Place this glove into the palm of the gloved hand.

15. Put the fingers of the ungloved hand *inside* the cuff of the gloved hand. Pull the glove off inside out. The first glove removed should be inside the second glove.

16. Discard the gloves into a covered container or trash, according to facility policy.

17. Wash your hands.

FIGURE 51-20
Use sterile transfer forceps to add sterile items to a sterile field. Do not allow the tips of the forceps to touch unsterile surfaces or objects. Wash the forceps after use and return them for sterilization according to facility policy. Do not use them for more than one procedure.

Transfer Forceps. Some facilities use sterile transfer forceps to add supplies to the sterile field (Figure 51-20). When the sterile tray is packaged, the cup for liquids is turned on its side. The transfer forceps are also used to turn the cup without contaminating the sterile tray. The forceps are used for one procedure, then sterilized after use. Using transfer forceps eliminates the need to use sterile gloves to handle sterile supplies.

The handle of the sterile forceps is contaminated because you have touched it with your hands. Avoid touching the end of the forceps. The tips must be kept sterile to contact sterile items. After using the forceps, the tips must rest on a sterile surface to keep them sterile until the end of the procedure.

INTRODUCTION TO ADVANCED AIRWAY MANAGEMENT

If you work in the subacute or critical care units, you will work with various patients who have advanced airways and those who need airway support to prevent or treat hypoxemia (Unit 39). Advanced health care providers, nurses, and RCPs will be responsible for managing patients' airways and ventilation devices. You must be able to identify the airways and ventilation devices and understand basic patient care. You must also be able to identify a patient who is in distress and needs immediate attention.

Oropharyngeal Airway

An **oropharyngeal airway** (Figure 51-21), or oral airway, is a curved plastic device that is inserted into the mouth to the posterior pharynx. The most common cause of airway obstruction is the tongue. The oral airway prevents the tongue from falling to the back of the throat and obstructing the airway. The airway has a flange at the end, which fits between the patient's lips. The curve of the airway holds the tongue forward. It is not the airway of choice for patients with recent oral surgery or those with loose teeth. The oral airway is used to keep the airway open in unconscious patients.

Difficult SITUATIONS

Conscious patients cannot tolerate the oropharyngeal (oral) airway. Inserting this airway into a conscious or semiconscious patient will induce vomiting. *If the patient is awake enough to spit the airway out, he or she does not need it.* ■

When caring for a patient with an oral airway, apply gloves and other personal protective equipment as needed to apply the principles of standard precautions. If the patient is known to cough, gag, or choke, make sure you wear a mask and eye protection. The patient may move the hand to the face to remove the airway. If he does this, do not attempt to stop him. Even if the patient is not

PROCEDURE

132

USING TRANSFER FORCEPS

1. Wash your hands.
2. Open the package of sterile supplies in the normal manner.
3. Grasp the needed item with the tips of the forceps.
4. Pick the item up, moving it to the sterile field.
5. Lay the tips of the forceps within the sterile field. Keep the handles on the outside of the field. If the forceps are needed again during the procedure, you can pick them up by the handles to use them again.

FIGURE 51-21 Various types and sizes of oral airways are available. The oral airway is used only for unresponsive patients.

FIGURE 51-22 The nasal airway may be used for responsive patients. Advanced nursing assistants are permitted to insert and care for the nasal airway in many facilities. This airway must be removed once every shift to provide nasal care and check for irritation in the nose.

fully awake, if he can pull it out, he does not need the airway.

 Note: This applies only to an oral airway, not an endotracheal tube.)

Check the patient's respirations immediately after the airway is removed to ensure that they are adequate. If you have concerns about the patient's ability to maintain the airway, discuss them with the nurse. When doing patient care, make sure the patient's tongue and lips are not positioned between the airway and the teeth. Make sure the airway remains in the correct position.

Nasopharyngeal Airway

A **nasopharyngeal airway** (Figure 51-22) is a curved, soft rubber device that is inserted through one nostril. It extends from the nostril to the posterior pharynx area, keeping the tongue off the back of the throat. This airway may be used in responsive patients. It is the airway of choice for patients with recent oral surgery, loose teeth, trauma of the mouth, and those who need frequent nasal suctioning. In many facilities, the airway is removed once every shift to provide nasal care and check for irritation in the nose. The airway is cleaned before it is reinserted. Follow your facility policies. You may hear this airway called a "nasal trumpet." This airway is not used for patients receiving anticoagulant (blood-thinning) medications or for those who have nasal deformity, bleeding disorders, or sepsis.

If the patient gags or coughs after the airway has been inserted, it may be too long. Notify the nurse or RCP promptly. If the patient is gagging and coughing, it may be necessary to wear a mask and eye protection in addition to gloves when providing patient care. A gown is needed if the patient cannot contain the secretions.

Endotracheal Intubation

Endotracheal intubation is a measure that provides complete control over the airway. It is commonly called "intu-

bation." An **endotracheal tube (ET tube)** is passed through the mouth, or less commonly the nose, into the patient's lungs (Figure 51-23). The patient is ventilated and suctioned through the tube. Patients are routinely intubated for many surgical procedures. Intubation is also commonly performed in some emergencies, including code (CPR) situations or when complete airway control is needed. Intubating the patient has many advantages over other methods of controlling the airway.

The endotracheal tube is inserted by a qualified health professional who is certified in advanced cardiac life support (ACLS). Although you will provide many aspects of patient care, only a licensed nurse, RCP, or physician should care for the endotracheal tube.

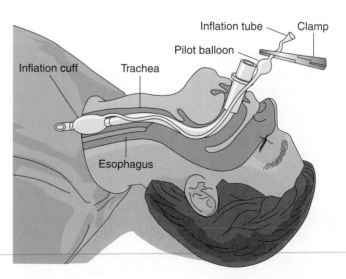

FIGURE 51-23 The endotracheal tube provides complete airway control. Patients cannot talk when this method of airway management is used.

Difficult SITUATIONS

Some bariatric surgery patients (Unit 31) require prolonged intubation, and continued mechanical ventilation is sometimes necessary after surgery. The airway can be difficult to manage in these patients because of the configuration of the head and neck. An emergency tracheostomy tube and tray should be kept at the bedside and be readily available at all times. Morbidly obese patients often cough more forcefully than smaller persons. The force of the cough can cause the endotracheal tube to migrate out of position. Select and wear the correct PPE if the patient is coughing or you will be exposed to oral, nasal, or airway secretions. To prevent accidental removal of the tube, be cautious and consider having extra staff available to help with:

- Transporting the morbidly obese patient who has an endotracheal tube

- Turning the patient and providing routine personal care

- Assisting with portable chest X-rays ∎

Caring for the Patient with an Endotracheal Tube. Patients who are intubated need a great deal of care, comfort measures, and reassurance. Because of the position of the tube, the patient will be unable to speak. Patients who are intubated are ventilated mechanically. This often involves using a **ventilator**, a positive-pressure mechanical device that forces air into the patient's lungs. The RCP and nurse will care for the ventilator, and will suction through the endotracheal tube, if needed. The patient may be restrained to prevent her from removing the endotracheal tube. A patient who is restrained will need total nursing care, including turning and repositioning, and restraint care and observation. The care plan or critical pathway will provide instructions.

Caring for a Patient Who Is Mechanically Ventilated

A ventilator is a mechanical device that facilitates breathing in patients with impaired respiratory or diaphragm function. The ventilator is connected to an endotracheal tube or the tracheostomy. Ventilators are used primarily in critical care and subacute care units. Patients who are using ventilators usually have serious medical problems, and may be very unstable. Most of the skilled services will be provided by the nurse or RCP. You will assist with ADLs and routine nursing care, as directed by the nurse.

The risk of infection is a great concern for patients who are mechanically ventilated. Use good handwashing (or alcohol-based hand cleaner) and be conscientious in using standard precautions and aseptic technique. Your job description and facility policy and procedure manuals will list your specific responsibilities.

GUIDELINES *for*

Guidelines and Nursing Assistant Responsibilities for Caring for Mechanically Ventilated Patients

- Monitor the patient frequently and anticipate his needs.

- Make sure the alarm is on at all times. It should never be turned off. Respond to alarms immediately. Remember, if an alarm sounds, check the patient first, not the machine.

- If an oral or nasal airway is used, the care plan may instruct you to keep the patient's head turned to the side to prevent aspiration.

- Monitor the patient's tolerance to the ventilator by checking pulse oximetry, vital signs, cardiac monitor, anxiety, ability to sleep, and mental status.

- Observe for changes in respiratory rate and depth, shortness of breath, and use of accessory muscles in breathing.

- When monitoring the vital signs of patients using mechanical ventilation, count spontaneous respirations as well as ventilator-delivered breaths.

- Visually inspect the chest when monitoring respirations. If it does not appear symmetrical (both sides expand equally) upon breathing, inform the nurse.

- Check for tube displacement or misplacement each time you are in the room. The endotracheal tube is usually marked at the lips, teeth, or nares, so you can see if the tube has moved.

continues

GUIDELINES *continued*

- Make sure the endotracheal tube is taped securely. Inform the nurse promptly if the tape is loose or comes off.

- Inform the nurse or RCP if the patient requires suctioning (is unable to manage oral or nasal secretions, is coughing or choking, or has loose or rattling respirations).

- Provide frequent oral and nasal care. Monitor the mucous membranes for signs of pressure, irritation, and breakdown from the breathing apparatus.

- Keep the lips and mucous membranes moist.

- Monitor the patient regularly for complaints of pain, and report to the nurse.

- Elevate the head of the bed 60° to 90°, or as directed in the care plan.

- Remember that elevation of the head of the bed increases the risk of skin breakdown. Reposition the patient every 2 hours or more often. Provide preventive skin care with lotion. Apply a therapeutic mattress, if ordered.

- Elevate the heels off the surface of the bed to prevent pressure ulcers. Heel protectors relieve friction and shearing. They do not prevent pressure.

- Condensation in the ventilator tubing causes resistance to air flow and increases the risk of aspiration. Condensate must be drained into a collection trap, or the patient must be disconnected from the ventilator long enough to empty the tubing. Inform the nurse or RCP if condensation forms. Do not attempt to perform this procedure. Never empty condensation in the ventilation tubing backward into the humidifier or in a way that causes you to get sprayed in the face with contaminated fluid.

- Make sure that adequate sterile supplies are available in the room in case they are needed quickly. Get a list of supplies from the care plan or nurse and restock the room every shift and as needed.

- Items needed for emergency care, such as a Kelly clamp, clean airway, or tracheostomy tray, may be stored in plain view in close proximity to the patient. Small items may be taped to the headboard, over the head of the bed, or in another convenient location. Make sure these items remain in view. Do not store them in a drawer or cupboard.

- Monitor the patient for constipation; inform the nurse if the patient has not had a BM in 3 days.

- Provide active and passive range of motion, according to the plan of care. Use positioning aids as necessary to support the patient's position, promote comfort, and reduce the risk of contractures.

- Monitor restraints, if used; release restraints according to facility policy.

- Monitor bony prominences for signs of redness, irritation, or breakdown.

- Be compassionate and empathetic to the patient's circumstances; reassure the patient and family.

- Use nursing comfort measures, such as a backrub or supporting the patient's position, to promote comfort.

- Develop a means for communicating with the patient, such as using a magic slate or writing.

Clinical Information ALERT

In some facilities, personnel are instructed to bring extra supplies to the room in anticipation of needing them during a procedure. For example, personnel commonly contaminate sterile gloves or sterile urinary catheters. Once supplies have been brought to a patient's room, they cannot be returned to stock and used in the care of another patient. Thus, if the "extra" sterile supplies are not used, they must be discarded. This is costly, in terms of replacement supplies and waste disposal. Some of the patient conditions discussed in this chapter are unstable, making it necessary to keep some stock items in the room. Know and follow your facility policies for bringing extra supplies into patients' rooms in anticipation of needing them during sterile procedures. Bring only what is needed. Avoid overstocking. Do so only if permitted by facility policy, and obtain directions on how to dispose of unused sterile items. ■

Assisted Ventilation for a Patient with an Endotracheal Tube. There will be times when the patient with an endotracheal tube or tracheostomy is not connected to the ventilator, such as during transportation or when tracheostomy care is being done. When a mechanical ventilator cannot be used, the **bag-valve-**

mask device must be used to ventilate a patient who is completely without effective respirations. You may have seen the bag-valve-mask device used when CPR was being given. It is commonly used to support ventilation for patients in respiratory arrest. It consists of a face mask and a ventilation bag. When the patient is intubated or has a tracheostomy, the mask is removed and a sterile bag is connected directly to the endotracheal tube or tracheostomy cannula. The nurse and RCP will ventilate the patient. The nursing assistant may be responsible for cleaning the bag and ensuring that it is sterilized according to facility policy. Because of the importance of this device, if it is in a patient's room, do not put it away in a drawer. The bag-valve-mask should be visible and readily available in case it is needed for emergencies.

Suction

Suction is used to remove fluid, food, and secretions from a patient's nose, mouth, and airway, reducing the risk of aspiration. This keeps the airway clear in patients who are unable to cough effectively to maintain the airway on their own. There is usually no fixed interval for suctioning. It is done as often as necessary to remove secretions.

A flexible, plastic suction catheter (Figure 51-24A) or rigid plastic suction, called a **Yankauer catheter** (tonsil tip) (Figure 51-24B), are used for suctioning. The flexible catheter is inserted into the mouth or nose to remove secretions. The Yankauer is used only for oral suctioning (Figure 51-24C). Apply the principles of standard precau-

tions when caring for the patient and handling suction equipment. Wear a mask and face protection if this is your facility policy, or if there is a risk that the patient will cough in your face. In many facilities, oropharyngeal

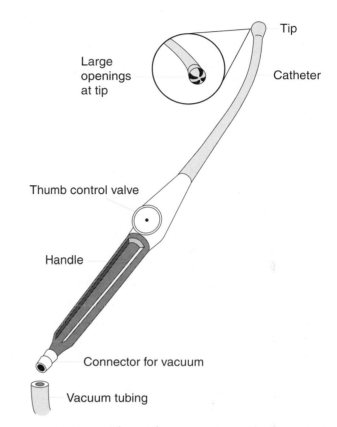

FIGURE 51-24B The Yankauer suction catheter may also be called a "tonsil tip."

FIGURE 51-24A The flexible suction tube may be used for nasal, oral, and tracheal suctioning. The patient cannot breathe during suction, so the duration of this procedure is limited to 10 seconds or less.

FIGURE 51-24C The Yankauer suction is used only for suctioning the mouth. It is never inserted beyond the base of the tongue.

suctioning is a sterile procedure because the catheter may inadvertently slip into the patient's trachea. Tracheal suctioning is always a sterile procedure, as is suctioning through a tracheostomy, laryngectomy (Unit 39), or endotracheal tube. Although an advanced care provider, nurse, or RCP will do the suctioning, you must understand the purpose of the procedure, keep sterile suction supplies stocked, and recognize when the patient needs suctioning.

REVIEW

A. True/False.

Mark the following true or false by circling T or F.

1. T F A stool with occult blood will appear bloody.

2. T F The Hemoccult test is used to determine the presence of bile in the feces.

3. T F Gloves must be used when doing tests on feces or urine.

4. T F The proper amount of time to observe a Hemoccult packet after placing a fecal smear and adding the developer is 5 minutes.

5. T F The urinary drainage tube should be clamped for half an hour before you collect a sample from a drainage port.

6. T F Odor control can be a problem when a patient has an ostomy.

7. T F Drainage from a colostomy is always watery.

8. T F Nursing assistants should follow established facility policies in carrying out assigned tasks.

9. T F Nursing assistants should not carry out any procedure they have not been taught and for which they have not received supervision.

10. T F It is impossible to safely collect a sample of urine from a closed urinary drainage system.

11. T F The nursing assistant should reinsert the catheter if the patient does not void within 4 hours of catheter removal.

12. T F Apply the principles of standard precautions when caring for an ostomy.

13. T F The patient may be asked to wear a mask during some sterile procedures.

14. T F The outside of a sterile package is always sterile.

15. T F Nonsterile items can be added to the edges of a sterile field.

16. T F You may handle sterile items if you are wearing sterile gloves.

17. T F You may reach across the sterile field to add supplies.

18. T F Waste products from ostomy care are discarded in the biohazardous trash.

B. Matching.

Choose the correct term from Column II to match each word or phrase in Column I.

Column I

19. _____ opening

20. _____ artificial opening in large intestine

21. _____ artificial opening in small intestine

22. _____ hidden

23. _____ drainage pouch

Column II

a. occult

b. ileostomy

c. stoma

d. appliance

e. colostomy

f. contamination

g. port

C. Multiple Choice.

Select the one best answer for each of the following.

24. An artificial opening in the colon is known as a/an
   a. tracheostomy.
   b. colostomy.
   c. ileostomy.
   d. proctostomy.

25. The reaction time for a Hemoccult test is
   a. 2 to 4 seconds.
   b. 30 to 60 seconds.
   c. 2 to 3 minutes.
   d. 90 to 120 seconds.

26. The port of a closed urinary drainage system should be cleaned before urine withdrawal with
   a. soap and water.
   b. a paper towel.
   c. alcohol.
   d. a sterile 4 × 4 gauze pad.

27. During routine care, the area around a colostomy should
    a. be cleaned with an alcohol sponge.
    b. be covered with petroleum jelly.
    c. be washed with soap and water.
    d. be cleaned with an antiseptic.

28. An ileostomy as compared to a colostomy
    a. has more formed stool.
    b. tends to be more irritating.
    c. has drainage containing blood clots.
    d. has a larger stoma.

29. You are giving routine stoma care to a patient with a colostomy and find the area surrounding the stoma red and irritated. You should
    a. complete the procedure.
    b. clean the area with alcohol.
    c. apply powder and attach the ostomy bag.
    d. cover the area and notify the nurse.

30. If the skin around an ileostomy stoma is broken, you should
    a. wipe it with alcohol.
    b. wash it with soap and water.
    c. seal it with appliance adhesive.
    d. inform the nurse.

31. Sterile technique is used for
    a. colostomy care.
    b. changing surgical dressings.
    c. routine Stage I pressure ulcer care.
    d. administering enemas and suppositories.

32. Which of the following statements are true?
    a. A sterile package may be used up to 30 days after the expiration date.
    b. Always wash your hands before applying sterile gloves.
    c. The sterile area of the sterile drape includes the top and area hanging over the edge.
    d. Regular exam gloves are worn when assisting with a sterile dressing change.

33. When pouring liquid into a cup on a sterile field, a small amount splashes onto the sterile drape. The drape is
    a. contaminated.
    b. clean.
    c. sterile.
    d. aseptic.

34. You are using transfer forceps to add supplies to a sterile field. You expect to add more supplies before the procedure is finished. Which of the following is true?

a. The handle to the forceps is sterile.
b. The forceps must be stored in liquid disinfectant solution so they remain sterile.
c. The tip of the forceps must be placed on a sterile area until the procedure is finished.
d. The forceps may be used for 24 hours after the package is opened.

35. When removing an indwelling catheter,
    a. cut the inflation port close to the catheter to remove fluid from the balloon.
    b. tell the patient to take a deep breath, then quickly remove the catheter with the balloon inflated.
    c. withdraw fluid from the inflation port with a needle and syringe.
    d. remove half the fluid from the balloon before removing the catheter.

36. When caring for a patient who is being mechanically ventilated, the nursing assistant should
    a. empty condensation in the tubing every hour.
    b. keep the head of the bed elevated.
    c. suction the mouth every 2 hours.
    d. restrain the hands and feet.

37. If a patient removes an oral airway with her hand, the nursing assistant should
    a. leave the airway out and inform the nurse.
    b. restrain both of the patient's hands right away.
    c. quickly reinsert the airway and tape it in place.
    d. insert an endotracheal tube promptly.

38. The Yankauer catheter is a/an
    a. nasal airway.
    b. three-way urinary catheter.
    c. sterile endotracheal catheter.
    d. oral suction device.

39. A patient in whom the RCP has just inserted a nasal airway is gagging and coughing. This suggests that
    a. the airway is too short.
    b. the patient needs suctioning.
    c. the airway is too long.
    d. the patient needs an oral airway.

40. A patient with an endotracheal tube has foamy mucus running from the nose and mouth. She makes a rattling sound when she breathes. This suggests that she
    a. should be ventilated using the bag-valve-mask.
    b. needs a different type of airway device.
    c. has too much condensation in the ventilator tubing.
    d. needs to be suctioned.

D. Nursing Assistant Challenge.

Mrs. Knight, who is 60 years old, was in an accident and received a broken right leg and two broken wrists. She has a long-standing colostomy, but because of her injuries cannot provide her own colostomy care. Answer the following questions about her care.

41. Will you need to wear gloves to give her colostomy care?

42. What will you use to remove feces from around the stoma?

43. What will happen if you apply lotion around the stoma?

44. How will the ostomy bag be held in place?

45. What are the three major problems associated with having a stoma?

SECTION **13**

Response to Basic Emergencies

UNIT 52

Response to Basic Emergencies

OBJECTIVES

After completing this unit, you will be able to:

- Spell and define terms.
- Recognize emergency situations that require urgent care.
- Evaluate situations and determine the sequence of appropriate actions to be taken.
- List and describe the 11 standardized types of codes.
- Describe how to maintain the patient's airway and breathing during respiratory failure and respiratory arrest.
- Recognize the need for CPR.
- List the benefits of early defibrillation.
- Identify the signs, symptoms, and treatment of common emergency situations such as:
  - Cardiac arrest
  - Choking
  - Bleeding
  - Shock
  - Fainting
  - Heart attack
  - Brain attack (stroke)
  - Seizure
  - Vomiting and aspiration
  - Thermal injuries
  - Poisoning
  - Known or suspected head injury
- Demonstrate the following procedures:
  - Procedure 133 Head-Tilt, Chin-Lift Maneuver
  - Procedure 134 Jaw-Thrust Maneuver
  - Procedure 135 Mask-to-Mouth Ventilation
  - Procedure 136 Positioning the Patient in the Recovery Position
  - Procedure 137 Heimlich Maneuver—Abdominal Thrusts
  - Procedure 138 Assisting the Adult Who Has an Obstructed Airway and Becomes Unconscious
  - Procedure 139 Obstructed Airway: Infant
  - Procedure 140 Child with Foreign Body Airway Obstruction

VOCABULARY

Learn the meaning and the correct spelling of the following words and phrases:

adjunctive devices	dislocation	Heimlich maneuver	shock
automatic external defibrillator (AED)	emergency	hemorrhage	sprain
	emergency care	jaw-thrust maneuver	strain
cardiac arrest	Emergency Medical Services (EMS)	pocket mask	vascular
cardiopulmonary resuscitation (CPR)		recovery position	ventilation
	first aid	respiratory arrest	victim
defibrillation	head-tilt, chin-lift maneuver	respiratory failure	

DEALING WITH EMERGENCIES

All emergency situations develop rapidly and unpredictably. Emergency situations can occur at any time to anyone. Examples include:

- Automobile accidents
- Brain attacks (strokes)
- Suddenly feeling weak

- Fainting and falling

An **emergency** is any unexpected situation that requires immediate action and medical attention. In a true emergency, prompt action is needed to prevent further complications and to save the life of the **victim** (person needing help). It is important that you know the signs and symptoms of an emergency and that you be able to take immediate action. The following guidelines are basic actions to remember for any emergency.

GUIDELINES *for*

Responding to an Emergency

- Always remember the priorities of any emergency as the ABCs:
  - **A**irway: obstructed or unobstructed?
  - **B**reathing: is the victim able to breathe?
  - **C**irculation: is the heart beating, is there bleeding?
- Stay calm. Nothing is accomplished and more problems will result if the people at the scene of the emergency become flustered and agitated. If you are calm, you will be a calming influence on the victim.
- Know what to do to summon immediate help; you need to get the nurse to the scene as soon as possible. Stay with the victim and call out for help. If you are out in the community, tell the closest person to call Emergency Medical Services (EMS).
- Do not move the victim unless the person will be endangered by staying where he is.
- Stay with the victim until the person in charge gives you permission to leave.
- Know your limitations. Be aware of what procedures you are qualified to perform in an emergency. Never attempt to render treatment unless you have received the appropriate training.
- Know the procedures to follow for emergencies. Health care facilities have code names for various emergencies. Know what these are and how to announce a code. If you are out in the community, know the appropriate first aid to apply in emergency situations.
- Know the procedures for activating the **Emergency Medical Services (EMS)** system (Figure 52-1). In most areas, this is done by dialing 911 (Figure 52-2). You will need to:
  - give the address
  - describe what happened (e.g., the person was burned or has no heartbeat)

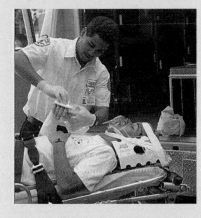

FIGURE 52-1 Know the procedure for activating the EMS system in your community.

  - give the person's name (if you know this information)
  - give the telephone number where the call is being made from
  - report the number of persons needing help
- Keep the person warm. Cover with blankets.
- Do not give the person any fluids or food.
- If the person starts to vomit, turn his head to one side to avoid aspiration.
- If the person is conscious, assure him that help has been called and is on the way.
- Protect the person's privacy. Keep other people away from the scene unless they are qualified to assist.
- In all situations, apply standard precautions to prevent exposure to blood, body fluids, mucous membranes, and nonintact skin during the emergency.

FIGURE 52-2 911 is the universal telephone number for obtaining professional help in an emergency in the United States.

BEING PREPARED

While working in the hospital or long-term care facility, you are always close to professional medical help. When you witness an accident away from the medical facility, however, professional help is not always readily available. Whatever course of action you choose, the victim should not be further endangered.

FIRST AID

First aid includes:

- Immediate care for victims of injuries or sudden illness
- Care needed thereafter if medical help is delayed or is not available

First aid will be needed for different conditions in a variety of situations. These conditions can range from the minor to the very severe. When you give first aid, you deal with the:

- Victim's emotional state
- Victim's physical injuries
- Management of the whole accident situation

Persons in life-threatening situations must be given immediate attention. Life-threatening situations include those in which a person:

- Has no airway
- Has stopped breathing
- Is in shock
- Has been poisoned
- Is choking
- Is bleeding profusely

Evaluating the Situation

At the scene of an accident, assess the situation and find out the extent of injuries. Quickly determine the number of victims, their potential injuries, and any dangerous factors at the scene.

For example, at the scene of an auto accident, there may be several victims. Some may be trapped in their vehicles, others may be lying on the highway. There may be cars burning and the danger of explosion. In this situation, you must first get yourself and the victims away from further danger.

In the medical facility, unless there is a fire, you usually will be dealing with a single victim. You will be able to focus on the needs of that individual. For example, you might enter a patient's room and find a patient lying on the floor, despite the fact that the bed side rails are up. Quickly evaluate the situation as you signal for help, giving the patient's name and location and describing the situation.

CODE EMERGENCIES

Most health care facilities call the various types of emergencies *codes*. They have code designations for many situations. The most common of these is a cardiac arrest, which has been designated as a *Code Blue* in many facilities.

In 1999, three employees of a California hospital were killed by an intruder. The intruder shot one employee near the lobby and one near the first-floor stairwell. He proceeded up the stairs and shot another employee on the second floor. Authorities investigating the situation questioned how the gunman was able to make his way to the second floor after a distress code had been paged. The employee who was shot on the second floor was at the nurses' station, not in hiding. This tragedy prompted a trade association to survey the hospitals in the state regarding how codes were identified and handled. The survey revealed that only two codes, *Code Blue* and *Code Red* (fire), were standardized, even though most hospitals had code designations, policies, and procedures for many other types of emergencies.

Most hospitals have a core group of personnel who work in more than one facility, such as doctors, nurses, nurse practitioners, and EMS personnel. It is very difficult for these workers to remember which codes are used by which facility. In some types of codes, all health care workers must respond. In others, workers on all units must implement specific safety measures when a code is called. The potential for error is great.

Because codes are high-risk, emergency situations, the California Hospital Association adopted the emergency code words listed in Table 52-1. Many long-term care facilities and hospitals in other states also adopted the standardized code words. As a result, these codes are being used in facilities throughout the United States. Make sure to learn the code words and designations used by your facility.

Assisting with a Code

The nursing assistant's responsibilities in a code will be determined by the employer, and are set out in the job description. Your responsibilities may also be outlined in the policy and procedure manual. In general, you must know how to function in a code situation, but your role and responsibility will vary according to facility policy and the nature of the code. Many facilities have "mock code" practices. These are not announced in advance. For example, when personnel respond to the mock cardiac arrest code, they find that a manikin is being used. However, the code is conducted as if it were a real patient. This provides all staff with an opportunity to practice their skills, learn their responsibilities, and become comfortable with and proficient in providing lifesaving care.

Always follow the directions of the nurse or other licensed health care professional in an emergency situation. For example, in a cardiac arrest code, you may be asked to act as a messenger by transporting blood samples to the labo-

TABLE 52-1 STANDARDIZED CODE WORDS

- Code Red: Fire
- Code Blue: Medical emergency—adult
- Code White: Medical emergency—pediatric
- Code Pink: Infant abduction
- Code Purple: Child abduction
- Code Yellow: Bomb threat
- Code Gray: Combative person
- Code Silver: Person with a weapon and/or hostage situation
- Code Orange: Hazardous material spill/release
- Code Triage Internal: An internal disaster
- Code Triage External: An external disaster

Note: *This list was originally developed for acute care hospitals, and there is no code word for a patient or resident who elopes (wanders away).* Some long-term care facilities have designated this a *Code Brown.* This omission was probably an oversight, so the code designation for an elopement may change in the future, or the color designation may be different in your facility. Facilities have been discouraged from changing the designation of the colors listed here, to prevent confusion.

ratory, record the times that CPR was started and stopped, or record the times defibrillation was delivered. A code is a very busy time for everyone. Many tasks must be accomplished in a rapid, orderly manner. However, accuracy is also very important. Become familiar with your facility policies and your responsibilities so that you are confident in your ability to perform your best in this highly critical situation.

EMERGENCY CARE

Emergency care is care that must be given right away to prevent loss of life.

- Whether you are out in the community or in the health care facility, ask someone nearby to summon help.
- Do not leave people who need urgent care to get help yourself. (Exception—CPR)
- As help is on the way, check, in the following order, for the victim's:
  - Degree of reponsiveness
  - Airway/breathing capability
  - Presence and rate of heartbeat
  - Signs of bleeding
  - Signs of shock
- Do not move the person if you do not have to.
- Do not allow the person to get up and walk around.
- Check for other injuries.

MAINTAINING THE PATIENT'S BREATHING

The normal respiratory rate is determined by age. Normal respiratory rates for various age groups are listed in Table 52-2.

Respiratory failure occurs when breathing is insufficient to sustain life. **Respiratory arrest** occurs when breathing stops. It is caused by many conditions, including heart attack, brain attack (stroke or CVA), overdose, drowning, electrocution, poisoning, and traumatic injuries. Follow the criteria in Table 52-3 to determine if the patient's breathing is adequate. Abnormal respirations are often a warning of an impending crisis. Stay with the patient and use the call signal or telephone to request assistance if the patient is in distress. Report problems to the nurse immediately. (Review Unit 39 for information on signs and symptoms to be reported immediately.)

Opening the Airway

If you discover a patient who is in respiratory failure or respiratory arrest, remain in the room and signal or call

Clinical Information ALERT

The respiratory rates listed in Table 52-2 are for normal individuals. During CPR, a lower-than-normal respiratory rate will maintain the patient with adequate oxygen and carbon dioxide elimination because blood flow to the lungs is less than usual. Rescuers must take care to avoid overinflating the lungs, because this interferes with return blood flow to the heart. Follow the CPR guidelines and disregard the various normal values you have learned that apply to nonemergency situations. ∎

TABLE 52-2 NORMAL RESPIRATORY RATES

Age	Normal Respiratory Rate per Minute
Infant	30–60
Toddler	24–40
Preschool child	22–34
School-age child	18–30
Teenager	12–24
Adult	12–20

TABLE 52-3 MONITORING FOR BREATHING ADEQUACY

- The patient can talk, respirations are between 12 and 20, and there is no apparent distress.
- The rhythm is regular.
- The patient's color is normal, with no cyanosis or gray coloration.
- Look at the patient's chest. It should expand equally with each inspiration.
- Listen for breath sounds, by placing your ear next to the patient's nose and mouth, if necessary. The sounds should be quiet, without gurgling, wheezing, gasping, or other abnormal sounds.
- Feel for breath movement on your cheek and ear.

for immediate help. You must open the patient's airway if she cannot do this independently. The most common cause of airway obstruction is the tongue falling back into the throat. Opening the airway lifts the tongue from the back of the throat, making breathing easier. This procedure, as well as some other emergency procedures in this unit, is most effective when the patient is lying in the supine position. Always remove the pillow. Position the patient on the back before beginning.

Because of the nature of the situation, you may not have time to wash your hands or perform other initial procedure actions. Immediately after the patient is safe, wash your hands well. Avoid contact with the patient's secretions if you are not wearing gloves or other personal protective equipment.

The **head-tilt, chin-lift maneuver** (Procedure 133) is the most common method of opening the airway. If the patient has a neck injury, do not perform this procedure. Instead, use the jaw-thrust maneuver.

The **jaw-thrust maneuver** (Procedure 134) is used to open the airway of patients with known or suspected neck injuries, and in those whose airways cannot be opened using the head-tilt, chin-lift method. In some facilities, this procedure is used for patients with head and facial injuries. This is because patients with injuries of the head and face often have neck injuries as well. The purpose of the procedure is to open the airway without moving the head or neck.

Mask-to-Mouth Resuscitation

When a patient stops breathing, his respirations must be sustained by artificial means to prevent brain damage and other complications. If you have taken a CPR class, you may have learned mouth-to-mouth **ventilation**. This is a technique of breathing for the patient. Most health care facilities discourage staff from using this method on patients because of the risk of disease transmission. Various **adjunctive devices** are used instead. An airway

adjunct (unit 50) is a secondary device used to maintain respirations. This is done by a trained and qualified health care professional.

Mask-to-mouth ventilation is performed using a **pocket mask** (Figure 52-3). This is a temporary measure until more advanced airway support is available. The mask has a special valve that prevents the patient's exhaled air and secretions from entering the caregiver's mouth. This infection control feature protects the user. Room air contains approximately 21% oxygen. You do not use all the oxygen you take in when you breathe. You exhale extra oxygen, so there is more than enough for the patient to use. He or she must be positioned in the supine position with the airway open for effective ventilation. The mask covers both the nose and the mouth. It can be turned upside down for infant resuscitation. (Refer to Procedure 135.)

Most pocket masks are clear plastic. This enables you to see the position of the patient's mouth. Monitoring the color of the patient's lips will help you see how well the patient is being oxygenated. Sometimes the patient will vomit during artificial ventilation. You will see this in the mask. If vomiting occurs, quickly turn the patient on his or her side, then clear the mouth and continue ventilation. A licensed professional will suction the patient when suction is available.

CARDIAC ARREST

A person may stop breathing but still have a heartbeat. This is called respiratory arrest. If the situation is not reversed, the heart will stop beating. **Cardiac arrest** is the term used when the heart has stopped beating and respirations have ceased. When the heart and lungs are not functioning, blood and oxygen are not circulated to the

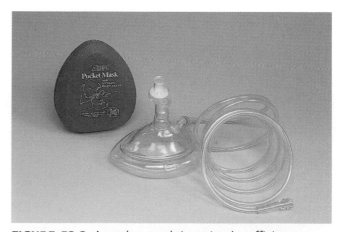

FIGURE 52-3 A pocket mask is a simple, efficient device that provides a one-way barrier if mouth-to-mouth (mask) ventilation is necessary. Supplemental oxygen may be added by connecting the tubing to the male adapter on the mask. However, do not delay resuscitation if oxygen is not available.

brain and the rest of the body. The person is clinically dead. Permanent damage to the brain and other organs occurs within 4 to 6 minutes. Indications of cardiac arrest are:

- No response from the victim
- No breathing can be detected
- No pulse

Cardiopulmonary resuscitation (CPR) is a procedure used to maintain blood circulation throughout the body until the EMS can respond to the emergency. *You must never perform CPR unless you have completed an approved course, taught by an approved instructor.* The American Heart Association and the American Red Cross both offer such courses in communities across the country. **The information in this book is not intended to take the place of an approved course.** Use the guidelines as a quick reference or refresher.

In the health care facility, you must know whether CPR is to be initiated. A patient who is very elderly or who has a terminal illness may not wish to be resuscitated if cardiac arrest occurs. In these cases the physician must write an order "do not resuscitate" (DNR) or "no code" (Figure 52-4). If there is no DNR order, full life support measures are given for cardiac arrest.

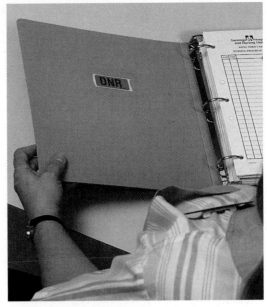

FIGURE 52-4 A DNR on the patient's chart means the patient does not wish to be resuscitated in the event of cardiac arrest. A physician's order is needed to place a patient on DNR status.

PROCEDURE

133

HEAD-TILT, CHIN-LIFT MANEUVER

1. Place one hand on the forehead. Place the fingers of the opposite hand below the center of the jaw bone, directly under the chin.

2. Tilt the head back gently.

3. With your fingertips, lift the lower jaw forward (Figure 52-5). The lower teeth should almost touch the upper teeth. Avoid pressing on the neck, which may worsen the airway obstruction.

4. Keep the patient's mouth open. If necessary, pull the patient's lower lip forward. Avoid inserting your fingers into the mouth.

5. If the patient cannot maintain this position, maintain the airway manually, by holding your hands in place, if necessary.

6. As soon as the patient is safe, and the nurse or other professionals have assumed responsibility for care, wash your hands well.

FIGURE 52-5 Use the head-tilt, chin-lift technique to open the airway unless head injury is suspected.

PROCEDURE

134

JAW-THRUST MANEUVER

1. Move the patient into the supine position as a single unit. Avoid twisting the neck, back, or spine during movement.

2. Pull the head of the bed away from the wall.

3. Position yourself above the patient's head.

4. Position your elbows on the mattress.

5. Using your forearms, stabilize the sides of the head to prevent movement.

6. Place one hand on each side of the lower jaw, just below the ears (Figure 52-6).

7. Use the tips of your index fingers to push the lower jaw forward.

8. Keep the patient's mouth open. If necessary, pull the patient's lower lip forward. Avoid inserting your fingers into the mouth.

9. If the patient cannot maintain this position, maintain the airway manually, by holding your hands in place, if necessary.

10. As soon as the patient is safe, and the nurse or other professionals have assumed responsibility for care, wash your hands well.

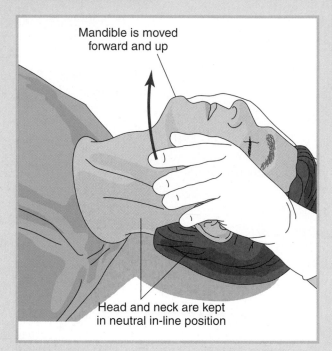

Mandible is moved forward and up

Head and neck are kept in neutral in-line position

FIGURE 52-6 Position your fingers at the angle of the jaw, pushing it upward and forward.

PROCEDURE

135

MASK-TO-MOUTH VENTILATION

1. Supplies needed:
   - Disposable exam gloves
   - Pocket mask with anti-reflux (one-way) valve

2. Pull the head of the bed away from the wall.

3. Apply gloves.

4. Open the patient's airway using the head-tilt, chin-lift method or the jaw-thrust maneuver.

5. Position yourself at the patient's head.

continues

PROCEDURE 135 CONTINUED

6. Position the mask on the patient's face, with the small end over the bridge of the nose and the wide end on the patient's chin. The ventilation port should be centered over the patient's mouth.

7. Seal the mask to the patient's face by positioning your thumbs on the top of the mask and fingers at the sides. Hold the airway in the open position.

8. Take a normal breath, then seal your mouth over the ventilation port, exhaling into the mask. The ventilation should take 1 second in adults. During the ventilation, look at the patient's chest. It should rise as you blow air in.

Note: Remember to take a normal breath, not a deep breath, before administering ventilation. Your objective is to avoid overinflating the patient's lungs or filling the stomach with air. During the ventilation, look at the patient's chest to be sure it rises as you blow air in. If it does not, reposition the airway and try again.

9. Remove your mouth from the mask and allow the patient to exhale passively. Continue to breathe into the mask once every 5 to 6 seconds.

GUIDELINES *for*
Performing CPR

Note: Perform CPR *only* if you have completed an approved course, taught by an approved instructor.

- Follow standard precautions if at all possible. Wear gloves and use a barrier device. If the victim is bleeding, a gown, mask, and eye protection may also be necessary. In a health care facility, these items should be readily available.
- Careful evaluation is required before CPR is administered.

Adult Victim

- Call for help, or have another person call the EMS system.
- For CPR to be effective, the victim must be lying on his back on a hard surface.
- Make sure the victim's airway is open. Look, listen, and feel for breathing.
- If the victim is not breathing, ventilate 2 times, taking 1 second for each ventilation.
- Check for a heartbeat. If there is a pulse, but no respirations, continue with ventilations at the rate of 1 every 6 to 8 seconds.
- If there is no pulse, begin chest compressions at the ratio of 30 compressions to 2 ventilations.

Compressions should be smooth, rhythmic, hard, and fast. Make sure hand placement on the sternum is correct, and compress the victim's chest straight down $1^1/_2$ to 2 inches.

- With 2 rescuers, one rescuer does chest compressions and the other checks for pulse and breathing and gives ventilations. The ratio remains 30 compressions to 2 ventilations.
- Two rescuers may switch positions and roles about every 2 minutes; try to complete the switch in 5 seconds or less.

Infant Victim

- The compression-to-ventilation ratio is the same as for adults: 30 compressions to 2 ventilations.
- If there are 2 rescuers, use a 15:2 ratio of compressions to breaths.
- Breaths are given with the rescuer's mouth covering the infant's nose *and* mouth.
- Breaths must be gentle because of an infant's small size; do not overinflate the lungs.
- Use your fingers to give chest compressions. Compress about $1/_3$ to $1/_2$ the depth of the chest. Do not compress over the xiphoid process.

THE RECOVERY POSITION

If the patient is unresponsive, but is breathing and has a pulse, he should be positioned in the **recovery position** to prevent complications. The recovery position is a modified lateral position (Figure 52-7). The patient's position must:

● Be stable
● Avoid pressure on the chest
● Avoid pressure on the lower arm
● Allow the airway to remain open

Continue to monitor the patient according to facility policy to ensure that the pulse and respirations remain adequate. Take vital signs according to the nurse's instructions.

EARLY DEFIBRILLATION

Public access to **defibrillation** has proven to be highly successful. Defibrillation is a method of treatment that uses an electric shock to reverse disorganized activity in the heart during cardiac arrest. Early defibrillation has proven to be critical to survival in a victim with cardiac arrest. Defibrillators are placed in various locations in the community and are used in the event of cardiac arrest. Some studies have shown that the chance of survival doubles when early access to defibrillation is available. The speed with which defibrillation is performed is the key to success. Early defibrillation (within 5 minutes) is a high-

FIGURE 52-7 If the victim is breathing but not conscious, place him in the recovery position.

priority goal in the community. In health care facilities, the goal is to defibrillate within 3 minutes.

Automatic external defibrillators (AEDs) are computerized devices that are simple to learn and operate. The AED is used *only* when a patient is unresponsive, not breathing, and pulseless. When the device is attached to the victim's chest, the unit determines if an electrical shock is necessary to reestablish or regulate the heartbeat. Several different models are available, and the operating instructions are slightly different for each. The four basic steps to using the AED are:

1. Turn the power to the unit on.
2. Apply the electrode pads to the patient's chest.
3. All rescuers stand back to allow the machine to analyze the heart rhythm.
4. All rescuers continue to stand back; the operator of the unit presses the shock button and/or follows the unit's instructions, which are usually audible through a voice-synthesized message.

PROCEDURE

136

POSITIONING THE PATIENT IN THE RECOVERY POSITION

1. Kneel beside the patient and straighten his legs.

2. Place the arm nearest you above the patient's head with the palm up and the elbow bent slightly.

3. Position his opposite arm across his chest.

4. Place your lower hand on the patient's thigh on the far side of the body. Pull the thigh up slightly, closer to the center of the patient's body.

5. Place your upper hand on the patient's shoulder on the opposite side of the body.

6. With one hand on the thigh and the other on the shoulder, roll the patient onto his side, facing you.

7. Move the patient's upper hand close to the cheek, bending the elbow. This hand should be close to the face, but not under the body. Adjust the upper body so that the hip and knee are at right angles.

8. Tilt the patient's head back slightly to keep the airway open. Now place his upper hand, palm facing down, under the cheek to maintain the head position.

9. Continue to monitor the patient closely for adequate breathing.

Hospitals normally use manual, portable defibrillators for caring for patients who are in cardiac arrest. These defibrillators are operated by qualified, licensed personnel. The AED is not routinely used in most hospitals. However, hospitals with large campuses have purchased AED units for public areas, such as the lobby and cafeteria. Some use semi-automatic AEDs, which can be used automatically and manually. If your facility uses AEDs, employees will be trained in their use. Although the AED is simple to operate, only those who are properly trained may use it. CPR and use of the AED are included in basic life support classes for health care professionals.

CHOKING

A person chokes when the throat is occluded (closed up or blocked) and air cannot get into the airway. In this situation, you must take quick, decisive action.

- The airway can be blocked by accumulation in the back of the throat of:
  - Any foreign body
  - Blood
  - Food
  - Vomitus
- Tilting the head back can sometimes clear the airway, because positioning in this way pulls the tongue forward.
- If the person can speak and is coughing vigorously, do not intervene. Coughing is the most effective way to

dislodge materials from the airway. Stay close by and encourage coughing.

- A complete blockage is signaled by the person being unable to speak, high-pitched sounds on inhalation, and grasping the throat in the universal distress signal (Figure 52-8).
- Apply standard precautions, if possible, when assisting a patient who is choking. This involves using gloves and a special mask during rescue breathing. Know where this equipment is kept and follow your facility policies for use of this equipment in an emergency.

FIGURE 52-8 The universal distress signal for choking is one or both hands about the throat.

PROCEDURE

HEIMLICH MANEUVER—ABDOMINAL THRUSTS

1. Ask the person if he is choking.

2. If the person starts to cough, wait.

3. If the person cannot speak, cough, or breathe, but is conscious, apply subdiaphragmatic abdominal thrusts (**Heimlich maneuver**) until the foreign body is expelled.

   a. Stand behind the victim and wrap your arms around the victim's waist.

   b. Clench your fist, keeping the thumb straight (Figure 52-9A).

   c. Place your fist, thumb side in, against the victim's abdomen slightly above the navel and below the tip of the xiphoid process.

FIGURE 52-9A Clench your fist, keeping the thumb straight.

   d. Grasp your clenched fist with your opposite hand (Figure 52-9B).

   e. Avoid pressing on the patient's ribs with your forearms. This could cause serious injury to the internal structures, including the liver.

continues

PROCEDURE 137 CONTINUED

FIGURE 52-9B Grasp the clenched fist with your opposite hand. Avoid pressing against the ribs with your forearms.

> **f.** Thrust forcefully with the thumb side of your fist against the midline of the victim's abdomen, slightly above his navel, inward and upward (Figure 52-9C). Keep your elbows bent and extended away from your body. You do not want to "hug" the victim because the thrust will not be as effective. Be sure you are below the tip of the sternum (xiphoid process). Deliver each thrust with the intention of freeing the obstruction.

4. Keep thrusting if the object is not dislodged. If the person begins to cough forcefully, wait.

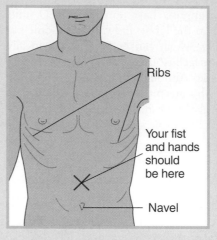

FIGURE 52-9C Thrust forcefully, inward and upward, with the thumb side of your fist just above the navel.

5. Activate the EMS system.

6. Continue the Heimlich maneuver until the obstruction is expelled or the victim becomes unconscious. If the victim becomes unconscious, place the victim in supine position. Proceed with Procedure 138.

Alternative Action: Chest thrusts are used when pressure to the abdomen would be harmful or impossible. Chest thrusts are used if the choking person is in late pregnancy or if the victim is so large you are unable to get your arms around him. Follow steps 1 and 2, then stand behind the victim, place arms directly under the victim's armpits, and around the victim's chest. Place the thumb side of your fist in the middle of the breastbone (avoid ribs and xiphoid process). Grab your fist with your other hand and perform thrusts until the foreign body is expelled or the victim becomes unconscious.

PROCEDURE

138

ASSISTING THE ADULT WHO HAS AN OBSTRUCTED AIRWAY AND BECOMES UNCONSCIOUS

1. Activate the EMS system.

2. Apply gloves.

3. Turn the victim on his back.

4. Begin CPR.

5. Each time you open the airway (using the head-tilt, chin-lift procedure), look in the patient's mouth to see if a foreign body is in the mouth or back of the throat. If you see a foreign body

continues

PROCEDURE 138 CONTINUED

in the mouth or throat, remove it. Take care to avoid pushing it farther down into the throat.

6. Continue CPR until the object is expelled, further help arrives, or you are exhausted and unable to continue.

 Note: A victim who is given mouth-to-mouth breathing or abdominal thrusts may vomit. Roll a victim who vomits away from you onto one side and clean out the mouth with your fingers. Then roll the victim back and continue the procedure.

CPR AND OBSTRUCTED AIRWAY PROCEDURES FOR INFANTS AND CHILDREN

The following procedures for infants and children are only guidelines for emergency treatment of an obstructed airway. An *infant* is a baby from birth to approximately 1 year of age. A *newly born* infant (newborn) is from the time of birth to approximately 1 month of age. A child is considered to be between 1 and 8 years of age. If the child is more than 8 years old, adult CPR and obstructed airway procedures are used. You *must* successfully complete an approved course before you perform these procedures.

PROCEDURE

139

OBSTRUCTED AIRWAY: INFANT

Perform this procedure only if the airway of the infant is completely obstructed and someone has witnessed or strongly suspects that there is a foreign body obstruction. If the infant cannot breathe because of an infection, the infant should be rushed to the nearest life support facility. Procedures to clear the airway *should not be performed*. Allow the infant with respiratory distress to find and maintain the most comfortable position.

1. Determine whether there is airway obstruction by observing breathing difficulties, weak or absent cry, or ineffective cough.

2. Supporting the infant's head and neck with one hand, position the infant face down with head lower than trunk, over one arm (support your arm on your thigh) and deliver up to 5 back blows (Figure 52-10A).

3. Supporting the infant on your arm, turn the infant face up and deliver up to 5 chest thrusts in the midsternal region (Figure 52-10B). Do chest thrusts at a rate of 1 per second.

4. Repeat steps 2 and 3 until the foreign body is expelled or the infant becomes unconscious.

FIGURE 52-10A Position the infant face down, with face lower than trunk. Deliver up to 5 back blows.

If the Infant Becomes Unconscious

5. Call out for help. If someone responds, have that person call the EMS system. Place the infant on her back.

6. Open the airway with the head-tilt, chin-lift method and try to give rescue breaths.

7. Reposition the infant's head and try again to give rescue breaths. If you see a foreign body in the

continues

PROCEDURE **139** CONTINUED

FIGURE 52-10B Turn the infant face up and deliver up to 5 chest thrusts.

mouth or throat, remove it. Take care to avoid pushing it farther down into the throat. Do not perform a finger sweep or attempt to remove an object you cannot see.

8. Check the brachial pulse. If the pulse is absent, begin CPR. Continue until further help arrives, you are exhausted and unable to continue, or the infant has respirations and a pulse above 60.

PROCEDURE

CHILD WITH FOREIGN BODY AIRWAY OBSTRUCTION

Conscious Child

1. Ask "Are you choking?"

2. Give abdominal thrusts, using the same hand placement as you would for an adult, slightly above the navel and well below the xiphoid process. Do not rest your forearms on the ribcage, as this can cause injury.

3. Repeat thrusts until the foreign body is removed or the victim becomes unconscious.

If the Child Becomes Unconscious

4. If another person is present, have that person activate the EMS system.

5. Open the airway and try to do rescue breathing. If still obstructed, reposition the child's head and try to do rescue breathing again. If you see a foreign body in the mouth or throat, remove it. Take care to avoid pushing it farther down into the throat. Do not perform a finger sweep or attempt to remove an object you cannot see.

6. Check the carotid pulse. If the pulse is absent, begin CPR.

7. If the airway obstruction is not relieved after about one minute, activate the EMS system, if this has not been done.

8. Continue until further help arrives, you are exhausted and unable to continue, or the child has respirations and a pulse.

OTHER EMERGENCIES

For some of the emergencies described here, a patient at home or in a long-term care facility may need to be transported to a hospital emergency room. If the patient is at home, be sure that you know:

• Initial emergency actions to perform

• How and when to notify the EMS system
• How and when to notify the nurse
• How, when, and which family members to notify in the event of emergency

If the patient is in a long-term care facility, know the initial emergency actions to perform and the procedure to follow for emergencies.

OSHA ALERT

Emergencies are often stressful and it is easy to become distracted. Remember to protect yourself from exposure to blood, body fluids, secretions, excretions, mucous membranes, and nonintact skin by applying the principles of standard precautions. If accidental contact occurs, wash the exposed skin area well with soap and water. If mucous membrane contact occurs, rinse thoroughly with running water. Inform your supervisor of the exposure as soon as the emergency is over. ∎

Clinical Information ALERT

The head and face are very **vascular** areas. A vascular area is one that contains many blood vessels. Because of this, bleeding may be copious and bruising extensive. The neck also contains some very large blood vessels. If these are severed, the threat to life is immediate. Because of the anatomy of the head and face, there is an increased risk of bleeding into the airway, so you must monitor for this potential emergency. ∎

BLEEDING

Remember that if the person is conscious, the extent of injuries is likely to be far less severe than if the person is unconscious. With the unconscious person, the next imminent threat to life is the loss of blood. Apply gloves and follow standard precautions if you see or suspect that the patient is bleeding. Bleeding is usually easy to see. Sometimes, however, the bleeding is internal. Internal

---

GUIDELINES *for*
Non-Cardiac Facility Emergencies

- Anticipate and prevent emergencies whenever possible. Think safety and evaluate the patient and environment for potential safety hazards when you enter the room and again when you leave the room.
- If you discover a patient who is ill or injured, stay with the patient and call for help. Your facility will teach you the procedure for getting help. Some facilities instruct employees to call out. Others instruct you to pull the call signal or bathroom emergency signal. Some instruct you to use the telephone in the patient's room.
- Know facility procedures, phone numbers, and names for various code situations for reporting emergencies and completing incident reports.
- Do not move patients who have fallen to the floor unless they are in immediate danger. Movement may worsen an injury. The nurse will check the patient and give permission for the move.
- Stay calm and do not panic. Reassure the patient.
- Start emergency measures that you are permitted to do while you are waiting for help to arrive.
- Do not give the patient anything to eat or drink.
- Know the location of emergency equipment and supplies on your unit. You may be instructed to get emergency supplies.

- Many emergencies involve bleeding. Remember that the potential for contact with blood, body fluid, secretions (except sweat), excretions, mucous membranes, and nonintact skin exists. Always remember and apply the principles of standard precautions (Figure 52-11). Carry extra gloves in your pockets if you are working in an area where they are not immediately available. Know where personal protective equipment is kept.
- Once the nurse arrives, do as he or she directs.

FIGURE 52-11 Know where protective equipment is kept and apply the principles of standard precautions when giving emergency care.

bleeding will only be shown by the signs of shock (described in the next section). Examine the person for evidence of bleeding. Take the following steps to prevent additional loss:

- Identify the area that is bleeding.
- Have the victim apply continuous pressure over the bleeding area, if able.
- If the victim is not able, apply continuous, direct pressure over the bleeding area with a pad and your gloved hand, if necessary (Figure 52-12).
- Call for help.
- If seepage occurs, increase the padding and pressure.
- If there are no broken bones and there is no pain, raise the wounded area above the level of the heart, but do not release pressure. This will help to reduce bleeding.
- Support the elevated area.
- Use binding of some kind to hold the padded pressure if there is bleeding from more than one area.
- If you have learned the location of the major blood vessels that control blood flow to an area, and direct pressure seems ineffective, apply pressure over the appropriate pulse point to control **hemorrhage** (heavy bleeding) (Figure 52-13).
- Keep the victim comfortably warm and quiet until help arrives.

Note: Persons who are bleeding are often very frightened. Their anxiety contributes to the development of shock. Continuous reassurance is essential.

FIGURE 52-12 Apply firm hand pressure over the bleeding area with a pad and your gloved hand.

Safety ALERT

Do not be distracted by copious bleeding in an unconscious patient. Always check the adequacy of the patient's airway first. If airway, breathing, and circulation are adequate, quickly apply gloves and take measures to stop the bleeding. ■

SHOCK

Shock is defined as a disturbance of the oxygen supply to the tissues and return of blood to the heart. It can follow:

- Any severe injury
- Cardiac arrest
- Acute hemorrhage
- Severe pain
- Excessive loss of body fluids (as in severe burns)
- Serious infection

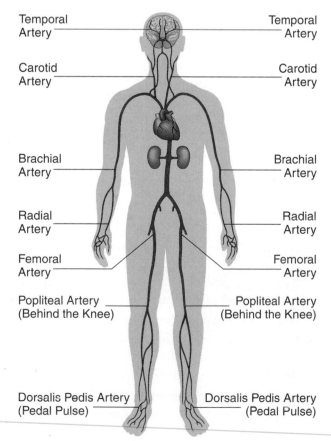

FIGURE 52-13 Pressure on the pulse points is effective for slowing or stopping bleeding.

Signs and Symptoms

Early signs and symptoms include:

- Pale, cold skin that is moist to the touch
- Complaints of weakness
- Weak, rapid pulse
- Rapid and irregular breathing
- Restlessness and anxiety
- Perspiration

Later signs of shock include:

- Mottled skin
- Lack of response
- Sunken eyes with pupils that are dilated, and vacant expression
- Loss of consciousness
- Drop in body temperature
- Low blood pressure

Preventive Measures

Anxiety aggravates the situation, but shock can be prevented if steps are taken early. Prevention of shock includes controlling situations that could trigger it.

- Call for help—activate the emergency medical system.
- Keep the person lying down and quiet.
- Maintain normal body temperature. Provide light warmth if needed.
- Position the person with the feet and legs slightly higher than body and head (Trendelenburg position), unless contraindicated by specific injury. This ensures improved circulation to vital organs.
  - Burned areas should be elevated unless it causes the person pain.
  - If fractures are involved, make sure the part is splinted (braced) before positioning the person, to prevent shock.
- The patient may complain of thirst. Do not give her anything to eat or drink.
- Intravenous fluids to improve circulatory volume and low volumes of oxygen will be given.
  - This equipment will be available in a care facility.
  - In the community, the emergency personnel answering the call will bring the supplies necessary to manage fluid and oxygenation.
- Continue to monitor pulse and respirations.

Unless shock is controlled, death can occur. Until help arrives, your care can often make the difference between life and death.

FAINTING

When the blood supply to the brain is reduced for a short time, the person loses consciousness. This is called faint-ing. Fainting is usually a temporary condition (Figure 52-14). It is corrected as soon as blood flow to the brain is restored.

Unfortunately, when consciousness is lost, the person is likely to fall and injuries can occur. Patients who are ambulating for the first time should be assisted. If fainting occurs and the patient falls, do not try to hold the patient upright. Ease the patient to the floor to prevent injury (Figure 52-15). Assist patients who are *feeling* faint to a safe position.

The patient who is sitting and feels faint, light-headed, dizzy, and nauseated should be encouraged to lower her head between her knees. Pallor, cold skin, perspiration, or visual changes also signal fainting. To provide assistance to a fainting person, the nursing assistant should:

- Help the patient to assume a protected position, sitting or lying down
- Loosen tight clothing
- Position head lower than heart to encourage cerebral blood flow

FIGURE 52-14 Fainting occurs when blood flow to the head is suddenly and temporarily decreased.

FIGURE 52-15 Do not try to hold the person up. Ease her to the floor, making sure the airway is open. Stay with the victim and call for help.

- Allow person to rest for at least 10 minutes
- Maintain normal body temperature
- Call for additional help
- Monitor pulse, respirations, and blood pressure
- Do not give the patient anything to eat or drink

HEART ATTACK

Heart attacks can occur in any age group, but the high-risk group includes those who:

- Are overweight
- Smoke
- Have atherosclerosis
- Remain immobile for long periods
- Are older
- Have diabetes
- Have a history of heart disease

Signs and Symptoms

Signs and symptoms of heart attack include:

- Crushing pain that can radiate up the jaw and down the arm, or heaviness in chest
- Perspiring, skin cold and clammy
- Nausea and vomiting
- Pale to grayish color of the face
- Difficulty breathing or absence of breathing
- Loss of consciousness
- Irregular pulse or loss of pulse (the loss of heart function is called cardiac arrest)

At other times, the pain of the attack may resemble indigestion and the person remains conscious. Do not be fooled into thinking that the degree of pain indicates the severity of the attack. Both victims need immediate attention.

Action

In the health care facility:

- Immediately signal for help
- Stay with the patient
- Have the patient stop any activity and assume a comfortable position
- Help keep the patient calm
- Elevate the head of the bed to assist breathing
- Provide oxygen, if available

If the patient is unconscious:

- Check for breathing and heartbeat
- If necessary, institute CPR (if you have been taught how) until a professional takes charge

In the community, and if the person is conscious, proceed as follows.

1. Evaluate the situation.

2. Activate the EMS.
3. Allow the person to sit up or assume a comfortable position. Loosen clothing about the neck.
4. Keep onlookers away.
5. Provide fresh air but keep the person comfortably warm.
6. Monitor pulse and respirations.
7. Be prepared to initiate CPR.

In the community, if the person is unconscious, follow steps 1 and 2. Then:

3. Check for breathing and heartbeat.
4. If heartbeat is present but breathing has ceased, establish an open airway and institute mask-to-mouth resuscitation.
5. If breathing and heartbeat have ceased (cardiac and respiratory arrest), institute CPR until a professional takes charge.

STROKE

A *brain attack* (cerebral vascular accident or CVA), also called a *stroke*, occurs when there is interference with normal blood circulation to the brain. It usually is caused by a clot that has lodged in a cerebral vessel or by a blood vessel that has ruptured (Figure 52-16).

Signs and Symptoms

The person with a severe brain attack usually:

- Experiences seizure activity
- Loses consciousness
- Experiences difficulty breathing
- Develops weakness or paralysis on one side of the body and of the muscles on either side of the face
- Has unequal pupil reaction

The patient with a less severe brain attack may experience:

- Disorientation
- Dizziness
- Headache
- Slurred speech
- Memory loss
- Loss of consciousness

Action

First aid includes:

- Maintaining an airway (Figure 52-17)
- Providing mask-to-mouth breathing as needed
- Administering CPR, if needed (by a trained, qualified individual)
- Positioning the victim on one side so fluids will drain from the mouth
- Maintaining normal body temperature

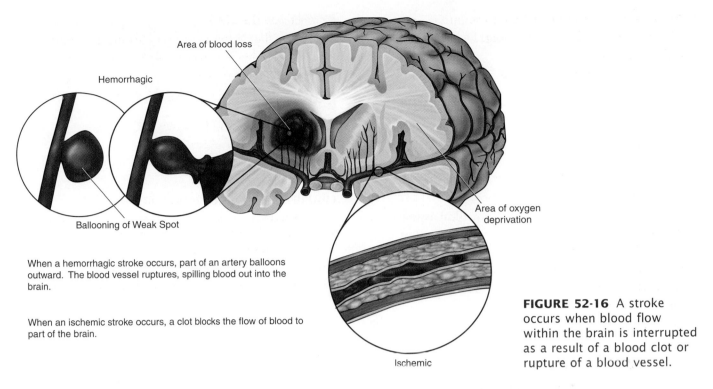

Hemorrhagic

Area of blood loss

Ballooning of Weak Spot

When a hemorrhagic stroke occurs, part of an artery balloons outward. The blood vessel ruptures, spilling blood out into the brain.

When an ischemic stroke occurs, a clot blocks the flow of blood to part of the brain.

Area of oxygen deprivation

Ischemic

FIGURE 52-16 A stroke occurs when blood flow within the brain is interrupted as a result of a blood clot or rupture of a blood vessel.

- Keeping the person quiet until help arrives or transportation to a medical facility can be arranged

SEIZURES

Seizures or convulsions are sometimes seen when there is:

- Drug overdose.
- Head injury.
- Degenerative brain disease.
- Stroke.
- Infectious disease and fevers.
- Tumors.
- Hypoglycemic reactions.
- Seizure disorder. Seizure disorder now is largely controlled with medication, but unusual stress, missed medication doses, and other factors can cause a convulsion.

FIGURE 52-17 Maintain the airway by holding it open manually, if necessary.

Signs and Symptoms

Seizures do not always follow the same pattern. Their range may be:

- A momentary loss of contact with the environment (absence seizure, or *petit mal*), in which there are no random or uncontrolled movements but the person seems to stare blankly.
- A generalized tonic-clonic seizure, or *grand mal* form in which:
  - consciousness is lost
  - the person falls
  - the person becomes rigid
  - uncontrolled voluntary movements occur
  - frothing at the mouth occurs
  - the person becomes cyanotic
  - the person loses control of bladder and/or bowel function

Gradually the seizure lessens and the person recovers. The person is usually:

- Confused
- Disoriented for a period of time
- Very tired

Action

If you witness a seizure, take the following steps:

- Wear gloves and apply standard precautions, because there is a high probability of contact with blood and body fluids when caring for a patient with a seizure.
- Do not restrain the person's movements.
- Protect the person from injury. For example, move any objects that might break or cause bruising.

- Loosen clothing around the neck.
- Maintain an airway by positioning. Do not try to put anything in the mouth.
- Protect the person's head (Figure 52-18).
- Observe the seizure.

After seizure activity stops:

- Turn the person to the side so fluid or vomitus can drain freely after the movements subside.
- Give mask-to-mouth resuscitation if breathing is not resumed following the seizure.
- Allow the person to rest undisturbed.
- Stay with the person but summon medical assistance.
- Report and record seizure activity: time, length of seizure, body parts or activity involved.

VOMITING AND ASPIRATION

Food and air are both taken into the body through the mouth. The passageway in which food and air enter is shared. The ability to swallow is made less efficient by some diseases and by aging. Occasionally food, water, vomitus, or other objects accidentally go down the trachea and into the lungs. This is called *aspiration*, and can occur when a patient is vomiting, bleeding, eating, or drinking. Thick secretions from the mouth may also enter the lungs. Aspiration can cause serious complications.

Signs and Symptoms

Signs and symptoms of aspiration include:

- Coughing
- Choking on food or liquid
- Cyanosis
- Vomiting, especially when lying flat in the supine position
- Inability to swallow
- Inability to spit out vomitus, blood, or secretions from the mouth

Action

If a patient has aspirated anything:

- Stay with the patient and call for help.
- Use standard precautions and select personal protective equipment appropriate to the procedure.
- Do not give the patient any liquids.
- Keep the patient's head elevated if allowed (Figure 52-19).
- Turn the patient's body to the side if she is vomiting while lying down. If turning the patient's body is not possible, turn the head to the side.
- Provide an emesis basin if the patient is vomiting (Figure 52-20).
- If the patient begins choking and an airway obstruction occurs, follow the procedure for clearing the obstructed airway.

FIGURE 52-18 Protect the patient's head.

FIGURE 52-19 Elevate the head of the bed.

FIGURE 52-20 Provide an emesis basin and assist the patient as necessary.

- After the episode, assist the patient with mouth care (Figure 52-21).

Make observations as possible and report to the nurse:

- Observe any vomitus for color, odor, presence of undigested food, blood, or coffee-ground appearance (coffee-ground appearance suggests blood in the stomach). Save the emesis for the nurse to inspect.
- Measure or estimate the amount of vomitus or blood, and record on the intake and output record.

ELECTRIC SHOCK

Electric shock can occur in the:

- Community, when high-tension wires are knocked down in accidents or storms, or when electrical appliances are misused or malfunction

FIGURE 52-21 Provide or assist with oral care when the patient has finished vomiting.

FIGURE 52-22 Perform CPR, if necessary.

- Health facility, because of frayed wires and faulty outlets or fixtures

Severe burns and cardiac and respiratory arrest can result from electric shock. You must protect yourself as you try to rescue the victim.

Action

- Turn off the electricity at the terminal source, such as at a fuse box, before touching the victim, if possible.
- If the source of electricity cannot be controlled, try to move the victim away with some nonconductive material. Dry wood (a broom handle, for example) is a good nonconductor.
- Once free of the electrical source, check the victim for breathing and pulse.
- Summon medical help.
- Administer CPR, if necessary (and you are permitted to do so) (Figure 52-22).
- Once breathing and heart function are restored, check for burns and other injuries. Keep the person lying down and comfortable.
- Give first aid for burns or other injuries.

> ## OSHA ALERT
>
> Evaluate the environment carefully. Make sure you are in a safe zone before approaching the patient, away from sources of electricity and water. ■

BURNS

Burns result in loss of skin integrity. They may be caused by heat, chemicals, or radiation. There is a high risk of infection with any burn. Burns are classified as partial thickness or full thickness, depending on the degree of injury. Partial-thickness burns are:

- First-degree burns—involve only the top layer (epidermis) of skin. There is redness, temporary swelling, and pain. There is usually no permanent scarring. This burn looks like a sunburn. The skin is not broken or blistered.
- Second-degree burns—involve both epidermis and dermis. The skin color may vary from pink or red to white or tan. Blistering, pain, and some scarring occur.

Full-thickness burns are:

- Third-degree burns—involve epidermis, dermis, and subcutaneous tissue. The tissue is bright red to tan and brown. There may be no pain initially because nerve endings have been destroyed. Later, pain and scarring will result.

> ## Infection Control ALERT
>
> Cool burns with cold water. Avoid ice, which will damage sensitive tissue. Never break blisters on a burn. Cover them loosely with material that will not stick to the tissue. ■

Emergency Treatment

1. Call the nurse immediately.
2. If the patient's clothing is on fire, use a coat or blanket to smother the flames.
3. Cool water may be applied to lower skin temperature and to stop further tissue damage. Remove wet clothing (follow nurse's instructions).
4. Third-degree burns usually require extensive treatment.

ORTHOPEDIC INJURIES

Orthopedic injuries include injuries to bones, joints, muscles, and ligaments.

- A fracture is a break in a bone.

- A **sprain** is an injury to a ligament caused by sudden overstretching. A sprained ankle may occur, for example, if a person falls and turns the ankle quickly while falling. Swelling may be noted shortly afterward.
- A **strain** is excessive stretching of a muscle that results in pain and swelling of the muscle. You may strain the muscles in your back if you use incorrect lifting and moving techniques.
- A **dislocation** occurs in a joint, when one bone is displaced from another bone. This can occur in a paralyzed arm that is allowed to hang without support. The weight of the arm pulls the upper arm bone out of position in the shoulder joint. A dislocation can also be caused by improperly lifting a patient under the arms.

Treatment

If you suspect a patient has suffered a fracture:

- Stay with the patient.
- Immobilize the injured extremity to prevent pain and possible worsening of a fracture and bleeding resulting from tissue damage.
- Do not attempt to move the patient.
- Call the nurse immediately.
- If the patient is on the floor and a fracture is suspected, the nurse will instruct you to put the patient to bed after the nursing assessment. Have plenty of help available. One staff member should be responsible for immobilizing and moving the fractured extremity while others move the rest of the body. Roll the patient onto a sheet, blanket, or backboard and then lift him into bed. This is less traumatic for the patient and reduces the risk of worsening the injury.
- Monitor the patient's vital signs as instructed. Report changes to the nurse.

If a fracture is suspected, X-rays will be taken of the injury. If a fracture is present, the physician will put a cast on the affected extremity, place the patient in traction, or do surgery.

If you suspect that a patient has suffered a sprain, strain, or dislocation, notify the nurse at once. You may be instructed to:

- Immobilize the injured extremity to prevent pain and possible worsening of a fracture and bleeding resulting from tissue damage
- Elevate the injured extremity
- Apply ice packs to the area
- After 24 hours, you may be instructed to apply warm packs to the area

HEAD INJURY

A patient with a known or suspected head injury always requires close observation and monitoring. Bleeding inside the skull commonly occurs when the head strikes a broad, hard object, such as the floor, causing internal bleeding. Some serious complications of head injuries may not be apparent until 72 hours (or more) after a head injury. This is particularly true in the elderly. As people age, the brain shrinks slightly. This does not affect the person mentally. The space between the brain and the skull allows extra room for swelling and bleeding. Signs and symptoms of an acute bleeding problem may not be apparent for several days until the problem progresses to a point where it increases pressure on the brain. It can take up to six weeks before the patient shows symptoms from a very tiny "bleed." This is usually long after the original injury has been forgotten.

Signs and Symptoms

Signs and symptoms of a possible head injury include:

- Change in the patient's level of alertness or consciousness
- Change in orientation (ability to recognize time, place, person)
- Memory loss
- Unequal pupils
- Visual disturbances
- Blood or clear fluid leaking from ears or nose
- Change in ability to speak or make self understood
- Change in ability to follow directions
- No response to verbal stimulation
- Weakness of arms or legs, difficulty maintaining balance
- Headache
- Nausea and/or vomiting

Remember that signs and symptoms of a problem may not occur for several days.

Action

If you think a patient has suffered a head injury:

- Stay with the patient and call for help
- Monitor pulse and respirations while waiting for the nurse to arrive
- Keep the environment quiet and calm
- Do not give the patient anything to drink
- Reassure and orient the patient
- Elevate the head on a pillow (Figure 52-23)
- Do not move the patient if he is on the floor
- Monitor vital signs regularly after the injury, as instructed

ACCIDENTAL POISONING

Immediate attention is needed if a patient is the victim of accidental poisoning. All potentially harmful substances

FIGURE 52-23 Keep the environment quiet and comfortable with the head slightly elevated on a pillow.

must be kept in locked cupboards. If you suspect that a poisoning has happened:

- Call the nurse immediately.
- Try to determine what the patient has taken and save the container.
- The nurse may administer a substance that will cause vomiting. (Not all substances can be safely removed from the patient's body by vomiting.)
- Know where to find the telephone number for the regional poison control center.

REVIEW

A. True/False.

Mark the following true or false by circling T or F.

1. T F You need no special training to give CPR.
2. T F CPR is needed if breathing and circulation fail.
3. T F The Heimlich maneuver is used to stop bleeding.
4. T F The person in shock should be kept quiet and lying down.
5. T F When controlling bleeding, the bleeding part should be elevated.
6. T F Vomiting should be induced for anyone who has swallowed a poisonous substance.
7. T F Immediate treatment for burns may include applying cool water to lower skin temperature.
8. T F A dislocation occurs when one bone is displaced from another bone.
9. T F For orthopedic injuries, immediate treatment includes the application of warm packs.
10. T F Third-degree burns only involve the epidermis.

B. Matching.

Choose the correct term from Column II to match each phrase in Column I.

Column I

11. _____ person needing first aid
12. _____ excessive bleeding
13. _____ care given when victim has no breathing or heartbeat
14. _____ signaled by a drop in blood pressure
15. _____ emergency care

Column II

a. arrest   **c.** victim

b. first aid   **d.** CPR

e. contraindicated   **g.** splintered

f. hemorrhage   **h.** shock

C. Multiple Choice.

Select the one best answer for each of the following.

16. An organization that offers instruction in CPR is the
    a. American Diabetes Association.
    b. American Association of Nurses.
    c. Association for Resuscitation.
    d. American Heart Association.

17. First aid is care given
    a. for nausea and vomiting.
    b. only upon a physician's order.
    c. if medical help is delayed.
    d. for cough, cold, or sore throat.

18. Which of the following is a life-threatening situation requiring intervention? A person who
    a. broke a finger.
    b. fell and bruised a knee.
    c. is in shock.
    d. is coughing.

19. The first step you should take when arriving on the scene of an accident is to
    a. stop a passerby.
    b. evaluate the situation.
    c. move the victims to one side.
    d. help the victims get up and walk.

20. To assist a person who has fainted,
    a. help the person to walk to circulate the blood.
    b. cover the person with several blankets.
    c. loosen tight clothing.
    d. position the person's head higher than the heart.

21. To assist the person who is experiencing a seizure, you should
    a. keep the person as active as possible.
    b. restrain the person's movements.
    c. keep the head straight.
    d. maintain an airway and protect the person from injury.

22. You suspect that a patient is in shock because the
    a. blood pressure is elevated.
    b. face is flushed.
    c. skin is cold and clammy.
    d. pulse is full and bounding.

23. Overstretching of a ligament can result in a
    a. fracture.
    b. sprain.
    c. strain.
    d. dislocation.

24. For one-person CPR, the ratio of chest compressions to ventilations is
    a. 30 compressions to 2 ventilations.
    b. 5 compressions to 1 ventilation.
    c. 15 compressions to 2 ventilations.
    d. 30 compressions to 1 ventilation.

25. If a victim of cardiac arrest resumes breathing but is unconscious, you should place the victim
    a. in recovery position.
    b. on his back.
    c. on his abdomen.
    d. in a chair.

26. The first action to take when an adult is choking and is conscious is to tell the person what you are going to do and then
    a. slap the person on the back.
    b. give abdominal thrusts.
    c. begin artificial respirations.
    d. begin chest compressions.

27. The first priority in an emergency is
    a. airway.
    b. bleeding.
    c. circulation.
    d. level of consciousness.

28. When a person suffers cardiac arrest,
    a. the heart has stopped beating.
    b. the respirations are less than 12 per minute.
    c. biological death has occurred.
    d. unconsciousness occurs in about 4 minutes.

29. In the health care facility, you would initiate CPR for cardiac arrest unless
    a. the patient has a DNR order.
    b. you think the patient would not want to be revived.
    c. the patient is very old.
    d. the death is unexpected.

30. If you are working in a patient's home and CPR is initiated, you must
    a. call the EMS system yourself if you are alone.
    b. drive the patient to the closest hospital.
    c. do CPR for 20 minutes and if the patient does not respond, call the EMS system.
    d. go next door to have the neighbor call the EMS system.

31. The procedure to clear an obstructed airway on a conscious infant is to position the infant and
    a. deliver 5 abdominal thrusts followed by 5 back blows.
    b. deliver 5 back blows followed by 5 chest thrusts.
    c. perform a blind finger sweep.
    d. perform 2 ventilations followed by 5 compressions.

32. When performing single rescuer CPR on an infant, the procedure is
    a. done with 5 back blows and 5 chest thrusts.
    b. done only with 2 rescuers.
    c. done with a ratio of 1 ventilation to 5 chest compressions.
    d. done with a ratio of 2 ventilations to 30 chest compressions.

33. Vomiting may be treated as an emergency because of the risk of
    a. airflow.
    b. aspiration.
    c. hemorrhage.
    d. cardiac arrest.

34. The preferred treatment for external bleeding is to apply
    a. continuous, direct pressure.
    b. a tourniquet.
    c. pressure to pulse points.
    d. a heat pack.

D. Nursing Assistant Challenge.

You and a friend are driving home from work. A car immediately ahead of you goes through a stop sign and is hit on the passenger side by a car going through the intersection. You and your friend park your car to see if your help is needed in this emergency. The people in the other car are conscious, alert, and deny having any injuries. The passenger in the car that ran the stop sign is unconscious and begins to vomit. You see blood coming from the person's right arm. The driver is conscious but dazed and seems to be disoriented. List, in sequence, the actions you will take.

Moving Forward

UNIT 53
Employment Opportunities
and Career Growth

UNIT 53

Employment Opportunities and Career Growth

OBJECTIVES

After completing this unit, you will be able to:

- Spell and define terms.
- List nine objectives to be met in obtaining and maintaining employment.
- Follow a process for self-appraisal.
- Name sources of employment for nursing assistants.
- Prepare a résumé and a letter of resignation.
- List the steps for a successful interview.
- List the requirements that must be met when accepting employment.
- List steps for continuing development in your career.

VOCABULARY

Learn the meaning and the correct spelling of the following words and phrases:

job interview	networking	reference	résumé

INTRODUCTION

Having completed a nursing assistant program, you are now ready to look for employment. You will want to be as successful as an employee as you were as a student. If you meet the objectives presented in this unit, the task will be made much easier.

Searching for and obtaining a job requires several steps:

- Completing a self-appraisal
- Searching for employment opportunities
- Assembling a résumé
- Validating your references
- Making specific applications for work
- Participating in interviews
- Deciding whether to take the job

OBJECTIVE 1: SELF-APPRAISAL

The first objective is to determine your personal assets and limitations that could influence your choice of employment. To do this:

- Divide a piece of paper into three columns.
- Title one column *assets*, one *limitations*, and one *solutions*.
- Review all the positive contributions you can make in an employment situation and list them. For example:
  - Your preference in the care of certain patients
  - Your caring attitude
  - Special skill you have with particular patients
  - Your personal appearance

- Honestly review all the limitations that might make certain employment less obtainable. For example, consider:
  - Home responsibilities
  - Specific hours you can work
  - Transportation problems
  - Physical limitations
- Think of possible solutions so that you reduce the number of limitations. The fewer limitations you have at the beginning of your job search, the more you can expand the possibilities for employment.

Make your lists, review them, and add to them over several days.

OBJECTIVE 2: SEARCH FOR ALL EMPLOYMENT OPPORTUNITIES

Having thought through your assets and limitations and found as many solutions to the limitations as possible, you are ready to search for employment. Possible sources for the search process are all the agencies or facilities that employ nursing assistants:

- Physicians' offices
- Blood banks
- Clinics
- Hospices
- Homes for aged or disabled, assisted living, or personal care facilities
- Long-term care facilities
- Hospitals
- Home health care agencies
- Rehabilitation centers
- Telephone directory—select facilities that meet your specific needs for available transportation or specific type of care
- Classified ads found in the newspaper
  - Look for facilities in your area.
  - Consider the type of work you are willing to do.
  - Consider the shifts that have openings.
  - Note the person to contact for an interview or additional information.
- Facility in which you received your clinical experience
  - Administrators sometimes offer jobs to new nursing assistants who trained in their facility.
  - Job openings may be posted on the employee bulletin board.
- Friends and colleagues
  - Friends may know of job openings.
  - Colleagues may put you in touch with others who have potential job connections (Figure 53-1).
  - A term for these activities is **networking**.

FIGURE 53-1 Friends and classmates are valuable sources of information about potential jobs.

Finding employment is a full-time job. You must wake up early and set a time to begin looking for work. It may be helpful to list the steps involved in looking for a job, and preparations you need to make, such as ironing a shirt, finding a babysitter, and preparing a résumé. Apply for jobs early in the day. This makes a good impression and gives you enough time to fill out applications, take tests, or have interviews. Applying at several facilities in the same area will help you organize your time and save time and travel. Follow up on all job leads right away. If you hear of a job opening late in the day, call and schedule an appointment for the next day.

OBJECTIVE 3: ASSEMBLE A PROPER RÉSUMÉ

A **résumé** is a written summary of work and educational history. You should:

- Prepare several copies
- Always keep a copy for yourself
- Type the résumé for a neat appearance
- Carry a copy whenever you seek employment
- Use the résumé as a ready reference when you fill out forms
- Update the résumé regularly

The résumé should be carefully prepared to include:

- Your name, address, and telephone number
- Your educational background
  - List your most recent education first.
  - Give dates.
  - Include a brief summary of the content.
- Your work history over the last five years, especially if it gives evidence of successful experiences in the same or related areas as the job for which you are applying
- Proof of being on the State Nurse Aide Registry

- List of any continuing education classes you have attended
- Other experiences you have had; include jobs that show initiative, reliability, trustworthiness, and worthwhile ways you have spent your time
- References—a list of three people who know you and can verify your abilities
- Some personal information that indicates your interests and activities

It is not necessary to include the following in your résumé, although some of this information may be shared during the interview:

- Age
- Marital status
- Religion
- Sex
- Height
- Weight

OBJECTIVE 4: VALIDATE REFERENCES

References are people who know you and who would be willing to comment, either in writing or verbally over the telephone, about you and your abilities. Be sure to include accurate titles, names, addresses, and telephone numbers when listing references.

Anyone you use as a reference:

- Should give you permission to use their names (Figure 53-2)
- Should know you well enough to make an honest evaluation
- Should not be related to you

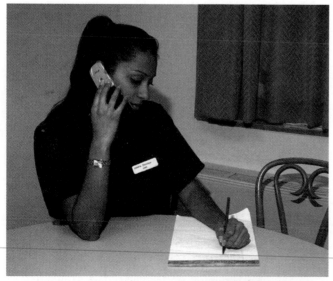

FIGURE 53-2 Get permission before using names for references.

- May need to have their memories refreshed about dates of employment or experiences you have stated in your résumé

OBJECTIVE 5: MAKE SPECIFIC APPLICATIONS FOR WORK

Handle this part of the job search process in a businesslike way:

- Select three facilities that interest you most.
- Call and ask for the director of nursing or personnel department.
- Tell the person who answers that you are interested in learning if there are any openings for a nursing assistant, and if so, what the application procedure is.
- Be prepared to answer questions about your preparation and experience. Have your résumé in your hand.
- Make an appointment for an interview, if possible. A **job interview** is an opportunity for the person applying for a job and the employer's representative to learn about each other. Each person has the opportunity to ask questions to determine if the job seeker has qualifications that match the needs of the job available.
- Fill out an application form. Use your résumé to be sure you complete the form. Read the directions on the application carefully. Fill out all information. If something on the application does not apply, put "N/A" (not applicable) in the space rather than leaving it blank. List all your previous employers, even if they were not health care providers. If you skip an employer, it looks as if you are hiding something. Complete the application in its entirety. Do not write "see résumé." Although you may attach your résumé to the application, there are legal reasons why you must complete the application. Make sure the information is accurate, spelled correctly, complete, and neat. Use a pen to complete the application. The application represents you on paper. A messy application sends a negative message.
- Learn the names of the persons to whom you speak.
- Thank the person speaking with you by name.

Repeat the steps until you land the job.

OBJECTIVE 6: PARTICIPATE IN A SUCCESSFUL INTERVIEW

After you have investigated job leads and completed applications, an employer may contact you to schedule an interview. You will be given a date and time to meet. The interview is very important. Most hiring decisions are made during the interview. How you present yourself in the interview is as important as your training, experience, and ability to do the job.

Approach the interview in three steps.

Preparation.

- Plan what you will wear.
- Do not overdress, but be neat and clean.
- Check your clothes for loose or lost buttons or stains.
- Be sure to take a bath and use deodorant.
- Brush your teeth.
- Make sure your fingernails are short and clean.
- Polish your shoes.
- Make sure your hair is neat.
- If you have a beard or a mustache, be sure it is trimmed.
- Do not chew gum.
- Prepare a list of questions you want to ask.
- Have your résumé in hand.

Actual Interview. Be prepared when going to an interview. Bring pens and pencils, papers, a map, reference information, and your résumé with you. You will also need a photo identification, such as a driver's license, and your Social Security card. If you have completed a CNA program, bring a copy of your certificate and state certification. Go to the interview alone. Arrange for babysitters and transportation ahead of time. It is a good idea to arrive a little early so you can complete paperwork, if requested.

- Offer a firm handshake (Figure 53-3).
- Stand until you are invited to sit.
- Remember that you are "selling" yourself.
- Make sure your body language sends a positive message
- Make good eye contact with the interviewer. Your eyes should send a message such as, "I like you."
- Listen carefully to the interview questions and be sure you understand them before you answer (Figure 53-4). If you do not understand, ask for clarification. Your answers to questions should reflect your positive features.
- Share information willingly with the interviewer.
- Use your list to learn information important to you such as:
  - responsibilities (ask for a job description)
  - hours of work
  - dress code
  - opportunities for future assistance or financial aid to further your education
  - starting salary
  - fringe benefits such as health insurance
  - schedule of raises

Sensitive Issues. Be honest but tactful when discussing former employers. Speak positively of them. Making negative comments about a previous employer is not a good practice. Your answers to questions should reflect your positive features. Avoid discussing negative traits

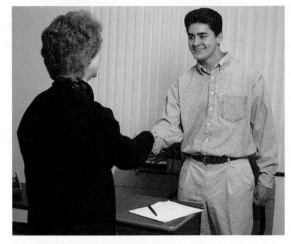

FIGURE 53-3 A firm handshake sends a positive message about you.

Sample Interview Questions	
Question:	Tell me about yourself.
Answer:	Briefly outline your strengths. Concentrate on your education and professional achievements. Avoid discussing marriage, family, and your personal life.
Question:	Describe your qualifications for this job.
Answer:	Describe your most recent education and experience. List your strongest skills and talents relating to job performance.
Question:	Why do you want this job?
Answer:	Know something about the employer and say something positive about the company. Avoid using money as the reason you want the position.
Question:	Tell me about your last job.
Answer:	Describe your duties and responsibilities. Discuss skills that apply to the position for which you are applying.
Question:	Why did you leave your last job?
Answer:	Be honest, but avoid making negative comments about your previous employer.
Question:	Tell me about your goals and ambitions.
Answer:	State that you look forward to learning new things, accepting challenges, and taking on new responsibilities. State your career goals.
Question:	What are your strengths?
Answer:	Describe strong personal qualities such as honesty, dependability, and caring about other people.
Question:	What are your weaknesses?
Answer:	Mention weaknesses or problems, but state how you have learned and grown from them.

FIGURE 53-4 Have a friend ask you typical interview questions so you can practice your presentation and gain confidence in your answers.

unless you are specifically asked to do so. Be honest with the interviewer. It is easier to defend the truth than it is to be caught in a lie. Avoid discussing your personal life or financial problems. Consider how you will respond to certain questions, such as "Are you available to work every other Sunday?" Avoid responding with excuses such as, "My husband will not let me work on Sundays." Your name is on the paycheck. Your husband's is not. A better way to respond would be, "My husband is a pastor and we are very involved in church activities on Sundays. Working will be a hardship in my personal life, but if it is a job requirement I will do my best to work it out." Remember that health care facilities are open 24 hours a day, 7 days a week. All workers are required to do some weekend, holiday, and shift work. This is one of the requirements of your chosen career.

Discussing Salary and Benefits. Salary and benefits can be sensitive issues. Asking questions about them early in the process gives the employer the impression that you are not really interested in working at the facility, but are instead shopping for the highest salary available. This sends a negative message. Save discussions about salary and benefits for late in the interview. Let the employer lead into them. If the interviewer has not discussed salary and benefits by the end of the interview, it is appropriate to ask.

At the end of the interview, thank the interviewer, whether you are hired or not (Figure 53-5).

After the Interview. When you get home:

- Write a short thank-you note to the person who interviewed you, thanking her for her time and the opportunity to be considered for the job.
- Review the interview in your mind. Plan changes you should make to improve future interviews.

OBJECTIVE 7: ACCEPT A JOB

Before accepting a job, think carefully about your employer's expectations of your abilities and job perfor-

mance. If you accept the job, you must be prepared to follow the policies and procedures of the facility. For example, if the interviewer told you that nursing assistants are scheduled to work every other weekend, do not take the job unless you are willing to do this. There are some additional requirements you will have to complete as you begin your job, as we discuss in this section.

Orientation

Orientation is designed to help you safely perform the duties listed in your job description. It is mandatory and all new employees are required to attend. Keep in mind that even if you were hired to work an evening or night shift, orientation classes may be held during the day. Orientation generally consists of two parts. You will spend at least a day in the classroom learning about the policies and procedures of the employer (Figure 53-6). You will be given employee

---

Legal ALERT

To work in the United States, you must complete an I-9 form, which proves your legal eligibility to work. To do this, you must provide a copy of your Social Security card and a picture identification. The employer may make a copy of these documents. He or she will also have to sign the form to verify that the facility has verified your identity and work eligibility. ■

---

1. Poor appearance (not dressed properly, poorly groomed).
2. Acting like a know-it-all.
3. Cannot express self clearly; poor voice, diction, grammar.
4. Lack of planning for work—no purpose or goals.
5. Lack of confidence or poise.
6. No interest in or enthusiasm for the job.
7. Not active in school extracurricular programs.
8. Interested only in the best dollar offer.
9. Poor school record (academic, attendance).
10. Unwilling to start at the bottom.
11. Making excuses, hedges on unfavorable record.
12. No tact.
13. Not mature.
14. No curiosity about the job.
15. Critical of past employers.

FIGURE 53-5 Employers were surveyed for reasons for not hiring applicants. The reasons are listed from 1 (most important) to 15 (least important).

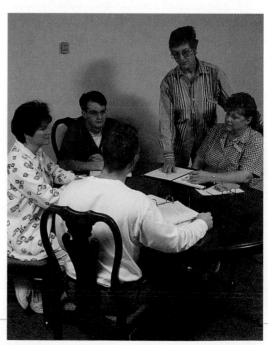

FIGURE 53-6 Orientation is an important part of your employment.

handbooks that you can refer to in the future. Information presented during the class may include:

- Policies for scheduling and making assignments
- What to do during fire and other emergencies
- How and when performance evaluations are completed
- The organizational chart of the facility
- Safety policies and procedures

A clinical orientation is provided on the nursing unit. An instructor, another nurse, or an experienced competent nursing assistant will work with you the first few days so that you may learn

- The routine of the unit
- The location of equipment and supplies
- How to do specific procedures as required by the employer

Health and Safety Requirements

State and federal regulations require new employees to:

- Obtain a physical examination within a specified number of days (some employers will require this before you begin work).
- Receive a two-step Mantoux (tuberculosis) test within a specified number of days (this too may be required before you begin work).
- Indicate whether they wish to receive the hepatitis B vaccine. Health care employers are required by law to offer this vaccination without cost to direct-care employees. It is the employee's choice whether to take the vaccine. If the employee refuses it at the time of orientation, it can be given at another time if she changes her mind.

Some employers require employees to wear back supports while working. These are generally issued to you by the employer.

Health Care Worker Background Check

Some states require that a criminal background check be performed on all health care workers. If you work in one of these states, the procedure should be explained to you during the interview.

Drug Testing

Many employers require that drug testing be performed before you begin work. This procedure too should be explained during the interview.

Uniform Requirements

Most health care employers have dress codes that indicate:

- Color and style of uniform to be worn on duty
- Acceptable jewelry that can be worn with the uniform

Legal ALERT

Drug testing is usually done by means of a urine sample. Some prescription drugs, foods, and vitamins may interfere with the urine test results. You will be asked to list prescription and nonprescription medications you are taking. Be honest, and list everything. Collection of the urine specimen is generally monitored to prevent tampering. Some agencies check the temperature of the urine immediately after the specimen is obtained, as a further safeguard. Some facilities will not allow you to take personal items into the bathroom when providing the specimen. Access to water may also be limited, because it is possible to dilute a sample. Some facilities seal the container with tamper-evident tape, which is signed by both the employee and the nurse who assists with specimen collection. Your employer may also have a policy requiring random drug testing if you are involved in a work-related injury, or if any use of illicit substances is suspected. ■

- Type of shoes and stockings that are safe to wear
- Acceptable hairstyles and makeup (including whether nail polish is permitted)

Remember that these policies are for purposes of safety and infection control. Some employers will issue the uniforms to you either at no charge or for a charge that is deducted from your paycheck over a period of time.

OBJECTIVE 8: KEEP THE JOB

You can make your new position secure if you:

- Arrive on time prepared to work. Good attendance is very important. Be at work when you are scheduled and avoid calling off unless you are ill. If you will be

Culture ALERT

You will work with people from other cultures. Remember, they also have cultural needs, beliefs, and practices. Use cultural competencies and show respect for your coworkers. Do your best to work well with everyone. When staff make the effort to work well together, everyone's job satisfaction increases and patients receive better care. ■

unable to work your next scheduled shift, notify your facility as far in advance as possible so they can find a replacement.

- Follow the policies and procedures outlined in your orientation.
- Follow the rules of ethical and legal conduct.
- Recognize your limitations and seek help.
- Have an open and positive attitude.

OBJECTIVE 9: CONTINUE TO GROW THROUGHOUT YOUR CAREER

You will continue to grow if you take advantage of each new experience and opportunity you find.

- Keep your certificate current
- Seek out knowledgeable staff members and watch and learn by their example
- Do not be afraid to ask questions at appropriate times
- Use the nursing literature to learn more about patients' conditions
- Participate in care conferences with an open mind so that each conference can be a learning experience for you
- Complete 12 hours of continuing education each year (Figure 53-7), or follow the requirements in your state
- Investigate the possibilities of advancing your formal education by:
  - enrolling in general education courses offered at the high school or college in your area
  - taking courses in communication, listening, English, and psychology
  - participating in in-service education programs at your facility or at nearby hospitals
  - enrolling in minicourses offered by hospitals on subjects of general public interest, such as hypertension, weight control, and diabetes
  - selecting books at the library that pertain to health issues
  - researching programs that can prepare you for professional advancement into the ranks of LVN or RN

Career Ladders

Many facilities have career ladders available for nursing assistants. The career ladder enables the assistant to progress to a higher position within the organization, such as a restorative assistant. One professional nursing organization has developed the End-of-Life Nursing Education Consortium (ELNEC) Project, which enables direct caregivers, including nursing assistants, to achieve advanced status in providing end-of-life care. Additional education is usually required to move up the career ladder. Complet-

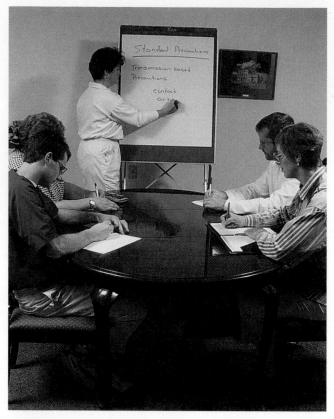

FIGURE 53-7 Take advantage of staff development programs to further your knowledge.

ing specialized certificate programs is an excellent way to advance in your career. Explore the possibilities within your facility. Community and junior colleges in your area may also have classes available.

OBJECTIVE 10: RESIGN PROPERLY FROM EMPLOYMENT

When you are ready to leave your present position, you should do so pleasantly and properly.

- Give as much notice as possible—usually equal to the length of one pay period.
- Submit a letter of resignation and include:
  - date
  - salutation (greeting) to the director of nursing
  - brief explanation of your reasons for leaving

 Note: Even if you feel upset by something that happened, make your reasons positive in nature.

  - date your resignation is to be effective
  - thanks for the opportunity to have worked and grown by working in that facility
  - your signature

REVIEW

A. True/False.

Mark the following true or false by circling T or F.

1. T F The employer may ask your religion during an interview.

2. T F In making a self-appraisal, you only need to list the things you could offer an employer.

3. T F What you wear to an interview is not important.

4. T F The availability of transportation should be considered when you are choosing a job.

5. T F The interview should provide you with information about the exact responsibilities you will have.

6. T F Checking for job possibilities with the facility in which you had your clinical experience is proper.

7. T F If you fail to get the job after the interview, there is nothing left for you to do about the situation.

8. T F At the end of every interview, you should thank the interviewer, even if you did not get the job.

9. T F Participation in care conferences can be a way to continue to grow.

10. T F When resigning, give ample notice.

B. Multiple Choice.

Select the one best answer for each of the following.

11. The first step in finding a job is
    a. making phone calls.
    b. doing a self-assessment.
    c. looking in the paper.
    d. writing letters to friends.

12. A self-appraisal includes
    a. reading classified ads.
    b. networking with friends.
    c. caring for patients.
    d. listing assets, limitations, and solutions.

13. A compilation of your work history is called a/an
    a. résumé.
    b. interview.
    c. summary.
    d. application.

14. Which of the following would you include in your résumé?
    a. Marital status
    b. Religion
    c. Weight
    d. Address

15. Before putting a reference name down,
    a. ask permission.
    b. call the prospective employer.
    c. tell the person you are going to use his name.
    d. get the phone number and birth date.

C. Nursing Assistant Challenge.

You have made it! You have completed your course and are eagerly looking forward to employment. Answer these questions.

16. What information will you need to have when completing an application for employment?

17. What items do you need to have with you when you go for your interview?

18. How will you dress for the interview?

19. The interview comes to a close and the interviewer has not given you any information concerning wages and benefits. How would you handle this?

90-90-90 position a method of positioning the patient in good posture with the feet at a 90° angle to the lower legs, the lower legs at a 90° angle to the thigh, and the thighs at a 90° angle to the torso.

AII (A2) room an isolation room with an anteroom and negative-pressure ventilation that may be used for patients in airborne precautions.

abbreviation shortened form of a word or phrase.

abdominal distention a condition in which the abdomen is bloated and enlarged.

abduction movement away from midline or center.

abduction pillow pillow used to maintain separation between the legs of a patient who has had hip surgery.

ablutions the practice of removing sins and diseases and cleansing negative energy from body, mind, and spirit through the use of ritual washing.

abrasion injury that results from scraping the skin.

abscess a collection of pus in the tissue, usually in a confined space; abscesses can occur anywhere in the body.

absence seizure another name for a petit mal seizure.

abuse improper treatment or misuse.

accelerated increased or faster motion, as in pulse or respiration.

acceptance coming to terms with a situation and awaiting the outcome calmly; final stage of dying which some people, but not all, reach.

acetone colorless liquid produced during the metabolism of fats because glucose cannot be oxidized in the blood; has a sweet, fruity odor; appears in blood and urine of persons with diabetes.

acquired immune deficiency syndrome (AIDS) a progressive disease of the immune system caused by the human immunodeficiency virus; initially an extremely high mortality rate was the norm for the disease; now combination drug therapy can slow the disease process and lengthen life expectancy of those infected with HIV.

activities of daily living (ADLs) the activities necessary to fulfill basic human needs.

acupuncture insertion of tiny, thin needles in various parts of the body to correct imbalances in energy and treat disease.

acute disease disease that comes on suddenly, requires urgent treatment, and is usually resolved.

acute exacerbation an increase in the severity of signs and symptoms of a chronic disease.

acute illness illness that comes on suddenly; requires intensive, immediate treatment.

adaptation adjustment.

adaptive device item altered to make it easier to use by those with functional deficits to perform any activity of daily living.

Addison's disease disease caused by underfunctioning of the adrenal glands.

adduction movement toward midline or center.

adjunctive devices secondary devices used to maintain the airway and respirations.

ADLs *See* **activities of daily living**

admission procedure carried out when a patient first arrives at a facility.

adolescence teenage years.

adoptive parent person who is a parent through a legal adoption procedure.

adrenal glands endocrine glands; one is located on the top of each kidney; secrete hormones, including epinephrine.

advance directive document signed before the diagnosis of a terminal illness, when the individual is still in good health, indicating the person's wishes regarding care during dying.

advocate a person who speaks on behalf of the patient.

AED *See* **automatic external defibrillator**

AEM *See* **Anthroposophically Extended Medicine**

affective disorders a group of mental disorders characterized by a disturbance in mood. They may also be called *mood disorders*, and are usually marked by a profound and persistent sadness.

afterbirth *See* **placenta**

agitation mental state characterized by irregular and erratic behavior.

aiding and abetting not reporting dishonest acts that are observed.

AIDS *See* **acquired immune deficiency syndrome**

airborne precautions procedures used to prevent the spread of airborne pathogens.

airborne transmission method of spreading disease by breathing tiny pathogens that remain suspended in the air for long periods of time.

akinesia difficulty and slowness in carrying out voluntary muscular activities.

alcoholism a dependency on alcohol.

alignment *See* **body alignment**

allergen substance that causes sensitivity or allergic reactions.

allergy abnormal and individual hypersensitivity.

alopecia absence of hair where hair normally grows.

alternative choice; option.

alternative medical systems therapeutic or preventive health care practices that are used instead of conventional health care; often involves the use of natural products rather than those derived from chemicals. These systems do not follow generally accepted methods and may not have a scientific explanation for their effectiveness.

alveoli tiny air sacs that make up most of the lungs.

Alzheimer's disease neurological condition in which there is a gradual loss of cerebral functioning.

AM care care given in the early morning when the patient first awakens.

ambulate to walk.

ambulation the process of walking.

amenorrhea without menstruation.

amino acids basic components of proteins.

amniocentesis transabdominal perforation of the amniotic sac to obtain a sample of the amniotic fluid.

amniotic fluid fluid in which the fetus floats in the mother's womb.

amniotic sac sac enclosing the fetus and amniotic fluid.

amputation removal of a limb or other body appendage.

amulet charm used to ward off evil.

amyotrophic lateral sclerosis (ALS) a progressive neuromuscular disease that causes muscle weakness and paralysis.

analgesic pain-relieving medication.

anaphylactic shock extreme, sometimes fatal, sensitivity or allergic reaction to a specific antigen.

anatomic position standing erect, facing observer, feet flat on floor and slightly separated, arms at sides, palms forward.

anatomy study of the structure of the human body.

anemia deficiency of quality or quantity of red blood cells in the blood.

aneroid gauge device for measuring and registering blood pressure.

anesthesia loss of feeling or sensation.

anger feeling of hostility, rage.

angina pectoris acute pain in the chest caused by interference with the supply of oxygen to the heart.

animal-assisted therapy pet therapy; pets visiting in a health care facility for a therapeutic purpose.

anorexia lack or loss of appetite for food.

anorexia nervosa an eating disorder in which the patient has a disturbed body image; despite appearing skeletal, he or she views the body as being fat.

anterior in anatomy, in front of the coronal or ventral plane.

anteroom a small room just inside the entrance to the isolation room that usually has a sink and containers for trash disposal.

Anthroposophically Extended Medicine (AEM) a holistic system of natural medicine that treats the whole person and not just the disease or symptoms; treatment is designed to harmonize the relationship of body, mind, and spirit.

antibiotic medication used to treat bacterial infection.

antibodies proteins produced in the body in response to invasion by a foreign agent (antigen); react specifically with the foreign agent.

anticoagulant medication that thins the blood and increases the risk of bleeding.

anti-embolism hose elasticized stockings used to support the leg blood vessels.

antigen marker on cells that identifies a cell as self or nonself; antigens on foreign substances that enter the body, such as pathogens, stimulate the production of antibodies by the body.

anxiety fear, apprehension, or sense of impending danger that is often marked by vague physical symptoms, such as tension, restlessness, and rapid heart rate.

anxiety disorder one of a group of recognized mental illnesses involving anxiety reactions in response to stress.

Apgar score method for determining an infant's condition at birth by scoring heart rate, respiratory effect, muscle tone, reflex irritability, and color.

aphasia language impairment; loss of ability to comprehend normally.

apical pulse pulse rate taken by placing a stethoscope over the tip of the heart.

apnea period of no respiration.

appliance device used with colostomy or ileostomy to collect drainage from a stoma.

approaches actions used by the health care team to help resolve a patient's problems; steps taken to reach a goal.

Aquamatic K-Pad brand name of a unit for applying heat or cold.

aromatherapy use of natural scents and smells to promote health and well-being.

art therapy using art and the various senses to express oneself.

artery vessel through which oxygenated blood passes away from the heart to various parts of the body.

arthritis joint inflammation.

ascites fluid accumulation in the abdomen.

asepsis without infection.

aspirate to withdraw.

aspiration a very serious condition in which food, water, gastric contents, or other materials enter the trachea and lungs. It is usually accidental, such as when the patient "swallows down the wrong tube" or accidentally inhales food or fluids. If you suspect that a patient has aspirated, inform the nurse promptly.

assault attempt or threat to do violence to another.

assessment act of evaluating.

assignment specific list of duties; tells you which patients you will care for during your shift and the specific procedures to be performed.

assimilate to absorb.

assisted living situation in which a person primarily cares for himself or herself but has some help in meeting health care needs; may reside in a facility that provides health care supervision.

assistive devices equipment used to help people be more effective in their physical activity.

asthma chronic respiratory disease characterized by bronchospasms and excessive mucus production.

atelectasis decreased or absent air in all or part of a lung, resulting in loss of lung volume and inability to expand the lung fully.

atheroma degeneration or thickening of artery walls due to formation of fatty plaque and scar tissue.

atherosclerosis degenerative process involving the lining of arteries, in which the lumen eventually narrows and closes; a form of arteriosclerosis.

atrium one of the two upper chambers of the heart.

atrophy shrinking or wasting away of tissues.

attitude an external expression of inner feelings about oneself or others.

aura peculiar sensation preceding the appearance of more definite symptoms in a convulsion or seizure.

auscultatory gap sound fadeout for 1–15 mm Hg (mercury) pressure, after which sound begins again; sometimes mistaken for the diastolic pressure.

autoclave machine that sterilizes articles.

autoimmune presence of antibodies against component(s) of body.

automatic external defibrillator (AED) computerized device that uses an electric shock to reverse disorganized activity in the heart during cardiac arrest.

autonomic dysreflexia potentially life-threatening complication of spinal cord injury; indicates uncontrolled sympathetic nervous system activity.

autonomy self-determination.

autopsy examination of body after death to determine cause of death.

avulsion fracture fracture caused by a bone fragment pulling off at the point of ligament or tendon attachment.

axilla armpit.

axon extension of neuron that conducts nerve impulses away from the cell body.

Ayurveda a natural system of medicine based on the belief that disease is due to an imbalance in the consciousness. Uses lifestyle interventions, natural therapies, and rebalancing among the body, mind, and environment.

bacillus (plural **bacilli**) rod-shaped bacterium.

bacteremia bacterial infection in the bloodstream; also known as *septicemia*.

bacterium (plural **bacteria**) a form of simple microbes.

bag-valve-mask device used to support ventilation for patients in respiratory arrest; consists of a face mask and a ventilation bag.

balance bar section of an upright scale that holds the weights used to determine a patient's weight.

bandages fabric, gauze, net, or elasticized material used to cover dressings and keep them securely in place.

bargaining stage of the grieving process in which the individual seeks to make a deal or form a pact that will delay death.

bariatric surgery surgery on the stomach and/or intestines to help the patient with morbid or super obesity and a BMI over 40 lose weight. Sometimes used as a treatment for people with a BMI between 35 and 40 who have health problems and potentially serious comorbidities, such as heart disease or type 2 diabetes.

bariatrics a relatively new field of medicine that focuses on the treatment and control of obesity and diseases associated with obesity.

baseline measurement of patient's vital signs or other body functions upon admission; future measurements are compared to baseline measurements to track the patient's progress.

baseline assessment initial observations of the patient and his or her condition.

battery an unlawful attack upon or touching of another person.

bedbugs parasites that are difficult to eliminate and have been found throughout the world; they are active mainly at night, seeking a blood meal from a human or animal host.

belief idea based on commonly held opinions, knowledge, and attitudes.

benign nonmalignant (tumor).

benign prostatic hypertrophy noncancerous enlargement of prostate gland.

bile substance produced by the liver that prepares fats for digestion.

binders fabric or elastic wraps that encircle the abdomen; may be used to hold dressings in place or support a surgical site.

biofeedback a method of retraining the mind to control various physical problems and stresses that one would not normally be aware of.

biohazard waste items or laboratory specimens or materials, and their containers contaminated by body fluids; these have the potential to transmit disease. Discarded items must be labeled. Special precautions are taken to handle and contain this waste.

biological parent natural parent who contributed sperm or an ovum to the development of the fetus.

biological therapy biologically based practices using natural substances and products to promote or regain health.

biopsy removal and examination of a piece of tissue from a living body.

bioterrorism the use of biological agents, such as pathogenic organisms or agricultural pests, for terrorist purposes.

bipolar affective disorder a mood disorder in which the person has marked mood swings beyond what most people experience (also called *manic depression* or *bipolar depression*).

bisexuality having sexual interest in both genders.

blood pressure pressure of blood exerted against vascular walls.

BMI *See* **body mass index**

body alignment position of a human body in which the body can properly function.

body-based therapy practices based on direct body contact, such as manipulation or movement.

body core center of the body (internal).

body language use of facial expression, body positions, and vocal inflections to convey a message.

body mass index (BMI) a mathematical calculation used to determine whether a person is at a healthy, normal weight, is overweight, or is obese. The BMI measures body weight relative to a person's height by dividing a person's weight (in kilograms) by his or her height (in meters, squared).

body shell outer surface of the body.

bolus soft mass of food that is ready to be swallowed.

borderline personality disorder (BPD) a condition in which the patient feels very unstable. He or she may be impulsive, prone to self-injurious behavior, and fear abandonment.

Bowman's capsule tubule surrounding the glomerulus of the nephron.

box (square) corner one type of corner used in the making of a hospital bed.

BPD *See* **borderline personality disorder**

brachial artery main artery of the arm.

brachytherapy a form of radiation therapy in which tiny radioactive seeds or pellets are implanted directly inside the prostate gland or tumor site.

bradycardia unusually slow heartbeat.

braille method of communication used by persons with visual impairments, who use fingertips to feel a series of raised dots representing letters and numbers.

brain attack interference with the supply of blood to the brain; also known as *stroke* or *cerebral vascular accident*.

brain stem base of the brain; enlarged extension of the spinal cord, located in the cranium; includes medulla oblongata, diencephalon, pons, and midbrain.

bridging supporting the body on either side of an affected area to relieve pressure on the area.

bronchi tubal structures connecting the trachea to the lungs.

bronchioles smaller subdivisions or branches at end of the bronchi, located in the lungs.

bronchitis inflammation of the bronchi.

bruxism grinding of the teeth.

bulimia nervosa   a condition in which patients usually binge-eat in huge amounts, then vomit (*purge*) to undo the binge. The binge eating causes feelings of guilt, depression, and self-condemnation.

burn   traumatic injury to the skin and underlying tissues caused by heat, chemicals, or electricity. Burns are a very painful injury with a high risk of complications. Extensive treatment is often required.

burnout   loss of enthusiasm for and interest in an activity.

bursae   small sacs of fluid found around joints.

bursitis   condition in which the bursae become inflamed and the joint becomes very painful.

cachexia   state of malnutrition, emaciation, and debility, usually resulting from a prolonged illness.

CAM   *See* **complementary/alternative medicine**

cancer   a disease in which the normal mechanisms of cell growth are disturbed. Cells grow abnormally, invade surrounding tissues, and use nutrition targeted for normal cells.

cannula   an indwelling tube inserted through a stoma (or into the skin) to maintain patency.

CAPD   *See* **continuous ambulatory peritoneal dialysis**

capillary   hairlike blood vessel; link between arterioles and venules.

capillary refill   quick and painless method of checking a patient's peripheral circulation and oxygenation status; done by pressing on a fingernail and noting the time needed for skin color to return to normal when pressure is released.

carbohydrates   energy foods; used by the body to produce heat and energy for work.

carbon dioxide   gas that is a waste product in cellular metabolism.

carcinogen   a cancer-causing substance.

carcinoma   malignant tumor made up of connective tissue enclosing epithelial cells.

cardiac arrest   sudden and often unexpected stoppage of effective heart action.

cardiac cycle   all (mechanical and electrical) events that occur between one heart contraction and the next.

cardiac decompensation   another name for congestive heart failure.

cardiac muscle   muscle that forms the heart wall.

cardiopulmonary resuscitation (CPR)   emergency medical procedure undertaken to restart and sustain heart and respiratory functions.

care plan   nursing plan for care of a resident in a long-term care facility.

care plan conference   meeting of members of an interdisciplinary health care team to develop approaches and a plan of care.

caries   tooth decay or cavities.

carrier   person who hosts infectious organisms without having symptoms of disease. This person can give the disease to others. He or she may not know of the infection.

cartilage   type of connective tissue usually found between bones.

cataract   opacity of the lens of the eye, resulting in loss of vision.

catastrophic reaction   severe and unpredictable violent behavior of a person with dementia.

catheter   tube for evacuating or injecting fluids.

causative agent   etiology (cause) of a specific disease process.

cavity   enclosed area; space within the body that contains organs.

celibate   has no sexual intercourse.

cell   basic unit in the organization of living substances.

cellulose   basic substance of all plant foods, which can supply the body with roughage.

Celsius scale   centigrade scale for measuring temperature.

centimeter   one-hundredth of a meter.

central venous (CV) catheter   tube inserted into a large vein in the area of the clavicle.

cerebellum   portion of the brain lying beneath the occipital lobe; coordinates muscular activities and balance.

cerebrospinal fluid (CSF)   water cushion protecting the brain and spinal cord from shock.

cerebrovascular accident (CVA)   more commonly called *brain attack* or *stroke*; disorder of the blood vessels of the brain resulting in impaired cerebral circulation and often causing motor and cognitive deficits.

cerebrum   largest part of the brain, consisting of two hemispheres separated by a deep longitudinal fissure; controls all mental activities.

certification   an inspection process for facilities that accept state or federal funds as payment for health care.

cervical traction   use of weights to apply traction in the area of the cervical vertebrae.

cesarean   method of delivering fetus through a surgical incision in the abdominal wall and uterus.

chain of infection   process of events involved in the transmission and development of an infectious disease.

chancre   shallow, craterlike lesion; primary lesion of syphilis.

charting   entering information (documentation) in a patient's medical record (chart).

chelation therapy   intravenous injection of an amino acid by a licensed professional; commonly used to treat serious circulatory problems, heavy metal poisoning, and reduced blood flow in the legs.

chemical burn   injury (burn) caused by exposure to chemicals that damage the skin and mucous membranes.

chemical restraint   use of medications to control behavior.

chemotherapy   use of medications to treat disease.

chest tubes   sterile, clear plastic tubes that are inserted through the skin of the chest, between the ribs, and into the space between the lung and chest wall; used after surgery to drain bloody fluid from the chest and allow air to escape if there is a small leak of air at the suture line after lung surgery.

Cheyne-Stokes respirations   periods of apnea alternating with periods of dyspnea.

CHF   *See* **congestive heart failure**

chiropractic care   manual adjustments to keep the vertebrae in good alignment, relieving pressure on nerves, muscles, and joints.

chlamydia   type of sexually transmitted disease.

cholecystectomy   surgical removal of a diseased gallbladder and stones.

cholecystitis   inflammation of the gallbladder.

cholelithiasis   formation of stones in the gallbladder.

chorea   abnormal, spastic movements that are the primary sign of Huntington's disease.

chronic disease or **illness**   incurable illness or disease, but treatable; requires ongoing care.

chronic obstructive pulmonary disease (COPD)   any condition, such as emphysema or bronchitis, that interferes with normal respiration over a long period of time.

chronologic   in sequential order by date or age.

chyme   semiliquid form of food as it leaves the stomach.

circumcision   removal of the end of the prepuce by a circular incision.

citation   written notice that informs a facility of violations of OSHA rules.

clear liquid diet   diet of water and high-carbohydrate fluids given every 2 to 4 hours.

client   person receiving care; depending on the health care setting, also known as *patient* or *resident*.

client care record   documentation of care provided in the home situation.

Clients' Rights   document spelling out rights of persons receiving home health care.

climacteric   menopause; the combined phenomena accompanying cessation of the reproductive function in the female or reduction of testicular activity in the male.

clinical thermometer   instrument used to measure body temperature.

clitoris   small, cylindrical mass of erotic tissue; part of the external female reproductive organs analogous to the penis in the male.

closed bed   bed with sheets and spread positioned to the head of the bed; unoccupied.

closed (simple) fracture   fracture in which bones remain in proper alignment.

coccus   (plural **cocci**)   round bacteria.

cochlea   spiral-shaped organ in the inner ear that receives and interprets sounds.

coercion   forcing a patient to do something against his or her wishes.

cognitive impairment   deficit in intellect, memory, or attention.

coitus   sexual intercourse; copulation.

cold pack   a type of thermal application used to lower the temperature of a portion of the body; often a commercially prepared, disposable item.

colon   large intestine.

colony   group of organisms derived from a single organism.

color therapy   alternative health care practices that use color to affect mood, emotions, relationships, and sense of well-being.

colostomy   artificial opening in the abdomen for the purpose of evacuation of feces.

colostrum   secretion from the lactiferous glands of the mother before the onset of true lactation two or three days after delivery of a baby.

colporrhaphy   suturing of the vagina; surgical procedure used to tighten vaginal walls.

combining form   word part that can be used with other word parts to form a variety of new words.

comfort   a state of well-being in which the patient is calm and relaxed, and is not in pain or upset.

comminuted fracture   fracture in which the bone is broken or crushed into small pieces.

communicable disease   disease caused by pathogenic organism; can be transmitted from person to person, either directly or indirectly.

communication   exchange of messages.

community   people who live in a common area and share common health needs.

comorbidities   diseases and medical conditions that are either caused by or contributed to by morbid obesity or another medical problem.

compartment syndrome   a painful condition that occurs when pressure within the muscles builds up, preventing blood and oxygen from reaching muscles and nerves; a very serious complication that may develop following an injury or surgical procedure.

compensate   to seek a substitute for something unattainable or unacceptable.

complementary/alternative medicine (CAM)   a group of diverse systems, practices, and products that are not presently considered part of conventional medicine.

complementary medicine   a treatment regimen in which alternative practices are combined with conventional health care.

complete fracture   a break across the entire cross-section of the bone.

complication   situation that makes the original medical condition more serious.

compound (open) fracture   fracture in which part of the broken bone protrudes through the skin.

compression fracture   break in a bone with crushing of the bone fragments.

compulsion   a purposeful, repetitive behavior that is done many times each day and problematic enough to cause distress, be time-consuming, or interfere with the person's normal routine, occupation, social activities, or relationships.

concurrent cleaning   daily, routine cleaning of patient unit.

condom catheter   latex sheath that fits over the penis; used for urinary drainage when connected to a urinary collection bag.

confidential   keeping what is said or written to oneself; private; not shared.

congenital   condition present at birth.

congestive heart failure (CHF)   condition resulting from cardiac output inadequate for physiological needs, with shortness of breath, edema, and abnormal retention of sodium and water in body tissues.

conjunctiva   mucous membrane that lines the eyelids and covers the eye.

connective tissue   tissue that holds other tissues together and provides support for organs and other body structures.

connective tissue cells   cells that form connective tissue.

constipation   difficulty in defecating.

contact precautions   practices used to prevent spread of disease by direct or indirect contact.

contact transmission   spread of disease by direct or indirect contact with infected person or contaminated objects.

contagious   communicable or easily spread.

contagious disease   disease that is communicable; disease that is caused by a pathogenic organism.

contaminated   unclean; impure; soiled with microbes.

continuous ambulatory peritoneal dialysis (CAPD)   a form of dialysis that removes waste products from the patient's blood; performed in subacute care centers and at home.

continuous passive motion (CPM) a therapy that prevents stiffness and improves circulation by delivering a form of passive range-of-motion exercise so that the joint is moved without the patient's muscles being used.

continuous positive airway pressure (CPAP) oxygen therapy in which a mask is placed on the patient's face, then connected to a device that creates low levels of pressure.

continuum continuous related series of events or actions.

contracture permanent shortening or contraction of a muscle due to immobility spasm, or paralysis.

contraindicated not recommended; disallowed; situation in which a remedy or treatment is not called for because of the patient's condition.

contraindication situation in which a treatment or action is inappropriate.

contusion mechanical injury (usually caused by a blow) resulting in hemorrhage beneath the unbroken skin.

convulsion a seizure or change in electrical brain function.

COPD *See* **chronic obstructive pulmonary disease**

coping handling or dealing with stress.

core body temperature the normal operating temperature of the body center, or *core*. This value reflects the temperature in deep structures of the body such as the liver.

cornea transparent portion of the eye through which light passes.

coronary embolism blood clot lodged in a coronary artery.

coronary occlusion closing off of a coronary artery.

coronary thrombosis blood clot within a coronary vessel.

corporal punishment use of painful treatment to change or correct behavior.

cortex outer portion of a kidney.

countertraction providing opposing balance to traction; used in reduction of fractures.

Cowper's glands pair of small glands that open into the urethra at the base of the penis; part of the male reproductive system.

CPAP *See* **continuous positive airway pressure**

CPM *See* **continuous passive motion**

CPR *See* **cardiopulmonary resuscitation**

critical list list that patients are placed on when they are dangerously or terminally ill.

critical (clinical) pathways written documents that detail the expected course of treatment and expected outcomes for a DRG.

cross-trained educated in many different skills across (health care) disciplines.

crust scab made of dried exudate.

CSF *See* **cerebrospinal fluid**

culture views and traditions of a particular group.

culture and sensitivity test to determine type of microorganisms causing a disease and the specific antibiotics that can be used to treat the disease.

cupping use of warmed glass jars to create suction on certain points of the body.

Cushing's syndrome condition that results from an excess level of adrenal cortex hormones.

cutaneous membrane skin.

cuticle base of the fingernail.

CV catheter *See* **central venous catheter**

CVA *See* **cerebrovascular accident**

cyanosis dusky, bluish discoloration of skin, lips, and nails caused by inadequate oxygen.

cyanotic relating to the condition of cyanosis.

cystitis inflammation of the urinary bladder.

cystocele bladder hernia.

cystoscopy procedure that uses an instrument (cystoscope) for visualization of the urinary bladder, and urethra.

D & C *See* **dilatation and curettage**

dance therapy use of dance to express oneself.

dangling sitting up with legs hanging over the edge of the bed.

debilitating weakening.

debride to remove foreign material and necrotic tissue.

decubitus ulcer older term for a pressure ulcer; open area that develops on the skin over a bony prominence as the result of pressure.

deep vein thrombosis (DVT) blood clot that commonly occurs in the femoral vein, the large blood vessel in the groin.

defamation something harmful to the good name or reputation of another person; slander.

defecation bowel movement that expels feces.

defense mechanism psychological reaction or technique for protection against a stressful environmental situation or anxiety.

defibrillation using an electric shock to reverse disorganized activity in the heart during cardiac arrest.

degenerative joint disease (DJD) deterioration of the tissues of the joints.

dehydration excessive water loss.

delirium acute, reversible mental confusion due to illness and medical problems.

delirium tremens (DTs) part of a serious withdrawal syndrome seen in persons who stop drinking alcohol following continuous and heavy consumption; signs and symptoms commonly begin 48 to 96 hours after taking the last drink.

delusion false belief.

dementia progressive mental deterioration due to organic brain disease.

dendrite branch of a neuron that conducts impulses toward the cell body.

denial unconscious defense mechanism in which an occurrence or observation is refused recognition as reality in order to avoid anxiety or pain.

dentures artificial teeth.

depilatory substance used to remove body hair.

depressant drug that slows down body functions.

depressed fracture fracture in which the bone is depressed and fragments are driven inward; seen only in fractures of the skull and face.

depression morbid sadness or melancholy.

dermal ulcer pressure sore; pressure ulcer.

dermis layer of tissue that lies under the epidermis.

development gradual growth.

developmental milestones achievement of specific skills at a particular age level.

developmental tasks   in psychology, normal steps in personality development.

diabetes mellitus   disorder of carbohydrate metabolism.

diagnosis related groups (DRGs)   method used by Medicare to determine the number of hospital days required for specific illnesses.

dialect   local terminology and usage of a group's common language.

dialysis   movement of dissolved materials through a semipermeable membrane, passing from an area of higher concentration to an area of lower concentration; means of cleansing waste or toxic materials from the body.

diaphoresis   profuse sweating.

diarrhea   a condition in which the patient has multiple, watery stools.

diastole   period during which the heart muscle relaxes and the chamber fills with blood.

diastolic pressure   blood pressure during period of cardiac ventricular relaxation.

diathermy   treatment with heat.

digestion   process of converting food into a form that can be used by the body.

digital thermometer   hand-held, battery-operated device that registers temperature and displays reading as numbers.

dilatation and curettage (D & C)   procedure in which the cervical canal is expanded and tissue is scraped from the lining of the uterus.

dilation stage   stage of labor in which the opening to the cervix enlarges.

diplegia   paralysis affecting the same region on both sides of the body (such as both arms).

diplo-   arranged in pairs, such as diplococci (bacteria that are arranged in groups of two).

dirty   anything that has potentially been exposed to pathogens.

disability   persistent physical or mental deficit or handicap.

discectomy   a minimally invasive surgery to repair a back injury.

discharge   procedure carried out as a patient leaves the facility.

disease   definite, marked process of illness having characteristic symptoms.

disinfection   process of eliminating pathogens from equipment and instruments.

dislocation   displacement of the ends of a joint.

disorientation   loss of recognition of time, place, or people.

disposable   not reusable after one use.

disruption   interference with the normal progress of events.

distal   farthest away from a central point, such as point of attachment of muscles.

distended   condition in which a body part, particularly the abdomen, becomes very large and tender.

distention   the state of being stretched out (distended).

diuresis   increase in output of fluids by the kidneys.

diverticula   small blind pouches that form in the lining and wall of the colon.

diverticulitis   inflammation of diverticula.

diverticulosis   presence of many diverticula.

DJD   *See* **degenerative joint disease**

DNR   do not resuscitate order; used when cardiac and respiratory arrest occur.

Doctor of Osteopathy (D.O.)   a physician who receives a complete medical education similar to that of a medical doctor (MD). Additionally, the D.O. learns how to manipulate the spine for a therapeutic response in the body.

document   legal record; recording observations and data about a patient's condition.

dorsal   posterior or back.

dorsal lithotomy position   position in which the patient is on the back with knees flexed and well separated; feet are usually placed in stirrups.

dorsal recumbent position   position in which the patient is flat on the back with knees flexed and slightly separated, with feet flat on the bed.

dorsiflexion   toes pointed up.

dosimeter   a small, personal monitoring instrument that measures the radiation dose received by each individual working with patients receiving radiation therapy or brachytherapy.

douche   irrigation of the vaginal canal with medicated or normal saline solution.

doula   person who accompanies the mother during the childbirth process; he or she is responsible for supporting and comforting the mother and enhancing communication between the mother and medical professionals.

drainage   systematic withdrawal of fluids and discharges from wounds, sores, or body cavities.

draw sheet   sheet folded under the patient, extending from above the shoulder to below the hips.

dressings   gauze, film, or other synthetic substances that cover a wound, ulcer, or injury.

DRGs   *See* **diagnosis related groups**

droplet precautions   procedures used to prevent spread of disease by droplets in air.

droplet transmission   a method of spreading infection by inhaling pathogens from the droplets of a patient's respiratory secretions. The droplets do not travel more than 3 feet from the source patient.

DTs   *See* **delirium tremens**

duodenal resection   surgical removal of a portion of small intestine (duodenum).

duodenal ulcer   ulcer on the mucosa of the duodenum due to the action of gastric juice.

durable power of attorney for health care   document stating that a person appointed by the patient can make health care decisions when the patient is unable to do so for himself or herself.

DVT   *See* **deep vein thrombosis**

dyscrasia   abnormality or disorder of the body.

dysentery   infection in lower bowel.

dysmenorrhea   difficult or painful menstruation.

dysphagia   difficulty swallowing food and liquids.

dyspnea   difficult or labored breathing.

dysuria   painful voiding.

eating disorders   a group of disorders characterized by disturbances in appetite or food intake.

ecchymosis   bruising.

edema   excessive accumulation of fluid in the tissues.

efface   thinning of the cervix during labor.

ejaculatory duct   part of the male reproductive system extending down from the seminal vesicles to the urethra.

elasticity   ability to stretch.

electric bed   bed operated by electricity.

electrical burn   injury (burn) caused by contact with electricity and lightning. Typically deep; the electricity charts an unpredictable path through the body, causing major damage along the pathway from entrance to exit.

electromagnetic therapy   use of various forms of electrical energy to correct imbalances in the electric and magnetic fields, which are believed to cause illness and disease.

electronic thermometer   battery-operated clinical thermometer that uses a probe and records the temperature on a viewing screen in a few seconds.

eloping   wandering away from the health care facility.

embolus   mass of undissolved material carried in the bloodstream; frequently causes obstruction of a vessel.

emergency   situation requiring immediate attention or medical treatment.

emergency care   medical treatment and nursing care provided to emergency patients.

Emergency Medical Services (EMS)   treatment and care provided by specially trained health care personnel during emergencies.

emesis   vomiting.

emotional lability   unstable emotional status with frequent changes in emotions and mood.

empathy   understanding how someone else feels.

emphysema   chronic obstructive pulmonary disease in which the alveolar walls are destroyed.

EMS   *See* **Emergency Medical Services**

enabler   a device that empowers patients and assists them to function at their highest possible level.

enabling   reacting to a patient in a manner that shields the patient from experiencing the full impact or consequences of his or her actions or behavior.

endocardium   lining of the heart.

endocrine gland   gland that secretes hormonal substances directly into the bloodstream; ductless gland.

endometrium   mucous membrane lining the inner surface of the uterus.

endoscope   instrument for examining the interior of the body.

endotracheal intubation   inserting a large tube through the trachea and into the lungs to provide complete control over the airway; the procedure is commonly called *intubation*.

endotracheal tube (ET tube)   a large tube that is passed through the mouth, or less commonly the nose, into the patient's lungs to control the airway; the patient is ventilated and suctioned through the tube.

enema   injection of water and/or medications into the rectum and colon; commonly used to help the bowels eliminate feces.

energy therapy   alternative and complementary practices that involve working with the energy field that reportedly surrounds and penetrates the body.

engagement   time when the fetus moves downward in the uterus in preparation for delivery (dropping).

enteral feeding   giving nutrition through a tube inserted into the digestive tract.

enuresis   bedwetting.

environmental safety   adaptation of the environment to prevent incidents and injuries.

epidermis   top layer of skin.

epididymis   elongated, cordlike structure along the posterior border of the testes, in the ducts of which sperm is stored.

epidural catheter   tube inserted into spinal area for delivery of medication.

epilepsy   A disorder in which temporary abnormal activity occurs in brain cells, causing mild, episodic loss of attention, sleepiness, convulsions with loss of consciousness, and various other symptoms.

episiotomy   incision of the perineum at the end of the second stage of labor to avoid tearing of the perineum.

epithelial cells   structures that form protective coverings (epithelial tissue) and sometimes produce body fluids.

epithelial tissue   structure formed from epithelial cells; protects, absorbs, and produces fluids, excretes wastes.

ergonomics   process of adapting the environment and using techniques and equipment to prevent worker injuries.

erythrocyte   red blood cell.

eschar   slough of tissue produced by burning or by a corrosive application.

Escherichia coli **(*E. coli 0157:H7*)**   a strain of bacteria (not found in humans); a pathogen that multiplies rapidly and produces large amounts of toxins that cause serious illness and death.

essential nutrients   foods required for normal growth and development and to maintain health.

estrogen   hormone produced by the ovaries.

ethical standards   guides to moral behavior.

ethnic   relating to customs, languages, and traditions of specific groups of people.

ethnicity   special groupings within a race.

etiology   cause of a disease.

eustachian tube   auditory tube; leads from the middle ear to the pharynx.

evaluation   judgment.

eversion   turning outward.

exacerbation   worsening of a chronic medical condition.

exchange list   list of measured foods that allows equivalent exchanges between foods within a designated food group.

excoriation   superficial injury, such as that produced by scratching the skin.

excrete   to eliminate wastes from body.

expanded precautions   another term for *transmission-based precautions*.

expectorate   to spit (to bring up sputum).

expiration   exhalation.

exposure incident   an occurrence during which there is possible personal contact with infectious material.

expressive aphasia   inability to use verbal speech.

expulsion stage   stage of labor and delivery during which the fetus is expelled.

extension   movement by which the two ends of any jointed part are drawn away from each other.

face shield   type of personal protective equipment; protects mucous membranes of eyes, nose, and mouth from pathogens.

facility (health care)   an agency that provides health care.

Fahrenheit scale   system used in the United States to express temperature.

fallopian tube   *See* **oviduct**

false imprisonment   unlawfully restraining another.

family   group of persons (usually related by blood or marriage) with common values and traditions.

fasting   not eating.

fat   nutrient used to store energy.

fecal impaction   the most serious form of constipation, in which stool is retained in the rectum, where water is absorbed. Over time, the stool becomes hard and dry, and the patient is unable to pass it.

fecal material   another term for feces, stool, or solid body waste (bowel movement or BM). Normally brown, but color can be affected by certain foods, medications, and diseases. A BM is normally soft and formed.

feces   stool; semisolid waste eliminated from the body.

feedback   confirmation that a message was received as intended.

fetal monitor   device used to register activity and health status of the unborn fetus during labor.

fetoscopy   examination of the fetus while in the uterus.

fetus   child in the uterus from the third month to birth.

fibromyalgia   a common pain syndrome for which there is no known cause.

fingerstick blood sugar (FSBS)   a method of checking blood sugar by collecting a sample of capillary blood with a lancet.

first aid   emergency care and treatment of an injured person before complete medical and surgical care can be secured.

fistula   abnormal communication between two hollow organs or between a hollow organ and the exterior.

flaccid paralysis   loss of muscle tone and absence of tendon reflexes.

flagged   marked in a special way to call attention to it.

flatulence   excessive gas in the stomach and intestines.

flatus   gas or air in the stomach or intestines; air or gas expelled by way of any body opening.

flexion   decreasing the angle between two bones.

flora   normal population of organisms found in a given area.

flow sheet   clinical record of ongoing patient care and progress.

fluid balance   balance between fluid intake and fluid output.

Foley catheter   indwelling catheter placed in the urinary bladder to remove urine continuously.

fomite   any object contaminated with germs and thus able to transmit disease.

foot drop   a neurological problem that causes the foot to point downward.

footboard   appliance placed at the foot of the bed so the feet rest firmly against it and are kept at right angles to the legs.

force fluids   notation meaning that the patient must be encouraged to take as much fluid as possible.

foreskin   prepuce; loose tissue covering the penis and clitoris.

foster parent   parent figure assigned by an agency.

Fowler's position   position in which the patient lies on the back with backrest elevated 45 to 60°.

fracture   break in the continuity of bone.

friction   rubbing of the skin against another surface, such as bed linen.

FSBS   *See* **fingerstick blood sugar**

full liquid diet   diet consisting of all types of fluids.

full weight-bearing   able to stand on both legs.

fundus   portion of the uterus above the point of entrance of the oviducts.

fungus (plural fungi)   class of organisms to which molds and yeasts belong.

fusion   combination into a single unit.

gait   manner of walking.

gait belt   belt placed around the patient's waist to assist in ambulation.

gait training   teaching the patient to walk.

gastrectomy   surgical removal of part or all of the stomach.

gastric bypass   the most common of the 6 accepted bariatric surgical techniques. In this procedure, the surgeon creates a 2-inch-long pouch at the top of the patient's stomach and attaches a portion of small intestine to the stomach pouch.

gastric resection   surgical removal of part of the stomach.

gastric ulcer   erosion of the lining of the stomach.

gastroscopy   procedure to examine the inside of the stomach, using a scope for visualization.

gastrostomy feeding   nutrition given through a tube inserted into the stomach through the abdominal wall.

gatch bed   bed fitted with a jointed backrest and knee rest; patient can be raised to a sitting position and kept in that position by manually adjusting the bed.

general anesthetic   medication that induces a state of unconsciousness and reduces or eliminates ability to feel pain.

generalized tonic-clonic seizure   another name for grand mal seizure.

genetic   pertaining to or carried by a gene or genes.

genitalia   external reproductive organs.

geriatric   relating to age or the elderly.

gestational age   age of development of a new individual within the uterus from conception to birth.

Glasgow Coma Scale   a system used to monitor neurologic problems after trauma, stroke, and other illnesses and injuries; uses a point score to rank the patient's responses to stimuli.

glaucoma   a condition in which the pressure is increased within the eye. Untreated, it will lead to blindness.

global aphasia   loss of all language ability.

glomerulus   blood vessels that branch to form a ball of capillaries in the cortex of the kidney.

glucagon   hormone produced by pancreas that increases blood sugar level.

glucose   simple sugar; also called *dextrose*.

glycated hemoglobin (A1C)   a series of stable minor blood components formed from hemoglobin and glucose. The A1C test is a measurement of glucose levels in the blood over a prolonged period of time.

glycogen   polysaccharide that is the chief carbohydrate storage material.

glycosuria   sugar in the urine.

goal   an outcome resulting from implementation of a care plan.

goggles   type of personal protective equipment used with standard precautions to protect the eyes.

gonads   reproductive organs; ovaries and testes.

gonorrhea   sexually transmitted disease that causes an acute inflammation.

gout   a metabolic disease that results in increased uric acid deposits in the joints, which causes pain.

graduate   container marked for milliliters, used to measure liquids.

graft   body tissue used for transplantation.

grand mal seizure   major epileptic seizure attended by loss of consciousness and convulsive movements.

greenstick fracture   breaking of a bone on one side only; most often seen in children.

grievance   situation in which a consumer feels there are grounds for complaint.

growth   physical changes that take place in body during development.

guided imagery   a practice in which the patient focuses on and visualizes positive changes, so as to cause the changes to occur.

halitosis   bad breath.

handicap   inability of person to fulfill a normal role due to disability.

hand-off communication   essential communication that must occur when patient care is transferred from one worker or department to another worker or department.

hand-over-hand technique   method in which an instructor or caregiver places his or her hand over the hand of a learner or patient to guide an activity.

hantavirus   a virus spread by contact with rodents (rats and mice) or their excretions; causes serious illness or death.

harvest   to remove donor organs.

HD   *See* **Huntington's disease**

head lice   parasites that live in the hair and scalp and feed on blood; spread primarily by direct contact with an infected person.

head-tilt, chin-lift maneuver   a procedure used to open a patient's airway if no neck injury is suspected; pressure is placed on the forehead while the jaw is lifted up.

health   state of physical, mental, and social well-being.

health care consumer   person requiring health care services.

Health Insurance Portability and Accountability Act (HIPAA)   a law passed in 1996 that protects privacy, confidentiality, and medical records and other individually identifiable patient information.

health maintenance organization (HMO)   a group of health care providers and hospitals paid by an insurance company. HMO members must see only certain doctors and go only to designated hospitals, except in emergencies.

heart block   condition in which conduction of electrical impulses from atrium to ventricles is impaired and pumping action of heart is slowed down (change in rhythm of heart).

Heimlich maneuver   procedure that uses abdominal thrusts to relieve obstruction in the trachea.

hematoma   a localized mass of blood that is confined to one area.

hematuria   blood in the urine.

hemianopsia   visual impairment due to stroke; affects one-half of visual field in one or both eyes.

hemiparesis   weakness on one side of the body; usually the result of a stroke.

hemiplegia   paralysis on one side of the body.

hemodialysis   method for circulating blood through semipermeable membranes to remove liquid body wastes.

hemoptysis   expectoration of blood.

hemorrhage   escape of blood from blood vessels.

hemorrhoids   varicose veins in the rectum.

HEPA   *See* **high efficiency particulate air filter mask**

hepatitis   inflammation of the liver.

herbal therapy   use of herbs to treat pain and illness.

herbs   medicines made from plants.

hernia   protrusion or projection of a stomach organ through the wall or cavity that normally contains it.

herniorrhaphy   surgical operation for hernia.

herpes simplex II   the virus that causes genital herpes.

heterosexuality   sexual attraction between persons of opposite genders.

high efficiency particulate air (HEPA) filter mask   a mask used by health care workers that prevents the spread of airborne infection.

high Fowler's position   position in which backrest of bed is elevated to 90°, with patient on back.

HIV   *See* **human immunodeficiency virus**

HMO   *See* **health maintenance organization**

holistic care   practices that consider the whole person, including mind, body, and spirit.

home health assistant   nursing assistant who practices under supervision in a client's home.

homemaker aide   person hired to perform light housekeeping tasks in a client's home.

homemaker assistant   person who provides home management help to a client in the client's home.

homeopathy   alternative medicine system that uses a wide range of natural (plant and mineral) substances to stimulate the body's immune system to fight disease.

homosexuality   sexual attraction between persons of the same gender.

hormone   secretion of endocrine gland; chemical messenger carried to other parts of the body where it alters activity.

hospice   special facility or arrangement to provide care of terminally ill persons.

hospice care   health care for persons who are dying.

hospital   facility for care of the sick or injured.

host   animal or plant that harbors another organism.

human immunodeficiency virus (HIV)   virus that causes acquired immune deficiency disease (AIDS).

humidifier   a water bottle that moistens oxygen for comfort and prevents drying of the mucous membranes in the nose, mouth, and lungs; used when oxygen is administered at flow rates of 5 liters a minute and over.

Huntington's disease (HD)   (also called *Huntington's chorea*) a hereditary disease that usually begins when an individual is in the 40s or 50s, although some may be younger. The disease is progressive, and is marked by involuntary, spastic movements called *chorea*; the condition progresses until the person is totally dependent, with cognitive decline or dementia.

hydrochloric (HCl) acid   acid produced by the stomach.

hydronephrosis   increased pressure of urine on the kidney cells that results in their destruction.

hyperalimentation   technique in which high-density nutrients are introduced into a large vein.

hypercalcemia   excess calcium in the bloodstream.

hyperglycemia   excessive level of blood sugar.

hyperpyrexia   abnormally high body temperature of 104°F (rectal) or above.

hypersecretion   excessive secretion.

hypersensitivity   state of altered reactivity in which the body reacts to a foreign agent more strongly than normal or in an abnormal way.

hypersomnia   disorder characterized by sleeping very late in the morning and napping during the day; causes can be physical or psychological.

hypertension   high blood pressure.

hyperthermia   hyperpyrexia.

hyperthyroidism   excessive functioning of the thyroid gland.

hypertrophy   increase in the size of an organ or structure that does not involve tumor formation.

hyperventilation   breathing abnormally fast and deep, resulting in excessive amounts of oxygen in the lungs and reduced carbon dioxide levels in the bloodstream.

hypnotherapy   practice used to create an altered state of consciousness in which the patient is more open to suggestion.

hypoallergenic tape   tape that reduces the incidence of skin reactions in patients who are allergic to adhesive backing.

hypochondriasis   abnormal concern about one's health.

hypoglycemia   abnormally low level of sugar in the blood.

hyposecretion   less than normal production of secretions.

hypotension   low blood pressure.

hypothermia   lowering of core body temperature to 95°F or below.

hypothermia-hyperthermia blanket   a fluid-filled blanket, the temperature of which can be raised or lowered.

hypothyroidism   condition due to deficiency of thyroid secretion, resulting in a lower basal metabolism.

hypoxemia   a condition in which there is insufficient oxygen in the blood.

hypoxia   lack of adequate oxygen supply.

hysterectomy   surgical removal of the uterus.

ice bag   type of cold treatment.

IDDM   *See* **insulin-dependent diabetes mellitus**

ideal body weight   a mathematical formula. The concept of ideal body weight developed from life insurance statistics related to life span or longevity and health.

ileostomy   incision in the ileum.

immune response   response of the body to elements recognized as nonself, with the production of antibodies and rejection of the foreign material.

immunity   ability to fight off infectious disease; state of being protected from a disease.

immunization   process of making a person more resistant to an infectious agent.

immunosuppression   condition in which the immune system is unable to respond to the challenge of infectious disease.

immunotherapy   a cancer treatment that alters the patient's immune response to eliminate the cancer.

impacted fracture   a fracture that occurs when the fragment from one bone is wedged into another bone.

impaction   *See* **fecal impaction**

implementation   putting into effect.

incarcerated (strangulated) hernia   abnormal constriction of part of the intestinal tract that has herniated.

incentive spirometer   apparatus used to encourage better ventilation.

incident   an occurrence or event that interrupts normal procedures or causes a crisis.

incident report   summary of information about an incident.

incomplete fracture   a partial break in a bone.

increment   amount of increase in measurements.

incubation   development of bacteria in body between time of exposure and onset of signs and symptoms.

indwelling catheter   Foley catheter that remains in the patient's bladder to drain urine.

infarction   death of tissue.

infection   invasion and multiplication of any organism and the damage this causes in the body.

infectious   capable of transmitting disease.

inferior   below another part.

infiltration   passage of fluid into the tissues surrounding a vein that occurs when an IV needle or catheter comes out of the vein.

inflammation   a localized protective reaction of tissue to irritation, injury, or infection; characterized by pain, redness, swelling, and sometimes loss of function.

informed consent   permission given after full disclosure of the facts.

initiative   action of taking the first step or initial action.

insertion   distal point of attachment of skeletal muscle.

insomnia   a chronic deprivation of quality or quantity of sleep because sleep is ended or interrupted prematurely.

inspiration   drawing of air into the lungs; inhalation.

insulin   active antidiabetic hormone secreted by the islets of Langerhans in the pancreas.

insulin-dependent diabetes mellitus (IDDM)   form of diabetes mellitus that requires insulin administration as part of the therapy.

intake and output (I&O)   recording of the amount of fluid ingested and the amount of fluid expelled by a patient.

integrative (integrated) health care   using both mainstream medical treatments and CAM therapies to treat a patient.

integument   the skin.

intention tremor   involuntary movement of muscles (particularly hands) that increases when the patient attempts to use the muscles.

interdisciplinary health care team   group of professionals from different health care disciplines who each contribute their expertise to the care of a single patient.

intermediate care   health care provided to persons with medically stable conditions.

intermittent care   care given periodically, at intervals.

interpersonal relationships   how people interact with each other.

interpreter a communication professional who mediates between speakers of different languages.

intervention actions that influence the eventual outcome of a situation.

intimacy feelings of closeness and familiarity.

intracranial pressure pressure exerted within the cranium.

intravenous (IV) infusion nourishment given through a sterile tube into a vein.

intravenous pyelogram (IVP) X-ray of urinary tract following injection of dye into vein.

invasion of privacy taking liberties with the person or personal rights of another.

invasive characterized by invading (penetrating into) or spreading.

inversion turning inward.

involuntary muscle muscle not under conscious control, mainly smooth muscle.

involuntary seclusion separation of patient from other patients and people, against the patient's will.

involution reduction in the size of the uterus following delivery.

I&O *See* **intake and output**

iodine element needed for proper function of the thyroid gland.

iris colored portion of the eye.

ischemia deficient blood supply to body tissues.

ischemic having inadequate blood flow to an area.

islets of Langerhans cells in the pancreas that produce insulin.

isolation place where a patient with easily transmitted disease is separated from others.

isolation technique special procedures carried out to prevent the spread of infectious organisms from an infected person.

isolation unit used for patients with communicable illness, for protection of other patients, staff, and visitors.

isolette environmentally controlled unit used to house a newborn infant.

IVP *See* **intravenous pyelogram**

jaundice a yellow color of the skin and sclera.

jaw-thrust maneuver a method of opening the airway of patients with known or suspected neck injuries; involves pushing the jaw forward and upward.

jejunostomy tube (J-tube) a long, small-bore tube that is threaded through the GI tract until the tip reaches the small intestine. These tubes may be placed through the nose (nasojejunostomy), or surgically through an incision in the abdominal skin. Used for providing enteral nutrition for patients who do not have a stomach and those in whom recurrent formula aspiration is a problem.

job interview discussion between employer and potential employee.

Joint Commission an organization that inspects and accredits health care agencies that meet high quality standards.

Kaposi's sarcoma a cancer that usually occurs in persons with HIV disease and men over 60 years of age.

Kardex type of file in which nursing care plans are kept.

Kelly a special clamp used to close tubes quickly.

kidney glandular, bean-shaped organ, purplish-brown, situated in back of the abdominal cavity, one on each side of the spinal column; excretes waste matter in the form of urine.

kilogram metric unit of weight measurement, equal to 1,000 grams or 2.2 pounds.

knee-chest position position in which the patient is on the abdomen with knees drawn up toward the abdomen and legs separated; arms are brought up and flexed on either side of the head, which is turned to one side.

labia majora two large, hair-covered, liplike structures that are part of the vulva.

labia minora two hairless, liplike structures found beneath the labia majora.

labor physiologic process by which the fetus is expelled from the uterus at term.

laceration accidental break in skin, an injury.

lacrimal gland produces tears.

lactation secretion of milk.

laminectomy surgical excision of the rear part of one or more vertebrae, usually to remove a herniated disk or lesion.

lancet a tiny needle.

laryngectomee a person who has had a laryngectomy (voice box removal); the patient breathes through an artificial opening in the neck and trachea.

laryngectomy surgical removal of the larynx. The airway is separated from the mouth, nose, and esophagus; there is no longer a connection between the upper and lower airways.

larynx organ located at upper end of trachea; part of airway and organ of voice (voice box).

lateral away from the midline.

lateral transfer *See* **sitting transfer**

legal custody condition of having the responsibility for another person (including the right to consent to hospitalization and to give permission for procedures).

legal guardian person who has the legal right to make decisions for another person.

legal standards guides to lawful behavior.

lesions abnormal changes in tissue formation.

leukemia malignant disease of the blood-forming organs, characterized by abnormal proliferation and distortion of the leukocytes in the blood and bone marrow.

leukocyte white blood cell.

leukorrhea white vaginal discharge.

Lhermitte's sign sharp, electrical-type sensation felt down spine when head is flexed; found in patients with multiple sclerosis.

liable legally responsible.

libel any written defamatory statement.

license a state permit allowing a facility to operate.

licensed practical nurse (LPN); licensed vocational nurse (LVN) graduate of a certificate nursing program, who must pass a state exam before being permitted to practice nursing.

life-sustaining treatment treatment given to a critically ill or injured patient to maintain life and prevent death.

ligament band of fibrous tissue that holds joints together.

light therapy treatment in which patients are exposed to special lights covered with a plastic screen to block ultraviolet rays; used to treat mood and sleep disorders, jet lag, and depression.

Listeriosis an illness caused by ingesting the *Listeria monocytogenes* bacterium in contaminated food. The bacterium is found in some raw foods, such as uncooked meats and vegetables, hot dogs, cold cuts, and soft cheeses.

lithotripsy   the crushing of calculi such as kidney stones.

living will   document describing the wishes of a terminally ill person, relating to health care.

local anesthetic   substance that blocks pain receptors or sensation in a specific area.

lochia   discharge from the uterus of blood, mucus, and tissue during the puerperal period.

long-term acute care hospital (LTACH)   hospital in which a lengthy stay is anticipated; the patients accepted have medically complex problems but have a good chance of improvement.

long-term care   health care given to a person in a facility or the person's home for an extended period of time.

low bed   bed in which the frame is 4 to 6 inches from the floor to the top of the frame deck; reduces the risk of injury if the patient falls from the bed.

LPN   *See* **licensed practical nurse**

lumpectomy   excision of abnormal tissue, such as a "lump" in the breast.

LVN   *See* **licensed vocational nurse**

lymph   fluid found in lymphatic vessels.

lymphatic vessel   vessel that conveys electrolytes, water, and proteins.

macular degeneration   vision impairment due to damage to the macula located at the back of the eye, generally related to aging.

macule   flat, discolored spot on the skin.

Magnet Program for Excellence in Nursing Services   a voluntary program that recognizes hospitals for nursing excellence.

maladaptive behavior   inappropriate reaction due to mental breakdown.

malignant   cancerous.

malodorous   having a bad or foul odor.

malpractice   improper, negligent, or unethical conduct that results in harm, injury, or loss to a patient.

mammogram   X-ray examination of the breasts.

managed care   methods used by insurance companies to reduce health care costs.

manual patient handling   moving a patient by hand or bodily force, including pushing, pulling, carrying, holding, or supporting the patient or a body part.

massage therapy   rubbing various areas of the body to stimulate circulation, promote relaxation, and provide pain relief. Massage increases feelings of well-being and reduces stress and fatigue.

mastectomy   excision of the breast.

masturbation   sexually stimulating self.

Material Safety Data Sheet (MSDS)   information provided by manufacturers about hazardous products; includes health hazards, safe use guidelines, and emergency procedures for chemical exposure.

mechanical lift   a manually-operated hydraulic lift, electrically (or battery-) operated lift, or a ceiling-mounted lift. Used to transfer dependent or heavy patients from one surface to another.

mechanical soft diet   a diet that includes ground meats; served to patients with no teeth, or those with serious dental problems.

mechanically altered diet   diet in which the consistency and texture of food are modified, making it easier to chew and swallow.

medial   close to the midline of the body or structure.

Medicaid   federal- and state-funded program that pays medical expenses for those whose income is below a certain level.

medical asepsis   procedures followed to keep germs from being spread from one person to another.

medical chart   patient record containing all information about that patient.

medical diagnosis   name of disease; determination made by a physician.

Medicare   federal program that assists persons over 65 years of age with hospital and medical costs.

meditation   calming and quieting the mind by focusing attention.

medulla   forms part of the brain stem; also, the middle area of the kidney.

membranes   tissue sheets that line the body cavities.

memo   brief, written communication to relay information.

meninges   three-layered serous membranes covering the brain and spinal cord.

meningitis   inflammation of the meninges.

menopause   period when ovaries stop functioning and menstruation ceases; female climacteric.

menorrhagia   excessive bleeding during menstruation.

menstruation   loss of an unneeded part of the endometrium following the release of an ovum and lack of conception.

mental illness   behavioral maladaptations.

message   the information the sender wants to communicate.

metabolism   sum total of the physical and chemical processes and reactions taking place in the body.

metastasis   spreading of cancer to other body parts or locations.

metastasize   to spread (cancer) to other body parts.

methicillin-resistant *Staphylococcus aureus* **(MRSA)**   bacteria resistant to most antibiotics.

metrorrhagia   abnormal discharge from the uterus.

MI *See* **myocardial infarction**

microbe   *See* **microorganism**

microorganism   tiny organism that can be seen only with a microscope, particularly bacteria.

mind-body therapy   practices that use various techniques to enhance the mind's ability to affect bodily function and symptoms.

mineral   inorganic chemical compound found in nature; many minerals are important in building body tissues and regulating body fluids.

minimally invasive surgery   any surgical procedure that does not require a large incision. It can be done by entering the body through a small cut or incision on the skin, or through a body cavity or other anatomical opening. Miniature scopes and instruments are used to visualize and repair the organs on the inside of the body.

mite   microscopic organism that cannot be seen with the naked eye.

mitered corner   one type of corner used in making a facility bed.

mobility   ability to move or to be moved easily from place to place.

mobility skills ability to move about in bed, out of bed, and walking.

modalities forms of treatment or uses of therapeutic agents or regimens.

mold organism in fungus family.

monoplegia paralysis affecting one limb only.

Montgomery straps long strips of adhesive attached to the skin on either side of a wound, then tied to hold a dressing in place.

morbid obesity being 100 pounds or more over ideal body weight, or having a BMI of 40 or higher; this condition usually qualifies for surgical treatment.

mores customs of ethnic groups.

moribund dying.

movement therapy treatment that combines nonaerobic exercise and breath control to give patients an awareness of how the body moves; alters posture and motion to reduce pain and stress.

moxibustion burning of herbal substances on or near the body.

MRSA *See* **methicillin-resistant *Staphylococcus aureus***

MS *See* **multiple sclerosis**

MSDS *See* **Material Safety Data Sheet**

mucous membrane epithelial tissue that produces fluid called mucus; lines body cavities that open to the outside of the body.

mucus secretion of mucous membranes; thick, sticky fluid.

multiple sclerosis (MS) disease characterized by hardened patches scattered throughout the brain and spinal cord that interfere with the nerves in those areas.

multisensory stimulation intense stimulation of sight, sound, touch, smell, pressure, pain, and touch to help the patient to awaken and use previously unused portions of the brain.

muscle cells form muscle tissue; have ability to shorten or lengthen and to change their shape and the position of parts to which they are attached.

muscle tissue tissue that has the ability to shorten and lengthen.

music therapy therapeutic use of music to address physical, psychological, or cognitive needs and/or social functioning.

myocardial infarction (MI) formation of an infarct in the heart muscle due to interruption of the blood supply to the area.

myocardium heart muscle.

N95 respirator mask with small, tightly woven pores that protects the wearer from airborne infection.

NACEP *See* **Nurse Aide Competency Evaluation Program**

narcolepsy condition in which the patient has sudden, uncontrollable, unpredictable urges to fall asleep during daytime hours.

narcotic drug that relieves pain and produces sleep.

nasal cannula tubing inserted into nostrils to administer oxygen.

nasogastric feeding (NG feeding) nourishment given through a tube inserted through the nose into the stomach.

nasogastric (NG) tube soft rubber or plastic tube that is inserted through a nostril into the stomach.

nasopharyngeal airway (nasal airway) a curved, soft-rubber device that is inserted through one nostril and extends to the posterior pharynx, keeping the tongue off the back of the throat. May be used in responsive patients, including those with recent oral surgery, loose teeth, or trauma of the mouth, and those who need frequent nasal suctioning.

National Institute of Occupational Safety and Health (NIOSH) federal agency responsible for conducting research and making recommendations for the prevention of work-related disease and injury.

naturopathic medicine a medical system that focuses on whole-person wellness, emphasizing prevention and self-care. The doctor looks for the cause of illness, rather than strictly treating symptoms.

nebulizer device used to apply a liquid in the form of a fine spray or mist; may be used to administer medication.

necrosis tissue death.

necrotizing fasciitis a serious condition that may be called "flesh-eating" or "man-eating" strep. It occurs when bacteria enter the body through minor trauma or a break in the skin, resulting in shock and systemic infection, organ failure, and the need for amputation.

negative air pressure room a room with a special ventilation system in which the room air is drawn upward into the ventilation system and is either specially filtered or exhausted directly to the outside of the building.

neglect failing to provide services to patients to prevent physical harm or mental anguish.

negligence failure to exercise the degree of care considered reasonable under the circumstances, resulting in an unintended injury to a patient. Negligence is carelessness that may be caused by hurrying or not focusing on the task at hand.

neonate newborn baby.

neoplasm new growth; tumor.

nephritis inflammation of the kidney.

nephron microscopic kidney unit that produces urine.

nerve bundle of nerve processes (axons and dendrites) that are held together by connective tissue.

nerve cells carry electrical messages to and from different parts of body.

nervous tissue highly specialized tissue capable of conducting nerve impulses.

networking communication between individuals with a common interest or goal.

neuron cell of the nervous system.

neurotransmitter chemical compound that transmits a nervous impulse across cells at a synapse.

NG *See* **nasogastric feeding; nasogastric tube**

NIDDM *See* **non–insulin-dependent diabetes mellitus**

NIOSH *See* **National Institute of Occupational Safety and Health**

nits tiny, oval-shaped eggs of head lice; are yellow-white and adhere to the hair. They look like dandruff, but are firmly attached to the hair and are very difficult to remove.

no-code order an order not to resuscitate a patient.

nodule a small, knotlike protrusion; a small mass of tissue.

non–insulin-dependent diabetes mellitus (NIDDM) diabetes controlled by diet and sometimes oral medication, for which insulin is not needed.

noninvasive remaining localized and not spreading; not penetrating.

nonpathogen microorganism that does not produce disease.

nonrapid eye movement (NREM) sleep   the phase that accounts for 75% of the sleep cycle, in which sleep progresses from light to deep.

nonverbal communication   communication transmitted without spoken words, such as by facial expression and body language.

nonweight-bearing   unable to stand or walk on one or both legs.

nosocomial   pertaining to or originating in a facility.

nosocomial infection   infection acquired in a facility.

nourishments   substantial food items given to patients to increase nutrient intake; often planned and ordered by the facility dietitian.

NPO   nothing by mouth.

nucleoplasty   *See* **discectomy**

Nurse Aide Competency Evaluation Program (NACEP)   test taken by the nursing assistant which, when passed successfully, entitles the nursing assistant to certification.

nurse's notes   section of medical record in which nursing staff records procedures, medications, and observations.

nursing assistant   person who provides personal care and assists with ADLs under nursing supervision.

nursing diagnosis   statement of a patient's problems leading to nursing interventions.

nursing process   framework for nursing action.

nursing team   members of the nursing staff who provide patient care.

nutrient   nourishing substance or food.

nutrition   process by which the body uses food for growth and repair and to maintain health.

nutrition therapy   evaluation and modification of the patient's diet and nutrient intake to promote optimal nutrition for health, wellness, and healing.

nystagmus   constant involuntary movement of the eyeball.

obese   overweight.

obesity   being overweight by 20 to 30% of the ideal body weight. Being overweight or obese increases the risk for many health conditions, including diabetes, heart disease, and stroke.

objective observation   observation made through the senses of the observer.

oblique fracture   *See* **closed fracture**

OBRA   *See* **Omnibus Budget Reconciliation Act**

observation   noticing something.

obsession   a frequent idea, impulse, or thought that usually does not make sense. However, the person cannot suppress or eliminate it.

obsessive-compulsive disorder (OCD)   an anxiety disorder in which the patient has recurrent obsessions, frequent thoughts, ideas, impulses, or compulsions, resulting in repeated ritualistic activity over which the person has no control.

obstetric, obstetrical   pertaining to pregnancy, labor, and delivery.

obstruction   blockage in a passageway.

occult blood   small quantity of blood that can be detected only by microscope or chemical means.

occupational exposure   coming into contact with infectious materials during the performance of a person's job.

Occupational Safety and Health Administration (OSHA)   federal agency that makes and enforces regulations to protect workers.

occupational therapy   therapeutic use of work and activities to help patients regain self-care skills.

OCD   *See* **obsessive-compulsive disorder**

OJD   *See* **osteoarthritic joint disease**

Omnibus Budget Reconciliation Act (OBRA)   law that regulates the education and certification of nursing assistants in acute care and long-term care facilities.

OMT   *See* **osteopathic manipulative treatment**

oncology   study of cancer.

oophorectomy   surgical excision of an ovary.

open bed   bed with top bedding fanfolded to bottom, ready for occupancy.

open (compound) fracture   fracture in which part of the broken bone protrudes through the skin.

open reduction/internal fixation (ORIF)   surgical procedure to reduce a fractured bone. The skin is opened and the fracture realigned and held in place by screws, plates, and pins.

operative   pertaining to an operation.

oral hygiene   care of the mouth and teeth.

oral report   verbal report.

orchiectomy   excision of one or both of the testes.

organ   any part of the body that carries out a specific function or functions, such as the heart.

organism   any living thing, plant, or animal.

organizational chart   guide for communication; spells out lines of authority.

ORIF   *See* **open reduction/internal fixation**

orifice   body opening such as the nose or mouth.

origin   proximal point of attachment to skeletal muscle.

oropharyngeal airway (oral airway)   a curved plastic device that is inserted into the mouth to the posterior pharynx to prevent the tongue from falling to the back of the throat and obstructing the airway.

orthopedic   concerning the prevention or correction of deformities (orthopedics).

orthopnea   need to sit upright in order to breathe without difficulty.

orthopneic position   a position in which the patient must sit up to breathe comfortably. The patient sits as upright as possible and leans slightly forward, supporting herself with the forearms.

orthotic devices (orthoses)   devices that restore or improve function and prevent deformity.

OSHA   *See* **Occupational Safety and Health Administration**

ossicles   any small bones, such as one of the three bones in the ear.

osteoarthritic joint disease (OJD)   degenerative disease of joints.

osteopathic manipulative treatment (OMT)   a passive, thrusting motion used to restore normal body movement and enhance blood and oxygen flow; used in combination with regular medical treatment.

osteoporosis   a metabolic disorder of the bones in which bone mass is lost, causing them to become porous and spongy; affected bones are at very high risk for fracture.

ostomy suffix meaning "to create a new opening"; for example, colostomy.

otitis media inflamed condition of the middle part of the ear.

otosclerosis formation of bone in the inner ear that causes the ossicles to become fixed.

ovaries (singular **ovary**) endocrine glands located in the female pelvis; female gonads.

overweight a condition in which a person weighs more than he or she should, according to standards set according to the person's height and bone (frame) size.

oviduct tube in the body between the ovary and the uterus through which an ovum travels; part of the female reproductive system.

ovulation lunar monthly ripening and discharge of an ovum from the cortex of the ovary.

ovum (plural **ova**) female egg.

oxygen gas that is essential to cellular metabolism and life.

oxygen concentrator device that removes impurities from room air and concentrates oxygen to be delivered to a patient.

oxygen mask device to administer oxygen through nose and mouth; placed over patient's face.

oxygenation movement of oxygen from the lungs into the blood, which carries the oxygen to body cells.

pacemaker artificial device placed in the body to regulate the heartbeat.

PACU *See* **postanesthesia care unit**

pain a state of discomfort; a warning signal that something is wrong.

palliative care comfort care; care that treats the symptoms of discomfort, but not the underlying disease.

pallor less color than normal for the skin.

panhysterectomy removal of the entire uterus.

panic disorder a condition characterized by unexpected, chronic *panic attacks* (bouts of overwhelming fear). The person usually feels that he is in danger, but there is no specific cause for the fear. The person may be so fearful that she is unable to function.

panniculus the fatty apron of abdominal skin seen in most bariatric patients.

pannus a large, hanging flap of skin; usually seen in the abdomen of people who have recently lost a significant amount of weight.

Pap smear simple test used to detect cancer of the cervix.

papule solid, elevated lesion of the skin.

PAR *See* **post-anesthesia recovery**

paralysis loss or impairment of the ability to move parts of the body.

paranoia state in which one has delusions of persecution and/or grandeur.

paraphrasing providing communication feedback by restating one's understanding of what was said.

paraplegia paralysis of the lower portion of the body and of both legs.

parasite organism that lives within, upon, or at the expense of another organism known as the *host*.

parathormone hormone produced by parathyroid glands that regulates calcium and phosphorus levels in the blood.

parathyroid glands two pairs of endocrine glands situated on posterior of thyroid gland; produce the hormone parathormone.

paresis weakness of an extremity.

Parkinson's disease neurological disorder due to deficiency of dopamine, a neurotransmitter; progressive disease characterized by stiffness of muscles and tremors.

partial weight-bearing unable to bear full weight on one or both legs.

partners in practice a method of providing care in which a registered nurse works with a nursing assistant as a team.

PASS acronym for fire extinguisher use meaning: *P*ull the pin; *A*im the nozzle; *S*queeze the handle; *S*weep back and forth.

passive range of motion (PROM) exercises performed for the patient by the nursing assistant when independent movement is not possible. Maintains movement and prevents deformities, but does not strengthen muscles.

pathogen microorganism or other agent capable of producing a disease.

pathologic fracture fracture in a diseased bone that occurs as a result of osteoporosis, a tumor, or cancer.

pathology disease.

patient person who needs care; *see also* **resident** and **client**.

patient-controlled analgesia (PCA) administration of pain-relieving medication controlled by the patient, using a special device; amount of medication to be delivered is preset by the nurse.

patient-focused care attention given to mental, physical, and emotional aspects of a person's being.

Patients' Bill of Rights document developed by the American Hospital Association that describes the basic rights to which each patient is entitled.

PCA *See* **patient-controlled analgesia**

PDA *See* **personal digital assistant**

pediatric patient from birth to 18 years of age.

pediculosis body lice; parasites that feed on humans and animals.

PEG *See* **percutaneous endoscopic gastrostomy**

pelvic belt traction form of traction in which a belt that is secured around a patient's hips is attached to weights.

pelvic inflammatory disease (PID) inflammation of the pelvic organs.

pelvis lower portion of the trunk of the body; basin-shaped area bounded by the hip bones, the sacrum, and the coccyx.

penis male organ of copulation and urinary elimination.

pepsin enzyme produced in the stomach that begins protein digestion.

perceptual deficit inability to reason, think systematically, make judgments, or use common items.

percutaneous endoscopic gastrostomy (PEG) a gastrostomy tube that is surgically placed by a physician by threading the tube through the mouth, then out an incision in the abdominal wall over the stomach.

pericardium membrane that surrounds the heart.

perineal care cleansing of genital and rectal areas.

perineum in the male, the area between the anus and the scrotum; in the female, the area between the anus and the vagina.

perioperative occurring in association with an operative procedure.

perioperative hypothermia   hypothermia that develops in the operating room as a result of anesthesia and some other drugs, open body cavities, cold environment, and administration of cold fluids.

peripheral   pertaining to the outside or outer part.

peripheral intravenous central catheter (PICC)   intravenous line inserted into a vein in the arm and threaded through to a larger vein.

peristalsis   progressive, wavelike movement that occurs involuntarily in hollow tubes of the body, especially the alimentary canal.

peritoneal dialysis   removal of liquid waste by washing chemicals through the abdominal cavity.

peritoneum   serous membrane that lines the walls of the abdominal and pelvic cavities.

personal digital assistant (PDA)   small, hand-held computer that operates on battery. May be used for documentation and storing research information and personal data.

personal protective equipment (PPE)   equipment such as waterproof gowns, masks, gloves, goggles, and other equipment needed to protect a person from infectious material.

personal space   physical closeness that a person is comfortable with during interactions with others.

personality   sum of the behavior, attitudes, and character traits of an individual.

petechiae   small purplish spots on the body surface, caused by minute hemorrhages.

petit mal seizure   type of epileptic attack that is generally short in nature; "absence" attack.

PFR95 respirator   mask with very tiny pores that prevents the wearer from breathing in infectious airborne microorganisms.

phagocyte   white blood cell that destroys substances such as bacteria, protozoa, and cells.

phantom pain   pain experienced in a body part that has been removed from the body, as if the part were still attached.

pharynx   muscular, membranous tube between mouth and esophagus; throat.

phlebitis   inflammation of a vein.

phobia   an unfounded, recurring fear that causes the person to feel panic.

physiatrist   medical doctor specializing in rehabilitation.

physical abuse   mistreatment by hitting or other physical contact.

physical restraint   device used to prevent a patient from moving about or having access to his or her own body.

physical therapy   structured exercise that assists patients to regain mobility skills.

physiology   the science that deals with the functioning of living organisms.

PICC   *See* **peripheral intravenous central catheter**

PID   *See* **pelvic inflammatory disease**

piggyback   procedure used to administer medication through a vein.

pigmentation   coloration of an area by pigment.

pineal body   pea-sized endocrine gland located in the brain.

pituitary gland   "master" endocrine gland located in brain at base of skull (attached to hypothalamus); produces hormones that regulate growth and reproduction.

pivot   to twist or turn in a swiveling motion.

placenta   structure within the womb through which the unborn child is nourished; the afterbirth.

placental stage   period of the delivery process during which the afterbirth is expelled from the uterus.

planning   establishing possible solutions for a patient's problems (as determined by nursing diagnoses).

plantar flexion   extending the foot in a downward movement.

plasma   liquid portion of blood.

Platinum Rule   "Treat others the way they want to be treated." Think about how this affects feelings and relationships. This rule shifts the focus from treating everyone alike to providing individualized care and treating patients as they want to be treated, in keeping with their plans of care.

pleura   membranes that surround the lungs.

pleural effusion   fluid that collects around the lungs in patients who have cancer.

PM care   care given to prepare a patient for sleep.

pneumonia   inflammation and infection of the lungs.

pocket mask   a barrier device used for providing "mouth"-to-mouth resuscitation that prevents the patient's exhaled air and secretions from entering the caregiver's mouth.

polydipsia   excessive thirst.

polyphagia   excessive ingestion of food.

polyuria   excessive excretion of urine.

port   opening.

portal of entry   area of body through which microbes enter and cause disease.

portal of exit   area of body through which disease-producing organisms leave the body.

position sense   ability to know one's position in space, including how extremities are positioned.

postanesthesia care unit (PACU)   room where patients receive immediate care following surgery.

post-anesthesia recovery (PAR)   area where patients are taken after surgery to recover from anesthesia.

posterior   back or dorsal.

postmortem   after death.

postmortem care   care given to the body after death.

postoperative   after surgery.

postpartum   after parturition; after birth.

post polio syndrome (PPS)   a neurologic disorder marked by increased weakness and/or abnormal muscle fatigue in persons who had paralytic polio many years earlier.

posttraumatic stress disorder (PTSD)   the development of unusual symptoms, such as nightmares or flashbacks, after a psychologically traumatic event.

postural support   device used as an enabler that maintains body position and alignment.

potentially infectious material   material or equipment that could be a source of disease-producing organisms.

pound   unit of measurement of weight, equivalent to 16 ounces or 453.6 grams.

PPE   *See* **personal protective equipment**

PPS   *See* **post polio syndrome**

prayer   a connection with a person's higher power.

preadolescence   years between the ages of 12 and 14.

predisposing factor   condition that contributes to the development of disease.

prefix word part that is placed before a word root that changes or modifies the meaning of the word root.

prenatal before birth.

preoperative period before surgery.

pressure ulcer ulceration due to ischemia; pressure sore.

private room room in a health care facility that contains only one patient at a time.

probe as used in this text, a long, slender part of an instrument; that portion of the electronic or tympanic thermometer placed into the patient.

procedure the practices and processes used when following facility policies in patient care. A procedure prioritizes and orders your responsibilities when doing the task.

proctoscopy inspection of the rectum using a proctoscope.

professional boundaries limits on how a health care worker interacts with patients.

progesterone hormone produced by female ovaries.

prognosis probable outcome of a disease or injury.

projection unconscious defense mechanism by which an individual denies his or her own emotionally unacceptable traits and sees them as belonging to another.

PROM *See* **passive range of motion**

pronation placing or lying in a face-downward position; as applied to the hand, indicates the palms facing backward.

prone position in which the patient is on the abdomen, spine straight, legs extended, and arms flexed on either side of the head.

prostate gland gland of male reproductive system that surrounds the neck of the urinary bladder and the beginning of the urethra.

prostatectomy removal of all or part of the prostate gland.

prosthesis artificial substitute for a missing body part, such as dentures, hand, leg.

protein basic material of every body cell; an essential nutrient.

protocol standards of procedure and care developed for preparation of a patient for diagnostic tests.

protozoan (plural **protozoa**) microscopic unicellular organism.

proximal closest to the point of attachment.

pseudomembranous colitis disease caused by overgrowth of *Clostridium difficile*, often after antibiotic therapy has depleted normal bowel flora; results in severe diarrhea and may cause dehydration.

psychiatric relating to mental illness.

psychological abuse mistreatment by threatening, belittling, or otherwise causing mental or emotional harm or upset.

PTSD *See* **posttraumatic stress disorder**

puberty condition or period of becoming capable of sexual reproduction.

pubic relating to or near the pubis.

pulmonary embolism blood clot in the lungs.

pulse wave of blood pressure exerted against the walls of the arteries in response to ventricular contraction.

pulse deficit difference between contractions of the heart and pulse expansions of the radial artery.

pulse oximetry procedure for measuring level of oxygen in arterial blood.

pulse pressure difference between the systolic and diastolic pressures.

pupil circular opening in the center of the iris; regulates light entering the eye.

pureed diet diet in which foods are blended with gravy or liquid until they are the consistency of pudding.

push fluids to encourage a patient to drink additional fluids.

pustule circumscribed, pus-containing lesion of the skin.

pyelogram *See* **intravenous pyelogram (IVP)**

pyloric sphincter muscle at the exit point of the pylorus.

QA *See* **quality assurance**

qigong physical and mental activities to teach the patient to channel the *chi* (life force or energy), thereby improving health.

quadrant one of the four imaginary sections of the surface of the abdomen.

quadriplegia *See* **tetraplegia**

quality assurance (QA) an internal review done by facility staff to identify problems and find solutions for improvement.

quickening first movement of the fetus in the uterus that is felt by the mother.

RA *See* **rheumatoid arthritis**

race classification of people according to shared physical characteristics.

RACE acronym relating to fire emergency procedure, meaning: *R*emove patient from danger; *A*ctivate alarm; *C*ontain fire; *E*xtinguish fire.

radial deviation wrists are turned toward the thumb side.

radial pulse pulse that can be measured by palpating the radial artery.

radiation isolation sign a sign that lists where to find special safety precautions, including the maximum length of time to remain in the room; posted on the door to a patient's room after radioactive material has been given to the patient.

radiation therapy treatment of cancer with radiation.

radical mastectomy removal of entire breast and adjacent lymph nodes.

rales abnormal respiratory sound heard in auscultation of the chest.

range-of-motion (ROM) exercises series of exercises specifically designed to move each joint through its full range.

rapid eye movement (REM) sleep the part of the sleep cycle in which dreams occur.

rate valuation based on comparison with a standard.

RCP *See* **respiratory care practitioner**

reaction formation repressing the reality of an anxiety-producing situation; the individual exhibits behaviors that are exactly opposite to the real feelings.

reality orientation techniques used to help a person remain oriented to environment, time, and self.

receiver person for whom a communication is intended.

receptive aphasia inability to understand written or spoken language.

recovery position a modified lateral position used when the patient is recovering from certain emergencies, such as unconsciousness.

recovery room location where surgical patients are taken after surgery; they return to their rooms when their conditions stabilize.

rectocele   protrusion of part of the rectum into the vagina.

references   in a résumé, statements about abilities and characteristics; persons who give such statements.

reflex   activity performed without conscious thought.

reflexology   stimulating reflex areas in the hands and feet to reduce stress, stabilize body functions, and correct health problems.

reflux   the backflow of fluid, such as when stomach juices and food flow back from the stomach into the esophagus and mouth; typically the cause of heartburn.

registered nurse (RN)   specially educated person who is licensed to plan and direct the nursing care of patients.

regress   to move in a backward fashion.

rehabilitation   process of assisting ill or injured person to attain optimal level of well-being and function.

Reiki   using touch on various areas of the body to promote health and well-being, restore energy, and enhance the body's natural healing ability.

relaxation   techniques and methods of reducing stress.

reminiscing   thinking and talking about the past.

remission   times in which a chronic disease appears stable.

renal calculi   kidney stones.

renal colic   spasm in an area near the kidney, accompanied by pain.

repression   involuntary exclusion from awareness of a painful experience or conflict-creating memory, feeling, or impulse.

reservoir   storage area; biologically, an animal or source that maintains infectious organisms that periodically can be spread to others.

resident   person being cared for in a long-term care facility; *see also* **client** and **patient**.

Residents' Rights   document that spells out rights of residents receiving care in long-term care facilities.

respiration   process of taking oxygen into the body and expelling carbon dioxide.

respiratory arrest   cessation of breathing.

respiratory care practitioner (RCP)   a licensed professional who specializes in care of patients with disorders of the cardiopulmonary system, respirations, and sleep disorders that affect the patient's breathing.

respiratory failure   a condition that occurs when breathing is insufficient to sustain life.

respiratory therapy   the department that provides care for patients with disorders of the cardiopulmonary system, respirations, and sleep disorders.

rest   state of comfort, calmness, and relaxation.

restoration   basic nursing care measures designed to maintain or improve a patient's function and assist the patient to return to self-care.

restorative   returning to preexisting level or status.

résumé   short account of a job applicant's career and qualifications.

retention   inability to excrete urine that has been produced.

retinal degeneration   breakdown and functional loss of the nervous layer of the eye.

retrograde pyelogram   backward-moving X-ray picture of ureter and renal pelvis.

rheumatoid arthritis (RA)   autoimmune response that results in inflammation of the joints.

rhythm   the repeat interval of measured time or movement.

rigor mortis   rigidity of skeletal muscles, developing 6 to 10 hours after death.

risk factor   condition indicating that a problem may develop, causing the patient's health to worsen.

ritual   ceremonial acts that reinforce faith.

RN   *See* **registered nurse**

ROM   *See* **range-of-motion exercises**

rooming-in   practice of having mother and baby share a single room after delivery.

rotation   act of turning about the axis of the center of a body, as in rotation of a joint.

rubra   unusual redness or flushing of the skin.

Sacrament of the Sick   last rites given by clergy to a person who is terminally ill (dying).

SAD   *See* **seasonal affective disorder**

salpingectomy   surgical removal of the fallopian tubes.

sarcoma   connective tissue tumor, often highly malignant.

SARS   *See* **severe acute respiratory syndrome**

scabies   a parasitic disease of the skin that causes a rash and severe itching.

schizoaffective disorder   a condition that is believed to be a combination of schizophrenia and a mood disorder. This chronic, disabling mental illness has symptoms of schizophrenia, alternating with times when the patient also has symptoms of major depression or a manic episode.

scope of practice   extent or range of permissible activities.

scrotum   saclike pouch that holds the male gonads.

seasonal affective disorder (SAD)   a depression that recurs each year at the same time, usually starting in fall or winter and ending in spring or early summer. The cause is not known, but it is believed to be related to lack of exposure to sunlight or abnormal melatonin levels.

sebaceous gland   gland that produces a lubricating substance for hairs.

seizure   a convulsion; a condition characterized by severe, involuntary shaking and jerking of the body.

self-care deficit   inability to perform an activity of daily living.

self-esteem   feeling of confidence about oneself.

self-identity   personal knowledge of who one is; personal view of self.

semicircular canal   three tubes in the inner ear containing fluid; the function is concerned with balance and detecting motion.

semi-Fowler's position   position in which the patient is on the back with knees slightly flexed, and the head of the bed is elevated 30 to 45°.

seminal vesicles   pair of accessory male sex glands that open into the vas deferens before it joins the urethra; they secrete fluid into seminal fluid.

semiprivate room   room in a health care facility that is shared by two patients.

semiprone   patient is positioned between the side and the abdomen.

semisupine   patient is positioned between the side and the back.

sender   the person who originates a communication.

senile purpura   dark purple bruises on the forearms and back of hands, common in elderly individuals.

sensitivity   ability to be aware of and appreciate personal characteristics of others; state of acute or abnormal response to stimuli or allergens.

sepsis   presence of pus-forming and other pathogens or their toxins in the blood.

sequential compression therapy   postoperative procedure in which pneumatic boots are applied to massage the legs using a milking, wavelike motion. Prevents blood clots.

seropositive   state in which antibodies to HIV exist in the bloodstream.

serous membrane   tissue that produces serous fluid, covers organs, and lines closed body cavities.

severe acute respiratory syndrome (SARS)   a serious, highly infectious viral respiratory illness caused by a coronavirus.

sexual abuse   use of physical means or verbal threats to force a person to perform sexual acts.

sexual harassment   unwelcome sexual advances, requests for sexual favors, and other verbal or physical conduct of a sexual nature. The action may be physical, verbal, or nonverbal.

sexuality   maleness or femaleness of an individual.

sexually transmitted disease (STD)   disease that is passed from one individual to another through sexual contact.

shaman   a traditional spiritual leader, healer, or medicine man. In some societies, the shaman is expected to heal the sick, escort the souls of the dead into heaven, and meet with gods by taking on the shape or language of an animal or bird.

sharps   needles, knife blades, etc.; items that can cut or puncture skin.

shearing   force on skin over bone when the skin remains at the point of contact while the bone moves; causes damage to skin.

shift report   information about patients passed from outgoing shift to oncoming shift.

shock   condition in which there is a disruption of circulation that results in dangerously low blood pressure and an upset of all bodily functions.

side rails   sliding metal bars that may be pulled up on each side of the bed to prevent the patient from falling out of bed.

sigmoidoscopy   direct examination of the interior of the sigmoid colon.

sign   any objective evidence of an abnormal nature in the body or its organs.

sign language   communication for persons with hearing impairment; uses gestures and signs made with the fingers and hands.

simple fracture   fracture that does not produce an open wound in the skin. *See also* **closed fracture**

simple goiter   thyroid gland hyperplasia unaccompanied by other signs or symptoms.

simple mastectomy   removal of the breast tissue without removal of the underlying muscles.

Sims' position   position in which the patient is on the left side with left leg extended and right leg flexed; left arm is extended and brought behind the back; right arm is flexed and brought forward.

singultus   hiccup.

sitting (lateral) transfer   moving patient from one surface to another with patient sitting.

sitz bath   a method of bathing in which only the pelvic area is immersed; a cleansing or therapeutic bath in a small tub that holds enough water for the patient to sit with the hips covered and the legs and torso above water. Usually done to relieve discomfort following childbirth, perineal, and rectal surgery.

skeletal muscle   muscle that is attached to bone and provides voluntary movement.

skilled care   health care provided to persons who require professional services over a period of time.

skilled care facility   long-term care facility. Skilled nursing facilities provide the most intensive level of care on the residential care continuum. Residents of these facilities have complex medical care and rehabilitation demands. Some are chronically ill and can no longer live independently.

skin tear   shallow injuries in which the epidermis is ripped or torn.

slander   false oral statement that injures the reputation of another person.

sleep   a period of continuous or intermittent unconsciousness in which physical movements are decreased.

sleep apnea   a potentially serious condition in which airflow stops for 10 seconds or more while a person is sleeping.

sleep deprivation   prolonged sleep loss (inadequate quality or quantity of REM or NREM sleep).

sliding board   a plastic or wooden board that is about 2 feet long with a slippery surface. Used for a sitting, *lateral* transfer.

smooth muscle   muscle located in internal organs, responsible for involuntary movement.

soft diet   intake consisting of low-residue, mildly flavored, easily digested foods.

somnambulism   sleepwalking.

source   person who has an infection that can be spread to others.

spastic paralysis   paralysis in which there is no voluntary movement. The extremities move in an involuntary pattern, similar to muscle spasms. The patient is aware of the movements, but cannot stop or control them.

spasticity   sudden, frequent, involuntary muscle contractions that impair function.

spatial-perceptual deficit   inability to distinguish between left and right and up and down.

speech therapy   treatment to assist a patient to regain communication skills.

sperm   male reproductive cell.

sphygmomanometer   instrument for determining arterial pressures; blood pressure gauge.

spica cast   body cast.

spinal anesthesia   technique of providing anesthesia by introducing drugs into the spinal canal.

spiral fracture   a fracture that twists around the bone.

spirillum (plural spirilla)   spiral-shaped bacteria.

spirituality   feeling of wholeness resulting from filling the human need to feel connected to the world and to a power greater than oneself.

splint   type of orthosis used to maintain position and prevent contractures of the arm and hand.

spores   microscopic reproductive bodies that spread infection and are very difficult to eliminate. They can survive in a dormant form until conditions are ideal for reproduction. The spores then multiply and continue to spread infection.

sprain   injury to ligament, resulting in pain and swelling.

sputum   matter brought up from the lungs; phlegm.

square corner   *See* **box corner**

stable   health condition is steady, predictable, without complications.

staff development   process used to educate staff in health care facilities.

standard   a basis for comparison; a reference point against which performance can be evaluated.

standard precautions   practices used in health care facilities to prevent the spread of infection via blood, body fluids, secretions, excretions, mucous membranes, and nonintact skin.

standing transfer   patient is moved from one surface to another while standing.

staphylo-   prefix meaning "in clusters."

status   condition or state of health.

status epilepticus   a seizure that lasts for a long time, or repeats without recovery; a very serious medical emergency.

STD   *See* **sexually transmitted disease**

stenosis   *See* **stricture**

stent   device that keeps the arteries open.

stepparent   person who is married to a child's natural parent.

stereotype   rigid beliefs based on generalizations.

sterile   absence of all microorganisms; incapable of reproducing sexually.

sterile field   area considered free of all microbes.

sterility   inability to produce offspring.

sterilization   process that renders an individual incapable of reproduction; process of cleaning equipment to remove all microbes and make equipment sterile.

stertorous   snoring-type respirations.

stethoscope   instrument used in auscultation to make audible the sounds produced in the body.

stimulant   agent that produces stimulation or elicits a response.

stimulus   anything that provokes a response in a cell, tissue, or other structure.

stoma   artificial, mouthlike opening.

stool   another name for feces.

strain   injury to a muscle, resulting in pain.

strepto-   prefix meaning "in chains."

Streptococcus **A**   a bacterium that produces very powerful enzymes that destroy tissue and blood cells. Causes a skin condition that may be called "flesh-eating strep" or "man-eating strep."

stressors   situations, feelings, or conditions that cause a person to be anxious about his or her well-being.

stricture   the narrowing of a passageway in the body, often caused by inflammation or scar tissue.

stroke   cerebrovascular accident or brain attack; damage to the blood vessels of the brain.

subacute care   comprehensive, goal-oriented care for individuals with acute illness, injury, or worsening of a chronic medical problem.

subcutaneous tissue   connective tissue located under the dermis; attaches skin to muscle.

subjective observation   observation based on ideas perceived only by the individual involved.

substance abuse   a disorder characterized by the use of one or more substances (such as alcohol or drugs) that alter mood or behavior, resulting in impairment.

sudoriferous gland   gland that secretes perspiration.

suffix   word part added to the end of a word root that changes or modifies the meaning of the word root.

suicide   self-destruction; killing oneself.

suicide precautions   checks and practices a facility follows if a patient states that he or she no longer wishes to live and intends to harm himself or herself. May involve modifying the physical environment and securing the assistance of mental health professionals. The facility maintains these procedures until the patient is discharged or believed to be out of danger.

sundowning   behavior in which a person becomes more agitated and disoriented during the evening hours.

superior   toward the head; upward.

supination   act of turning the palm upward.

supine position   lying with the face upward.

supplement   to add.

supplements   nutritional substances used to make up a deficiency or strengthen the whole.

supportive care   care given to a dying patient that avoids prolonging life but provides comfort measures only.

supportive device   used to help maintain a patient's body in a specific position.

suppository   medication used to help the bowels eliminate feces.

suppression   consciously refusing to acknowledge unacceptable feelings and thoughts.

suprapubic catheter   a urinary catheter that is inserted surgically through the abdominal wall directly into the bladder.

surgical bed   bed prepared for a patient returning from surgery.

surgical mask   mask worn by health care workers during surgery, sterile procedures, and work in a droplet precautions room.

survey   a review and evaluation to ensure that the facility maintains acceptable standards of practice and quality of care.

surveyor   a representative of a private or governmental agency who reviews facility policies, procedures, and practices for quality of care.

symbols   signs, pictures, or other characters used to communicate.

symmetry   matching or correspondence in size, form, and arrangement.

symptom   any perceptible change in the body or its function that indicates disease or the phases of disease.

synapse   space between the axon of one cell and the dendrites of others.

synovial membranes   tissues that produce synovial fluid and line joint cavities.

syphilis   infectious, chronic, venereal disease characterized by lesions that may involve any organ or tissue; usually exhibits cutaneous manifestations; relapses are frequent; may exist asymptomatically for years.

system   group of organs organized to perform a specific body function or functions; for example, the respiratory system.

systole   contraction or period of contraction of cardiac muscle.

systolic pressure   blood pressure exerted by the ventricles during the heart's contraction phase.

tablet PC (TPC)   *See* **personal digital assistant**

tachycardia   unusually rapid heartbeat.

tachypnea pattern of rapid, shallow respirations.

talisman object used to ward off evil.

tasks accomplishments throughout life that lead to healthy participation in society; work to be done.

tasks of personality development growing stages through which personality is formed, as described by Erickson.

TCM *See* **traditional Chinese medicine**

TED hose support hose.

tendon fibrous band of connective tissue that attaches skeletal muscle to bone.

TENS *See* **transcutaneous electrical nerve stimulation**

tepid lukewarm.

terminal final; life-ending stage.

testes male gonads; reproductive glands located in the scrotal sac.

testosterone hormone produced by the testes.

tetany nervous condition characterized by intermittent toxic spasms that are usually paroxysmal and involve the extremities.

tetraplegia paralysis of the arms, legs, and trunk below the level of spinal cord injury.

THA *See* **total hip arthroplasty**

theft taking anything that does not belong to you; stealing.

therapeutic diet treatment through specifically planned nutrition.

therapeutic touch (TT) use of the hands to exchange energy and stimulate healing by restoring the energy field in the body. The practitioner's hands do not touch the patient.

therapy treatment designated to eliminate disease or other bodily disorder.

thermal blanket large, fluid-filled blanket used to raise or lower a patient's temperature.

thermal burn injury (burn) caused by heat, fire, or flame.

thrombocyte blood platelet that is formed in the bone marrow and is important in blood clotting.

thrombophlebitis development of venous thrombi in the presence of inflammatory changes in the vessel wall.

thrombus (plural **thrombi**) blood clot.

throcalcitonin thyroid hormone that lowers calcium in blood.

thyroid gland endocrine gland situated in base of neck; has two lobes, one on either side of trachea; produces hormones thyrocalcitonin and thyroxine.

thyroxine hormone of the thyroid gland that contains iodine.

TIA *See* **transient ischemic attack**

time/travel records records kept of the time spent with clients and the distance traveled between client locations.

tissue collection of specialized cells that perform a particular function; piece of paper used for cleansing (for example, toilet tissue, facial tissue).

toddler stage of childhood from 1 to 3 years of age.

toe pleat an extra space made by folding the top linen over 2 to 3 inches at the end of the bed to keep the linen from pulling the feet downward. This is more comfortable for the patient and reduces the risk of contractures, such as foot drop.

tonsil tip *See* **Yankauer catheter**

total hip arthroplasty (THA) surgical replacement of hip joint with a prosthesis.

total parenteral nutrition (TPN) also called *hyperalimentation*. A complete IV solution containing proteins, carbohydrates, and fats; given to a patient who cannot digest food normally and whose bowel needs complete rest.

toxin microbe that produces poisons that travel to the central nervous system and cause damage.

TPC *See* **tablet PC; personal digital assistant**

TPN *See* **total parenteral nutrition**

trachea windpipe.

tracheostomy opening made into anterior trachea.

traditional Chinese medicine (TCM) a complete health care system that treats disease by restoring the balance between the internal body organs and the external elements of earth, fire, water, wood, and metal.

traditions customs and practices followed by a culture and passed from generation to generation.

transcutaneous electrical nerve stimulation (TENS) use of electrical stimulation to relieve pain.

transfer procedure followed when changing a patient's location.

transfer belt gait belt used to assist and support patients during ambulation.

transient ischemic attack (TIA) temporary reduction of flow of blood to the brain.

transitional care subacute care given after acute care.

transmission transfer from one place or person to another.

transmission-based precautions isolation practices that prevent the spread of infection by interrupting the way in which the disease is spread.

transverse fracture a fracture that breaks completely across the bone.

trapeze horizontal cross bar suspended over the bed to enable patient to move in bed.

trauma wound or injury.

tremor involuntary trembling.

Trendelenburg position position in which the patient has the head lower than the feet.

trichomonas vaginitis inflammation of vaginal tissues with vaginal discharge caused by a protozoan.

trimester period of three months.

tripod position a sitting position that makes the thorax larger on inspiration, enabling the patient to inhale more air.

trochanter roll rolled sheet or bath blanket placed under the patient extending from waist to mid-thigh; positioned against the hip to prevent lateral hip rotation.

TT *See* **therapeutic touch**

tubercle small, rounded nodule formed by infection with *Mycobacterium tuberculosis*.

tuberculosis disease condition occurring when tuberculosis bacteria enter body and damage tissue.

tuberculosis infection condition in which tuberculosis bacteria enter body but are walled off and contained and do not cause disease.

tumor neoplasm.

turning (moving) sheet *See* **draw sheet**

tympanic membrane membrane serving as the lateral wall of the tympanic cavity and separating it from the external acoustic meatus (outer ear).

tympanic thermometer device used to measure temperature at the tympanic membrane in the ear.

ulcer   open sore caused by inadequate blood supply and broken skin.

ulcerative colitis   inflammation of the colon resulting in the formation of ulcers.

ulnar deviation   with hand in supination, lateral movement of the wrist.

ultrasound   high-frequency sound waves (mechanical radiant energy of a frequency greater than 20,000 cycles per second) used for noninvasive imaging and other procedures.

ultraviolet germicidal irradiation (UVGI)   special lights used to irradiate an isolation room to eliminate pathogens.

umbilical cord   attachment connecting the fetus with the placenta. It is severed artificially at the birth of the child.

umbilicus   depressed scar marking the site of entry of the umbilical cord in the fetus.

unilateral neglect   patient ignores one side of body, such as the affected side after a stroke.

upper respiratory infection (URI)   infection involving the organs of the upper respiratory tract.

ureter   narrow tube that conducts urine from the kidney to the urinary bladder.

urethra   mucus-lined tube conveying urine from the urinary bladder to the exterior of the body; in the male, the urethra also conveys the semen.

urgency   need to urinate.

URI   *See* **upper respiratory infection**

urinalysis   laboratory analysis of urine.

urinary bladder   receptacle for urine before it is voided.

urinary incontinence   inability to control urination.

urinary meatus   external opening to urethra.

uterus   organ of gestation; womb.

UVGI   *See* **ultraviolet germicidal irradiation**

vaccine   artificial or weakened antigens that help the body develop antibodies to prevent infectious disease.

vagina   tube that extends from the vulva to the uterine cervix; female organ of copulation that receives the penis during sexual intercourse.

vaginal examination   examination of vaginal and pelvic organs.

validation therapy   techniques used to help individuals feel good about themselves.

vancomycin-resistant enterococci (VRE)   type of bacteria resistant to most antibiotics.

varicose vein   enlarged vein in the leg due to an impaired valve in the vein.

vas deferens   tube that carries sperm from the epididymis to the junction of the seminal vesicle; ductus deferens.

vascular   an area of the body that contains many blood vessels and bleeds readily.

vasoconstriction   decrease in the inner diameter of the blood vessels.

vasodilation   dilation of the blood vessels.

vector   carrier, such as an arthropod, that transmits disease.

vein   vessel through which blood passes on its way back to the heart.

venereal wart   viral condition that can be sexually transmitted.

ventilation   process of breathing in oxygen and breathing out carbon dioxide; also, a means of breathing for another person.

ventilator   a positive-pressure mechanical device that forces air into the patient's lungs; used to facilitate breathing in patients with impaired respiratory or diaphragm function. The ventilator is connected to an endotracheal tube or the tracheostomy.

ventral   front; anterior.

ventricle   small cavity or chamber, as in the brain or heart.

verbal abuse   use of speech to humiliate, threaten, or cause fear or anxiety in another person.

verbal communication   transmitting messages using words.

vertebrae   bones surrounding the spinal cord; the backbone or spine.

vertigo   sensation of rotation or movement of or about the person.

vesicle   blister-like skin lesion.

victim   someone who is injured unexpectedly, as in an accident.

virus   tiny living organisms by which some infectious diseases are transmitted.

visceral muscle   muscle that operates without conscious control.

visualization   a form of guided imagery that uses the imagination to form mental pictures to reduce the stress, pain, and symptoms associated with many medical conditions.

vital signs   measurements of temperature, pulse, respiration, and blood pressure.

vitamin   general term for various, unrelated organic substances, found in many foods in small amounts, that are necessary for normal metabolic function of the body.

vocal cords   tissue that stretches across the larynx and produces vocal sounds.

void   to release urine from the bladder.

volume   capacity or size of an object or of an area; measure of the quantity of a substance.

voluntary muscle   *See* **skeletal muscle**

VRE   *See* **vancomycin-resistant enterococci**

vulva   external female genitalia.

vulvovaginitis   inflammation of the external female reproductive structures (vulva and vagina).

ward   multiple-bed room, usually with 3 or 4 beds.

warm soak   method of applying moist heat.

weight-bearing   able to stand on one or both legs.

wet compress   method for applying moist heat or cold.

wheal   localized area of edema on the body surface, often associated with severe itching.

word root   word form with a basic meaning; used in forming new words by combining it with prefixes or suffixes.

work practice controls   procedures used to prevent the spread of disease.

workplace violence   any physical assault, threatening behavior, or verbal abuse occurring in the workplace.

Yankauer catheter (tonsil tip)   a rigid, plastic suction catheter; used only for oral suctioning.

yeast   one type of fungus.

yoga   system to promote union between mind and body; involves a combination of breath control, postures, relaxation, and meditation.

(**bolding** indicates nursing assistant procedure)

StudyWare™ to Accompany [title]
Minimum System Requirements
- Operating System: Microsoft Windows 2000, Windows XP, Vista
- Processor: Pentium PC 500 MHz or higher (750 Mhz recommended)
- Memory: 64 MB of RAM (128 MB recommended)
- Screen Resolution: 800 x 600 pixels
- Color Depth: 16-bit color (thousands of colors)
- Macromedia Flash Player 9. The Macromedia Flash Player is free, and can be downloaded from *http://www.adobe.com/products/flashplayer/*

Installation Instructions
1. Insert disc into CD-ROM drive. The StudyWare™ installation program should start automatically. If it does not, go to step 2.
2. From My Computer, double-click the icon for the CD drive.
3. Double click the *setup.exe* file to start the program.

Technical Support
Telephone: 1-800-648-7450, 8:30 A.M.-5:30 P.M. Eastern Time
Fax: 1-518-881-1247
E-mail: *delmarhelp@thomson.com*
StudyWare™ is a trademark used herein under license.
Microsoft® and Windows® are registered trademarks of the Microsoft Corporation.
Pentium® is a registered trademark of the Intel® Corporation.

IMPORTANT! READ CAREFULLY: This End User License Agreement ("Agreement") sets forth the conditions by which Thomson Delmar Learning, a division of Thomson Learning Inc. ("Thomson") will make electronic access to the Thomson Delmar Learning-owned licensed content and associated media, software, documentation, printed materials, and electronic documentation contained in this package and/or made available to you via this product (the "Licensed Content"), available to you (the "End User"). BY CLICKING THE "I ACCEPT" BUTTON AND/OR OPENING THIS PACKAGE, YOU ACKNOWLEDGE THAT YOU HAVE READ ALL OF THE TERMS AND CONDITIONS, AND THAT YOU AGREE TO BE BOUND BY ITS TERMS, CONDITIONS, AND ALL APPLICABLE LAWS AND REGULATIONS GOVERNING THE USE OF THE LICENSED CONTENT.

1.0 SCOPE OF LICENSE
1.1 <u>Licensed Content.</u> The Licensed Content may contain portions of modifiable content ("Modifiable Content") and content which may not be modified or otherwise altered by the End User ("Non-Modifiable Content"). For purposes of this Agreement, Modifiable Content and Non-Modifiable Content may be collectively referred to herein as the "Licensed Content." All Licensed Content shall be considered Non-Modifiable Content, unless such Licensed Content is presented to the End User in a modifiable format and it is clearly indicated that modification of the Licensed Content is permitted.
1.2 Subject to the End User's compliance with the terms and conditions of this Agreement, Thomson Delmar Learning hereby grants the End User, a nontransferable, nonexclusive, limited right to access and view a single copy of the Licensed Content on a single personal computer system for noncommercial, internal, personal use only. The End User shall not (i) reproduce, copy, modify (except in the case of Modifiable Content), distribute, display, transfer, sublicense, prepare derivative work(s) based on, sell, exchange, barter or transfer, rent, lease, loan, resell, or in any other manner exploit the Licensed Content; (ii) remove, obscure, or alter any notice of Thomson Delmar Learning's intellectual property rights present on or in the Licensed Content, including, but not limited to, copyright, trademark, and/or patent notices; or (iii) disassemble, decompile, translate, reverse engineer, or otherwise reduce the Licensed Content.

2.0 TERMINATION
2.1 Thomson Delmar Learning may at any time (without prejudice to its other rights or remedies) immediately terminate this Agreement and/or suspend access to some or all of the Licensed Content, in the event that the End User does not comply with any of the terms and conditions of this Agreement. In the event of such termination by Thomson Delmar Learning, the End User shall immediately return any and all copies of the Licensed Content to Thomson Delmar Learning.

3.0 PROPRIETARY RIGHTS
3.1 The End User acknowledges that Thomson Delmar Learning owns all rights, title and interest, including, but not limited to all copyright rights therein, in and to the Licensed Content, and that the End User shall not take any action inconsistent with such ownership. The Licensed Content is protected by U.S., Canadian and other applicable copyright laws and by international treaties, including the Berne Convention and the Universal Copyright Convention. Nothing contained in this Agreement shall be construed as granting the End User any ownership rights in or to the Licensed Content.
3.2 Thomson Delmar Learning reserves the right at any time to withdraw from the Licensed Content any item or part of an item for which it no longer retains the right to publish, or which it has reasonable grounds to believe infringes copyright or is defamatory, unlawful, or otherwise objectionable.

4.0 PROTECTION AND SECURITY
4.1 The End User shall use its best efforts and take all reasonable steps to safeguard its copy of the Licensed Content to ensure that no unauthorized reproduction, publication, disclosure, modification, or distribution of the Licensed Content, in whole or in part, is made. To the extent that the End User becomes aware of any such unauthorized use of the Licensed Content, the End User shall immediately notify Thomson Delmar Learning. Notification of such violations may be made by sending an e-mail to delmarhelp@thomson.com.

5.0 MISUSE OF THE LICENSED PRODUCT
5.1 In the event that the End User uses the Licensed Content in violation of this Agreement, Thomson Delmar Learning shall have the option of electing liquidated damages, which shall include all profits generated by the End User's use of the Licensed Content plus interest computed at the maximum rate permitted by law and all legal fees and other expenses incurred by Thomson Delmar Learning in enforcing its rights, plus penalties.

6.0 FEDERAL GOVERNMENT CLIENTS
6.1 Except as expressly authorized by Thomson Delmar Learning, Federal Government clients obtain only the rights specified in this Agreement and no other rights. The Government acknowledges that (i) all software and related documentation incorporated in the Licensed Content is existing commercial computer software within the meaning of FAR 27.405(b)(2); and (ii) all other data delivered in whatever form, is limited rights data within the meaning of FAR 27.401. The restrictions in this section are acceptable as consistent with the Government's need for software and other data under this Agreement.

7.0 DISCLAIMER OF WARRANTIES AND LIABILITIES

7.1 Although Thomson Delmar Learning believes the Licensed Content to be reliable, Thomson Delmar Learning does not guarantee or warrant (i) any information or materials contained in or produced by the Licensed Content, (ii) the accuracy, completeness or reliability of the Licensed Content, or (iii) that the Licensed Content is free from errors or other material defects. THE LICENSED PRODUCT IS PROVIDED "AS IS," WITHOUT ANY WARRANTY OF ANY KIND AND THOMSON DELMAR LEARNING DISCLAIMS ANY AND ALL WARRANTIES, EXPRESSED OR IMPLIED, INCLUDING, WITHOUT LIMITATION, WARRANTIES OF MERCHANTABILITY OR FITNESS FOR A PARTICULAR PURPOSE. IN NO EVENT SHALL THOMSON DELMAR LEARNING BE LIABLE FOR: INDIRECT, SPECIAL, PUNITIVE OR CONSEQUENTIAL DAMAGES INCLUDING FOR LOST PROFITS, LOST DATA, OR OTHERWISE. IN NO EVENT SHALL THOMSON DELMAR LEARNING'S AGGREGATE LIABILITY HEREUNDER, WHETHER ARISING IN CONTRACT, TORT, STRICT LIABILITY OR OTHERWISE, EXCEED THE AMOUNT OF FEES PAID BY THE END USER HEREUNDER FOR THE LICENSE OF THE LICENSED CONTENT.

8.0 GENERAL

8.1 Entire Agreement. This Agreement shall constitute the entire Agreement between the Parties and supercedes all prior Agreements and understandings oral or written relating to the subject matter hereof.

8.2 Enhancements/Modifications of Licensed Content. From time to time, and in Thomson Delmar Learning's sole discretion, Thomson Delmar Learning may advise the End User of updates, upgrades, enhancements and/or improvements to the Licensed Content, and may permit the End User to access and use, subject to the terms and conditions of this Agreement, such modifications, upon payment of prices as may be established by Thomson Delmar Learning.

8.3 No Export. The End User shall use the Licensed Content solely in the United States and shall not transfer or export, directly or indirectly, the Licensed Content outside the United States.

8.4 Severability. If any provision of this Agreement is invalid, illegal, or unenforceable under any applicable statute or rule of law, the provision shall be deemed omitted to the extent that it is invalid, illegal, or unenforceable. In such a case, the remainder of the Agreement shall be construed in a manner as to give greatest effect to the original intention of the parties hereto.

8.5 Waiver. The waiver of any right or failure of either party to exercise in any respect any right provided in this Agreement in any instance shall not be deemed to be a waiver of such right in the future or a waiver of any other right under this Agreement.

8.6 Choice of Law/Venue. This Agreement shall be interpreted, construed, and governed by and in accordance with the laws of the State of New York, applicable to contracts executed and to be wholly preformed therein, without regard to its principles governing conflicts of law. Each party agrees that any proceeding arising out of or relating to this Agreement or the breach or threatened breach of this Agreement may be commenced and prosecuted in a court in the State and County of New York. Each party consents and submits to the nonexclusive personal jurisdiction of any court in the State and County of New York in respect of any such proceeding.

8.7 Acknowledgment. By opening this package and/or by accessing the Licensed Content on this Web site, THE END USER ACKNOWLEDGES THAT IT HAS READ THIS AGREEMENT, UNDERSTANDS IT, AND AGREES TO BE BOUND BY ITS TERMS AND CONDITIONS. IF YOU DO NOT ACCEPT THESE TERMS AND CONDITIONS, YOU MUST NOT ACCESS THE LICENSED CONTENT AND RETURN THE LICENSED PRODUCT TO DELMAR LEARNING (WITHIN 30 CALENDAR DAYS OF THE END USER'S PURCHASE) WITH PROOF OF PAYMENT ACCEPTABLE TO THOMSON DELMAR LEARNING, FOR A CREDIT OR A REFUND. Should the End User have any questions/comments regarding this Agreement, please contact Thomson Delmar Learning at delmarhelp@thomson.com.